Dietary Reference Intakes (DRIs): Recommended Intakes for Individuals, Minerals
Food and Nutrition Board, Institute of Medicine, National Academies

Life-Stage Group	Calcium (mg/day)	Chromium (µg/day)	Copper (µg/day)	Fluoride (mg/day)	Iodine (µg/day)	Iron (mg/day)	Magnesium (mg/day)	Manganese (mg/day)	Molybdenum (µg/day)	Phosphorus (mg/day)	Selenium (µg/day)	Zinc (mg/day)	Potassium (g/day)	Sodium (g/day)	Chloride (g/day)
Infants															
0-6 mo	210*	0.2*	200*	0.01*	110*	0.27*	30*	0.003*	2*	100*	15*	2*	0.4*	0.12*	0.18*
7-12 mo	270*	5.5*	220*	0.5*	130*	11	75*	0.6*	3*	275*	20*	3*	0.7*	0.37*	0.57*
Children															
1-3 yr	500*	11*	340	0.7*	90	7	80	1.2*	17	460	20	3	3.0*	1.0*	1.5*
4-8 yr	800*	15*	440	1*	90	10	130	1.5*	22	500	30	5	3.8*	1.2*	1.9*
Males															
9-13 yr	1300*	25*	700	2*	120	8	240	1.9*	34	1250	40	8	4.5*	1.5*	2.3*
14-18 yr	1300*	35*	890	3*	150	11	410	2.2*	43	1250	55	11	4.7*	1.5*	2.3*
19-30 yr	1000*	35*	900	4*	150	8	400	2.3*	45	700	55	11	4.7*	1.5*	2.3*
31-50 yr	1000*	35*	900	4*	150	8	420	2.3*	45	700	55	11	4.7*	1.5*	2.3*
51-70 yr	1200*	30*	900	4*	150	8	420	2.3*	45	700	55	11	4.7*	1.3*	2.0*
>70 yr	1200*	30*	900	4*	150	8	420	2.3*	45	700	55	11	4.7*	1.2*	1.8*
Females															
9-13 yr	1300*	21*	700	2*	120	8	240	1.6*	34	1250	40	8	4.5*	1.5*	2.3*
14-18 yr	1300*	24*	890	3*	150	15	360	1.6*	43	1250	55	9	4.7*	1.5*	2.3*
19-30 yr	1000*	25*	900	3*	150	18	310	1.8*	45	700	55	8	4.7*	1.5*	2.3*
31-50 yr	1000*	25*	900	3*	150	18	320	1.8*	45	700	55	8	4.7*	1.5*	2.3*
51-70 yr	1200*	20*	900	3*	150	8	320	1.8*	45	700	55	8	4.7*	1.3*	2.0*
>70 yr	1200*	20*	900	3*	150	8	320	1.8*	45	700	55	8	4.7*	1.2*	1.8*
Pregnant															
≤18 yr	1300*	29*	1000	3*	220	27	400	2.0*	50	1250	60	12	4.7*	1.5*	2.3*
19-30 yr	1000*	30*	1000	3*	220	27	350	2.0*	50	700	60	11	4.7*	1.5*	2.3*
31-50 yr	1000*	30*	1000	3*	220	27	360	2.0*	50	700	60	11	4.7*	1.5*	2.3*
Lactating															
≤18 yr	1300*	44*	1300	3*	290	10	360	2.6*	50	1250	70	13	5.1*	1.5*	2.3*
19-30 yr	1000*	45*	1300	3*	290	9	310	2.6*	50	700	70	12	5.1*	1.5*	2.3*
31-50 yr	1000*	45*	1300	3*	290	9	320	2.6*	50	700	70	12	5.1*	1.5*	2.3*

Data from Food and Nutrition Board, Institute of Medicine: *Dietary Reference Intakes for calcium, phosphorus, magnesium, vitamin D, and fluoride* (1997); *Dietary Reference Intakes for thiamin, riboflavin, niacin, vitamin B₆, folate, vitamin B₁₂, pantothenic acid, biotin, and choline* (1998); *Dietary Reference Intakes for vitamin C, vitamin E, selenium, and carotenoids* (2000); *Dietary Reference Intakes for vitamin A, vitamin K, arsenic, boron, chromium, copper, iodine, iron, manganese, molybdenum, nickel, silicon, vanadium, and zinc* (2001), and *Dietary Reference Intakes for water, potassium, sodium, chloride, and sulfate* (2004), Washington, DC, National Academies Press (www.nap.edu).

NOTE: This table presents Recommended Dietary Allowances (RDAs) in **bold type** and Adequate Intakes (AIs) in ordinary type followed by an asterisk (*). RDAs and AIs may both be used as goals for individual intake. RDAs are set to meet the needs of almost all (97% to 98%) individuals in a group. For healthy breast-fed infants, the AI is the mean intake. The AI for other life-stage and gender groups is believed to cover needs of all individuals in the group, but lack of data or uncertainty in the data prevent being able to specify with confidence the percentage of individuals covered by this intake.

Dietary Reference Intakes (DRIs): Tolerable Upper Intake Levels (UL[a]), Minerals
Food and Nutrition Board, Institute of Medicine, National Academies

Life-Stage Group	Arsenic[b]	Boron (mg/day)	Calcium (g/day)	Chromium	Copper (µg/day)	Fluoride (mg/day)	Iodine (µg/day)	Iron (mg/day)	Magnesium (mg/day)[c]	Manganese (mg/day)	Molybdenum (µg/day)	Nickel (mg/day)	Phosphorus (g/day)	Selenium (µg/day)	Silicon[d]	Vanadium (mg/day)[e]	Zinc (mg/day)	Potassium	Sulfate	Sodium (g/day)	Chloride (g/day)
Infants																					
0-6 mo	ND[f]	ND	ND	ND	ND	0.7	ND	40	ND	ND	ND	ND	ND	45	ND	ND	4	ND	ND	ND	ND
7-12 mo	ND	ND	ND	ND	ND	0.9	ND	40	ND	ND	ND	ND	ND	60	ND	ND	5	ND	ND	ND	ND
Children																					
1-3 yr	ND	3	2.5	ND	1000	1.3	200	40	65	2	300	0.2	3	90	ND	ND	7	ND	ND	1.5	2.3
4-8 yr	ND	6	2.5	ND	3000	2.2	300	40	110	3	600	0.3	3	150	ND	ND	12	ND	ND	1.9	2.9
Males, Females																					
9-13 yr	ND	11	2.5	ND	5000	10	600	40	350	6	1100	0.6	4	280	ND	ND	23	ND	ND	2.2	3.4
14-18 yr	ND	17	2.5	ND	8000	10	900	45	350	9	1700	1.0	4	400	ND	ND	34	ND	ND	2.3	3.6
19-70 yr	ND	20	2.5	ND	10,000	10	1100	45	350	11	2000	1.0	4	400	ND	1.8	40	ND	ND	2.3	3.6
>70 yr	ND	20	2.5	ND	10,000	10	1100	45	350	11	2000	1.0	3	400	ND	1.8	40	ND	ND	2.3	3.6
Pregnant																					
≤18 yr	ND	17	2.5	ND	8000	10	900	45	350	9	1700	1.0	3.5	400	ND	ND	34	ND	ND	2.3	3.6
19-50 yr	ND	20	2.5	ND	10,000	10	1100	45	350	11	2000	1.0	3.5	400	ND	ND	40	ND	ND	2.3	3.6
Lactating																					
≤18 yr	ND	17	2.5	ND	8000	10	900	45	350	9	1700	1.0	4	400	ND	ND	34	ND	ND	2.3	3.6
19-50 yr	ND	20	2.5	ND	10,000	10	1100	45	350	11	2000	1.0	4	400	ND	ND	40	ND	ND	2.3	3.6

Data from Food and Nutrition Board, Institute of Medicine: *Dietary Reference Intakes for calcium, phosphorus, magnesium, vitamin D, and fluoride* (1997); *Dietary Reference Intakes for thiamin, riboflavin, niacin, vitamin B₆, folate, vitamin B₁₂, pantothenic acid, biotin, and choline* (1998); *Dietary Reference Intakes for vitamin C, vitamin E, selenium, and carotenoids* (2000); *Dietary Reference Intakes for vitamin A, vitamin K, arsenic, boron, chromium, copper, iodine, iron, manganese, molybdenum, nickel, silicon, vanadium, and zinc* (2001), and *Dietary Reference Intakes for water, potassium, sodium, chloride, and sulfate* (2004), Washington, DC, National Academies Press (www.nap.edu).

[a]UL = The maximum level of daily nutrient intake that is likely to pose no risk of adverse effects. Unless otherwise specified, the UL represents total intake from food, water, and supplements. Due to lack of suitable data, ULs could not be established for arsenic, chromium, and silicon. In the absence of ULs, extra caution may be warranted in consuming levels above recommended intakes.

[b]Although the UL was not determined for arsenic, there is no justification for adding arsenic to food or supplements.

[c]The ULs for magnesium represent intake from a pharmacologic agent only and do not include intake from food or water.

[d]Although silicon has not been shown to cause adverse effects in humans, there is no justification for adding silicon to supplements.

[e]Although vanadium in food has not been shown to cause adverse effects in humans, there is no justification for adding vanadium to food, and vanadium supplements should be used with caution. The UL is based on adverse effects in laboratory animals, and this data could be used to set a UL for adults but not children and adolescents.

[f]ND = Not determinable due to lack of data of adverse effects in this age-group and concern with regard to lack of ability to handle excess amounts. Source of intake should be from food only to prevent high levels of intake.

Dietary Reference Intakes (DRIs): Recommended Intakes for Individuals, Macronutrients
Food and Nutrition Board, Institute of Medicine, National Academies

Life-Stage Group	Protein RDA/AI (g/day)[a]	Protein AMDR[b]	Carbohydrate RDA/AI (g/day)	Carbohydrate AMDR	Fiber RDA/AI (g/day)	Fiber AMDR	Fat RDA/AI (g/day)	Fat AMDR	n-6 Polyunsaturated Fatty Acids (Linoleic Acid) RDA/AI (g/day)	n-6 AMDR	n-3 Polyunsaturated Fatty Acids (α-Linolenic Acid) RDA/AI (g/day)	n-3 AMDR[c]	Saturated and trans Fatty Acids and Cholesterol RDA/AI (g/day)[e]	Sat AMDR
Infants														
0-6 mo	9.1	ND[d]	60	ND	ND		31		4.4	ND	0.5	ND		
7-12 mo	**11**	ND	95	ND	ND		30		4.6	ND	0.5	ND		
Children														
1-3 yr	**13**	**5-20**	**130**	45-65	19			30-40	7	5-10	0.7	0.6-1.2		
4-8 yr	**19**	**10-30**	**130**	45-65	25			25-35	10	5-10	0.9	0.6-1.2		
Males														
9-13 yr	**34**	**10-30**	**130**	45-65	31			25-35	12	5-10	1.2	0.6-1.2		
14-18 yr	**52**	**10-30**	**130**	45-65	38			25-35	16	5-10	1.6	0.6-1.2		
19-30 yr	**56**	**10-35**	**130**	45-65	38			20-35	17	5-10	1.6	0.6-1.2		
31-50 yr	**56**	**10-35**	**130**	45-65	38			20-35	17	5-10	1.6	0.6-1.2		
51-70 yr	**56**	**10-35**	**130**	45-65	30			20-35	14	5-10	1.6	0.6-1.2		
>70 yr	**56**	**10-35**	**130**	45-65	30			20-35	14	5-10	1.6	0.6-1.2		
Females														
9-13 yr	**34**	**10-30**	**130**	45-65	26			25-35	10	5-10	1.0	0.6-1.2		
14-18 yr	**46**	**10-30**	**130**	45-65	26			25-35	11	5-10	1.1	0.6-1.2		
19-30 yr	**46**	**10-35**	**130**	45-65	25			20-35	12	5-10	1.1	0.6-1.2		
31-50 yr	**46**	**10-35**	**130**	45-65	25			20-35	12	5-10	1.1	0.6-1.2		
51-70 yr	**46**	**10-35**	**130**	45-65	21			20-35	11	5-10	1.1	0.6-1.2		
>70 yr	**46**	**10-35**	**130**	45-65	21			20-35	11	5-10	1.1	0.6-1.2		
Pregnant														
≤18 yr	**71**	**10-35**	**175**	45-65	28			20-35	13	5-10	1.4	0.6-1.2		
19-30 yr	**71**	**10-35**	**175**	45-65	28			20-35	13	5-10	1.4	0.6-1.2		
31-50 yr	**71**	**10-35**	**175**	45-65	28			20-35	13	5-10	1.4	0.6-1.2		
Lactating														
≤18 yr	**71**	**10-35**	**210**	45-65	29			20-35	13	5-10	1.3	0.6-1.2		
19-30 yr	**71**	**10-35**	**210**	45-65	29			20-35	13	5-10	1.3	0.6-1.2		
31-50 yr	**71**	**10-35**	**210**	45-65	29			20-35	13	5-10	1.3	0.6-1.2		

Data from *Dietary Reference Intakes for energy, carbohydrate, fiber, fat, fatty acids, cholesterol, protein, and amino acids (macronutrients),* Washington, DC, 2002, The National Academies Press.

NOTE: This table presents Recommended Dietary Allowances (RDAs) in **bold type** and Adequate Intakes (AIs) in ordinary type. RDAs and AIs may both be used as goals for individual intake. RDAs are set to meet the needs of almost all (97% to 98%) individuals in a group. For healthy breast-fed infants, the AI is the mean intake. The AI for other life-stage and gender groups is believed to cover the needs of all individuals in the group, but lack of data prevents being able to specify with confidence the percentage of individuals covered by this intake.

[a]Based on 1.5 g/kg/day for infants, 1.1 g/kg/day for 1-3 yr, 0.95 g/kg/day for 4-13 yr, 0.85 g/kg/day for 14-18 yr, 0.8 g/kg/day for adults, and 1.1 g/kg/day for pregnant (using prepregnancy weight) and lactating women.

[b]Acceptable Macronutrient Distribution Range (AMDR) is the range of intake for a particular energy source that is associated with reduced risk of chronic disease while providing intakes of essential nutrients. If an individual has consumed in excess of the AMDR, there is a potential of increasing the risk of chronic diseases and insufficient intakes of essential nutrients.

[c]Approximately 10% of the total can come from longer-chain, n-3 fatty acids.

[d]ND = Not determinable due to lack of data of adverse effects in this age-group and concern with regard to lack of ability to handle excess amounts. Source of intake should be from food only to prevent high levels of intake.

[e]Keep intake as low as possible while consuming a nutritionally adequate diet.

WILLIAMS'

ESSENTIALS
of Nutrition & Diet Therapy

Ninth Edition

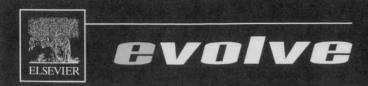

WILLIAMS'
ESSENTIALS
of Nutrition & Diet Therapy

Ninth Edition

Eleanor D. Schlenker, PhD, RD
Professor and Extension Specialist
Department of Human Nutrition, Foods, and Exercise
College of Agriculture and Life Sciences
Virginia Polytechnic Institute and State University
Blacksburg, Virginia

Sara Long, PhD, RD
Professor and Assistant Chair
Director, Didactic Program in Dietetics
Department of Animal Science, Food, and Nutrition
Southern Illinois University Carbondale
Carbondale, Illinois

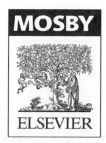

MOSBY

ELSEVIER

MOSBY
ELSEVIER

11830 Westline Industrial Drive
St. Louis, Missouri 63146

WILLIAMS' ESSENTIALS OF NUTRITION & DIET THERAPY   ISBN-13: 978-0-323-03764-8
Copyright © 2007, 2003, 1999, 1994, 1990, 1986, 1982, 1978, 1974   ISBN-10:0-323-03764-X
by Mosby, Inc., an affiliate of Elsevier Inc.

Notice

Knowledge and best practice in this field are constantly changing. As new research and experience broaden our knowledge, changes in practice, treatment and drug therapy may become necessary or appropriate. Readers are advised to check the most current information provided (i) on procedures featured or (ii) by the manufacturer of each product to be administered, to verify the recommended dose or formula, the method and duration of administration, and contraindications. It is the responsibility of the practitioner, relying on their own experience and knowledge of the patient, to make diagnoses, to determine dosages and the best treatment for each individual patient, and to take all appropriate safety precautions. To the fullest extent of the law, neither the Publisher nor the Authors assumes any liability for any injury and/or damage to persons or property arising out of or related to any use of the material contained in this book.

The Publisher

ISBN-13: 978-0-323-03764-8
ISBN-10: 0-323-03764-X

Senior Editor: Yvonne Alexopoulos
Developmental Editor: Kristin Hebberd
Editorial Assistant: Sarah Vales
Publishing Services Manager: John Rogers
Senior Project Manager: Cheryl A. Abbott
Interior Designer: Paula Ruckenbrod
Cover Design Direction: Paula Ruckenbrod

Printed in Canada

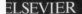
Last digit is print number: 9   8   7   6   5   4   3   2   1

*This edition is dedicated to Sue Rodwell Williams, who created
the first eight editions and will continue to be a source of inspiration.*
The Authors

*To my parents, Harold and Nora, who taught me
to appreciate the opportunity to learn.*
Eleanor D. Schlenker

*To my mother, Ruth:
Thank you for giving me life and supporting me in whatever I do.
I love you. From your Favorite Daughter. Thanks,*
Sara

Contributors

Ethan Bergman, PhD, RD, CD, FADA

Associate Dean
College of Education and Professional Studies
Professor of Food Science and Nutrition
Department of Family and Consumer Sciences
Central Washington University
Ellensburg, Washington

George A. Bray, MD

Boyd Professor
Pennington Biomedical Research Center
Louisiana State University
Baton Rouge, Louisiana

Nancy Buergel, MS

Assistant Professor of Food Science and Nutrition
Dietetic Internship Coordinator
Department of Family and Consumer Sciences
Central Washington University
Ellensburg, Washington

Catherine M. Champagne, PhD, RD

Chief, Nutritional Epidemiology
Professor, Dietary Assessment and Counseling
Pennington Biomedical Research Center
Louisiana State University
Baton Rouge, Louisiana

M. Patricia Fuhrman, MS, RD, LD, FADA, CNSD

Area Clinical Nutrition Marketing Manager
Advanced Nutrition Services
Coram Healthcare
Saint Louis, Missouri

Staci Nix, MS, RD, CD

Instructor and Lecturer
Division of Nutrition
College of Health
University of Utah
Salt Lake City, Utah

Sharon M. Nickols-Richardson, PhD, RD

Associate Professor
Department of Human Nutrition, Foods, and Exercise
Virginia Polytechnic Institute and State University
Blacksburg, Virginia

Meredith Catherine Williams

New Haven, Connecticut

Reviewers

Peter L. Beyer, MS, RD

Associate Professor
Dietetics & Nutrition
University of Kansas Medical Center
Kansas City, Kansas

Liz Friedrich, MPH, RD, LDN

Nutrition and Health Promotion Consultant
Salisbury, North Carolina

Delaine Curtis Furst, MS, EdS

Associate Professor
Foods and Nutrition
Indian River Community College
Fort Pierce, Florida

Kathy A. Hammond, MS, RN, CNSN, RD, LD, CNSD

Coordinator, Continuing Education
Clinical Nutrition Specialist
Chartwell Diversified Services, Inc.
Lilburn, Georgia;
Adjunct Assistant Professor
Department of Foods and Nutrition
University of Georgia
Athens, Georgia

Debra A. Indorato, RD, LDN

Owner, Nutrition Therapist
Approach Nutrition and Fitness
Chesapeake, Virginia;
Patient Services Manager
Morrison Healthcare Management
Norfolk, Virginia

Betty (Elizabeth) Kenyon, BS, RD, LMNT

Consultant Dietitian
Panhandle Community Services
Gering, Nebraska;
Adjunct Faculty
Western Nebraska Community College
Scottsbluff, Nebraska

Bridget Klawitter, PhD, RD, CD, FADA

Director
Clinical Nutrition and Diabetes Services
All Saints Healthcare
Racine, Wisconsin;
Nutrition Consultant
Nutritional Management and Consultations
Salem, Wisconsin

Kelly Kohls, PhD, RD, LD

Owner
Kelko Consultants, Inc. (dba) Able Weight and Wellness
    Services
Lebanon, Ohio;
Consultant
ABC Pediatric Therapy
North East Pediatrics
Miami University
Oxford, Ohio

Jane Kufus-Krump, MS, LRD

Associate Professor
North Dakota State College of Science
Wahpeton, North Dakota

Diane T. Kupensky, RN, MSN, CNS

Trauma-Clinical Nurse Specialist
Saint Elizabeth Health Center
Youngstown, Ohio

Edith Lerner, PhD

Associate Professor and Vice-Chair
Department of Nutrition
School of Medicine
Case Western Reserve University
Cleveland, Ohio

Jaimette A. McCulley, MS, RD

Assistant Professor
Human Environmental Sciences Department
Fontbonne University
Saint Louis, Missouri

Jessie Pavlinac, MS, RD, CSR, LD

Clinical Nutrition Manager
Food & Nutrition Services
Oregon Health & Science University
Portland, Oregon

Rena Quinton, PhD

Nutritionist
Health Promotion Council of Southeastern Pennsylvania
Philadelphia, Pennsylvania

Jennifer M. Williams, MS, RD, CNSD, LDN

Senior Clinical Dietitian Specialist
Clinical Nutrition Support Service
Hospital of the University of Pennsylvania
Philadelphia, Pennsylvania

Preface

Through eight highly successful editions, this nutrition textbook has presented a sound basis for student learning and clinical practice in the health professions. It has provided both a strong research base and a person-centered approach to the study and application of nutrition in human health. We have appreciated the suggestions and positive reception of this text by users in colleges, community colleges, and clinical settings throughout the United States and in other parts of the world.

Rapid changes are occurring in nutrition. New regulations are being proposed and debated. The science base in biology, biotechnology, and health is expanding. Social problems and structures are changing. Patient populations are more culturally diverse. Healthcare systems and practices are very different from a generation or even a decade ago. Public interest and concern with nutrition and healthcare are increasing. Nutrition has become more prominent in the marketplace of competing ideas and products. It is small wonder then that these changes are being reflected in nutrition education and professional practice because nutrition is fundamentally a very human applied science and art.

This new ninth edition reflects these far-reaching changes. As always, its guiding principle continues to be our commitment to sound nutrition principles rooted in basic science and their application to human health and well-being. We have built on previous editions to produce this new book—updated and rewritten—incorporating a new design and format with reliable content to meet the expectations and changing needs of students, faculty, and practitioners in the health professions.

NEW TO THIS EDITION

To accommodate the demands of a rapidly developing science and the needs of an increasingly diverse society, the entire text has been updated and rewritten. Changes and additions based on input from many teachers, students, and clinicians were incorporated to increase its usefulness.

Chapter Changes

With the retirement of Dr. Sue Rodwell Williams, the founder and primary author of the first eight editions of this textbook, we have shared the responsibility for the preparation of this ninth edition. Part 1, *Introduction to Human Nutrition,* provides the foundation for under-standing the basic science of nutrition, which is applied to human nutritional needs in *Part 2, Community Nutrition: The Life Cycle.* Part 3, *Introduction to Clinical Nutrition,* addresses the nutritional care needs within specific illnesses and conditions and associated clinical therapies and interventions.

Since the preparation of the eighth edition, the problem of obesity has emerged as a growing health crisis among all age-groups and in all parts of the world. To address this topic adequately, we have introduced a new chapter on obesity, providing readers with a comprehensive review of this public health problem, its causes, and possible solutions. We welcome contributing authors Dr. George A. Bray, an internationally recognized expert in the field of obesity, and his associate Dr. Catherine M. Champagne, who prepared Chapter 15: "The Complexity of Obesity: Beyond Energy Balance." Dr. Sharon M. Nickols-Richardson has updated Chapters 11 and 12, which focus on nutrition in pregnancy and lactation and normal growth and development. Ms. Staci Nix, author of *Williams' Basic Nutrition & Diet Therapy,* contributed Chapter 14, which addresses nutrition and physical fitness. Ms. M. Patricia Fuhrman, returning contributor for Chapter 18, discusses concerns surrounding enteral and parenteral nutrition. Finally, Dr. Ethan Bergman and Ms. Nancy Buergel have updated the discussion of Chapter 26, which tackles nutrition therapy of individuals with chronic debilitating conditions and those undergoing rehabilitation.

New material has been incorporated throughout this edition, including not only recent scientific research findings and clinical treatment therapies, but also coverage of significant developments in nutrition and public policy. The new edition of *Dietary Guidelines for Americans,* released in 2005, and MyPyramid—the new USDA food guidance system also released in 2005—have replaced earlier versions of these nutrition materials. An emphasis on health promotion is a recurring theme throughout the text, and students are encouraged to look for the *Health Promotion* heading in each chapter to direct them toward special information to assist in the nutrition education of clients and patients.

Several new feature boxes have been added to address contemporary issues in human nutrition and disease intervention. *Complementary and Alternative Medicine (CAM)* boxes—found in all chapters in Part 3—review and evaluate new therapies relevant to chapter topics. *Focus on Culture* boxes, also new to the ninth edition, introduce students to the concept of cultural competence and the special nutritional needs, problems, and appropriate interventions applicable to various cultural, ethnic, racial, and age-groups. *Focus on Food Safety* boxes alert readers to food safety issues related to the nutrient, age-group, or medical condition being discussed. *Perspectives in Practice* boxes contain practical applications of nutrition principles to the care and well-being of healthy individuals, as well as those at risk or diagnosed with chronic or acute diseases. Tools for nutrition education have been included in various sections. Finally, *To Probe Further* boxes, continued from the eighth edition, help students explore in greater depth new research findings or issues of controversy within the public or professional community. In addition to these features, a new section, "Websites of Interest," has been added to each chapter's *Further Readings and Resources* section to connect students with Internet sources of accurate and appropriate information useful in finding answers to client or patient inquiries.

Illustrations and Design

Numerous illustrations—anatomic figures, graphic line drawings, and photographs—most all in full color, enhance the overall design and help students better understand the concepts and clinical practices presented.

Enhanced Readability and Student Interest

Increasing attention has been given to the issues of student interest and comprehension. Efforts have been made to enhance this text's readability and to enliven it stylistically with greater use of boxes, illustrations, and recurring themes. New material has been added, and remaining sections have been rewritten. Recent advances in basic and clinical science are explained and applied. Issues of public-professional controversy of interest to students are discussed.

LEARNING AIDS WITHIN THE TEXT

This new edition continues to include many learning aids throughout the text.

Chapter Openers

To alert students to the content of each chapter and draw them into its study, each chapter opens with an illustration and a preview of the chapter topics. In addition, an outline of the major chapter headings is included on this page.

Key Terms

Key terms important to the student's understanding and application of the chapter content are presented in three steps. They are first identified in green type in the body of the text. These terms are then grouped and defined in boxes in the lower corners of the pages close to their men-

tion. Finally, all key terms are collected in a comprehensive glossary for easy reference at the end of the book. This three-level approach to vocabulary development greatly improves the overall study and usefulness of the text.

Pedagogy Boxes: *To Probe Further, Perspectives in Practice, Focus on Culture, Complementary and Alternative Medicine (CAM),* and *Focus on Food Safety*

Special features throughout the text are these boxes introducing supplemental material—brief information on chapter-related issues or controversies, a deeper look at chapter topics, and illustrations of practical application of nutrition concepts. These interesting and motivating studies help the student comprehend the importance of scientific thinking and develop sound judgment and openness to varied points of view.

Case Studies

In Parts 2 and 3 realistic case studies lead the student to apply the text material to related nutrition care problems. Each chapter contains one case accompanied by questions for analysis and decision making. These case studies help students learn to apply nutrition therapy and intervention to the patients they will encounter in their clinical assignments.

Chapter Summaries

To assist the student in drawing the chapter material together as a whole, each chapter concludes with a summary of the key concepts presented and their significance or application. The student can then return to any part of the material for repeated study and clarification as needed.

Review Questions

To help the student understand and learn to think critically about key parts of the chapter and apply it to patient needs or problems, review questions are provided at the end of each chapter.

Chapter References

A strength of this text is its range of current documentation for the topics presented, drawn from a wide selection of pertinent journals. To provide immediate access to all references cited in the chapter text, a full list of these key references is given at the end of each chapter rather than collected at the end of the book.

Further Readings and Resources

In addition to referenced material in the text, an annotated list of suggestions for further reading for added interest and study is provided at the end of each chapter. These selections extend or apply the text material according to student needs or areas of special interest. The annotations improve the student's ability to use them by identifying the pertinent topics of the reference. A new addition to each chapter is a list of reliable websites for further reference or study.

Appendixes

The revised appendixes include a number of materials for use as reference tools and guidelines in learning and practice. The recently updated CDC growth charts are included, as well as the most recent edition of the *Exchange Lists for Meal Planning.* New appendixes containing updated standards for physical assessment and resources for planning restricted diets have been added.

SUPPLEMENTARY MATERIALS

Several available supplements enhance the teaching and learning process.

Instructor's Manual and Test Bank

Prepared by experienced nutrition writer, editor, and project coordinator Gill Robertson, MS, RD, this convenient electronic resource (available both on CD-ROM and on the Evolve website) contains the following:

- *Instructor's Manual* with chapter overviews, objectives, chapter outlines with teaching notes, and individual/group activities
- Extensive *Test Bank* of more than 1250 NCLEX-style multiple-choice examination questions
- *Image Collection* of approximately 100 images from the text
- *PowerPoint presentations* per chapter, each containing approximately 30 to 50 text slides to guide classroom lecture

Evolve Website

Designed to provide supplemental online learning opportunities that complement the material in the book, this site contains sections for both instructor and student resources. The abovementioned *Instructor's Resource, Test Bank, Image Collection,* and *PowerPoint presentations* are available in the instructor portion of this site, whereas the student section introduces a variety of new learning enhancements—*Crossword Puzzles* created from the book's key terms; *Practice Questions* (10 per chapter) with instant feedback useful for exam preparation; a *Food Composition Table* containing a detailed listing of the more than 3700 foods featured within the *Nutritrac Nutrition Analysis Software* CD-ROM at the back of this book; and *WebLinks,* an extensive listing of hyperlinked online resources organized by chapter and part topics.

Mosby's Nutritrac Nutrition Analysis Software CD-ROM, Version IV

This innovative and completely revised and updated program, packaged with every copy of this text, gives users the hands-on, interactive tools to perform a complete nutrition analysis of food intake and energy expenditure for an unlimited number of individuals. Data are tied to personal profiles that the user creates, allowing for a customized analysis each time. The program generates helpful nutrient reports, calorie and fat content charts, DRI graphs, running tallies of energy expenditure, and much more. This latest version features a database of more than 3700 foods in 18 different food categories—including cultural food items and those used in a variety of diet plans, such as the Atkins and South Beach diets and Weight Watchers. The expanded activities database contains more than 175 various daily/common, sporting, recreational, and occupational activities. An ideal body weight (IBW) calculator is new to this version, as is a feature that uses the Harris-Benedict formula to calculate total daily energy needs.

PERSONAL APPROACH

The person-centered approach that has been a hallmark of previous editions continues to be emphasized in this new edition. The authors and contributors have continued to write in a personal style, use materials and examples from personal research and clinical experience, and present scientific knowledge in human terms as a tool to develop practical solutions to individual problems.

ACKNOWLEDGMENTS

A textbook of this sort is never the work of just authors and contributors. It develops into the planned product through the committed hands and hearts of a number of persons. It would be impossible to name all of the individuals involved, but several groups deserve special recognition.

First, the authors are grateful to the reviewers who gave their valuable time and skills to strengthen the manuscript: Peter L. Beyer, Liz Friedrich, Delaine Curtis Furst, Kathy A. Hammond, Debra A. Indorato, Betty (Elizabeth) Kenyon, Bridget Klawitter, Kelly Kohls, Jane Kufus-Krump, Diane T. Kupensky, Edith Lerner, Jaimette A. McCulley, Jessie Pavlinac, Rena Quinton, and Jennifer M. Williams.

Second, we are indebted to Elsevier and the many persons there who had a part in this extensive project. We especially thank our editor of nutrition publications, Yvonne Alexopoulos, whose skills and support have always been invaluable, and our developmental editor,

Kristin Hebberd, whose creative and energetic talents helped shape the book's pages. We also thank our production project manager, Cheryl Abbott, for essential guidance, and our design manager, Paula Ruckenbrod, who helped to bring a new look to this ninth edition. To our marketing managers and the many fine Elsevier sales representatives throughout the country, we owe great appreciation for their help in ensuring the book's success with users.

Finally, we would like to thank Brian K. Jones for his help with several chapters in Part 3—you will make SIUC proud and be an asset to the profession of dietetics.

Eleanor D. Schlenker
Blacksburg, Virginia

Sara Long
Carbondale, Illinois

Contents

APPENDIXES

WILLIAMS'
ESSENTIALS
of Nutrition & Diet Therapy

Ninth Edition

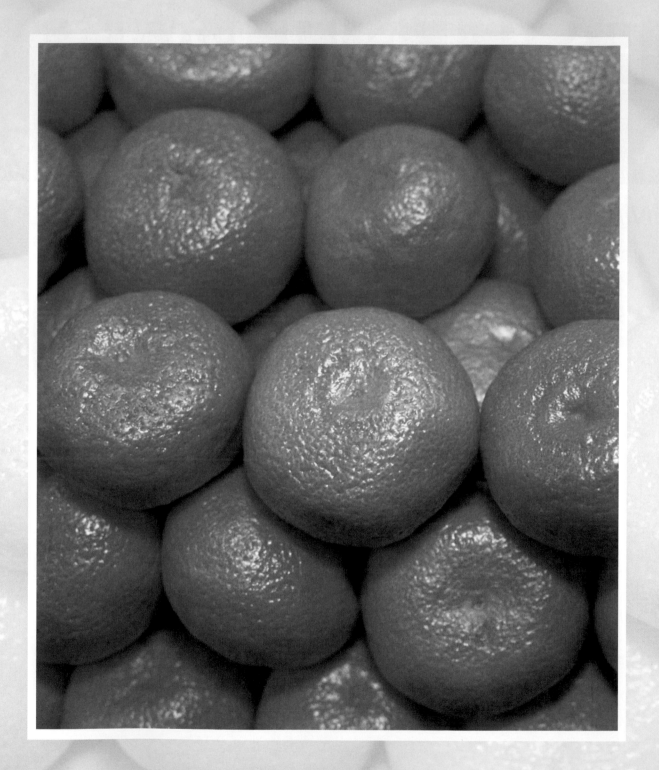

Introduction to Human Nutrition

CHAPTER 1

Nutrition and Health

Eleanor D. Schlenker

With this chapter we begin our study of nutrition and human health. Sound nutrition principles along with skills in food selection are the cornerstone for personal health and teaching others. Current knowledge in nutrition founded in basic science reflects the new food patterns, emerging health problems, and growing understanding of the relationships between food and health in our rapidly changing world. Nutrition is receiving growing attention from government agencies charged with the enormous task of lowering chronic disease rates and containing healthcare costs. A primary means of promoting health and well-being is a wholesome food supply and the nutrition it provides. In our study we will emphasize a person-centered approach for nutrition education and intervention, keeping in mind individual needs, differences, and goals.

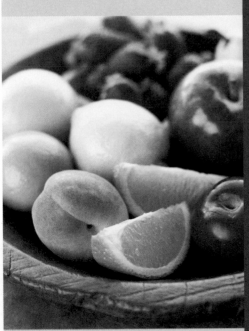

NUTRITION AND HUMAN HEALTH

New Directions for Nutrition

Emerging Health Issues: The Obesity Epidemic

The most alarming health problem worldwide is the growing obesity. Changes in food and lifestyle patterns over the past 25 years have resulted in tremendous changes in body weights across the United States (Figure 1-1). Body weights have increased by 10%, even when corrected for increases in body height.[1] Currently 65% of adults are overweight or obese, and 31% of children are either overweight or at risk for overweight.[2] The "obesity epidemic" as it has been called, includes children and adults from all regions of the country and all social and ethnic groups.[1] The obesity among children and adolescents is of special concern. In recent years the number of overweight adolescents has tripled[3]—and overweight adolescents have an 80% chance of being overweight or obese adults.[4] Higher body weights in children and teens are leading to accelerating rates of type 2 diabetes in these age-groups—a situation almost unheard of 20 years ago.

This rise in obesity, a first for the United States, is related to environmental not biologic factors.[1] In contrast to early times when humans survived as "hunter-gatherers," today we have a plentiful supply of good-tasting, relatively inexpensive food with no energy expenditure required to obtain it.[3] The ever-present vending machine, special offers of two hamburgers for the price of one, and accessible food at most sporting and social events all contribute to food intake (Box 1-1).

Portions served at restaurants or eaten at home often equal three to four times the serving size referred to in meal planning guides (Figure 1-2). As energy intake is rising, energy expenditure is falling, accelerating weight gain. For children sedentary pastimes such as watching television or playing video games or surfing the Internet have replaced active games, and most ride rather than walk to school. Many new residential developments and

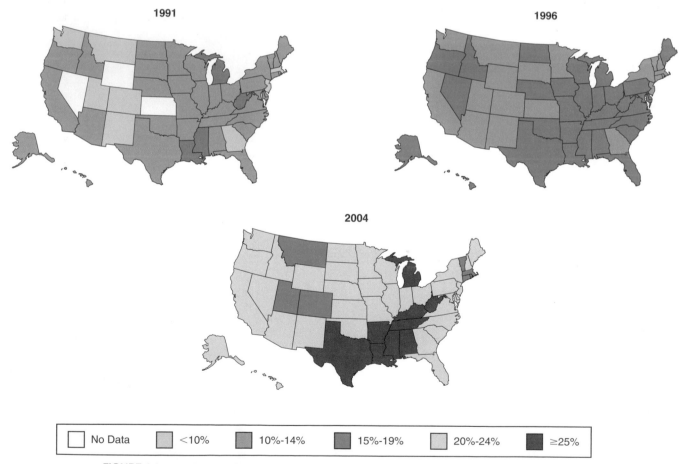

FIGURE 1-1   The obesity epidemic among U.S. adults. Notice the rise since the early 1990s in the number of states in which at least one fifth (20%) or more of the residents are obese. Obesity is defined as a body mass index of 30 or greater. This is approximately 30 lb overweight for a person 64 inches tall. *(Map data from the Behavioral Risk Factor Surveillance System, Centers for Disease Control and Prevention: U.S. obesity trends: 1995-2004, Atlanta, 2005, Author. Retrieved November 22, 2005, from* www.cdc.gov/nccdphp/dnpa/obesity/trend/maps/index.htm.*)*

most rural localities lack sidewalks, making it difficult to walk, and other neighborhoods are unsafe for walking. Collaborative efforts among government agencies, schools, community planners, the food service industry, and health professionals to discourage overeating and promote physical activity will be required to solve this problem.

Rise in the Aging Population

Over the past 100 years improvements in sanitation and public health have raised life expectancy at birth from 45 years to nearly 80 years. Infectious diseases such as influenza and pneumonia have been replaced by chronic diseases, heart disease, cancer, and stroke, as leading causes of death.[5] As life expectancy has increased, so has the number of persons age 65 and over, and this will continue in the coming decades. In fact, the number of older individuals is increasing twice as rapidly as the general population (Figure 1-3).[6] Although the 65-and-older group makes up only 13% of the population, they incur nearly 30% of all healthcare costs.[6] Education and intervention programs putting emphasis on appropriate food intake and physical activity minimize chronic disease and required treatment.

Growth in Ethnic and Racial Diversity

The racial, ethnic, and cultural diversity within the United States continues to expand. Diverse racial and ethnic groups now make up one third of the general population, and this proportion is expected to rise.[6] Hispanic Americans, Asian Americans, and Pacific Islander Americans are increasing at a more rapid rate than other groups. The number of Hispanic Americans now surpasses the number of African Americans, making them the largest minority group.

As a health professional you should become familiar with the eating patterns and favorite foods of racial, ethnic, and cultural groups outside of your own. When helping an individual plan a diet you need to recommend grains or vegetables or protein foods that are familiar and will be accepted. The *Focus on Culture* box, "Diversity in Food Patterns," introduces the food patterns and typical food group choices of various diverse groups; however, it should represent only the beginning of your study of cultural and ethnic foods.

Portion Distortion

CHEESEBURGER

20 Years Ago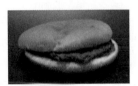

Today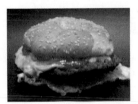

260 calories   850 calories

FIGURE 1-2 Change in portion size of common foods. Over the last 20 years, portion sizes of many common foods have almost tripled. As described on the educational website of the National Heart, Lung, and Blood Institute, a hamburger and roll that supplied 260 kcal may now contain as many as 850 kcal. Visit the website of the National Heart, Lung, and Blood Institute, National Institutes of Health (*http://hin/nhlbi.nih.gov/portion/*) to view photographs of many other food items that have changed in size and kcalorie content, and take the quiz to learn how many minutes you would need to exercise to burn the extra kcalories. (*Concept from U.S. Department of Health and Human Services, National Institutes of Health, National Heart, Lung and Blood Institute, Obesity Education Initiative: Portion distortion! Bethesda, Md, 2004, Author. Available at* http://hin.nhlbi.nih.gov/portion/.)

BOX 1-1	Factors Contributing to Increased Food Intake

Advertising of high-sugar and high-calorie foods targeted at children and adults
Vending machines selling high-sugar drinks and high-fat snacks
Greater number of meals eaten in restaurants
Increase in number of "all-you-can-eat" restaurant buffets
Increase in food portion sizes—both at home and in restaurants
Continuous snacking
"Supersize" portions in fast-food restaurants costing only a fraction more than the "normal" portion

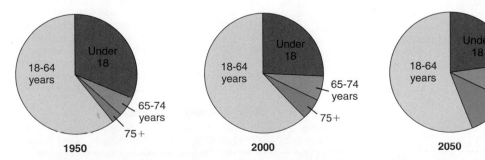

FIGURE 1-3 Projected increases in persons over age 65 between 1950 and 2050. The population age 65 and over grew twice as rapidly and the population age 75 and over grew three times as rapidly as the general population. During the next 50 years older groups will continue to increase twice as fast as younger groups. (*From National Center for Health Statistics:* Health, United States, 2004: with chartbook on trends in the health of Americans with special feature on drugs, *Hyattsville, Md, 2004, U.S. Department of Health and Human Services.*)

◆ FOCUS ON CULTURE

Diversity in Food Patterns

Development of Food Patterns

Foods are the substances that provide the nutrients to sustain life, but for most of us that is not why we choose to eat what we do. Food habits—what we eat and when we eat it—have evolved over thousands of years in the many different cultural and ethnic groups living around the world. In all cultures and societies several factors influence food patterns, as follows:

- *Religion:* Religious beliefs point to not only what is appropriate food but also when it may be eaten. Fasting can restrict certain foods or set periods when no foods should be eaten.
- *Agriculture:* The available land for raising crops or animals led to the evolution of food patterns based on plant foods or animal foods. Raising cattle requires land for grazing.
- *Climate:* When persons raised all of their own food, the length of the growing season, amount of rainfall, and general temperature defined what they ate.
- *Proximity to water:* Those living near water included fish or seafood in their diets as compared to those living inland.

Food Patterns and Food Groups

Regardless of their location and the types of foods available, people survived the world over, receiving their nourishment from different forms of meat or fish, cereals, grains, fruits, vegetables, or milk. In your work as a nutrition and health professional you will see many different food patterns followed by the various cultural and ethnic groups living in the United States.

Religious Dietary Laws

For many groups religious laws set standards for the foods to be eaten and their methods of preparation.

Judaism

The observance of Jewish food laws differs among the three groups within Judaism: (1) the Orthodox follow a strict observance, (2) the Conservative are less strict, and (3) the Reformed have the least emphasis on food laws. The body of dietary laws is called the *Rules of Kashruth.* Foods selected and prepared according to these laws are called *kosher,* from the Hebrew word meaning "fit or proper." Jewish dietary laws govern the slaughter, preparation, and serving of meat, the combining of meat and milk, and the eating of fish and eggs with the following food restrictions:

- *Meat:* Pork is forbidden. Forequarters of other meats and common forms of poultry are allowed. Meat must be rigidly cleansed of all blood, and supervision by a rabbi certifies that correct procedures were followed.
- *Meat and milk:* Meat and milk may not be combined. Orthodox homes maintain two sets of dishes and cooking utensils—one for serving meat and the other for meals containing dairy products. These dishes and cookware must be washed and stored separately.
- *Fish:* Fish with fins and scales are allowed in the diet and may be eaten with either meat or dairy foods. No shellfish or eels are used.
- *Eggs:* Eggs may be eaten with either meat or dairy foods, but eggs with a blood spot must be discarded.

Many traditional Jewish foods such as matzo, a type of unleavened bread, relate to observances that commemorate significant events in Jewish history. Others are used on the Sabbath. Although bagels are a traditional Jewish food, they have become a popular item in the general population.

Islam

Muslim dietary laws are derived from Islamic teachings in the Koran. Food is considered to be a form of worship, and Muslims are urged to avoid self-indulgence. The Koran offers guidance for particular foods, as follows:

- *Milk products:* Permitted at all times
- *Fruits and vegetables:* Permitted unless fermented or poisonous
- *Breads and cereals:* Permitted unless contaminated or harmful
- *Meats:* Pork is strictly forbidden; all other land animals and seafood, including fish, shellfish, eels, and sea animals are permitted. Animals must be slaughtered under the supervision of a religious leader to ensure appropriate procedures. In the United States many Muslims use kosher meats.
- *Alcohol:* Strictly forbidden

Foods may be eaten in any combination as long as no prohibited items are included. The Koran mentions certain foods as being of special value: these include figs, olives, dates, honey, milk, and buttermilk. Prohibited foods may be eaten when no other sources of food are available.

Muslims celebrate Ramadan, a 30-day period of daylight fasting that occurs during the ninth month of the Islamic lunar calendar. During Ramadan Muslims take in no food or beverages from dawn to sunset, but celebrate special meals after sundown. Traditionally these meals start with an appetizer such as dates or a fruit drink, followed by the family's "evening breakfast," the *iftar.* At the end of Ramadan a feast with special foods climaxes the observance.

Latino Food Patterns

The early Spanish explorers to the New World merged their food patterns with those of the people in the lands they settled. The heritage of Latinos can be Mexican, Puerto Rican, or Cuban. Each group has somewhat different food patterns, so when working with Latinos it is important to determine their background.

Mexican

Three foods are basic to the traditional Mexican food pattern: (1) dried beans, (2) chili peppers, and (3) corn. Relatively small amounts of meat are included, and eggs are used occasionally. Corn is the basic grain, and bread takes the form of tortillas, flat cakes baked on a hot griddle. Rice and oats are other grains. Cheese is the primary dairy food because most Mexican Americans are lactose intolerant. Coffee is the main beverage. The cooking fat is lard.

Puerto Rican (Caribbean Islanders)

Puerto Rican families share a common heritage with Mexican families, so some of their foods are the same. Puerto Rican Americans include in their diets tropical fruits and vegetables that often are found in neighborhood markets in the United States. *Viandas,* starchy vegetables and fruits such as plantain and green bananas, are dietary staples along with rice, beans, and dried codfish. Milk, meat, and dark yellow and green vegetables are used in limited amounts. Lard is used in cooking.

Native American Food Patterns

The Native American populations include the Native Americans in the North Central and Southwest regions of the United States, as well as the Alaska Natives. These groups share an attachment to the land and a determination to retain their culture. Food has great religious and social significance and is integral to both celebrations and everyday hospitality. Among Native Americans in the Southwest, traditional dietary staples are combined with food products from supermarkets and fast-food restaurants.

FOCUS ON CULTURE—cont'd

Diversity in Food Patterns

Meat is eaten daily and can be fresh, smoked, or in processed items. Bread tortillas or fry bread, blue cornbread, and cornmeal mush are the usual grain foods. Coffee, soft drinks, and fruit-flavored drinks are popular. Corn, potatoes, green beans, and tomatoes are the usual vegetables, along with fresh or canned fruit. Most foods are fried using lard or shortening.

Southern United States

Traditional African-American Diet

Food dishes of the Southern African Americans, often referred to as "soul food," were created when the early slaves adapted their African recipes to the food staples available in this country. Traditional hot breads were made with corn, and included spoon bread, cornmeal muffins, and skillet cornbread. Cooked cereals such as cornmeal mush and hominy grits along with rice were staple foods. Many Southern African Americans in rural areas had gardens, and okra, sweet potatoes, green beans, tomatoes, potatoes, and black-eyed peas or red beans were plentiful. Leafy greens—turnip greens, collards, mustard greens, and spinach—were cooked with bacon or salt pork. Pork, beef, poultry, organ meats, and fish were popular. Foods were usually fried. Beverages included coffee, apple cider, lemonade, sweet tea, and buttermilk.

French Americans

The Cajun people are descendants of early French colonists who settled in Nova Scotia and eventually relocated to southern Louisiana. They made use of the seafood nearby and blended their French culinary background with the Creole cookery found around New Orleans. Cajun foods are strong flavored and spicy with seafood as a base and are usually cooked as a stew and served over rice. Tabasco sauce evolved from Cajun cookery. Crawfish, catfish, red snapper, shrimp, and oysters are used frequently. Vegetables include onions, bell peppers, okra, squash, yams, and tomatoes. Seafood and chicken gumbo, jambalaya, red beans and rice, blackened catfish, and boiled crawfish are typical Cajun foods. Breads and cereals include French bread, hush puppies, cornbread muffins, cush-cush, grits, and rice.

Asian Food Patterns

Chinese

Chinese cooks believe that refrigeration diminishes natural flavors, so they select the freshest foods available, hold them for the shortest time possible, and cook them quickly at a high temperature. Most foods are prepared in a wok with small amounts of fat and liquid. This stir-fry method preserves natural flavor, color, and texture. Meat is used in small amounts in combined dishes rather than as a main entree. Eggs and soybean foods such as tofu add protein. Dried, salted, pickled, spiced, and candied foods are added as relishes. Rice is the staple grain served at most meals. The traditional beverage is unsweetened green tea. Peanut oil is the main cooking fat.

Japanese

Japanese and Chinese food patterns share some similarities because both use rice as a basic grain and emphasize fresh ingredients; however, the Japanese use less oil. Vegetables are usually boiled with vinegar and soy sauce. The Japanese meal includes steamed rice along with grilled, broiled, or pan-cooked fish or shellfish and a wide variety of vegetables. Poultry, pork, and beef are eaten frequently. A large bowl of noodles combined with meat and vegetables is a popular, quick, and easy meal. Soy sauce and rice vinegar are used as flavorings. Sushi made with very fresh raw fish and tempura,

battered and deep-fried shrimp and vegetables, have become popular in the United States.

Southeast Asian Food Patterns

Hmong, Cambodian, and Laotian

The Hmong from Vietnam are the largest ethnic group from Southeast Asia in the United States. Rice is the core food of the Vietnamese, and plain rice served in a separate bowl is included at most meals. Fish and shellfish are popular as are chicken, duck, pork, and beef. Foods are often stir-fried with a small amount of lard or peanut oil. Mixed dishes containing vegetables and seasonings with small amounts of seafood or meat form the basis of most meals. Since coming to the United States, these groups have increased their use of eggs, beef, and pork.

East Asian Indians and Pakistanis

Rice, lentils, beans, and peas are diet staples. Main dishes consist of vegetables cooked with a small amount of chicken, beef, pork, or fish. Yogurt sauces and milk-based desserts are milk sources for adults. Breads are unleavened. Potatoes, spinach, eggplant, tomatoes, carrots, and collard greens are common vegetables. Spicy deep-fried turnovers filled with meat, fish, or vegetables are popular. Clarified butter, peanut oil, and sesame seed oil are used in cooking. Beverages include water flavored with sweet syrups, along with coffee and tea.

Mediterranean Influences

Italian

The sharing of food is an important part of Italian life. Bread and pasta are served at most meals. Cheese is a favorite food with many popular varieties. Meat, poultry, and fish are used in various ways, along with Italian sausages and cold meats. Vegetables are ingredients in mixed main dishes and soups, in sauces, in salads, or served plain. In mixed dishes vegetables are browned and seasoned in olive oil; meat or fish is added and covered with wine, broth, or tomato sauce; and all is simmered slowly for several hours. Fresh fruit is often a dessert or snack.

Greek

Everyday meals are simple with bread at the center. Milk is seldom used as a beverage but eaten in the fermented form of yogurt. Cheese is a favorite food, especially feta cheese, made from goat's milk. Lamb is a favorite meat, although fish is served frequently. Eggs are sometimes a main dish, but never a breakfast food. Vegetables are served as an entree cooked with broth, tomato sauce, onions, olive oil, and parsley. A typical salad consists of thinly sliced raw vegetables and feta cheese, dressed with olive oil and vinegar. Rice is the major grain. Fruit is an everyday dessert, but rich pastries such as baklava are served on special occasions.

Changes in Ethnic Patterns

Over time individuals living in the United States begin to adapt to the food patterns around them and place less emphasis on their traditional foods. The foods adopted from the American pattern are often less nutritious than their native foods. Traditional meal patterns usually emphasize rice, legumes, and vegetables high in nutrients and fiber, with small amounts of meat or fish. Those foods are replaced with soft drinks, fast foods, highly processed foods, and snack foods high in sugar and fat, resulting in rapid weight gain and increased risk of diabetes. A balance between the old and the new is the best way to preserve one's heritage and health.

Continued

FOCUS ON CULTURE—cont'd

Diversity in Food Patterns

References

Diabetes Care and Education Dietetic Practice Group of the American Dietetic Association: *Ethnic and regional food practices: A series. Alaska native food practices, customs, and holidays,* Chicago/Alexandria, VA, 1998, American Dietetic Association/American Diabetes Association.

Diabetes Care and Education Dietetic Practice Group of the American Dietetic Association: *Ethnic and regional food practices: A series. Chinese American food practices, customs, and holidays,* Chicago/Alexandria, VA, 1998, American Dietetic Association/American Diabetes Association.

Diabetes Care and Education Dietetic Practice Group of the American Dietetic Association: *Ethnic and regional food practices: A series. Filipino American food practices, customs, and holidays,* Chicago/Alexandria, VA, 1994, American Dietetic Association/American Diabetes Association.

Diabetes Care and Education Dietetic Practice Group of the American Dietetic Association: *Ethnic and regional food practices: A series. Hmong American food practices, customs, and holidays,* Chicago/Alexandria, VA, 1999, American Dietetic Association/American Diabetes Association.

Diabetes Care and Education Dietetic Practice Group of the American Dietetic Association: *Ethnic and regional food practices: A series. Indian and Pakistani food practices, customs, and holidays,* ed 2, Chicago/Alexandria, VA, 2000, American Dietetic Association/American Diabetes Association.

Diabetes Care and Education Dietetic Practice Group of the American Dietetic Association: *Ethnic and regional food practices: A series. Jewish food practices, customs, and holidays,* Chicago/Alexandria, VA, 1998, American Dietetic Association/American Diabetes Association.

Diabetes Care and Education Dietetic Practice Group of the American Dietetic Association: *Ethnic and regional food practices: A series. Mexican American food practices, customs, and holidays,* Chicago/Alexandria, VA, 1998, American Dietetic Association/American Diabetes Association.

Diabetes Care and Education Dietetic Practice Group of the American Dietetic Association: *Ethnic and regional food practices: A series. Navajo food practices, customs, and holidays,* Chicago/Alexandria, VA, 1998, American Dietetic Association/American Diabetes Association.

Diabetes Care and Education Dietetic Practice Group of the American Dietetic Association: *Ethnic and regional food practices: A series. Soul and traditional southern food practices, customs, and holidays,* Chicago/Alexandria, VA, 1995, American Dietetic Association/American Diabetes Association.

Kittler PG, Sucher KP: *Cultural foods: traditions and trends,* Belmont, Calif, 2000, Wadsworth/Thomson Learning.

The Science of Nutrition

Nutrition builds on two areas of science. The life sciences of biochemistry and physiology help us see how nutrition relates to our physical health and well-being. The behavioral sciences help us understand how nutrition is interwoven with our psychosocial needs. Both of these are at work in our lives.

The principles of biochemistry teach us that human organisms are highly complex groupings of chemical compounds constantly at work in an array of reactions that sustain life. Nutrients participate in and help to control these chemical reactions. Various physiologic systems integrate the activities of the millions of individually functioning cells and organs, uniting them into a functioning whole. This highly sensitive internal control is called homeostasis.

As humans we also have social and emotional qualities rooted in our earliest awareness of psychosocial interactions and life experiences. Our eating patterns and attitudes toward food develop over our lifetime based on the acculturating influences of our primary family and friends, ethnic or cultural group, community, nation, and world. How we perceive our food, what we choose to eat, why we eat what we do, and the manner in which we eat are all integral parts of human nutrition.

Food and Nutrients

The term nutrition means to nourish. Nutrition is both a science and an art, focusing on the food people eat and how it nourishes their lives physically, socially, and personally. From the moment of conception until death, an appropriate supply of food supports optimum growth and maturation, mental and physical well-being, and resistance to disease. Good nutrition promotes health and reduces the risk of adverse conditions ranging from low birth weight to cardiovascular disease and cancer.[7] Food supplies the energy to carry out physical functions such as inhaling and exhaling, maintaining body temperature, and engaging in physical activity. But food also nourishes the human spirit. We all have our particular "soul foods," those comfort foods that connect us to our family and provide a sense of psychologic and emotional well-being.

Working Definitions

To study nutrition we need to define the terms that describe this body of knowledge and the health professionals that work within it. *Nutrition* refers to the food people eat and how it nourishes their bodies, whereas nutrition science is the scientific knowledge that defines nutrient requirements for body maintenance, growth, activity, and reproduction. Dietetics is the health profession with primary responsibility for the practical application of nutrition science to persons and groups in various conditions of health and disease. The registered dietitian (RD) is the nutrition expert on the healthcare team. The RD, in collaboration with the physician and nurse, carries the major responsibility for patients' nutritional care. Public health nutritionists oversee the care of high-risk groups in the community such as pregnant teenagers or older adults, assessing needs and developing intervention programs. Other RDs collaborate with school nurses to teach weight management classes for children and their parents, assist day care providers in planning menus and snacks, or help clients at fitness centers improve their body composition or athletic performance.

Functions of Food and Nutrients

Food serves as the vehicle for bringing nutrients into the body. However, it is the specific chemical compounds and elements in foods—the nutrients—that the body requires. We must do away with the myth that any particular food or food combination is required to ensure health. The human race has survived for centuries on wide varieties of foods, depending on what was available and what the culture designated as appropriate food. Approximately 50 nutrients have been found to be essential to human life and health, although countless other elements and molecules are being studied and may be essential. The identification of all essential nutrients is particularly important to those who develop formulas for enteral and parenteral feeding of critically ill patients.

Essential nutrients include the macronutrients—carbohydrates, fats, and proteins—and the micronutrients—vitamins and minerals. The macronutrients supply energy and build tissue. The micronutrients are used in much smaller amounts to form specialized structures and regulate and control body processes. Water is the often forgotten nutrient that sustains all of our life systems. The sum of all chemical reactions that use nutrients is referred to as metabolism. The first section of this text describes these important nutrients. In later chapters we look at how they participate in growth, maturation, aging, and health and evaluate nutrient-based interventions for acute and chronic diseases.

Nutrient Interrelationships

An important principle in nutrition is *nutrient interaction,* a concept that is made up of the following two parts:

1. Individual nutrients participate in many different metabolic functions; in some functions a nutrient has a primary role, and in others it has a supporting role.
2. No nutrient ever works alone.

The human body is made up of many parts and processes. Intimate and ongoing metabolic relationships exist among all the basic nutrients and their metabolites. Although we separate the nutrients to simplify our study, they do not exist that way in the body. Nutrients are always working together as an integrated whole, providing energy, building and rebuilding tissue, and regulating metabolic activities. This synergy and interaction among nutrients is important in carrying out body functions and may be overlooked when we examine the effects of one nutrient at a time.[8] In the next section we look at the various classes of nutrients as a prelude to our detailed study of their roles. Nutrients have three general functions in the body, as follows:

1. They provide energy.
2. They build and repair body tissues and structures.

3. They regulate all the metabolic processes that maintain homeostasis and support life.

Energy Sources

The energy-yielding nutrients—carbohydrates, fats, and proteins—provide primary and alternate sources of energy.

homeostasis State of dynamic equilibrium within the body's internal environment; a balance achieved through the operation of various interrelated physiologic mechanisms.

nutrition The sum of the processes involved in taking in food, releasing the nutrients it contains, and assimilating and using these nutrients to provide energy and maintain body tissue; a foundation for life and health.

nutrition science The body of scientific knowledge developed through controlled research that relates to all aspects of nutrition—national, international, community, and clinical.

dietetics Management of diet and the use of food; the science concerned with the nutritional planning and preparation of foods and diets.

registered dietitian (RD) A professional dietitian who has completed an accredited academic program and 900 hours of postbaccalaureate supervised professional practice and has passed the National Registration Examination for Dietitians administered by the Commission on Dietetic Registration.

public health nutritionist A professional nutritionist who has completed an academic program and special graduate study (MPH, DrPH) in a school of public health accredited by the American Association of Public Health and is responsible for nutrition components of public health programs in varied community settings—county, state, national, international.

nutrients Substances in food that are essential for energy, growth, normal body function, and maintenance of life.

macronutrients The three energy-yielding nutrients: carbohydrates, fats, and proteins.

micronutrients The two classes of small non–energy-yielding elements and compounds—the minerals and the vitamins. Minerals and vitamins are essential for regulation and control functions in cell metabolism and for building certain body structures.

metabolism Sum of all the various biochemical and physiologic processes by which the body grows and maintains itself (anabolism) and breaks down and reshapes tissue (catabolism) and transforms energy to do its work. Products of these various reactions are called metabolites.

metabolites Any substance produced by metabolism or by a metabolic process.

Carbohydrates

Dietary carbohydrates, starch and sugar, are the body's primary source of fuel for heat and energy. *Glycogen* is a storage form of carbohydrate used for quick energy. It is sometimes called *animal starch* because its structure is similar to that of plant starch. Each gram of carbohydrate when metabolized in the body yields 4 kilocalories (kcalories or kcal), referred to as its *fuel factor*. In a well-balanced diet for a healthy person 45% to 65% of total kcalories are supplied by carbohydrate.[9] The majority of these kcalories should come from complex carbohydrates (starch) and a smaller amount from simple carbohydrates (sugars). Another form of complex carbohydrate known as *fiber* is non-energy yielding but has other important body functions. Although the general public uses the word *calorie* to refer to the energy value of food, nutritionists use the technical term *kilocalorie* (kcalorie). Later in this chapter you will notice that MyPyramid, the food guidance system developed for the general public, and the *Dietary Guidelines for Americans* use the term *calorie* when indicating the energy value of foods or diets. We will learn more about these terms in Chapter 5.

Fats

Dietary fats from animal and plant sources provide the body's alternate or storage form of energy. Fat is a more concentrated fuel with a fuel factor of 9, yielding 9 kcal/g. It is recommended that fats supply no more than 20% to 35% of total kcalories.[9] Less than 10% of dietary fat should be saturated fat with the remainder coming from unsaturated fats.

Proteins

The primary function of protein is tissue building, although it can be used for energy if needed. The body draws on dietary or tissue protein when the fuel supply from carbohydrates and fats is not sufficient to meet body needs. Protein yields 4 kcal/g, making its fuel factor 4. Protein can provide 10% to 35% of total kcalories in a well-balanced diet for healthy individuals.[9]

Tissue Building and Repair

Proteins, vitamins, and minerals help form body structures. Minerals and vitamins have important roles in various specialized tissues.

Protein

Protein provides the building blocks for body tissues. Protein foods are broken down into amino acids, the building units necessary for making and repairing tissues. Body tissues are constantly being broken down and rebuilt to ensure growth and maintenance of body structure. Proteins also form vital substances that regulate body systems.

Minerals

Minerals are used to build tissues with very specific functions. The major minerals calcium and phosphorus give strength to bones and teeth. The trace element iron is a component of hemoglobin and binds oxygen for transport to cells.

Vitamins

Vitamins are complex molecules needed in very minute amounts, but they are essential in certain tissues. Vitamin C helps produce the intercellular ground substance that cements tissues together and prevents tissue bleeding. Vitamin A in the rods and cones of the eye is needed for vision in dim light.

Metabolic Regulation

Minerals and vitamins act as regulators to keep the body functioning efficiently and maintain homeostasis. Water provides the fluid environment in which all chemical reactions take place.

Minerals

Minerals serve as coenzyme factors in cell metabolism. Iron controls the enzyme actions in the cell mitochondria that produce and store high-energy compounds.

Vitamins

Vitamins are components of cell enzyme systems and govern reactions that produce energy and synthesize important molecules. Thiamin helps control the release of energy to carry on the work of the cell.

Water

Water forms the blood, lymph, and intercellular fluids that transport nutrients to cells and remove waste. Water also functions as a regulatory agent, providing the fluid environment in which all metabolic reactions take place.

Nutritional Status

The nutritional health of an individual is referred to as his or her *nutritional status* and describes how well nutrient needs are being met.[10] Nutritional status is influenced by one's living situation, available food supply, food choices, and state of health or disease. A complete evaluation of nutritional status requires a combination of dietary, biochemical, anthropometric, and clinical measurements (Box 1-2). It is important to know not only what an individual is eating but also whether the body is absorbing and using the nutrients in that food. Blood nutrient levels can help to identify a nutrient deficiency or excess brought about by overuse of highly fortified foods or supplements. Body weight for height and other anthropometric measurements provide estimates of body fat and muscle mass. We will discuss nutritional assessment in greater detail in Chapter 16 and review disease conditions that adversely affect nutritional status.

Optimal Nutrition

Individuals with optimal nutritional status have neither a deficiency nor an excess of nutrients. Nutrient reserves are at the upper end of the normal range and are not being used to meet daily metabolic needs. General evidence of optimal nutrition includes appropriate weight for height (ratio of muscle mass to fat) and good muscle development and tone. The skin is smooth and the eyes are clear and bright. Appetite, digestion, and elimination are normal. Detailed characteristics of good and poor nutritional status are listed in Table 1-1. Think about these signs, and begin to look for them so you may become a more skilled observer. Well-nourished persons are more likely to be alert, both mentally and physically. They are not only meeting their day-to-day needs but also keeping nutrient stores to resist disease and extend their years of normal function.

Undernutrition

Undernutrition may take various forms ranging from marginal nutritional status to the famine victim with kwashiorkor or marasmus. Persons with *marginal nutritional status* are meeting their minimum day-to-day nutritional needs but lack the nutrient reserves to cope with any added physiologic or metabolic demand arising from injury or illness, the need to sustain a healthy pregnancy, or a childhood growth spurt. Marginal nutritional status results from poor eating habits, stressed environments, or insufficient resources to obtain appropriate types or amounts of food. Meals at fast-food restaurants, a matter of convenience for families with busy lifestyles, can lead to higher intakes of fat and lower intakes of calcium, vitamins A and C, and fiber in both children and adults.[11] Three food categories—(1) sweets and desserts, (2) soft drinks, and (3) alcoholic beverages—provide almost one fourth of all the kcalories in the diets of Americans.[12] Pastries and baked goods, candy, and soft drinks and other sweetened beverages are replacing nutrient-dense foods such as fruits, vegetables, whole grain breads and cereals, and milk. Individuals with higher intakes of sugar have lower intakes of vitamins and minerals.[13] Although persons with poorer intakes of the micronutrients may not be undernourished, they are at greater risk of physical illness than those who are well nourished, and they lack nutrient stores. The body can adapt to marginal nutrition, but even limited physiologic stress can result in overt malnutrition.

Overt Malnutrition

When nutrient intake is not sufficient to meet day-to-day needs and nutrient reserves are depleted, signs of malnutrition will begin to appear. Individuals and families with incomes below the poverty threshold often have diets lacking in both quantity and quality of food. Approximately 10% of U.S. households (10.5 million) report some level of food insecurity. Single-parent families, families without health insurance, and families headed by a person with less than a high school diploma are most likely to be food insecure.[14] Even if energy needs are met, foods high in micronutrients—fruits, vegetables, whole grains, and fish—may not be accessible to low-income families.[15]

Hunger influences health in all age and sex groups, but the most vulnerable are infants, children, pregnant women, and older adults. Prenatal care for women who are poor, young, or lack education is often inadequate, resulting in poor pregnancy outcomes. Toddlers from

---

BOX 1-2	Measurements Used to Evaluate Nutritional Status

Dietary Intake

Where and when food is eaten
Use of dietary supplements
Food resources
Special diet, if any
Cooking facilities

Biochemical Measurements

Blood vitamin levels
Blood protein levels
Blood lipid levels

Anthropometric Measurements

Body weight for height (Body Mass Index)
Skinfold thicknesses
Waist circumferences

Clinical Measurements

Skin
Hair
Eyes

---

kilocalorie The general term *calorie* refers to a unit of heat measure and is used alone to designate the small calorie. The large calorie, 1000 calories of kilocalorie, is used in the study of metabolism to avoid the use of very large numbers in calculations.

amino acid An acid containing the essential element nitrogen (in the chemical group NH_2). Amino acids are the structural units of protein and the basic building blocks of body tissue.

synthesize To form new compounds in the body for use in building tissues or carrying out metabolic or physiologic functions.

anthropometric Measurement of the human body to determine height, weight, skinfold thickness, or other dimensions that provide estimates of the relative proportion of body fat and body muscle; such measurements can be used to evaluate health status and risk of chronic disease.

TABLE 1-1	Clinical Signs of Nutritional Status	
Feature(s)	**Good Nutritional Status**	**Poor Nutritional Status**
General appearance	Alert, responsive	Listless, apathetic, cachectic
Hair	Shiny, lustrous, healthy scalp	Stringy, dull, brittle, dry, depigmented
Neck glands	No enlargement	Thyroid enlarged
Skin—face, neck	Smooth, slightly moist	Greasy, scaly
Eyes	Bright, clear, no fatigue circles	Dryness, signs of infection, increased vascularity, glassiness, thickened conjunctivae
Lips	Good color, moist	Dry, scaly, swollen, angular lesions (stomatitis)
Tongue	Good pink color, surface papillae present, no lesions	Papillary atrophy, smooth appearance, swollen, red, beefy (glossitis)
Gums	Good pink color, no swelling or bleeding, firm	Marginal redness or swelling, receding, spongy
Teeth	Straight, no crowding, well-shaped jaw, no discoloration	Unfilled cavities, absent teeth, worn surfaces, mottled, malpositioned
Skin, general	Smooth, slightly moist	Rough, dry, scaly, irritated; petechiae, bruises
Abdomen	Flat	Swollen
Legs, feet	No tenderness, weakness, swelling	Edema, tender calf, tingling, weakness
Skeleton	No malformations	Bowlegs, chest deformity at diaphragm, beaded ribs, prominent scapulas
Weight	Normal for height, age, body build	Overweight or underweight
Posture	Erect, arms and legs straight, abdomen in, chest out	Sagging shoulders, sunken chest, humped back
Muscles	Well-developed, firm	Flaccid, poor tone, undeveloped, tender
Nervous control	Good attention span for age, does not cry easily, not irritable or restless	Inattentive, irritable
Gastrointestinal function	Good appetite and normal digestion, regular elimination	Anorexia, indigestion, constipation or diarrhea
General vitality	Endurance, energetic, sleeps well at night, vigorous	Easily fatigued, no energy, falls asleep in school, looks tired, apathetic

families who are food insecure are twice as likely to have health problems as those from families that have a good food supply.[16] Children with chronically inadequate diets develop anemia with lower resistance to infection, impaired learning ability, and less energy. Food banks that serve homeless and low-income families have limited supplies of nutrient-dense items such as dairy foods and fruit.[17]

We also find malnutrition in hospital patients and residents of long-term care facilities. Hypermetabolic diseases and prolonged illness in older persons with low nutrient reserves leads to nutrient depletion and debilitating weight loss.[18] Both prescription and over-the-counter drugs have adverse effects on nutritional status. (Malnutrition in clinical care will be discussed in Part 3.)

Overnutrition

Excessive energy intake and low physical activity will, over time, result in unwanted weight gain and *overnutrition.* In contrast to colonial times when a portly appearance was a sign of prosperity, it is now recognized as a health risk. Childhood or adolescent obesity sets the

stage for premature development of type 2 diabetes and cardiovascular disease.[19] *Overnutrition* also occurs with excessive intakes of micronutrients. Inappropriate use of vitamin or mineral supplements can damage tissues and interfere with the absorption and metabolism of other nutrients. Herbal preparations growing in popularity carry the potential for harmful interactions with nutrients or prescribed medications.

We continue to learn more about the relationship between our genes and our nutrient needs and the specific actions of particular components in foods that influence our health (see the *To Probe Further* box, "Emerging Trends in Nutrition").

NUTRITION POLICY AND NATIONAL HEALTH PROBLEMS

Diet, Health, and Public Policy

Need for Public Policy

Public policy refers to the laws, regulations, and government programs around a certain topic or issue. Examples

TO PROBE FURTHER

EMERGING TRENDS IN NUTRITION

New research is directing our attention beyond the basic nutrients and their general functions in growth and health to gene-nutrient interactions and how they influence both the well-being of individuals and the development and maintenance of our food supply. We discuss some of these new research findings in this box.

Nutrigenomics: Nutrition and Our Genes

Over the past 100 years researchers have discovered more than 50 nutrients known to be required for human health. We have studied the actions of these nutrients on the body as a whole and on particular cells and tissues. New developments in the world of biology are making it possible for nutrition researchers to examine life at the molecular level and look at interactions between nutrients and the genetic code.[1] These studies will help us learn why some individuals cannot produce the enzyme needed to break down lactose or why others are allergic to certain proteins in wheat flour. Persons with particular gene types appear to have a greater or smaller need for a particular nutrient or respond to a health intervention in a different way. For example, a change in the amount or type of dietary fat that decreases blood lipid levels in most people may actually worsen the blood lipid levels in another.[2] Individuals who appear to be physically similar may have very different nutrient requirements. Race and ethnicity may influence health and nutrient responses. In time we may be able to individualize diets based on genetic predisposition to specific diseases. In the meantime we need to recognize that patients or clients may respond differently to nutrition interventions.

Nutrition and Plant Genetics

New biotechnology also influences our food supply. Agricultural scientists are developing new crop varieties resistant to particular viruses or plant diseases or adaptable to less fertile soils.[3] The introduction of certain genes into a plant to improve its nutritional quality can improve human health, particularly in parts of the world where the food supply is limited.[4] Addressing the concerns of the general public regarding the safety of genetically engineered foods is a new responsibility for nutrition and health professionals. Health workers, farmers, and food processors must work together to support sustainable agricultural practices that conserve natural resources and reduce water and air pollution.[5]

Products in the Marketplace

The growing concern about obesity and chronic disease among public health agencies, the healthcare community, and the general public has attracted the attention of food scientists and food processors. We know that many foods promote health in ways over and above the actions of the known nutrients they contain. Such foods have come to be called *functional foods*. Plant chemicals called *phytochemicals* found in fruits and vegetables have cancer-fighting properties.[6] One food industry response to consumer interest in disease-fighting foods is a margarine fortified with plant sterols, shown to help lower blood cholesterol levels. Some brands of orange juice have calcium and vitamin D added to prevent bone loss and provide an alternative source for these nutrients. Even dark chocolate, formerly considered a food to be avoided, is now known to contain health-promoting phytochemicals and in moderation has a role in a healthy diet.[7] Health researchers are also discovering new therapeutic uses of certain nutrients in common foods. Particular fatty acids found in fatty fish may help to control inflammatory conditions such as asthma.[8] Herbs and other alternative medicines are competing for the public's attention.

New Sources of Nutrition Information

The Internet and other technology-based materials are an expanding source of health and nutrition advice for the eager consumer. Although Internet sites maintained by government agencies, universities, and nonprofit health organizations provide appropriate information and direct readers to other reputable resources, commercial sites devoted to sales often make misleading health claims. Internet sales of herbs, drugs, or health devices are not monitored by government regulatory agencies, and such products can be intrinsically harmful along with delaying a visit to a trained health professional. At the close of each chapter in our text is a list of websites recommended for clients or patients wishing additional information.

References

1. Ordovas JM, Corella D: Nutritional genomics, *Annu Rev Genomics Hum Genet* 5:71, 2004.
2. Hoolihan LE: Individualization of nutrition recommendations and food choices, *Nutr Today* 38:225, 2003.
3. Mackey M, Montgomery J: Plant biotechnology can enhance food security and nutrition in the developing world, part 1, *Nutr Today* 39:52, 2004.
4. Mackey M, Montgomery J: Plant biotechnology can enhance food security and nutrition in the developing world, part 2, *Nutr Today* 39:221, 2004.
5. American Dietetic Association: Position of the American Dietetic Association: Dietetics professionals can implement practices to conserve natural resources and protect the environment, *J Am Diet Assoc* 101(10):1221, 2001.
6. Food and Nutrition Board, National Research Council: *Dietary reference intakes for vitamin C, vitamin E, selenium, and carotenoids*, Washington, DC, 2000, National Academies Press.
7. Steinberg FM, Bearden MM, Keen CL: Cocoa and chocolate flavonoids: implications for cardiovascular health, *J Am Diet Assoc* 103:215, 2003.
8. Stephensen CB: Fish oil and inflammatory disease: is asthma the next target for n-3 fatty acid supplements? *Nutr Rev* 62:486, 2004.

of public policy affecting our food system include nutrition labeling, use of food additives, and food service sanitation standards in healthcare facilities. Nutrition policies are concerned with food guidance for the public, nutrition standards for government food programs, and the health and well-being of our population. In recent years nutrition policy has focused on obesity and how we can reduce chronic disease. As a future health professional you need to stay informed and participate in public policy making in your community and at state and national levels.

National Nutrition Monitoring and Related Research Program

Developing and implementing national nutrition policy falls under the broad heading of the National Nutrition Monitoring and Related Research Program (NNMRRP). This program has the following three objectives[20]:

1. *Developing nutrition policy:* The *Dietary Guidelines for Americans* and the food stamp program for limited-resource families fall under the NNMRRP. Nutrition policy influences agricultural production, what foods are grown, and what fertilizers may be used.

2. *Monitoring the nutritional well-being of the population:* Several ongoing surveys collect information that tells us about the nutritional status of different age, race, and ethnic groups in the United States. The National Health and Nutrition Examination Surveys (NHANES) look at health measures including nutrient intake, body weight status, bone health, iron deficiency anemia, and blood lipid levels. The Continuing Survey of Food Intake by Individuals (CSFII) monitors food intake and knowledge and attitudes about food and nutrition.

3. *Conducting nutrition research:* Researchers in government and university laboratories are learning more about nutrient requirements and the effects of nutrient deficiencies or excesses on health. A current research priority is the effect of obesity on the development of chronic diseases in youth and adults. Government laboratories study the nutrient content of food and provide the values for nutrient analysis programs, as found on the CD-ROM included with your text.

These three activities, working together, give a unified approach to our nation's nutrition and health needs. In policy making we set standards for nutrient intake and pass laws regulating the development of new food products. The nutrition-monitoring system gives feedback on whether our policies are appropriate and successful: are the *Dietary Guidelines for Americans* helping people choose a healthy diet? As new questions arise in food and health, the research arm of the program provides answers that serve as a basis for changes or additions to nutrition policy. In this chapter we look at nutrition policy surrounding food intake and nutrition monitoring. In Chapter 9 we will discuss nutrition labeling and food safety.

Development of Nutrition Policy

Up until the mid-1900s government policy and programs were intended to eradicate hunger and malnutrition. Deficiency diseases such as rickets and pellagra still existed in various parts of the United States in the early part of the century, and a law passed in the 1930s required the addition of vitamin D to milk. The enrichment of grains with several of the B vitamins and iron began sometime later. The development of the School Nutrition Program with policies for free or reduced-cost lunches responded to concerns about hunger among certain population groups. By the 1970s and 1980s, however, the focus shifted to overnutrition as new research linked dietary habits to the growing prevalence of cardiovascular disease. Congressional committees began to discuss the role of government in setting dietary guidelines to improve health.

The first major policy report issued by the U.S. government linking nutrition and chronic disease was the *Surgeon General's Report on Nutrition and Health*[21] released in 1988. This report established the connection between the typical American diet high in fat and salt and both morbidity and early death from cardiovascular disease. The American people were urged to cut down their use of foods high in fat and salt and increase their use of foods high in complex carbohydrates and fiber. In 1989 the Food and Nutrition Board of the National Academy of Sciences issued its extensive research report, *Diet and Health: Implications for Reducing Chronic Disease Risk.*[22] Their dietary recommendations agreed with those of the Surgeon General and advised persons to (1) reduce total fat to 30% or less of total kcalories, (2) reduce saturated fat and cholesterol, (3) increase fiber and complex carbohydrates, (4) avoid excessive sodium and protein, and (5) maintain appropriate levels of calcium.

Healthy People 2010

In 1990 the U.S. Department of Health and Human Services (USDHHS) developed a public health initiative addressing diet, physical activity, and other health-related lifestyle factors. This program outlined specific objectives and health goals to be reached by the year 2000.[23] Although some goals were achieved by the target date, others, including lowering the prevalence of obesity and improving intakes of appropriate foods and levels of physical activity, fell short of their objectives. *Healthy People 2010* has continued this work with a new set of objectives and target indicators.[24] The overall goals for 2010 are (1) to increase the years of healthy life and (2) to reduce the disparities in healthcare that exist among individuals of different races, ethnic groups, and income levels.

NUTRITION GUIDES FOR A HEALTHY DIET

Since the early 1900s food and nutrient guides have been in place to help Americans meet their nutritional needs. The underlying assumptions used in developing these guides reflected not only the growing body of nutrition science, but also social, political, and economic events occurring at the time including wars and national emergencies. Over time the focus of these guides also shifted from preventing undernutrition to controlling chronic diseases related to overnutrition. These guides are of three types:

(1) nutrition standards, (2) dietary guidelines, and (3) food guides. Each has a different purpose and target audience.

Nutrition Standards

U.S. Standards

Most countries have standards for nutrient intakes of healthy persons according to age and gender. These standards are not intended to define the nutrient needs of a particular individual or set nutrient goals in illness or disease. Rather, nutrient standards are intended for use by professionals in making decisions about the nutritional health of individuals and groups.

In the United States these nutrient and energy standards are called the Dietary Reference Intakes (DRIs) and include several categories of recommendations. The first set of nutrient standards, however, included only one category called the Recommended Dietary Allowances (RDAs).

Development of the Recommended Dietary Allowances

The first set of RDAs grew out of a national nutrition conference held in 1941.[25] These nutrient and energy recommendations were published in 1943 as a guide for nutrition workers planning food supplies for national defense and general population needs. Revised editions followed every 4 to 5 years to update the standards as needed. The last edition to follow this format was issued in 1989 by the Food and Nutrition Board of the National Research Council.[27]

During the 1990s nutrition experts recommended the framework of the RDAs be expanded to address the following three emerging issues:

1. The growing population of older adults
2. The health benefits that might be achieved with higher intakes of certain nutrients even though research information was limited
3. The dangers of inappropriately high intakes of specific nutrients

The expanded set of standards that evolved was given the working title of Dietary Reference Intakes (DRIs).

Dietary Reference Intakes

The categories included in the DRIs are described in Box 1-3. The first set of DRIs released in 1997 provided us with new standards for calcium, phosphorus, magnesium, and vitamin D and emphasized the role of calcium and vitamin D in bone health.[26] Reports that followed established DRIs for the B complex vitamins (1998);[27] important antioxidant nutrients and carotenoids (2000);[28] vitamins A and K and the trace minerals (2001);[29] the energy-yielding macronutrients, energy, and fiber (2002);[9] and electrolytes and water (2004).[30]

Each category within the DRIs is useful to the health professional. The Recommended Dietary Allowance (RDA) serves as an intake goal for all healthy people. The

Adequate Intake (AI) sets a dietary goal when new research suggests a health benefit. The AIs for calcium and vitamin D support bone health. The Tolerable Upper Intake Level (UL) is an important guide for practitioners advising individuals on the use of dietary supplements. The Estimated Average Requirement (EAR) is used to evaluate the nutrient intakes of population groups. The DRIs also recognize the changes in nutrient requirements that occur as persons grow older. The two categories for older adults group those ages 51 to 70 years and those ages 71 years and over. The Acceptable Macronutrient Distribution Range (AMDR) guides the division of kcalories among carbohydrate, fat, and protein in ranges supportive of health. (The DRIs for vitamins, minerals, and macronutrients can be found on the inside front cover of this textbook.)

Other Standards

Canadian and British standards are similar to United States standards. In underdeveloped countries where the supply of protein and other nutrient sources may be limited, workers refer to standards set by the Food and Agriculture Organization (FAO) of the World Health Organization (WHO). These standards provide nutrient and energy guidelines to help workers in various locations promote physical well-being through sound nutrition.

Dietary Guidelines

Dietary guidelines are the second type of nutrition guide. Dietary guidelines are useful for health professionals, nutrition educators, and the general public in planning a nutritious diet. Dietary guidelines focus on health and call attention to food, nutrients, and lifestyle practices that prevent chronic disease and promote health. Since first published in 1980, the *Dietary Guidelines for Americans* has reflected the growing health concerns of government agencies, health providers, and professional groups. By law the *Dietary Guidelines for Americans* are updated every 5 years and are intended for all healthy people ages 2 and older. They represent a cooperative effort between the USDHHS, the federal agency concerned with health,

---

anemia Condition of abnormally low blood hemoglobin levels caused by too few red blood cells or red blood cells with an abnormally low hemoglobin content.
Dietary Reference Intake (DRI) See Box 1-3.
Recommended Dietary Allowance (RDA) See Box 1-3.
Adequate Intake (AI) See Box 1-3.
Tolerable Upper Intake Level (UL) See Box 1-3.
Estimated Average Requirement (EAR) See Box 1-3.
Acceptable Macronutrient Distribution Range (AMDR) See Box 1-3.

BOX 1-3 | Defining the Dietary Reference Intakes

Dietary Reference Intakes (DRIs)

The framework of nutrient standards now in place in the United States, the DRIs, include the Recommended Dietary Allowance, the Adequate Intake, the Tolerable Upper Intake Level, and the Estimated Average Requirement. They provide reference values for use in planning and evaluating diets for healthy people.

Recommended Dietary Allowance (RDA)

The Recommended Dietary Allowance is the average daily intake of a nutrient that will meet the requirement of nearly all (97% to 98%) healthy people of a given age and gender. The RDAs are established and reviewed periodically by an expert panel of nutrition scientists and amended as needed based on new research. When planning diets it is best to aim for this level of intake.

Adequate Intake (AI)

The Adequate Intake is the suggested daily intake of a nutrient to meet daily needs and support health and is used when there is not a sufficient amount of research available to develop an RDA. The AI also serves as a guide for intake when planning diets.

Tolerable Upper Intake Level (UL)

The Tolerable Upper Intake Level is the highest amount of a nutrient that can be safely consumed with no risk of toxicity or adverse effects on health. This standard can be used to evaluate dietary supplements or review total nutrient intake from food and supplements. Intakes exceeding the UL usually occur from the use of concentrated dietary supplements, not from food intake.

Estimated Average Requirement (EAR)

The Estimated Average Requirement is the average daily intake of a nutrient that will meet the requirement of half of the healthy people of a given age and gender. This standard is used to plan and evaluate the nutrient intakes of groups, not individuals.

Acceptable Macronutrient Distribution Range (AMDR)

The Acceptable Macronutrient Distribution Range is the suggested distribution of kcalories across the macronutrients; carbohydrate should provide 45% to 65% of total kcalories, fat should provide 20% to 35% of total kcalories, and protein should provide 10% to 35% of total kcalories.

Data from Food and Nutrition Board, Institute of Medicine: *Dietary Reference Intakes for energy, carbohydrate, fiber, fat, fatty acids, cholesterol, protein, and amino acids (macronutrients),* Washington, DC, 2002, National Academies Press.

and the U.S. Department of Agriculture (USDA), the federal agency concerned with food.

The Dietary Guidelines are developed from the DRIs and other research evidence describing the types and amounts of food we should eat and the physical activity we need for optimum health and growth. Every edition has addressed the problems of overweight and obesity and advocated a healthy weight. The importance of safe food-handling practices to prevent foodborne illness has been included in these materials. The Dietary Guidelines provide the basis for federal nutrition policy and give direction to government programs involving food and nutrition such as Head Start, school meals, and nutrition programs for older adults.

Health Promotion

Dietary Guidelines for Americans 2005

The *Dietary Guidelines for Americans* released in 2005 included two publications: (1) a technical report for use by health professionals (Figure 1-4)[31,32] and (2) a brochure for the general public. The 2005 edition is organized around the following three questions:

1. What should Americans eat?
2. How should we prepare our food to keep it safe and wholesome?
3. How should we be active to stay healthy?

The Dietary Guidelines help Americans choose diets that meet nutrient requirements, promote health, support active lives, and reduce chronic disease. The key recommendations of the 2005 edition are presented in Box 1-4.

The *Dietary Guidelines for Americans* stress making smart choices from every food group, finding a balance between food and activity, and getting the most nutrition out of your calories. They provide helpful advice for choosing whole grains, fruits, vegetables, meats, and milk-based foods rich in protein, vitamins, and minerals but low in fat and sodium. Although the Dietary Guidelines provide positive goals for food selection, they do not include a food pattern for the day that advises consumers as to the specific types of food they should eat and how much. Providing help with meal planning is the role of the third type of nutrition guide—the food guide.

Food Guides

Food guides are intended to assist individuals in day-to-day meal planning. They give a practical interpretation of both nutrition standards and dietary guidelines that is useful in daily food selection. Most food guides group foods into particular categories based on their nutrient content and recommend a certain number of servings from each group. The most commonly used food group guides are the MyPyramid from the USDA and the *Exchange Lists for Meal Planning* from the American Diabetes Association and the American Dietetics Association. These guides group foods differently and serve different needs.

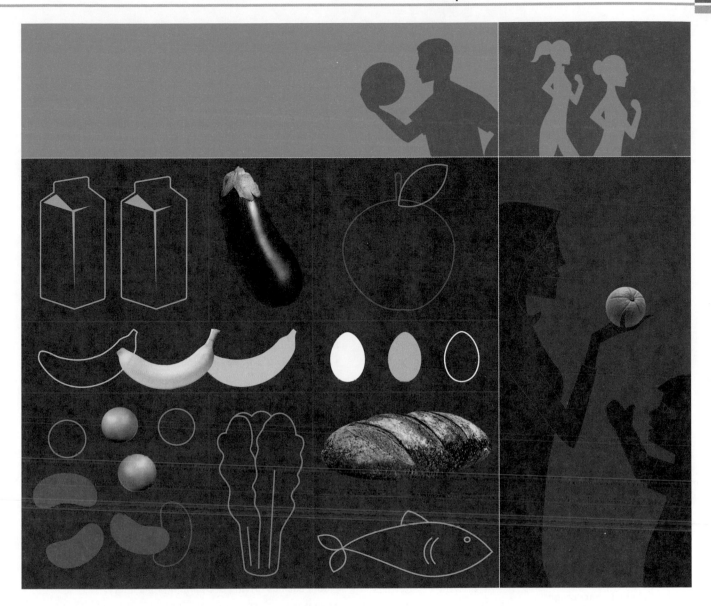

Dietary Guidelines for Americans 2005

U.S. Department of Health and Human Services
U.S. Department of Agriculture
www.healthierus.gov/dietaryguidelines

FIGURE 1-4 **Dietary Guidelines for Americans 2005.** *(From U.S. Department of Health and Human Services, U.S. Department of Agriculture:* Dietary guidelines for Americans 2005, *ed 6, Washington, DC, 2005, U.S. Government Printing Office* [www.healthierus.gov/dietaryguidelines]*.)*

BOX 1-4 | *Dietary Guidelines for Americans 2005*—Key Recommendations for the General Population

Adequate Nutrients Within Calorie Needs

- Consume a variety of nutrient-dense foods and beverages within and among the basic food groups while choosing foods that limit the intake of saturated and *trans* fats, cholesterol, added sugars, salt, and alcohol.
- Meet recommended intakes within energy needs by adopting a balanced eating pattern, such as the U.S. Department of Agriculture (USDA) Food Guide or the Dietary Approaches to Stop Hypertension (DASH) Eating Plan.

Weight Management

- To maintain body weight in a healthy range, balance calories from foods and beverages with calories expended.
- To prevent gradual weight gain over time, make small decreases in food and beverage calories and increase physical activity.

Physical Activity

- Engage in regular physical activity and reduce sedentary activities to promote health, psychological well-being, and a healthy body weight.
  - To reduce the risk of chronic disease in adulthood, engage in at least 30 minutes of moderate-intensity physical activity, above usual activity, at work or home on most days of the week.
  - For most people, greater health benefits can be obtained by engaging in physical activity of more vigorous intensity or longer duration.
  - To help manage body weight and prevent gradual, unhealthy body weight gain in adulthood, engage in approximately 60 minutes of moderate- to vigorous-intensity activity on most days of the week while not exceeding caloric intake requirements.
  - To sustain weight loss in adulthood, participate in at least 60 to 90 minutes of daily moderate-intensity physical activity while not exceeding caloric intake requirements. Some people may need to consult with a healthcare provider before participating in this level of activity.
- Achieve physical fitness by including cardiovascular conditioning, stretching exercises for flexibility, and resistance exercises or calisthenics for muscle strength and endurance.

Food Groups to Encourage

- Consume a sufficient amount of fruits and vegetables while staying within energy needs. Two cups of fruit and 2½ cups of vegetables per day are recommended for a reference 2000-calorie intake, with higher or lower amounts depending on the calorie level.
- Choose a variety of fruits and vegetables each day. In particular, select from all five vegetable subgroups (dark-green, orange, legumes, starchy vegetables, and other vegetables) several times a week.
- Consume three or more ounce-equivalents of whole grain products per day, with the rest of the recommended grains coming from enriched or whole grain products. In general, at least half the grains should come from whole grains.
- Consume 3 cups per day of fat-free or low-fat milk or equivalent milk products.

Fats

- Consume less than 10% of calories from saturated fatty acids and less than 300 mg/day of cholesterol, and keep *trans* fatty acid consumption as low as possible.
- Keep total fat intake between 20% to 35% of calories, with most fats coming from sources of polyunsaturated and monounsaturated fatty acids, such as fish, nuts, and vegetable oils.
- When selecting and preparing meat, poultry, dry beans, and milk or milk products, make choices that are lean, low-fat, or fat-free.
- Limit intake of fats and oils high in saturated and/or *trans* fatty acids, and choose products low in such fats and oils.

Carbohydrates

- Choose fiber-rich fruits, vegetables, and whole grains often.
- Choose and prepare foods and beverages with little added sugars or caloric sweeteners, such as amounts suggested by the USDA Food Guide and the DASH Eating Plan.
- Reduce the incidence of dental caries by practicing good oral hygiene and consuming sugar- and starch-containing foods and beverages less frequently.

Sodium and Potassium

- Consume less than 2300 mg (approximately 1 tsp salt) of sodium per day.
- Choose and prepare foods with little salt. At the same time, consume potassium-rich foods, such as fruits and vegetables.

Alcoholic Beverages

- Those who choose to drink alcoholic beverages should do so sensibly and in moderation—defined as the consumption of up to one drink per day for women and up to two drinks per day for men.
- Alcoholic beverages should not be consumed by some individuals, including those who cannot restrict their alcohol intake, women of childbearing age who may become pregnant, pregnant and lactating women, children and adolescents, individuals taking medications that can interact with alcohol, and those with specific medical conditions.
- Alcoholic beverages should be avoided by individuals engaging in activities that require attention, skill, or coordination, such as driving or operating machinery.

Food Safety

- To avoid microbial foodborne illness, do the following:
  - Clean hands, food contact surfaces, and fruits and vegetables. Meat and poultry should not be washed or rinsed.
  - Separate raw, cooked, and ready-to-eat foods while shopping, preparing, or storing foods.
  - Cook foods to a safe temperature to kill microorganisms.
  - Chill (refrigerate) perishable food promptly and defrost foods properly.
  - Avoid raw (unpasteurized) milk or any products made from unpasteurized milk, raw or partially cooked eggs or foods containing raw eggs, raw or undercooked meat and poultry, unpasteurized juices, and raw sprouts.

  NOTE: The *Dietary Guidelines for Americans 2005* contains additional recommendations for specific populations. The full document is available at *www.healthierus.gov/dietaryguidelines*.

From U.S. Department of Health and Human Services, U.S. Department of Agriculture: *Dietary guidelines for Americans 2005,* ed 6, Washington, DC, 2005, U.S. Government Printing Office.

USDA Food Guides

USDA issued its first food guide for children and adults in the 1940s, and food guides released since then, reflecting new scientific understanding and nutritional concerns, have had various formats. The Food Guide Pyramid made available in 1991 visually represented the relative amounts of each food group to be included in the daily diet. However, the need to provide the public with a motivational tool that would translate the DRIs and the *Dietary Guidelines for Americans* into a format easily understood and followed required a new graphic and a new slogan. MyPyramid: Steps to a Healthier You, the new USDA food guidance system, provides "one-stop shopping" for advice on food intake and physical activity.[33]

MyPyramid Food Guidance System

MyPyramid is an interactive system that promotes a personalized approach to healthy eating and physical activity (Figure 1-5).[34] The symbol, still a pyramid, was designed to be simple but remind consumers to make healthy food choices and be active every day. The food bands portrayed vertically rather than horizontally are grains, vegetables, fruits, milk, and meat and beans, with oils as a new category. The oils band brings attention to the need for good fats supplying important nutrients. Consumers are reminded to eat servings from various categories of food that each supply specific nutrients (Table 1-2). MyPyramid recommendations indicate both foods to be added and foods to be reduced to improve the typical American diet. Following are the overall goals of the *MyPyramid Food Guidance System*:

- Increase intakes of vitamins, minerals, and dietary fiber.
- Lower intakes of saturated fats, *trans* fats, and cholesterol.
- Increase intakes of fruits, vegetables, and whole grains.
- Balance energy intake with energy needs to prevent weight gain and/or promote a healthy weight.

Using the MyPyramid interactive website, consumers can obtain a food plan that indicates both the amounts and types of food needed for a person of their age, gender, and activity level, and a goal for physical activity. Figure 1-6 displays the reference food intake pattern providing 2000 calories. (As noted earlier, MyPyramid uses the term calories, which is well known to the public, rather than the technical term kcalories used by nutrition scientists.) Consumers are urged not only to eat more vegetables but also to "vary your veggies" over a week's time. In addition to food portions, each plan contains a number of discretionary calories that can be used for solid fats, added sugars, alcohol, or more food from any group. For less active persons, however, discretionary calories are rather limited. MyPyramid provides food plans ranging from 1000 calories to 3200 calories to cover the needs of individuals from age 2 across the life span (Table 1-3). Notice that only 267 discretionary calories are available within the 2000-calorie food plan. There is also a *MyPyramid for Kids* that we will look at in Chapter 12.

Two concepts poorly understood by the general public are serving size and activity level. In a recent survey consumers described a serving size as "what I have on my plate."[35] Confusion about serving size has contributed in part to the inappropriate weight gain that is occurring across all age-groups. To avoid overconsumption food amounts are given in household measures, and consumers might be encouraged to measure their food servings for several meals at home to gain an idea of what a ½-cup serving looks like. The MyPyramid website contains illustrations of various serving sizes and advice on how to divide the ingredients of mixed dishes such as pizza into the appropriate food group portions. Figure 1-7 illustrates a simple tool that can be carried in a wallet or school pack to help with estimating serving size.

Describing your activity level—sedentary, low active, or active—is also difficult. MyPyramid provides definitions and offers suggestions for increasing your physical activity to include at least 30 minutes on most days. As we see in Figure 1-6, 60 minutes of physical activity may be needed each day to prevent weight gain and more than 60 minutes a day to sustain weight loss. When using the MyPyramid, think about the stepwise progression found on the graphic. You need not make all your recommended changes in food choices and activity level in one day.[36]

To develop effective health messages behavioral and communication experts must work side by side with nutrition and biologic scientists. Nutrition messages that are easy to understand and implement and attractively presented are less likely to be ignored. Government agencies and nutrition and health educators must join forces to produce practical materials in media formats and languages appropriate to all segments of our society.

The Exchange Lists for Meal Planning

The *Exchange Lists for Meal Planning* was first introduced in 1950 by the American Diabetes Association and the American Dietetic Association as a meal-planning tool for persons with diabetes. The Exchange Lists groups foods on the basis of macronutrient content and equivalent energy values. This makes it useful for planning any diet in which control of carbohydrate, fat, protein, and total kcalories is the goal. Because the foods in each exchange list are equal to one another when eaten in the portions indicated, items can be freely exchanged within each list and food values and kcalories remain constant. The freedom to exchange within groups promotes greater variety and satisfaction with meals and snacks.

The most recent edition of the *Exchange Lists for Meal Planning* is found in Appendix G.[37] Foods are arranged into the following three groups:

1. *Carbohydrates:* This group includes starches (grains and starchy vegetables), fruits, nonstarchy vegeta-

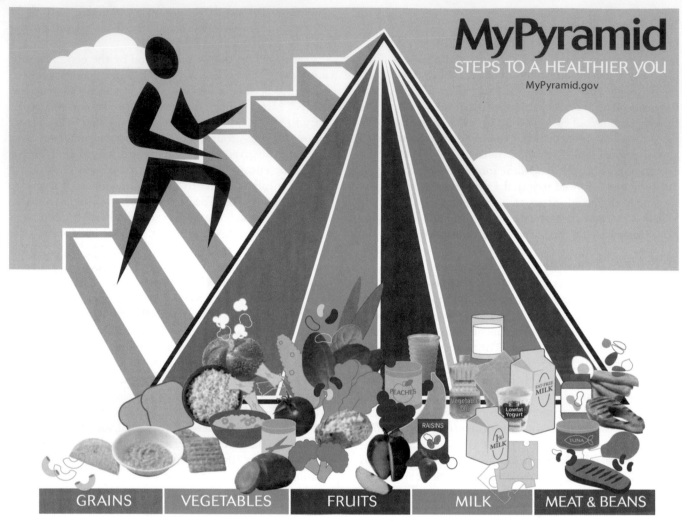

GRAINS   VEGETABLES   FRUITS   MILK   MEAT & BEANS

One size doesn't fit all

USDA's new MyPyramid symbolizes a personalized approach to healthy eating and physical activity. The symbol has been designed to be simple. It has been developed to remind consumers to make healthy food choices and to be active every day. The different parts of the symbol are described below.

Activity

Activity is represented by the steps and the person climbing them, as a reminder of the importance of daily physical activity.

Moderation

Moderation is represented by the narrowing of each food group from bottom to top. The wider base stands for foods with little or no solid fats or added sugars. These should be selected more often. The narrower top area stands for foods containing more added sugars and solid fats. The more active you are, the more of these foods can fit into your diet.

Personalization

Personalization is shown by the person on the steps, the slogan, and the URL. Find the kinds and amounts of food to eat each day at MyPyramid.gov.

Proportionality

Proportionality is shown by the different widths of the food group bands. The widths suggest how much food a person should choose from each group. The widths are just a general guide, not exact proportions. Check the Web site for how much is right for you.

Variety

Variety is symbolized by the 6 color bands representing the 5 food groups of the Pyramid and oils. This illustrates that foods from all groups are needed each day for good health.

Gradual Improvement

Gradual improvement is encouraged by the slogan. It suggests that individuals can benefit from taking small steps to improve their diet and lifestyle each day.

FIGURE 1-5   MyPyramid: Steps to a Healthier You. The MyPyramid graphic emphasizes activity, moderation, personalization, proportionality, variety, and gradual improvement. *(From Center for Nutrition Policy and Promotion: MyPyramid food guidance system mini-poster, Washington, DC, 2005, U.S. Department of Agriculture. Retrieved November 22, 2005, from* www.mypyramid.gov/downloads/MiniPoster.pdf.*)*

TABLE 1-2	**Nutrient Contributions of the Food Groups and Daily Amounts Needed**

Food Group	Major Nutrients*	Other Nutrient Contributions†‡	Daily Amount Needed (2000-kcal diet)	Serving Equivalents
Fruit group	Vitamin C	Thiamin Vitamin B$_6$ Folate Magnesium Potassium Carbohydrate Fiber	2 cups	1 cup fruit or 1 cup 100% fruit juice or ½ cup dried fruit equals 1 cup from the fruit group
Vegetable group	Vitamin A Potassium	Vitamin E Vitamin C Thiamin Niacin Vitamin B$_6$ Folate Calcium Phosphorus Magnesium Iron Zinc Carbohydrate Fiber Alpha-linolenic acid	2½ cups	1 cup raw or cooked vegetables or 1 cup vegetable juice or 2 cups raw leafy greens equal 1 cup from the vegetable group
Grains group			Total of 6 oz	1 slice of bread, 1 cup ready-to-eat cereal, or ½ cup cooked rice, pasta, or cooked cereal equals 1 oz from the grains group
Whole grains	Folate Magnesium Iron Carbohydrate Fiber	Thiamin Riboflavin Niacin Vitamin B$_6$ Phosphorus Zinc Protein	At least 3 oz	
Enriched grains	Folate Thiamin Carbohydrate	Riboflavin Niacin Iron	3 oz	
Meat, poultry, fish, eggs, beans, and nut group	Niacin Vitamin B$_6$ Zinc Protein	Vitamin E Thiamin Riboflavin Vitamin B$_{12}$ Phosphorus Magnesium Iron Potassium Linoleic acid (Nutrients differ according to the particular food item within the group.)§	5 ½ oz	1 oz lean meat, poultry, or fish, 1 egg, 1 Tbsp peanut butter, ¼ cup cooked dry beans, or ½ oz nuts or seeds equals 1 oz from the meat and beans group

Modified from Dietary Guidelines Advisory Committee, 2005: *Report of the dietary guidelines advisory committee on the dietary guidelines for Americans 2005,* U.S. Department of Agriculture, Agricultural Research Service, Beltsville, Md, 2004 (August).

*Major nutrient means that this food group supplies more of this nutrient than any other single food group in the food plan. For example, fruit supplies more of the vitamin C in the MyPyramid diet plan than any other food group.

†Other nutrient contributions means that this food group supplies more than 10% of this nutrient in the food plan. For example, vegetables supply at least 10% of the vitamin C in the MyPyramid food plan. Most foods supply a major nutrient but also add smaller amounts of other nutrients to the daily diet. It is most important to remember the major nutrient contributions for each food group.

‡Linoleic acid and alpha-linolenic acid are the essential fatty acids that we obtain from dietary fats.

§As an example of the differences among foods in this group, vitamin B$_{12}$ is found only in animal foods.

Continued

TABLE 1-2	Nutrient Contributions of the Food Groups and Daily Amounts Needed—cont'd

Food Group	Major Nutrients*	Other Nutrient Contributions†‡	Daily Amount Needed (2000-kcal diet)	Serving Equivalents
Milk group	Riboflavin Vitamin B_{12} Calcium Phosphorus	Vitamin A Thiamin Vitamin B_6 Magnesium Zinc Potassium Carbohydrate Protein	3 cups (2 cups for children ages 2 to 8)	1 cup milk, 1 cup yogurt, 1½ oz natural cheese or 2 oz processed cheese equals 1 cup from the milk group
Oils and soft margarine	Vitamin E Linoleic acid Alpha-linolenic acid		6 tsp	

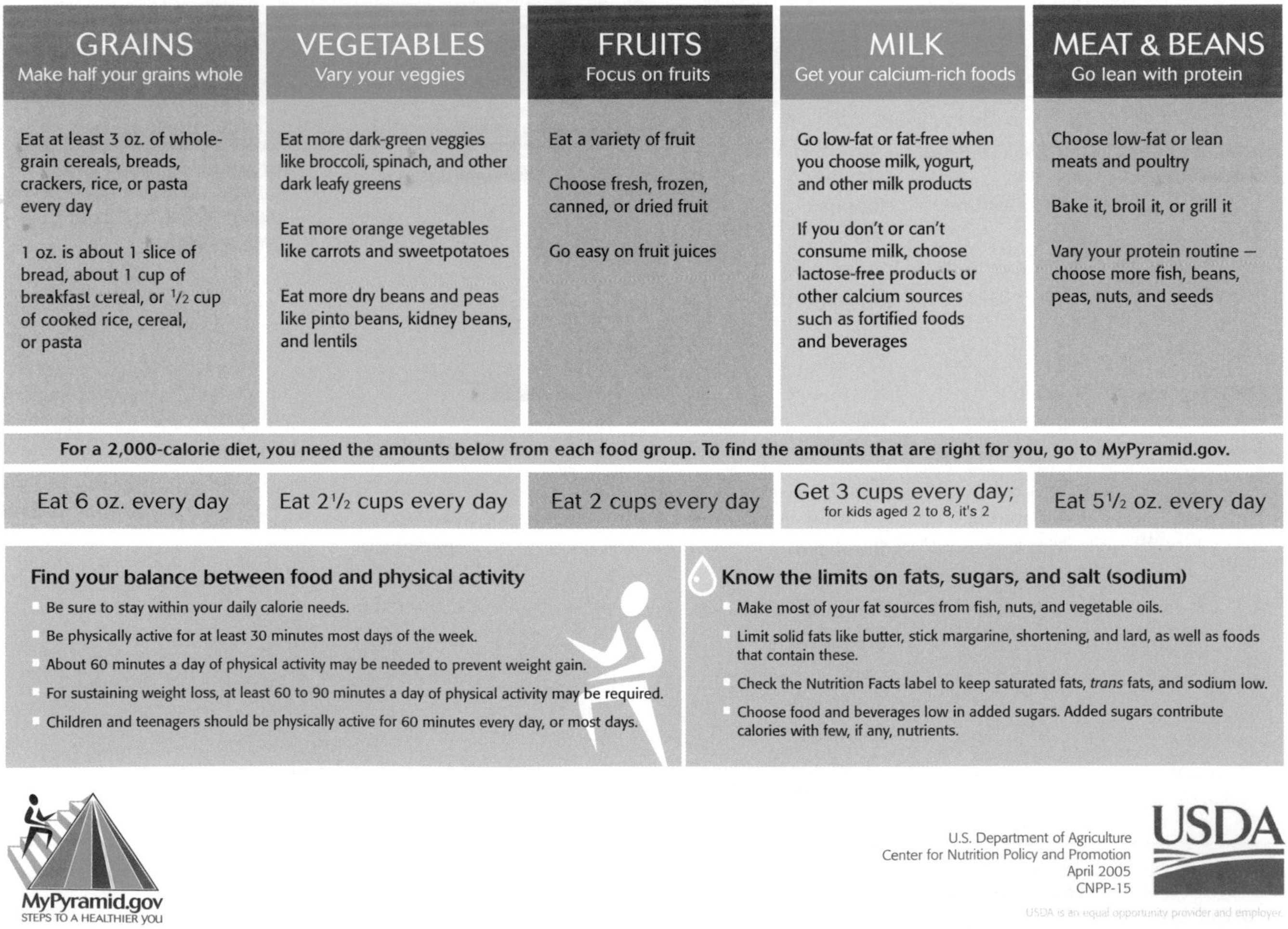

GRAINS Make half your grains whole	VEGETABLES Vary your veggies	FRUITS Focus on fruits	MILK Get your calcium-rich foods	MEAT & BEANS Go lean with protein
Eat at least 3 oz. of whole-grain cereals, breads, crackers, rice, or pasta every day 1 oz. is about 1 slice of bread, about 1 cup of breakfast cereal, or ½ cup of cooked rice, cereal, or pasta	Eat more dark-green veggies like broccoli, spinach, and other dark leafy greens Eat more orange vegetables like carrots and sweetpotatoes Eat more dry beans and peas like pinto beans, kidney beans, and lentils	Eat a variety of fruit Choose fresh, frozen, canned, or dried fruit Go easy on fruit juices	Go low-fat or fat-free when you choose milk, yogurt, and other milk products If you don't or can't consume milk, choose lactose-free products or other calcium sources such as fortified foods and beverages	Choose low-fat or lean meats and poultry Bake it, broil it, or grill it Vary your protein routine — choose more fish, beans, peas, nuts, and seeds

For a 2,000-calorie diet, you need the amounts below from each food group. To find the amounts that are right for you, go to MyPyramid.gov.

Eat 6 oz. every day	Eat 2½ cups every day	Eat 2 cups every day	Get 3 cups every day; for kids aged 2 to 8, it's 2	Eat 5½ oz. every day

Find your balance between food and physical activity
- Be sure to stay within your daily calorie needs.
- Be physically active for at least 30 minutes most days of the week.
- About 60 minutes a day of physical activity may be needed to prevent weight gain.
- For sustaining weight loss, at least 60 to 90 minutes a day of physical activity may be required.
- Children and teenagers should be physically active for 60 minutes every day, or most days.

Know the limits on fats, sugars, and salt (sodium)
- Make most of your fat sources from fish, nuts, and vegetable oils.
- Limit solid fats like butter, stick margarine, shortening, and lard, as well as foods that contain these.
- Check the Nutrition Facts label to keep saturated fats, *trans* fats, and sodium low.
- Choose food and beverages low in added sugars. Added sugars contribute calories with few, if any, nutrients.

MyPyramid.gov
STEPS TO A HEALTHIER YOU

U.S. Department of Agriculture
Center for Nutrition Policy and Promotion
April 2005
CNPP-15

USDA is an equal opportunity provider and employer.

FIGURE 1-6 MyPyramid food intake pattern for a 2000-kcal diet. Consumers can obtain a food intake pattern based on their age, gender, and level of physical activity that will assist them in their daily food selection. (*From Center for Nutrition Policy and Promotion:* MyPyramid food guidance system mini-poster, *Washington, DC, 2005, U.S. Department of Agriculture. Retrieved November 22, 2005, from* www.mypyramid.gov/downloads/MiniPoster.pdf.)

TABLE 1-3	MyPyramid Food Intake Patterns for Different Kcalorie Levels

Daily Amount of Food From Each Group

Calorie Level[1]	1000	1200	1400	1600	1800	2000	2200	2400	2600	2800	3000	3200
Fruits[2]	1 cup	1 cup	1½ cups	1½ cups	1½ cups	2 cups	2 cups	2 cups	2 cups	2½ cups	2½ cups	2½ cups
Vegetables[3]	1 cup	1½ cups	1½ cups	2 cups	2½ cups	2½ cups	3 cups	3 cups	3½ cups	3½ cups	4 cups	4 cups
Grains[4]	3 oz-eq	4 oz-eq	5 oz-eq	5 oz-eq	6 oz-eq	6 oz-eq	7 oz-eq	8 oz-eq	9 oz-eq	10 oz-eq	10 oz-eq	10 oz-eq
Meat and Beans[5]	2 oz-eq	3 oz-eq	4 oz-eq	5 oz-eq	5 oz-eq	5½ oz-eq	6 oz-eq	6½ oz-eq	6½ oz-eq	7 oz-eq	7 oz-eq	7 oz-eq
Milk[6]	2 cups	2 cups	2 cups	3 cups	3 cups	3 cups	3 cups	3 cups	3 cups	3 cups	3 cups	3 cups
Oil[7]	3 tsp	4 tsp	4 tsp	5 tsp	5 tsp	6 tsp	6 tsp	7 tsp	8 tsp	8 tsp	10 tsp	11 tsp
Discretionary calorie allowance[8]	165	171	171	132	195	267	290	362	410	426	512	648

1. **Calorie Levels** are set across a wide range to accommodate the needs of different individuals. Another table found on the MyPyramid website "Estimated Daily Calorie Needs" can be used to help assign individuals to the food intake pattern at a particular calorie level.

2. **Fruit Group** includes all fresh, frozen, canned, and dried fruits and fruit juices. In general, 1 cup of fruit or 100% fruit juice, or ½ cup of dried fruit can be considered as 1 cup from the fruit group.

3. **Vegetable Group** includes all fresh, frozen, canned, and dried vegetables and vegetable juices. In general, 1 cup of raw or cooked vegetables or vegetable juice, or 2 cups of raw leafy greens can be considered as 1 cup from the vegetable group.

4. **Grains Group** includes all foods made from wheat, rice, oats, cornmeal, barley, such as bread, pasta, oatmeal, breakfast cereals, tortillas, and grits. In general, 1 slice of bread, 1 cup of ready-to-eat cereal, or ½ cup of cooked rice, pasta, or cooked cereal can be considered as 1 ounce equivalent from the grains group. **At least half of all grains consumed should be whole grains.**

5. **Meat and Beans Group** in general, 1 ounce of lean meat, poultry, or fish, 1 egg, 1 Tbsp. peanut butter, ¼ cup cooked dry beans, or ½ ounce of nuts or seeds can be considered as 1 ounce equivalent from the meat and beans group.

6. **Milk Group** includes all fluid milk products and foods made from milk that retain their calcium content, such as yogurt and cheese. Foods made from milk that have little to no calcium, such as cream cheese, cream, and butter, are not part of the group. Most milk group choices should be fat-free or low-fat. In general, 1 cup of milk or yogurt, 1½ ounces of natural cheese, or 2 ounces of processed cheese can be considered as 1 cup from the milk group.

7. **Oils** include fats from many different plants and from fish that are liquid at room temperature, such as canola, corn, olive, soybean, and sunflower oil. Some foods are naturally high in oils, like nuts, olives, some fish, and avocados. Foods that are mainly oil include mayonnaise, certain salad dressings, and soft margarine.

8. **Discretionary Calorie Allowance** is the remaining amount of calories in a food intake pattern after accounting for the calories needed for all food groups—using forms of foods that are fat-free or low-fat and with no added sugars.

From Center for Nutrition Policy and Promotion: *MyPyramid food intake patterns,* Washington, DC, 2005, U.S. Department of Agriculture. Retrieved November 23, 2005, from *www.mypyramid.gov/downloads/MyPyramid_Food_Intake_Patterns.pdf.*
    oz-eq, Ounce-equivalents.

bles, milk, and other carbohydrates (e.g., cakes, cookies, and other sweets).

2. *Meat and meat substitutes:* This group includes protein foods arranged according to fat content (very lean, lean, medium-fat, and high-fat).

3. *Fats:* These foods are divided into three lists— monounsaturated, polyunsaturated, and saturated fats.

Other sections give serving size and macronutrient content for fat-modified, vegetarian, and fast-food items. A similar resource, the *Exchange Lists for Weight Management,* is also available.[38]

Nutrition Monitoring and Assessment

Early Background

As early as 1909 the federal government began tracking the food intake of the American people. In the 1960s concerns about existing malnutrition and hunger led to the development of the NHANES and CSFII monitoring

SERVING SIZE CARD:

Cut out and fold on the dotted line. Laminate for longtime use.

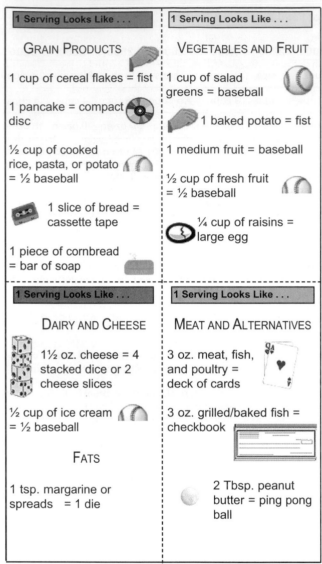

FIGURE 1-7   Serving size card. This pocket-sized guide can be useful when choosing serving sizes at home and when eating away from home. *(From U.S. Department of Health and Human Services, National Institutes of Health, National Heart, Lung and Blood Institute, Obesity Education Initiative:* Keep an eye on portion size, *Bethesda, Md, 2004, Author. Retrieved November 22, 2005, from* http://hp2010.nhlbihin.net/portion/servingcard7.pdf.)

lected included comparisons of food eaten at home or away from home, knowledge of nutrition and food safety, and attitudes about how nutrition and health are related.[39]

Integration of Nutrition Surveys

In 2000 it was decided that these two surveys would be combined into one survey, the National Food and Nutrition Survey, and the USDHHS and the USDA would work together on it. (Remember that these two government departments also work cooperatively in developing the *Dietary Guidelines for Americans* and preparing nutrition education materials for the public.) The new survey will be continuous, with groups of people examined every year.

Use of Nutrition Survey Data

Nutrition experts depend on the data from nutrition monitoring to make decisions about nutrition programs and set priorities for research. In future chapters we will refer to the NHANES and CSFII surveys in our discussion of nutrient intakes and nutrition problems. These survey data are used for various purposes, as follows:

- Develop and update the Dietary Reference Intakes
- Evaluate the prevalence of dieting and types of diets followed
- Monitor the acceptance of new foods such as fat-modified items
- See relationships between dietary intake and health
- Revise child growth charts to reflect current patterns and differences among race and ethnic groups

Look for new releases of information from the nutrition monitoring system to guide your future work in nutrition and health promotion.

PERSONAL ASSESSMENT OF FOOD PATTERNS

Personal Perceptions of Food

Each of us develops ways of eating based on our ethnic background, cultural or religious beliefs, family habits, socioeconomic status, health status, geographical location, and personal likes and dislikes. However, the growing ethnic and cultural diversity in our society has brought about a greater intermingling of foods and ideas about food. How people perceive themselves in relation to food and food patterns also plays an important role in their attitudes toward food and personal eating behavior.

A simple way to get an idea of your own food pattern is to look at what you actually eat. Keeping a record of everything you eat and drink noting the time, place, activity, and persons with you gives important insight into your true perception of food. Most of us eat by habit, according to where we are and what we are doing, and not because of any serious thought or plan. Evaluating what you eat and drink

programs that we mentioned earlier. The NHANES program directed by the USDHHS began in the early 1970s and collected dietary, clinical, biochemical, and anthropometric data along with health information on disease risk. The NHANES program carried out between 1988 and 1994 reached about 34,000 people over 2 months of age nationwide. Ethnic and racial minorities and people over the age of 60 were targeted in recent evaluations.[39]

The CSFII program began in the mid-1980s under the supervision of the USDA. It was conducted about every 3 years and had a special focus on high-risk families with incomes at or below the poverty level. Information col-

PERSPECTIVES IN PRACTICE
Perceptions and Analysis of Personal Food Patterns

What do you usually eat? What are your attitudes and values toward food? Do you eat regular meals or snack most of the time? Do you make an effort to choose nutritious foods or eat mostly whatever is around? To find the answers, check yourself for a few days using the following directions:

• *Keep a detailed record of everything you eat and drink for 3 days: 2 weekdays and 1 weekend day.* Make it as complete as possible. Keep a small pocket pad with you, and jot down what you eat or drink throughout the day and evening while you are still clear on details. Be sure to note the type of food or ingredients, how much you ate using household measures such as cups or tablespoons, how the food was prepared, and brand name, if applicable. Be specific: for example, was the milk you drank nonfat, 1% fat, 2% fat, or whole, or what type of milk did they use to make your latte? Do not miss the butter or margarine or mayonnaise on your bread, fats added when preparing foods, salad dressings and condiments added at the table, and additions to coffee or tea.

Notice the factors that influenced your food choices such as where you ate and at what time. Did you eat alone or with someone, and how were you feeling at the time? Just this recording process alone may tell you some things about your eating habits that you were not aware of before. You are going to analyze this record, so make it as readable, accurate, and detailed as possible, as follows.

• *Using MyPyramid, list the foods you ate and drank under their respective food group.* For mixed dishes such as pasta with tomato sauce and meatballs you may need to list ingredients separately. Compare what you ate with the number of servings and portion sizes recommended for a person of your age, gender, and level of physical activity (see the MyPyramid website at *www.mypyramid.gov*). Estimate how closely you met the recommended servings or what portions, if any, were missing.

• *Go through the same process of listing each food and beverage in its respective group using the Exchange Lists for Meal Planning (Appendix G).* Look at your total amounts of fat (g), carbohydrate (g), protein (g), and kcalories. Do your intakes of the macronutrients fall within the AMDR listed below?

Acceptable Macronutrient Distribution Ranges
Carbohydrate: 45% to 65% of total kcalories
Fat: 20% to 35% of total kcalories
Protein: 10% to 35% of total kcalories

• *Using the CD-ROM that came in the back of your textbook, enter your foods in the dietary analysis program.* Calculate your intakes of both the macronutrients and important micronutrients. Are your kcalories partitioned appropriately? If not, suggest some changes that would help you move toward the recommended ranges. How do your intakes compare with the DRIs for a person of your age and gender? If you are not consuming at least 70% of the DRI for important vitamins and minerals, suggest foods that you could add to your daily meal pattern that would supply these nutrients.

• *Compare your results using the three methods of dietary evaluation: (1) MyPyramid, (2) the Exchange Lists for Meal Planning, and (3) the computer-assisted analysis program.* Were you meeting your recommended amounts of food or nutrients by all three methods, one or two of the methods, or none of the methods? If your diet had a different level of nutritional adequacy when evaluated by one method versus another, what factors might have contributed to this difference? If you were a public health nutritionist working in a clinic serving pregnant women and their preschool children, which dietary assessment method would be most applicable to your work?

Now that you have thought about it, how do you see yourself as an eater? Are there food behaviors that you need or want to modify to promote good health? Also, give yourself a pat on the back for those categories where you are meeting current recommendations.

---

each day using the MyPyramid reference 2000-calorie diet plan (see Figure 1-6) will provide an estimate of your use of foods from each group. The energy provided by the macronutrients in your foods can be calculated using the Exchange Lists in Appendix G. The simple approach of analyzing food records by food groups and food exchange lists can increase awareness of our personal food patterns and assess the food intake of those we counsel in community or healthcare settings. (See the *Perspectives in Practice* box, "Perceptions and Analysis of Personal Food Patterns," for a general guide to evaluating your dietary intake.)

Nutritional Analysis by Nutrients and Energy Values

A more comprehensive nutritional analysis of food intake records is accomplished using a computer-assisted nutrient analysis program as included on the CD-ROM with your text. A computer-assisted program enables you to evaluate individual vitamins and minerals, specific fats, fiber, and energy as compared to the DRIs. Such a nutri-

tional analysis is used by government agencies to evaluate dietary information obtained in national surveys and identify nutrition problems existing among various age, gender, race, or ethnic groups.

TO SUM UP

The role of nutrition in human health has evolved in response to our changing society. A plentiful supply of food coupled with limited physical activity has produced an epidemic of obesity among all population groups in the United States. Discoveries of new substances in food beneficial to health have attracted the attention of nutrition experts and food technologists and have led to the definition of functional foods. Despite the availability of foods high in vitamins and minerals, some persons choose a diet high in sugar and fat, compromising their nutritional status. Others may be chronically undernourished as a result of illness or disease or limited resources for purchasing appropriate amounts or types of food. Undernourished individuals are vulnerable to infection, poor growth, and nutrition-related diseases. Overnutrition results from excessive energy intake or inappropriate use of high-potency nutritional supplements.

Various resources are used by health professionals and the general public in planning and evaluating diets. The Dietary Reference Intakes are used by professionals in planning intervention programs and evaluating the nutrient intakes of individuals and groups. MyPyramid helps individuals select a healthy diet. The *Dietary Guidelines for Americans* speaks to health-related aspects of nutrition and suggests food patterns to reduce chronic disease. Together, these materials provide a framework for public policy that directs federally funded meal programs and health education messages reaching people of all ages.

QUESTIONS FOR REVIEW

1. Visit the following page on the website of the U.S. Centers for Disease Control and Prevention *(www.cdc.gov/nccdphp/dnpa/obesity/trend/maps/)*, and follow the link to the obesity statistics. What is the prevalence of obesity in your state as compared to the national average?
2. Describe the two major disciplines that provide the foundation for nutrition. What contribution does each make toward our understanding of human nutrition needs?
3. Define the terms *nutrition* and *dietetics*. Identify work-related roles of professionals in human nutrition.
4. Compare the four levels of nutritional status: optimal nutrition, marginal nutrition, malnutrition, and overnutrition. Describe an individual or a situation that would illustrate each level and the physical or clinical signs that you would use to identify it.
5. List the six major nutrient groups. What is the primary function of each?
6. Define each of the categories in the Dietary Reference Intakes.
7. Compare nutrient standards, dietary guidelines, and food guides. List (a) an example of a standard or guide now in use, (b) the intended audience (professional or consumer), (c) the type of information included, and (d) a professional situation in which you would use it.
8. Visit the *Healthy People 2010* website at *www.health.gov/healthypeople/*. List five measurable objectives that pertain to diet or nutrition.
9. Visit your local library, and research the food patterns of a cultural or ethnic group different from your own. Using MyPyramid *(www.mypyramid.gov/)*, develop a 1-day menu for a child or adult in the group.

REFERENCES

1. Jeffery RW, Utter J: The changing environment and population obesity in the United States, *Obes Res* 11(suppl):12S, 2003.
2. Hedley AA et al: Prevalence of overweight and obesity among U.S. children, adolescents, and adults, 1999-2002, *JAMA* 291:2847, 2004.
3. Butchko HH, Petersen BJ: The obesity epidemic: stakeholder initiatives and cooperation, *Nutr Today* 39:235, 2004.
4. Dietz WH: Overweight in childhood and adolescence, *N Engl J Med* 350:855, 2004.
5. Federal Interagency Forum on Aging-Related Statistics: *Older Americans 2004: key indicators of well-being*, Washington, DC, 2004, U.S. Government Printing Office.
6. National Center for Health Statistics: *Health, United States, 2004: with chartbook on trends in the health of Americans with special feature on drugs*, Hyattsville, Md, 2004, U.S. Department of Health and Human Services.
7. American Dietetic Association: Position of the American Dietetic Association: the role of dietetics professionals in health promotion and disease prevention, *J Am Diet Assoc* 102:1680, 2002.
8. Messina M et al: Reductionism and the narrowing nutrition perspective: time for reevaluation and emphasis on food synergy, *J Am Diet Assoc* 2001(12):1416, 2001.
9. Food and Nutrition Board, Institute of Medicine: *Dietary Reference Intakes for energy, carbohydrate, fiber, fat, fatty acids, cholesterol, protein, and amino acids, (macronutrients)*, Washington, DC, 2002, National Academies Press.
10. Mahan LK, Escott-Stump S, eds: *Krause's food, nutrition, and diet therapy*, ed 11, St. Louis, 2004, Saunders/Elsevier.
11. Paeratakul S et al: Fast-food consumption among U.S. adults and children: dietary and nutrient intake profile, *J Am Diet Assoc* 103:1332, 2003.
12. Block G: Foods contributing to energy intake in the U.S.: data from NHANES III and NHANES 1999-2000, *J Food Comp Anal* 17:439, 2004.
13. Murphy SP, Johnson RK: The scientific basis of recent U.S. guidance on sugars intake, *Am J Clin Nutr* 78(suppl):827S, 2003.
14. Drewnowski A, Specter SE: Poverty and obesity: the role of energy density and energy costs, *Am J Clin Nutr* 79:6, 2004.
15. Drewnowski A, Barratt-Fornell A: Do healthier diets cost more? *Nutr Today* 39:161, 2004.
16. Cook JT et al: Food insecurity is associated with adverse health outcomes among human infants and toddlers, *J Nutr* 134:1432, 2004.
17. Akobundu UO et al: Vitamins A and C, calcium, fruit, and dairy products are limited in food pantries, *J Am Diet Assoc* 104:811, 2004.
18. Thomas DR: Distinguishing starvation from cachexia, *Clin Geriatr Med* 18:883, 2002.
19. Diabetes in Children Adolescents Work Group, National Diabetes Education Program: An update on type 2 diabetes in youth from the National Diabetes Education Program, *Pediatrics* 114:259, 2004.
20. Briefel RR: Nutrition monitoring in the United States. In Bowman BA, Russell RM, eds: *Present knowledge in nutrition*, ed 8, Washington, DC, 2001, International Life Sciences Institute.
21. U.S. Department of Health and Human Services, Public Health Service: *The Surgeon General's report on nutrition and health*, PHS publication No. 88-50210, Washington, DC, 1988, U.S. Government Printing Office.
22. Food and Nutrition Board, Institute of Medicine: Committee on Diet and Health: *Diet and health: implications for reducing chronic disease risk*, Washington, DC, 1989, National Academies Press.
23. U.S. Department of Health and Human Services, Public Health Service: *Healthy People 2000: national health promotion and disease prevention objectives*, Washington, DC, 1990, U.S. Government Printing Office.

24. U.S. Department of Health and Human Services: *Healthy People 2010: understanding and improving health,* Washington, DC, 2000, U.S. Government Printing Office (for full report, *www.health.gov/healthypeople/*).

25. Food and Nutrition Board, National Research Council: *Recommended Dietary Allowances,* ed 10, Washington, DC, 1989, National Academies Press.

26. Food and Nutrition Board, Institute of Medicine: *Dietary Reference Intakes for calcium, phosphorus, magnesium, vitamin D, and fluoride,* Washington, DC, 1997, National Academies Press.

27. Food and Nutrition Board, Institute of Medicine: *Dietary Reference Intakes for thiamin, riboflavin, niacin, vitamin B_6, folate, vitamin B_{12}, pantothenic acid, biotin, and choline,* Washington, DC, 1998, National Academies Press.

28. Food and Nutrition Board, Institute of Medicine: *Dietary Reference Intakes for vitamin C, vitamin E, selenium, and carotenoids,* Washington, DC, 2000, National Academies Press.

29. Food and Nutrition Board, Institute of Medicine: *Dietary Reference Intakes for vitamin A, vitamin K, arsenic, boron, chromium, copper, iodine, iron, manganese, molybdenum, nickel, silicon, vanadium, and zinc,* Washington, DC, 2001, National Academies Press.

30. Food and Nutrition Board, Institute of Medicine: *Dietary Reference Intakes for sodium, potassium, sulfur, chloride, and water,* Washington, DC, 2004, National Academies Press.

31. U.S. Department of Health and Human Services, U.S. Department of Agriculture: *Dietary guidelines for Americans 2005,* ed 6, Washington, DC, 2005, U.S. Government Printing Office *(www.healthierus.gov/dietaryguidelines).*

32. U.S. Department of Health and Human Services, U.S. Department of Agriculture: *Finding your way to a healthier you: based on the Dietary Guidelines for Americans,* HHS Publication Number HHS-ODPHP-2005-01-DGA-B, USDA Publication Number Home and Garden Bulletin No. 232-CP, Washington, DC, 2005, U.S. Government Printing Office *(www.healthierus.gov/dietaryguidelines).*

33. McDermott AY: MyPyramid.gov, *Nutr Clin Care* 8:103, 2005.

34. U.S. Department of Agriculture, Center for Nutrition Policy and Promotion: *MyPyramid food guidance system,* Washington, DC, 2005, Author *(www.mypyramid.gov/).*

35. U.S. Department of Agriculture, Center for Nutrition Policy and Promotion: *MyPyramid—USDA's new food guidance system* peer-to-peer PowerPoint presentation, Washington, DC, 2005, Author. Retrieved November 22, 2005, from *www.mypyramid.gov/professionals/index.html.*

36. Anonymous: Special report: rebuilding the pyramid, *Tufts Univ Health & Nutr Letter* 23(4, June):1, 2005.

37. Daly A et al: *Exchange lists for meal planning,* Alexandria, Va/Chicago, 2003, American Diabetes Association/American Dietetic Association.

38. Daly A et al: *Exchange lists for weight management,* Alexandria, Va/Chicago, 2003, American Diabetes Association/American Dietetic Association.

39. Boyle MA: *Community nutrition in action: an entrepreneurial approach,* ed 3, Belmont, Calif, 2003, Thomson/Wadsworth.

FURTHER READINGS AND RESOURCES

Readings

Tillotson JE: Pandemic obesity: what is the solution, *Nutr Today* 39:6, 2004.

Prince JR: Why all the fuss about portion size, *Nutr Today* 39:59, 2004.

> *These authors give us their views on what has contributed to the obesity epidemic and how health professionals can help to solve this problem.*

Hoolihan LE: Individualization of nutrition recommendations and food choices, *Nutr Today* 38:225, 2003.

> *This article introduces the concept of the gene-nutrient relationship and tells how we might be individualizing diets in the future based on an individual's genetic background.*

Hogbin M, Lyon L, Davis C: Comparison of dietary recommendations using the Dietary Guidelines for Americans as a framework, *Nutr Today* 38:204, 2003.

> *Dr. Hogbin and her co-workers trace the development of dietary recommendations over the past 50 years and show us how they have changed according to new needs and nutrition problems.*

Websites of Interest

- U.S. Centers for Disease Control and Prevention; this site provides an overview of nutrition and health problems in the United States, along with consumer health information and materials: *www.cdc.gov.*

- U.S. Department of Agriculture, Agricultural Research Service, Food Surveys Research Group, Beltsville Human Nutrition Research Center; this website provides an overview of the National Nutrition Monitoring and Related Research Program and the types of food and nutrition survey data that have been collected: *www.barc.usda.gov/bhnrc/foodsurvey/pdf/Tronm.pdf.*

- U.S. Department of Health and Human Services, U.S. Department of Agriculture; the site of the *Dietary Guidelines for Americans 2005* includes materials for both health professionals and consumers: *www.healthierus.gov/.*

- U.S. Department of Agriculture, Center for Nutrition Policy and Promotion; the MyPyramid website offers materials for use by professionals, as well as practical tips for consumers to use in planning their meals: *http://www.mypyramid.gov/.*

- U.S. Department of Health and Human Services, National Heart, Lung and Blood Institute; look for consumer materials on portion size on this website: *http://hin.nhlbi.nih.gov/portion/.*

CHAPTER 2

Carbohydrates

Eleanor D. Schlenker

With this chapter we begin a three-chapter sequence on the macronutrients—carbohydrates, fats, and proteins. These three nutrients share a unique capacity, the ability to yield energy.

Carbohydrates are of prime importance in the human diet. Over the ages they have nurtured cultures throughout the world as the major fuel for sustaining work and growth. We look first at the nature of this macronutrient and then its function as the primary body fuel.

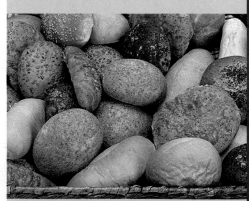

THE NATURE OF CARBOHYDRATES

Basic Fuels: Starches and Sugars

Two forms of carbohydrate occurring naturally in plant foods are (1) starches and (2) sugars. Energy on planet Earth comes ultimately from the sun and its action on plants. Using their internal process of photosynthesis, plants transform the sun's energy into the stored fuel form of carbohydrate (Figure 2-1). By this important process plants use carbon dioxide from the air and water from the soil—with the plant pigment *chlorophyll* as a chemical catalyst—to manufacture starch and sugars.[1] The starch that plants store for their own energy needs becomes a source of fuel for humans who eat those plants. Because our body can rapidly break down starch and sugars to obtain energy for immediate needs, carbohydrates are often referred to as "quick energy" foods. They are our primary source of energy.

Dietary Importance

Carbohydrates comprise a major portion of the diets of people all over the world. Fruits and vegetables along with grains and cereals supply carbohydrate, and in some countries carbohydrate-containing foods make up 85% of the diet.[1] Rice is one of the world's most important sources of carbohydrate, feeding 3 billion people in the developing world.[2] In the typical American diet about half of total kilocalories (kcalories) come from carbohydrates.[3] Carbohydrate foods are generally available, relatively low in cost, and easily stored. Compared with food items that require refrigeration or have a short shelf life, many carbohydrate foods can be kept in dry storage for fairly long periods without spoiling. Modern processing and packaging methods have extended the shelf life of carbohydrate products almost indefinitely.

CLASSIFICATION OF CARBOHYDRATES

The term *carbohydrate* comes from the chemical nature of these molecules. Carbohydrates contain the elements carbon, hydrogen, and oxygen with the hydrogen/oxygen ratio usually that of water—CH_2O. Carbohydrates are classified according to the number of basic sugar or saccharide units

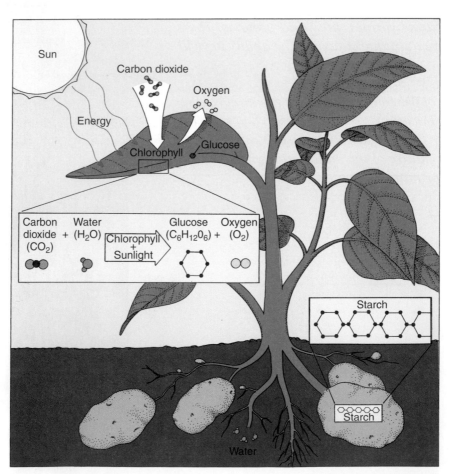

FIGURE 2-1   Photosynthesis. In the presence of sunlight and the green leaf pigment chlorophyll, green plants use water and carbon dioxide to produce glucose and starch by capturing the sun's energy and transforming it into chemical energy in the food products stored in their roots, stems, and leaves; through this process oxygen is returned to the atmosphere. *(Credit: Medical and Scientific Illustration.)*

that make up their structure. The monosaccharides and disaccharides are referred to as simple carbohydrates because of their relatively small size and structure. The polysaccharides, starches and certain forms of fiber, are called complex carbohydrates based on their larger size and complicated structure.

Monosaccharides

The simplest form of carbohydrate is the monosaccharide, or simple (single) sugar. The three monosaccharides important in human nutrition are (1) glucose, (2) fructose, and (3) galactose.

Glucose

Glucose is a moderately sweet sugar found naturally in only a few foods, one being corn syrup. Glucose is the common body fuel oxidized by cells to provide energy. It is supplied to the body directly from the digestion of starch but also can be obtained from other simple sugars in food that are converted to glucose for immediate use or storage. Glucose (called by its older name, *dextrose,* in hospital intravenous solutions) is the form in which carbohydrates circulate in the blood. Fasting plasma glucose levels normally range from 3.9 to less than 5.6 mmol/L (70 to less than 100 mg/dl).

After a high-carbohydrate meal, plasma glucose levels will temporarily rise but should return to a level less than 7.8 mmol/L (less than 140 mg/dl) within 2 hours.[4] *Hyperglycemia* refers to an elevated blood glucose level, and *hypoglycemia* refers to a blood glucose level below the normal range. We will discuss both hyperglycemia and hypoglycemia in more detail in Chapter 21.

Fructose

Fructose, the sweetest of the simple sugars, is found in fruits and other natural substances such as honey (see the *Focus on Food Safety* box, "Honey"). Fructose intake has escalated since high-fructose corn syrup was introduced for use in food processing. High-fructose corn syrup is the sweetener in many soft drinks, fruit drinks, commercial baked products, and dessert mixes. It accounts for 16% of the total energy intake of Americans 2 years of age and older.[5] In human metabolism fructose is converted to glucose to be burned for energy.

FOCUS ON FOOD SAFETY
Honey

Honey is a natural sweetener but in fact contains no more vitamins or minerals than table sugar. Honey should never be given to infants younger than 1 year of age because it may contain small amounts of the bacteria spores that produce botulism, a form of food poisoning that is often fatal.

Fructose is absorbed less efficiently than glucose, and amounts of 50 g or more can cause gastrointestinal distress in some individuals.[6,7] (A 12-oz container of sweetened soft drink or fruit drink can supply as much as 22 g of fructose.[7])

Galactose

The simple sugar galactose is not found free in foods but is released through the digestion of lactose (milk sugar) and then converted to glucose in the liver. This reaction is reversible, and in lactation glucose is reconverted to galactose for use in milk production.

The physiologic and nutritional importance of the monosaccharides (sometimes referred to as *hexoses* because of their six-carbon structure) is summarized in Table 2-1.

Disaccharides

The disaccharides are double sugars made up of two monosaccharides linked together. The three disaccharides of physiologic importance are sucrose, lactose, and maltose. Their monosaccharide components are as follows:

Sucrose = one glucose + one fructose

Lactose = one glucose + one galactose

Maltose = one glucose + one glucose

Notice that glucose is found in each of the disaccharides.

Sucrose

Sucrose is common "table sugar" and is made commercially from sugar cane and sugar beets. It is found in molasses and

carbohydrate Compound of carbon, hydrogen, and oxygen; starches, sugars, and dietary fiber made and stored in plants; major energy source in the human diet.

photosynthesis Process by which plants containing chlorophyll are able to manufacture carbohydrate by combining CO_2 from air and water from soil. Sunlight is used as energy; chlorophyll is a catalyst.

$$6\,CO_2 + 6\,H_2O + Energy + Chlorophyll = C_6H_{12}O_6 + 6\,O_2$$

monosaccharide Simple single sugar; a carbohydrate containing a single saccharide (sugar) unit. The most common monosaccharides are glucose, galactose, and fructose.

disaccharide Class of compound sugars composed of two molecules of monosaccharide. The three most common disaccharides are sucrose, lactose, and maltose.

| TABLE 2-1 | Summary of Physiologic and Nutritional Significance of Monosaccharides |

Hexose	Source	Significance
D-Glucose*	Fruit juices; hydrolysis of starch, cane sugar, maltose, and lactose	Form of sugar used by the body; found in blood and tissue fluids; fuel source for body cells
D-Fructose	Fruit, juices, honey; hydrolysis of sucrose from cane sugar	Changed to glucose in the liver and intestine to serve as fuel source for body cells
D-Galactose	Hydrolysis of lactose (milk sugar)	Changed to glucose in the liver to be used as fuel source for body cells; synthesized in the mammary gland to make lactose for milk; constituent of glycolipids and glycoproteins

*Monosaccharides can exist in D or L forms depending on the position of the hydroxyl group on the right (D) or the left (L) side of a specific carbon. Digestive enzymes are stereospecific and act only on D sugars.

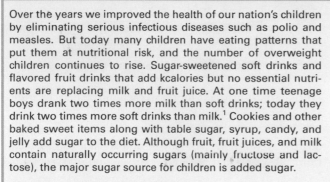

PERSPECTIVES IN PRACTICE

Sugar in the Diets of Children: The Case for Moderation

Over the years we improved the health of our nation's children by eliminating serious infectious diseases such as polio and measles. But today many children have eating patterns that put them at nutritional risk, and the number of overweight children continues to rise. Sugar-sweetened soft drinks and flavored fruit drinks that add kcalories but no essential nutrients are replacing milk and fruit juice. At one time teenage boys drank two times more milk than soft drinks; today they drink two times more soft drinks than milk.[1] Cookies and other baked sweet items along with table sugar, syrup, candy, and jelly add sugar to the diet. Although fruit, fruit juices, and milk contain naturally occurring sugars (mainly fructose and lactose), the major sugar source for children is added sugar.

How Much Sugar Is Appropriate?

The Dietary Reference Intakes suggest that no more than 25% of total kcalories come from added sugars.[2] Foods with added sugar displace more nutrient-dense foods in the diet, reducing intakes of nutrients important for health and growth. Researchers looked at this effect among children ages 4 to 8. When no more than 10% of their kcalories came from sugar, 95% of the children met their goal for calcium. But when added sugar rose above 25% of their kcalories, only 41% met their Adequate Intake for calcium. About one in five children exceeds the 25% limit for sugar.[3]

What Are the Problems With Sugar?

Excess Energy Intake

Children who drink more soft drinks or other sugar sweetened beverages have higher body weights and more body fat than children who drink less.[4,5] Many high-sugar items are eaten away from home when parents are not available to supervise. Children who eat more meals with a parent drink less soft drinks.[6]

Greater Risk of Dental Caries

Sugars are fermentable carbohydrates. Bacteria in the mouth feed on the simple sugars released by the action of salivary amylase and produce acids that attack the surface of the tooth. The longer this situation continues, the greater the formation of dental caries and tooth loss.

Loss of Important Nutrients

The greater the use of foods such as pies, cookies, and pastries, high in kcalories and low in essential nutrients, the fewer the portions of fruits, vegetables, nonsweetened grains, and dairy foods. Children in middle school and high school who used more high-sugar foods and sweetened beverages had lower intakes of vitamin A, folate, calcium, and iron.[7]

Goals for Intervention

What can we do to turn this around? First we might look at items available in vending machines frequented by children. Fruit juice and ultrapasteurized milk rather than fruit drinks or soft drinks with added sugar should be an option. (Ultrapasteurized milk has a longer shelf life than milk pasteurized by usual methods.) Plain popcorn, peanuts, and other high-fiber snacks could replace the high-sugar, high-fat cookies and cakes. Parents, school officials, school nurses, and nutritionists must work together to influence food industry advertising that promotes high-sugar foods.

References

1. Lytle LA: Nutritional issues for adolescents, *J Am Diet Assoc* 102(suppl):S8, 2002.
2. Food and Nutrition Board, Institute of Medicine: *Dietary Reference Intakes for energy, carbohydrate, fiber, fat, fatty acids, cholesterol, protein, and amino acids (macronutrients)*, Washington, DC, 2002, National Academies Press.
3. American Dietetic Association: Position of the American Dietetic Association: dietary guidance for healthy children ages 2 to 11 years, *J Am Diet Assoc* 104:660, 2004.
4. Novotny R et al: Dairy intake is associated with lower body fat and soda intake with greater weight in adolescent girls, *J Nutr* 134:1905, 2004.
5. Gillis LJ, Bar-Or O: Food away from home, sugar-sweetened drink consumption and juvenile obesity, *J Am Coll Nutr* 22:539, 2003.
6. Neumark-Sztainer DN et al: Family meal patterns: associations with sociodemographic characteristics and improved dietary intake among adolescents, *J Am Diet Assoc* 103:317, 2003.
7. Kant AK: Reported consumption of low-nutrient-density foods by American children and adolescents, *Arch Pediatr Adolesc Med* 157:789, 2003.

TABLE 2-2	Summary of Physiologic and Nutritional Significance of Disaccharides	
Disaccharide	**Source**	**Significance**
Sucrose	Cane and beet sugar, sorghum cane, carrots, pineapple	Hydrolyzed to glucose and fructose; fuel source for cells
Lactose	Milk	Hydrolyzed to glucose and galactose; fuel source for cells; constituent of milk production during lactation
Maltose	Starch digestion by amylase or commercial hydrolysis; malt and germinating cereals	Hydrolyzed to glucose; fuel source for cells; metabolite formed in digestion; can be fermented

certain fruits and vegetables such as peaches and carrots. Sucrose is also an added sweetener in many processed foods.

Lactose

Lactose is the sugar found in milk. It is the least sweet of the disaccharides, only about one sixth as sweet as sucrose. Although milk is relatively high in lactose, one of its main products—cheese—has little or none. When milk sours in the initial stage of cheese making, the lactose dissolves in the liquid whey that separates from the solid curd. The curd is processed into cheese, but the whey is discarded. Up to 75% of adults worldwide are lactose intolerant, but many are able to digest lactose-free milk products such as cheese.[8] (We will learn more about lactose intolerance and use of milk in Chapter 8.)

Maltose

Maltose results from the breakdown of starch and is found in commercial malt products and germinating cereal grains. Maltose occurs naturally in relatively few foods but is formed in the body as an intermediate product in starch digestion.

The physiologic and nutritional significance of the disaccharides is summarized in Table 2-2. Although sugars occur naturally in fruits and milk, the preponderance of sugars in the U.S. diet are added sugars.[3] These are sugars or syrups added to food in preparation or processing. We add sugar when we pour syrup on pancakes or use table sugar to sweeten coffee, tea, or cereal. Various forms of sugar are added to pies, cakes, cookies, candy, soft drinks, fruit drinks, breakfast cereals, and snack items. Researchers from the U.S. Department of Agriculture found that children take in about 24 tsp of added sugar every day and adults take in about 20 tsp.[9] One third of all added sugar comes from soft drinks.[10] The current Nutrition Label does not distinguish between naturally occurring and added sugars.[3] Box 2-1 lists examples of foods containing sugar. (The *Perspectives in Practice* box, "Sugar in the Diets of Children: The Case for Moderation," describes the effects of added sugars on the nutrient intakes of children.)

Sugar Alcohols

Sugar alcohols (sometimes referred to as *polyols*) are other forms of carbohydrate with sweetening power. Sugar alcohols such as sorbitol, mannitol, and xylitol occur in nature but are also used by food industry. Foods in which sugar alcohols replace sugar can be labeled as sugar free. Some sugar alcohols are incompletely absorbed in the small intestine, adding only 1.6 to 2.6 kcal/g to energy intake as compared to 4 kcal/g for other sugars.[7]

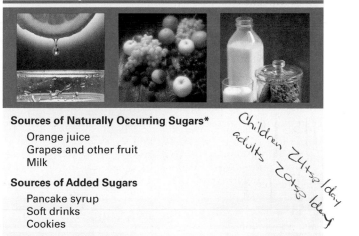

BOX 2-1 | Food Sources of Sugar

Sources of Naturally Occurring Sugars*
  Orange juice
  Grapes and other fruit
  Milk

Sources of Added Sugars
  Pancake syrup
  Soft drinks
  Cookies

*Foods such as fruits and milk that contain naturally occurring sugars also supply the body with many other important nutrients; added sugars supply kcalories only.
  Images copyright 2006 JupiterImages Corporation.

sugar alcohol An alcohol formed from a simple sugar; many sugar alcohols are used as sweetening agents by food manufacturers because they do not react with bacteria in the mouth to form dental caries.

These sweeteners are used in many low-fat foods such as ice cream and baked goods advertised as being artificially sweetened and lower in kcalories. Sugar alcohols are attractive to food processors because they are not attacked by the bacteria in the mouth that form dental caries. Because they do not require insulin for their metabolism, these sweeteners may offer an alternative for diabetics, although it is important to remember they do add kcalories to the diet. At high intakes, sugar alcohols can cause abdominal distress or exert a laxative effect, so foods with these sweeteners are best used in moderation.[11]

 Polysaccharides

Complex carbohydrates are called polysaccharides because they are made up of many *(poly)* single glucose (saccharide) units. Starch is the most important energy-yielding polysaccharide; others are glycogen and dextrins. Nondigestible polysaccharides such as cellulose provide important bulk to the diet and are categorized as dietary fiber. We will discuss the nondigestible polysaccharides later in this chapter. Box 2-2 lists some food sources of complex carbohydrates.

– *Starch*

Starch is a complex carbohydrate made of many coiled and branching chains of single glucose units and yields only glucose on complete digestion. Cooking not only improves the flavor of starch but also softens and ruptures the starch cells, making digestion easier. Starch mixtures thicken when cooked because the substance encasing the starch granules has a gel-like quality that thickens mixtures in the same way as pectin causes jelly to set.

– *Resistant Starch*

At one time we thought all starch was completely digested and absorbed in the small intestine. Now we know that some of the starch in particular foods such as cereals, potatoes, bananas, and legumes escapes digestion in the small intestine and enters the large intestine generally intact.[12,13] This starch, called *resistant starch,* can make up as much as 10% of the total starch in the typical Western diet.[3] Three types of resistant starch are found in food: (1) physically trapped starch in coarsely ground or chewed cereals; (2) ungelatinized starch granules in uncooked potato and green banana; and (3) starch polymers, mainly amylose, produced when starch is cooled after gelatinization (as in cooled cooked potato).[12]

Undigested starch that moves into the colon has an important role in health.[12,13] Bacterial fermentation of resistant starch produces three short-chain fatty acids, acetic, butyric, and propionic. Butyric acid is the preferred energy source of the cells lining the colon, and when it is not available, the risk of colonic diseases such as ulcerative colitis and colon cancer increases.[3] Resistant starch has other health benefits similar to those of dietary fiber that will be discussed in a later section. Based on its health-related properties, food product researchers are looking for new ways of processing grain foods to maximize their content of resistant starch.

Importance of Complex Carbohydrates

The major source of energy in the diet should be complex carbohydrates found in vegetables, legumes, and grains that also supply fiber and micronutrients. In the United States the major food sources of starch are bread, potatoes, ready-to-eat cereals, pasta, and rice.[14] Fruits add energy-yielding carbohydrate in the form of naturally occurring sugars but also contain fiber and important vitamins and minerals. Added sugars in processed foods provide energy but add little else to the diet and should represent only a small fraction of carbohydrate intake. The 2005 *Dietary Guidelines for Americans* recommends that added sugars be limited to 8 tsp (120 kcal) or less each day.[15]

BOX 2-2 | Food Sources of Complex Carbohydrates

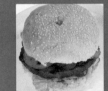 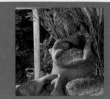 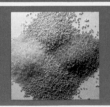 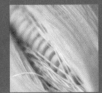 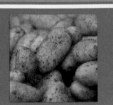 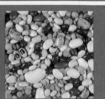

Hamburger bun
Whole wheat bread
Corn flakes
Baked potato with skin
Beans

- Grain foods such as bread, cereal, rice, and pasta; legumes; and certain vegetables such as potatoes contain large amounts of starch.
- Whole grain breads and cereals, legumes, vegetables, and whole fruits supply fiber.

Glycogen

The storage form of carbohydrate in animals is glycogen, whereas in plants it is starch. Glycogen is synthesized in liver cells and stored in relatively small amounts in the liver and muscle. Liver stores help sustain normal blood glucose levels during fasting periods such as sleep hours, and muscle glycogen provides immediate fuel for muscle action, especially during athletic activity. Sometimes athletes practice pregame "glycogen loading" to add fuel stores for athletic competition (see Chapter 14). Dietary carbohydrate is required to maintain normal glycogen stores and prevent the stress symptoms of low carbohydrate intake—fatigue, dehydration, weakness, and light-headedness. When carbohydrate is not available in sufficient amounts, the body breaks down protein and converts the released amino acids to an energy form. A severe lack of carbohydrate to support energy needs leads to undesirable metabolic effects such as ketoacidosis (see Chapter 21).

Dextrins

Dextrins are polysaccharide compounds formed as intermediate products in the breakdown of starch. Starch breakdown is ongoing in the process of digestion (Box 2-3).

Oligosaccharides

Oligosaccharides are small fragments of partially digested starch ranging in size from 3 to 10 glucose units. They are formed through digestion and produced commercially by acid hydrolysis. These small starch molecules are used in special formulas for infants and others with gastrointestinal problems because they are so easy to digest. Oligosaccharides are also used in sports drinks, in which they may contribute almost half of the total glucose (see Chapter 14).

Some naturally occurring oligosaccharides are formed with bonds that cannot be broken by human enzymes and remain undigested. Two of these—(1) stachyose and (2) raffinose—are found in legumes such as beans, peas, and soybeans. These small starch fragments provide a feast for bacteria in the colon, producing large amounts of gas that bring discomfort and embarrassment.

Glycemic Index

Various food carbohydrates are broken down and enter the bloodstream at different rates. These differences become important in the management of diabetes, hypoglycemia, or other conditions in which it is important to prevent a rapid elevation or drop in blood glucose levels. Attention to the rise in blood glucose levels following a meal is also important to general health as a moderate and prolonged rise in blood glucose promotes extended satiety[16] and could assist in weight management.

The glycemic index is a measure of the effect of a carbohydrate-containing food on blood glucose levels. It compares the rise in blood glucose levels that occurs over 2 hours after eating a test food containing 50 g of carbohydrate with the response obtained from a reference food or carbohydrate, usually white bread or a glucose solution. White bread is digested quickly, producing a rapid rise in blood glucose, and has been given the reference value of 100. Foods are generally categorized as follows[17]:

- Low glycemic index: less than 50
- Intermediate glycemic index: 55 to 70
- High glycemic index: greater than 70

Common foods differ greatly in their glycemic index (Table 2-3). Foods high in starch or refined carbohydrate and low in fiber have a high glycemic index with rapid digestion and release of glucose into the blood. Highly processed and overcooked foods have a high glycemic index. High-fiber foods that are firm and raw or in discrete hard pieces are digested more slowly, moderating the rise in blood glucose. The presence of protein or fat in a mixed meal slows the glucose response.[18] Plant-based foods containing dietary fiber can help prevent wide fluctuations in blood glucose levels.

Prediabetes

Type 2 diabetes, a complicated metabolic disorder characterized by inappropriately high blood glucose levels, can have devastating effects on life expectancy, morbidity, and quality of life. Risk factors for type 2 diabetes include

---

BOX 2-3	Breakdown of Starch in Digestion

Starch + Water → Soluble starch → Dextrins → Maltose → Glucose

---

glycogen A polysaccharide made up of many saccharide (sugar) units. Glycogen is the body storage form of carbohydrate found mostly in the liver, with lesser amounts stored in the muscle.

dietary fiber Nondigestible carbohydrates and lignin found in plants; dietary fiber is eaten as an intact part of the plant in which it is found.

oligosaccharides Intermediate products of polysaccharide digestion that contain from 3 to 10 glucose units.

raffinose A colorless crystalline trisaccharide composed of galactose and sucrose joined by bonds that human enzymes cannot break; raffinose is found in legumes and in the intestine is attacked by bacteria, producing the gas associated with eating these foods.

obesity and a sedentary lifestyle. But growing evidence suggests that a regular diet with a high glycemic index that taxes the capacity of the beta cells of the pancreas to produce insulin may hasten the development of this disease in those at risk.[16] An expert panel has set standards for blood glucose levels that identify individuals at high risk for diabetes, and this condition has been termed prediabetes. It is estimated that more than 12 million overweight middle-age adults and older adults in the United States have prediabetes.[19] Lifestyle changes focusing on diet and physical activity slow the progression from prediabetes to type 2 diabetes, preserving quality of life and reducing the staggering economic costs associated with this disease. (In later chapters we will touch on intervention strategies.)

FUNCTIONS OF CARBOHYDRATES

Energy

The primary function of starches and sugars is to provide energy to cells, especially brain cells that depend on glucose. When carbohydrate is lacking, fats can provide fuel for most organ systems, but to function most efficiently body tissues require a constant supply of carbohydrate.

The amount of carbohydrate stored in the body, although relatively small, is an important energy reserve.

TABLE 2-3	Glycemic Index of Common Foods*

Food	Glycemic Index
Baked potato (without skin)	121
Corn flakes	119
Jelly beans	114
White bread	101
Soft drink	97
Angel food cake	95
Cheese pizza	86
Spaghetti	83
Banana	76
Orange juice	74
Converted long grain rice	72
Green peas	68
All Bran cereal	60
Pumpernickel bread	58
Apple	52
Skim milk	46
Kidney beans	42
Fructose	32

Data from Foster-Powell K, Miller JB: International tables of glycemic index, *Am J Clin Nutr* 62:871S, 1995.

*White bread as reference food = 100

An adult man has about 300 to 350 g of carbohydrate stored in his liver and muscle in the form of glycogen, and another 10 g of glucose is circulating in his blood (Table 2-4). Together, this glycogen and glucose will supply the energy needed for only a half day of moderate activity. To meet the body's constant demand for energy, carbohydrate foods must be eaten regularly and at reasonably frequent intervals.

Special Functions of Carbohydrates in Body Tissues

Carbohydrates have specialized roles in body tissues in addition to their general function as an energy source.

Glycogen Reserves

Liver and muscle glycogen are in constant interchange with the body's overall energy system. These energy reserves protect cells, especially brain cells, from depressed metabolic function and injury and support urgent muscle responses as needed.

Protein-Sparing Action

Carbohydrates help to regulate protein metabolism. An adequate supply of carbohydrates to satisfy ongoing energy demands prevents the channeling of protein for energy. This protein-sparing action of carbohydrate allows protein to be used for tissue building and repair.

Antiketogenic Effect

Carbohydrates influence fat metabolism. The supply of dietary carbohydrate determines how much fat must be broken down to meet energy needs, thereby controlling the formation and disposal of *ketones*. Ketones are intermediate products of fat metabolism that are normally produced in only small amounts as fats are oxidized. However, under extreme conditions when available carbohydrates are inadequate to meet energy needs, as occurs in starvation or uncontrolled diabetes or very low-carbohydrate diets, fat is oxidized at excessive rates. Ketones accumulate and the result is *ketoacidosis* (see Chapter 21). Sufficient amounts of dietary carbohydrates prevent any damaging excess of ketones.

TABLE 2-4	Carbohydrate Storage in Normal Adult Man (70 kg [154 lb])

	Glycogen (g)	Glucose (g)
Liver (weight 1800 g)	72	
Muscles (weight 35 kg [77 lb])	245	
Extracellular fluids (10 L)		10
Component totals	317	10
TOTAL STORAGE	327	

Heart Action

Heart action is a life-sustaining muscular exercise. Although fatty acids are the preferred fuel for the heart, the glycogen stored in cardiac muscle is an important emergency source of contractile energy.

Central Nervous System

The brain and central nervous system (CNS) depend on carbohydrate as an energy source. However, these tissues have very low carbohydrate reserves—enough to last only 10 to 15 minutes—so they are especially dependent on a minute-to-minute supply of glucose from the blood. Sustained hypoglycemic shock causes irreversible brain damage. A practical application of the need for a constant supply of glucose to the brain is the finding that individuals who eat breakfast do better in school than those who skip breakfast.[20] Glucose increases the synthesis of acetylcholine, a neurotransmitter that acts on areas of the brain involved with memory and cognitive functions.[21]

Recommended Intake of Carbohydrate

Dietary Reference Intake

The Recommended Dietary Allowance (RDA) for carbohydrate is the same for all persons over 1 year of age. Children, adolescents, and adults should take in a minimum of 130 g/day.[3] This will ensure a sufficient amount of glucose to supply the energy needs of the brain for 1 day. Most people consume a greater amount of carbohydrate to meet their overall energy requirement and keep fat and protein intakes at acceptable levels.

Acceptable Macronutrient Distribution Range

A diet rich in plant-based foods lowers the risk of heart disease and some cancers, but it is unwise to take in an excessive amount of carbohydrate, just as it is not prudent to severely limit carbohydrate. To provide guidance for appropriate diet patterns nutrition experts developed the Acceptable Macronutrient Distribution Ranges (AMDR) (Box 2-4) that set a range for each of the macronutrients as a proportion of total kcalorie intake.[3] Diet patterns falling within the AMDRs will (1) lower

---

BOX 2-4 | Acceptable Macronutrient Distribution Ranges

Carbohydrate: 45% to 65% of total kcalories
Fat: 20% to 35% of total kcalories
Protein: 10% to 35% of total kcalories

Data from Food and Nutrition Board, Institute of Medicine: *Dietary Reference Intakes for energy, carbohydrate, fiber, fat, fatty acids, cholesterol, protein, and amino acids (macronutrients),* Washington, DC, 2002, National Academies Press.

---

the risk of chronic disease, (2) promote optimum intakes of all essential nutrients, and (3) support energy balance and weight management. The adult AMDR for carbohydrate is 45% to 65% of total energy with no more than 25% of total kcalories from added sugar.[3] This range of acceptable intake allows for differences in cultural or ethnic food patterns or particular health needs. The AMDRs enable us to individualize diets to meet specific situations and encourage sound nutrition practices.

Nonnutritive Sweeteners

Most of us have an inborn desire for foods that are sweet, yet we are faced with the dilemma of moderating our energy intakes to avoid unwanted weight gain or bring about a moderate weight loss. Nonnutritive sweeteners allow persons to indulge their taste for sweets while limiting their kcalorie intake. Sweeteners are grouped as nutritive or nonnutritive depending on the kcalories they contain. Sucrose (table sugar) and other natural sugars contain 4 kcal per gram. Nonnutritive sweeteners yield no energy or an insignificant amount of energy.[7] Because of their intense sweetening power, very small amounts of these substances are needed to produce the desired level of sweetness, so the added kcalories are negligible (aspartame is such a nonnutritive sweetener).

Five nonnutritive sweeteners have been approved by the Food and Drug Administration (FDA) for use in the United States. They sweeten beverages, baked products, soft drinks, fruit drinks, and candy marketed as low or reduced calorie, and some are available for use in homemade products. The nonnutritive sweetener aspartame contains the amino acid phenylalanine, and these food products must carry a label indicating that phenylalanine is present.[7] This protects persons with phenylketonuria who lack the enzyme needed to metabolize phenylalanine and must eliminate it from their diet. Table 2-5 reviews the properties of nonnutritive sweeteners.

The nonnutritive sweetener most recently approved by the FDA is sucralose marketed under the trade name of Splenda. This substance is 600 times sweeter than sucrose and provides virtually no energy. Only 3.8 oz of sucralose has the sweetening power of 2 lb of sugar.[7] Kcalories contributed by an added bulking agent are insignificant at the level added. Sucralose is poorly absorbed (on average approximately 15%), and what is absorbed is excreted in the urine unchanged.[22] Because it is heat stable and available in granular form, this product

---

nonnutritive sweetener A substance with sweetening power that is not efficiently absorbed by the body or cannot be metabolized to provide energy; these substances are used in small amounts, and in most cases the kcalories added to the food product are negligible.

TABLE 2-5	Properties and Applications of Common Nonnutritive Sweeteners

Name	Sweetening Power (compared with sucrose)	Effect of Heat	Trade Names	Applications
Aspartame	160 to 220 times sweeter	Decomposes with high heat and loses sweetening power	Nutrasweet, Equal, Sugar Twin (blue box)	Beverages, table sweetener, gelatin, pudding, chewing gum, cold breakfast cereal
Acesulfame-K	200 times sweeter	Not affected by heating	Sweet One, Sweet & Safe	Beverages, table sweetener, baked goods, all-purpose sweetener
Saccharin	200 to 700 times sweeter	Not affected by heating	Sweet and Low, Sweet Twin, Necta Sweet, Sweet 'N Low Brown	Beverages, table sweetener, chewing gum, baked goods, pudding
Sucralose	600 times sweeter	Not affected by heating	Splenda	Beverages, desserts, baked goods, candy, table sweetener, all-purpose sweetener
Neotame	8,000 times sweeter	Not affected by heating	(Currently being evaluated by the Food and Drug Administration)	Beverages, table sweetener, frozen desserts, chewing gum, candy, baked goods, sauces, cereals

Data from American Dietetic Association: Position of the American Dietetic Association: use of nutritive and nonnutritive sweeteners, *J Am Diet Assoc* 104:255, 2004.

has application for both commercial and home-prepared baked items or other desserts.

Imbalances in Carbohydrate Intake

High-Carbohydrate Diets

In an effort to lower their intakes of fat and kcalories or achieve reductions in blood lipoprotein levels, persons have adopted diets containing 65% to 75% carbohydrate.[23] Carbohydrate intakes above the AMDR of 65% carry health risks. Such increases in carbohydrate often bring proportionate decreases in fat, jeopardizing intakes of the essential fatty acids and vitamins and minerals associated with higher-fat foods. Dramatic increases in dietary carbohydrate lead to a rise in plasma triglycerides and a drop in high-density lipoprotein (HDL) cholesterol in certain individuals.[3] (HDL is the lipoprotein that helps remove cholesterol from the body.) Diets exceeding the AMDR for carbohydrate can elevate blood glucose levels, putting heavy demands on the beta cells of the pancreas for insulin. Disproportionate intakes of carbohydrate also are likely to include higher than desirable intakes of added sugar. These issues will continue to arise in succeeding chapters.

Low-Carbohydrate Diets

Diets very low in carbohydrate (and often very high in fat) have been popularized as efficient ways to lose weight. Two such diets, the Atkins diet and the South Beach diet, restrict carbohydrate to 10% to 30% of total kcalories. These regimens result in weight loss over the short term *if* energy intake is sufficiently reduced but carry nutritional risk when extended for weeks or months.[24,25] Diets very low in carbohydrate are unlikely to contain the minimum servings of fruits, vegetables, and whole grains recommended by MyPyramid.[26] These plant-based carbohydrate foods supply health-promoting phytochemicals and fiber and assist in controlling blood pressure.[27] Low-carbohydrate diets often replace carbohydrate foods with high-fat foods and may provide as much as 46% of total kcalories as fat, adding to cardiovascular risk.[28] Low-carbohydrate diets that replace carbohydrate with protein exceeding recommended levels increase the burden on the kidneys.

Researchers have compared the success of weight loss diets equal in kcalories but with different amounts of carbohydrate. Over the short term, high-carbohydrate diets lead to more rapid weight loss, likely the result of a shift in body water.[24] High levels of protein in low-carbohydrate diets increase feelings of satiety that may help to limit food intake.[29] However, the real measure of effectiveness of any weight loss regimen is what happens over the long term. When various popular diets—low to moderate in carbohydrate—were compared after 1 year, total weight loss related to how well individuals adhered to their diet, not to the particular diet they followed.[30] Weight reduction diets with a moderate amount of carbohydrate protect lean body mass, with more of the weight loss coming from fat tis-

◆ FOCUS ON CULTURE

Cross-Cultural Competence: A Goal for the Health Professional

Consider the following situations:

- You are counseling pregnant and lactating mothers in a public health clinic and using MyPyramid to evaluate their food intake. A Hmong (Vietnamese) mother tells you that she never eats bread, and you express concern about her servings from the grains group.
- You are working with an older adult African-American man, and he tells you that his favorite meal is his daughter's homemade Brunswick stew. What foods are included?

As a nation we are becoming increasingly diverse. In another 10 to 15 years one of every three Americans will be an African American, Hispanic American, Asian American, Hmong American, Native American, or Pacific Islander American. To be effective nutrition educators we need to understand the food patterns of different ethnic, race, and cultural groups, not just our own. We must acknowledge the health beliefs and values that influence a person's food choices and nutritional status. The Hmong mother may not eat bread but is likely to have rice at every meal and more than meet her recommended servings of grains. However, she may be reluctant to take the vitamin and mineral supplements her doctor recommended in the belief that they will cause her to have a large infant and difficult delivery. The African-American man obtains important vitamins, fiber, and protein from his Brunswick stew made with chicken, carrots, tomatoes, white beans, and greens. We must learn about the foods enjoyed by various groups and the important nutrients found in those foods.

Value Diversity

The United States is made up of people from many different countries and cultures with many different customs. At one time we referred to our society as a "melting pot," in which newcomers were expected to blend their customs and beliefs with the mainstream culture. Healthcare providers imposed their beliefs and values on patients from other ethnic or cultural backgrounds. Today we strive to become a "salad bowl," with each individual adding a special quality to the mix. Individual differences are important and enhance the lives of us all. As health professionals we must respect different customs and beliefs and give counseling and support consistent with the values of the person we are helping, not our own.

Cross-Cultural Situations

Throughout our professional lives we will continue to experience cross-cultural situations in which we belong to a different race, cultural, or ethnic group than our supervisor or our colleagues or the persons for whom we provide nutritional care.

We can begin to develop cross-cultural competence in various ways, as listed below:

- *Learn about other cultures by reading, observing, and sharing experiences.* A potluck meal provides an opportunity to share foods and the cultural aspects surrounding food choices.
- *Examine your own beliefs and feelings about other cultures.* Identify and resolve any stereotypes that you may hold about groups other than your own.
- *Assess how other cultures view you, and make an effort to present yourself in a positive light.* Develop verbal and nonverbal communication skills applicable to various cultural groups.
- *Value the differences among people.* Do away with the attitude that your way is best.

References

Curry KR: Multicultural competence in dietetics and nutrition, *J Am Diet Assoc* 100:1142, 2000.

Kittler PG, Sucher KP: *Food and culture*, ed 4, Belmont, Calif, 2004, Brooks/Cole, a division of Thomson Learning.

Other Resources

Diabetes Care and Education Dietetic Practice Group of the American Dietetic Association: *Ethnic and regional food practices: A series. Alaska native food practices, customs, and holidays*, Chicago/Alexandria, VA, 1998, American Dietetic Association/American Diabetes Association.

Diabetes Care and Education Dietetic Practice Group of the American Dietetic Association: *Ethnic and regional food practices: A series. Chinese American food practices, customs, and holidays*, Chicago/Alexandria, VA, 1998, American Dietetic Association/American Diabetes Association.

Diabetes Care and Education Dietetic Practice Group of the American Dietetic Association: *Ethnic and regional food practices: A series. Filipino American food practices, customs, and holidays*, Chicago/Alexandria, VA, 1994, American Dietetic Association/American Diabetes Association.

Diabetes Care and Education Dietetic Practice Group of the American Dietetic Association: *Ethnic and regional food practices: A series. Hmong American food practices, customs, and holidays*, Chicago/Alexandria, VA, 1999, American Dietetic Association/American Diabetes Association.

Diabetes Care and Education Dietetic Practice Group of the American Dietetic Association: *Ethnic and regional food practices: A series. Indian and Pakistani food practices, customs, and holidays*, ed 2, Chicago/Alexandria, VA, 2000, American Dietetic Association/American Diabetes Association.

Diabetes Care and Education Dietetic Practice Group of the American Dietetic Association: *Ethnic and regional food practices: A series. Jewish food practices, customs, and holidays*, Chicago/Alexandria, VA, 1998, American Dietetic Association/American Diabetes Association.

Diabetes Care and Education Dietetic Practice Group of the American Dietetic Association: *Ethnic and regional food practices: A series. Mexican American food practices, customs, and holidays*, Chicago/Alexandria, VA, 1998, American Dietetic Association/American Diabetes Association.

Diabetes Care and Education Dietetic Practice Group of the American Dietetic Association: *Ethnic and regional food practices: A series. Navajo food practices, customs, and holidays*, Chicago/Alexandria, VA, 1998, American Dietetic Association/American Diabetes Association.

Diabetes Care and Education Dietetic Practice Group of the American Dietetic Association: *Ethnic and regional food practices: A series. Soul and traditional southern food practices, customs, and holidays*, Chicago/Alexandria, VA, 1995, American Dietetic Association/American Diabetes Association.

---

sue.[31] Establishing a kcalorie deficit between energy intake and energy expenditure using a combination of foods that support nutritional well-being is the only effective means of long-term weight management.[32]

As we help persons make positive food choices for health and well-being, we need to consider their accustomed food patterns and recommend appropriate foods that are familiar to them. The *Focus on Culture* box, "Cross-Cultural Competence: A Goal for the Health Professional," presents some ideas on how to work effectively with individuals whose dietary patterns may differ from our own.

Dietary and Functional Fiber

Up to this time we have discussed those carbohydrates in our food supply that are digestible and provide energy to carry on the work of body cells. Now we turn to the indigestible complex carbohydrates usually referred to as *fiber* that also have important body functions.

Fiber is the nondigestible material found in whole grain cereals, fruits, vegetables, and legumes that our grandmothers referred to as roughage. Because humans lack the necessary enzymes to break down these complex carbohydrates into forms that can be absorbed, they travel the length of the gastrointestinal tract and are eliminated in the feces. Their ability to promote regular bowel function has been recognized for generations. All types of fiber are beneficial to health, but different fibers have different physiologic effects, so it is necessary to consume a variety of foods containing different forms of fiber. Most foods contain more than one type of fiber, although they likely have more of one kind than another.

There are two general categories of fiber: (1) dietary fiber and (2) functional fiber.[3]

Dietary Fiber

Dietary fiber includes nondigestible carbohydrates and lignin that are intact in plant foods. Dietary fiber can be divided into soluble and insoluble fiber (Box 2-5). These designations are based on their chemical properties in the laboratory, but insoluble and soluble fibers also have different functions in our bodies (Table 2-6).

Insoluble Fiber.   Various plant components contain insoluble fibers, as follows:

- *Cellulose:* Cellulose is the material in plant cell walls that provides the structure for most plants. We find it in the stems and leaves of vegetables, the coverings of seeds and grains, and in skins and hulls. Because humans are unable to break down cellulose, it remains in the digestive tract and contributes important bulk to the food mass.
- *Hemicellulose:* This polysaccharide is found in plant cell walls and often surrounds cellulose. Some hemicelluloses help to regulate colon pressure by providing bulk for normal muscle action.

BOX 2-5 | Sources of Soluble and Insoluble Fiber

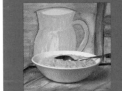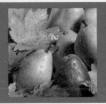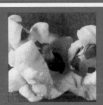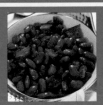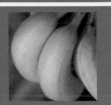

Soluble Fiber
- Oatmeal
- Orange
- Kidney beans
- Carrots
- Apple

Insoluble Fiber
- Whole wheat bread
- Popcorn
- Baked beans
- Banana
- Pear

Images copyright 2006 JupiterImages Corporation.

TABLE 2-6 | Dietary Fiber: Properties and Sources

Types of Dietary Fiber	Functions	Sources*
Insoluble fibers: Cellulose, some hemicelluloses, lignin	Holds water, increases fecal bulk, reduces intraluminal pressure in the colon; promotes growth of helpful bacteria in the colon	Wheat bran, bran cereals, whole grains (wheat and barley), popcorn, peanuts, apples, pears, berries, bananas, peaches, legumes, peas, cabbage family, corn, spinach, sweet potato, sunflower seeds
Soluble fibers: Pectin, beta glucans, some hemicelluloses, gums	Binds cholesterol and bile acids; slows gastric emptying; provides fermentable materials for colonic bacteria with production of volatile fatty acids and gas; slows absorption of glucose, preventing rapid rise in blood glucose levels	Oat bran, oat cereal, barley, pumpernickel bread, apples, citrus fruits, pears, broccoli, brussels sprouts, carrots, sweet potato, white potato, peas, legumes, (gums and psyllium used as thickeners or stabilizers in processed foods)

*Food source data from Duyff RL: *American Dietetic Association complete food and nutrition guide*, ed 2, Hoboken, NJ, 2002, John Wiley & Sons.

- *Lignin:* Lignin is the only dietary fiber that is not a carbohydrate. It is a large molecule that forms the woody part of plants. In the intestine it combines with bile acids and prevents their reabsorption. Lignin contributes the sandy texture to pears and lima beans.

Good food sources of insoluble fiber are whole grain cereals, especially wheat and wheat bran, nuts, root vegetables, vegetables of the cabbage family, and fruits with edible seeds.[11,33]

Soluble Fiber. The following list describes types of soluble fiber:

- *Pectin:* This water-soluble fiber is found in the cell walls of plants. It forms a viscous, sticky gel that binds cholesterol and prevents its absorption. Pectin also helps to slow gastric emptying and extend feelings of satiety.
- *Gums:* Gums are secreted by plants in response to plant injury. They bind cholesterol and prevent its absorption. Gums are fermented by bacteria in the colon to form short-chain fatty acids (this action was also noted earlier for resistant starch).

TABLE 2-7	Dietary Fiber and Kilocalorie Content of Selected Foods		
Food Group	**Serving Size**	**Dietary Fiber (g)**	**Kilocalories**
Grains Group			
All Bran	¾ cup	8.5	70
Bran Buds	⅓ cup	7.9	75
Oatmeal	1 cup	2.5	144
Air-popped popcorn	1 cup	2.2	25
Whole wheat bread	1 slice	1.4	60
Vegetable Group			
Kidney beans	½ cup	7.3	110
Green peas	½ cup	3.6	55
Corn	½ cup	2.9	70
Potato, with skin	1 medium	2.5	95
Carrots	½ cup	2.3	25
Broccoli	½ cup	2.2	20
Lettuce, fresh	1 cup	0.8	7
Fruit Group			
Apple	1 medium	3.5	80
Raisins	¼ cup	3.1	110
Strawberries	1 cup	3.0	45
Orange	1 medium	2.6	60
Banana	1 medium	2.4	105

Nutrient data from U.S. Department of Agriculture, Nutrient Data Laboratory: *National nutrient database for standard reference, Release 18,* Washington, DC, 2005, USDA Agricultural Research Service. Retrieved August 22, 2005, from *www.nal.usda.gov/fnic/foodcomp/.*

- *Hemicellulose:* Some forms of hemicellulose are water soluble and like gums are fermented by bacteria in the colon.
- *Beta glucans:* These water-soluble fibers are found in oats and oat bran, foods that carry a health claim on the label indicating their benefit for reducing risk of heart disease. (Beta glucans interfere with the absorption of cholesterol.)

Soluble fibers are found in legumes, oats, nuts, fruits, and some vegetables.[11,33] (See Appendix B for food contents of soluble and insoluble fibers.)

Functional Fiber

Functional fibers are nondigestible polysaccharides that have been isolated from plants or commercially produced and added to foods.[3] The term *functional fiber* was developed to indicate those fibers that were separated from plants or commercially produced as compared to those that are intact in plants and eaten in that form. Functional fibers are used as supplements or added to processed foods to improve their nutritional quality. Some fibers can be both dietary and functional depending on how they are eaten or used. The pectin in the apple you ate at lunch is considered a dietary fiber. On the other hand, pectin that was isolated from fruit sources and added to homemade and commercial jellies or used as an ingredient in patient tube feedings to provide fiber is classed as a functional fiber.[33] Functional fibers added in food processing must be listed on the food label.

A person's total fiber intake includes both dietary fiber and functional fiber. Food sources of dietary fiber and their energy content are listed in Table 2-7. Notice that many foods high in fiber are low to moderate in kcalories.

Health Promotion

Health Benefits of Fiber

Dietary fiber has various effects on the food mix in the gastrointestinal tract and its fate in the body. These physiologic actions have measurable influences on health, as follows:

- *Increase in fecal mass:* The capacity of insoluble fiber to hold water and associated bacteria contributes to its bulk-forming and laxative effects. The added mass

---

functional fiber Nondigestible carbohydrates isolated from plant foods or manufactured that are added to foods to increase their fiber content.

total fiber Dietary fiber plus functional fiber; the total amount of fiber in an individual's diet from all sources.

helps the food bolus move more rapidly through the small intestine, promoting normal bowel action. Dietary fiber prevents and alleviates constipation and is effective in reducing diarrhea.[34] A larger food mass in the colon averts the development of diverticulosis. When the food residue entering the colon is low in bulk, the muscles must contract more forcefully to move it forward, which over time forms diverticula with risk of inflammation and infection.

- *Binding of bile acids and cholesterol:* Soluble fibers and lignin lower blood cholesterol levels through their ability to bind both cholesterol and bile acids. When cholesterol is bound to fiber, it cannot be absorbed and is carried through the intestinal tract and eliminated in the feces. Certain fibers also bind bile salts and prevent their reabsorption. When bile acids are lost in the feces, the liver must remove cholesterol

from circulating blood lipoproteins to use in making more bile acids to replace those that were lost.[34,35] Flaxseed has particular value for reducing cardiovascular risk because it contains not only soluble fiber but also n-3 fatty acids.[36] (We will learn more about n-3 fatty acids in Chapter 3.)

- *Effect on colonic microflora:* Dietary fiber along with resistant starch is fermented by bacteria living in the colon. This fermentation produces gas and short-chain fatty acids that nourish the cells lining the colon and stimulate their growth.[13] The positive effect of fiber on the bifidobacteria population may prevent ulcerative colitis[37] and help protect against colon cancer.[13]

- *Positive effect on blood glucose and insulin levels:* Foods rich in fiber have a low glycemic index and slow the rise in blood glucose following a meal. This blunting

TO PROBE FURTHER

PHYTOCHEMICALS AND FUNCTIONAL FOODS: WHAT'S THE CONNECTION?

A new term—*phytochemical*—is being used to describe special nonnutrient health-promoting substances found in plant foods. It comes from the Greek word *phyton* meaning "plant" and refers to the tens of thousands of naturally occurring chemicals found in plants that have biological effects in the body.[1] Plants produce phytochemicals to protect themselves against bacteria and viruses. When the plants are eaten, these substances are absorbed and act as protective factors for humans. Most plant foods contain many different phytochemicals; tomatoes, for example, may contain as many as 10,000 different ones.[1] Men and women who eat recommended amounts of fruits, vegetables, and whole grains reduce their risk of death from all causes by more than 20% as compared to individuals who eat fewer plant foods.[2] Various categories of phytochemicals have important roles in human health and many act as antioxidants.

Phytoestrogens

The phytoestrogens have effects on the body that mimic the female hormone estrogen. The phytoestrogens help protect bone in postmenopausal women[3] and may lower the risk of heart disease in both women and men by their favorable effects on blood cholesterol levels.[4] The major phytoestrogens are genistein, daidzein, and other isoflavones. Their primary food sources are soybeans and other soy foods.

Polyphenols

Polyphenols are the largest group of phytochemicals and are widely distributed in fruits, vegetables, grains, legumes, herbs, tea, and spices. The formation of polyphenols is light dependent, so they are found in highest amounts in the leaves and outer parts of plants.

Polyphenols have many actions in the body, as follows:
- They prevent the oxidation of low-density lipoprotein (LDL) cholesterol; oxidized LDL cholesterol is especially harmful to the lining of the coronary arteries.
- They attack compounds that act on cells to form cancers and interrupt the steps in the development of tumors.
- They protect proteins, lipids, and carbohydrates from oxidation and damage during digestion.

The following list contains several important polyphenols and their food sources:
- *Phenolic acids:* grape juice, apples, citrus fruit, berries, coffee bean
- *Anthocyanins:* cocoa beans, berries, red wine
- *Tannins:* nuts, cocoa beans
- *Catechins:* green tea, pear, wine, apples
- *Isothiocyanates:* cruciferous vegetables such as broccoli, cabbage, and cauliflower
- *Diallyl disulfide and allicin:* garlic, onions

Some phytochemicals extracted from their plant sources are being sold as supplements. Phytochemicals like nutrients work best in combination with one another, so eating foods that contain a mixture of these substances offers the best protection against chronic disease.[5] Also, phytochemicals are found in foods in very small amounts, and not much is known about the safety of using concentrated amounts as found in supplements. Phytochemicals are lost in food processing, so it is best to use whole grain breads and cereals and eat fruits and vegetables without removing the skins or peels. Including a variety of fruits, vegetables, grains, and nuts in our daily diet provides an ample supply of these important substances.

References

1. Gropper SS, Smith JL, Groff JL: *Advanced nutrition and human metabolism*, ed 4, Belmont, Calif, 2005, Thomson/Wadsworth.
2. Kant AK, Graubard BI, Schatzkin A: Dietary patterns predict mortality in a national cohort: The National Health Interview Surveys, 1987 and 1992, *J Nutr* 134:1793, 2004.
3. Zhang X et al: Prospective cohort study of soy food consumption and risk of bone fracture among postmenopausal women, *Arch Intern Med* 165:1890, 2005.
4. Zhan S, Ho SC: Meta-analysis of the effects of soy protein containing isoflavones on the lipid profile, *Am J Clin Nutr* 81:397, 2005.
5. Liu RH: Health benefits of fruits and vegetables are from additive and synergistic combinations of phytochemicals, *Am J Clin Nutr* 78(suppl):517S, 2003.

of blood glucose levels lowers the amount of insulin needed to move this glucose into muscle and fat cells, reducing the work of the beta cells of the pancreas. A diet high in fiber assists in both preventing and managing type 2 diabetes.[16]

Health Benefits of Phytochemicals

Fruits, vegetables, legumes, and whole grain foods rich in carbohydrate and fiber also contain phytochemicals (plant chemicals) beneficial to health. These foods are often referred to as *functional foods* because their positive effects on body function and health cannot be explained solely by the known nutrients they contain.[38] Those who eat these plant foods regularly have a lower risk of heart disease, cancer, and diabetes. It is likely that fiber and phytochemicals work together to bring about these effects on health. This is why it is best to obtain your fiber by eating a variety of whole foods that supply both phytochemicals and fiber rather than choosing fiber supplements or highly processed foods with added functional fiber (see the *To Probe Further* box, "Phytochemicals and Functional Foods: What's the Connection?").

Dietary Reference Intake for Fiber

The Adequate Intake (AI) for total fiber is expected to reduce the risk of coronary heart disease and type 2 diabetes. Men below age 51 should consume 38 g/day and those ages 51 and over need 30 g/day. The AIs for younger and older women are 25 g/day and 21 g/day, respectively.[5] The Nutrition Label lists the amount of fiber per serving and recommends a daily fiber intake of 25 g in a diet of 2000 kcal. This is considerably lower than the current AI.

Fiber intakes in the United States are much below the Dietary Reference Intake. Median daily intake ranges from about 16 to 18 g/day for men and 12 to 14 g/day for women.[3] The *MyPyramid* goals of 4½ cups of fruits and vegetables and three whole grain servings each day as part of a 2000-kcal diet provides 31 g of fiber.[26]

DIGESTION-ABSORPTION-METABOLISM PREVIEW

We discuss the digestion, absorption, and metabolism of the macronutrients in greater detail in Chapter 8, but a brief outline of this process for carbohydrate will set the scene for the larger picture to follow.

Digestion

Starches and sugars in carbohydrate foods must be converted to glucose for use by cells. The process by which this change occurs is digestion. Digestion involves two types of actions: (1) mechanical or muscle actions that break the food mass into smaller particles and (2) chemical actions by which specific enzymes break down food components into smaller, usable metabolic products.

Mouth

Chewing breaks food into fine particles and mixes it with the salivary secretions. A salivary amylase (ptyalin) from the parotid gland acts on starch to begin its breakdown into dextrins and maltose.

Stomach

Successive wavelike contractions of the muscle fibers in the stomach wall continue the mechanical action of digestion. This muscle action is called *peristalsis*. It mixes the food particles with gastric secretions to help chemical digestion take place more efficiently. There is no specific enzyme in the stomach to break down carbohydrate, and the hydrochloric acid in the gastric secretions stops the action of salivary amylase. However, before the food mass is completely mixed with gastric acid, as much as 20% to 30% of the starch is changed to maltose. By the time the food mass reaches the lower section of the stomach it has been transformed into a thick creamy chyme, ready to pass through the pyloric valve into the duodenum, the first section of the small intestine.

Small Intestine

Peristalsis continues to aid digestion in the small intestine by mixing and moving the chyme along the intestinal lumen. Chemical digestion of carbohydrate is completed by enzymes from two sources: (1) the pancreas and (2) the small intestine, as follows:

- *Pancreatic secretions:* Secretions from the pancreas enter the duodenum through the common bile duct. One is pancreatic amylase, which continues the breakdown of starch to maltose.
- *Intestinal secretions:* Cells within the brush border of the small intestine secrete three disaccharidases—sucrase, lactase, and maltase. These enzymes act on

---

lumen The cavity or channel within a tube or tubular organ such as the intestines.

sucrase Enzyme that splits the disaccharide sucrose, releasing the monosaccharides glucose and fructose.

lactase Enzyme that splits the disaccharide lactose, releasing the monosaccharides glucose and galactose.

maltase Enzyme that splits the disaccharide maltose, releasing two units of the monosaccharide glucose.

their respective disaccharides to release the monosaccharides—glucose, galactose, and fructose—for absorption. The disaccharidases are integral proteins of the brush border and break down the disaccharides as absorption takes place.

Table 2-8 summarizes carbohydrate digestion.

Absorption

The monosaccharides are now ready to be absorbed and carried to the cells. Glucose is absorbed by an active transport or pumping system requiring sodium as a carrier. Of the total carbohydrate absorbed, 80% is in the form of glucose and absorbed by the sodium transport mechanism; the remaining 20% is in the form of galactose and fructose.[39]

Absorbing Structures

The absorbing surface of the small intestine is enhanced by three structures: the mucosal folds, the villi, and the microvilli. Together they greatly expand the absorbing surface, enabling 90% of the digested food material to move across the intestinal wall and enter the blood.

Route of Absorption

Via the capillaries in the villi, the monosaccharides—glucose, galactose, and fructose—enter the portal blood circulation and are transported to the liver. Here fructose and galactose are converted to glucose. Glucose can be used immediately for fuel or converted to glycogen for short-term storage. Glycogen constantly reconverts to glucose as needed.

Metabolism

Definition

The term metabolism refers to the sum of the various chemical activities in a living organism that sustain life. These include reactions by which energy is produced and tissues are built, carry out their function, and are broken down and replaced. The products of specific metabolic processes are called metabolites.

Metabolism of Carbohydrates

Cells are the functional units in the human body. The most important carbohydrate for cell nutrition is glucose. In the cell glucose is burned to produce energy through a series of chemical reactions requiring specific enzymes. This energy is used by the cell to do its work. Glucose not needed immediately is converted to glycogen or adipose tissue for storage as a reserve fuel.

Metabolic Concept of Unity

A central principle pervading all of our discussions is the unity of the human organism. Our bodies are made up of many parts and processes having unequaled specificity and flexibility. Intimate metabolic relationships exist among all the nutrients and their metabolites, making it impossible to understand any one metabolic process without viewing it in relation to the whole.

Keep in mind that all nutrients do their best work in partnership with other nutrients. Thus the emphasis in nutrition education should be a balanced dietary pattern avoiding undue emphasis on one nutrient or group of nutrients to the exclusion of others.

TO SUM UP

Carbohydrates produced by photosynthesis in plants supply most of the world's population with its primary source of energy. Simple carbohydrates, the monosaccharides and disaccharides, are easily digested and provide quick energy. Starch, a digestible complex carbohydrate, requires greater breakdown to become available for use. Carbohydrates serve special functions through their ability to spare protein, prevent the build-up of ketones, and supply energy for the central nervous system. Fiber, nondigestible carbohydrates found in the structural walls, hulls, seeds, skins of fruits and vegetables, and whole grains affect the digestion and absorption of food in ways that are beneficial to health. Carbohydrates should provide 45% to 65% of total kcalories.

QUESTIONS FOR REVIEW

1. Differentiate among the terms *monosaccharide*, *disaccharide*, and *polysaccharide*. List two food sources of each.
2. What is resistant starch? Where is it found? Name two health benefits of resistant starch.

TABLE 2-8	Summary of Carbohydrate Digestion	

Digestive Area	Enzyme	Action
Mouth	Salivary amylase: ptyalin	Starch → Dextrins → Maltose
Stomach	None	Starch hydrolysis continues briefly
Small intestine	Pancreatic amylase	Starch → Dextrins → Maltose
	Intestinal disaccharidases	
	Sucrase	Sucrose → Glucose + Fructose
	Lactase	Lactose → Glucose + Galactose
	Maltase	Maltose → Glucose + Glucose

3. For breakfast you had a piece of whole grain bread with jelly, a banana, and a glass of low-fat milk. List both the digestible and nondigestible forms of carbohydrate included in this meal. Make a table of the digestible carbohydrates, indicating the site of digestion, the required enzymes, and the products formed.
4. Using the CD-ROM included with your text, determine the daily energy need of a 25-year-old woman who is 5 ft 4 in tall, weighs 125 lb, and is relatively sedentary. How many grams of carbohydrate should be included in her diet, and how many kcalories should it supply? What is her upper limit for grams of sugar? How much fiber is recommended? Develop a 3-day menu that provides the appropriate amounts of carbohydrate and dietary fiber and does not exceed the limit for sugar.
5. Describe the clinical effects of fiber in the prevention or treatment of the following conditions: diverticular disease, hyperlipidemia, and type 2 diabetes.
6. Your client Mr. B wants to lose 20 lb before his high school reunion next month. He has decided to eat only meat and other fried foods for the next 4 weeks because he believes a very low-carbohydrate diet will help him lose weight. What are the dangers of the diet he has proposed? How would you explain why he needs carbohydrate?
7. Describe five special functions of carbohydrate in the body.
8. Visit your local grocery store, and find two fruit juices, two fruit drinks, and two carbonated beverages available in single-serving, easy-to-carry containers. Use the Nutrition Label to construct a table indicating the kcalories, total carbohydrate (g), sugar (g), vitamins, and minerals per 8-oz serving. Check the list of ingredients, and note which products contain added sugar. Which are most appropriate for daily use, and which should be limited?

REFERENCES

1. Englyst HN, Hudson GJ: Carbohydrates. In Garrow JS, James WPT, Ralph A, eds: *Human nutrition and dietetics,* ed 10, Edinburgh, 2000, Churchill Livingstone.
2. Mackey M, Montgomery J: Plant biotechnology can enhance food security and nutrition in the developing world, part 1, *Nutr Today* 39(2):52, 2004.
3. Food and Nutrition Board, Institute of Medicine: *Dietary Reference Intakes for energy, carbohydrate, fiber, fat, fatty acids, cholesterol, protein, and amino acids, (macronutrients),* Washington, DC, 2002, National Academies Press.
4. The Expert Committee on the Diagnosis and Classification of Diabetes Mellitus: Follow-up report on the diagnosis of diabetes mellitus, *Diabetes Care* 26:3160, 2003.
5. Bray G, Nielsen SJ, Popkin BM: Consumption of high-fructose corn syrup in beverages may play a role in the epidemic of obesity, *Am J Clin Nutr* 79:537, 2004.
6. Skoog SM, Bharucha AE: Dietary fructose and gastrointestinal symptoms, *Am J Gastroenterol* 99:2046, 2004.
7. American Dietetic Association: Position of the American Dietetic Association: use of nutritive and nonnutritive sweeteners, *J Am Diet Assoc* 104:255, 2004.
8. Solomon NW: Fermentation, fermented foods and lactose intolerance, *Eur J Clin Nutr* 56(suppl 4):550, 2002.
9. Sigman-Grant M, Morita J: Defining and interpreting intakes of sugars, *Am J Clin Nutr* 78(suppl):815S, 2003.
10. Murphy SP, Johnson RK: The scientific basis of recent U.S. guidance on sugars intake, *Am J Clin Nutr* 78(suppl):827S, 2003.
11. Duyff RL: *American Dietetic Association complete food and nutrition guide,* ed 2, Hoboken, NJ, 2002, John Wiley & Sons.
12. Muir JG et al: Combining wheat bran with resistant starch has more beneficial effects on fecal indexes than does wheat bran alone, *Am J Clin Nutr* 79:1020, 2004.
13. Slavin J: Why whole grains are protective: biological mechanisms, *Proc Nutr Soc* 62:129, 2003.
14. Cotton PA et al: Dietary sources of nutrients among U.S. adults, *J Am Diet Assoc* 104:921, 2004.
15. U.S. Department of Health and Human Services, U.S. Department of Agriculture: *Dietary Guidelines for Americans 2005,* ed 6, Washington, DC, 2005, Authors. Retrieved July 18, 2005, from *www.healthierus/gov/dietaryguidelines.*
16. Roberts SB, Pittas AG: The role of glycemic index in type 2 diabetes, *Nutr Clin Care* 6(2):73, 2003.
17. Anonymous: The glycemic index: principle vs. practice, *Nutr Clin Care* 6(1):41, 2003.
18. Roberts SB: Glycemic index and satiety, *Nutr Clin Care* 6(1):20, 2003.
19. Benjamin SM et al: Estimated number of adults with prediabetes in the U.S. in 2000: opportunities for prevention, *Diabetes Care* 26:645, 2003.
20. Rampersaud GC et al: Breakfast habits, nutritional status, body weight, and academic performance in children and adolescents, *J Am Diet Assoc* 105:743, 2005.
21. Benton D, Nabb S: Carbohydrate, memory, and mood, *Nutr Reviews* 61(5, part 2):S61, 2003.
22. Binns NM: Sucralose—all sweetness and light, *Nutr Bull* 28.53, 2003 (British Nutrition Foundation).
23. Schneeman BO: Carbohydrate: friend or foe? Summary of research needs, *J Nutr* 131:2764S, 2001.
24. Astrup A, Larsen TM, Harper A: Atkins and other low-carbohydrate diets: hoax or an effective tool for weight loss? *Lancet* 364:897, 2004.
25. Jequier E, Bray GA: Low-fat diets are preferred, *Am J Med* 113(suppl 9B):41S, 2002.
26. U.S. Department of Agriculture, Center for Nutrition Policy and Promotion: MyPyramid food guidance system, Washington, DC, 2005, Author. Retrieved July 17, 2005, from *www.mypyramid.gov.*

portal An entryway, usually referring to the portal circulation of blood through the liver. Blood is brought into the liver via the portal vein and moves out via the hepatic vein.

metabolism Sum of all the various biochemical and physiolgic processes by which the body grows and maintains itself (anabolism) and breaks down and reshapes tissue (catabolism) and transforms energy to do its work. Products of these various reactions are called metabolites.

27. Bowman SA, Spence JT: A comparison of low-carbohydrate vs. high-carbohydrate diets: energy restriction, nutrient quality and correlation to body mass index, *J Am Coll Nutr* 21:268, 2002.

28. Kennedy ET et al: Popular diets: correlation to health, nutrition, and obesity, *J Am Diet Assoc* 101(4):411, 2001.

29. Schoeller DA, Buchholz AC: Energetics of obesity and weight control: does diet composition matter, *J Am Diet Assoc* 105:S24, 2005.

30. Dansinger ML et al: Comparison of the Atkins, Ornish, Weight Watchers, and Zone diets for weight loss and heart disease risk reduction: a randomized trial, *JAMA* 293:43, 2005.

31. Meckling KA, O'Sullivan C, Saari D: Comparison of a low-fat diet to a low-carbohydrate diet on weight loss, body composition, and risk factors for diabetes and cardiovascular disease in free-living, overweight men and women, *J Clin Endocrinol Metab* 89:2717, 2004.

32. Eckel RH: The dietary approach to obesity: is it the diet or the disorder? *JAMA* 293:96, 2005.

33. Gropper SS, Smith JL, Groff JL: *Advanced nutrition and human metabolism,* ed 4, Belmont, Calif, 2005, Thomson/Wadsworth.

34. American Dietetic Association: Position of the American Dietetic Association: health implications of dietary fiber, *J Am Diet Assoc* 102:993, 2002.

35. Bazzano LA et al: Dietary fiber intake and reduced risk of coronary heart disease in U.S. men and women, *Arch Intern Med* 163:1897, 2003.

36. Bloedon LT, Szapary PO: Flaxseed and cardiovascular risk, *Nutr Reviews* 62:18, 2004.

37. Nyman EM: Importance of processing for physico-chemical and physiological properties of dietary fibre, *Proc Nutr Soc* 62:187, 2003.

38. American Dietetic Association: Position of the American Dietetic Association: functional foods, *J Am Diet Assoc* 104:814, 2004.

39. Marsh MN, Riley SA: Digestion and absorption of nutrients and vitamins. In Feldman M, Scharschmidt BF, Sleisenger MH, eds: *Gastrointestinal and liver disease,* ed 6, vol 2, Philadelphia, 1998, WB Saunders.

FURTHER READINGS AND RESOURCES

Readings

Jones JM, Elam K: Sugars and health: is there an issue? *J Am Diet Assoc* 103:1058, 2003.

Grimm GC, Harnack L, Story M: Factors associated with soft drink consumption in school-aged children, *J Am Diet Assoc* 104:1244, 2004.

These authors present the nutritional problems related to excessive sugar intake and what influences use of sugar-sweetened soft drinks by children. This background information can help us develop nutrition education programs to influence this behavior.

McNutt K: What clients need to know about sugar replacers, *J Am Diet Assoc* 100:466, 2000.

This article evaluates nonnutritive sweeteners and provides information to guide us in educating our patients about their appropriate use in a balanced diet.

Jones JM et al: Becoming proactive with the whole-grains message, *Nutr Today* 39(1):10, 2004.

These writers give important reasons for why consumers need to increase their intakes of fiber and provide ideas on how we can help them be successful.

Roberts SB, Pittas AG: The role of glycemic index in type 2 diabetes, *Nutr Clin Care* 6:73, 2003.

These researchers describe the benefits of complex carbohydrates and fiber in preventing and treating type 2 diabetes.

Websites of Interest

- U.S. Department of Agriculture, Center for Nutrition Policy and Promotion: *MyPyramid food guidance system; MyPyramid* offers suggestions on how to increase your intakes of healthy carbohydrate foods: *www.mypyramid.gov.*

- U.S. Department of Health and Human Services, U.S. Department of Agriculture: *Dietary Guidelines for Americans 2005;* the *Dietary Guidelines for Americans 2005* provides guidance on increasing intakes of complex carbohydrates and decreasing intakes of sugar: *www.healthierus.gov/dietaryguidelines/.*

- Produce for Better Health Foundation; this organization is the sponsor of the 5 A Day Campaign encouraging everyone to eat at least five fruits and vegetables each day: *www.5aday.com/.*

- Office of Disease Prevention, U.S. Department of Health and Human Services; these websites for children and adults provide materials and good suggestions for helping people improve their selection of carbohydrate foods: *www.healthfinder.gov/kids/; www.healthfinder.gov/.*

CHAPTER 3

Lipids

Eleanor D. Schlenker

Lipids, the second of the energy-yielding macronutrients, continue to receive mixed publicity. Although we hear about the dangers of a high-fat diet and the added risk of heart disease, we also read about the health benefits of the Mediterranean diet that is moderately high in fat. A recent consumer survey explored the reasons why the general public craves fast-food hamburgers and received such answers as "Has a taste you can't duplicate," "Is warm and inviting," and "Fills that empty spot."[1] In large part these attributes come from fat. Fats add taste and pleasant mouth feel to our food and contribute to our "feeling full." Fat itself is an essential nutrient.

Traditionally, fat held a prominent place in the American diet. However, spurred by justified health concerns, our attitudes toward dietary lipids have changed. We need to assess not only how much fat we eat, but also what type, because different fats have different effects on our body and our health. As health professionals we need to focus on the total diet, not on a single nutrient.[2] In our study of lipids and their role in nutrition we will learn why we need fat for energy and overall good health.

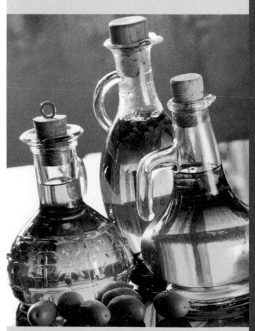

LIPIDS IN NUTRITION AND HEALTH

Functions of Lipids

Food Lipids

Lipids found in food carry out important body functions. They provide energy, supply the essential fatty acids necessary for survival, and add to our enjoyment of food. These important functions are described below.

- *Provide fuel for energy:* Lipids are a concentrated source of fuel to store and use as needed. Food lipids yield 9 kilocalories (kcalories or kcal) per gram when oxidized in the body as compared with carbohydrates and protein which yield only 4 kcal/g.
- *Supply essential fatty acids:* Food lipids contain the essential fatty acids linoleic acid and alpha-linolenic acid. Food lipids from animal sources also provide cholesterol, supplementing the body's endogenous supply.
- *Support absorption of the fat-soluble vitamins:* Lipid must be present in the food mix in the small intestine to provide a vehicle for absorption of the fat-soluble vitamins.
- *Add to food palatability:* Lipids add flavor and a certain mouth feel to food and heighten the feeling of satisfaction that comes with eating. Our food choices are strongly influenced by tastes and textures from lipids that enhance our eating pleasure.
- *Promote satiety:* A meal containing lipids brings a longer period of satiety than a meal containing only carbohydrate and protein. Particular brain cells respond to the mouth feel of fat and influence the region of the brain controlling appetite.[3] Fat contributes texture and body to food mixtures that slows their movement out of the stomach and helps prolong the feeling of fullness.

Body Lipids

Lipids are stored in the body as adipose tissue. This lipid tissue has a number of functions essential to life and health, as follows:

- *Ready source of energy:* Lipids provide an efficient form of fuel for all tissues except the brain and central nervous system. In fact, fatty acids are the preferred fuel of the heart muscle.
- *Thermal insulation:* The layer of lipid deposited directly beneath the skin helps maintain body temperature.
- *Protection of vital organs:* A weblike padding of adipose tissue surrounds vital organs such as the kidneys, protecting them from mechanical shock and providing structural support.
- *Transmission of nerve impulses:* Lipid layers surrounding nerve fibers provide electrical insulation and transmit nerve impulses.
- *Membrane structure:* Lipids are structural components of cell membranes and help to transport nutrients, metabolites, and waste molecules in and out of cells.

- *Carriers of fat-soluble materials:* Lipoproteins, molecules made of lipids and protein, carry lipids from the liver to body tissues. Lipids transport the fat-soluble vitamins A, D, E, and K to the cells for metabolic use.
- *Precursors of other substances:* Lipids supply fatty acids and cholesterol for the synthesis of various materials required for tissue integrity and metabolic function. For example, brain tissue and the retina of the eye contain many fatty acids.

Health Issues and Lipids

It is evident that lipids perform many essential functions in the body. Yet there continue to be questions about the amounts and types of fat that we should eat.[4-6] As with many things you need what you need, but you do not need more than you need. Health concerns related to dietary fat generally focus on two issues: (1) the high energy intake associated with a diet high in fat and (2) the negative health effects of saturated and *trans* fatty acids. As we will learn in future sections, different types of fat have different effects on body tissues and functions.

Amount of Fat

Fat contains over twice as many kcalories per gram as do protein and carbohydrate (9 kcal/g versus 4 kcal/g). Too much fat in the diet supplies an excess of kcalories, more than required for immediate use. Excess kcalories are stored as adipose tissue and over time add to body weight. Inappropriate increases in body weight—or more precisely, inappropriate increases in body fat—are associated with such health problems as type 2 diabetes, hypertension, and heart disease.[7] Watch for specific relationships between increased body weight and body fat and these health problems in later chapters.

Type of Fat

Saturated fats from animal sources when eaten in excessive amounts have negative effects on health. High intakes of saturated fats and cholesterol promote atherosclerosis, the buildup of fatty deposits on the interior walls of the major arteries that increase risk of heart attack or stroke. In contrast to saturated fats, fats in vegetable oils, olive oil, and fatty fish, eaten in moderation, can reduce our risk of cardiovascular disease.[8] So it is important to help people learn to recognize the different sources and types of fats and how they affect health. Recently nutrition scientists have alerted us to the health risks from *trans* fats found in processed foods.

THE PHYSICAL AND CHEMICAL NATURE OF LIPIDS

Physical Characteristics

The term *lipid* includes fats, oils, and related compounds that are insoluble in water and greasy to the touch. Some food lipids—butter, margarine, or cooking oil—are easily recognized as fats. Other foods that may appear to be mainly carbohydrate (bakery items)[9] or protein (beef patty) often contain significant amounts of fat. We refer to this fat as *hidden fat.*

Chemical Characteristics

The chemical name for fats and fat-related compounds is *lipids.* Lipids are organic compounds consisting of a carbon chain as a "backbone," with hydrogen and oxygen atoms and other radicals or groups of elements attached. The fatty acids and their related compounds are the lipids important in human nutrition. Lipids have something in common with carbohydrates. The same chemical elements that make up carbohydrates—carbon, hydrogen, and oxygen—also make up the fatty acids. However, carbohydrates and lipids have the following two important differences:

1. Lipids are more complex in structure, with more carbon (C) and hydrogen (H) atoms and fewer oxygen (O) atoms.
2. The common structural units of lipids are fatty acids, whereas the common structural units of carbohydrates are simple sugars.

We will look first at the unique characteristics of fatty acids—their saturation, chain length, and essentiality—before focusing on the nature of the lipids (triglycerides) that are built from fatty acids.

BASIC LIPIDS: FATTY ACIDS AND TRIGLYCERIDES

Characteristics of the Fatty Acids: Saturation

The degree of saturation or unsaturation gives lipids their physical characteristics. Saturated lipids are hard, less saturated are soft, and unsaturated are liquid at room temperature (Box 3-1). These physical differences relate to the ratio of hydrogen atoms to carbon atoms in the fatty acids in the lipid. If a fatty acid has a hydrogen atom attached at each available space, the fatty acid is said to be completely saturated. If, however, the fatty acid has some hydrogen spaces unfilled, it is less saturated. The following three terms are used to designate saturation in fats.

1. *Saturated:* Food lipids composed of saturated fatty acids are called *saturated fats.* The most saturated lipids are two tropical oils: coconut oil, which is 88% saturated, and palm kernel oil, which is 80% saturated.[10] Other saturated fats are of animal origin and are found in meat, butter, and whole milk dairy products.
2. *Monounsaturated:* Food lipids made up of fatty acids with one hydrogen space unfilled, creating one double bond, are called *monounsaturated fats.* These lipids are generally from plant sources. Canola oil obtained from rapeseed and olive oil are monounsaturated fats.

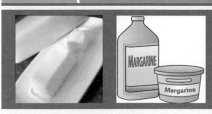

BOX 3-1 | **Food Fats With Different Degrees of Saturation**

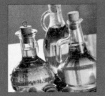

Highly Saturated Fat (solid at room temperature)
   Stick margarine
   Butter
   Beef fat

Less-Saturated Fat (very soft at room temperature)
   Tub margarine
   Squeeze margarine

Unsaturated Fat (liquid at room temperature)
   Salad oil

Images copyright 2006 JupiterImages Corporation.

3. *Polyunsaturated:* When fatty acids have two or more spaces unfilled with hydrogen, creating two or more double bonds, they are called *polyunsaturated fats.* Many of these fats come from plant sources. Common polyunsaturated fats are corn oil and safflower oil. Polyunsaturated fatty acids with two or more double bonds are also referred to as *n-3* or *n-6 fatty acids.* The number refers to the position in the carbon chain where the first double bond appears. An important n-6 fatty acid is linoleic acid, an essential fatty acid found in vegetable oils. The n-3 fatty acids in fatty fish have a role in cardiovascular health.[8]

---

lipids Chemical group name for fats and fat-related compounds such as cholesterol, lipoproteins, and phospholipids; general group name for organic substances of a fatty nature including fats, oils, waxes, and related compounds.

fatty acid The building block or structural component of fats.

adipose Cells and tissues that store fat.

organic Carbon-based chemical compounds.

saturated Term used for a substance that is united with the greatest possible number of other atoms or chemical groups through solution, chemical combination, or the like. A fatty acid is saturated if all available chemical bonds of its carbon chain are filled with hydrogen. A fat is saturated if the majority of fatty acids making up its structure are saturated.

Characteristics of Fatty Acids: Chain Length

A second characteristic of fatty acids important in human nutrition is the length of the carbon chain forming their structure. Fatty acids in foods range from 4 carbons to 22 carbons (Box 3-2). Chain length affects absorption. Long-chain fatty acids are more difficult to absorb and require a helping carrier. Short- and medium-chain fatty acids are soluble in water and can be absorbed directly into the bloodstream. When intestinal diseases injure the absorbing mucosal surface of the small intestine, short- or medium-chain fatty acids are preferred. A commercial product called MCT (medium-chain triglycerides), an oil made of short- and medium-chain fatty acids, can replace ordinary vegetable oil in food preparation.

The Essential Fatty Acids

The terms *essential* and *nonessential* are applied to nutrients according to their relative necessity in the diet. A nutrient is essential if the body cannot make it or cannot make it in the amount needed. In that case the substance must be supplied in food. If a sufficient amount of the nutrient is not obtained from the diet, signs of deficiency will begin to appear.

Two kinds—(1) linoleic acid (an n-6 fatty acid) and (2) alpha-linolenic acid (an n-3 fatty acid)—are essential fatty acids for humans. Arachidonic acid, a fatty acid important in human nutrition, can be made from linoleic acid; eicosapentaenoic acid and docosahexaenoic acid can be made from alpha-linolenic acid. Box 3-3 lists some food sources of these fatty acids.

Linoleic acid and alpha-linolenic acid, the essential fatty acids, have the following important roles in the body:

- *Skin integrity:* The essential fatty acids strengthen cell membranes and prevent a harmful increase in skin permeability. Essential fatty acid deficiency causes a breakdown in skin tissue with characteristic eczema and skin lesions.
- *Blood cholesterol regulation:* Linoleic and alpha-linolenic acids participate in both the transport and metabolism of cholesterol and help to lower blood cholesterol levels.
- *Growth:* Normal growth requires an adequate supply of the essential fatty acids and is impaired in essential fatty acid deficiency. Alpha-linolenic acid is especially important for the development of brain tissue before and after birth.
- *Gene expression:* The essential fatty acids regulate the production of enzymes needed for synthesis of nonessential fatty acids by the liver.[11]

BOX 3-2 | Chain Length of Fatty Acids

Short-chain fatty acids have 4 to 6 carbons.
Medium-chain fatty acids have 8, 10, or 12 carbons.
Long-chain fatty acids have 14, 16, 18 or more carbons.

BOX 3-3 | Food Sources of n-3 and n-6 Fatty Acids

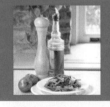 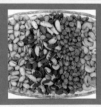 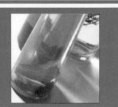 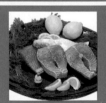 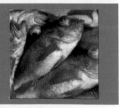

Linoleic Acid: n-6 Fatty Acid (essential)

Safflower oil
Corn oil
Cottonseed oil
Soybean oil
Nuts
Wheat germ

Alpha-Linolenic Acid: n-3 Fatty Acid (essential)

Soybean oil
Flaxseed oil
Canola oil
Walnuts
Wheat germ

Fatty Acids From Fish: n-3 Fatty Acids (can also be synthesized by the body)

All of the following supply eicosapentaenoic acid and docosahexaenoic acid:
- Herring
- Mackerel
- Halibut
- Salmon
- Canned tuna

- *Immune function:* Persons with essential fatty acid deficiency have a higher rate of infection.[11]
- *Blood platelet aggregation:* Eicosapentaenoic acid and docosahexaenoic acid, n-3 fatty acids made from alpha-linolenic acid, prevent unwanted aggregation of blood platelets that block the flow of blood in a major artery causing a heart attack or stroke.[11]
- *Synthesis of hormonelike agents:* Linoleic acid and alpha-linolenic acid are the metabolic precursors of a group of physiologically and pharmacologically active compounds known as prostaglandins (Figure 3-1). They were first identified in human semen and named prostaglandins because they were thought to originate in the prostate gland. Prostaglandins exist in virtually all body tissues and act as local hormones to direct and coordinate biologic functions. Their activities influence blood pressure, blood clotting, and cardiovascular function.[12]

Dietary Reference Intakes

Adequate Intakes (AIs) have been established for both linoleic and alpha-linolenic acids. (See inside front cover to review the various categories of the Dietary Reference Intakes.) The AI for linoleic acid (an n-6 fatty acid) is 17 g/day for men and 12 g/day for women ages 19 to 50 years. Men ages 51 years and over should take in 14 g/day of linoleic acid, and women of that age should take in 11 g/day. The AI for alpha-linolenic acid (an n-3 fatty acid) is 1.6 g/day for all adult men and 1.1 g/day for all adult women.[6] (Review Box 3-3 for good sources of the two essential fatty acids.)

Special Needs of Infants

Breast milk is high in fat, with more than 50% of kcalories coming from fat. The essential fatty acids along with preformed arachidonic and docosahexaenoic acids are found in breast milk in higher amounts than were formerly included in infant formulas. Although arachidonic acid can be made from linoleic acid and docosahexaenoic acid from alpha-linolenic acid, we are not sure if infants have the ability to produce these acids in the amounts needed for optimum development.[13] Infant formulas with added arachidonic and docosahexaenoic acids are now available in the United States.

Food Sources

The best sources of the two essential fatty acids, linoleic and alpha-linolenic acids, are vegetable oils. Corn oil, safflower oil, soybean oil, cottonseed oil, sunflower oil, and peanut oil all contain linoleic acid (an n-6 acid). Alpha-linolenic acid (an n-3 acid) is found in canola oil, soy oil, linseed oil, and rapeseed oil, and dark green leafy vegetables. Although the body can make eicosapentaenoic acid and docosahexaenoic acid from alpha-linolenic acid, these n-3 fatty acids can also be obtained from fish and shellfish.[6] (Review Box 3-3 for food sources.)

Triglycerides

Structure

Fatty acids are stored in the body in the form of triglycerides. Triglycerides are made of three fatty acids attached to a glycerol base. They are named glycerides because they contain glycerol and fatty acids. When glycerol is combined with one fatty acid it is called a *monoglyceride;* with two fatty acids it is a *diglyceride;* and with three fatty acids, a *triglyceride.* Glycerides are found in food and also formed in the body. Most natural lipids from either animal or plant sources are triglycerides. They are seen in body cells as oily droplets and circulate in the water-based blood plasma encased in a covering of water-soluble protein. These lipid-protein complexes are called *lipoproteins.* Triglycerides serve multiple functions throughout the body.

Food Lipids and Health

Degree of Saturation

Food lipids contain both saturated and unsaturated fats. Foods from animal sources—such as meat, milk, and eggs—contain more saturated fats. Most food lipids from plant sources, primarily vegetable oils, are unsaturated.

---

linoleic acid An essential fatty acid for humans; an n-6 polyunsaturated fatty acid.

alpha-linolenic acid An essential fatty acid for humans; an n-3 polyunsaturated fatty acid.

essential fatty acid A fatty acid that must be supplied in the diet because the body cannot make it or cannot make it in sufficient amounts.

prostaglandins Group of naturally occurring substances derived from long-chain fatty acids that have multiple local hormonelike actions; they regulate gastric acid secretion, blood platelet aggregation, body temperature, and tissue inflammation.

triglyceride Chemical name for fat that indicates the structure of three fatty acids attached to a glycerol base. A neutral fat synthesized from carbohydrate and stored in adipose tissue; it releases free fatty acids into the blood when hydrolyzed by enzymes.

glycerol An alcohol that is esterified with fatty acids to produce fats and released when fats are hydrolyzed; a colorless, odorless, syrupy sweet liquid.

glyceride Group name for fats; any of a group of esters obtained from glycerol by the replacement of one, two, or three hydroxyl (OH) groups with a fatty acid. Monoglycerides contain one fatty acid; diglycerides contain two fatty acids; and triglycerides contain three fatty acids. Glycerides are the principal constituent of adipose tissue and are found in animal and plant fats and oils.

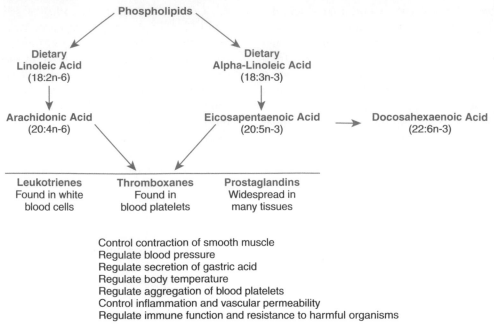

FIGURE 3-1   Synthesis, sites, and functions of eicosanoids. Various eicosanoids such as leukotrienes, thromboxanes, and prostaglandins are made from the essential fatty acids. The individual substances made from each of the two essential fatty acids work together to regulate body functions. For some functions they have opposing actions that help maintain homeostasis or coordinate responses to new situations.

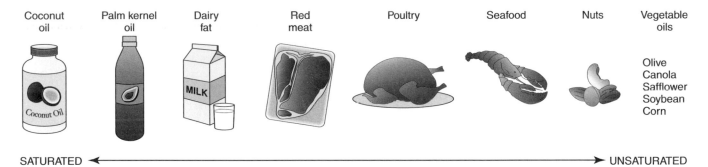

FIGURE 3-2   Spectrum of food fats according to degree of saturation of their component fatty acids. Note that the two food fats with the highest degree of saturation are plant fats, followed by various animal fats in decreasing order of saturation. In general, plant fats are more unsaturated.

The spectrum of food fats—from saturated to unsaturated—is illustrated in Figure 3-2. The fats on the saturated end of the spectrum, mostly animal fats, are solid at room temperature; those toward the center are somewhat less saturated and softer at room temperature. The plant lipids on the unsaturated end are free-flowing oils that do not solidify even at low temperatures. But the *exceptions* to the usual pattern of saturation can be injurious to human health. Coconut oil and palm kernel oil—highly saturated plant lipids—are used extensively in products such as nondairy creamers and baked goods because they are generally cheaper oils.

The Nutrition Label can guide a consumer's choice of fats. The Nutrition Label indicates the number of grams of both saturated and unsaturated fats per serving. Added fats such as coconut oil and palm kernel oil can be found in the list of ingredients on the food label. Both the general distinction in saturation between animal and plant fats and the Nutrition Label will assist in food selection.

Cis *Versus* Trans *Fats*

To meet the demand for inexpensive solid fats for use as table fats or food ingredients the process of hydrogenation was developed. This procedure changes unsaturated liquid oils into solid fats such as margarine and shortening. When unsaturated oils are surrounded with hydrogen gas, hydrogen ions attach at available sites, producing a more saturated (or solid) fat. However, a particular type of unsaturated fatty acid formed in this process, a *trans* fatty acid, is detrimental to health.

In Figure 3-3 we compare the two possible structures of an unsaturated fatty acid. When double bonds occur in

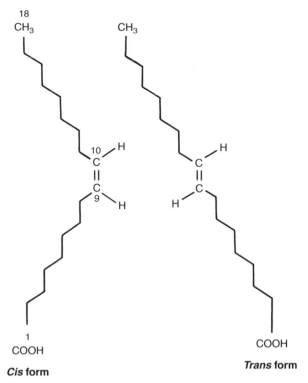

FIGURE 3-3 The *cis* and *trans* forms of a fatty acid.

nature, the fatty acid chain bends in such a way that both parts are on the same side of the bond. In this case the fatty acid is called a *cis* fatty acid, meaning "same side." The fatty acids occurring naturally in vegetable oils are in the *cis* form. But when oils are partially hydrogenated to produce more solid fats, the normal bend can change such that the two structural parts are on opposite sides of the bend. This form is called a *trans* fatty acid, meaning "opposite side." Commercially hydrogenated lipids used in soft margarine and other food products often contain *trans* fatty acids.

Trans fatty acids have been implicated in the development of both coronary artery disease and type 2 diabetes.[14,15] They decrease high-density lipoprotein (HDL) cholesterol levels and increase low-density lipoprotein (LDL) cholesterol levels. Even more importantly they disrupt essential fatty acid functions in cells.[6,16] It is estimated that *trans* fatty acids provide 4% to 7% of total kcalories in the United States diet.[9] *Trans* fatty acids are found in breads, cakes, cookies, crackers, margarine, and frozen potato products.[17] Oils used for frying at fast-food restaurants contain *trans* fats.[9] Beginning in 2006, food processors will be required to include *trans* fatty acid content on the Nutrition Label.[17]

Visible and Hidden Fat

Fat enters the diet in many different forms and foods. Fats are quite visible in butter, margarine, vegetable oils, salad dressing, bacon, and other added fats, which account for over 30% of the fat in the American diet.[18] But less obvious are the fats in milk (unless it is nonfat), egg yolk, cheese, nuts, seeds, and olives, often referred to as hidden fats. Other major sources of hidden fats are bakery items, including cake, cookies, crackers, and muffins, and frozen entrees such as baked lasagna (Box 3-4). Meat has both visible and hidden fat. Even when the visible fat has been trimmed away, the lean portion still contains hidden fat in the marbling—tiny fat deposits within the muscle tissue. This is especially true for beef. Pastries, desserts, candy, ice cream, chocolate, grain foods with added fat, and high-fat meats along with fats added to food during preparation or at the table account for almost 25% of the kcalorie intake of U.S. adults.[19] When evaluating the food and nutrient intake of various cultural and ethnic groups it is important to consider potential sources of hidden fat in recipes or fats added in food preparation (see the *Focus on Culture* box, "Developing a Food-Frequency Questionnaire for Use with Different Cultural or Ethnic Groups").

Acceptable Macronutrient Distribution Range

The Acceptable Macronutrient Distribution Range (AMDR) for fat is 20% to 35% of total kcalories.[6] This range allows an appropriate intake of the essential fatty acids along with fat-containing foods that are rich sources of other important nutrients, yet limits energy intake to avoid unwanted weight gain. The lower end of the range helps reduce the energy density of the diet, assisting in weight management for less active individuals or in weight loss. The upper intake level of 35% could promote weight gain in underweight individuals or ensure sufficient kcalories to support an active lifestyle or growth. Fat intakes falling below 10% of total energy intake may not supply the needed amounts of essential fatty acids. In future chapters we will continue to see how the AMDR is used in diet planning.

Appropriate Intakes of Fat and Carbohydrate

The AMDR for fat (20% to 35% of total kcalories) and the AMDR for carbohydrate (45% to 65% of total kcalories) set a balance between these two energy sources.[6] Several popular weight loss regimens severely limit

---

eicosanoids Long-chain fatty acids composed of 20 carbon atoms.

hydrogenation Process used to produce margarine and shortening from vegetable oil; when vegetable oils are exposed to hydrogen gas, hydrogen atoms are added at many of the double bonds of the polyunsaturated fatty acids, forming a solid fat.

BOX 3-4 | Visible and Hidden Fats

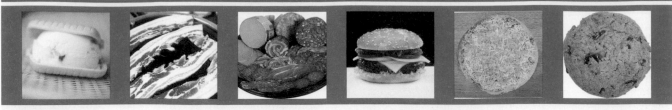

Visible-Fat Foods
   Butter
   Salad dressings
   Bacon
   Fat attached to meat

Hidden-Fat Foods
   Hamburger
   Peanuts
   Cheese
   Potato chips
   Chocolate chip cookie

Images copyright 2006 JupiterImages Corporation.

carbohydrate and replace carbohydrate with fat and protein to the extent that fat supplies 46% or more of total kcalories.[20] At the other extreme, if fat provides less than 20% of total kcalories, carbohydrate or protein intakes can rise disproportionately. Carbohydrate intake exceeding 65% of total kcalories can adversely affect blood triglyceride levels. The appropriate range for protein intake will be discussed in Chapter 4.

Health Promotion

Lowering Fat Intake

Despite public health campaigns urging Americans to limit their dietary fat as a way of lowering their total energy intake and risk of chronic disease, only small changes have occurred. Over the past decade fat intake as a proportion of total kcalories dropped approximately 1%, but obesity rates continue to go up.[21] In fact energy intake actually rose over this period, so the apparent drop in kcalories from fat is a result of the rise in kcalories from carbohydrate,[22] not a decrease in total fat. The popularity of fast-food restaurants adds to fat intake. On days that include a fast-food meal adults obtain 34.4% of their total kcalories from fat; on days when all meals are eaten at home or elsewhere fat supplies only 32.2% of total kcalories.[23]

There are various ways to lower dietary fat. Attempting to eliminate all foods high in fat not only reduces intakes of many important nutrients such as iron, zinc, vitamin E, and the essential fatty acids, but also is unlikely to be sustained over time. Alternatively, eating a mix of high-fat and modified-fat foods effectively lowers fat intake,[24,25] yet maintains appropriate levels of those nutrients found in higher-fat foods (Box 3-5). Including a higher-fat food at mealtime also adds to satiety and can help curb the urge to eat between meals. Limiting portion size is another effective way to reduce both fat and kcalories. Balancing the

BOX 3-5 | Ways to Lower Fat Intake

1. Reduce the fat you add.
   - Use less margarine on your toast.
   - Be stingy when adding salad dressing.
2. Reduce the portion size.
   - Order the smallest portion rather than the "supersize" portion of french fries.
3. Reduce the frequency of use.
   - Have ice cream as a snack only once or twice a week; choose fresh fruit on other days.
4. Choose a lower-fat version of a food.
   - Use low-fat milk or skim milk in place of whole milk.
   - Choose a broiled chicken breast with no skin rather than a fried chicken leg with skin.
   - Trim all visible fat from meats.
5. Substitute modified foods lower in fat.
   - Look for reduced-fat mayonnaise and reduced-fat or nonfat salad dressings.
6. Eliminate fat when preparing foods.
   - Eat raw carrots without salad dressing.
   - Season cooked vegetables with lemon juice, orange juice, or beef broth rather than margarine or butter.

diet with a variety of both higher-fat and lower-fat foods is the best strategy for overall good health.

Fat Replacers

Fats have many different functions in food recipes and food preparation. In cooking and baking fats (1) absorb flavors from various ingredients and help to blend them throughout the food; (2) assist in heat transfer necessary for browning or crispiness; and (3) create a velvety mouth feel in foods such as ice cream, pudding, and cheese.[26] Fat replacers are ingredients that can fulfill these functions but are lower in kcalories than fat. Fruit purees made from

✦ FOCUS ON CULTURE

Developing a Food Frequency Questionnaire for Use With Different Cultural or Ethnic Groups

Using a Food Frequency Questionnaire

Persons coming to the United States from other countries can be at high risk for cardiovascular disease based on changes that occur in their food patterns. Both body weight gain and increases in dietary fat contribute to chronic disease risk among all race and ethnic groups. Food frequency questionnaires (FFQs) are one way of finding out what people eat and provide a tool to evaluate an individual's diet and follow up with any nutritional advice that may be needed. An FFQ contains a list of common foods from all the major food groups, and persons are asked to respond how often they eat each food. There is also an effort to obtain some indication of the portion size that is usually eaten. The FFQ can be completed in writing or administered by an interviewer. There are special considerations when collecting dietary information from individuals who may not speak or read English. It will be necessary to translate the FFQ into their language or hire an interviewer who is not only fluent in their language but also familiar with their dietary patterns.

Developing a Food Frequency Questionnaire

To obtain an accurate response from individuals regarding their food intake, it is necessary to provide them with a list of foods they commonly eat. The daily food pattern of an East Indian or Chinese or Latino family that recently emigrated to the United States will include many different foods than are found in the typical U.S. diet.

Several researchers who developed an FFQ for use with Southeast Asian families have provided us with a framework that can be applied to any ethnic or cultural group with which you may work.

Step 1

Talk with those who are doing the cooking about the types of foods that they prepare for their families. Collect recipes for specific dishes to be sure that you understood what grains, fruits, vegetables, meats, and fats are included in each dish. Foods such as certain vegetables may be consumed only as components of mixed dishes and not eaten separately.[1] Check to see what ingredients may be available in local shops and what substitutions the homemakers may need to make when preparing their native dishes.

Step 2

Group foods together according to their nutrient content (e.g., putting grain foods, protein foods, or calcium-containing foods together).

Step 3

Assign the food name that is familiar to your target group. For example, families from Southeast Asia may recognize broccoli by the name Chinese broccoli, or Kai lan or Fai lan.[2]

Step 4

Compile a database that includes the specific nutrient content of each food item that will appear on your FFQ. Many foods will likely be available from the USDA Nutrient Data Base for Standard Reference used to calculate the nutrient content of diet records obtained in U.S. surveys. Using these food values, calculate the nutrient content of mixed food dishes that are common to your group.

Special Problems With Fats

Based on the high energy density of fat and its relationship to cardiovascular disease, it is important that we obtain good estimates of the types and amounts of fat eaten regularly. Hidden fats in foods and fats used in cooking are especially important. Food preparation methods strongly influence fat intake across national groups and require particular attention. Food researchers found that Southeast Asian families obtained about 40% of their kcalories from fat, with much of it coming from oil-based curry sauces, although Chinese families took in only 34% of their total kcalories as fat—yet both added about the same amounts of oil to their stir-fried foods.[2] When the researchers looked at the actual foods being prepared, they found their answer. For the stir-fried foods much of the fat remained in the pan when the food was served; with the thick curry sauces, most of the sauce was eaten along with the other ingredients. It may be helpful to visit a family at mealtime to fully appreciate their food intake patterns.

As groups become more health conscious, it may be necessary to include on a food intake questionnaire food items being marketed for their specific nutrient content. Health professionals developing an FFQ questionnaire for African American women who were trying to lower their intakes of fat included not only traditional foods but also the low-fat and modified-fat foods popular with individuals trying to reduce fat intake.[3]

Food intake questionnaires must be individualized for different race, ethnic, or cultural groups. Think about your own cultural or ethnic group. If you were to develop a food frequency questionnaire to determine the food intake of individuals in the group, what foods should you include?

References

1. Tseng M, Hernandez T: Comparison of intakes of U.S. Chinese women based on food frequency and 24-hour recall data, *J Am Diet Assoc* 105:1145, 2005.
2. Kelemen LE et al: Development and evaluation of cultural food frequency questionnaires for South Asians, Chinese, and Europeans in North America, *J Am Diet Assoc* 103:1178, 2003.
3. Schlundt DG, Hargreaves MK, Buchowski MS: The Eating Behavior Patterns Questionnaire predicts dietary fat intake in African American women, *J Am Diet Assoc* 103:338, 2003.

apples or prunes are used as fat replacers in cookies and moist cakes. Food technologists have developed other fat replacers for use in processed foods. In the United States, 79% of consumers buy foods containing fat replacers.[26]

Most fat replacers are carbohydrates—plant polysaccharides, celluloses, or gums—although protein and fat provide the structure for some products. Fat replacers act as thickeners and emulsifiers and provide the mouth feel associated with fat. Because they are poorly digested or absorbed, most add fewer kcalories than would fat (Table 3-1). One concern is their safety when used over long periods of time. Although studies reviewed by the U.S. Food and

TABLE 3-1	Fat Replacers in Common Food Products			
Type	**Ingredients**	**Energy Value**	**Trade Names**	**Applications**
Carbohydrate	Cellulose, pectin, gums, starches, dextrins, polydextrose, fruit-based fiber (dried plum or prune paste)	Typically provide only 1-2 kcal/g; cellulose or pectin provides 0 kcal/g	Just Fiber, WonderSlim, Betatrim, Maltrin, Splendid, Litesse	Frozen desserts, salad dressings, baked goods, dry mixes, dairy type of products, snack foods, cereal products, candy
Protein	Modified whey protein, milk and egg protein blends, micro-protein particles, protein-starch mixtures	1 kcal/g to 4 kcal/g (often usable in amounts less than fat; 1 g of such a protein-based substance can replace 3 g of fat in cream)	Simplesse, Dairy-Lo	Fat-free ice cream, frozen desserts; reduced-fat butter, sour cream, and cheese; baked products; salad dressing; coffee creamers
Fat	Sucrose polyesters bonded with long-chain fatty acids; emulsifiers; triglycerides with short-chain fatty acids	0 kcal/g to 9 kcal/g (those providing 9 kcal/g can often be used in smaller amounts than fat)	Benefat (salatrim) provides 9 kcal/g Olean (olestra) provides 0 kcal/g	Cake mixes, icing, vegetables, dairy products, fried snack foods

Data from American Dietetic Association: Position of the American Dietetic Association: fat replacers, *J Am Diet Assoc* 105:266, 2005.

Drug Administration indicate that fat replacers do not pose health risks for adults, little is known about the long-term effects of their use in children. Olestra interferes with the absorption of the fat-soluble vitamins, so olestra-containing food products have added amounts of vitamins A, D, E, and K to compensate for what may be lost.[27] Fat replacers that are not digested and remain in the stomach longer may add to satiety[28] and assist in appetite control.

Unfortunately, the general public assumes that baked goods, frozen desserts, and salad dressings made with fat replacers are lower in kcalories than those made with fat—and this is not always true. In fact a food that is made with a fat replacer and is lower in fat may contain the same number of kcalories or even more kcalories than its higher-fat counterpart if more sugar has been added to maintain flavor and mouth feel. People may assume they can eat a larger portion of a lower-fat item made with a fat replacer and be taking in even more kcalories than if they chose a smaller portion of the higher-fat food. It would be to a consumer's benefit to select less-processed desserts or snacks—fruits, whole grains, or low-fat dairy items—that are not only lower in fat but also rich in nutrients.

LIPID-RELATED COMPOUNDS

Cholesterol

Structure

Cholesterol is usually discussed in connection with dietary lipids; however, it is not a fat or a triglyceride. Rather, it belongs to a family of substances called steroids and travels in the blood attached to long-chain fatty acids. These cholesterol transport compounds are cholesterol esters. Many people confuse cholesterol with saturated fat because both substances are believed to promote atherosclerosis.

Functions

Cholesterol is required for normal body function[29] and can be synthesized in the liver. If a person obtained no cholesterol whatsoever from food, the body would still have an adequate supply. Cholesterol plays the following broad roles in body structure and function:

- *Precursor to steroid hormones:* A cholesterol compound in the skin, *7-dehydrocholesterol,* is converted to vitamin D when the ultraviolet rays of the sun pass into the skin; cholesterol is also a precursor of estrogen and testosterone.
- *Formation of bile acids:* Cholesterol is used to form bile acids, which emulsify fats and facilitate their digestion; bile acids serve as carriers in fat absorption.
- *Component of brain and nerve tissue:* Cholesterol helps form the structure of the brain and nerves.
- *Component of cell membranes:* Cell membranes contain cholesterol.

A constant supply of cholesterol is required to perform these critical roles.

Food Sources

Cholesterol occurs naturally in animal foods but not plant foods. Egg yolk, meat, whole and low-fat milk, and cheese add cholesterol to the diet; liver and organ meats are particularly high in content. Animal fats (but *not* plant fats) are rich sources.

PERSPECTIVES IN PRACTICE
Plant Sterols: New Weapon for Lowering Blood Cholesterol Levels

Plant sterols, also known as *phytosterols,* are found in small amounts in vegetable oils and grains such as corn, rye, and wheat. The chemical structure of plant sterols is much like that of cholesterol, and, based on this similarity, plant sterols compete with cholesterol for absorption in the small intestine. For some time nutrition researchers speculated that plant sterols in the diet would lower the amount of cholesterol that would be absorbed and delivered to the liver. When less cholesterol is available, the liver produces fewer lipoproteins, and blood levels of low-density lipoprotein (LDL) cholesterol drop.[1] Unfortunately, plant sterols occur naturally in food in very small amounts—too small to make a difference in cholesterol absorption.

Recently, food technologists found ways to incorporate plant sterols into food products to help persons increase their dietary intake. Table fats and orange juice with added plant sterols are available in food stores and are examples of new functional foods. Adding 1.5 g to 3 g of plant sterols to the daily diet can lower blood LDL cholesterol levels by as much as 15%[1] and reduce the tendency of blood platelets to form unwanted blood clots.[2] The Food and Drug Administration has approved a health claim for sterol-containing foods, so the Nutrition Label may carry a statement indicating that regular use of the item along with a diet that is low in saturated fat and cholesterol may reduce the risk of heart disease.[3]

Although plant sterols may support heart health, we must help persons understand that these foods should replace the conventional item in their daily meal pattern and not add to to-

tal fat and kcalorie intake. An 8-oz serving of orange juice that provides 1 g of plant sterols also contains 110 kcal but meets the MyPyramid equivalent of one serving of fruit. Additional fruit servings, however, should be selected from whole fruits that will add fiber to the diet. Table spreads containing about 0.7 g of plant sterols per tablespoon (1 tbsp being the recommended serving size) add 70 kcal and 8 g of fat per serving. Products advertised as "light" spreads usually contain about 50 kcal/tbsp and 5 g of fat. Two tablespoons per day are needed to reach the suggested intake of plant sterols.

Sterol-containing foods appear to be safe for use over long periods of time.[4] (We will examine health claims on nutrition labels in greater detail in Chapter 9.)

References

1. Castro IA, Barroso LP, Sinnecker P: Functional foods for coronary heart disease risk reduction: a meta-analysis using a multivariate approach, *Am J Clin Nutr* 82:32, 2005.
2. Kozlowska-Wojciechowska M et al: Impact of margarine enriched with plant sterols on blood lipids, platelet function, and fibrinogen level in young men, *Metabolism* 52:1378, 2003.
3. Food and Drug Administration: *FDA talk paper: FDA authorizes new coronary heart disease health claim for plant sterol and plant stanol esters,* Rockville, Md, 2000 (September 5), U.S. Department of Health and Human Services. Retrieved October 2, 2005, from *www.fda.gov/bbs/topics/ANSWERS/ANS01033.html.*
4. Hendriks HFJ et al: Safety of long-term consumption of plant sterol esters-enriched spread, *Eur J Clin Nutr* 57:681, 2003.

Suggested Cholesterol Intake

Because the body can synthesize as much cholesterol as it needs, there is no Dietary Reference Intake.[6] Persons are encouraged to limit their intake, keeping in mind that eliminating cholesterol entirely would also eliminate meat, eggs, and some dairy products that contain vitamins and minerals important to health. The American Heart Association recommends that dietary cholesterol be held to 300 mg/day or less, an intake associated with appropriate blood cholesterol levels.[7] Through genetic selection the cholesterol content of eggs and meat has been lowered, reducing the cholesterol present in the food supply. Nevertheless, intake averages about 350 mg in men and 240 mg in women.[30] Eggs, beef, poultry, cheese, and milk add most to cholesterol intake.[18] Certain plant sterols interfere with the absorption of cholesterol and help lower blood cholesterol levels (see the *Perspectives in Practice* box, "Plant Sterols: New Weapon for Lowering Blood Cholesterol Levels").

Lipoproteins
Function

The liver serves as the body's clearing house for fatty acids and cholesterol whether obtained from the diet or produced or released from body tissues. When received

by the liver, fatty acids and cholesterol are (1) packaged into lipoproteins and (2) released into the circulation for transport to cells.[12]

Lipid Transport

Lipids are insoluble in water, a characteristic that poses a problem when they need to be carried to cells in a water-based circulatory system. The body solves this problem

cholesterol A fat-related compound; a sterol ($C_{27}H_{45}OH$) that is normally found in bile and is a principal constituent of gallstones. Cholesterol is synthesized by the liver and is a precursor of various steroid hormones, such as sex hormones and adrenal corticoids. It is found in animal tissues such as meat, egg yolk, and milk fat.

steroids Group name for lipid-based sterols including hormones, bile acids, and cholesterol.

ester A compound produced by the reaction between an acid and an alcohol with elimination of a molecule of water. This process is called esterification. A triglyceride is a glycerol ester, and cholesterol forms esters by combining with fatty acids, largely linoleic acid.

by producing lipoproteins, packages of lipids wrapped in water-soluble protein. Chemically, lipoproteins are really *complexes* (noncovalent structures) of lipids and lipidlike substances surrounded by protein. Special compounds called phospholipids have an important role in the structure of lipoproteins. Phospholipids are molecules in which one of the three fatty acids attached to a glycerol base is replaced with a phosphate (PO_4^{-3}) group. The phosphate end of these molecules is water soluble, and phospholipids on the surface of lipoproteins help make possible their transport in the blood. Phospholipids in cell membranes help lipid molecules move from the circulatory system into the cell.

Lipoproteins contain fatty acids, triglycerides, cholesterol, phospholipids, and traces of other materials such as fat-soluble vitamins and steroid hormones. The lipoproteins—together with their attached apolipoprotein—serve as the major vehicle for lipid transport in the blood.

TO PROBE FURTHER

HEALTH BENEFITS OF UNSATURATED FATTY ACIDS: WHAT'S IN A DOUBLE BOND?

Over the years we have learned that excessive amounts of saturated fatty acids are harmful to health. Saturated fatty acids raise blood low-density lipoprotein (LDL) cholesterol levels and the risk of heart disease and stroke.[1] This is why we recommend that saturated fats provide less than 10% of total energy intake.[2] On the other hand, monounsaturated fatty acids with one double bond and polyunsaturated fatty acids with two or more double bonds have very different effects on health. Unsaturated fatty acids in moderation may help prevent cardiovascular disease through their effects on blood cholesterol and blood clotting factors.

Monounsaturated Fatty Acids
Monounsaturated fatty acids are plentiful in olive oil, canola oil, nuts, and seeds. In fact olive oil is credited with some of the positive effects associated with the Mediterranean diet, a plant-based eating pattern rich in legumes and grains. Monounsaturated fatty acids bring about a slight decrease in LDL cholesterol levels and other blood fats while raising high-density lipoprotein (HDL) cholesterol levels. Monounsaturated fatty acids have this favorable effect on blood fats even when the diet contains as much as 34% fat, as long as one third or more is monounsaturated.

Polyunsaturated Fatty Acids
Polyunsaturated fatty acids contain at least two double bonds. They include the n-6 fatty acids and the n-3 fatty acids. The n-6 fatty acids include linoleic acid and arachidonic acid. These fatty acids help to regulate blood cholesterol levels and reduce the risk of cardiovascular disease. They do this by lowering blood LDL cholesterol levels through the following actions[3]:
- They lower the amounts of LDL cholesterol produced by the liver.
- They enhance the clearing of LDL cholesterol from the blood by promoting the movement of cholesterol into the cells.

It is important that we obtain appropriate amounts of these fats in our diets.

The n-3 fatty acids include alpha-linolenic acid and two fatty acids found in fish—eicosapentaenoic acid and docosahexaenoic acid. Flaxseed oil, canola oil, and oily fish are good sources of the n-3 fatty acids. Eicosapentaenoic acid and docosahexaenoic acid were first identified in the diets of Eskimos from Greenland who had low rates of heart disease despite their high intakes of fat from fish. We have since learned that these fatty acids have various effects in the body that lower the risk of heart disease, as follows:
- They lower the ability of blood platelets to form a clot; this reduces the risk of an unwanted clot in the coronary arteries or arteries of the brain.

- They lower blood fats; blood triglyceride levels are lower in persons who eat fish regularly.
- They dilate the major arteries; this lowers blood pressure and prevents cardiac arrhythmias. Men who eat at least one fish meal each week lower their risk of sudden cardiac death by more than half.[3]

Despite the positive health benefits of polyunsaturated fatty acids, there are risks if we consume too large an amount. Fatty acids containing double bonds can undergo oxidation reactions that change their structure and lead to destructive actions against other fatty acids and molecules with double bonds found in membranes and other tissues. Nutrition experts recommend that *polyunsaturated* fatty acids make up no more than 10% of total kcalories.[2] We also need to remember that no matter how beneficial certain fatty acids may be, our total intake of fat should stay within the Acceptable Macronutrient Distribution Range of 20% to 35% of total kcalories.[4]

The greatest improvement in blood cholesterol levels occurs when unsaturated fatty acids *replace* some of the saturated fat in the diet rather than being added to the total fat already being consumed.[5]

Fish Oil Supplements
With health experts encouraging the general public to increase their intakes of n-3 polyunsaturated fatty acids, companies have begun to sell fish oil supplements designed to meet our need for these nutrients. Fish oil isolated from the livers of ocean fish may harbor pollutants concentrated in that body organ, and at present dietary supplements are not tested for purity or content by the U.S. Food and Drug Administration. (We will learn more about this situation in Chapter 9.) It is always best to obtain your nutrients from real food that will supply a variety of important nutrients (see Box 3-3).

References

1. German JB, Dillard CJ: Saturated fats: What dietary intake? *Am J Clin Nutr* 80:550, 2004.
2. Wylie-Rosett J: Fat substitutes and health: an advisory from the Nutrition Committee of the American Heart Association, *Circulation* 105:2800, 2002.
3. Wijendran V, Hayes KC: Dietary n-6 and n-3 fatty acid balance and cardiovascular health, *Annu Rev Nutr* 24:597, 2004.
4. Food and Nutrition Board, Institute of Medicine: *Dietary Reference Intakes for energy, carbohydrate, fiber, fat, fatty acids, cholesterol, protein, and amino acids (macronutrients),* Washington, DC, 2002, National Academies Press.
5. Karmally W: Balancing unsaturated fatty acids: what's the evidence for cholesterol lowering? *J Am Diet Assoc* 105:1068, 2005.

Classes of Lipoproteins

Lipoproteins are classified according to their density. The density of a lipoprotein is determined by its relative content of lipid and protein. The higher the proportion of protein, the higher the density. The amount of each lipoprotein in the blood is influenced by time since the last meal and the quantity and type of fat that a person consumes on a regular basis. The following list contains a discussion of the five lipoprotein classes:

1. *Chylomicrons:* These relatively large particles are formed in the intestinal wall after a meal and carry the digested and absorbed fat to the liver for conversion to other lipoproteins.
2. *Very low-density lipoproteins (VLDLs):* The VLDLs are formed in the liver during the fasting interval between meals. When there is no food in the digestive tract and chylomicrons are not entering the circulatory system, VLDLs transport endogenous triglycerides from the liver to tissue cells.
3. *Intermediate-density lipoproteins (IDLs):* IDLs are formed from VLDLs and continue the delivery of endogenous triglycerides to the cells.
4. *Low-density lipoproteins (LDLs):* LDLs are formed from VLDLs and IDLs and carry primarily cholesterol, because most of the triglyceride has moved into the cells.
5. *High-density lipoproteins (HDLs):* HDLs return cholesterol from the cells to the liver for breakdown and elimination.

Cholesterol, Lipoproteins, and Cardiovascular Risk

All of the individual lipoproteins carry some cholesterol, but the two major carriers are the LDLs and the HDLs. Approximately half of the cholesterol circulating in the blood is contained in the LDLs,[31] so one's LDL level has important implications for health. Elevated blood cholesterol in the form of LDL cholesterol is related to *atherosclerosis,* the underlying pathologic condition in coronary heart disease. High LDL cholesterol levels cause a buildup of fatty plaque on the walls of the vessels supplying blood to the heart muscle. Over time these plaques narrow the lumen of the coronary arteries, decreasing the delivery of both oxygen and other nutrients to the cells of the heart. An interruption of the blood supply to the heart, as a result of a blood clot or built-up plaque, causes a heart attack, and a similar occurrence in an artery in the brain results in a stroke (cerebral hemorrhage). Elevated LDLs increase the risk of heart attack or stroke whereas higher HDLs slow or prevent the progression of atherosclerosis. HDLs gather up free cholesterol from the cells and return it to the liver for elimination. Individuals with higher levels of HDLs have lower cardiovascular risk.

Although it would seem that cholesterol intake would be the major influence on blood LDL cholesterol levels, it is not this simple. Some people absorb cholesterol to a greater extent than others or synthesize greater amounts regardless of dietary intake. Genetic factors affect the production of HDLs and the rate at which cholesterol is eliminated from the body.[31] LDL and HDL levels are influenced by the types and amounts of dietary fat. (See the *To Probe Further* box, "Health Benefits of Unsaturated Fatty Acids: What's in a Double Bond?," to learn more about these effects.) Chapter 20 will tell us about lifestyle interventions and medications that help individuals maintain appropriate blood lipoprotein levels.

DIGESTION-ABSORPTION-METABOLISM PREVIEW

We will discuss the digestion, absorption, and metabolism of the macronutrients in greater detail in Chapter 8, but a brief outline of fat digestion is also included here.

Digestion

The triglycerides that occur naturally in animal and plant foods must be broken down into individual fatty acids, the form the cells can burn for energy. This is accomplished through the process of digestion.

Mouth

There is no chemical breakdown of lipids in the mouth. Here the action is mechanical as lipids are broken up into smaller particles and moistened for passage into the stomach.

---

lipoprotein Noncovalent complexes of fat with protein. The lipoproteins function as major carriers of lipids in the plasma; this combination of fat surrounded by protein makes possible the transport of fatty substances in a water medium such as plasma.

phospholipid A class of fat-related substances that contain phosphorus, fatty acids, and a nitrogenous base. The phospholipids are important components of cell membranes, nerve tissues, and lipoproteins.

apolipoprotein A protein compound that attaches to a specific receptor site on a particular lipoprotein and activates certain functions, such as synthesis of a related enzyme. An example is apolipoprotein C II, an apolipoprotein of chylomicrons and very low-density (VLD) lipoproteins that activates the enzyme lipoprotein lipase, which helps move fats into the cell.

endogenous Originating from within the body; an example is endogenous cholesterol, which is produced by cells in the liver.

TABLE 3-2	Summary of Fat Digestion	
Organ	**Enzyme**	**Activity**
Mouth	None	Mechanical, mastication
Stomach	No major enzyme	Mechanical separation of fats as protein and starch are digested out
	Small amount of gastric lipase (tributyrinase)	Butterfat (tributyrin) to fatty acids and glycerol
Small intestine	Gallbladder bile salts (emulsifier)	Emulsifies fats
	Pancreatic lipase	Triglycerides to diglycerides and monoglycerides in turn, then fatty acids and glycerol

Stomach

Little chemical digestion of lipids occurs in the stomach. The only enzyme in the gastric secretions specific to lipids is gastric lipase (tributyrinase), which acts on emulsified butterfat. General peristalsis continues the mechanical mixing of lipids with the stomach contents. As gastric enzymes act on the carbohydrates and proteins in the food mix, the lipids begin to separate out, making them more accessible to their own enzymes upon entering the small intestine.

Small Intestine

The chemical changes necessary for lipid digestion begin in the small intestine. Digestive secretions for lipid breakdown come from three sources: (1) the biliary tract, (2) the pancreas, and (3) the small intestine, as follows:

1. *Bile from the liver and gallbladder:* The presence of lipids in the duodenum (the upper section of the small intestine) stimulates the secretion of cholecystokinin (CCK), a local hormone produced by glands in the intestinal wall. In turn cholecystokinin initiates the contraction of the gallbladder, the relaxation of the sphincter muscle, and the flow of bile into the small intestine via the common bile duct. The liver produces a large amount of dilute bile, and the gallbladder concentrates and stores it, ready for use as needed. Bile acts as an emulsifier. Although *emulsification* does not in itself bring about a chemical change, it prepares lipids for further digestion by (1) breaking them into smaller particles or globules to enlarge the surface area accessible for action by digestive enzymes and (2) lowering the surface tension of the finely dispersed and suspended lipid globules, enabling enzymes to penetrate more easily. This process is similar to the wetting action of detergents.

   Bile also provides the alkaline medium needed for the action of pancreatic lipase. When bile secretion is low, as in gallbladder disease, fat is not digested and absorbed efficiently and as much as 40% of dietary fat is lost in the feces.[12]

2. *Enzymes from the pancreas:* Pancreatic juice contains one enzyme that acts on lipids and one that acts on cholesterol. *Pancreatic lipase,* the lipid enzyme, breaks off one fatty acid at a time from the glycerol base of triglycerides. The initial action on a triglyceride yields one fatty acid plus a diglyceride, and continuing action yields another fatty acid plus a monoglyceride. Each successive step in this breakdown becomes more difficult. In fact separation of the final fatty acid from the remaining monoglyceride is such a slow process that less than one third of the total fat in the food mass breaks down completely. The final products of lipid digestion ready to be absorbed are fatty acids, diglycerides, monoglycerides, and glycerol. Some remaining lipids pass into the large intestine for elimination in the feces.

   The pancreas also secretes the enzyme *cholesterol esterase.* In preparation for absorption this enzyme forms cholesterol esters by combining free cholesterol and fatty acids

3. *Enzyme from the small intestine:* The small intestine secretes an enzyme in the intestinal juice called *lecithinase.* As its name indicates it acts on lecithin, a *phospholipid,* to break it down into its components for absorption.

Table 3-2 summarizes lipid digestion.

Absorption

Lipid absorption is complicated. Because lipids are not soluble in water and blood is basically water, lipids always require some type of carrier. The task of transporting lipids from the small intestine into the bloodstream takes place in three stages.

Stage I: Initial Lipid Absorption

In the small intestine bile salts combine with the products of lipid digestion to form a micellar bile-lipid complex. This unique carrier system described in Figure 3-4 moves the lipid molecules from the lumen of the intestine into the intestinal wall.

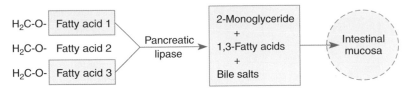

FIGURE 3-4 Micellar complex of fats with bile salts for transport of fats into the intestinal mucosa. The fatty acid in the 2 position of the triglyceride is the most difficult to remove, and some fat is absorbed in the monoglyceride form.

Stage II: Absorption Within the Intestinal Wall

Once inside the wall of the small intestine the bile salts separate from the lipid complex, are absorbed, and return to the liver via the *enterohepatic circulation,* ready to carry out their task again. As the lipid products are released from the micellar-complex, the following two important actions take place:

1. *Enteric lipase digestion:* A lipase within the intestinal wall completes the digestion of any remaining diglycerides and monoglycerides, releasing fatty acids and glycerol.
2. *Triglyceride synthesis:* The available fatty acids and glycerol form new human triglycerides, ready for final absorption and transport.

Stage III: Final Absorption and Transport

The newly formed human triglycerides—along with any other lipid materials present—are given a protein covering to form the lipoproteins called chylomicrons. These lipid packages, in a milklike liquid called *chyle,* cross the cell membrane into the lymphatic system and then drain into the portal blood. Here a final lipid-clearing enzyme, *lipoprotein lipase,* helps remove the large meal load of lipids from the blood. In the liver the lipids are converted into new lipoproteins for transport to body cells. Figure 3-5 illustrates lipid absorption through its three stages.

Metabolism

Fatty acids are a concentrated source of fuel for body cells having more than twice the energy value of glucose. As we will see in Chapter 8, the metabolism of lipids is closely interrelated with the metabolism of carbohydrate and protein.

TO SUM UP

Lipids are the most energy dense of all the energy-producing nutrients. Lipids provide insulation to assist in temperature regulation, protect vital organs from damage, and contribute flavor and texture to foods. They also have a part in the transmission of nerve impulses, production of steroid hormones, formation of cell membranes, and transport of the fat-soluble vitamins. The building blocks of lipids are fatty acids. Fatty acids are classified on the basis of

chain length and degree of saturation. Two polyunsaturated fatty acids—(1) linoleic acid, an n-6 acid, and (2) alpha-linolenic acid, an n-3 acid—cannot be made by humans and must be supplied in food. These essential fatty acids are important for skin integrity, growth (especially the development of brain and neural tissue), control of blood cholesterol levels, and immune function. Several n-3 fatty acids found in fish control platelet aggregation and reduce the risk of heart attack and stroke. Both the type and amount of lipids in the diet affect health. Inappropriately high intakes of fat, especially saturated fat, increase cardiovascular risk. The Acceptable Macronutrient Distribution Range for fat is 20% to 35% of total kcalories. When lipids provide less than 10% of total kcalories, supplies of linoleic and alpha-linolenic acids may not be adequate to meet body needs.

---

lipase Group of fat enzymes that cut the ester linkages between the fatty acids and glycerol in triglycerides (fats).

cholecystokinin (CCK) A peptide hormone secreted by the duodenal mucosa when fat is present. Cholecystokinin causes the gallbladder to contract and propel bile into the duodenum, where it is needed to emulsify the fat and prepare it for digestion and absorption.

bile A fluid secreted by the liver and transported to the gallbladder for concentration and storage. It is released into the duodenum on entry of fat and acts as an emulsifier to facilitate enzymatic fat digestion.

emulsifier An agent that breaks down large fat globules to smaller, uniformly distributed particles. This action is accomplished in the intestine by bile acids, which lower the surface tension of the fat particles. Emulsification increases the surface area of fat, facilitating contact with digestive enzymes.

micellar bile-lipid complex A combination of bile and fat that carries fat into the wall of the small intestine in preparation for the final stage of absorption into the circulation.

chylomicrons Lipoproteins formed in the intestinal wall after a meal that carry food fats into the lymph and then the general circulation for transport to body cells.

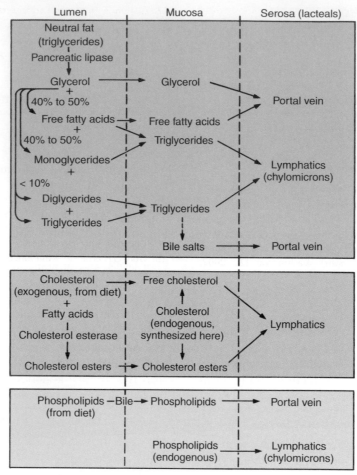

FIGURE 3-5   Absorption of fat, cholesterol, and phospholipids.

QUESTIONS FOR REVIEW

1. What is a lipid? Name several members of this nutrient class.
2. Compare saturated, monounsaturated, and polyunsaturated fatty acids based on their (a) chemical structure, (b) effects on health, and (c) usual food sources.
3. List several roles of the prostaglandins.
4. Name the two essential fatty acids. Why are they called essential? What happens when they are not available in the amounts needed? What foods will supply the essential fatty acids?
5. You are counseling a patient who has been told that he should lose 10 to 15 lb. His usual fat intake is about 35% of his total energy intake. He has agreed to lower his intake of fat to 30% in an effort to reduce his daily kcalories. What are some strategies that might help him lower his dietary fat? He and his co-workers eat their lunch at fast-food restaurants. Develop three lunch menus that include fast food but limit fat and kcalories.
6. Two persons with strong family histories of cardiovascular disease are concerned about their heart health. Both lower their cholesterol intake and avoid butter. One person started to use a stick margarine made from corn oil and the other a soft tub corn oil margarine. Which person made the better choice? Why?
7. A woman runner has decided to remove all fat from her diet. If she is successful in doing this, what health problems might she encounter?
8. Go to the grocery store and identify five crackers or cookies that offer both a regular and a "reduced-fat" version. Using the Nutrition Label, make a chart indicating the (a) serving size, (b) total kcalories per serving, (c) grams of total fat per serving, (d) grams of saturated fat per serving, (e) grams of unsaturated fat per serving, (f) grams of *trans* fat per serving, (g) grams of sugar per serving, and (h) cost per serving. What nutritional differences did you observe between the regular and reduced-fat versions? Was there a difference in price, and, if so, was the reduced-fat version worth the difference in terms of nutritional benefit? How do the regular and reduced-fat versions compare in serving size, kalories, fat, and sugar?

REFERENCES

1. Moskowitz H, Beckley J, Adams J: What makes people crave fast foods? *Nutr Today* 37:237, 2002.
2. American Dietetic Association: Position of the American Dietetic Association: total diet approach to communicating food and nutrition information, *J Am Diet Assoc* 102(1):100, 2002.
3. Rolls ET: Smell, taste, texture, and temperature multimodal representations in the brain, and their relevance to the control of appetite, *Nutr Rev* 62(11, part 2):S193, 2004.
4. Wahrburg U: What are the health effects of fat?, *Eur J Nutr* 43(March-suppl 1):I/6, 2004.
5. Hu FB, Manson JAE, Willett WC: Types of dietary fat and risk of coronary heart disease: a critical review, *J Am Coll Nutr* 20(1):5, 2001.
6. Food and Nutrition Board, Institute of Medicine: *Dietary Reference Intakes for energy, carbohydrate, fiber, fat, fatty acids, cholesterol, protein, and amino acids (macronutrients),* Washington, DC, 2002, National Academies Press.
7. Krauss RM et al: Revision 2000: a statement for healthcare professionals from the Nutrition Committee of the American Heart Association, *J Nutr* 131:132, 2001.
8. Herder R, Demmig-Adams B: The power of a balanced diet and lifestyle in preventing cardiovascular disease, *Nutr Clin Care* 7:46, 2004.
9. Elias SL, Innis SM: Bakery foods are the major dietary source of trans-fatty acids among pregnant women with diets providing 30% energy from fat, *J Am Diet Assoc* 102(1):46, 2002.
10. Jones PJH, Kubow S: Lipids, sterols, and their metabolites. In Shils ME et al, eds: *Modern nutrition in health and disease,* ed 10, Baltimore, 2006, Lippincott, Williams & Wilkins.
11. Sampath H, Ntambi JM: Polyunsaturated fatty acid regulation of gene expression, *Nutr Rev* 62(9):333, 2004.
12. Guyton AC, Hall JE: *Textbook of medical physiology,* ed 10, Philadelphia, 2000, WB Saunders.
13. Heird WC, Lapillonne A: The role of essential fatty acids in development, *Annu Rev Nutr* 25:549, 2005.
14. Mozaffarian D et al: Dietary intake of trans fatty acids and systemic inflammation in women, *Am J Clin Nutr* 79:606, 2004.
15. Clifton PM, Keogh JB, Noakes M: Trans fatty acids in adipose tissue and the food supply are associated with myocardial infarction, *J Nutr* 134:874, 2004.
16. Stachowska E et al: Dietary trans fatty acids and composition of human atheromatous plaques, *Eur J Nutr* 43:313, 2004.
17. Satchithanandam S et al: Trans, saturated, and unsaturated fat in foods in the United States prior to mandatory trans-fat labeling, *Lipids* 39:11, 2004.
18. Cotton PA et al: Dietary sources of nutrients among U.S. adults, *J Am Diet Assoc* 104:921, 2004.
19. Food Surveys Research Group, Beltsville Human Nutrition Research Center, Agricultural Research Service: *Data tables: food and nutrient intakes by individuals in the United States, by Race, 1994-1996,* Washington, DC, 1998, U.S. Department of Agriculture. Retrieved October 9, 2005, from *www.ars.usda.gov/SP2UserFiles/Place/12355000/pdf/Race.PDF.*
20. Kennedy ET et al: Popular diets: correlation to health, nutrition, and obesity, *J Am Diet Assoc* 101(4):411, 2001.
21. U.S. Centers for Disease Control and Prevention: Trends in intake of energy and macronutrients—United States, 1971-2000, *Morb Mortal Wkly Rep* 53(04):80, Feb 6, 2004.
22. Chanmugam P et al: Did fat intake in the United States really decline between 1989-1991 and 1994-1996? *J Am Diet Assoc* 103:867, 2003.
23. Paeratakul S et al: Fast-food consumption among U.S. adults and children: dietary and nutrient intake profile, *J Am Diet Assoc* 103:1332, 2003.
24. Sigman Grant M, Warland R, Hsieh G: Selected lower-fat foods positively impact nutrient quality in diets of free-living Americans, *J Am Diet Assoc* 103:570, 2003.
25. Patterson RE et al: Changes in food sources of dietary fat in response to an intensive low-fat dietary intervention: early results from the Women's Health Initiative, *J Am Diet Assoc* 103:454, 2003.
26. American Dietetic Association: Position of the American Dietetic Association: fat replacers, *J Am Diet Assoc* 105:266, 2005.
27. Food and Drug Administration: Olestra labeling change, *FDA Consumer,* Nov-Dec 2003.
28. Bray GA et al: A 9-mo randomized clinical trial comparing fat-substituted and fat-reduced diets in healthy obese men: the Ole Study, *Am J Clin Nutr* 76:928, 2002.
29. U.S. National Heart, Lung and Blood Institute: High blood cholesterol, *Nutr Clin Care* 6:108, 2003.
30. Ervin RB et al: *Dietary intake of fats and fatty acids for the United States population: 1999-2000, Advance data, No 348,* Washington, DC, 2004 (November 8), U.S. Dept of Health and Human Services.
31. Grundy SM: Nutrition in the management of disorders of serum lipids and lipoproteins. In Shils ME et al, eds: *Modern nutrition in health and disease,* ed 10, Baltimore, 2006, Lippincott, Williams & Wilkins.

FURTHER READINGS AND RESOURCES

Readings

Cheng C, Graziani C, Diamond JJ: Cholesterol-lowering effect of the Food for Heart Nutrition Education Program, *J Am Diet Assoc* 104:1068, 2004.

Fitzgerald CM et al: Effect of a promotional campaign on heart-healthy menu choices in community restaurants, *J Am Diet Assoc* 104:429, 2004.
These two articles provide examples of community intervention programs to build awareness and provide nutrition education to help persons lower their dietary fat. It is important that local restaurants offer healthy choices to support individuals trying to make dietary changes.

Kelley C et al: Dietary intake of children at high risk for cardiovascular disease, *J Am Diet Assoc* 104:222, 2004.
This article focuses on the cultural aspects of fat intake and the need to work with families as we develop diet intervention programs.

Fulkerson JA, French SA, Story M: Adolescents' attitudes about and consumption of low-fat foods: associations with sex and weight control behaviors, *J Am Diet Assoc* 104:233, 2004.
Body image is very important to adolescents. Dr. Fulkerson and her colleagues help us understand factors that influence food choices and practices in this age group.

Websites of Interest

- National Cancer Institute, National Institutes of Health, *The color guide;* this site offers educational materials that assist with low-fat eating: *http://app1-ws1b-2.nci.nih.gov/color/.*

- National Heart, Lung, and Blood Institute, National Institutes of Health, Information for . . . Patients and the Public, Heart and Vascular Diseases; this government agency provides information on interventions for lowering blood cholesterol levels: *www.nhlbi. nih.gov/health/public/heart/index.htm#chol.*

- National Heart, Lung, and Blood Institute, National Institutes of Health, The Antihypertensive and Lipid-Lowering Treatment to Prevent Heart Attack Trial (ALLHAT); this current clinical study is evaluating the benefits of lifestyle changes on cardiovascular risk: *www.nhlbi.nih.gov/health/allhat/index.htm.*

CHAPTER 4

Proteins

Eleanor D. Schlenker

This chapter describing protein completes our sequence on the macronutrients. Protein is quite different from its partners, carbohydrate and fat. First, it is the body's major source of nitrogen, the essential element of all living things. Second, its main task is forming body tissues using its individual building units, the amino acids.

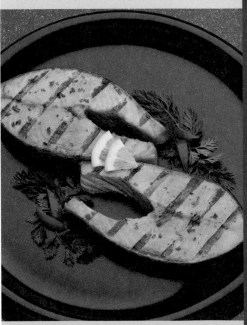

PHYSICAL AND CHEMICAL NATURE OF PROTEINS

General Definition

In 1838 when Dutch chemist Johann Mulder first identified protein as a prime substance in all life forms, it is unlikely he realized how far-reaching his work would become. Proteins are associated with all living things, and the effort to determine how life began has centered on how proteins were first produced.[1]

Proteins shape our lives. They act as structural units to build our bodies. Protein enzymes break down our food into nutrients the cells can use. As antibodies they shield us from disease. Peptide hormones carry messages that coordinate continuous body activity. And proteins do much more: they guide our growth in childhood and maintain our bodies throughout adulthood. They make us the unique individuals that we are.

Chemical Nature

The proteins we eat do none of this work as proteins. Rather, their structural units—the amino acids—are the working currency in body cells. Amino acids are composed of the elements carbon, hydrogen, oxygen, and nitrogen—the special element of all living matter. Several amino acids also contain sulfur.

THE NATURE OF AMINO ACIDS

Amino acids carry out the life-sustaining task of building and rebuilding body tissues. The name amino acid tells us they have a dual nature. The word *amino* refers to a base or alkaline substance, so at once we have a contradiction. How can a chemical substance be both a base and an acid, and why is this important? Consider the significance of this fact as we examine the structure of amino acids.

General Pattern and Structure

A common structural pattern holds for all amino acids. This pattern is built around a central alpha-carbon with several attached chemical groups (Figure 4-1), as described below:

- *Amino (base, NH_2) group:* The amino group contains the essential nitrogen and as an ion carries a positive charge.

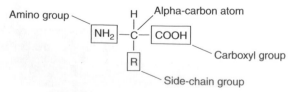

FIGURE 4-1 Basic structure of an amino acid.

- *Carboxyl (acid, COOH) group:* The carboxyl (COOH) group is a characteristic of all acids and as an ion carries a negative charge.

- *An attached radical (R) group:* The R stands for *radical,* a general term referring to a group of elements attached to a chemical compound. In this case it refers to the attached side chains on amino acids, each one different. The distinctive side chain on an amino acid gives it a unique size, shape, and set of properties.[2] Note the structure of the two simplest amino acids, glycine and alanine, based on the core amino acid pattern (Figure 4-2). Now compare the larger and more complex amino acid arginine (Figure 4-3) with its extended carbon chain (R) and three additional amino groups.

Amino acids contain the same three elements—carbon, hydrogen, and oxygen—that make up carbohydrates and fats. But amino acids and their proteins have an important additional element—nitrogen—as the base (alkaline [NH_2]) portion of their structure. Twenty amino acids are used to build body proteins.[3] They all have the same core pattern, but each has a specific and different side group attached.

The dual chemical structure of amino acids combining both acid (carboxyl [COOH]) and base (amino [NH_2]) groups gives them a unique amphoteric nature. This means that an amino acid can behave as either an acid or a base depending on the pH of the solution in which it is found, and can act as a buffer, important in clinical care.

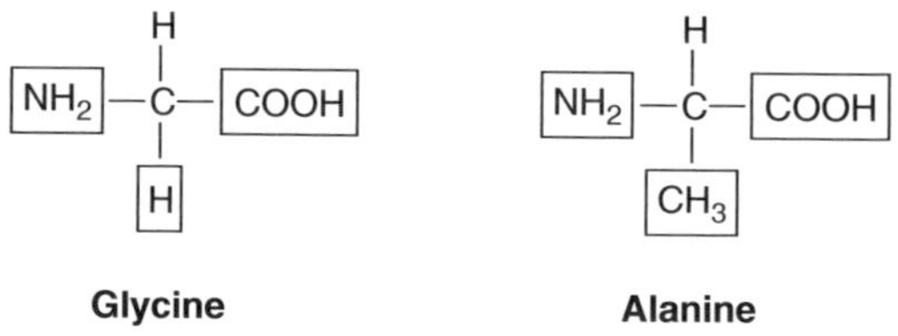

FIGURE 4-2 Structure of glycine and alanine.

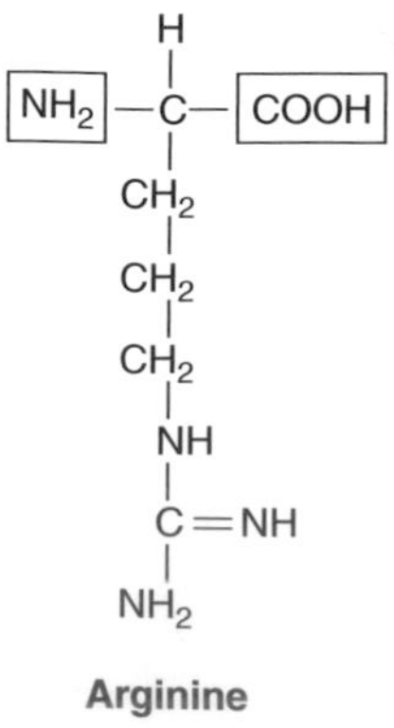

Glycine

Alanine

Arginine

FIGURE 4-3 Structure of arginine.

Essential Amino Acids

Of the 20 amino acids used to build body proteins, 9 cannot be synthesized by the body and must be supplied in food. These 9 amino acids are designated as *indispensable (essential) amino acids*. Another five of the 20 can be synthesized by the body in adequate amounts and are termed *dispensable (nonessential) amino acids*. Another 6 fall in between and are known as *conditionally indispensable* amino acids (Box 4-1).[3] Although the body is able to synthesize these amino acids, it cannot meet the demand when tissue needs are elevated or the supply of necessary precursors is inadequate. Arginine is such an amino acid. The amount that can be produced in the liver is not sufficient to meet the needs of the newborn.

At one time amino acids were classified as essential and nonessential, and you may see these terms being used. Nutrition experts recommended that we stop using those designations because the term *nonessential* implies that those amino acids are not really necessary for human health.[3] Nevertheless, the concept of *dietary essentiality* for the indispensable and conditionally indispensable amino acids is important when assessing protein quality.

THE BUILDING OF PROTEINS

The ability of amino acids to form peptide linkages and arrange themselves into peptide chains is basic to all body tissues.

Tissue Protein Structure

Peptide Bond

The dual chemical nature of amino acids—the presence of a base (amino [NH₂]) group on one end and an acid (carboxyl [COOH]) group on the other—enables them to form the unique chain structure found in all proteins. The end amino group of one amino acid joins with the end carboxyl group of the amino acid beside it. This joining of amino acids is called a *peptide bond*. Specific amino acids are joined in a particular sequence to form long chains of amino acids called *polypeptides,* and specific polypeptides come together to form proteins. Polypeptides vary in length from relatively short chains of 3 to 15 amino acids called *oligopeptides* to medium-sized polypeptides with chains of 21 to 30 amino acids such as insulin. Larger still are complex proteins made up of several hundred amino acids.

Large-Complex Proteins

New technology is helping us learn how protein chains fold and twist in space and interact with other body molecules. To build a compact structure, long polypeptide chains coil or fold back on themselves in a spiral shape

---

BOX 4-1 | Categories of Amino Acids

Indispensable (Essential)
Histidine
Isoleucine
Leucine
Lysine
Methionine
Phenylalanine
Threonine
Tryptophan
Valine

Conditionally Indispensable (Essential)
Arginine
Cysteine
Glutamine
Glycine
Proline
Tyrosine

Dispensable (Nonessential)
Alanine
Aspartic acid
Asparagine
Glutamic acid
Serine

Data from Food and Nutrition Board, Institute of Medicine: *Dietary Reference Intakes for energy, carbohydrate, fiber, fat, fatty acids, cholesterol, protein, and amino acids (macronutrients),* Washington, DC, 2002, National Academies Press.

---

amino acid An acid containing the essential element nitrogen (in the amino group—NH₂). Amino acids are the structural units of protein and the basic building blocks of the body.

carboxyl (COOH) group The monovalent radical, COOH, found in organic acids.

amphoteric Having opposite characteristics; capable of acting either as an acid or a base or combining with an acid or a base.

buffer Mixture of acid and alkaline components that when added to a solution is able to protect it against large changes in pH, even when strong acids and bases are added. If an acid is added, the alkaline partner reacts to counteract the acidic effect. If a base is added, the acid partner reacts to counteract the alkalizing effect. A solution to which a buffer has been added is called a buffered solution. This process keeps important body fluids at the pH levels required for life.

indispensable (essential) amino acid An amino acid that the body cannot synthesize or cannot synthesize in sufficient amounts to meet body needs so must be supplied by the diet. The nine indispensable amino acids are histidine, isoleucine, leucine, lysine, methionine, phenylalanine, threonine, tryptophan, and valine. Six amino acids are conditionally indispensable because the body cannot synthesize sufficient amounts under certain conditions.

peptide bond The characteristic joining of amino acids to form proteins. Such a chain of amino acids is termed a peptide. Depending on the number of amino acid units, it may be a dipeptide or a large polypeptide.

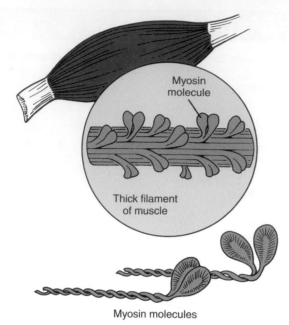

FIGURE 4-4   Myosin is a globulin in muscle that in combination with actin forms actomyosin, the fundamental contractile unit of muscle active with ATP.

called a helix. Other proteins form a pleated sheet held together by strengthening cross-links of sulfur and hydrogen bonds. Learning more about the structure of body proteins helps medical researchers develop effective medications and gain an understanding of how our genes influence disease risk.

Types of Proteins

Proteins are a widely diverse group of compounds. They have important roles in body structure and metabolism made possible by their specific content and placement of amino acids. Consider several examples detailed in the following sections.

Myosin

This fibrous protein found in muscle fiber (Figure 4-4) is built from chains of 153 amino acids that coil and unfold as the muscle contracts and relaxes. Shaped into long rods, these fibers end in two-headed bundles so they can change their shape and bend, making it possible to tighten and contract muscles and then relax them.

Collagen

This structural protein contains three separate polypeptide chains that wind around each other to produce a triple helix (Figure 4-5). Thus reinforced, collagen is shaped into long rods and bundled into stiff fibers to do its job of strengthening bone, cartilage, and skin to maintain body form.

Hemoglobin

This globular type of protein (Figure 4-6) includes four globin polypeptide chains per molecule of hemoglobin. Each chain has several hundred amino acids conjugated with a nonprotein—the iron-containing pigment called *heme.* The globin wraps around the heme and forms protective pockets to secure the iron. The iron in heme has a special ability to bind oxygen and as part of the red blood cell delivers oxygen to the tissues.

Albumin

Albumin is the major plasma protein and has a compact globular shape. It consists of a single polypeptide chain of 584 amino acids, twisted and coiled into helix structures held together by 17 disulfide bridges.[4] Albumin helps maintain fluid balance by exerting colloidal pressure in the capillaries that forces the flow of fluid and nutrients into the cells and the return of fluid and waste products out of the cells. In severe illness albumin is broken down to supply amino acids for the synthesis of new proteins needed to meet the body emergency.

Other Proteins With Special Roles

Other proteins with special structural or metabolic roles include the antibodies of the immune system and the blood protein fibrinogen, important in blood clotting. Hormones such as insulin and thyroxin and the enzymes that regulate our day-to-day metabolic activities such as the digestion of our food are proteins.[2]

FUNCTIONS OF PROTEINS

Growth, Tissue Building, and Maintenance

Dietary protein supplies building material for the growth and maintenance of body tissues. It furnishes amino acids in the appropriate patterns and amounts for efficient synthesis of specific structural molecules. Nitrogen is a vital element in our body's structure. Unlike carbohydrates and fats, which contain no nitrogen, protein is about 16% nitrogen. Dietary protein also supplies amino acids for making other nitrogen-containing substances such as the lipoproteins that transport fats in the blood (see Chapter 3) and growth hormone that controls the growth of the long bones.

Physiologic Roles

All amino acids participate in tissue growth and maintenance. Some, however, have important metabolic roles of their own, as follows:

- *Produce neurotransmitters for brain and nerve function*[5]: Methionine assists in the formation of choline, a precursor of acetylcholine, and *tyrosine* is used to synthesize

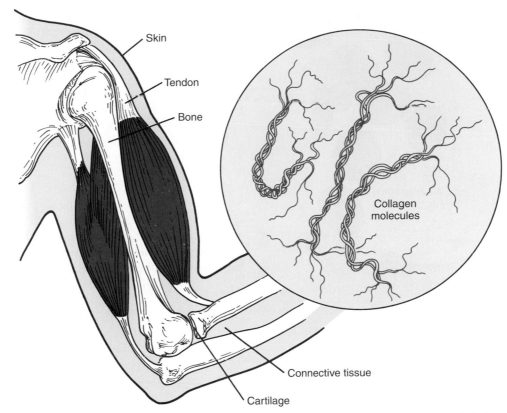

FIGURE 4-5 Tissues that contain collagen, a structural protein forming connective tissue throughout the body.

the neurotransmitters dopamine and norepinephrine; tryptophan is the precursor of the neurotransmitter serotonin. Age-related decreases in the neurotransmitter dopamine are associated with Parkinson's disease, a disorder in older adults causing muscle tremors and muscle rigidity.[6] These patients have difficulty with motor functions such as eating and walking.

- *Produce other amino acids:* Methionine is the precursor of the conditionally indispensable amino acid *cysteine;* methionine is also the precursor of carnitine and taurine; carnitine transports long-chain fatty acids into the mitochondria for energy production, and taurine, found in bile salts, also regulates fluid pressure in the eye.[5]
- *Produce hormones: Phenylalanine* is the precursor of the conditionally indispensable amino acid tyrosine needed to form thyroxin and epinephrine.
- *Support immune function:* Protein is used to make antibodies for the immune system.
- *Maintain fluid balance:* Plasma proteins control the flow of fluids, nutrients, and waste products back and forth between the capillaries and the cells.

Role in Critical Care

Particular amino acids are receiving attention for their possible advantages in treating illness or disease. Recovery from severe infection, trauma, or life-threatening malnutrition may be improved with specific amino acid supplements. Glutamine derived from the dispensable amino acid *glutamic acid* is the most abundant free amino acid in the body, and it can serve two roles: (1) because it has two amino (NH_2) groups, it can donate an amino group for the synthesis of another amino acid or (2) it can be an important energy source for liver and immune cells when its amino groups are removed.[7] Glutamine protects the mucosal surface of the intestine from invasion of harmful

helix A coiled structure found in protein. Some are simple chain coils; others are made of several coils, as in a triple helix.

precursor A substance from which another substance is derived.

carnitine A naturally occurring amino acid ($C_{17}H_{15}NO_3$) formed from methionine and lysine; carnitine is required to transport long-chain fatty acids into the mitochondria, where they are oxidized for energy.

taurine A sulfur-containing amino acid, $NH_2(CH_2)_2 \cdot SO_2OH$, formed from the indispensable amino acid methionine. It is found in lung and muscle tissues and in bile and breast milk.

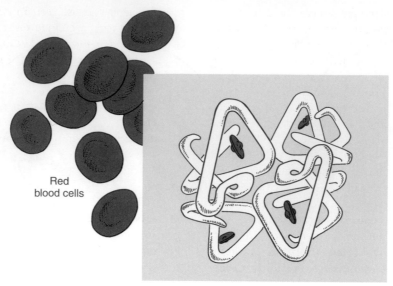

Red
blood cells

Hemoglobin molecule

FIGURE 4-6   Hemoglobin is an oxygen-carrying protein of red blood cells.

bacteria and enhances the production of white cells and other immune factors, giving it special importance in critical care. Glutamine works with the kidney in responding to acidosis as occurs in uncontrolled diabetes. Arginine, a conditionally dispensable amino acid, has a role in immune response and assists in wound healing. Burn patients may have an increased need for arginine.[1]

In kwashiorkor and wasting diseases, decreased protein synthesis coupled with rapid tissue breakdown leads to the stark consequences of protein deficiency on growth, development, and resistance to disease. At these times cysteine becomes an indispensable amino acid for the production of proteins to assist in recovery.[8-10] The branched-chain amino acids leucine, isoleucine, and valine improve nitrogen retention and appetite in patients with liver disease.[11] Although we are learning new ways in which amino acids can improve patient status, self-medication with amino acid supplements is dangerous in both sickness and health. For example, glutamine supplementation is not appropriate for cancer patients because it promotes the growth of tumor cells.[1] (The hazards of amino acid supplements for body building are discussed in Chapter 14.)

Energy Source

Protein contributes to overall energy metabolism as needed, particularly during aerobic exercise[12] or in the fasting state. Protein is not used for energy in the fed state, when glucose is readily available. Before amino acids can be burned for energy, the nitrogen-containing amino (NH_2^+) group is removed. The carbon skeleton that remains, called a *keto-acid,* can be converted to either glucose or fat. For every 100 g of high-quality protein consumed by an adult, 17 g to 25 g are oxidized for

energy.[5] Adequate supplies of carbohydrate spare protein for its primary purpose of tissue building.

Protein and Nitrogen Balance

The Concept of Balance

Many interdependent checks and balances throughout the body keep it in working order. There is constant ebb and flow with tissue building and breakdown, and storage and release of body materials. These coordinated activities enable the body to respond to any situation that disturbs its normal function. This state of dynamic equilibrium is called homeostasis, and the various mechanisms that preserve it are called *homeostatic mechanisms.*

The concept of balance as related to protein balance refers to the steady state that exists between protein synthesis (anabolism) and protein breakdown (catabolism). In periods of growth the rate of protein synthesis exceeds protein breakdown, resulting in a net gain of new tissue. When food intake is drastically reduced as in famine, or extreme voluntary food restriction, or serious illness, tissue breakdown exceeds protein synthesis and the body loses protein. In healthy individuals adjustments in protein balance on a day-to-day basis manage the daily variations in protein intake or short-term emergencies.

Body Protein Reserves

The average man contains about 11 kg of protein.[3] Nearly half this protein (43%) is found in skeletal muscle with the remainder in skin, blood, kidney, liver, brain, and other organs. Body distribution of protein changes with growth and development. The newborn has relatively little skeletal muscle with proportionately more protein in the brain and visceral organs.

In contrast to the extensive fat reserves held by most people, body protein reserves are quite limited. What are referred to as the *labile protein reserves,* meaning they are easily broken down to meet immediate needs, make up only about 1% of total body protein and like glycogen are sufficient to maintain body functions for only a very short period of time.[3] Labile protein reserves are intended to provide amino acids for an emergency; if the condition continues, as in chronic illness or body wasting, these reserves are rapidly depleted and skeletal muscle is broken down to furnish amino acids as needed.

Protein Balance

Finely tuned mechanisms control protein balance and regulate protein synthesis and breakdown across all body tissues. When less protein is supplied in the diet, protein is conserved and protein losses minimized to adjust to the reduced intake. When fighting infection the body breaks down available protein reserves to obtain amino acids for making immune cells or other proteins necessary to preserve life. When more protein is available than is needed for body growth or repair, amino acids are broken down and used for energy or stored as fat. Various body systems and protein compartments participate in overall control of protein metabolism, as follows:

- *Protein turnover:* Protein turnover is the process by which body proteins are continuously broken down and the amino acids released are made into new proteins.[3] New proteins are formed to replace worn-out proteins, and different proteins are formed to meet changing needs. When an amino acid labeled with a radioactive carbon atom is incorporated into a protein food and eaten, it can be traced—that is, we can follow its journey through the body. By these studies we learned that amino acids are rapidly incorporated into body proteins and then, when these proteins are broken down, are used again to form new proteins. Protein turnover varies among tissues. Turnover rates are higher in the intestinal mucosa, liver, pancreas, kidney, and plasma, tissues that are more metabolically active, and lower in muscle, brain, and skin. Protein turnover is very slow in structural tissues such as collagen. Total body protein turnover is higher in infants and children who are growing rapidly and lower in older adults.
- *Protein compartments:* Body protein is divided between two compartments—tissue protein and plasma protein. Protein from one compartment may be drawn to supply a need in the other. Plasma proteins such as prealbumin and albumin have very rapid turnover and respond quickly to changes in protein intake or an increase in protein catabolism. Levels of these proteins are used to identify patients needing added nutrition.[13,14] A low plasma albumin level is characteristic of children with kwashiorkor, the protein-energy

deficiency disease seen in countries with food shortages. Plasma protein levels are restored to normal when protein and additional kcalories become available.
- *Metabolic amino acid pool:* Amino acids derived from tissue breakdown and amino acids supplied by dietary protein both contribute to a common metabolic "pool." Amino acids from this pool are used to synthesize body proteins as needed. Figure 4-7 summarizes the many aspects of protein metabolism.

Nitrogen Balance

Protein balance is sometimes described as nitrogen balance. Total nitrogen balance involves all sources of nitrogen in the body—protein nitrogen as well as nonprotein nitrogen in compounds such as urea, uric acid, and ammonia. Nitrogen balance is the net result of nitrogen gain and loss across all body tissues. A harmful state of negative nitrogen balance exists when the loss of body nitrogen exceeds the nitrogen input from food; this occurs in long-term illness, hypermetabolic wasting disease, and starvation.

Protein Quality

Evaluating Food Proteins

The nutritional quality of a protein is based on its ability to provide nitrogen and amino acids for the growth, maintenance, and repair of body tissues. In general, protein quality depends on the following two characteristics:

1. *Protein digestibility:* To be of use to the body, amino acids must be released from other food components and made available for absorption. If nondigestible components prevent this breakdown, valuable amino acids are lost in the feces.

homeostasis State of dynamic equilibrium within the body's internal environment; a balance achieved through the operation of various interrelated physiologic mechanisms.
protein balance The balance between the building up (anabolism) and the breaking down (catabolism) of body tissues, necessary to maintain positive growth and maintenance.
synthesis The making of a substance or compound by the body.
anabolism Metabolic process for building body tissues.
catabolism Metabolic process for breaking down body tissues; the opposite of anabolism.
labile Easily changed or modified; unstable.
nitrogen balance The metabolic balance between nitrogen intake in dietary protein and nitrogen losses in urine, feces, sweat, and cells; 6.25 g dietary protein contains 1 g of nitrogen.

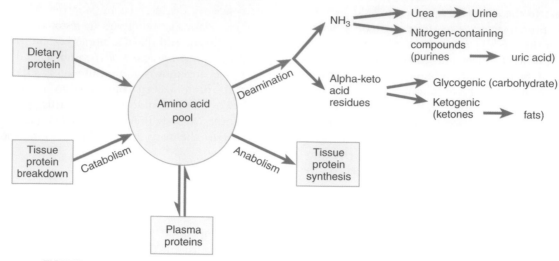

FIGURE 4-7   Balance between protein compartments and the amino acid pool. Amino acids are constantly entering and leaving the body's amino acid pool. These amino acids can form new proteins or other nitrogen-containing compounds, be converted to carbohydrate and used for energy, or be converted to fat for storage.

2. *Amino acid composition:* All 20 amino acids used in the synthesis of body proteins must be available at the same time for new tissues to be formed. Thus a food protein must supply each of the indispensable, or essential, amino acids in the amount required along with other sources of amino (NH_2^+) groups to synthesize the dispensable amino acids needed.

Comparing Food Proteins

The nutritive value of a food protein is often expressed as its *amino acid score,* a value based on both its digestibility and amino acid composition. The Amino Acid Reference Pattern used to evaluate proteins is quite similar to the pattern of egg white, the reference protein often used in nutrition studies. When evaluating an amino acid score it is important to identify the limiting amino acid(s). The limiting amino acid(s) is any indispensable amino acid present in a lower amount than recommended in the Amino Acid Reference Pattern. For protein synthesis to take place, all indispensable amino acids must be available in the required amount. Thus the limiting amino acid "limits" or hinders the body from effectively using the other amino acids in the food regardless of their adequacy. When one or two limiting amino acids are identified in a food protein containing optimal levels of other indispensable amino acids, that protein can be combined with another food protein that will supply the limiting amino acid(s).

The following other methods have been used in animal studies to evaluate protein digestibility and composition:

- *Biologic value (BV)* is based on nitrogen balance and the ability of a protein to replace daily nitrogen losses or support growth.
- *Net protein utilization (NPU)* is based on biologic value and degree of digestibility.
- *Protein efficiency ratio (PER)* is based on weight gain of a growing test animal divided by its protein intake.

| TABLE 4-1 | Comparative Protein Quality of Selected Foods According to Amino Acid Score, Biologic Value (BV), Net Protein Utilization (NPU), and Protein Efficiency Ratio (PER) |

Food	Amino Acid Score	BV	NPU	PER
Egg	100	100	94	3.92
Cow's milk	95	93	82	3.09
Beef	69	74	67	2.30
Soybeans	47	73	61	2.32
Peanuts	65	55	55	1.65
Polished rice	57	64	57	2.18
Whole wheat	53	65	49	1.53
Sesame seeds	42	62	53	1.77
Peas	37	64	55	1.57

Data from Committee on Amino Acids, Food and Nutrition Board: *Improvement of protein nutriture,* Washington, DC, 1974, National Academy of Sciences.

A comparison of the scores and nutritive values of various protein foods based on these measures is shown in Table 4-1. In general, proteins from animal sources have higher scores than those from plant sources across all measures.

Amino Acid Content of Plant and Animal Foods

Plant and animal foods differ in their content of indispensable amino acids. Animal foods contain all of the indispensable amino acids in the amounts and ratio needed to support protein synthesis and are referred to as *complete proteins.* These foods include eggs, milk, cheese, meat, poultry, and fish (Box 4-2). Plant proteins vary in quality but are incomplete proteins (Box 4-3). Individual plant proteins supply less than the required amount of

BOX 4-2	Complete Proteins

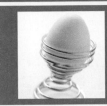 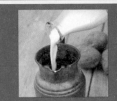 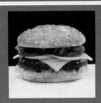 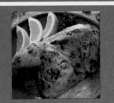 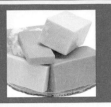

Animal foods, such as the following, contain complete proteins:

- Egg
- Milk
- Cheese
- Hamburger
- Chicken
- Fish fillet

Images copyright 2006 JupiterImages Corporation.

BOX 4-3	Incomplete Proteins

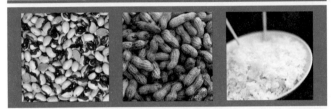

Plant foods, such as the following, contain incomplete proteins:
- Meat analogue
- Beans
- Peanuts
- Rice
- Tofu
- Sesame seeds

Images copyright 2006 JupiterImages Corporation.

BOX 4-4	Plant Sources of Protein

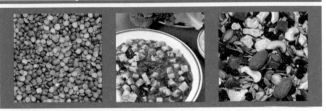

Each of the following servings provides at least 4 to 6 g of protein:*
- Cooked beans, peas, or lentils: ½ cup
- Tofu or tempeh: ½ cup
- Nut butter: 2 tbsp
- Nuts: ¼ cup
- Tahini (sesame seed butter): 2 tbsp
- Meat (soy) analogue: 1 oz

Data from Messina V, Melina V, Mangels AR: A new food guide for North American vegetarians, *J Am Diet Assoc* 103:771, 2003.

Images copyright 2006 JupiterImages Corporation.

*A plant protein can be combined with a small amount of animal protein to form a complete protein, or two different plant protein foods can be combined to form a complete protein (see Figures 4-8 and 4-9).

one or more indispensable amino acids or are missing an indispensable amino acid. But a mixture of plant proteins can together supply the required amounts of indispensable amino acids to support tissue growth and maintenance.[3,15] Soy protein, although lower in methionine than animal protein, meets the amino acid needs of adults. Figure 4-8 illustrates examples of complementary proteins, and Box 4-4 lists the total protein in various plant foods. Complementary proteins have played a role in the traditional food patterns of individuals and families worldwide (see the *Perspectives in Practice* box, "Increase Your Variety: Exploring Complementary Proteins").

PROTEIN REQUIREMENTS

Dietary Reference Intake

Protein

The Recommended Dietary Allowance (RDA) for adults furnishes the protein and amino acids needed to maintain body tissues and replace nitrogen lost via the urine, feces, and sweat. This amount is 0.8 g/kg body weight or 56 g/day for men and 46 g/day for women.[3] An additional 25 g/day is needed for pregnancy and lactation. The protein requirements of infants and children vary according to age and growth patterns.

A Tolerable Upper Intake Level (UL) has not been established for protein, yet the safety of very high protein intakes in excess of two times the RDA is a concern. Waste products from protein breakdown are excreted in the urine, and high protein intakes can lead to dehydration if fluid intake is not sufficient. Accelerated loss of bone calcium and excessive stress on the kidneys have

---

limiting amino acid The indispensable amino acid in a food found in the smallest amount as related to the Reference Amino Acid Pattern.

incomplete protein A protein with a lower amount of one or more of the indispensable amino acids or missing an indispensable amino acid needed to form body proteins.

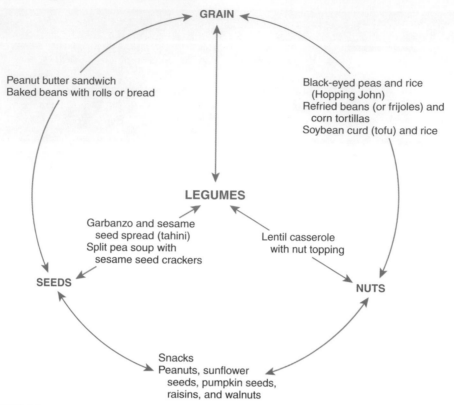

FIGURE 4-8 Complementary vegetable proteins. Examples of common plant foods eaten together that supply the essential amino acids. (*Redrawn from Stanfield PS, Hui YH: Nutrition and diet therapy: self-instructional modules, ed 4, Sudbury, Mass, 2003, Jones & Bartlett.*)

TABLE 4-2	Amino Acid Requirements of Different Age-Groups

	Recommended Dietary Allowance by Age-Group (mg/kg/day)				
			Children, Age 9-13 yr		
Amino Acid	Infants, Age 0-6 mo	Children, Age 4-8 yr	Boys	Girls	Adults
Histidine	23	16	17	15	14
Isoleucine	88	22	22	21	19
Leucine	156	49	49	47	42
Lysine	107	46	46	43	38
Methionine plus cysteine	59	22	22	21	19
Phenylalanine plus tyrosine	135	41	41	38	33
Threonine	73	24	24	22	20
Tryptophan	28	6	6	6	5
Valine	87	28	28	27	24

Data compiled from Food and Nutrition Board, Institute of Medicine: *Dietary Reference Intakes for energy, carbohydrate, fiber, fat, fatty acids, cholesterol, protein, and amino acids, parts 1 and 2,* Washington, DC, 2002, National Academies Press.

been suggested as possible consequences of protein intakes more than twice the RDA, but further study is needed.[3]

Amino Acids

Individuals meeting the RDA who eat both animal and plant protein will have an adequate supply of the indispensable amino acids. If no animal foods are included in the diet, an intake of mixed plant proteins obtained from legumes (including soy), grains, nuts, seeds, and vegetables can supply amino acids in the pattern needed for health and growth.[3] Table 4-2 lists the amino acid requirements for different age-groups.

ULs have not been set for individual amino acids, although imbalances can result from supplements that

PERSPECTIVES IN PRACTICE
Increase Your Variety: Exploring Complementary Proteins

In many parts of the world, animal proteins are not as plentiful as in the United States and populations have survived and thrived on diets emphasizing complementary proteins. Traditional diets the world over have been plant based, emphasizing cereals, legumes, vegetables, and fruit. In many cultures the main dish served at mealtime is a stew containing a variety of plant foods. Some recipes use plant foods with a small amount of added animal protein in the form of meat, fish, poultry, eggs, or cheese. In Chapter 1 we discussed the need to become familiar with the food patterns of different cultural and ethnic groups. Exploring complementary protein dishes is a perfect way to do this. Visit your local library and review some ethnic cookbooks, or visit a website that provides ethnic recipes. Better yet, seek out a member of a cultural or ethnic group different from your own, and learn more about their food and the customs that it represents. Try a new recipe, and calculate the amounts of protein coming from both animal and vegetable sources.

Some traditional food patterns based on plant proteins can help you get started, as follows:

- *Mexican:* The traditional Mexican diet is founded on beans, corn, and rice. Corn tortillas combined with beans and vegetables provide a complete protein, as do beans and rice. The addition of cheese to stews or tortillas adds some complete animal protein to complement the incomplete proteins of the grain foods. Eggs accompanied by beans are a favorite Mexican breakfast.
- *East Indian:* The Hindu religion forbids the slaying of animals for meat, so many East Indians are vegetarians but may eat eggs, yogurt, and cheese. Traditional East Indian meals are based on stews with a variety of accompaniments. A stew containing rice, vegetables, and beans might be served with yogurt, cheese, and peanuts. Bread is made from wheat flour or flour from ground peas or beans, which adds good-quality protein.
- *Hmong (Vietnamese):* The traditional pattern of this family emphasizes rice and vegetables; in fact rice is served at every meal including breakfast. Rice mixed with green vegetables and small amounts of fish and peanuts are typical of

this region of the world. Rice rather than bread is the basic grain in this dietary pattern.

- *African American soul food: Soul food* is the term used to refer to the food patterns that developed among the African slaves brought to America. Food played an important role in preserving their traditions and nourishing their spirits. Beans and rice provided some protein along with the corn used to make a variety of breads such as corn bread or hoe cakes. Fish, pork, and chicken were popular sources of animal protein when available and were used to flavor both stews and cooked vegetables.
- *Traditional American:* Don't forget some of the typical American dishes that represent the use of complementary proteins. A peanut butter sandwich, a ready-to-eat cereal and milk, macaroni and cheese, and pinto beans and corn bread all represent the concept of complementary proteins.

References

Diabetes Care and Education Dietetic Practice Group of the American Dietetic Association: *Ethnic and regional food practices: A series. Hmong American food practices, customs, and holidays,* Chicago/Alexandria, VA, 1999, American Dietetic Association/American Diabetes Association.

Diabetes Care and Education Dietetic Practice Group of the American Dietetic Association: *Ethnic and regional food practices: A series. Indian and Pakistani food practices, customs, and holidays,* ed 2, Chicago/Alexandria, VA, 2000, American Dietetic Association/American Diabetes Association.

Diabetes Care and Education Dietetic Practice Group of the American Dietetic Association: *Ethnic and regional food practices: A series. Mexican American food practices, customs, and holidays,* Chicago/Alexandria, VA, 1998, American Dietetic Association/American Diabetes Association.

Diabetes Care and Education Dietetic Practice Group of the American Dietetic Association: *Ethnic and regional food practices: A series. Soul and traditional southern food practices, customs, and holidays,* Chicago/Alexandria, VA, 1995, American Dietetic Association/American Diabetes Association.

Kittler PG, Sucher KP: *Cultural foods: traditions and trends,* Belmont, Calif, 2000, Wadsworth/Thompson Learning.

exaggerate the intake of one or more of the amino acids. Such imbalances interfere with protein synthesis and lead to urinary amino acid losses.[3] Methionine, cysteine, and histidine supplements in particular can have adverse effects if taken over long periods.[16] It is important to recognize that amino acid imbalances or toxicity are not a hazard when amino acids are obtained from food. (See Chapter 14 for more on amino acid supplements.)

Acceptable Macronutrient Distribution Range

The Acceptable Macronutrient Distribution Range (AMDR) for protein is 10% to 35% of total kcalories.[3] Protein needs are generally met if 10% of energy intake is supplied by protein; however, if total energy intake is low, it may be necessary to obtain more kcalories from protein to meet the RDA. The suggested range for protein kcalories is intended to provide some flexibility in balancing the suggested proportions of fat and carbohydrate. (The AMDRs for carbohydrate and fat are discussed in Chapters 2 and 3, respectively.)

Factors Influencing Protein Requirements

Tissue Growth

Protein requirements reflect the growth patterns of infancy, childhood, and adolescence. Periods of rapid growth—as for fetal and maternal tissues in pregnancy—require added protein.

Protein Quality

Protein requirements are influenced by the quality of dietary protein and its amino acid pattern. There are no special recommendations for persons consuming some animal protein along with plant protein. Those who eat no animal protein should emphasize a wide variety of complementary plant foods to ensure an adequate supply of all indispensable amino acids.

Protein Digestibility

Amino acid availability is affected by food preparation. Heat causes chemical bonding between some sugars and amino acids, forming compounds that cannot be digested. Digestibility and absorption is influenced by the time interval between meals, with longer intervals lowering the competition for available enzymes and absorption sites.

Energy Content of the Diet

Sufficient amounts of carbohydrates must be available to meet energy needs, so dietary protein can be used exclusively for tissue building (protein-sparing action of carbohydrate). Dietary carbohydrates also support protein synthesis by stimulating the release of insulin. (Insulin promotes the use of amino acids for tissue building rather than energy.)

Health Status

Critical illness and diseases that increase the rate of protein turnover and tissue breakdown (catabolism) raise the protein requirement. After trauma or surgery amino acids are needed for tissue formation and wound healing and producing infection-fighting immune factors. Extensive tissue destruction as occurs with serious burns substantially increases protein needs (see Chapter 23). In critically ill patients, protein requirements may reach 1.5 to 2.0 g/kg of body weight.[17] Increased protein and carbohydrate may help limit the loss of muscle protein associated with immobilization and bed rest.[18] Muscle protein synthesis is influenced not only by the amount of protein available but also by when it is consumed. Older adults, those recovering from burns, or human immunodeficiency virus (HIV) patients may benefit from eating some protein immediately following training exercises.[19]

Protein Intake

Amount and Type

Protein intake differs widely among population groups with some getting far more and others far less than they need. Protein-energy malnutrition (PEM) is a major health problem in many developing countries where protein intakes are low in both quantity and quality. More than 6 million children die each year from protein-related deficiencies.[3] Plant researchers are working to improve the indispensable amino acid content of grains such as rice that are dietary staples for millions of people.[20] At the other extreme, many in the United States eat two or three times as much protein as they need with most coming from animal sources.[21] Foods of animal origin contribute at least 60% of the protein intake of U.S. adults, with 42% coming from meat, poultry, and fish; 15% from dairy products; and 3% from eggs.

Clinical Implications: Low and High Protein Intakes

Low-Protein Diets

We often associate low-protein diets with the severe PEM we see in underfed children and adults in famine-ravaged countries. But those individuals lack not only quality protein but also kcalories and essential vitamins and minerals. Children with PEM have poor growth with wasting (low weight for height) and stunting (low height for age).[3] Immune function is impaired in PEM and likely contributes to the chronic respiratory infections and diarrhea in many poorly nourished children and adults. Low protein intake during pregnancy increases risk of a low-birth-weight infant.

Other concerns may limit protein intake regardless of the available supply. In certain clinical situations, it is prudent to limit protein to levels below the usual intake; in those cases it is especially important to choose protein high in biologic value. Individuals may also choose to limit their protein intake for personal reasons. The following list presents a few examples of these conditions and situations:

- *Parkinson's disease:* Protein intake is controlled, so excessive amino acids do not compete with the treatment drug levodopa for passage across the blood-brain barrier.[22]
- *Chronic kidney disease (CKD):* When kidney function declines, protein intake is controlled to minimize the burden of excreting urea and other nitrogen-containing waste,[23] yet sufficient amounts of protein are provided to prevent development of PEM. Resistance training and regular exercise help preserve muscle mass in renal patients.[24]
- *Vegan diets:* Individuals who consume no animal foods and obtain all of their protein from plant sources can have marginal protein intakes resulting in part from the added bulk of plant protein foods. In some cases protein provides only 10% of total kcalories (10% is the minimum AMDR level).[3,15]

High-Protein Diets

High-protein diets are in the spotlight with the current media attention to weight loss regimens that restrict carbohydrate with preference to protein and fat. Diets in which protein provides 30% or more of total kcalories promote weight loss, add satiety, and can restore effective energy regulation.[25] Protein suppresses hunger to a greater extent than carbohydrate and might reduce energy intake.[26] Protein also increases energy expenditure to a small degree as compared to carbohydrate and fat based on the extra kcalories needed to break down protein for use as a fuel source; however, this by itself is unlikely to produce significant weight loss (see Chapter 5).[25] Reducing kcalorie intake and increasing energy expenditure are key, regardless of the proportion of specific macronutrients in the diet.[27]

Although high-protein diets have been successful in promoting weight loss, there are risks with protein intakes exceeding the upper limit of the AMDR (greater than 35% of total kcalories). Animal protein is rich in sulfur-containing amino acids that increase calcium loss in the urine and deplete bone mineral if not compensated with optimum calcium intakes.[3,25] High protein intakes from animal sources often include large amounts of saturated fat. Clinicians are raising concerns about the effects of excessive protein intakes on kidney function. Protein intakes more than three times the RDA aggravate kidney problems in those with even mild renal impairment,[28] and many adults in the early stages of kidney disease are unaware of their condition. Those with hypertension or diabetes risk kidney impairment if protein intake reaches this level.[29] Current nutrition standards for diabetes management recommend that protein intake not exceed 20% of total kcalories.[30]

Health Promotion

Health Benefits of Plant Foods

Soy foods and legumes supply good-quality protein and may help to prevent certain chronic diseases.[15] Soy foods appear to lower blood levels of total cholesterol and low-density lipoprotein (LDL) cholesterol, reducing cardiovascular risk.[31-33] The regular use of soy-based foods such as tofu and tempeh may play a part in the lower rates of some cancers in Asian countries.[31] Two phytochemicals in soy protein, genistein and daidzein, have estrogen-like activity and may help prevent bone loss in postmenopausal women.[34] (See the *Focus on Culture* box, "A Protein Source for Thousands of Years," to learn more about traditional soy-based foods.)

Beans, members of the legume family, are good sources of fiber and other complex carbohydrates (see Chapter 2). Adults eating legumes at least 4 times a week have a lower risk of cardiovascular disease than those eat-

---

 FOCUS ON CULTURE

A Protein Source for Thousands of Years

Soybeans have been used for centuries by millions of people throughout Asia. In China, Japan, Vietnam, Indonesia, the Philippines, Cambodia, and Laos, soybeans eaten in various forms are a dietary staple and a major source of protein. In many of these countries population density and limited land for agriculture restricted the number of cattle, making meat or milk-based foods costly and relatively uncommon. Traditional soy foods, including tofu, tempeh, and soy milk, were introduced to Americans by newcomers to the United States and over time have gained acceptance. Vegetarians, those unable to tolerate cow's milk, and others looking to expand their food horizons have adopted soy foods. The growing interest in Asian cooking, fueled by the increasing number of ethnic restaurants, has encouraged more people to try these foods.

The most important soy-based foods adding protein to Asian food patterns are tofu and tempeh, as described below:

- *Tofu:* In Chinese *fu* means "riches," so tofu is usually served during New Year celebrations to bring good luck in the following months. In China soybeans were referred to as the "poor man's cow" because they could be made into cheese and milk, similar to dairy foods. Tofu, often called the "cheese of Asia," is made by a process similar to cheese making. A coagulating agent such as calcium sulfate, vinegar, or lemon juice is added to pureed soybeans. After the curd has formed, it is placed in molds to form cakes and the liquid whey is discarded. If the tofu is made with calcium sulfate, it will have a higher calcium content. Some types of tofu look much like farmer cheese, although they are very different in flavor. Although most cheeses have strong flavors, tofu is very bland and absorbs the flavors of other foods. This makes it an excellent addition to cooked mixed dishes with a variety of seasonings or highly spiced ingredients. Tofu is available in two forms: soft and firm. Soft tofu can be mashed and used in recipes in the place of ground beef or ricotta cheese; firm tofu can be grilled or stir-fried. Tofu has a limited shelf life, so consumers should check the

expiration date on the package and be sure to keep it refrigerated.
- *Tempeh:* This soy food originated in Indonesia and is a mixture of soy and grain. When fermented, it becomes a firm mass that can be sliced or made into patties. Tempeh has more flavor than tofu and is a rich source of protein.

Soybeans are mixed with other ingredients to make sauces and seasonings used in Asian cooking, as follows:

- *Hoisin sauce:* This sauce is used in Chinese cooking and is a combination of fermented soybeans, water, flour, sugar, and garlic.
- *Miso:* Miso originated in Japan and is a fermented mixture of soybeans and rice or barley. It is a pungent, salty paste used as a seasoning or as a soup base; however, it is very high in sodium. It may contain 900 mg of sodium or more per tablespoon.
- *Soy sauce:* This seasoning is made from a mixture of steamed rice, roasted soybeans, and salt and fermented. Based on its high sodium content, it should be used in moderation.

Tofu and tempeh are available in many supermarkets and Asian food stores and add both variety and nutrition to the meal pattern. If you have not tasted these foods, look for an Asian cookbook in your local library and find a recipe to try.

References

Diabetes Care and Education Dietetic Practice Group of the American Dietetic Association: *Ethnic and regional food practices: A series. Hmong American food practices, customs, and holidays,* Chicago/Alexandria, VA, 1999, American Dietetic Association/American Diabetes Association.

Kittler PG, Sucher KP: *Cultural foods: traditions and trends,* Belmont, Calif, 2000, Wadsworth/Thompson Learning.

Margen S, ed: *The wellness encyclopedia of food and nutrition,* New York, 1992, Health Letter Associates.

BOX 4-5	Reasons for Following a Plant-Based Diet

Religious preferences
Cultural patterns
Protection of animals
Environmental concerns
Health
Extension of the world food supply

ing legumes less than once a week.[35] Beans along with nuts (a good source of essential fatty acids) are important foods in the Mediterranean diet and likely contribute to the lower risk of chronic disease among people following that diet pattern.[36]

Nutritional Contributions of Animal Foods

Proteins from animal sources, including meat, fish, poultry, eggs, and milk, provide all the indispensable amino acids in the appropriate amounts, and used singly or in combination with vegetable proteins meet the needs of children and adults. Various animal foods supply trace minerals that can be difficult to obtain in sufficient amounts from plant foods based on their lower content and interfering substances such as phytates and oxalates that can bind minerals and prevent their absorption. Both iron and zinc are more easily absorbed from animal foods. Dairy foods are rich in calcium and riboflavin and provide preformed vitamin A.[37] Vitamin B_{12} and vitamin D occur naturally in animal foods only.

Mixing Animal and Plant Proteins

For persons choosing to eat animal foods, mixing plant and animal proteins can benefit overall nutrition and health. Calcium is well absorbed from dairy foods, and the vitamin D in milk and other fortified milk products supports calcium absorption and promotes bone density. Iron and zinc, important for growth and body functions, are more easily absorbed from meats than plant foods. Vitamin B_{12} is found naturally in animal sources only. At the same time, plant protein foods such as legumes add important fiber, and phytochemicals and nuts contribute essential fatty acids in addition to the amino acids they contain. Fortified soy milk is an important source of calcium and vitamin D for those avoiding dairy products. Look to include both types of protein in your meal patterns as seems appropriate for you.

Vegetarian Diets

There are various reasons why people choose to follow a plant-based diet and limit or exclude animal foods (Box 4-5). Although such diet patterns are generally referred to as vegetarian diets, they are not all the same.[38] Vegetarian diets are generally categorized as follows:

- Ovolactovegetarian (includes all plant foods, dairy, and eggs)
- Lactovegetarian (includes all plant foods and dairy)
- Vegan (includes plant foods only)[15]
- Flexitarian (includes predominantly plant foods with nonvegetarian foods such as fish or poultry on occasion)[39]

Vegetarian diets are planned as any diet is planned, to include essential nutrients and sufficient kcalories for energy. A *Vegetarian Food Guide* published by the American Dietetic Association offers helpful advice for selecting nutritionally sound plant-based diets[40] (Figure 4-9).

Well-planned plant-based diets supply appropriate amounts of protein, vitamins, and minerals along with fiber and phytochemicals. Vegetarians have lower body weights[41] and blood pressures[42] than nonvegetarians. Vegetarians also have a lower risk of cardiovascular disease, possibly related to lesser intakes of saturated fat. Overall rates of various cancers are lower in vegetarians. Both diabetes and renal disease can be well managed using plant-based diets.[43] Easy-to-prepare recipes for vegetarian meals are widely available as public interest has given rise to many popular cookbooks. (See the *To Probe Further* box, "Vegetarian Diets: Implications for Nutrition and Health," for more ideas on planning diets based on plant foods.)

DIGESTION-ABSORPTION-METABOLISM PREVIEW

The food proteins taken into the body must be broken down into ready-to-use building units—the amino acids. We outline below the mechanical and chemical processes of digestion by which this is accomplished. (See Chapter 8 for a more detailed discussion of digestion, absorption, and metabolism.)

Mouth

The only digestive action on protein taking place in the mouth is the mechanical effect of chewing. Here the food is broken into particles, mixed with saliva, and passed on as a semisolid mass into the stomach.

Stomach

Because proteins are large complex structures, a series of reactions is necessary to release their amino acids. These chemical changes begin in the stomach. In fact the major digestive function of the stomach is the partial enzymatic breakdown of protein. The following three chemical agents in the gastric secretions help with this task: (1) pepsin, (2) hydrochloric acid, and (3) rennin.

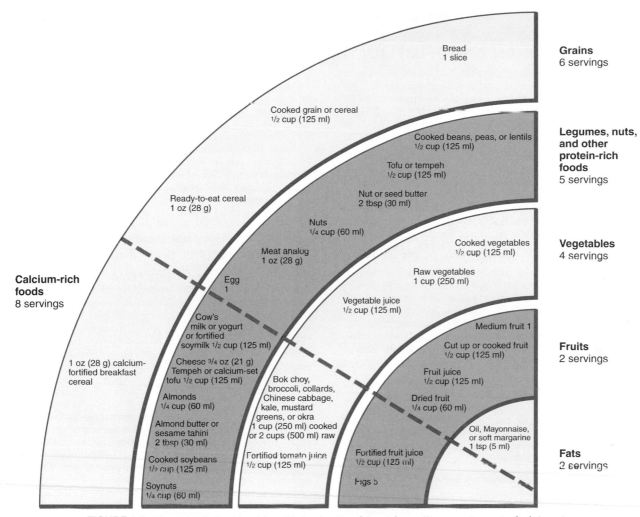

FIGURE 4-9 Vegetarian food guide rainbow. Notice the slice of the rainbow calling attention to the foods in each group that are good sources of calcium. *(Redrawn from Messina V, Melina V, Mangels AR: A new food guide for North American vegetarians,* J Am Diet Assoc *103:771, 2003; with permission from the American Dietetic Association.)*

1. *Pepsin:* The major gastric enzyme specific for proteins is pepsin. It is produced as the inactive proenzyme pepsinogen by the chief cells in the stomach wall. Pepsinogen requires hydrochloric acid to be transformed into the enzyme pepsin. The active pepsin then begins splitting the peptide linkages between amino acids, breaking the large polypeptides into successively smaller peptides. If protein remained in the stomach longer, pepsin would complete the breakdown to individual amino acids. However, with normal gastric emptying time, only the beginning stage is completed by the action of pepsin.

2. *Hydrochloric acid:* Gastric hydrochloric acid is an important catalyst in protein digestion, providing the acid medium necessary to convert pepsinogen to pepsin.

3. *Rennin:* This gastric enzyme (not to be confused with the renal enzyme renin) is present only in infancy and childhood. It has a special role in helping infants digest milk. Rennin acts on casein, the major protein in milk, to produce a curd. By coagulating milk, rennin prevents too rapid passage of food out of the infant's stomach.

Small Intestine

Protein digestion, beginning in the acid environment of the stomach, is completed in the alkaline environment of the small intestine. A number of enzymes secreted by the pancreas and glands in the wall of the intestine take part, as follows:

---

pepsin A gastric enzyme specific for proteins. Pepsin breaks large protein molecules into shorter chain polypeptides, proteases, and peptones. Gastric hydrochloric acid is necessary to activate pepsin.

proenzyme An inactive precursor converted to the active enzyme by the action of an acid or other enzyme.

TO PROBE FURTHER

VEGETARIAN DIETS: IMPLICATIONS FOR NUTRITION AND HEALTH

Vegetarian diets have existed since ancient times. The Greeks first developed the vegetarian diet, and Benjamin Franklin, the famous American inventor, was a vegetarian. Approximately 5 million people in the United States consistently follow a vegetarian diet, eating no meat, fish, or poultry, but less than 1% of these are vegans.[1] In general the more restrictive the diet, the more careful must be the planning to avoid nutrient deficiencies.

Why Choose a Vegetarian Diet?

There are various reasons why an individual may follow a vegetarian diet. Several major world religions, including Hinduism and Buddhism, advocate avoidance of meat and the preservation of animal life. Some members of the Seventh Day Adventist church do not eat meat, fish, or poultry but include dairy foods and eggs in their meal plans. Sustainability of the food supply and protection of the environment are growing concerns in many parts of the world. Land requirements for producing meat protein are about 10 times greater than for producing plant protein. About 40% of the world's supply of grain is used to feed animals sold for meat.[2] These facts have led some persons to adopt a plant-based diet with the intent that direct consumption of grains will assist in reducing food shortages in many parts of the world. Finally, well-planned vegetarian diets support health and diminish the risk of certain diseases.[1]

Nutritional Implications of a Vegetarian Diet

Vegetarian diets, including vegan diets that exclude all animal foods, will support nutrition needs throughout the life cycle *if* they are well planned. On the other hand, vegetarian and vegan diets, as well as diets that include all types of animal foods, can be inadequate if items high in fat and sugar and low in important nutrients are emphasized. For those vegetarians who consume eggs and dairy products, protein, calcium, vitamin D, and vitamin B_{12} are not a problem. Eggs also may supply small amounts of n-3 fatty acids obtained from animal feeds. The growing availability of fortified vegan foods is making it easier for pregnant women, young children, and adolescents to meet their elevated needs for these nutrients.

Vegans will need to seek out fortified foods to obtain their vitamin D and vitamin B_{12}. Some brands of soy milk and breakfast cereals are fortified with both of these vitamins. Vitamin supplements or products such as vegetarian formula nutrition yeast can supply these important nutrients. Some of the meat analogues prepared from soy protein have added vitamin B_{12}. It is important that vegans read the labels of these products to ensure their nutrition. The n-3 fatty acids can be obtained in flaxseed oil, canola or soybean oil, or walnuts.[3,4]

Although iron and zinc are found in many plant foods, they are not absorbed as efficiently from plant foods as from animal foods. Plant foods often contain phytates, substances that bind iron and prevent its absorption. Having a source of vitamin C at the same meal with the iron-containing plant food facilitates absorption, and vegetarians generally have high intakes of vitamin C coming from their frequent use of fruits and vegetables. Soaking beans before cooking makes the iron more available for absorption.[1] Fortified grains and cereals add iron to the diet. It may be the case that individuals adapt to lower iron intakes over the long term, because iron deficiency anemia is no more prevalent among vegetarians than nonvegetarians.[1] Zinc absorption from plants can also be a problem based on plant phytate content. Zinc-fortified cereals are an alternative source of this mineral.

Calcium can be low in the diets of vegetarians avoiding dairy foods. Calcium is found in many vegetables, although oxalates in certain vegetables interfere with the absorption of calcium as phytates interfere with the absorption of iron and zinc. However, the calcium found in broccoli, cabbage, collards, kale, and bok choy, vegetables low in oxalate, is well absorbed. In fact the calcium in these vegetables may be better absorbed than the calcium in tofu or fortified juices.[1] In contrast, vegetables such as spinach and Swiss chard are poor sources of calcium despite their relatively high content. Fortified soy milk and fortified breakfast cereals supply calcium. Although calcium intakes of lactovegetarians are about the same as for nonvegetarians, vegans often fall below the DRI and require special attention. The vegetarian food guide rainbow (see Figure 4-9) offers many alternative food sources of calcium.[3]

In recent years health professionals have had a paradigm shift in their attitudes about the healthfulness of vegetarian diets. Rather than associating vegetarian diet patterns with health risks, we have come to recognize the benefits of plant-based foods and are encouraging greater use of cereals, legumes, fruits, and vegetables.[5] Carefully planned plant-rich and plant-only diets support nutrient needs at all stages of the life cycle. New fortified foods make diet planning easier for those consuming plant-only diets.

Practical advice for vegetarian meal planning can be found in references 1 and 3.

References

1. American Dietetic Association: Position of the American Dietetic Association and Dietitians of Canada: vegetarian diets, *J Am Diet Assoc* 103:748, 2003.
2. Leitzmann C: Nutrition ecology: the contribution of vegetarian diets, *Am J Clin Nutr* 78(suppl):657S, 2003.
3. Messina V, Melina V, Mangels AR: A new food guide for North American vegetarians, *J Am Diet Assoc* 103:771, 2003.
4. Kris-Etherton P: Essential fatty acids and vegetarians: the missing link in long-chain omega-3 fatty acid recommendations, *Nutr & the MD* 31(8):1, 2005.
5. Sabate J: The contribution of vegetarian diets to health and disease: a paradigm shift, *Am J Clin Nutr* 78(suppl):502S, 2003.

- *Pancreatic secretions:* The following three enzymes from the pancreas continue breaking down proteins to smaller and simpler units:
  1. Trypsin is secreted first as inactive trypsinogen and then activated by the hormone enterokinase produced in the duodenal wall. Trypsin acts on proteins and large polypeptide fragments carried over from the stomach, yielding smaller polypeptides and dipeptides.
  2. Chymotrypsin is secreted by special cells in the pancreas as inactive chymotrypsinogen and then activated by the trypsin already present. Chymotrypsin continues the same protein-splitting action of trypsin.
  3. Carboxypeptidase, as its name implies, attacks the carboxyl end (acid [COOH]) of the peptide chain. The action of carboxypeptidase produces smaller peptides and some free amino acids.

TABLE 4-3	**Summary of Protein Digestion**			
Organ	**Inactive Precursor**	**Enzyme Activator**	**Active Enzyme**	**Digestive Action**
Mouth			None	Mechanical only
Stomach (acidic)	Pepsinogen	Hydrochloric acid	Pepsin	Protein $\Rightarrow$ polypeptides
			Rennin (infants) (calcium necessary for activity)	Casein $\Rightarrow$ coagulated curd
Intestine (alkaline) Pancreatic secretions	Trypsinogen	Enterokinase	Trypsin	Protein, polypeptides $\Rightarrow$ polypeptides, dipeptides
	Chymotrypsinogen	Active trypsin	Chymotrypsin	Protein, polypeptides $\Rightarrow$ polypeptides, dipeptides
			Carboxypeptidase	Polypeptides $\Rightarrow$ simpler peptides, dipeptides, amino acids
			Aminopeptidase	Polypeptides $\Rightarrow$ peptides, dipeptides, amino acids
Intestinal secretions			Dipeptidase	Dipeptides $\Rightarrow$ amino acids

- *Intestinal secretions:* Glands in the intestinal wall produce the following two protein-splitting enzymes:
  1. Aminopeptidase releases amino acids one at a time from the nitrogen-containing amino end (base [NH$_2$]) of the peptide chain. By this cleavage aminopeptidase produces smaller short-chain peptides and free amino acids.
  2. Dipeptidase breaks any remaining dipeptides into two free amino acids.

Through this system large complex proteins are broken down into progressively smaller peptide chains and finally into free amino acids ready for absorption. A summary of the steps in protein digestion is found in Table 4-3.

Absorption

Absorption of Amino Acids

Amino acids are water soluble, so they can be absorbed directly into the water-based bloodstream. They are absorbed rapidly from the small intestine through the fine network of villus capillaries and enter the portal blood. Amino acids require active transport to pass through the intestinal mucosa, as follows:

- *Active transport system:* Most amino acids are absorbed in the first section of the small intestine, the duodenum. An energy-dependent active transport mechanism, coupled with sodium transport, moves the amino acids into the blood circulation for delivery to the cells.
- *Competition for absorption:* When we eat a mixed diet containing a variety of amino acids, they compete with each other for absorption. The amino acid present in the largest amount retards the absorption of

the others. In the plasma, circulating amino acids compete for entry receptor sites on cell membranes that control transport into the cell.

Absorption of Peptides and Whole Proteins

A few short-chain peptides and smaller intact proteins escape digestion and are absorbed in that form. Most undergo hydrolysis within the cells of the intestinal mucosa and yield their amino acids. However, those

---

trypsin A pancreatic enzyme activated in the intestine from its precursor trypsinogen; it acts on proteins and polypeptides to yield smaller peptides and dipeptides.

chymotrypsin A pancreatic enzyme activated in the intestine from its precursor chymotrypsinogen. It breaks peptide linkages, forming smaller polypeptides and dipeptides.

carboxypeptidase A protein-splitting enzyme that cuts the peptide bond at the carboxyl (COOH) end of the chain, producing smaller peptide chains and free amino acids.

aminopeptidase A protein-splitting enzyme that cuts the peptide bond at the amino end of the chain, producing smaller peptide chains and free amino acids.

dipeptidase Final enzyme in the protein-splitting series that cleaves dipeptides to yield two free amino acids.

hydrolysis Process by which a chemical compound is split into simpler compounds by taking up molecules of water. This process occurs naturally in digestion.

protein molecules that pass into the blood intact may play a part in the development of immunity and protein sensitivity. We know that antibodies in the mother's colostrum, the first milk secreted after birth, are passed on to her nursing infant. Inadvertent absorption of intact proteins has been implicated in the development of some food allergies.[44]

Metabolism

The construction sites for building tissue proteins are in the cells. Each cell, depending on its nature and function, has a particular task to perform and requires a unique mix of amino acids to build the specific proteins needed. The amino acids are the "metabolic currency" of protein, and it is with these compounds that protein metabolism is ultimately concerned. The metabolic activities of protein are interwoven with those of carbohydrate and fat, which provide the energy to drive ongoing tissue building. We will look at these interrelationships more closely in Chapter 8.

TO SUM UP

The primary function of protein is to build and maintain body tissues. Amino acids are the building blocks that make up body tissues and the regulatory proteins that carry out important metabolic tasks. Of the 20 amino acids that build body proteins, 9 cannot be synthesized by the body and are referred to as indispensable, or essential, amino acids; another 6 cannot be synthesized in adequate amounts under conditions of stress or accelerated growth and are referred to as conditionally indispensable. The remaining 5 amino acids can be produced by the body and are termed the dispensable amino acids. Both the indispensable and conditionally indispensable amino acids must be supplied in the diet. Animal proteins are considered complete proteins because they contain all the indispensable amino acids in appropriate amounts. Plant proteins or incomplete proteins are missing one or more indispensable amino acids or contain less than the amount needed. Plant proteins can be mixed with animal proteins or with each other to provide the necessary proportions of all amino acids for body growth and maintenance. Protein requirements are influenced by growth, food protein quality, health status, and the availability of carbohydrate as an energy source. In many countries of the world, protein shortages lead to malnutrition with body wasting disease, stunted growth, chronic infection, and disease. In the United States overconsumption rather than underconsumption of protein is demanding our attention.

QUESTIONS FOR REVIEW

1. What is the difference between an indispensable, a dispensable, and a conditionally indispensable amino acid? List the names of each.

2. What is protein turnover? How does it relate to nitrogen balance?

3. Distinguish between protein anabolism and protein catabolism. Describe a clinical situation in which protein anabolism exceeds protein catabolism and one in which the opposite is true.

4. Explain the term *protein-sparing effect.* Which nutrient has this effect?

5. Describe the factors that influence dietary protein needs.

6. Visit a grocery store or drugstore, and examine five high-protein supplements. Make a chart that includes (a) the number of grams of protein provided in the container, (b) the cost of the entire container, and (c) the calculated cost for 8 g of protein. How does the cost of the protein supplement compare with the cost of 1 cup of milk or ½ cup of cooked kidney beans, which also provide about 8 g of good-quality protein? What are the better choices for supplying an individual's protein needs?

7. A vegan couple was told by their 2-year-old daughter's pediatrician that she was falling behind in her growth rate. What dietary factor(s) is likely related to her poor growth? What advice would you offer these parents to improve their child's nutritional status? Plan 1 day of meals for this family indicating food amounts for the child that would meet her protein needs and respect the vegan food pattern.

8. Protein intakes two to three times the RDA are not uncommon in the United States. Using the food values found on the CD-ROM that accompanied your textbook calculate the energy value and the number of grams of protein in a fast-food meal that includes one double-patty cheeseburger, a large serving of french fries, and a 12-oz milkshake. Compare the total grams of protein and the total kcalories with the protein and energy RDAs for a 16-year-old boy. What proportion of his daily protein and energy needs are provided by this one meal?

9. Describe the process of protein digestion and absorption including the (a) site in the gastrointestinal tract where each action occurs, (b) the enzymes responsible and their source, and (c) the resulting products.

REFERENCES

1. Matthews DE: Proteins and amino acids. In Shils ME et al, eds: *Modern nutrition in health and disease,* ed 10, Baltimore, 2006, Lippincott Williams & Wilkins.

2. Gropper SS, Smith JL, Groff JL: *Advanced nutrition and human metabolism,* ed 4, Belmont, Calif, 2005, Thomson/Wadsworth.

3. Food and Nutrition Board, Institute of Medicine: *Dietary Reference Intakes for energy, carbohydrate, fiber, fat, fatty acids, cholesterol, protein, and amino acids (macronutrients),* Washington, DC, 2002, National Academies Press.

4. Guyton AC, Hall JE: *Textbook of medical physiology,* ed 10, Philadelphia, 2000, WB Saunders.

5. Young VR: Protein and amino acids. In Bowman BA, Russell RM, eds: *Present knowledge in nutrition,* ed 8, Washington, DC, 2001, International Life Sciences Institute.

6. Timiras PS: *Physiological basis of aging and geriatrics,* ed 3, Boca Raton, Fla, 2003, CRC Press.

7. van de Poll MCG et al: Renal metabolism of amino acids, *Am J Clin Nutr* 79:185, 2004.

8. Badaloo A et al: Cysteine supplementation improves the erythrocyte glutathione synthesis rate in children with severe edematous malnutrition, *Am J Clin Nutr* 76:646, 2002.

9. Jackson AA: Glutathione in kwashiorkor, *Am J Clin Nutr* 76:495, 2002.

10. Wu G et al: Glutathione metabolism and its implications for health, *J Nutr* 134:489, 2004.

11. Mascarenhas R, Mobarhan S: New support for branched-chain amino acid supplementation in advanced hepatic failure, *Nutr Rev* 62(1):33, 2004.

12. Williams MH: Sports nutrition. In Shils ME et al, eds: *Modern nutrition in health and disease,* ed 10, Baltimore, 2006, Lippincott Williams & Wilkins.

13. Logan S, Hildebrandt LA: The use of prealbumin to enhance nutrition-intervention screening and monitoring of the malnourished patient, *Nutr Today* 38:134, 2003.

14. Fuhrman MP, Charney P, Mueller CM: Hepatic proteins and nutrition assessment, *J Am Diet Assoc* 104:1258, 2004.

15. American Dietetic Association: Position of the American Dietetic Association and Dietitians of Canada: vegetarian diets, *J Am Diet Assoc* 103:748, 2003.

16. Garlick PJ: The nature of human hazards associated with excessive intake of amino acids, *J Nutr* 134:1633S, 2004.

17. Hoffer LJ: Protein and energy provision in critical illness, *Am J Clin Nutr* 78:906, 2003.

18. Paddon-Jones D et al: Essential amino acid and carbohydrate supplementation ameliorates muscle protein loss in humans during 28 days bed rest, *J Clin Endocrinol Metab* 89:4351, 2004.

19. Tipton K: Postexercise nutrition: importance of protein and amino acids, *Nutr & the MD* 29(1):1, 2003.

20. Potrykus I: Nutritionally enhanced rice to combat malnutrition disorders of the poor, *Nutr Rev* 61(6,II):S101, 2003.

21. Cotton PA et al: Dietary sources of nutrients among U.S. adults, *J Am Diet Assoc* 104:921, 2004.

22. Holdern K: Reducing fracture risk in patients with Parkinson disease, *Nutr & the MD* 27(4):1, 2001.

23. Coulston AM: New name, old problem: chronic kidney disease, formerly known as chronic renal failure, *Nutr Today* 39:139, 2004.

24. Cupisti A et al: Skeletal muscle and nutritional assessment in chronic renal failure patients on a protein-restricted diet, *J Intern Med* 255:115, 2004.

25. Eisenstein J et al: High-protein weight-loss diets: are they safe and do they work? A review of the experimental and epidemiologic data, *Nutr Rev* 60(7,I):189, 2002.

26. Westerterp KR: Diet induced thermogenesis, *Nutr Metab* 1(1):5, 2004.

27. Dansinger ML et al: Comparison of the Atkins, Ornish, Weight Watchers, and Zone diets for weight loss and heart disease risk reduction, *JAMA* 293:43, 2005.

28. Knight EL et al: The impact of protein intake on renal function decline in women with normal renal function or mild renal insufficiency, *Ann Intern Med* 138:460, 2003.

29. Lentine K, Wrone EM: New insights into protein intake and progression of renal disease, *Curr Opin Nephrol Hypertens* 13:333, 2004.

30. American Diabetes Association: Nutrition principles and recommendations in diabetes, *Diabetes Care* 27(suppl I):S36, 2004.

31. Demonty I, Lamarche B, Jones PJH: Role of isoflavones in the hypocholesterolemic effect of soy, *Nutr Rev* 61:189, 2003.

32. Rosell MS et al: Soy intake and blood cholesterol concentrations: a cross-sectional study of 1033 pre- and postmenopausal women in the Oxford arm of the European Prospective Investigation in Cancer and Nutrition, *Am J Clin Nutr* 80:1391, 2004.

33. Omoni AO, Aluko RE: Soybean foods and their benefits: potential mechanisms of action, *Nutr Rev* 63(8):272, 2005.

34. Setchell KD, Lydeking-Olsen E: Dietary phytoestrogens and their effect on bone: evidence from in vitro and in vivo, human observational, and dietary intervention studies, *Am J Clin Nutr* 78(suppl 3):593S, 2003.

35. Bazzano LA et al: Legume consumption and risk of coronary heart disease in U.S. men and women: NHANES I Epidemiologic Follow-up Study, *Arch Intern Med* 161:2573, 2001.

36. Esposito K et al: Effect of a Mediterranean-style diet on endothelial dysfunction and markers of vascular inflammation in the metabolic syndrome: a randomized trial, *JAMA* 292:1440, 2004.

37. Murphy SP, Allen LH: Nutritional importance of animal source foods, *J Nutr* 133:3932S, 2003.

38. Weinsier R: Use of the term vegetarian, *Am J Clin Nutr* 71(5):1211, 2000.

39. Aronson D: Vegetarian nutrition: what every dietitian should know, *Today's Dietitian* 7(3):32, 2005.

40. Messina V, Melina V, Mangels AR: A new food guide for North American vegetarians, *J Am Diet Assoc* 103:771, 2003.

41. Willett W: Lessons from dietary studies in Adventists and questions for the future, *Am J Clin Nutr* 78(suppl):539S, 2003.

42. Liu RH: Health benefits from fruits and vegetables are from additive and synergistic combinations of phytochemicals, *Am J Clin Nutr* 78(suppl):517S, 2003.

43. Johnston PK, Sabate J: Nutritional implications of vegetarian diets. In Shils ME et al, eds: *Modern nutrition in health and disease,* ed 10, Baltimore, 2006, Lippincott Williams & Wilkins.

44. Taylor SL, Hefle SL: Food allergy. In Bowman BA, Russell RM, eds: *Present knowledge in nutrition,* ed 8, Washington, DC, 2001, International Life Sciences Institute.

FURTHER READINGS AND RESOURCES

Readings

Lupien J: Let's get our priorities straight in world nutrition, *Nutr Today* 39:227, 2004.

Although obesity is a growing problem in many parts of the world, Dr. Lupien does not want us to lose sight of the food shortages and low nutrient intake among people in many developing countries.

Spear BA: Adolescent growth and development, *J Am Diet Assoc* 102:S23, 2002.

Dr. Spear traces the importance of protein in the growth and development of adolescents.

Messina V, Melina V, Mangels AR: A new food guide for North American vegetarians, *J Am Diet Assoc* 103:771, 2003.

These authors tell us how they went about developing criteria to set up a new vegetarian food guide that would meet nutritional requirements for all age and gender groups.

Grivetti LE, Corlett JL, Lockett CT: Food in American history, part 3: beans, *Nutr Today* 36(3):172, 2001.

Grivetti LE et al: Food in American history, part 6: beef (part 2)—reconstruction and growth into the 20th century, *Nutr Today* 39:128, 2004.

> *Dr. Grivetti, a noted food historian, and his coauthors tell us about the use of two major sources of protein in America. Vegetable protein from legumes was an important part of the diet among various cultural groups in the early years of the American colonies. Within the last century beef has grown in popularity in the United States.*

Websites of Interest

- U.S. Department of Agriculture, Food and Nutrition Information Center, information and resource lists for vegetarian diets; these sites provide general diet information for protein nutrition along with ideas for plant-based and vegetarian meal planning: *www.nal.usda.gov/fnic/etext/000058.html; www.nal.usda.gov/fnic/pubs/bibs/gen/vegetarian.htm.*

- U.S. Department of Health and Human Services, U.S. Department of Agriculture: *Dietary guidelines for Americans 2005, ed 6: www.healthierus.gov/dietaryguidelines/.*

- U.S. Department of Agriculture, Center for Nutrition Policy and Promotion: *MyPyramid food guidance system;* these websites describe healthy choices and portion sizes of animal and plant protein foods: *www.mypyramid.gov/pyramid/meat.html; www.mypyramid.gov/pyramid/milk_tips.html; http://www.mypyramid.gov/tips_resources/vegetarian_diets.html.*

- American Dietetic Association, Vegetarian Nutrition Dietetic Practice Group; this site is a source of general information on healthy eating with vegetarian and plant-based diets: *http://www.vegetariannutrition.net/.*

CHAPTER 5

Energy Balance

Eleanor D. Schlenker

In Chapters 2, 3, and 4 we reviewed the three energy-yielding nutrients—carbohydrate, fat, and protein. In this chapter we look at the relationship between energy intake and energy expenditure and their combined effect on body composition and body weight.

Energy balance is not a simple matter. We are all different, and energy needs vary under different circumstances and for different body types. Each of us is unique, and our varying body weights reflect this. Physiologic, psychologic, environmental, metabolic, and genetic influences add to the complexities of energy balance and weight management.[1] We will take a positive approach based on healthy eating and regular physical activity, lifestyle patterns important to healthy weights in people of all ages.

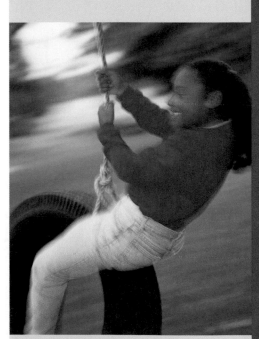

THE HUMAN ENERGY SYSTEM

Energy Cycle and Energy Transformation

Forms of Human Energy

In our physical world energy, like matter, is neither created nor destroyed. When we speak of energy being produced, what we really mean is energy being *transformed.* Energy is constantly being changed in form and recycled through a system. In the human body, metabolic reactions convert the stored chemical energy in our food to other forms of energy to carry out the body's work. Our bodies use four forms of energy: *chemical, electrical, mechanical,* and *thermal.* The ultimate source of energy is the sun with its vast reservoir of heat and light (Figure 5-1). Through the process of photosynthesis (see Figure 2-1), plants use water and carbon dioxide to transform the sun's energy into food storage forms of chemical energy. In the body these food fuels are converted to glucose, the energy unit that together with fatty acids is metabolized to release energy for use by body systems. Water and carbon dioxide, the materials used by plants, are the end products of energy metabolism in the body and become available to carry out the process once again. And so the cycle goes on.

Transformation of Energy

When food with its stored chemical energy is taken into the body, it undergoes many metabolic changes that convert it to other forms of stored chemical energy that the body can use. This chemical energy is then changed still further to other forms of energy as work is performed. In the brain chemical energy is changed to electrical energy for transmitting nerve impulses and carrying out brain activities. Chemical energy is changed to mechanical energy when muscles contract. It is changed to thermal energy in the regulation of body temperature. Chemical energy is used to form new tissues and proteins for growth and metabolism. In all of this work heat is given off to the surrounding atmosphere and larger biosphere.

In human *metabolism* as in other energy systems, energy is present as either *free energy* or *potential energy.* Free energy is the energy being used at any given moment in the performance of a task. It is unbound and in motion. Potential energy is energy that is stored or bound in a chemical compound and available for conversion to free energy when needed. For example, the energy stored in sugar is potential energy. When we eat it and it is metabolized, free energy is released for body work such as contraction of the muscles lining the gastrointestinal tract.

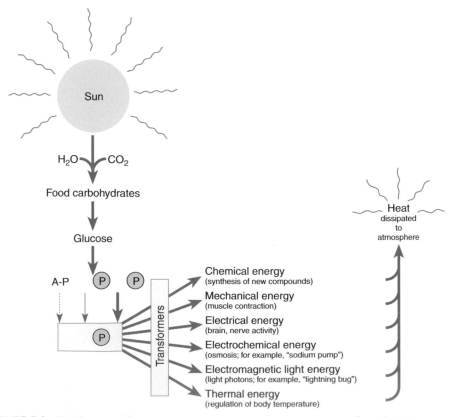

FIGURE 5-1 Transformation of energy from its primary source (the sun) to various forms for biologic work by means of metabolic processes ("transformers").

As the work is completed, this energy, now in the form of heat or thermal energy, is given off into the air. This makes it possible for us to express body energy consumption in kcalories or units of heat.

Energy Balance: Input and Output

The body demands a constant supply of available energy to sustain the activities essential for life. Energy is required to support internal needs along with the added expectations of physical activity. Whether the energy used is electrical, mechanical, thermal, or chemical, the supply of free energy and the reservoir of potential energy decrease as the metabolic and physical work of the body continue. Therefore the system must be constantly refueled from an outside source. For the human energy system this outside fuel source is food.

Energy Control in Human Metabolism

If the energy produced in the body through its many chemical reactions were "exploded" all at once, it would be destructive. So there needs to be a mechanism by which energy release can be controlled, so it may support life and not destroy it. Two means of control—chemical bonding and controlled reaction rates—make this possible.

Chemical Bonding

The main mechanism controlling energy in the human system is chemical bonding. The chemical bonds that hold together the elements in compounds are energy bonds. As long as the compound stays intact, energy is being exerted to maintain it. When the compound enters the body and is broken into its parts, this energy is released and becomes available for work. The following three types of chemical bonds transfer energy in the body:

1. *Covalent bonds:* These bonds are based on the relative valence of the elements making up a compound. Covalent bonds hold the carbon atoms together in organic compounds such as glucose.
2. *Hydrogen bonds:* Weaker than covalent bonds, hydrogen bonds are nonetheless significant because they are formed in large numbers. Also, the very fact that they are less strong and easily broken makes them important because they can transfer energy readily from one substance to another to form still another substance. The hydrogen attached to the oxygen molecule in the carboxyl group ($COOH^-$) of amino and fatty acids is an example of this type of bond.
3. *High-energy phosphate bonds:* A high-energy phosphate bond at work is the compound adenosine triphosphate (ATP), the substance the body uses to store energy for its work. Like storage batteries for electrical energy, these bonds are the controlling force of energy metabolism in the human cell.

Controlled Reaction Rates

The many chemical reactions that make up the body's energy system must have controls. Some reactions that break down protein, if left to themselves—as in sterile decomposition of plants—would span several years. Such reactions must be accelerated, or getting needed energy from the foods in a meal could take years. At the same time chemical reactions must be regulated so that too rapid a reaction will not produce a destructive burst of energy in a single "explosion." Energy reactions in cells are regulated by enzymes, coenzymes, and hormones, as follows:

- *Enzymes:* Specific enzymes in each cell control specific cell reactions. All enzymes are proteins and are produced in the cells under the direction of specific

---

energy The capacity of a system for doing work; available power. Energy is manifest in various forms—motion, position, light, heat, and sound. Energy is interchangeable among these various forms and is constantly being transformed and transferred among them.

chemical bonding Process of linking chemical elements or groups of elements in a chemical compound.

valence Power of an element or a radical to combine with or to replace other elements or radicals. Atoms from various elements combine in definite proportions. The valence number of an element is the number of atoms of hydrogen with which one atom of the element can combine.

adenosine triphosphate (ATP) A high-energy phosphate compound important in energy exchange within the cell. ATP is formed from the nucleotide adenosine with three attached phosphoric acid groups. The splitting off of the terminal phosphate bond (PO_4) to produce adenosine diphosphate (ADP) releases bound energy that is transformed to free energy and available for body work. ATP is then reformed as an energy store for use when needed.

enzyme Complex proteins produced by living cells that act as catalysts to speed the rate of chemical reactions. Enzymes facilitate chemical changes in other substances without themselves being changed in the process. Digestive enzymes act on food substances to break them down into simpler compounds. An enzyme is usually named according to the substance (substrate) on which it acts, with the common suffix *-ase;* for example, sucrase is the enzyme that breaks down sucrose to glucose and fructose.

genes. One gene controls the making of one enzyme, and there are thousands of enzymes in each cell. Each enzyme acts on its own particular substance, which is called its substrate. The enzyme and its substrate lock together to produce a new reaction product while the enzyme itself remains unchanged, ready to do its work over and over again (Figure 5-2).

- *Coenzymes:* Many reactions require a partner to assist the enzyme in completing the reaction. These coenzyme partners in many instances are vitamins, especially B-complex vitamins, or particular minerals. It may be helpful to think of the coenzyme as another substrate, because in receiving the material being transferred, the coenzyme is changed or reduced.
- *Hormones:* In energy metabolism hormones act as messengers to trigger or control enzyme action. The rate of oxidation reactions in the tissues—the body's metabolic rate—is controlled by *thyroxin* from the thyroid gland. Another familiar example is the controlling action of insulin on glucose utilization in the tissues. Various steroid hormones regulate the cell's ability to synthesize enzymes.

Types of Metabolic Reactions

There are two types of reactions constantly going on in body metabolism—anabolism and catabolism. Each requires energy. The process of *anabolism* synthesizes new and more complex substances. The process of *catabolism* breaks down more complex substances to simpler ones. Both activities release free energy, but the work performed also uses up some free energy. This creates a constant energy deficit to be met by food.

Sources of Stored Energy

When food is not available, as in fasting or starvation, the body must draw on its own stores for energy. Sources of stored energy can meet short-term or long-term needs, as follows:

- *Glycogen:* Only a 12- to 36-hour reserve of glycogen exists in liver and muscle and is quickly depleted.

- *Muscle mass:* Energy stores in the form of muscle protein exist in limited amounts but in greater volume than glycogen stores. Breakdown of muscle protein for energy should be a last resort when glycogen and adipose stores are depleted.
- *Adipose (fat) tissue:* Although fat storage is likely the largest source of stored energy, the supply varies from person to person.

Measurement of Energy Balance

The Kilocalorie

Because the body performs work only as energy is released and all work produces heat, energy expenditure can be measured in heat equivalents. Such a measure of heat is the calorie. To avoid using very large numbers nutritionists and biochemists use the kilocalorie—equal to 1,000 calories—abbreviated as *kcalorie* or *kcal.* This is the amount of heat required to raise 1 kg of water 1° C.

The Joule

The international (*Système International d'Unités* [SI]) unit of energy measurement is the joule. It equals the amount of energy expended when 1 kg of a substance is moved 1 m by a force of 1 Newton (N). It was named for James Prescott Joule (1818-1889), an English physicist who discovered the first law of thermodynamics. The conversion factor for changing kcalories to kilojoules (kJ) is 4.184; therefore 1 kcal equals 4.184 kJ. Because the energy content of diets given in kilojoules are very large numbers, the more common term is the *megajoule (MJ)*; 1 MJ equals 239 kcal. Some nutrition research journals use kilojoules rather than kcalories to describe energy intakes, so it is important to keep these conversion factors in mind.

Food Energy Measurement

The energy value of a particular food can be measured using two methods: calorimetry or calculation of approximate composition.

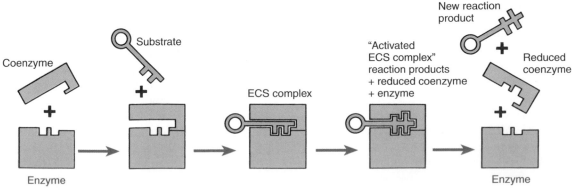

FIGURE 5-2   Lock-and-key concept of the action of enzyme, coenzyme, and substrate to produce a new reaction product.

Calorimetry

The kcalorie values of foods given in food tables (as found on the CD-ROM that accompanied your text) were determined by a method called direct calorimetry.[2] This method uses a metal container called a *bomb calorimeter,* named from its long tubular shape. A weighed amount of food is placed inside, and the bomb calorimeter is immersed in water. The food is then ignited by an electric spark in the presence of oxygen and burned to ash. The increase in the temperature of the surrounding water indicates the number of kcalories given off by the oxidation of the food sample. It is important to remember when you use food tables that these values represent averages from a number of samples of the given food, so the kcalorie value of a particular serving varies around that average.

Approximate Composition

An alternative method of estimating the energy value of a food is calculating the kcalories contributed by the carbohydrate, fat, and protein content as listed in food tables. These calculations are based on the average kcalorie value per gram of each of the energy-yielding macronutrients. These values are known as their respective fuel factors (Table 5-1). Note that 1 g of fat contains more than twice the number of kcalories as 1 g of carbohydrate or protein. The fuel factor for alcohol (7 kcal/g) falls about midway between fat and carbohydrate and protein.

TOTAL ENERGY REQUIREMENT

The total energy expended by an individual comes from three energy needs: (1) basal metabolism, (2) food intake effect, and (3) physical activity.

Basal Metabolic Needs

Basal Metabolic Rate

The basal metabolic rate (BMR) is a measure of the energy required to maintain the body at rest. This is the sum of all of the internal chemical activities that go on in the body plus the energy needed to fuel the brain, heart, lungs, kidneys, and other vital organs whose work continues even when the body rests.[3] Certain small but vitally active tissues—brain, liver, gastrointestinal tract, heart, and kidneys—make up less than 5% of the total body weight but contribute approximately 60% of the total basal metabolic activity. The BMR is the largest energy need, accounting for 60% to 75% of the daily energy expenditure of most persons.[4] The BMR is influenced not only by the physical characteristics of an

substrate The specific organic substance on which a particular enzyme acts to produce a new metabolic product.

hormones Internally secreted substances from the endocrine organs that are carried in the blood to another organ or tissue on which they act to stimulate functional activity or secretion. This tissue or organ is called its target tissue.

calorie The amount of heat energy needed to raise the temperature of 1 g of water from 14° C to 15° C. Because this is a small unit, we usually use the term *kilocalorie,* which is 1000 of these small calories, in the study of metabolism. A kilocalorie is the amount of heat required to raise the temperature of 1 kg of water 1° C (see also joule).

kilocalorie The general term *calorie* refers to a unit of heat measure and is used alone to designate the *small calorie.* The *large calorie,* 1000 calories or kilocalorie, is used in the study of metabolism to avoid the use of very large numbers in calculations.

joule A unit of energy. The International System of Units uses joules in place of calories to refer to food energy, and most nutrition journals require its use instead of calories (1 kcal = 4.184 kilojoules [kJ], often rounded to 4.2 kJ for ease in calculation.) A 1000-kcal diet would be equivalent to a 4200 kJ or 4.2 megajoule (MJ) diet.

calorimetry Measurement of amounts of heat absorbed or given off. *Direct method:* measurement of the heat produced by a subject enclosed in a small chamber. *Indirect method:* measurement of heat produced by a subject based on the quantity of nitrogen and carbon dioxide eliminated.

fuel factor The kilocalorie value (energy potential) of food nutrients; the number of kilocalories that 1 g of the nutrient yields when oxidized. The kilocalorie fuel factor is 4 for carbohydrate and protein, 9 for fat, and 7 for alcohol. Fuel factors are used in computing the energy values of foods and diets. (For example, 10 g of fat yields 90 kcal.)

basal metabolic rate (BMR) Amount of energy required to maintain the resting body's internal activities after an overnight fast with the subject awake. See also resting metabolic rate (RMR).

TABLE 5-1	Fuel Factors

Energy Source	Kcalories per Gram
Carbohydrate	4
Protein	4
Fat	9
Alcohol	7

BOX 5-1	Required Conditions for Measuring Basal Metabolic Rate

Overnight fast (12 to 14 hours after food intake)
Comfortably resting in a supine position
Relaxed state (no activity up to 1 hour before)
Awake but motionless
Normal body temperature
Comfortable room temperature (neither hot nor cold)

individual but also by the pretesting environment (Box 5-1).[3] In practice the BMR is seldom measured because of the many practical problems involved. Instead, the resting metabolic rate (RMR) is often used in clinical settings because it does not require the individual to be in a fasting state. It is important to recognize, however, that the RMR may be as much as 10% to 20% higher than the BMR because of energy being expended in the digestion, absorption, or metabolism of food or the delayed effect of recent physical activity.[3]

Measuring Basal Metabolic Rate

The BMR can be measured by both direct and indirect methods of calorimetry, as follows:

- *Direct calorimetry:* By the direct method a person is placed in an enclosed chamber having the capacity to measure the body's heat production while at rest. This instrument is large and costly and usually found only in research facilities.[2]
- *Indirect calorimetry:* With the indirect method a portable instrument called a *respirometer* is brought to the side of the bed or chair. In a clinical situation the complete apparatus is often called the *metabolic cart.* As the person breathes through a mouthpiece or ventilated hood, the exchange of gases in respiration, the *respiratory quotient* (CO_2/O_2), is measured. The BMR can be calculated from the rate of oxygen utilization, because more than 95% of the body's energy comes from oxidation (oxygen-related) reactions.[5] The oxygen used in the production of energy is equivalent to the heat released and so can be converted to kcalories.
- *Indirect laboratory tests:* Because the BMR is regulated by the thyroid hormone thyroxin, thyroid function tests can provide indirect measures of BMR and thyroid activity. These tests include measurements of serum *thyroid-stimulating hormone (TSH)* from the anterior pituitary gland and triiodothyronine (T_3) and thyroxin (T_4) levels. T_3 and T_4 are produced in the final stages of thyroid hormone synthesis and reflect the levels of hormones influencing the BMR. Thyroid hormone levels within the normal range indicate that cell metabolism is occurring at normal rates but cannot be used to calculate BMR.

Factors Influencing Basal Metabolic Rate

Major factors influencing BMR are body size and composition, growth, fever or disease, climate, and genetics, as explained below:

- *Body size and body composition:* The fat-free mass (FFM) is the body compartment containing muscle cells and vital body organs. It is the major factor influencing BMR because of the high metabolic activity of these tissues compared with the less active tissues of fat and bone. Differences in resting energy requirements between women and men relate to the generally lower muscle mass and higher body fat in women. The loss of organ and muscle tissues as we age lowers the BMR in older adults.[3]
- *Growth:* The increased anabolic work supported by growth hormone adds to the BMR in childhood, adolescence, pregnancy, and lactation.
- *Fever and disease:* Fever increases BMR approximately 7% for each 0.83° C (1° F) rise in body temperature. Diseases that increase cell activity such as cancer, certain anemias, cardiac failure, and chronic obstructive pulmonary disease increase BMR. Type 2 diabetes[6] and associated renal disease[7] increase the metabolic work of the body and the BMR. The involuntary muscle tremors of Parkinson's disease increase energy needs.[4] Standard prediction equations may underestimate the BMR of children with cystic fibrosis.[8] Conversely, starvation and protein-energy malnutrition lower BMR as cell metabolism slows in response to the drop in energy intake and FFM is lost.
- *Climate:* BMR rises in response to lower environmental temperatures as the body takes action to increase heat production and minimize heat loss. Opposite responses to reduce heat production and increase heat loss as environmental temperatures rise also increase the BMR. Unless weather conditions are extreme, these changes in BMR are temporary while the individual adapts to the new environment.
- *Genetics:* Race may influence BMR. Blacks appear to have a lower BMR per unit of FFM than whites, possibly related to differences in tissue composition.[9] Intrafamily differences in BMR, unrelated to age, gender, or FFM, may contribute to higher weight gain in some groups.[3]

Food Intake Effect (Thermic Effect of Food)

Taking in food stimulates body metabolism, and energy is needed to carry out the digestion, absorption, metabolism, and storage of nutrients. This overall metabolic stimulation is called the thermic effect of food (TEF). Approximately 10% of the kcalories in a meal or snack are used to process and metabolize that food, although this varies depending on the food. Macronutrients differ in their TEFs. The TEF for fat is 0% to 5%; for carbohydrate, 5% to 10%; for protein, 20% to 30%; and for alcohol, 10% to 30%.[3] The energy needed to metabolize amino acids and synthesize new proteins raises the TEF of this nutrient and may explain why a high-protein diet helps with weight maintenance.[10] The very low TEF of fat along with its high fuel factor (9 kcal/g) will accelerate weight gain on a high-fat diet.

Physical Activity Needs

Physical activity related to employment, housekeeping, recreation, organized sports, or physical training brings about wide individual variations in energy requirements. In sedentary individuals the kcalories expended in physical activity may be less than half the BMR, whereas in very active persons physical activity may require twice as many kcalories as the BMR.[3] The energy expenditures for several common activities for a person weighing 154 lb

TABLE 5-2	Calories per Hour Expended in Common Physical Activities

Activity	Approximate Calories Per Hour (154-lb Person)*
Moderate	
Hiking	370
Light gardening/yard work	330
Dancing	330
Golf (walking and carrying clubs)	330
Bicycling (<10 mph)	290
Walking (3.5 mph)	280
Weight lifting (general light workout)	220
Stretching	180
Vigorous	
Running/jogging (5 mph)	590
Bicycling (>10 mph)	590
Swimming (slow freestyle laps)	510
Aerobics	480
Walking (4.5 mph)	460
Heavy yard work (chopping wood)	440
Weight lifting (vigorous effort)	440
Basketball (vigorous)	440

From U.S. Department of Health and Human Services, U.S. Department of Agriculture: *Dietary guidelines for Americans 2005,* ed 6, Washington, DC, 2005, Authors. Accessible at *www.healthierus.gov/dietaryguidelines.*

*Calories burned per hour will be higher for persons who weigh more than 154 lb (70 kg) and lower for persons who weigh less.

This table presents examples of common physical activities and the average number of calories a 154-lb individual will expend by engaging in each activity for 1 hour. The expenditure value given includes both resting metabolic rate calories and activity expenditure. Some of the activities can be either moderate- or vigorous-intensity physical activity depending on the speed at which they are carried out (for walking and bicycling).

are given in Table 5-2, and additional listings can be found on the CD-ROM that accompanied your text. It is important to remember that the energy cost of weight-bearing movements such as walking is proportional to body weight. Thus the activity will require more kcalories for those whose body weight is higher than average and fewer kcalories for those whose body weight is lower (Figure 5-3). Regular physical activity not only supports energy balance but also reduces the risk of chronic disease.[11]

Total Energy Expenditure

Components of Energy Expenditure

The three components of energy expenditure when body weight remains constant are (1) the BMR, approximately 60% to 70% of the total energy expenditure in sedentary persons; (2) the TEF, approximately 10% of the total; and (3) the variable requirement of physical activity. Another factor sometimes added is called *nonshivering thermogenesis.* This is a response to cold that occurs in a special tissue called brown fat and increases the BMR in an effort to produce more heat.

Estimating Energy Balance

Estimating the total energy requirement for a given individual is difficult. It will be influenced by the BMR or RMR, TEF, body size and composition, age, gender, and physical activity. An expert panel defined the Estimated Energy Requirement (EER) as the energy intake that will maintain energy balance in a healthy adult of a certain age, gender, weight, height, and level of physical activity and be consistent with good health.[3] Typical ranges for energy expenditure at rest are 0.8 to 1.0 kcal/min for women and 1.1 to 1.3 kcal/min for men. (One kilocalorie per minute is about equal to the heat released by a burning candle or

supine **Lying down**

resting metabolic rate (RMR) Amount of energy required to maintain the resting body's internal activities when in a comfortable environmental temperature and awake. Because of small differences in measuring techniques, an individual's RMR and BMR (basal metabolic rate) differ slightly. In practice, however, RMR and BMR measurements are used interchangeably.

thermic effect of food (TEF) Body heat produced by food; the amount of energy required to digest and absorb food and transport nutrients to the cells. This work accounts for about 10% of the day's total energy (kcalorie) requirement.

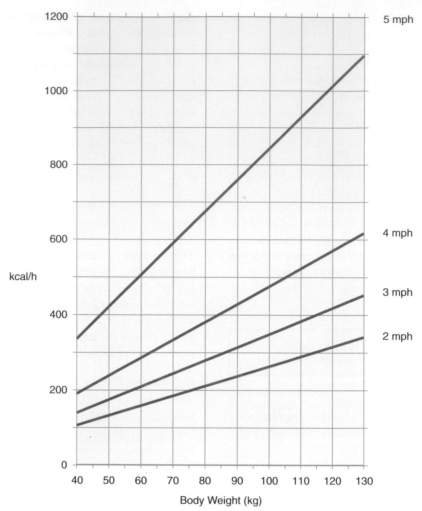

FIGURE 5-3   Effect of body weight on energy expenditure while walking at different speeds. Both body weight and walking speed influence the kcalories needed. Persons with a higher body weight use more kcalories in weight-bearing activities than persons with a lower body weight; also, the faster you walk the more kcalories you will use. *(Redrawn from Food and Nutrition Board, Institute of Medicine:* Dietary reference intakes for energy, carbohydrate, fiber, fat, fatty acids, cholesterol, protein, and amino acids (macronutrients), *Washington, DC, 2002, National Academies Press.)*

75-watt bulb over the course of a minute.[3]) Differences in body dimensions and the proportion of body fat versus muscle influence the EER. Individuals with a higher amount of body fat and a lower proportion of muscle and other active tissues will likely need fewer kcalories. Table 5-3 describes how age and physical activity influence the EER. Both persons within each gender have the same body weight and height. Long-term energy balance may be favorably influenced by particular foods or their components. Higher intakes of whole grain foods contributing fiber, phytochemicals, and trace minerals to the diet were associated with lower weight gain among middle-age and older men.[12] Energy requirements rise in pregnancy, lactation, and other periods of rapid growth and elevated metabolism. (In the clinical setting, standard prediction equations are often used to estimate energy requirements. We will learn about these methods in Chapter 18.)

TABLE 5-3	**Estimated Energy Requirements (EERs) Based on Activity Level and Age**

	Male (178 lb, 71 in*) Kcalories		Female (132 lb, 61 in*) Kcalories	
Activity Level	**Age 25**	**Age 65**	**Age 25**	**Age 65**
Very sedentary	2685	2285	1869	1589
Low active	2934	2534	2072	1792
Active	3250	2850	2325	2045
Very active	3770	3370	2628	2348

Calculations based on data presented in Food and Nutrition Board, Institute of Medicine: *Dietary Reference Intakes for energy, carbohydrate, fiber, fat, fatty acids, cholesterol, protein, and amino acids (macronutrients),* Washington, DC, 2002, National Academies Press.

*An individual of this height and weight has a BMI of approximately 25 kg/m².

BODY COMPOSITION: FATNESS AND LEANNESS

Individuals have different body shapes and sizes depending on their age, gender, genetic background, state of health, and body type. Ectomorphs have a body type that is generally slender and fragile, mesomorphs have prominent muscle and bone development, and endomorphs have a soft, round physique with some accumulation of body fat (Figure 5-4). Although each person's body type has a genetic base, dietary intake and physical activity influence how that body type is expressed. Particular body types are associated with better health, whereas others carry increased risk of chronic disease. We need to be sensitive to different body types when developing strategies to improve body composition and health status.

Body Weight and Body Fat

Overweight Versus Overfat

Because body weight and body height are easily measured, they are commonly used to evaluate health status. We need to recognize what these measurements do and do not tell us. The terms *overweight* and obesity have distinct meanings as related to body composition and health, and these distinctions are important. A football player in peak physical condition can be markedly "overweight" according to standard height-weight charts. That is, he weighs more than the average man of his height, but his body tissues are likely to be very different than might be expected. A sedentary man above average weight likely has an excess amount of body fat that is adding to his total body weight. The athlete above average weight likely has an exceptionally large amount of muscle. In fact the athlete above average weight may have a lower proportion of body fat than a sedentary individual of normal weight. When overweight is the result of excessive body fat rather than enhanced muscle or skeletal tissue, the term *overfat* or obese is the appropriate word to be used. In a later section we will learn how to evaluate the body weight of a given individual.

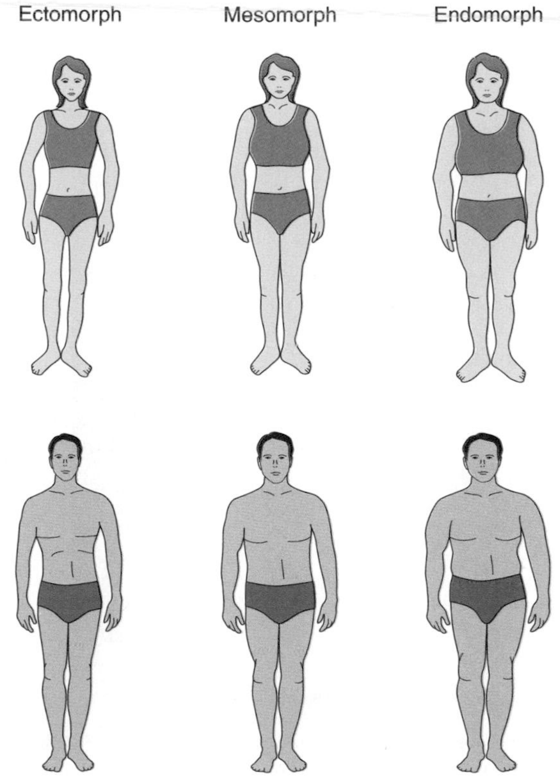

Body Composition

The critical element when evaluating body build and health is body composition. What we really need to know is how much of a person's body weight is fat and how much is FFM. It is more precise to think in terms of *fatness* and *leanness* rather than body weight or overweight. When speaking of body weight we need to ask for whom, under what circumstances, and by what measures. We need to consider individual body composition when developing a plan of care.

Body compartments are often defined on the basis of their comparative size and level of metabolic activity. The four-compartment model for evaluating body composition includes lean body mass (LBM), body fat, body water, and mineral mass (mainly bone), as follows:

1. *Lean body mass:* This compartment made up of active, fat-free cells from muscle and vital organs largely determines the BMR and related energy and nutrient needs. It changes through the life cycle and in adulthood constitutes 30% to 65% of the total body weight. In sedentary individuals it accounts for almost the entire energy requirement. When persons lose weight by lowering their energy intake, the weight lost reflects changes in both body fat and LBM. Physical activity and weight-bearing exercise are essential for maintaining muscle mass across the adult years.
2. *Body fat:* Total body fat reflects both the number and the size of fat cells (the adipocytes) that form the

Ectomorph   Mesomorph   Endomorph

FIGURE 5-4 Body types: the ectomorph, the mesomorph, and the endomorph.

obesity Fatness; an excessive accumulation of fat in the body.

body composition The relative sizes of the four body compartments that make up the total body: lean body mass (muscles and organs), fat, water, and mineral.

adipocyte A fat cell. All cell names end in the suffix *-cyte,* with the type of cell indicated by the root word to which it is added.

adipose tissue. In an adult male of normal weight, fat makes up 13% to 21% of body weight. In a woman of normal weight the range is 23% to 31%. These amounts vary with age, body type, level of exercise, and fitness, and as we will see later in this chapter, many persons have body fat levels markedly above or below these ranges. About half of all body fat is located in the subcutaneous fat layers under the skin, where it serves as insulation. In children and young adults the subcutaneous fat provides a useful measure—the triceps skinfold—for estimating body fat. As individuals grow older, more body fat is deposited on the trunk and less on the extremities, so waist or hip circumference is more representative of body fatness and health risk.[13]

3. *Body water:* Body water varies with relative leanness or fatness, age, hydration status, and health status. Generally water makes up approximately 50% to 65% of body weight. Muscle tissue has high water content, whereas adipose tissue contains relatively little water. Infants have a relatively high proportion of body water, which drops to adult levels by age 2.[8]

4. *Mineral mass:* The mineral mass, found largely in the skeleton, accounts for only 4% to 6% of body weight. The major minerals are calcium and phosphorus, located in bone as well as in other body cells and fluids.

The following various factors influence the relative sizes of the body compartments[14]:

- *Gender:* Women have more fat tissue, and men have more lean tissue, particularly muscle.
- *Age:* Younger adults have more LBM and less fat than older adults.
- *Physical exercise:* Persons who have a high level of physical activity have less fat and more LBM than persons with a sedentary lifestyle.
- *Race:* Black men and women have greater bone mineral than white and Hispanic men and women.
- *Climate:* Individuals living in very cold climates develop more subcutaneous fat to insulate against body heat loss.

Need for Body Fat

Although an excess of body fat is detrimental to health, some body fat is necessary for survival. In times of human starvation, victims die from fat loss, not protein depletion. For mere survival men require about 3% body fat and women require about 12%. However, for the human race to continue we must be able to work and reproduce. For reproductive capacity women require a body fat of about 20%. The initiation of menstruation or menarche occurs when the female body reaches a certain size or, more precisely, this critical proportion of body fat. The

body fat gained during pregnancy serves as an important energy reserve for lactation. The production of breast milk with a high energy cost usually brings about a gradual loss of these body fat stores. Ill-advised dieting during pregnancy in an attempt to avoid normal weight gain interferes with the development of the fetus and can result in a low-birth-weight infant at risk for various health problems.

Measuring Body Composition

Specialized Equipment

Estimating the relative proportions of body fat and LBM is useful for evaluating health status. Some methods that accurately estimate body fat and LBM involve very costly equipment and specialized procedures applicable only to a research setting. The classic method for determining body composition was hydrostatic weighing using Archimedes' principle. The individual was first weighed in air and then weighed under water, and the volume of water displaced was measured. In a new application of this principle an individual is weighed in air and then introduced to an air-controlled chamber, referred to as a "pod," in which the air displaced by the volume of the body can be measured (Figure 5-5).[15] Both methods take advantage of the fact that body fat and lean tissue differ in density, and standard calculations can be applied. The air displacement method offers an opportunity for measuring individuals who could not be weighed under water.

Other methods used to evaluate body composition include dual-energy x-ray absorptiometry (DEXA) that dif-

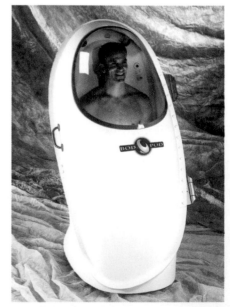

FIGURE 5-5 A "pod" for measuring body composition. The BOD POD uses air displacement technology to measure body composition. *(Courtesy Life Measurement, Inc., Concord, Calif.)*

ferentiates among muscle, fat, and bone.[14] DEXA is an effective way to measure bone mineral density and age-related bone loss. Bioelectrical impedance systems that pass a very small current of electricity through the body can distinguish water, fat, and bone, and are sometimes used in clinical settings. Body fat and muscle can be estimated from measurements of body circumferences and skinfold thicknesses. (These methods will be discussed in more detail in Chapter 16.)

Reference Height-Weight Tables

In many situations body height and weight are the only measurements available for estimating body composition. In that case these measurements can be compared to reference tables that suggest an appropriate body weight for a person of a given height and gender.

The first height-weight tables were constructed in the 1930s by the Metropolitan Life Insurance Company using information obtained from their life insurance policyholders, mostly white middle-age men. Desirable weights were based on the body weights of the policyholders that lived the longest. Early height-weight tables also provided adult reference weights according to age based on the assumption that weight gain continued throughout adult life. In recent years several new concepts have emerged regarding height-weight tables. First, body weight (and body fat) should not increase as individuals move into middle and older ages. Second, body build and body fat patterns may differ among racial and ethnic groups, such that height weight tables based on white populations may not be appropriate for black, Hispanic, or Asian groups.[16-19]

Height-weight tables are the method of choice for health screening in the clinical setting. Reference tables for evaluating body weight and body fat include (1) height-weight tables established by government agencies and (2) body mass index (BMI) standards.

Height-Weight Tables From Government Agencies

Nutrition and health professionals from the U.S. Department of Health and Human Services and the U.S. Department of Agriculture have developed appropriate reference standards for the general public.[3,20,21] The *Dietary Guidelines for Americans 2005* (Table 5-4) suggests appropriate ranges of body weight for adults of a given height as related to the BMI.[21] These reference weights, however, exceed those from earlier height-weight tables because they are based on measurements obtained from U.S. adults in recent national surveys. Americans are becoming taller and heavier, but body weights are rising at a faster rate than body heights.[22,23] Since 1960 the average body weight of adult females increased by 24 lb (from 140 to 164 lb), although body height increased less than 1 inch. Men increased in average weight from 166 lb to 191 lb (a

gain of 25 lb) with about an inch increase in height. Age becomes a factor when evaluating the risk associated with a rise in body weight. Moderate obesity has a drastic effect on cardiovascular risk in younger men, but body fat does not add substantially to mortality risk in older adults.[24]

Body Mass Index

The BMI developed by Quetelet in 1871 has become the medical standard to define obesity. Although based on body weight and body height measurements, BMI provides a better estimate of body fat than do simple height-weight tables. BMI values correlate well with estimates of total body fat obtained by underwater weighing and effectively predict the rise in health risk associated with excessive body fat. The BMI can be calculated as follows:

$$\text{BMI} = \text{Weight (kg)} \div \text{Height (m)}^2$$
Weight: 1 kg = 2.2 lb
Height: 1 m = 39.37 inches

The desirable BMI range for adults is 18.5 to 24.9 kg/m². Health risks associated with overweight begin at 25 kg/m² and become apparent at 30 kg/m². Values above 35 kg/m² indicate severe obesity (Table 5-5).[3] (See the *Focus on Culture* box, "Evaluating Body Composition: One Size Really Doesn't Fit All," which points to the influence of race and ethnicity on body build and implications for using standard measures such as BMI and waist circumference.)

Waist-to-Hip Ratio

Not only the amount of body fat but also where it is positioned can influence health. Over the years researchers have defined the *apple* versus the *pear* shape (Figure 5-6). The pear shape with a smaller waist and larger hip (gynoid shape) is characteristic of women and controlled to some extent by the female sex hormone estrogen. The apple shape with fat around the abdomen (android shape) is more commonly found in men and postmenopausal women. Because abdominal (visceral) fat contributes to high blood lipid levels and increases the risk of cardiovascular disease, the waist-to-hip ratio has been used to evaluate health risk. An appropriate ratio is 0.9 or less (indicating a smaller waist and larger hip measurement).

---

menarche The first menstruation with the onset of puberty.

visceral Referring to the organs in the abdominal cavity.

TABLE 5-4 | Adult BMI Chart

To determine BMI, locate the height of interest in the left-most column and read across the row for that height to the weight of interest. Follow the column of the weight up to the top row that lists the BMI. A BMI of 18.5 to 24.9 is the healthy-weight range, BMI of 25 to 29.9 is the overweight range, and BMI of 30 and above is in the obese range.

BMI	19	20	21	22	23	24	25	26	27	28	29	30	31	32	33	34	35
Height									Weight in Pounds								
4'10"	91	96	100	105	110	115	119	124	129	134	138	143	148	153	158	162	167
4'11"	94	99	104	109	114	119	124	128	133	138	143	148	153	158	163	168	173
5'	97	102	107	112	118	123	128	133	138	143	148	153	158	163	158	174	179
5'1"	100	106	111	116	122	127	132	137	143	148	153	158	164	169	174	180	185
5'2"	104	109	115	120	126	131	136	142	147	153	158	164	169	175	180	186	191
5'3"	107	113	118	124	130	135	141	146	152	158	163	169	175	180	186	191	197
5'4"	110	116	122	128	134	140	145	151	157	163	169	174	180	186	192	197	204
5'5"	114	120	126	132	138	144	150	156	162	168	174	180	186	192	198	204	210
5'6"	118	124	130	136	142	148	155	161	167	173	179	186	192	198	204	210	216
5'7"	121	127	134	140	146	153	159	166	172	178	185	191	198	204	211	217	223
5'8"	125	131	138	144	151	158	164	171	177	184	190	197	203	210	216	223	230
5'9"	128	135	142	149	155	162	169	176	182	189	196	203	209	216	223	230	236
5'10"	132	139	146	153	160	167	174	181	188	195	202	209	216	222	229	236	243
5'11"	136	143	150	157	165	172	179	186	193	200	208	215	222	229	236	243	250
6'	140	147	154	162	169	177	184	191	199	206	213	221	228	235	242	250	258
6'1"	144	151	159	166	174	182	189	197	204	212	219	227	235	242	250	257	265
6'2"	148	155	163	171	179	186	194	202	210	218	225	233	241	249	256	264	272
6'3"	152	160	168	176	184	192	200	208	216	224	232	240	248	256	264	272	279
	Healthy Weight						Overweight					Obese					

From U.S. Department of Health and Human Services, U.S. Department of Agriculture: *Dietary guidelines for Americans 2005,* ed 6, Washington, DC, 2005, Authors. Accessible at *www.healthierus.gov/dietaryguidelines.*

Source: National Institutes of Health, National Heart, Lung, and Blood Institute: *Evidence report of clinical guidelines on the identification, evaluation, and treatment of overweight and obesity in adults,* Bethesda, Md, 1998, Author.

TABLE 5-5 | Body Mass Index and Percent Body Fat

BMI (kg/m^2)	Body Weight Status	Body Fat (%): Men	Body Fat (%): Women
<18.5	Underweight	<13	<23
18.5-24.9	Normal	13-21	23-31
25-29.9	Overweight	21-25	31-37
30-34.9	Obese	25-31	37-42
≥35	Severely obese	>31	>42

From Food and Nutrition Board, Institute of Medicine: *Dietary Reference Intakes for energy, carbohydrate, fiber, fat, fatty acids, cholesterol, protein, and amino acids (macronutrients),* Washington, DC, 2002, National Academies Press.

◆ FOCUS ON CULTURE

Evaluating Body Composition: One Size Really Doesn't Fit All

When assessing a person's nutritional status and chronic disease risk, an important piece of information is the relative size of each body compartment. Lean body mass gives us an estimate of body protein and muscle mass, and the amount of body mineral can tell us if bone mineral is at an appropriate level or if this person is at risk for bone fracture. Finally, the proportion of body fat indicates the future risk of such conditions as diabetes or heart disease. Over the years researchers have developed sensitive equipment and standards for physical measurements that are used to obtain information on body composition useful in health assessment. However, the body relationships used as standards in these calculations were derived mostly from evaluations of white populations.

Recent studies tell us that various races and ethnic groups differ in both their body composition and their risk for chronic disease based on a specific proportion of body fat. We have known for some time that black persons have higher bone mineral than white persons, and Asians have the lowest amount of bone mineral per unit of body weight.[1] Total body potassium is sometimes used as a marker to assess the amount of lean body mass that an individual has. Blacks have the highest proportion of body potassium per unit of height followed by white persons and Hispanic persons. Asians have the lowest amount of body potassium for a given height.[2] Based on these differences, standard equations used to calculate lean body mass or body mineral need to be adjusted to reflect these different body proportions.

Estimates of body fat using the body mass index (BMI) have been compared with estimates obtained by x ray methods in men and women of different races and ethnicities. In women the BMI underestimated the proportion of body fat in Hispanic American women and overestimated the proportion of body fat in white women at BMI levels indicating overweight or obesity. There were no differences among the white, African American, or Hispanic American men.[3]

There are also differences in the disease risk associated with certain BMI and waist circumference measurements among persons of different genetic backgrounds.[4] Even slight increases in body weight and body fat carry greater health risks for Chinese men and women than for other groups. Chinese adults with a BMI below 25, the U.S. standard for normal weight, had increased risk of hypertension, hyperlipidemia, and diabetes. Of those considered to be normal weight, 40% had one of these conditions and almost 15% had two of the three. The World Health Organization defines overweight or obesity as a waist circumference greater than 94 cm in men and greater than 80 cm in women. In the Chinese adults the prevalence of chronic disease was also high in men whose waist circumference was below 94 cm.

It is apparent that common measurements and standards now used to evaluate body fat content are not equally appropriate for all population groups. Groups may differ in their genetically determined amounts and locations of total body fat. Different relationships among the various body compartments may interfere with some of these standard measurements. It is important that we define assessment methods and standards for each race and ethnic group that will accurately target disease risk and early intervention.

References

1. Sun AJ et al: Is there an association between skeletal muscle mass and bone mineral density among African-American, Asian-American, and European-American women, *Acta Diabetol* 40:S309, 2003.
2. He Q et al: Total body potassium differs by sex and race across the adult age span, *Am J Clin Nutr* 78:72, 2003.
3. Fernandez JR et al: Is percentage of body fat differentially related to body mass index in Hispanic Americans, African-Americans, and European Americans, *Am J Clin Nutr* 77:71, 2003.
4. Wildman RP et al: Appropriate body mass index and waist circumference cutoffs for categorization of overweight and central adiposity among Chinese adults, *Am J Clin Nutr* 80:1129, 2004.

Waist circumference measurements also serve as a tool for evaluating an individual's abdominal fat and health status.[20] Alcohol intake influences abdominal obesity. Individuals having four or more drinks at a drinking session have increased abdominal fat.[25]

Health Promotion

Finding a Healthy Weight

The basic problem with the concept of normal body weight is that it cannot be defined for many people. Body weight is influenced by a number of factors including age, body type, metabolic rate, genetic makeup, gender, and physical activity. One's amount of body fat and its location on the body can differ based on age, gender, and race.[1,26] In the traditional sense overweight (or an excess of body fat) represents an energy imbalance coming from a surplus in energy input (fuel from food) over energy output (total energy expenditure). However, it is not that simple. Our genetic makeup influences weight gain and body weight. Certain individuals have an exceptionally low RMR caused by an inherited obesity gene.[5] Fidgeting increases energy expenditure and helps some persons resist weight gain even if overfed.[27]

Just as weight gain results from a surplus of kcalories, weight loss should result from a deficit of kcalories. A deficit of 3500 kcal is expected to bring about the loss of 1 lb of body fat. But body mechanisms designed to preserve body mass may act to decrease spontaneous activity (e.g., fidgeting) or reduce BMR, making weight loss more difficult. There may be individuals for whom the weight loss required to move them into a more appropriate weight range will not be possible. So what should be our approach to a healthy weight?

Developing a Healthy Lifestyle

Successful weight management to improve overall health requires a lifelong commitment to positive lifestyle behaviors emphasizing sustainable and enjoyable eating habits and daily physical activity.[1] A sound food and activity pattern should be the goal rather than weight loss at all costs. The loss of even 10 to 15 lb can bring about functional improvements in blood glucose levels and blood pressure.[1] Following a meal plan lower in fat and sodium and rich in fruits, vegetables, whole grains, and fiber at an energy level that prevents weight gain improves well-being regardless of weight loss. A stable weight supported by a positive diet plan and regular physical activity, even if above one's recommended weight, is desired over regular cycles of weight loss followed by even greater weight gain. (See Chapter 1 for examples of sound eating plans.)

The *Dietary Guidelines for Americans 2005* recommends that all adults obtain at least 30 minutes of physical activity most days of the week and 60 minutes or more may be necessary to achieve or maintain weight loss. Walking for even 15 minutes a day and gradually increasing to longer periods is a safe way to get started and promotes fitness. Dividing physical activity across the day may work better for some people. Regular activity to achieve physical fitness (the ability to walk or jog at 5 mph) lowers the risk of heart attack by 20% even when individuals remain obese.[11] An added benefit of physical activity is the increase in energy expenditure that can continue up to 15 hours after the activity is completed.[3] (We will learn to develop activity programs in Chapter 14.) (See the *Focus on Food Safety* box, "Safe Snacking," for snacks to carry with you on hikes or bicycle trips.)

Evaluating Your Energy Balance

Where do you stand in your own energy balance? Try estimating your energy requirement and evaluate your body weight using the (1) BMI and (2) a height-weight table (see the *Perspectives in Practice* box, "Evaluating Your Energy Expenditure and Body Weight").

FATNESS, THINNESS, AND HEALTH

Rise in Obesity

Attitudes regarding obesity have undergone many changes over the years. In colonial times obesity was a sign of eco-

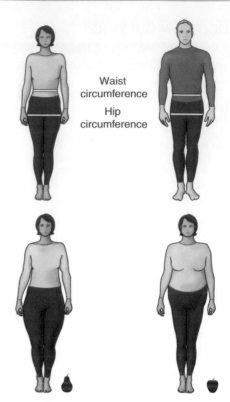

FIGURE 5-6   The pear versus the apple shape. Those with an apple shape and a larger amount of abdominal fat have a greater risk of chronic disease than those with a pear shape. (*From Grodner M, Long S, DeYoung S:* Foundations and clinical applications of nutrition: a nursing approach, *ed 3, St. Louis, 2004, Mosby, An Affiliate of Elsevier.*)

FOCUS ON FOOD SAFETY
Safe Snacking

Hiking, bicycle trips, an active game of soccer, or an hour workout at a fitness center can make you hungry. It is a good idea to take a snack with you to provide the energy you need, but be sure to choose foods that can be carried safely in a backpack or gym bag. Foods high in carbohydrate that will replenish your energy supply and do not need to be kept cold are bottled or boxed juices; fruit such as oranges, apples, or bananas; or crackers and peanut butter. Trail or granola mix also supplies energy but can be high in fat. Don't take a chance on spoiling your outing with an attack of food-borne illness. Always read the label to be sure that a food does not require refrigeration.

nomic well-being and identified a family that was prosperous. In recent years we have come to recognize the health risks associated with obesity, and 16.5% of adults are dieting for health reasons.[28] Yet the number of persons with a BMI of 25 or over continues to rise. Only 43% of U.S. adults have a healthy weight.[29] Limited-resource families[29] who have poor diets, hazardous living conditions, and limited access to healthcare are also more likely to be obese.

PERSPECTIVES IN PRACTICE
Evaluating Your Energy Expenditure and Body Weight

As a health professional you will be assisting others in defining their energy needs and evaluating their body weight and body fat using established standards. This exercise will give you experience in carrying out these activities and help you assess your own energy expenditure and weight status. Remember: underweight is as needful of intervention as overweight or obesity.

A. Calculate Your Total Energy Output per Day

Your total energy output in kcalories per day is the sum of your body's three uses of energy, as follows:
1. Resting metabolic rate (RMR)
2. Thermic effect of food (TEF)
3. Physical activity

1. Resting Metabolic Rate

Calculate your RMR using the following general formula[1]:
a. Select one of the following:
   Women: 0.9 kcal/kg/hr
   Men: 1.0 kcal/kg/hr
b. Convert your body weight (lb) to kg: 1 kg =
   2.2 lb Body wt (lbs) ÷ 2.2 = _____
c. RMR (kcalories) = 0.9 or 1.0 × kg Body weight ×
   24 (Hours in day) = _____

2. Thermic Effect of Food (TEF)

The TEF is the energy the body uses in digesting and absorbing the food you eat. TEF equals about 10% of the kcalorie value of our food intake. The factors we will use to estimate our energy expenditure in physical activity take into consideration the kcalories required for the TEF, so we will not add those kcalories in our calculation. But you need to be aware of this component as part of your total energy expenditure.

3. Physical Activity

Estimate your average level of physical activity. Energy expended in physical activity varies with both the time and intensity of the activity. There are two methods that you can use to estimate the kcalories used in physical activity. You can calculate activity kcalories using a 24-hour activity record or approximate your activity kcalories from your RMR.

Calculating Your Physical Activity Kcalories Using an Activity Record

Recording your physical activity over a 24-hour period is much like recording your food intake. Prepare a chart that allows you to record the time you start and stop each activity and the type of activity. Review the activities expenditure database on the CD-ROM that accompanied your textbook to become familiar with the various activities listed so you can be sure to indicate the appropriate amount of detail when keeping your record. Carry a notebook with you as you did when recording your food intake for the day (see Chapter 1). Using the energy expenditures assigned to your body weight (in pounds), calculate your total energy expenditure over a 24-hour period. Keep in mind when performing your calculations that the energy expenditures given in the activities expenditure database indicate the *kcalories used per hour* and include *the total kcalories expended for RMR needs, TEF needs, and physical activity needs for the given period of time and body weight;* thus you must sum only the time-corrected values obtained from that table to estimate your total energy expenditure for the day.

Approximating Your Physical Activity Kcalories Using Your RMR

Because your RMR is based on your body weight, your energy expenditure in physical activity can be calculated using a factor that estimates your level of activity.

Nutrition experts have defined several levels of physical activity and developed factors that estimate the kcalories required.[1] Look at the definitions below, and see which meets your general level of activity. If your only physical activity for the day involves the casual walking and activities we all perform as part of our daily living, you are a sedentary individual. Additional activity involving walking at a brisk pace, running, sports, dancing, or use of some type of fitness equipment is needed for the higher categories of activity.

Usual Activity Pattern	Definition	Physical Activity Factor*
Sedentary	Normal activities required for independent living	0.2
Low active	Normal activities required for independent living plus at least 30 to 60 minutes of moderately intensive activity	0.5
Active	Normal activities required for independent living plus *more* than 60 minutes of moderately intensive activity or a mix of moderately intensive and vigorous activity	0.7
Very active	Normal activities required for independent living plus 2 hours or more of vigorous activity	1.2

For numerous examples of moderate and vigorous activities, see the document entitled "General Physical Activities Defined by Level of Intensity," which is accessible on the website of the Centers for Disease Control and Prevention (CDC): *www.cdc.gov/nccdphp/dnpa/physical/measuring/index.htm.*

Calculate the energy cost of your physical activity using the physical activity factor that is the best fit with your current activity level.

Physical activity kcalories = RMR × Physical activity factor

For example, if you are sedentary, you would multiply your RMR by 0.2, as follows:

Physical activity kcalories = _____ (RMR) × 0.2 = _____

4. Calculate Your Total Energy Expenditure

Total energy expenditure (kcalories) = RMR + Physical activity kcalories (calculated using a physical activity factor as above)

Total energy expenditure = _____ RMR kcalories +
_____ Physical activity kcalories = _____

Refer to the dietary intake record that you completed as part of the *Perspectives in Practice* box in Chapter 1, and consider the following questions:
- How does your energy intake compare with your estimated total energy expenditure completed above? Are you taking in more kcalories, less kcalories, or about the same number of kcalories as you are using each day?
- What will be the effect on your body weight if you continue this pattern? What will be the effect on your health status?

*The physical activity factors used in this assignment represent the midpoint of the range given for each activity level.

Continued

PERSPECTIVES IN PRACTICE—cont'd
Evaluating Your Energy Expenditure and Body Weight

B. Evaluate Your Body Weight Status According to the Body Mass Index

1. Calculate Your Body Mass Index

Body mass index (BMI) is usually calculated in metric terms as follows:

BMI = Weight (kg) ÷ Height (m)^2

BMI can also be calculated using weight in pounds and height in inches, using calculation factors as follows:

Step 1: Body weight (lb) × 705 = _____
Step 2: Result from step 1 ÷ Height (in) = _____
Step 3: Result from step 2 ÷ Height (in) = BMI _____

You can also determine your BMI using Table 5-4 on p. 96. Health risks associated with overweight begin at a BMI of 25, and individuals with a BMI of 30 or above have growing levels of risk (see Table 5-5 on p. 96).

Based on your calculated BMI, consider the following questions:
- What is your assessment of your body weight status using the BMI? Are you underweight, overweight, or in the healthful range?
- If you are not in the healthful range, how might you begin to improve your health status?

Reference

1. Food and Nutrition Board, Institute of Medicine: *Dietary Reference Intakes for energy, carbohydrate, fiber, fat, fatty acids, cholesterol, protein, and amino acids (macronutrients)*, Washington, DC, 2002, National Academies Press.

Obesity and Health

Obesity and overweight have important implications for health. Weight-related problems can be divided into four categories: (1) metabolic, (2) degenerative, (3) neoplastic, and (4) anatomic, as described below:

1. *Metabolic problems:* Type 2 diabetes, hypertension, and elevated blood lipids often accompany obesity. Regardless of total body fat, abdominal fat raises the risk of metabolic disorders.[30]
2. *Degenerative problems:* Obesity and physical disability are strongly linked.[31] Osteoarthritis and joint problems, atherosclerotic changes, and pulmonary diseases are more serious in obese persons.[1]
3. *Neoplastic problems:* Many forms of cancer including colorectal, breast, prostate, esophageal, and ovarian cancer are more frequent in higher weight categories.
4. *Anatomic problems:* Individuals exceeding a healthy weight have greater risk of gastroesophageal reflux disease (GERD) and obstructive sleep apnea.

The growing prevalence of obesity among children and youth will have an impact on future health care costs.[32] Cumulative Medicare expenditures for the treatment of diabetes and related diseases are more than doubled in women with a BMI of 35 or over as compared to those with a BMI below 25. The rise in obesity-related type 2 diabetes in children, who will require lifetime care for this dangerous disease, will add to such costs.

Emerging Attitudes About Obesity and Its Treatment

A major shift in treatment goals that promotes *shared responsibility* rather than *control*[1] has emerged from our growing understanding of the psychologic and social factors surrounding fatness. We must involve our patients in setting treatment goals that emphasize physical health rather than cosmetic appearance. The *Dietary Guidelines for Americans 2005*[21] underscores the importance of developing food and exercise patterns that will support life-long weight management. (Chapter 15 will help us focus on the environmental factors in our society that favor the development of obesity.)

Obsession With Thinness

A trend opposite to obesity but equally harmful to health is the model of thinness directed toward women in our society. Fueled by advertising dollars, an image of thinness drives the marketing of clothes, cosmetics, and food to teenagers and young adults. Social pressures have created an abnormally thin and unrealistic ideal to the point that even fashion models express dissatisfaction with their overall body shapes.[33] Fears of fatness develop as early as elementary school. Fifty-one percent of girls ages 9 and 10 said they felt better about themselves when they were on a diet.[34] When parents restrict food intake to prevent overweight, children may overeat when those restricted foods are available.[35,36] Guilt feelings after eating certain foods and distorted perceptions of body size often form the basis for serious eating disorders that threaten nutritional and physical health. School programs, voluntary community programs, and sports programs can offer primary prevention for disordered eating.

The family setting can help youth develop positive attitudes toward food. Adolescents who eat more meals with their family are less likely to take on extreme weight control practices such as diet pills, laxatives or diuretics, or forced vomiting.[37] Parents should be encouraged to set schedules that allow family members to eat their evening meal together at least several times during the week.

Chronic Dieting

The ongoing quest for the perfect body has given rise to the chronic dieter who constantly tries to restrict food intake.[38] Although restrained eating is most often seen in women trying to lose weight, dieting is a concern for boys and girls. In a study of 4144 adolescents from diverse racial and socioeconomic backgrounds, only 12% of the girls and about 30% of the boys were *not* trying to either lose or avoid gaining weight.[39] While dieting most often involves efforts to lose weight, adolescent boys may follow inappropriate diets in an attempt to gain weight or increase muscle mass.

Eating Disorders

The pursuit of thinness may lead adolescents or adults to restrict their food intake to the point where it becomes life-threatening and requires medical intervention. Eating disorders include anorexia nervosa, bulimia nervosa, and binge eating disorder, as follows[40,41]:

- *Anorexia nervosa:* This form of self-induced starvation is more common in females than in males. Individuals with anorexia nervosa are terrified of gaining weight and refuse to eat, even though they may be hungry. They see themselves as overweight or obese, even when they are severely underweight or emaciated. A small percentage of these young victims die from this disorder.
- *Bulimia nervosa:* This gorging-purging syndrome involves both emotional and physical concerns. Patients with bulimia nervosa are likely to be normal weight or moderately overweight and use laxatives or self-induced vomiting to lose or keep from gaining weight.[42]
- *Eating disorders not otherwise specified (EDNOS):* Some eating disorders do not meet the criteria of any specific one. For example, eating behavior may be similar to anorexia nervosa, but body weight remains normal.[40]
- *Binge eating disorder (an EDNOS):* Binge eating is eating very large amounts of food in a short period of time. This differs from bulimia nervosa in that binge eating is not followed by purging using self-induced vomiting or laxatives.

The *To Probe Further* box, "Eating Disorders: A High Price for Thinness," describes these conditions in more detail.

Successful intervention of eating disorders requires a team approach including a nurse, physician, dentist, dietitian, psychologist, and psychiatrist. Patients with eating disorders need assessment and treatment for their medical and nutritional health, as well as counseling for the emotional and psychologic issues that first led to the problem.[41] Extensive and specialized training and experience are necessary for working with these patients.

THE PROBLEM OF UNDERWEIGHT

Up to this point we discussed the problem of excess body weight and body fat and situations in which individuals deliberately limit their food intake. Now we consider the causes and effects of underweight as related to lack of food or serious illness.

Definition

Extreme underweight can lead to or accompany serious health problems in both adults and children.[43,44] *Underweight,* defined as a BMI of less than 18.5, is uncommon in the United States but does occur in a small percentage of people.[29] Although a national survey identified only 2.3% of adults as underweight, the numbers were higher among women between the ages of 18 and 24, women over age 74, and Asian/Pacific Islanders. Nearly 5% of low-income children between the ages of 2 and 4 are underweight.[45] Underweight springs from poverty, poor living conditions, long-term illness, or physiologic changes. Infants and young children and older adults are at greatest risk. Low weight-for-age (a measure of malnutrition) causes more than 50% of the child deaths in developing countries.[44] Very underweight children can experience long term growth retardation. Resistance to infection is lower, general health is poor, and physical strength is reduced in seriously underweight individuals of all ages. Underweight older adult veterans scored lower on quality-of-life measures relating to physical function, health perception, and mental and emotional well-being than normal weight or overweight adults of the same age.[46]

---

neoplastic Describing abnormal growth of tissue, usually associated with the formation of tumors.

anorexia nervosa Extreme psychophysiologic aversion to food resulting in life-threatening weight loss. A psychiatric eating disorder caused by a morbid fear of fat in which a distorted body image is reflected as fat when actually the body is malnourished and thin from self-starvation.

bulimia nervosa A psychiatric eating disorder in which cycles of gorging on large quantities of food are followed by self-induced vomiting and use of diuretics and laxatives to maintain a "normal" body weight.

binge eating An eating disorder in which individuals consume large amounts of food in a short period of time, but without the purging behavior of bulimia nervosa.

TO PROBE FURTHER

EATING DISORDERS: A HIGH PRICE FOR THINNESS

More than 5 million Americans have eating disorders, and about 85% begin in adolescence.[1] Although eating disorders are classified as psychiatric disorders, they lead to nutritional deficiencies and medical complications and, if continued, eventual disability and death. We associate eating disorders with our society's current emphasis on thinness, but physicians in Great Britain and France described anorexia nervosa in the 1800s.

What Leads to Eating Disorders?

Biologic, psychologic, and social forces all play a part in producing the behavior that we associate with eating disorders.[2] In some cases hormonal changes associated with puberty are involved. Social pressures and perceived difficulty in meeting expectations of family or others may be a cause. Prior history of substance abuse[2] or physical abuse[1] are risk factors for disordered eating. For every individual who develops an eating disorder, a particular factor may be more important or less important. Eating disorders are found in all social classes and demographic groups. Adolescent females are thought to be especially vulnerable, although the incidence is increasing in adolescent males. The males often have a history of obesity, which may have led them to begin dieting.[3]

The growing interest in athletics among children and youth can either increase risk or assist in prevention. Those participating in activities in which thinness is expected, such as gymnastics or dance, are at higher risk for developing an eating disorder. Students who take part in school or recreational sports that do not require a thin body are at lower risk. Self-esteem and activities that help young people feel good about themselves and their accomplishments help protect against eating disorders.

The general characteristics of eating disorders are as follows[4]:

- A disturbed body image in which an individual perceives herself or himself as fat, even if body weight is normal or below normal
- An intense fear of gaining weight
- An unrelenting desire to be thinner

The following three forms of eating disorders are recognized by the American Psychiatric Association[4]:

1. Anorexia nervosa (AN)
2. Bulimia nervosa (BN)
3. Eating disorders not otherwise specified (EDNOS)

Each has distinctive diagnostic criteria and symptoms.

Anorexia Nervosa

The term *anorexia nervosa (AN)* means "appetite loss from nervous disease." AN is a form of starvation with excessive weight loss self-imposed at great physical and psychologic cost. Although these patients may have a body weight only 85% of average or a BMI of less than 17.5, they do not see themselves as underweight and emaciated, but always as fat. This distorted body image often persists during recovery. AN can lead to suicide[2] or sudden death from cardiac arrest.[1] Low bone mass is a frequent complication. With treatment, 76% of adolescent AN patients recover, but 30% continue to struggle with body weight and require repeated intervention for as long as 6½ years.[1]

Diagnostic Criteria*

According to the *Diagnostic and Statistical Manual of Mental Disorders,* fourth edition text revision, the following criteria are diagnostic of AN[4]:

- Refusal to eat sufficient food to maintain a body weight at least 85% of average

- Intense fear of gaining weight or becoming fat, even though current weight is below average
- Disturbed perception of one's body weight, size, or shape; the patient claims to be fat even if emaciated and refuses to recognize the seriousness of the underweight or emaciated condition
- In females the absence of at least three consecutive menstrual cycles when otherwise expected to occur

Bulimia Nervosa

Bulimia nervosa (BN), from the word meaning "ox-hunger," is descriptive of the massive amounts of food consumed by patients with this condition, sometimes called the binge-and-purge syndrome. Because this individual is eating, body weight is usually normal or even above normal, but he or she is ridden with guilt. BN is often associated with depression or difficulty in meeting social or role expectations. When large amounts of food are consumed, the eating episode is followed by purging through self-induced vomiting, use of laxatives or diuretics, or excessive exercise. Repeated vomiting of the highly acid stomach contents can be harmful to the teeth and tissues of the mouth.

Diagnostic Criteria*

According to the *Diagnostic and Statistical Manual of Mental Disorders,* fourth edition text revision, the following criteria are diagnostic of BN[4]:

- Recurrent episodes of binge eating—rapid consumption of a large amount of food in a single and relatively short period
- Lack of control over eating behavior during the binges; the feeling that one cannot stop eating or control how much is being eaten
- Regular self-induced vomiting, use of laxatives or diuretics, strict dieting or fasting, or vigorous exercise as compensatory behavior to prevent weight gain
- Minimum average of two binge eating episodes a week for at least 3 months
- Persistent overconcern with body shape and weight

Eating Disorder Not Otherwise Specified

About 50% of the persons with eating disorders fall under the category of eating disorder not otherwise specified (EDNOS). If their problems remain untreated and the behavior continues, they may progress to the conditions of either AN or BN.[4]

Diagnostic Criteria*

This category, as its name indicates, includes eating behaviors that do not meet the conditions for either AN or BN. According to the *Diagnostic and Statistical Manual of Mental Disorders,* fourth edition text revision, the following criteria are diagnostic of EDNOS[4]:

- It is like AN except the regular menses continue and, despite substantial weight loss, body weight is normal.
- It is like BN except that binges occur less often than twice a week and the pattern lasts for fewer than 3 months.
- The person maintains a normal weight by self-induced vomiting after eating even small amounts of food such as two cookies or by chewing and then spitting out the food.

Binge Eating Disorder

This eating disorder includes binge eating episodes without the purging behavior of BN. Binge eating may occur in response to stress or anxiety or to soothe or relieve painful feelings. Many of these patients are overweight and have the same medical problems as obese individuals who do not binge eat.

*Diagnostic criteria from American Psychiatric Association: *Diagnostic and statistical manual of mental health disorders,* ed 4, text revision, Washington, DC, 2000, The Association, with permission of American Psychiatric Association (DSM) in the format Textbook via Copyright Clearance Center.

EATING DISORDERS: A HIGH PRICE FOR THINNESS

Diagnostic Criteria*

According to the *Diagnostic and Statistical Manual of Mental Disorders,* fourth edition text revision, the following criteria are diagnostic of binge eating disorder[4]:

- Recurrent episodes of binge eating—rapid consumption of a large amount of food in a single, relatively short period of time to the point of feeling uncomfortably full
- Lack of control over eating behavior during the binges; the feeling that one cannot stop eating or control how much is being eaten
- Eating large amounts of food when not feeling hungry and eating alone to hide embarrassment over the amount
- Feelings of self-disgust, depression, or guilt after a bingeing episode, which occurs at least twice a week
- Marked distress about the binge eating, but no compensatory behaviors such as purging, fasting, or excessive exercise

Treatment Approaches

Eating disorders take a high toll on both physical and psychologic health and require individualized care. The best chance for success lies with a sensitive, experienced team of health professionals including a physician, clinical psychologist or psychiatrist, clinical nutritionist, and nurse. Outpatient services may provide the care needed in less advanced cases, but for life-threatening AN intense inpatient care is essential.[1]

The care plan should include nutritional, medical, and cognitive therapy. A meal plan that provides a framework for meals, snacks, and food choices must be implemented on a gradual basis to address the underweight or overweight. Medical complications arising from severe malnutrition, dehydration, habitual vomiting, or excessive use of diuretics or laxatives require immediate attention. The psychologist or psychiatrist on the healthcare team can address the personal or social issues that contributed to the distorted body image and eating disorder and help develop healthy behavior patterns that will sustain the nutritional and medical recovery. Unfortunately, many cases of eating disorders go undetected, delaying or preventing the intervention that is urgently needed.[3]

References

1. American Dietetic Association: Position of the American Dietetic Association: nutrition intervention in the treatment of anorexia nervosa, bulimia nervosa, and eating disorders not otherwise specified (EDNOS), *J Am Diet Assoc* 101:810, 2001.
2. Polivy J, Herman PC: Causes of eating disorders, *Annu Rev Psychol* 53:187, 2002.
3. Rees L, Clark-Stone S: Can collaboration between education and health professionals improve the identification and referral of young people with eating disorders in schools? A pilot study, *J Adolesc* 29(1):137, 2006.
4. American Psychiatric Association: *Diagnostic and statistical manual of mental disorders,* ed 4, text revision, Washington, DC, 2000, The Association.

BOX 5-2 | Causes of Underweight

Lack of sufficient amounts or quality of food (not enough money for food)
Loss of appetite (aging changes, certain medications)
Premature feeling of fullness
Physical disability (problems with food shopping, meal preparation, or self-feeding)
Long-term illness
    Cancer
    Cardiac failure
    Chronic obstructive pulmonary disease
    Sepsis
    End-stage renal disease
    Autoimmune deficiency disease
    Cystic fibrosis
Physical condition increasing energy needs (hyperthyroidism)

General Causes

Conditions that lead to general malnutrition contribute to underweight. These fall into three categories: (1) those that decrease food intake, (2) those that increase energy requirements, and (3) those that prevent optimum utilization of food intake (Box 5-2), as follows:

1. *Poor food intake:* Lack of sufficient amounts of appropriate food results in failure to thrive in both children and older adults. Anorexia and nausea are common side effects of digoxin and chemotherapeutic agents, frequently used with older patients. These negative effects on appetite and food intake when combined with the increased energy needs of heart disease and cancer bring about the devastating weight loss referred to as cachexia. Older people in poverty who live alone and lack transportation to a food store risk unwanted weight loss. Federal guidelines require monitoring of body weight in skilled nursing facilities where a patient's inability to self-feed can lead to significant weight loss. Self-imposed food restriction as in anorexia nervosa results in life-threatening underweight.

2. *Increase in energy requirements:* Long-term hypermetabolic diseases such as cancer, acquired immunodeficiency syndrome (AIDS), or infection with fever impose metabolic demands that drain the body's resources. Hyperthyroidism or other hormonal abnormalities can increase energy requirements. Large increases in physical activity without a sufficient increase in energy intake will over time lead to underweight.

---

cachexia A wasting condition marked by weakness, extreme weight loss, and malnutrition.

3. *Poor utilization of available nutrients:* Both malabsorption and the inflammatory response associated with chronic disease cause a wasting of nutrients. Malabsorption from prolonged diarrhea, gastrointestinal disease, or laxative abuse depletes nutrient stores. Cytokines produced by the immune system in cancer, chronic kidney disease, chronic obstructive pulmonary disease, congestive heart failure, and AIDS accelerate the breakdown of protein and fat.

Nutritional Care

Underweight persons require special nutrition attention to rebuild body tissues and nutrient stores. Any food plan must be adapted to the individual's unique situation because it involves personal preferences, financial issues, and household concerns, along with any underlying disease. The goal is to provide a diet that is (1) high in kcalories, at least 50% above standard needs; (2) high in protein, to rebuild tissue; (3) high in carbohydrates, to provide a primary energy source in an easily digested form; (4) moderate in fat, to add kcalories but not exceed recommended limits; and (5) optimum in vitamins and minerals, including supplements when deficiencies require them. Good food of wide variety that is well prepared and seasoned and attractively presented helps revive lagging appetites and the desire to eat. Nourishing meals and snacks spread through the day that include favorite foods increase interest in eating and promote the optimal use of foods and their nutrients. Food seasonings, such as margarine, butter, sauces, and dressings, or liquid nutritional supplements add kcalories and key nutrients. In extreme cases tube feeding or total parenteral nutrition (TPN) may be necessary (see Chapter 18).

The rehabilitation process requires creative counseling with the individual and caregivers and attention to underlying socioeconomic and disease conditions. Practical personal guides and ongoing support are needed to counteract the root causes of the malnutrition and build food patterns that can be maintained when the person is returned to health.

TO SUM UP

Energy is the force that enables the body to continue its life-sustaining physical and metabolic work. The energy provided by food is measured in kilocalories or joules. Through a series of on-going metabolic reactions, the chemical energy found in food is converted to thermal, electrical, and mechanical energy to carry out body work. When food is not available, the body draws on its energy stores: glucose from glycogen, fatty acids from adipose tissue, and amino acids from muscle to meet ongoing energy needs. The total energy requirement is the sum of (1) basal metabolic needs, (2) the food intake effect (TEF), and (3) physical activity needs. Physical activity is the most variable component of the energy requirement,

adding fewer kcalories for sedentary individuals but making up almost half or more of the total energy requirement for highly active persons.

The four major body compartments are (1) lean body mass (LBM), (2) body fat, (3) body water, and (4) mineral mass. Increasing proportions of body fat increase the risk of chronic disease. Interventions focusing on positive food and activity behaviors leading to a stable body weight, personal fitness, and an improvement in functional parameters such as improved blood pressure are of greater value than an emphasis on weight loss only. At the other extreme an obsession with thinness and self-imposed food restriction is a growing problem among children and youth. Poverty, chronic disease, and medications can be responsible for poor food intake, poor food utilization, or increased energy requirements, resulting in underweight. A nutrient- and energy-rich diet combined with ongoing counseling to help with the underlying causes and support the rehabilitation process can restore an underweight individual to a healthy weight.

QUESTIONS FOR REVIEW

1. Define the term *fuel factor.* What is the fuel value for each of the four energy-yielding nutrients?
2. List the three components that contribute to the total energy requirement. What is the *basal metabolic rate* and what factors influence it? Which body tissues contribute most to basal metabolic needs? Which is the most variable component of the total energy requirement and why?
3. What is the difference between the basal metabolic rate (BMR) and the resting metabolic rate (RMR)? Which is most often used in clinical practice? Why?
4. Name the four body compartments, and describe the tissues found in each. How can they be measured?
5. You are performing a nutritional assessment of a man who is 6 ft 2 in tall and weighs 248 lb. What is his BMI? Is he overweight, overfat, or both? Explain.
6. Describe the various eating disorders associated with an obsession for thinness or inappropriate attitudes toward food. What social factors contribute to disordered eating?
7. You are working with a single mother and her 3-year-old daughter who are both underweight. They live in a small apartment in a dilapidated building in the inner city. Their electricity was disconnected, so they have no working equipment for cooking and no refrigeration. They receive a noon and supper meal at a nearby food program for the homeless. Plan a breakfast, series of snacks, and food supplement plan that could increase their kcalorie and nutrient intake. (Remember, all foods you suggest must be safely stored at room temperature.)
8. You are working with an adolescent girl who wants to increase her energy expenditure by 250 kcal a day. Develop an activity plan that would mesh with her lifestyle and social time with friends.

9. Visit your local library, and review the magazines directed toward the teen audience. Look for three articles that suggest regimens for weight management. Evaluate each article in terms of (a) nutritional recommendations, (b) implications for health, (c) reliance on commercial weight loss products, and (d) safety for long-term use.

REFERENCES

1. American Dietetic Association: Position of the American Dietetic Association: weight management, *J Am Diet Assoc* 102: 1145, 2002.
2. Brody T: *Nutritional biochemistry,* ed 2, New York, 1999, Academic Press.
3. Food and Nutrition Board, Institute of Medicine: *Dietary Reference Intakes for energy, carbohydrate, fiber, fat, fatty acids, cholesterol, protein, and amino acids (macronutrients),* Washington, DC, 2002, National Academies Press.
4. Poehlman ET, Horton ES: Energy needs: assessment and requirements in humans. In Shils ME et al, eds: *Modern nutrition in health and disease,* ed 9, Philadelphia, 1999, Lippincott Williams & Wilkins.
5. Guyton AC, Hall JE: *Textbook of medical physiology,* ed 10, Philadelphia, 2000, WB Saunders.
6. Martin K et al: Estimation of resting energy expenditure considering effects of race and diabetes status, *Diabetes Care* 27:1405, 2004.
7. Nawata K et al: Increased resting metabolic rate in patients with type 2 diabetes mellitus accompanied by advanced diabetic nephropathy, *Metabolism* 53:1395, 2004.
8. Kleinman RE, ed: *Pediatric nutrition handbook,* ed 5, Washington, DC, 2004, American Academy of Pediatrics.
9. Jones A et al: Body-composition differences between African American and white women: relation to resting energy requirements, *Am J Clin Nutr* 79:780, 2004.
10. Westerterp KR: Diet induced thermogenesis, *Nutr Metab (Lond)* 1(1):5, 2004.
11. Wessel TR et al: Relationship of physical fitness vs body mass index with coronary artery disease and cardiovascular events in women, *JAMA* 292:1179, 2004.
12. Koh-Banerjee P et al: Changes in whole-grain, bran, and cereal fiber consumption in relation to 8-y weight gain among men, *Am J Clin Nutr* 80:1237, 2004.
13. Zhu P et al: Waist circumference and obesity-associated risk factors among whites in the third National Health and Nutrition Examination Survey: clinical action thresholds, *Am J Clin Nutr* 76:743, 2002.
14. Forbes GB: Body composition: role of nutrition, growth, physical activity, and aging. In Shils ME et al, eds: *Modern nutrition in health and disease,* ed 9, Philadelphia, 1999, Lippincott Williams & Wilkins.
15. Fields DA, Goran MI, McCrory MA: Body-composition assessment via air-displacement plethysmography in adults and children: a review, *Am J Clin Nutr* 75:453, 2002.
16. Fernandez JR et al: Waist circumference percentiles in nationally representative samples of African-American, European-American, and Mexican-American children and adolescents, *J Pediatr* 145:439, 2004.
17. Wildman RP et al: Appropriate body mass index and waist circumference cutoffs for categorization of overweight and central adiposity among Chinese adults, *Am J Clin Nutr* 80:1129, 2004.
18. World Health Organization Expert Consultation: Appropriate body-mass index for Asian populations and its implications for policy and intervention strategies, *Lancet* 363:157, 2004.
19. Deurenberg-Yap M, Deurenberg P: Is a re-evaluation of WHO body mass index cut-off values needed? The case of Asians in Singapore, *Nutr Rev* 61(5, part 2):S80, 2003.
20. National Heart, Lung, and Blood Institute/National Institute of Diabetes and Digestive and Kidney Diseases: *Clinical guidelines on the identification, evaluation, and treatment of overweight and obesity in adults: the evidence report,* NIH Publication No. 98-4083, Bethesda, Md, 1998, National Institutes of Health.
21. U.S. Department of Health and Human Services, U.S. Department of Agriculture: *Dietary guidelines for Americans 2005,* ed 6, Washington, DC, 2005, Authors. Accessible at *www.healthierus. gov/dietaryguidelines.*
22. Ogden CL et al: *Mean body weight, height, and body mass index, United States 1960-2002: advance data, vital and health statistics,* No. 347, Washington, DC, 2004 (October 27), U.S. Department of Health and Human Services.
23. Hedley AA et al: Prevalence of overweight and obesity among U.S. children, adolescents, and adults, 1999-2002, *JAMA* 291:2847, 2004.
24. Stevens J: Impact of age on associations between weight and mortality, *Nutr Rev* 58:129, 2000.
25. Dorn JM et al: Alcohol drinking patterns differentially affect central adiposity as measured by abdominal height in women and men, *J Nutr* 133:2655, 2003.
26. Ding J et al: The association of regional fat deposits with hypertension in older persons of white and African American ethnicity, *Am J Hypertens* 17:971, 2004.
27. Levine JA: Non-exercise activity thermogenesis (NEAT), *Nutr Rev* 62(7, part 2):S82, 2004.
28. Paeratakul S et al: Americans on diet: results from the 1994-1996 Continuing Survey of Food Intakes by Individuals, *J Am Diet Assoc* 102:1247, 2002.
29. Schoenborn CA, Adams PF, Barnes PM: *Body weight status of adults: United States, 1997-98—advance data, vital and health statistics,* No. 330, Washington, DC, 2002 (September 6), U.S. Department of Health and Human Services.
30. Pi-Sunyer FX: The epidemiology of central fat distribution in relation to disease, *Nutr Rev* 62(7, part 2):S120, 2004.
31. Larrieu S et al: Relationship between body mass index and different domains of disability in older persons: the 3C study, *Int J Obes* 28:1555, 2004.
32. Daviglus ML et al: Relation of body mass index in young adulthood and middle age to Medicare expenditures in older age, *JAMA* 292:2743, 2004.
33. Grivetti L: Psychology and cultural aspects of energy, *Nutr Rev* 59:S5, 2001.
34. Mathieu J: Disordered eating across the life span, *J Am Diet Assoc* 104:1208, 2004.
35. Birch LL, Fisher JO, Davison KK: Learning to overeat: maternal use of restrictive feeding practices promotes girls' eating in the absence of hunger, *Am J Clin Nutr* 78:215, 2003.
36. Shunk JA, Birch LL: Girls at risk for overweight at age 5 are at risk for dietary restraint, disinhibited overeating, weight concerns, and greater weight gain from 5 to 9 years, *J Am Diet Assoc* 104:1120, 2004.
37. Neumark-Sztainer D et al: Are family meal patterns associated with disordered eating behaviors among adolescents? *J Adolesc Health* 35:350, 2004.

38. American Dietetic Association/Dietitians of Canada: Position of the American Dietetic Association and Dietitians of Canada: nutrition and women's health, *J Am Diet Assoc* 104:984, 2004.

39. Neumark-Sztainer D et al: Weight-control behaviors among adolescent girls and boys: implications for dietary intake, *J Am Diet Assoc* 104:913, 2004.

40. American Psychiatric Association: *Diagnostic and statistical manual of mental health disorders,* ed 4, text revision, Washington, DC, 2000, The Association.

41. American Dietetic Association: Position of the American Dietetic Association: nutrition intervention in the treatment of anorexia nervosa, bulimia nervosa, and eating disorders not otherwise specified (EDNOS), *J Am Diet Assoc* 101:810, 2001.

42. Forman-Hoffman V: High prevalence of abnormal eating and weight control practices among U.S. high-school students, *Eat Behav* 5:325, 2004.

43. Thomas DR: Distinguishing starvation from cachexia, *Clin Geriatr* 18:883, 2002.

44. Caulfield LE et al: Undernutrition as an underlying cause of child deaths associated with diarrhea, pneumonia, malaria, and measles, *Am J Clin Nutr* 80:193, 2004.

45. Sherry B et al: Trends in state-specific prevalence of overweight and underweight in 2- through 4-year-old children from low-income families from 1989 through 2000, *Arch Pediatr Adolesc Med* 158:1116, 2004.

46. Arterburn DE et al: Association of body weight with condition-specific quality of life in male veterans, *Am J Med* 117:738, 2004.

FURTHER READINGS AND RESOURCES

Readings

Young LR, Nestle M: Expanding portion sizes in the U.S. marketplace: implications for nutrition counseling, *J Am Diet Assoc* 103:231, 2003.

Rolls BJ, Roe LS, Meengs JS: Increasing the portion size of a sandwich increases energy intake, *J Am Diet Assoc* 104:367, 2004.
These authors give us some insight into how larger portion sizes have influenced the growth of obesity in the United States.

Lake AJ, Staiger PK, Glowinski H: Effect of Western culture on women's attitudes to eating and perceptions of body shape, *Int J Eat Disord* 27:83, 2000.

Mathieu J: Beyond the headlines: disordered eating across the life span, *J Am Diet Assoc* 104:1208, 2004.
These articles explore the cultural differences in perceptions of the ideal body shape and how this has led to disordered eating among all age-groups.

Grivetti L: Psychology and cultural aspects of energy, *Nutr Rev* 59(1 Pt 2):S5, 2001.
This article provides an excellent overview of the social and cultural issues that contribute to both overeating and restrained eating in our society.

Bren L: Losing weight: more than counting calories, *FDA Consumer* 36:18, 2002.
This article appearing in the publication of the U.S. Food and Drug Administration gives us a perspective on both the appropriate and inappropriate treatments for obesity.

Websites of Interest

- U.S. Department of Health and Human Services, U.S. Department of Agriculture, *Dietary Guidelines for Americans 2005;* the *Dietary Guidelines for Americans 2005* provides information and nutrition education materials to assist with weight management: *www.usda.gov/cnpp/dietary_guidelines.html.*

- U.S. Department of Agriculture, National Agricultural Library, *Weight management;* this weight control site offers tips on food selection for weight management and links to sites that contain ideas for physical activity: *www.nutrition.gov/index.php?mode=subject&subject=ng_weight_control&d_subject=Weight%20Control.*

- National Institutes of Health and National Library of Medicine, Medline Plus, *Eating disorders;* this site offers comprehensive information on eating disorders, including causes, symptoms, treatment, and prevention: *www.nlm.nih.gov/medlineplus/eatingdisorders.html.*

- U.S. Department of Health and Human Services, Centers for Disease Control and Prevention, *Physical activity for everyone;* this site offers physical activity programs and information for all age-groups, as well as resources for health professionals: *www.cdc.gov/nccdphp/dnpa/physical/index.htm.*

CHAPTER 6

Vitamins

Eleanor D. Schlenker

Now we begin a two-chapter sequence on the non–energy-yielding micronutrients: the vitamins and minerals. First, we look at the vitamins.

No other group of nutritional elements has so captured the interest of scientists, health professionals, and the general public as the vitamins. Both research journals and the popular press describe how vitamins help to prevent chronic disease and support well-being in ways over and above their generally accepted roles. Opinions about vitamin needs vary widely, running the gamut from wise functional use to wild flagrant abuse.

In this chapter we review both the fat-soluble and water-soluble vitamins. We focus on why we need them and how we obtain them.

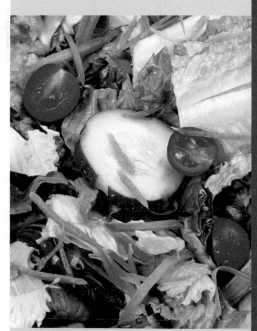

VITAMINS: ESSENTIAL NUTRIENTS

General Nature and Classification

Most of the vitamins we know about today were discovered between 1900 and 1950, and new scientific methods are helping us learn more about these molecules and what they do in the body. At the time of their discovery three key characteristics became evident: (1) they were not metabolized to yield energy as were carbohydrate, fat, and sometimes protein; (2) they were essential to life; and (3) often not a single substance but a group of related substances performed a particular metabolic activity. The name *vitamin* was adopted during the early research years when one of the scientists working with a nitrogen-containing chemical substance called an amine thought this was the common nature of all these vital molecules. So he named his discovery vitamine ("vital amine"). The final *e* was dropped when similar substances turned out to have different structures, but the name *vitamin* was retained for this class of nutrients. At first, a letter name was given to each vitamin as it was discovered. However, as the number of known vitamins grew, this created confusion, and scientific names based on the structure or function of each molecule were developed. For the fat-soluble vitamins the letter names have been retained because in each case a number of closely related compounds with similar properties and structures have been identified.[1]

Definition of a Vitamin

As the vitamins were discovered one by one and the list grew, several criteria were used to define a compound as a vitamin, as follows:

- It must be an organic dietary substance that is not an energy-producing carbohydrate, fat, or protein.
- It is needed in very small quantities to perform a particular metabolic function and prevent an associated deficiency disease.
- It cannot be manufactured by the body and therefore must be supplied in food.

These criteria form the basis for establishing that a vitamin is essential; however, new research has identified other vitamin-like substances in food that appear to promote health and increase resistance to chronic diseases. There have also been suggestions that certain vitamins that act as antioxidants might help prevent chronic diseases if used at levels higher than are required to prevent deficiency. But at this time we do not know what those intakes should be or how we can test for them.[2]

Later in this chapter we will discuss some of the newly discovered vitamin-like substances and their actions in the body. In time new substances may be added to the list of essential vitamins.[3]

Vitamins: Basic Concepts

As our understanding of the vitamins has expanded, the following important concepts have emerged:

- *Individual vitamins are multifunctional.* When the vitamins were first discovered, it was believed that each had one unique and essential role in maintaining body structure or function. In fact most vitamins have multiple roles or actions in the body, working independently or working cooperatively with other nutrients to regulate essential activities. Although we associate vitamin A with helping us to see in dim light, we will learn that this vitamin also maintains the mucous membranes that protect against infection.
- *One vitamin cannot substitute for another vitamin.* All vitamins must be available in sufficient amounts if the body is to function normally and tissues are to remain healthy. For example, vitamin C cannot protect the fetus of a folate-deficient mother from a neural tube defect.
- *Vitamins work together in carrying out body functions.* The formation and maturation of red blood cells require the actions of folate, pyridoxine, vitamin B_{12}, and ascorbic acid, along with several important minerals.
- *Vitamins function best when all are present in the appropriate proportions.* High-potency vitamin A supplements interfere with the action of vitamin D, decreasing calcium absorption and increasing the risk of hip fracture.

These functional truths underscore the importance of eating a variety of foods to supply our nutrients. A balanced diet contains not only the essential vitamins, but also other important substances that may contribute to well-being. A supplement containing one vitamin will not take the place of fruits and vegetables that supply many different vitamins along with fiber and phytochemicals. When vitamins are obtained from food as part of a balanced diet, we also are less likely to take in an excessive amount of any one vitamin that could interfere with the absorption or function of another.

Classification

As the vitamins were discovered, they were grouped according to their solubility in either fat or water, and this classification has continued (Box 6-1).

Fat-Soluble Vitamins

The fat-soluble vitamins are A, D, E, and K. They are closely associated with body lipids and are easily stored.

Their functions are generally related to structural activities with proteins.

Water-Soluble Vitamins

The water-soluble vitamins are vitamin C and the B-complex family. These vitamins are more easily absorbed and transported, but unlike the fat-soluble vitamins, they cannot be stored except in the general sense of tissue saturation. The B vitamins function mainly as coenzyme factors in cell metabolism. Vitamin C works with enzymes that support tissue building and maintenance.

Current Knowledge and Key Questions

In our study, we will answer the following key questions for each vitamin:

- *Chemical and physical nature:* What is the general structure of the vitamin?
- *Absorption, transport, and storage:* How does the body handle this particular vitamin?
- *Function:* What does this vitamin do?
- *Related deficiency symptoms or disease:* What occurs when this vitamin is absent or not available in sufficient amounts?
- *Clinical role in health:* Does this vitamin prevent or ameliorate a chronic disease?
- *Recommended intake and possible toxicity:* How much of this vitamin do we need, but how much is too much? What are the consequences of excessive intake?
- *Food sources:* Where do we obtain this vitamin?

We will review the four fat-soluble vitamins and the nine water-soluble vitamins (see Box 6-1), and answer the key questions above.

BOX 6-1	Classification of Vitamins

Fat-Soluble Vitamins

A
D
E
K

Water-Soluble Vitamins

Vitamin C (Ascorbic acid)
Thiamin
Riboflavin
Niacin
Vitamin B_6 (Pyridoxine)
Pantothenic acid
Biotin
Folate
Vitamin B_{12} (Cobalamin)

FAT-SOLUBLE VITAMINS

VITAMIN A

Chemical and Physical Nature

Vitamin A is the generic name for a group of compounds having similar biologic activity. These compounds are retinol, retinal, and retinoic acid. The term *retinoids* refers to both the natural forms of vitamin A and its synthetic copies. Chemically, retinol is a primary alcohol of high molecular weight ($C_{20}H_{29}OH$). Because of its specific function in the retina of the eye and its structure as an alcohol, vitamin A was given the chemical name retinol. It is soluble in fat and in ordinary fat solvents. Because it is insoluble in water, it is fairly stable in cooking.

Forms

There are two dietary forms of vitamin A: (1) preformed vitamin A and (2) provitamin A (Box 6-2), as described below:

1. *Preformed vitamin A: retinol:* This is the natural form of vitamin A found only in animal foods and usually associated with fat. Vitamin A compounds are deposited primarily in the liver but also in small amounts in the kidneys, lungs, and adipose tissue, so organ meats are a rich source. Other dietary sources are the fat portion of dairy foods, egg yolk, and fish.
2. *Provitamin A, or beta-carotene:* Plants cannot synthesize vitamin A but instead produce a family of compounds called carotenoids. These substances are found in plants, eaten by animals, and then

---

amine An organic compound containing nitrogen. Amino acids and pyridoxine are examples of amines.

retinol Chemical name for vitamin A derived from its function in the retina of the eye producing light-dark adaptation.

retinal The aldehyde form of retinol (vitamin A) derived from the enzymatic splitting of beta-carotene in the intestinal wall. In the retina of the eye, retinal combines with opsins to form visual pigments. In the rods it forms rhodopsin (visual purple), and in the cones it forms the pigments responsible for color vision.

carotenoids A group of yellow-red pigments widely distributed in plants that act as antioxidants protecting tissues from damage caused by free radicals; beta-carotene can be cleaved in the gastric mucosa to form one molecule of vitamin A.

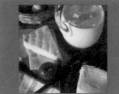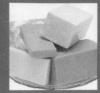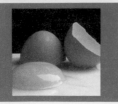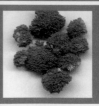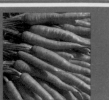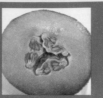

Preformed Vitamin A

2% Milk
Cheese
Egg yolk
Liver

Provitamin A

Broccoli
Carrots
Spinach
Cantaloupe
Tomato juice
Apricots

Images copyright 2006 JupiterImages Corporation.

converted to vitamin A. Thus humans can obtain their vitamin A directly by eating animal tissues or by converting carotenoids obtained from plant foods. The original plant source, beta-carotene ($C_{40}H_{56}$), was called carotene because a main source is the yellow and orange pigment in carrots and other vegetables and fruits. Other carotenoids found in plant foods include beta-cryptoxanthin, lutein, and zeaxanthin, but not all of these can be converted to vitamin A.

The carotenoids play an important role in human nutrition. Beta-carotene, converted to vitamin A in the body, provides about 21% of the total vitamin A intake in the United States.[4] Enzymes that split the carotenoid molecule to yield retinol are found in the mucosal cells lining the small intestine and in the liver. The yellow and red carotenoid pigments occurring in many fruits and vegetables and in red palm oil are the major food sources of vitamin A in most underdeveloped countries. Unfortunately, the conversion of the carotenes to retinol is much less efficient than we thought it was, casting doubt on the ability of plant foods to provide an adequate supply of vitamin A in regions of the world where animal foods are scarce (Table 6-1).[5]

Absorption, Transport, and Storage

Substances Needed for Absorption

Vitamin A enters the body as preformed vitamin A from animal sources or as the precursor beta-carotene from plant sources. Various materials are needed for the absorption of vitamin A or beta-carotene, as follows:

- *Bile salts:* Vitamin A joins with fat and other fat-related compounds and bile salts in the small intestine to form a micellar bile-lipid complex. Bile salts are needed to carry fats and fat-soluble materials into

TABLE 6-1 | **Conversion of Carotenoids to Vitamin A**

Amount in the Diet	Amount Available to the Body
1 μg retinol	1 μg retinol
12 μg beta-carotene	1 μg retinol
24 μg alpha-carotene or beta-cryptoxanthin	1 μg retinol

NOTE: Carotenoids can be converted to retinol (vitamin A) to help meet body needs, but greater amounts of these molecules are required to produce one molecule of vitamin A.

the intestinal wall for further breakdown. Clinical conditions affecting the biliary system such as obstruction of the bile ducts, infectious hepatitis, or liver cirrhosis that interfere with production or release of bile salts hinder vitamin A absorption.

- *Pancreatic lipase:* This fat-splitting enzyme released into the upper small intestine carries out the initial hydrolysis of fat emulsions or oil solutions containing vitamin A. Water-based preparations of retinol are available for use when the secretion of pancreatic lipase or absorption of fat is curtailed, as in cystic fibrosis or pancreatitis.[4]

- *Dietary fat:* The effective absorption of vitamin A requires the presence of fat to stimulate the release of bile and be absorbed along with the vitamin. Absorption is most efficient when fat intake is more than 10 g/day.[6]

Conversion of Beta-Carotene

Beta-carotene can be absorbed and utilized by the body in its original form or be converted to vitamin A. Some beta-carotene is converted to vitamin A in the intestinal wall during absorption, but other molecules of beta-carotene

TO PROBE FURTHER

THE CAROTENOIDS: NEEDED EVERY DAY

Carotenoids are the substances that form the rich yellow, orange, green, and red pigments in fruits and vegetables. As we learned in this chapter, beta-carotene and various other carotenoids have physiologic actions of their own completely separate from the actions of vitamin A. As researchers learn more and more about their positive effects on human health the most intriguing aspect is this: we must eat them in their natural form as they are found in fruits and vegetables. Supplements provide no particular health benefits and in fact can be harmful.[1] It may be that several of these substances must work together to bring about their protective effects.

The following list outlines some major carotenoids in the U.S. diet and their food sources:

- *Alpha-carotene:* carrots
- *Beta-carotene:* broccoli, cantaloupe, carrots, spinach
- *Beta-cryptoxanthin:* oranges and orange juice, peaches, tangerines, sweet peppers
- *Lutein:* broccoli, corn, green beans, green peas, spinach, and other greens
- *Lycopene:* tomatoes and tomato products

Although the carotenoids generally act as antioxidants and neutralize free radicals, it is likely they also act in other ways to bring about their observed benefits. Individuals who eat more fruits and vegetables and have higher blood carotenoid levels have a lower risk of death from all causes and fewer atherosclerotic lesions and conditions of heart disease, cancer, macular degeneration, and cataract.[1-2] Supplements of vitamins A, C, and E will not take the place of plant foods in providing this protection.

Food preparation practices can improve the absorption of carotenoids, as follows:

- Carotenoids are better absorbed from cooked vegetables than fresh vegetables. Lycopene, believed to reduce the risk of prostate cancer, is absorbed best from cooked tomato products such as catsup and pizza sauce.
- The carotenoids require the presence of fat for their absorption, so consider a salad dressing containing some fat when enjoying a salad rich in the carotenes and lycopene.[3]

References

1. Food and Nutrition Board, Institute of Medicine: *Dietary Reference Intakes for vitamin C, vitamin E, selenium, and carotenoids,* Washington, DC, 2000, National Academies Press.
2. Mares-Perlman JA et al: The body of evidence to support a protective role for lutein and zeaxanthin in delaying chronic disease, *J Nutr* 132:518S, 2002.
3. Brown MJ et al: Carotenoid bioavailability is higher from salads ingested with full-fat than with fat-reduced salad dressings as measured with electrochemical detection, *Am J Clin Nutr* 80:396, 2004.

are absorbed and transported intact. At one time we believed that carotenoids such as beta-carotene were biologically important only as precursors to vitamin A. New findings tell us that carotenoids perform roles in human health completely unrelated to the actions of vitamin A. Carotenoids are members of a broad category of phytochemicals that appear to promote well-being. To learn more about their health effects, see the *To Probe Further* box, "The Carotenoids: Needed Every Day."[5]

Transport and Storage

The route of absorption of both vitamin A and the carotenoids parallels that of fat. In the intestinal mucosa retinol from both preformed animal sources and plant carotenes is incorporated into the chylomicrons.[3] In this form it enters the bloodstream via the lymphatic system and is carried to the liver for storage or distribution to cells. The liver, an efficient storage organ for vitamin A, contains up to 85% of the body's total supply. Liver stores are usually sufficient to prevent deficiency for about 6 to 12 months and in some individuals for as long as 4 years.

The ability of the body to store a substantial amount of vitamin A has important application to areas of the world where vitamin A–containing foods are in short supply. A prophylactic dose of vitamin A administered every 6 months prevents mortality and blindness and supports normal growth in infants and young children.[7] Measles is a leading killer disease of malnourished children and is a target for vitamin A supplementation and immunization by the World Health Organization. Age is a factor in absorption. Newborns, especially premature infants, absorb vitamin A poorly. Persons using mineral oil as a laxative reduce their absorption of vitamin A.

Functions of Vitamin A

The role of vitamin A in visual adaptation to light and darkness is well known. However, vitamin A also has generalized actions that affect the integrity of body coverings and linings (epithelial tissues), growth, immune response, and reproductive function.

Vitamin A Deficiency and Clinical Applications

Vision

The ability of the eye to adapt to changes in light depends on a light-sensitive pigment, rhodopsin—commonly known as *visual purple*—in the rods of the retina (Figure 6-1). Rhodopsin is made up of the vitamin A compound retinal and the protein opsin (Figure 6-2). When the body lacks vitamin A, normal rhodopsin cannot be made and the rods and cones of the retina become

precursor A substance from which another substance is derived.

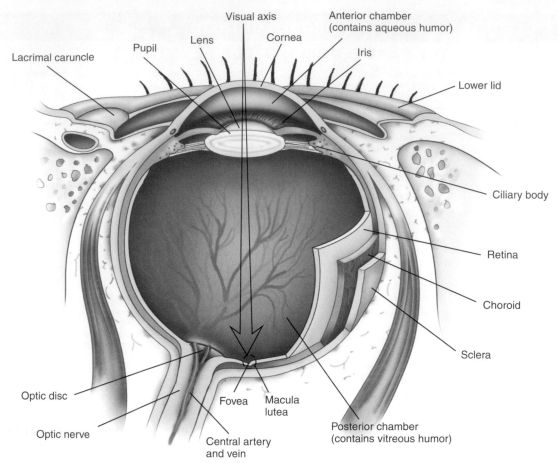

FIGURE 6-1   Structure of the eye, as viewed from the side. *(From Thibodeau GA, Patton KT:* Anatomy & physiology, *ed 5, St. Louis, 2003, Mosby/Elsevier.)*

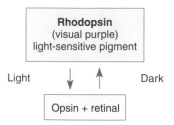

FIGURE 6-2   The vision cycle: light-dark adaptation role of vitamin A.

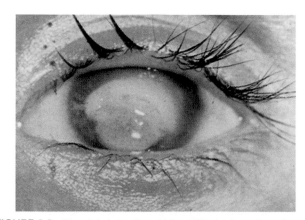

FIGURE 6-3   Xerophthalmia. *(From McLaren DS: A colour atlas and text of diet-related disorders, ed 2, London, 1992, Mosby-Year Book Europe Limited.)*

increasingly sensitive to changes in light, causing night blindness. This condition can be cured with an injection of vitamin A (retinol), which is readily converted to retinal and then rhodopsin.

Cell Differentiation

Vitamin A controls the differentiation of cells, or in other words, the types of specialized cells that are formed from basic stem cells. Vitamin A is needed to form and maintain healthy epithelial tissue, which provides our primary barrier to infection. The epithelium includes both the outer skin and the mucous membranes that line many body structures. Without vitamin A we form cells that are dry and flat rather than soft and moist. These dry, flat cells gradually harden to form keratin, a process called

keratinization. Keratin is a protein that creates dry, scaly tissue, normal for nails and hair but abnormal for skin and mucous membranes. In vitamin A deficiency such abnormal tissue changes occur in many body systems, as follows:

- *Eye:* The cornea dries and hardens, a condition called *xerophthalmia* (Figure 6-3). The tear ducts dry up, robbing the eye of its cleansing and lubricating fluid, and infection follows quickly. In extreme deficiency

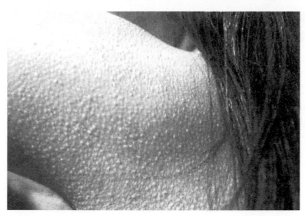

FIGURE 6-4 Follicular hyperkeratosis caused by vitamin A deficiency. *(From McLaren DS: A colour atlas and text of diet-related disorders, ed 2, London, 1992, Mosby-Year Book Europe Limited.)*

the keratinization progresses to blindness. Blindness related to vitamin A deficiency is a world public health problem; each year more than 350,000 preschool children lose their sight.[6]

- *Respiratory tract:* The ciliated epithelium in the nasal passages dry and the cilia are lost, removing a barrier to infectious organisms. Nasal secretions that trap invading particles and remove them from the body are absent.
- *Gastrointestinal tract:* The salivary glands dry, and the mouth becomes dry and cracked, open to invading bacteria. Mucosal secretions decrease throughout the digestive tract, and tissues dry and slough off, affecting digestion and absorption.
- *Genitourinary tract:* When epithelial tissue begins to break down, problems such as urinary tract infections, vaginal infections, and formation of calculi increase.
- *Skin:* As skin becomes dry and scaly, small pustules (hardened, pigmented, papular eruptions) appear around hair follicles, a condition known as *follicular hyperkeratosis* (Figure 6-4).
- *Tooth formation:* Specific epithelial cells surrounding tooth buds in fetal gum tissue that normally become specialized cup-shaped organs called *ameloblasts* do not develop properly. These little organs form the enamel of the developing tooth.

Growth

Vitamin A is essential for the growth of bones and soft tissues. Vitamin A controls protein synthesis and *mitosis* (cell division) and stabilizes cell membranes. The growth and maintenance of bone require constant remodeling, reshaping, and expansion. Vitamin A participates in the important job of tunneling out old bone to make way for new bone; then the tunnels are filled in to accommodate growth according to the pattern set in the initial embryonic cartilage model. Although inadequate supplies of vitamin A are detrimental to bone health so are excessive intakes that cause old bone to be lost more rapidly than it can be replaced, with a net loss of bone. Among postmenopausal

women intakes of preformed vitamin A in excess of the Dietary Reference Intake (DRI) were associated with a higher risk of hip fracture.[8] At the same time beta-carotene contributed by fruits and vegetables in the diet does not lead to excessive body levels of vitamin A or bone loss.

The changes in the mucosal lining of the gastrointestinal tract that occur in vitamin A deficiency result in poor absorption of many nutrients important to growth. This may explain in part why vitamin A supplementation of malnourished children brings about catch-up growth.[6] The action of vitamin A in controlling gene expression and the rate of cell division has led researchers to consider a possible role for vitamin A in cancer prevention.[9]

Reproduction

Vitamin A is needed to support normal sexual maturation and function. It participates in gene expression and plays an important role in fetal development, including development of the central nervous system.[4] A sufficient intake is required for successful lactation.

Immunity

Poor vitamin A status reduces resistance to infection in several ways. First, changes in epithelial and mucosal tissue allow disease organisms to enter the body more easily. Second, vitamin A has a direct effect on the immune system, and both cell-mediated and antibody-mediated immunity are impaired when intake is low. Measles is more likely to be fatal in vitamin A-deficient children in developing countries. Immune response returns to normal quite rapidly when vitamin A is restored.[10]

Vitamin A Requirement

Influencing Factors

A number of variables can modify the vitamin A needs of a given individual. These include:

- *Liver stores:* High vitamin A stores will supply body needs for an extended period; those with low body stores are dependent on day-to-day intakes.
- *Intake of preformed versus provitamin A:* Greater amounts of carotenoids are required to meet the DRI for vitamin A.
- *Illness and infection:* Needs are increased to support the production of immune cells and body defenses.
- *Gastrointestinal or hepatic defects:* Gallbladder or liver disease with the failure to produce adequate amounts of bile limits fat absorption and in turn the absorption of vitamin A and the carotenoids.

---

night blindness Inability to see well in diminished light, resulting from vitamin A deficiency.

keratinization The process of creating the protein keratin, a principal constituent of skin, hair, nails, and the matrix forming tooth enamel.

Causes of Vitamin A Deficiency

In the United States the primary cause of vitamin A deficiency is inadequate dietary intake, usually the result of poor food selection rather than unavailability of appropriate foods. The growing popularity of fast-food restaurants has influenced vitamin A status because both children and adults eat fewer carotene-containing fruits and vegetables and drink less milk on days that include a fast-food meal.[11] Vitamin A deficiency occurs as a result of poor absorption based on a lack of bile, lack of dietary fat, defective absorbing surface, inadequate conversion of beta-carotene, or liver or intestinal disease. A high alcohol intake causes a loss of vitamin A from the liver even if liver function remains normal.[4]

Dietary Reference Intake

The Recommended Dietary Allowance (RDA) for vitamin A is the amount required to maintain optimum liver stores. It is presented as micrograms of retinol,[4] and the term retinol activity equivalent (RAE) takes into account the ratios for converting carotenoids to vitamin A. Early on, vitamin A was measured in international units (IU), and some food composition tables still use those units. A major problem with the older tables is they overestimate the amount of vitamin A available from carotenoid-containing foods, such that intakes are calculated to be higher than is true. The RDA for men ages 19 and over is set at 900 μg, and the RDA for women of this age is 700 μg. To ensure sufficient vitamin A to support a successful pregnancy and production of milk with an appropriate vitamin A content, the RDA increases to 770 μg in pregnancy and 1300 μg in lactation.

Vitamin A Toxicity

Hypervitaminosis A

Because the liver can store very large amounts of vitamin A, it is possible for persons taking high-potency supplements to develop toxicity. Characteristic signs of hypervitaminosis A are listed in Box 6-3. Daily intakes above the Tolerable Upper Intake Level (UL) of 3000 μg of preformed vitamin A are especially dangerous for pregnant women, resulting in lower birth weights[12] or congenital malformations,[13] depending on intake. Increasing use of vitamin supplements and fortified foods are adding up to disturbing intakes of preformed vitamin A among some age-groups. Supplements often contain as much as two times the RDA and if combined with highly fortified food items bring both children and adults dangerously close to the UL.[14]

Food Sources of Vitamin A

Animal sources of preformed vitamin A include liver, milk, cheese, butter, egg yolk, and fish. Skim and low-fat

---

| BOX 6-3 | Signs of Vitamin A Toxicity |

Vomiting
Headache
Joint pain
Thickening of the long bones
Hair loss
Jaundice
Liver injury and ascites (if the condition continues)

---

milk are fortified with vitamin A to the level found naturally in whole milk. Nonanimal products such as margarine, ready-to-eat cereals, and cereal bars are being fortified with vitamin A. Dark yellow, orange, red, and green vegetables and fruits contain a variety of carotenoids and help meet the vitamin A requirement. Cooked vegetables can be better dietary sources of carotenoids than raw vegetables because cooking helps to release these substances from their plant sources, making them more available for absorption. The vitamin A contents of selected foods are listed in Box 6-4. (The *Focus on Culture* box, "Acculturation: Effect on Food Patterns," points to problems with low intakes of fruits and vegetables.)

VITAMIN D

Chemical and Physical Nature

When first discovered, vitamin D was classified as a vitamin. However, it is now clear that vitamin D is actually a prohormone and in its active form functions as a hormone. Chemically, vitamin D is a sterol, and its precursor found in human skin is the lipid molecule 7-dehydrocholesterol. All compounds with vitamin D activity are soluble in fat but not water. They are heat stable and not easily oxidized.

Forms

There are two forms of vitamin D that can be used by the body: (1) ergocalciferol (vitamin D_2) and (2) cholecalciferol (vitamin D_3). Vitamin D_2 is formed by irradiating ergosterol found in ergot (a fungus growing on rye and other cereal grains) and yeast. The more important form is vitamin D_3, cholecalciferol, formed by the action of ultraviolet light from the sun on the 7-dehydrocholesterol in the skin. Vitamin D_3 is the form occurring naturally in fish liver oils and used in the fortification of milk, other dairy products, cereal products, and juice.

Absorption, Transport, and Storage

Absorption

Vitamin D is absorbed in the small intestine along with fat. As with vitamin A, vitamin D joins the intestinal

BOX 6-4 | Food Sources of Vitamin A

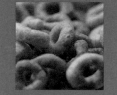 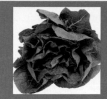 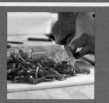 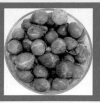 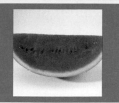

Food Source	Quantity	Vitamin A (μg RAE)*
Grains Group		
Fortified ready-to-eat cereals		
Instant oatmeal	packet	285
Special K	1 cup	230
Cheerios	1 cup	150
Wheaties	1 cup	150
Vegetable Group		
Sweet potato, baked in skin	1 medium	1403
Pumpkin, canned	½ cup	953
Spinach, frozen, cooked	½ cup	572
Collard greens, frozen, cooked	½ cup	488
Carrot, raw	1 medium	433
Chinese cabbage (bok choy), cooked	1 cup	360
Lettuce, dark green	1 cup	207
Peppers, sweet, chopped	½ cup	116
Broccoli, raw	6 flowerets	96
Brussels sprouts, cooked	1 cup	71
Fruit Group		
Cantaloupe	⅛ melon	117
Apricots, canned in juice	½ cup	104
Watermelon	1 wedge (4 × 8 inch)	80
Meat, Beans, Eggs, and Nuts Group		
Chicken livers, cooked	1	780
Clams, canned	3 oz	153
Milk Group		
Milk, skim, fortified	1 cup	148
Milk, low fat, fortified	1 cup	148
Soy milk, unfortified	1 cup	76
Cheddar cheese	1 oz	75
Milk, whole, unfortified	1 cup	68
Fats, Oils, and Sugar		
Margarine	1 tbsp	115
Butter	1 tbsp	97

Images copyright 2006 JupiterImages Corporation.

Recommended Dietary Allowances for adults: women, 700 μg; men, 900 μg.

*1 RAE (retinol activity equivalent) = 1 μg retinol.

retinol activity equivalent (RAE) Unit of measure for dietary sources of vitamin A, including both pre-formed retinol and the precursor provitamins beta-carotene, alpha-carotene, and beta-cryptoxanthin.

7-dehydrocholesterol A precursor cholesterol compound in the skin that is irradiated by sunlight to produce cholecalciferol (D_3).

cholecalciferol Chemical name for vitamin D in its inactive form. When the inactive cholecalciferol is consumed in food or synthesized in the skin, its first step in activation occurs in the liver and the final step is completed in the kidney to form the active vitamin D hormone calcitriol, 1,25-dihydroxychole-calciferol, or $1,25(OH)_2D_3$.

FOCUS ON CULTURE

Acculturation: Effect on Food Patterns

Acculturation describes the adoption of general customs and practices by persons entering a new country. Migration from one country to another and acculturation influence one's risk of certain diseases. Individuals who move from one part of the world to another quickly begin to develop the chronic diseases of their host country based on changes in their diet and environment. Those who move from Mexico to the United States are more likely to develop cardiovascular disease than their counterparts who remain in Mexico.[1] Unfortunately, newcomers to the United States often increase their intakes of sweetened soft drinks, sugary snacks, and fast food,[2] with possible weight gain and inappropriate changes in blood lipid levels. Children and adolescents are especially vulnerable to such changes in food habits.

Adolescence is an important time of life for developing healthy patterns. First, food habits established at this time are likely to be continued into adult life. Second, rapid growth and maturation require an optimum supply of nutrients. Fruits and vegetables supply important vitamins such as vitamin A, vitamin C, and folate, critical for physical development. Researchers evaluated the intakes of fruits and vegetables of 3200 boys and girls in California with an average age of 14.[3] These youth came from various race and ethnic groups, including white, black, Hispanic, and Asian. None of the groups were meeting the Food Guide Pyramid recommendation of at least three fruit servings and at least four vegetable servings every day. Hispanic adolescents ate the least amount of vegetables, and only 4% met the recommended intake. About 10% of black and Asian adolescents were eating the recommended number of vegetables. White adolescents ate the least amount of fruit compared with Hispanic, Black, and Asian groups.

About one third of the vegetables the youth selected came from the dark green/deep yellow group that supplies provitamin A. Less than half of their fruit was a citrus fruit or melon, good sources of vitamin C. Nevertheless, all groups met the DRI for vitamin A and vitamin C. Two thirds of these adolescents did not meet the DRI for folate, a matter of concern for girls approaching their childbearing years. Folate intake was lowest among Asian and Hispanic youth. However, all groups exceeded the recommended limit for sugar.

Family income and parents' level of education influenced fruit and vegetable intake. The greater the family income, the higher the intake of folate in all groups. When parents had a high school education or any years of college, their children were more likely to eat the recommended amounts of fruits and vegetables. Vegetables need to be encouraged among both Hispanic youth and their parents. Folate, although a problem in all adolescents, was especially low in Asian and Hispanic families. Nutrition educators should emphasize fruit and vegetable sources of vitamins A and C and folate that fall within the traditional food pattern and are compatible with the family food budget.

References

1. Neuhouser ML et al: Higher fat intake and lower fruit and vegetable intakes are associated with greater acculturation among Mexicans living in Washington State, *J Am Diet Assoc* 104:51, 2004.
2. Kittler PG, Sucher KP: *Cultural foods: traditions and trends,* Belmont, Calif, 2000, Brooks/Cole, a division of Thomson Learning.
3. Xie B et al: Effects of ethnicity, family income, and education on dietary intake among adolescents, *Prev Med* 36:30, 2003.

---

bile-fat complex known as the micelles and is absorbed. Malabsorption diseases such as celiac disease, cystic fibrosis, and Crohn's disease or pancreatic insufficiency hinder vitamin D absorption.

Active Hormone Synthesis

The active hormone form of vitamin D is 1,25-dihydroxycholecalciferol [$1,25(OH)_2D_3$] with the chemical name of calcitriol. Calcitriol is produced by the combined action of the skin, liver, and kidneys, an overall process referred to as the *vitamin D endocrine system.*[15]

We will look at each of the following three steps in this process (Figure 6-5):

1. *Skin:* When 7-dehydrocholesterol, the vitamin D precursor in the skin, is exposed to the ultraviolet rays of the sun, it is converted into vitamin D_3. The amount produced by this reaction depends on the length and intensity of sun exposure and the skin pigment. For those living in northern climates, sun exposure may not be sufficient to supply all of their vitamin D needs, especially in the winter months. Persons who are housebound or confined indoors and individuals residing in crowded city areas with high air pollution fail to receive adequate ultraviolet exposure to synthesize vitamin D. Heavy skin pigment prevents more than 95% of ultraviolet rays from reaching the deep layer in the skin where synthesis of vitamin D_3 occurs.[16] The use of sunscreen with a sun protection factor of 15 reduces vitamin D production by 99%.[15]

2. *Liver:* Vitamin D, whether produced in the skin or absorbed from dietary sources, is transported by a globulin protein carrier to the liver. Here a special liver enzyme converts vitamin D to 25-hydroxycholecalciferol [$25(OH)D_3$], the intermediate product in the vitamin D endocrine system. The same blood protein carrier transports this intermediate product to the kidneys for final activation.

3. *Kidneys:* In the kidneys a special renal enzyme, 1-alpha-hydroxylase, completes the last step in forming the physiologically active vitamin D hormone 1,25-dihydroxycholecalciferol [$1,25(OH)_2D_3$], or calcitriol.

Functions of Vitamin D Hormone

Vitamin D has been predominantly associated with calcium and phosphorus absorption and their metabolism and deposition in bone tissue. But we continue to learn of

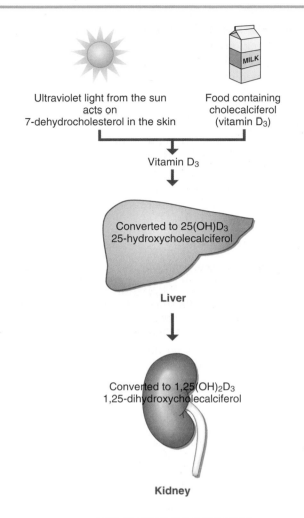

Ultraviolet light from the sun acts on 7-dehydrocholesterol in the skin

Food containing cholecalciferol (vitamin D₃)

Vitamin D₃

Converted to 25(OH)D₃ 25-hydroxycholecalciferol

Liver

Converted to 1,25(OH)₂D₃ 1,25-dihydroxycholecalciferol

Kidney

ACTIVE VITAMIN D HORMONE CALCITRIOL

FIGURE 6-5 Formation of the active vitamin D hormone. Vitamin D undergoes a conversion in the liver and then a second conversion in the kidney to form the vitamin D hormone calcitriol. Notice that vitamin D is handled the same whether it was synthesized in the skin or obtained from food.

many other functions of vitamin D important to our health and well-being.

Control of Calcium and Phosphorus Levels in Bone and Blood

The vitamin D endocrine system in cooperation with parathyroid hormone and calcitonin (1) stimulates the active transport of calcium and phosphorus in the small intestine, (2) promotes normal bone mineralization, and (3) maintains blood calcium at a normal level. Each hormone—calcitriol, parathyroid hormone, and calcitonin—has a specific role in controlling bone and blood calcium levels. Vitamin D acts primarily on the intestine to stimulate calcium and phosphorus absorption and facilitate their deposit in bone tissue. Parathyroid hormone and calcitonin are responsible for keeping blood calcium and phosphorus levels in the normal ranges.

Blood calcium must be maintained within very narrow limits to ensure proper function of the heart and nervous system. If blood calcium begins to fall, parathyroid hormone stimulates calcium withdrawal from the bone and excretion of phosphorus in the urine to help raise the calcium/phosphorus ratio to normal. If blood calcium levels begin to rise, calcitonin, a polypeptide hormone secreted by connective tissue cells in the thyroid gland, increases calcium excretion to lower blood calcium. Both parathyroid hormone and calcitonin are constantly secreted at low levels to prevent rapid fluctuations in blood calcium.

Optimum calcium intake and an adequate supply of vitamin D ensure the absorption of sufficient amounts of calcium to maintain normal blood calcium/phosphorus levels and prevent a rise in parathyroid hormone and mobilization of bone calcium. The limited hours of sunlight in northern climates during winter months has a detrimental effect on vitamin D status and bone health in all age-groups, including adolescents in peak bone growth.[17]

New Roles for Vitamin D

New research tells us that vitamin D acts on many tissues throughout the body and may have a role in preventing several chronic conditions. Vitamin D acts in the following ways:

- *Cell growth:* The rate of cell division in tissues such as the colon, breast, and lung is controlled by vitamin D. This ability to prevent abnormal cell proliferation assists in cancer prevention and is the basis for using vitamin D analogues to treat the skin disorder psoriasis.
- *Muscle strength:* Vitamin D participates in muscle metabolism and influences muscle strength and contraction. Individuals lacking in vitamin D are more likely to experience muscle weakness including weakness of the heart muscle. Falls are more frequent among older persons with poor vitamin D status.[18]
- *Immune function:* Inappropriate autoimmune responses contribute to the incidence of type 1 diabetes, multiple sclerosis, and inflammatory bowel disease. Vitamin D helps to control immune response.
- *Insulin levels:* The beta cells of the pancreas require vitamin D for normal secretion of insulin.[19]

micelle A particle made up of lipids and bile salts that carries digested lipids into the cells of the intestinal mucosa for absorption; the fat-soluble vitamins are also absorbed as part of this bile-lipid complex.

calcitriol Activated hormone form of vitamin D [1,25(OH)₂D₃]—1,25-dihydroxycholecalciferol.

25-hydroxycholecalciferol [25,(OH)D₃] Intermediate product formed in the liver in the process of developing the active vitamin D hormone.

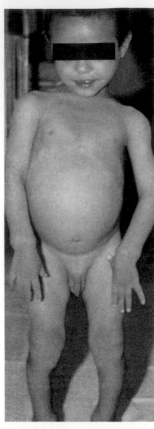

FIGURE 6-6   Bowlegs in rickets. *(From McLaren DS: A colour atlas and text of diet-related disorders, ed 2, London, 1992, Mosby-Year Book Europe Limited.)*

Vitamin D Deficiency and Clinical Applications

Role in Bone Disease

When the body does not have sufficient vitamin D, it cannot build normal bones. In children the vitamin D deficiency disease is called rickets and results in malformed skeletal tissue (Figure 6-6). Vitamin D–deficient adults develop osteomalacia, in which previously deposited bone mineral is mobilized, leading to bone pain and weak, brittle bones. Osteomalacia occurs in women of childbearing age who have little exposure to sunlight, diets low in calcium and vitamin D, and frequent pregnancies followed by periods of lactation. Older adults who use aluminum-containing antacids are at risk of osteomalacia because aluminum binds phosphorus and causes it to be excreted along with calcium. Osteomalacia is sometimes found along with osteoporosis, another bone disease common in older men and women and treated with vitamin D (see Chapter 7).

The widespread use of vitamin D–fortified milk and other foods had nearly eliminated rickets in the United States, but public health workers express concern that it is making a comeback. Increasing numbers of cases are being reported among breast-fed infants, especially African American breast-fed infants who were not given vitamin D supplements and whose mothers had poor

vitamin D status.[20,21] Rickets occurs more often in northern regions with limited winter sunlight and in individuals whose skin pigment inhibits passage of the sun's ultraviolet rays. African Americans with lactose intolerance are also likely to avoid vitamin D–fortified dairy foods. The vitamin D needs of breast-fed infants will be discussed in greater detail in Chapter 12.

Because of the active regulatory role of vitamin D in balancing bone mineral absorption and deposition, it has been used to treat the bone disease renal osteodystrophy. This condition is secondary to renal failure and results in defective bone formation.

Vitamin D Requirement

Influencing Factors

Setting dietary recommendations for vitamin D is complicated by the differing degrees of sun exposure and skin synthesis among individuals. Those working in offices must obtain more of their vitamin D from dietary sources than people who work outdoors. Individuals residing in northern climates with limited sun exposure are more vulnerable to vitamin D deficiency. Older adults are less able to synthesize vitamin D regardless of sun exposure because of aging changes in the skin.[15]

Dietary Reference Intake

Because very little research was available to help establish a DRI, the vitamin D recommendation is given as an Adequate Intake (AI) rather than an RDA (see Chapter 1 for a review of the DRI standards). The AI estimates the amount of dietary vitamin D required to sustain appropriate blood levels in the absence of sun exposure. The AI for persons between 6 months and 50 years of age is 5 μg (200 IU). For adults ages 51 to 70 years the AI is raised to 10 μg (400 IU), and for those ages 71 and older it increases to 15 μg (600 IU).[22] The elevated AI for those over age 70 points to their critical need to maintain bone mass and their limited ability to synthesize vitamin D in their skin.

Infant needs pose special problems and require the supervision of a physician. Vitamin D–fortified cereal and formula provide the current AI (5 μg or 200 IU) for this age-group. Breast-fed infants may need vitamin D supplementation.

Vitamin D Toxicity

Vitamin D is stored in the adipose tissue and released slowly, so toxic amounts can accumulate when intake is inappropriately high. Toxic levels come from self-administered doses of vitamin D supplements. There have been no reports of vitamin D toxicity resulting from fortified foods or long-term sun exposure. Adults taking daily megadoses of 1000 μg (40,000 IU) or more develop signs of severe intoxication.[22] In adults hypervitaminosis

D causes progressive weakness, bone pain, and hypercalcemia. Symptoms of toxicity in young children include failure to thrive and calcium deposits in soft tissues such as the kidneys. The UL is set at 50 μg.[22]

Health Promotion

Health Implications of Vitamin D Deficiency

Public health leaders continue to call attention to the numbers of persons of all ages who are vitamin D deficient. Medical advice for reducing the risk of skin cancer encourages people to limit their time in the sun or use sunscreen that interferes with skin production of vitamin D. Frail older people seldom venture outdoors. Youth are more likely to entertain themselves with video games or the Internet than outdoor activities. In a study of 307 healthy adolescents 24% were vitamin D deficient, and nearly 5% were severely deficient, putting them at risk of poor calcium absorption at a time when bone mineral deposition should be reaching its peak.[17] Older adults with poor vitamin D status have a greater number of falls,[18] and vitamin D deficiency can cause musculoskeletal pain.[23] Based on vitamin D intakes from food, a majority of Americans do not obtain sufficient amounts of this nutrient.[24] Less than 10% of adults ages 51 to 70 and only 2% of those above age 70 met the AI with food sources. Teenage girls and women have the lowest intakes. All of these groups are at risk of poor bone health, falls, and possibly chronic disease.

Food Sources of Vitamin D

Natural sources of vitamin D are very few. Vitamin D$_2$ is found only in yeast, and vitamin D$_3$ is found mostly in fish liver oils. Fatty fish such as mackerel contain reasonable amounts of vitamin D, and a small amount occurs in egg yolk. Major sources are foods fortified with crystalline vitamin D. Milk was selected as a practical carrier more than 50 years ago because it also contains calcium and phosphorus and was commonly used by children. The vitamin D content of milk is standardized at 10 μg (400 IU)/qt, and selected other dairy foods such as yogurt may have vitamin D added. The fortification of milk with vitamin D was credited with eradicating rickets in the United States; however, reduced use of milk in preference to soft drinks and fruit drinks has lowered intakes of both calcium and vitamin D. Margarine is fortified with 37.5 μg (1500 IU)/lb to serve as a butter substitute, and various ready-to-eat cereals have vitamin D added. Fortified juices are a potential source for the lactose intolerant. These juices also have added calcium at the level usually found in milk, and both nutrients are well absorbed from this food. Based on the need to increase vitamin D intakes in the general population, one nutrition expert proposed that it be added to the mandatory enrichment standards for grain and cereal products.[25] Good food sources are displayed in Box 6-5.

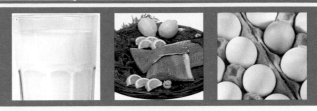

Vitamin D occurs naturally in eggs and fish. Fortified dairy foods, soy milk, juices, and cereals are other good sources for persons with limited exposure to sunlight.

Food Source	Quantity	Vitamin D (μg)
Grains Group		
Fortified ready-to-eat cereal	¾ cup	1.0
Fruit Group		
Orange juice*	1 cup	2.5
Meat, Beans, Eggs, and Nuts Group		
Tuna fish	3 oz	5.0
Egg yolk	1	0.5
Milk Group		
Milk	1 cup	2.5
Soy milk*	1 cup	2.5

Images copyright 2006 JupiterImages Corporation.
 Adequate Intake for adults: ages 19-50, 5 μg; 51-70, 10 μg; ≥71, 15 μg.
 *Consumers should check the Nutrition Label to ensure the brand they select is fortified with vitamin D.

VITAMIN E

Chemical and Physical Nature

Vitamin E was first discovered by researchers studying reproduction in laboratory animals. Because of its association with reproduction and its chemical structure as an alcohol, it was named *tocopherol* from the Greek word *tokos,* meaning "childbirth." Tocopherol came to be known as the antisterility vitamin, although this has been demonstrated only in laboratory animals and not in humans.

Forms

Vitamin E is the generic name given to a group of compounds with similar physiologic activity. These are eight

---

osteoporosis Abnormal loss of bone mineral and matrix leading to porous, fragile bone tissue with enlarged spaces that is prone to fracture or deformity; common disease of aging in both older men and women.
osteodystrophy Defective bone formation.
tocopherol Chemical name for vitamin E; it functions as an antioxidant to preserve structural membranes and other tissues with a high content of polyunsaturated fatty acids.

fat-soluble, 6-hydroxychroman compounds having some degree of the biologic activity of alpha-tocopherol, the most important in human nutrition.[26] Vitamin E is a pale yellow oil, stable to acids and heat and insoluble in water. It oxidizes very slowly, which gives it an important role as an antioxidant. As an antioxidant it inactivates free cell radicals that attack cell tissues and prevents the oxidation of unsaturated fats.[26]

Absorption, Transport, and Storage

Vitamin E is absorbed in the micelles with the aid of bile. Along with other lipids in the chylomicrons it is transported out of the intestinal wall into the lymph and then into the general circulation. Vitamin E is stored in the liver and adipose tissue, where it is held in bulk liquid droplets. The mobilization of alpha-tocopherol from these droplets is slow.

Functions of Vitamin E

Antioxidant Activity

As we study the vitamins, we will continue to hear the term *antioxidant* and the role antioxidants play in destroying molecules called free radicals. Free radicals have an unpaired electron and are constantly on the lookout for another molecule with an unpaired electron that they can join with. Free radicals are highly reactive, and the oxidation reactions they initiate are very damaging to body tissues. Free radicals are formed as byproducts of normal cell metabolism but also are found in tobacco smoke, car exhaust fumes, and other air pollutants.

Polyunsaturated fatty acids with several double bonds are especially vulnerable to attack. Cell membranes contain a high proportion of polyunsaturated fatty acids, and oxidation by free radicals alters their structure and destroys their ability to recognize harmful substances and prevent them from entering the cell. Brain cells and nerve fibers are high in unsaturated fatty acids. Deoxyribonucleic acid (DNA) and other proteins in the cell nucleus can be modified by unwanted oxidation reactions and produce molecules that are ineffective in carrying out body functions. Oxidation reactions may promote the development of various chronic conditions. Antioxidants such as vitamin E join with the unpaired electron of free radicals and break the chain of oxidation reactions that continue across tissues. Vitamin E is nature's most potent fat-soluble antioxidant, although particular tocopherol compounds differ in their degree of antioxidant activity.

Partnership With Selenium

Despite an adequate supply of vitamin E, some free radical damage may occur; therefore a second line of defense is needed to prevent a continuing chain of oxidation reactions. This added defense is an enzyme containing selenium. The trace mineral selenium can spare vitamin E and reduce the vitamin E requirement. In this partnership role, vitamin E can reduce the selenium requirement.

New Roles for Vitamin E

Researchers continue to evaluate potential therapeutic roles for vitamin E in preventing chronic disease and physiologic changes associated with aging (Box 6-6), but these efforts have been generally unsuccessful. Many age-related tissue changes are caused by oxidative damage; however, the ability of vitamin E to prevent these changes is still unclear. Vitamin E supplements do not appear to protect against cardiovascular disease,[27-29] and individuals relying on these supplements may avoid interventions of proven benefit such as adopting healthy lifestyle changes.[28] Also, vitamin E alone does not lower the incidence or progression of age-related cataracts or macular degeneration, major causes of blindness among older adults. It may be that appropriate intakes of a combination of nutrients with antioxidant activity are needed to bring about a preventive effect.[30-32]

Vitamin E Deficiency and Clinical Applications

Premature Infants

Inadequate vitamin E can have disastrous effects on red blood cells. When polyunsaturated fatty acids in the lipid membranes of red blood cells are exposed to oxidation, the membranes break, the cell contents are lost, and the cell is destroyed. Continued loss of red blood cells leads to anemia, and this vitamin E deficiency disease is called hemolytic anemia. Premature infants are especially vulnerable to hemolytic anemia because they miss the last month or two of fetal life when vitamin E stores are normally built up.

Children and Adults

In older children and adults vitamin E deficiency presents a different set of symptoms associated with the nervous system.[33] The nerves affected are (1) the spinal cord fibers that control physical movement such as walking and (2) the retina of the eye, which influences vision. Such problems were recognized in children with defective absorption of fat and fat-soluble vitamins caused by cystic fibrosis and pancreatic insufficiency. When the enzyme lipase produced by the pancreas and the emulsifying agent

---

| **BOX 6-6** | **Chronic Problems Associated With Free Radical Damage** |

Cancer: Changes in DNA can lead to uncontrolled growth of cells.
Cardiovascular disease: Oxidation of blood LDL cholesterol accelerates damage to the coronary arteries.
Cataracts and macular degeneration: Oxidation of proteins and lipids in the eye contributes to loss of sight.

bile are lost, fat and fat-soluble nutrients such as vitamin E cannot be absorbed and a chronic fatty diarrhea ensues. Vitamin E deficiency disrupts the making of myelin, the protective lipid covering of the nerve cell axons that helps pass messages along to the muscles. The neurologic complications from lack of vitamin E also cause degeneration of the pigment in the rods and cones of the retina. These light-sensitive cell membranes are rich in polyunsaturated fatty acids, and vitamin E is critical for preventing oxidation damage.

Vitamin E Requirement

Dietary Reference Intake

The RDA for vitamin E is expressed in milligrams of alpha-tocopherol because other forms of tocopherol are less effectively used by the body. Approximately 80% of the vitamin E from dietary sources, including fortified foods, is alpha-tocopherol, and about 20% comes from other forms.[26] The current RDA is 15 mg for both males and females ages 14 and older. Recent surveys tell us that many adults in the United States fall below this level.[34]

Special Clinical Needs

Vitamin E is important in the diets of pregnant and lactating women and especially urgent for newborns. An adequate intake during pregnancy can help ensure optimum vitamin E stores in the full-term infant. Hemolytic anemia, a medical problem in premature infants, responds positively to vitamin E therapy[33] and is avoided with vitamin E supplementation at birth. Optimum intakes of vitamin E and other antioxidants may benefit cystic fibrosis patients who have high tissue oxidation related to their disease.[34] Regular vitamin E replacement therapy is needed for those with chronic pancreatic insufficiency or other fat malabsorption syndromes.

Vitamin E Toxicity

Vitamin E is the only fat-soluble vitamin for which a toxicity syndrome has not been identified. Daily intakes up to 567 mg of alpha-tocopherol did not produce harmful effects, although individuals using daily supplements containing 1600 mg to 3000 mg experienced fatigue, gastrointestinal disturbances, altered blood lipoprotein patterns, and changes in thyroid function. The UL for vitamin E is 1000 mg of alpha-tocopherol per day.[26] Intakes exceeding the UL interfere with blood platelets and prevent normal blood clotting. This is particularly important for persons with low intakes of vitamin K or patients using anticlotting medications.

Food Sources of Vitamin E

The richest dietary sources of vitamin E are vegetable oils. Cottonseed, safflower, canola, and corn oil contain the highest amounts of alpha-tocopherol per serving, followed by olive oil.[35] Curiously, these oils are also rich sources of polyunsaturated fatty acids, which vitamin E protects from oxidation. Other food sources include peanut butter, nuts, and certain vegetables and fruits. Fortified ready-to-eat cereals make a significant contribution to vitamin E intake, and the vitamin is well absorbed from these foods.[36] Box 6-7 lists the major food sources of Vitamin E.

VITAMIN K

Chemical and Physical Nature

The studies of Henrik Dam, a biochemist at the University of Copenhagen working on a hemorrhagic disease in chicks, led to the discovery of vitamin K. He found that the missing factor was a fat-soluble vitamin. Because of its blood-clotting function, he called it the *koagulations vitamin,* or vitamin K, from the Swedish word for its physiologic action. For this discovery he received the Nobel Prize in physiology and medicine.

Chemical Nature

The form of vitamin K found in plants is named phylloquinone for its chemical structure. Phylloquinone is the major dietary form and is widely distributed in both animal and vegetable foods. Menaquinone, another form of vitamin K, is synthesized by intestinal bacteria. Both forms can be used by the body to meet its need for vitamin K. A water-soluble analogue of vitamin K, menadione, can be absorbed directly into the portal blood.[37] This

---

antioxidant A substance that prevents the formation and destructive actions of free radicals in the cells.

macular degeneration Destructive changes in the macula, a small spot in the center of the retina required for relay of the visual image; this condition is a major cause of blindness in older adults.

anemia Condition of abnormally low blood hemoglobin levels caused by too few red blood cells or red blood cells with an abnormally low hemoglobin content.

hemolytic anemia An anemia caused by breakdown of the outer membrane of red blood cells and loss of their hemoglobin.

myelin Substance made of fat and protein that forms a fatty sheath around the nerve axons; this covering protects and insulates the nerves and facilitates the transmission of neuromuscular impulses.

phylloquinone A fat-soluble vitamin of the K group found in green plants or prepared synthetically.

menaquinone Form of vitamin K synthesized by intestinal bacteria.

menadione A water soluble analogue of vitamin K.

BOX 6-7 | Food Sources of Vitamin E

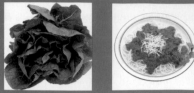 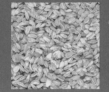 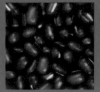 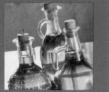

Food Source	Quantity	Vitamin E (mg)
Grains Group		
Fortified ready-to-eat cereal	¾-1 cup	13.5
Vegetable Group		
Spaghetti sauce, tomato	1 cup	5.1
Spinach, frozen, cooked	½ cup	3.3
Meat, Beans, Eggs, and Nuts Group		
Dry-roasted sunflower seeds	¼ cup	8.3
Peanut butter	2 tbsp	2.5
Sardines, canned	3 oz	1.7
Red kidney beans, canned	1 cup	1.5
Fats, Oils, and Sugar		
Corn oil	1 tbsp	1.9

Images copyright 2006 JupiterImages Corporation.
Recommended Dietary Allowance for adults: 15 mg.

makes it an important source for individuals with pancreatic insufficiency or fat malabsorption.

Absorption, Transport, and Storage

Both naturally occurring forms of vitamin K, phylloquinone and menaquinone, require pancreatic lipase and bile salts for absorption as do the other fat-soluble vitamins.[4] After entering the intestinal wall via the micelles, they are packaged into chylomicrons and travel by means of the lymphatic system and then the portal blood to the liver. In the liver vitamin K is stored in small amounts but excreted rapidly after administration of therapeutic doses.

Functional Roles of Vitamin K

Blood Clotting

The major function of vitamin K is to initiate the synthesis of four blood-clotting factors in the liver.[4] Each clotting factor is a specific protein in the form of an inactive precursor that depends on vitamin K for activation. Vitamin K works as a cofactor with a carboxylase enzyme to add a carboxyl (COOH) radical to the amino acid glutamic acid (Glu) to form gamma-carboxyglutamic acid (Gla). This activation step converts the precursor protein prothrombin to thrombin, which in turn acts on the precursor fibrinogen to form fibrin and complete the clotting process. Calcium ions as well as vitamin K are needed for normal blood clotting.

Vitamin K requires a functioning liver to carry out its tasks. When liver damage is the cause of low prothrombin levels leading to hemorrhage, vitamin K is ineffective as a therapeutic agent. Vitamin K also controls the liver synthesis of other proteins that regulate the speed and duration of coagulation. These regulatory proteins prevent the development of dangerous, unwanted blood clots or thromboses.[4,37]

Bone Metabolism

Vitamin K stimulates the synthesis of osteocalcin and other proteins that are important in bone.[38,39] Bone is constantly being remodeled (see Chapter 7), and these vitamin K–dependent proteins are necessary for the formation of bone matrix and mineral deposition. Children with higher blood vitamin K levels have higher bone mineral content than their peers.[38] Lettuce contributed the most vitamin K to the diet in one group of older women. Those who ate one serving of lettuce a day were less likely to have a hip fracture than those who ate lettuce only once a week.[40]

Clinical Applications

Cardiovascular Risk

Vitamin K–dependent proteins have been found in the walls of the major arteries. They appear to prevent the calcification of atherosclerotic plaques and may help to prevent coronary heart disease.[41]

Neonatology

The sterile intestinal tract of the newborn cannot supply vitamin K during the first few days of life until normal bacterial flora develop. During this immediate postnatal period, hemorrhage could occur. To prevent this a prophylactic dose of vitamin K is usually given to infants soon after birth.

COMPLEMENTARY AND ALTERNATIVE MEDICINE (CAM)
Vitamin K, Vitamin E, and Anticoagulant Drugs

Patients using medications such as Coumadin (warfarin), Plavix (clopidogrel), or Aggrenox (dipyridamole and aspirin) to prevent unwanted blood clots need to monitor their intakes of vitamin K. Too much vitamin K in the diet will counter the effect of the drug and reduce its effect. Several herbs used in cooking such as parsley, coriander, and mint contain vitamin K but are usually present in recipes in small amounts. At the other extreme, vitamin E, fish oil supplements, and flaxseed supplements oppose the action of vitamin K and can extend the anticoagulant action of these drugs, increasing the risk of bleeding. Vitamin E supplements should be avoided by patients on anticoagulant therapy without the prior advice of a physician.

Data from Herr SM: *Herb-drug interaction handbook,* ed 2, Nassau, NY, 2002, Church Street Books.

Malabsorption Problems

Any defect in fat absorption will impair vitamin K absorption, resulting in prolonged blood-clotting time. Thus there are several clinical situations in which supplemental vitamin K is required. Patients with bile duct obstruction are usually given vitamin K before surgery. Children with cystic fibrosis can become deficient in vitamin K.

Drug Therapy

Several drug-nutrient interactions involve vitamin K. Anticlotting drugs such as Coumadin (warfarin), Plavix (clopidogrel), or Aggrenox (dipyridamole and aspirin) act as antimetabolites, preventing the synthesis of blood-clotting factors in the liver, and so inhibiting the action of vitamin K (see the *Complementary and Alternative Medicine* [CAM] box, "Vitamin K, Vitamin E, and Anticoagulant Drugs"). When these drugs are used to prevent blood clots in the lungs or blood vessels, the dietary intake of vitamin K must be closely monitored. Too much vitamin K will oppose the action of the drug and neutralize its effect; too little vitamin K could lead to serious hemorrhage. Patients need help in choosing foods to maintain a constant intake of 65 to 85 µg/day.[42] Dark green leafy vegetables are rich in naturally occurring vitamin K, but other sources also need to be considered. Snack foods made with Olestra, a noncaloric fat substitute, are fortified with 80 µg of vitamin K per 1-oz serving, and vitamin K is also added to many multivitamin supplements. With extended use of antibiotics much of the intestinal bacterial flora is lost, eliminating one of the body's main sources of vitamin K.

Vitamin K Requirement

Dietary Reference Intake

It is difficult to set a DRI for vitamin K because part of the requirement can be met by intestinal bacterial synthesis. Moreover, reliable information is lacking as to the vitamin K content of many foods or its bioavailability. As a result, the expert committee established an AI rather than an RDA. The AI for men ages 19 and over is 120 µg/day, and the AI for women is 90 µg/day.[4] These values represent the median intakes of nearly 20,000 men and women participating in national nutrition and health surveys between 1988 and 1994. This amount of vitamin K is adequate to preserve blood clotting, but the intake needed for optimum bone health is unknown.

Newborns have a particular need for vitamin K and receive an injection shortly after birth. Persons who are taking antibiotics, being fed by enteral or parenteral nutrition, or have biliary obstruction or chronic malabsorption may require therapeutic supplementation. Toxicity has not been reported.

Food Sources of Vitamin K

Phylloquinone is found in many vegetables but is highest in dark green vegetables and liver. Menaquinones occur in milk, meat, and certain cheeses.[37] A list of good food sources can be found in Box 6-8.

For a complete summary of the fat-soluble vitamins see Table 6-2.

BOX 6-8 | Food Sources of Vitamin K

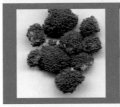

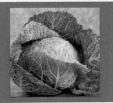

Spinach
Brussels sprouts
Broccoli
Lettuce

Cabbage
Canned tuna (packed in oil)
Spaghetti sauce

Images copyright 2006 JupiterImages Corporation.
Adequate Intake for adults: women, 90 µg; men, 120 µg.

---

prothrombin Blood-clotting factor synthesized in the liver from glutamic acid and CO_2; catalyzed by vitamin K.

antimetabolite A substance bearing a close structural resemblance to one required for normal physiologic function that interferes with the utilization of the essential metabolite.

TABLE 6-2	Summary of Fat-Soluble Vitamins

Vitamin	Physiologic Functions	Results of Deficiency	Dietary Reference Intake	Food Sources
Vitamin A Provitamin: beta-carotene Vitamin: retinol	Production of rhodopsin and other light-receptor pigments Formation and maintenance of epithelial tissue Growth Reproduction Toxic in large amounts	Poor dark adaptation, night blindness, xerosis, xerophthalmia Keratinization of epithelium Growth failure Reproductive failure	Adults Males ages ≥19: 900 μg Females ages ≥19: 700 μg Pregnancy Ages ≥19: 770 μg Lactation Ages ≥19: 1300 μg	Butter; fortified margarine Whole, fortified low-fat, and fortified nonfat cow's milk Fortified soy milk Dark green, deep yellow, and orange vegetables Yellow and orange fruits
Vitamin D Provitamins: ergosterol (plants); 7-dehydrocholesterol (skin) Vitamins: D_2 (ergocalciferol) and D_3 (cholecalciferol—used in food fortification)	Calcium and phosphorus absorption Calcitriol is major hormone regulator of bone mineral metabolism Possible roles in muscle function and control of cell growth Toxic in large amounts	Faulty bone growth; rickets (in children and youth); osteomalacia in adults	Adult males/females Ages 19-50: 5 μg Ages 51-70: 10 μg Ages ≥71: 15 μg Pregnancy All ages: 5 μg Lactation All ages: 5 μg	Fortified cow's milk Fortified soy milk Fortified orange juice Fortified margarine Oily fish (e.g., salmon, tuna) Sunlight on the skin
Vitamin E Tocopherols Most active form is alpha-tocopherol	Antioxidant Protects cell membranes including red blood cells Related to action of selenium	Anemia in premature infants Increased risk of oxidative damage to body tissues	Adults Males/females ages ≥19: 15 mg Pregnancy All ages: 15 mg Lactation All ages: 19 mg	Vegetable oils Fortified ready-to-eat cereals Nuts Dark green leafy vegetables Spaghetti sauce
Vitamin K K_1 (phylloquinone) K_2 (menaquinone) Analogue: K_3 (menadione)	Activates blood-clotting factors (e.g., converts prothrombin to thrombin) Participates in bone formation and remodeling Interferes with anticoagulant therapy	Hemorrhagic disease of the newborn Defective blood clotting Deficiency symptoms produced by anticoagulant and antibiotic therapy	Adults Males ages ≥19: 120 μg Females ages ≥19: 90 μg Pregnancy Ages ≥19: 90 μg Lactation Ages ≥19: 90 μg	Green leafy vegetables Canned tuna Spaghetti sauce Synthesized by intestinal bacteria

WATER-SOLUBLE VITAMINS

VITAMIN C (ASCORBIC ACID)

Chemical and Physical Nature

The discovery of vitamin C is associated with the search for the cause of the ancient hemorrhagic disease scurvy. Early observations of British sailors led to the discovery of an acid in lemon juice that could prevent or cure this disease. Its chemical name, ascorbic acid, is based on its antiscorbutic properties. The structure of vitamin C is similar to glucose, and most animals can convert glucose to ascorbic acid. Humans, however, lack this enzyme. So human scurvy could be called a disease of distant genetic origin, an inherited metabolic defect.

Vitamin C is an unstable, easily oxidized acid. It is destroyed by oxygen, alkali, and heat.

Absorption, Transport, and Storage

Vitamin C is easily absorbed from the small intestine but requires the presence of acid. When gastric hydrochloric acid is lacking, absorption is hindered. In contrast to vitamin A, vitamin C is not stored in a single site; instead it is generally distributed throughout the body, maintaining a limited tissue saturation level. Any excess is excreted in the urine. Tissue levels relate to intake. The total body pool in adults varies from about 2 g to as little as 0.3 g.[26] Optimum tissue saturation can meet day-to-day needs for as long as 3 months when intake is lacking. This explains why generally healthy people in isolated living situations can survive the winter without eating fresh fruits and vegetables.

Breast milk provides sufficient vitamin C for early infancy if the mother is eating a good diet. Cow's milk, however, contains very little vitamin C; this is to be expected because these animals have the enzymes to make their own vitamin C from glucose. Human infant formulas made from cow's milk are supplemented with ascorbic acid.

Functions of Vitamin C and Deficiency Conditions

Antioxidant Capacity

Vitamin C along with vitamin E is a powerful antioxidant. Vitamin C helps to take up the free oxygen arising from cell metabolism, making it unavailable to fuel the destructive actions of free radicals. This may define a role for vitamin C in preventing chronic diseases associated with oxidation (see Box 6-6).[43]

Formation of Intercellular Cement

Vitamin C helps build and maintain many body tissues, including bone matrix, cartilage, dentin, collagen, and connective tissue. Collagen is a protein found in the white fibers of connective tissue. When vitamin C is absent, an important ground substance is not formed and collagen fibers are defective and weak.[44] Blood vessels require this cementing substance to form firm capillary walls. In vitamin C deficiency capillaries are fragile and easily ruptured by blood pressure or trauma, and small hemorrhages occur in the skin and other tissues. When vitamin C is restored, the formation of normal collagen follows quickly.[42,44] Box 6-9 lists common signs of vitamin C deficiency.

Support of General Body Metabolism

Vitamin C is present in greater amounts in metabolically active tissues such as the adrenal and pituitary glands, brain, eyes, and leukocytes. The multiplying tissues of children contain more vitamin C than the resting tissues of adults. Vitamin C helps in the formation of hemoglobin and the development of red blood cells by (1) promoting iron absorption and (2) assisting in the removal of iron from the protein-iron complex called ferritin in which it is stored, making it available for use.

Vitamin C participates in other functions of metabolic importance, as follows:

- It aids the synthesis of carnitine, an amino acid that transports long-chain fatty acids into cell mitochondria, where they are burned for energy.
- It aids the synthesis of peptide hormones such as norepinephrine and receptors for the neurotransmitter acetylcholine.
- It supports the action of the mixed-function oxidase system that metabolizes drugs and breaks down carcinogens and other foreign molecules. This system sequesters lead and other heavy metals, so vitamin C may offer some protection against lead poisoning in children and adults exposed to this hazard.[45]

Clinical Applications

Wound Healing. The role of vitamin C in forming the cement for building supporting tissues makes it important in wound healing. This creates added demands for the vitamin in traumatic injury or surgery when extensive tissue regeneration is required. Formulas for parenteral feeding generally provide 100 mg of vitamin C per day. Protocols for burn patients with elevated needs for tissue growth and defense against infection call for 1000 mg/day.[46]

Fever and Infection. The body's response to infection depletes tissue stores of vitamin C. Fevers add to losses because they accompany infection and also produce a catabolic effect.

Growth. Additional vitamin C is required during periods of rapid growth in infants and children. An adequate

---

BOX 6-9 | **Signs of Vitamin C Deficiency**

Easy bruising
Pinpoint hemorrhages of the skin (petechiae)
Weak bones that fracture easily
Poor wound healing
Bleeding gums (often termed *gingivitis*)
Anemia

---

scurvy A hemorrhagic disease caused by lack of vitamin C; physical changes include diffuse tissue bleeding, painful and swollen limbs and joints, swollen and bleeding gums, loosening of teeth, and poor wound healing.
collagen The protein substance of the white fibers of skin, tendon, bone, cartilage, and all other connective tissue.

supply is critical in pregnancy to support fetal development and expansion of maternal tissues. Pregnant women who smoke may have elevated needs.[47]

Stress and Body Response.   Body stress arising from injury, general illness, debilitating disease, or emotional distress calls on vitamin C stores. The adrenal glands, which have a primary role in the stress response pattern, contain large amounts of vitamin C.

Chronic Disease Prevention.   Vitamin C may help to prevent cardiovascular disease[29,48,49] and cancer[50-52] through its action as an antioxidant, but we have much to learn. Food sources of vitamin C also contain other important nutrients and phytochemicals, making it difficult if not impossible to separate the effects of this vitamin from the other substances present. Some studies have found vitamin C supplements raise rather than lower disease risk.[50] The normally high concentration of vitamin C in the eye does suggests a possible role in the prevention of cataract or macular degeneration.[31]

Vitamin C Requirement

Dietary Reference Intake

At one time the RDA for vitamin C was set at the level required to prevent scurvy and maintain tissue saturation. The current DRI takes into account the need for antioxidant protection of body tissues. For men the RDA is 90 mg.[26] Because of their smaller lean body mass and body size, the RDA for women is only 75 mg. Cigarette smokers require an additional 35 mg each day. Additional vitamin C is necessary in pregnancy and lactation and to support gradual increases in growth.

Vitamin C Toxicity

Vitamin C intakes exceeding by far the recommended level have been promoted as effective in curing the common cold, protecting against heart disease or cancer, or delaying the signs of aging. Daily intakes of 1 g or more are not uncommon in the general population. A survey of nearly 3000 breast cancer survivors found that 24% were taking daily supplements of 1000 mg or more of vitamin C.[53] Health professionals should monitor supplement use to prevent potential interactions with ongoing drug therapy. The UL is set at 2 g; gastrointestinal symptoms and diarrhea are known to occur at higher levels.[26]

Food Sources of Vitamin C

The best known food sources of vitamin C are citrus fruits and tomatoes. Broccoli, salad greens, strawberries, watermelon, cabbage, and sweet potatoes are other good sources. (The *Focus on Food Safety* box, "Did You Wash That Orange?," offers some tips on proper handling of all fresh fruits and vegetables.) Vitamin C is easily oxidized when exposed to the air and heated, so storage, preparation, and cooking methods must be chosen carefully to preserve vitamin content (Box 6-10). Vitamin C is quite stable in an acid solution, so citrus and tomato products remain good sources even with heating. Box 6-11 lists the vitamin C content of a number of food sources. A summary of vitamin C functions and requirements is found in Box 6-12.

THE B VITAMINS

Deficiency Diseases and Vitamin Discoveries

The story of the B vitamins is a compelling one. It is a story of persons dying of a puzzling, age-old disease for which there was no cure. Eventually it was learned that common, everyday food held the answer. The paralyzing disease was beriberi, which plagued the Orient for centuries (Figure 6-7). It was named by the native words, "I can't, I can't," which describes its crippling effects. Early studies provided important clues, but the "vitamine" connection to this human sickness was needed. This was accomplished when an American chemist, R.R. Williams, used extracts of rice polishings to cure the epidemic infantile beriberi. The food factor that brought the cure was labeled water soluble B because it was thought to be a single vitamin. Now we know there are several vitamins in the B group, all water soluble but with unique metabolic functions. Each of the B vitamins has been given a specific chemical name.

Vital Coenzyme Role

The B vitamins have important metabolic functions. They serve as coenzyme partners with cell enzymes that control

---

BOX 6-10 | Food-Preparation Methods to Preserve Vitamin Content

Vitamins can be destroyed by heat, light, or the action of oxygen in the air. Water-soluble vitamins dissolve in cooking water and are lost if that water is discarded. The following practices will help consumers store and prepare their vegetables and fruits to retain the maximum vitamin content:

- Store vegetables, juices, and cut-up fruit in tightly covered containers to protect them from light and oxygen; when preparing fresh fruit or vegetables for salads or cooking, try to minimize the length of time they are exposed to the air.
- Avoid cutting food into very small pieces because this increases the surface area for loss of nutrients.
- Cook in a very small amount of water to minimize nutrient losses. (Vegetables need not be covered with water; the steam in the covered container will soften the food.)
- Cook in a tightly covered pan because this will speed cooking time and prevent loss of nutrients.
- Use the microwave to reduce both the time and amount of water needed for cooking and to help retain nutrients.
- Cook for the shortest amount of time possible (vegetable should be tender but still retain its original shape).
- Vary your menus to include both fresh and cooked vegetables. Broccoli, carrots, and cauliflower taste good eaten fresh or cooked.

BOX 6-11 | Food Sources of Vitamin C

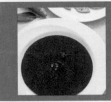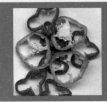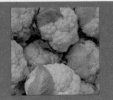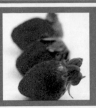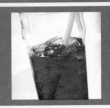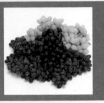

Food Source	Amount	Vitamin C (mg)
Vegetable Group		
Tomato soup	1 cup	68
Vegetable juice cocktail	1 cup	67
Pepper, chili, red	1	65
Peppers, sweet, green, chopped	½ cup	60
Broccoli, cooked	½ cup	51
Cole slaw, homemade	1 cup	39
Sweet potato, canned, cooked	½ cup	34
Cauliflower, frozen, cooked	½ cup	28
Fruit Group		
Strawberries	1 cup	105
Orange juice, frozen, reconstituted	1 cup	97
Cranberry juice	1 cup	90
Grape juice, fortified	1 cup	85
Orange	1 medium	70
Cantaloupe	⅛ melon	29
Watermelon	1 wedge (4 × 8 inch)	23
Other		
Fruit punch, fortified	1 cup	85

Images copyright 2006 JupiterImages Corporation.
Recommended Dietary Allowances for adults: women, 75 mg; men, 90 mg.

BOX 6-12 | Summary of Vitamin C (Ascorbic Acid)

Physiologic Functions

Antioxidant activity
Collagen synthesis
General metabolism
  Makes iron available for hemoglobin synthesis
  Controls conversion of the amino acid phenylalanine to tyrosine

Clinical Applications

Wound healing, tissue formation
Fevers and infections
Stress reactions
Growth
Scurvy (classic deficiency disease)

Dietary Reference Intake

Adults
  Males ages ≥19: 90 mg
  Females ages ≥19: 75 mg
Pregnancy
  Ages ≥19: 85 mg
Lactation
  Ages ≥19: 120 mg

Food Sources

Citrus fruits and berries
Vegetables: broccoli, cabbage, chili peppers, potatoes, tomatoes

FOCUS ON FOOD SAFETY
Did You Wash That Orange?

Fresh fruits and vegetables are good sources of vitamin C, folate, pyridoxine, and provitamin A. Oranges, apples, bananas, and tiny raw carrots are healthy snacks and travel well in a backpack or school bag. Fresh produce needs to be washed before you eat it or cook it to remove any remaining pesticides, any soil particles, and bacteria that accumulated as the foods were picked, shipped, and handled in the store. Fruits and vegetables to be peeled still need to be washed first. If your hands touch the banana peel that has not been washed, you will transfer those bacteria to the fruit as you peel it. It is also a good idea to wash all "prewashed" vegetables and salad greens to be sure that all soil particles have been removed.

beriberi A disease of the peripheral nerves caused by thiamin deficiency; characteristics include pain (neuritis), paralysis of the extremities, cardiovascular changes, and edema.

coenzyme A substance that is a necessary partner with a cell enzyme in carrying out a chemical reaction; vitamins and minerals are important coenzymes in energy, lipid, and protein metabolism.

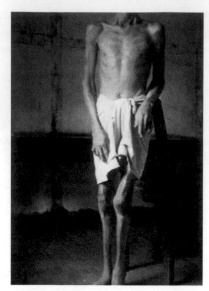

FIGURE 6-7 Beriberi is a thiamin deficiency disease characterized by extreme weakness, paralysis, anemia, and wasting away (e.g., decreased metabolic function in the liver). *(From McLaren DS: A colour atlas and text of diet-related disorders, ed 2, London, 1992, Mosby-Year Book Europe Limited.)*

energy metabolism and build tissues. There are eight vitamins in this group. First we look at the three associated with classic deficiency diseases—thiamin, riboflavin, and niacin; then the more recently discovered coenzyme factors—pyridoxine (vitamin B_6), pantothenic acid, and biotin; and finally, the important blood-forming factors—folate and vitamin B_{12} (cobalamin).

THIAMIN

The search for the cause of beriberi was successfully concluded with the identification of thiamin. Its nature and metabolic role were clarified in the early 1930s.

Chemical and Physical Nature

Thiamin is a water-soluble and fairly stable vitamin, although it is destroyed in alkaline solutions. Its name comes from its chemical ring–like structure; one of its major parts is a thiazole ring.

Absorption and Storage

Thiamin is absorbed most efficiently in the acid environment of the upper small intestine before the acidity of the food mass is buffered by the alkaline fluids in the intestine. Thiamin is not stored in large quantities, so a continuous dietary supply is needed.[54] Tissue thiamin responds rapidly to increased metabolic demand as in fever, high muscular activity, pregnancy, and lactation. Tissue stores depend on both the adequacy of the diet and its general composition. Carbohydrate increases the need for thiamin, whereas fat and protein spare thiamin. When the tissues are saturated, unused thiamin is excreted in the urine.

Function of Thiamin

Coenzyme Role

Thiamin functions as a control agent in energy metabolism. When combined with phosphorus to form thiamin pyrophosphate (TPP), thiamin serves as a coenzyme in key reactions involving glucose. About 90% of the body's thiamin is in the coenzyme form.[55] Depending on body need, glucose can be burned to provide energy or converted to fat for storage. The symptoms of beriberi—muscle weakness, gastrointestinal disturbance, and neuritis—can be traced to the loss of the energy function of thiamin and its control of glucose metabolism.

Thiamin Deficiency and Clinical Signs

When thiamin levels fall below what is needed to continue its actions in cellular energy metabolism, broad clinical effects become apparent, as follows:

- *Gastrointestinal system:* Anorexia, constipation, gastric atony, and poor hydrochloric acid secretion result from thiamin deficiency. When the cells of the smooth muscles and the secretory glands do not receive enough energy from the metabolism of glucose, they cannot perform their digestive work needed to supply still more glucose to meet body needs. This vicious cycle accelerates as the deficiency continues.
- *Nervous system:* The central nervous system depends on glucose to do its work. Without sufficient thiamin to provide this constant fuel, nerve activity is impaired, alertness and reflex responses are diminished, and general apathy and fatigue take over. If the deficiency continues, lipogenesis is hindered, followed by damage to the myelin sheaths—the lipid tissue covering the nerve fibers. This causes increasing nerve irritation, pain, and prickly or deadening sensations. If unchecked, paralysis results as in the classic thiamin deficiency disease beriberi.
- *Cardiovascular system:* The heart muscle weakens in thiamin deficiency, leading to cardiac failure. An outcome of cardiac failure is edema of the lower legs. The smooth muscle of the vascular system also deteriorates, causing dilation of the peripheral blood vessels.
- *Musculoskeletal system:* A chronic painful musculoskeletal condition results from inadequate amounts of TPP in muscle tissue. This widespread muscle pain responds to thiamin therapy.

The biochemical response to thiamin can be measured by the activity of the TPP-dependent enzyme transketolase found in red blood cells. This is a common test to evaluate thiamin status[55] and will help to determine whether a clinical observation is related to thiamin deficiency or another cause.

Thiamin Requirement

Dietary Reference Intake

The thiamin requirement is based on energy intake expressed in kcalories. The minimum requirement is 0.3 mg of thiamin/1000 kcal. To provide a margin of safety the RDA is set at 1.2 mg for adult men and 1.1 mg for adult women.[54] An intake of 1.4 mg/day is needed during pregnancy, and 1.5 mg/day is needed for lactation. Excess thiamin is excreted by the kidneys, so to date there have been no reports of toxicity from oral doses up to 50 mg. No UL has been established.

Clinical Applications

Several conditions influence thiamin needs, as follows:

- *Alcohol abuse:* Thiamin is an important vitamin when planning medical nutrition therapy for those with alcohol problems.[54] Both a primary deficiency (an inadequate diet) and a conditioned deficiency (the effect of alcohol itself) lead to thiamin malnutrition and over time serious neurologic disorders. Alcohol interferes with the active transport of thiamin across the intestinal wall, resulting in rapid depletion of tissue stores.
- *Acute illness or disease:* Fever and infection increase energy requirements and the need for thiamin. Patients on hemodialysis lose thiamin and require supplementation to prevent deficiency.
- *Normal growth and development:* Thiamin needs increase in pregnancy and lactation to meet the demands of rapid fetal growth, the elevated metabolic rate of pregnancy, and the production of milk. Continuing growth throughout infancy, childhood, and adolescence requires attention to thiamin intake. At any point in the life cycle the larger the body and its tissue mass, the greater the cellular energy requirements and thiamin needs.
- *Use of diuretics:* Diuretics used to manage hypertension and cardiac failure increase urinary losses of thiamin. If thiamin intake is low, these patients can develop a thiamin deficiency that worsens their cardiac symptoms.[56]
- *Gastric bypass surgery:* Thiamin supplementation may be necessary following a gastric bypass because energy intake is drastically reduced and absorption less efficient.[57]

Food Sources of Thiamin

Thiamin is widespread in plant and animal foods, although the amount in individual foods is usually small. This makes thiamin deficiency a distinct possibility when kcalories are markedly curtailed. Good food sources include lean pork, beef, and liver, but the major sources in the American diet are whole and enriched breads, ready-to-eat cereals, and legumes. Thiamin is extremely water soluble and readily lost in cooking water (see Box 6-10). Box 6-13 lists food sources of thiamin.

RIBOFLAVIN

Discovery

In 1897 a London chemist observed a water-soluble pigment with a peculiar yellow-green fluorescence in milk whey, but it was not until 1932 that riboflavin was actually discovered by researchers in Germany.[58] The vitamin was given the chemical name *flavin* from the Latin word for "yellow." Later when it was found to contain a sugar called ribose, the name *riboflavin* was officially adopted.

Chemical and Physical Nature

Riboflavin is a yellow-green fluorescent pigment that forms yellowish brown, needlelike crystals. It is water soluble and relatively heat stable but easily destroyed by light and irradiation.

Absorption and Storage

Riboflavin is easily absorbed in the upper section of the small intestine. Bulk fiber supplements such as psyllium, especially when taken with milk or near meals, can hinder riboflavin absorption and contribute to deficiency. Body stores are limited, although small amounts are found in the liver and kidney. Day-to-day tissue needs must be supplied by the diet.

Functions of Riboflavin

Coenzyme Role

Riboflavin is a part of the cell enzymes called flavoproteins. These enzymes—flavin mononucleotide (FMN) and flavin adenine dinucleotide (FAD)—are integral to both energy metabolism and deamination. *Deamination* is the removal of a nitrogen-containing amino group from an existing amino acid so a new amino acid can be

> pantothenic acid A member of the B vitamin complex widely distributed in nature and throughout body tissues; it functions as a part of coenzyme A, important in lipid and carbohydrate metabolism.
> thiamin pyrophosphate (TPP) Activating coenzyme form of thiamin key in carbohydrate metabolism.

BOX 6-13 | Food Sources of Thiamin

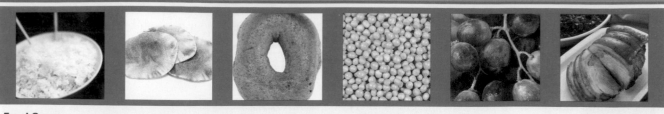

Food Source	Amount	Thiamin (mg)
Grains Group		
Ready-to-eat cereals		
Product 19	1 cup	1.50
Total Raisin Bran	1 cup	1.50
Rice Krispies	1¼ cup	0.87
Wheaties	1 cup	0.75
Corn flakes	1 cup	0.60
Instant oatmeal	1 packet	0.28
Rice, parboiled, cooked	1 cup	0.44
Pancakes	2	0.39
Bagel	3½ in	0.38
Macaroni/spaghetti	1 cup	0.29
Hamburger roll	1	0.17
Bread, enriched	1 slice	0.11
Vegetable Group		
Green peas, frozen, cooked	½ cup	0.23
Potatoes, mashed	½ cup	0.14
Tomato juice	1 cup	0.11
Fruit Group		
Orange juice	1 cup	0.20
Grapes	1 cup	0.11
Meat, Beans, Eggs, and Nuts Group		
Pork, roasted	3 oz	0.98
Ham, sliced, lean	2 oz	0.53
Kidney beans, cooked	1 cup	0.28
Baked beans, canned	1 cup	0.24
Milk Group		
Milk, whole, skim, low fat	1 cup	0.11

Images copyright 2006 JupiterImages Corporation.
   Recommended Dietary Allowances for adults: women, 1.1 mg; men, 1.2 mg.

formed. Accordingly, riboflavin is active in both energy production and tissue building.

Riboflavin Deficiency and Clinical Signs

Riboflavin deficiency results in the condition termed ariboflavinosis. This brings a combination of clinical signs that center on tissue inflammation and breakdown and poor healing of even minor injuries (Box 6-14 and Figure 6-8). Tissues subject to persistent abrasion that require continual replacement, such as the cells in the corners of the mouth, are affected first. Riboflavin deficiency seldom occurs alone; it is most likely to develop in combination with other B vitamin deficits. Riboflavin deficiency sometimes occurs in newborns. Because riboflavin is light sensitive, infants with elevated blood levels of bilirubin who are treated with phototherapy may require additional riboflavin.

Riboflavin Requirement

Dietary Reference Intake

The RDA for riboflavin is based on the amount needed to sustain optimum levels of the flavoprotein enzymes. Recommended intakes are 1.3 mg/day for adolescent and adult men and 1.1 mg/day for adolescent and adult women.[54] The higher level for men relates to their higher kcalorie intakes and larger body size. No UL has been set for riboflavin, but this does not mean that there is no danger in consuming supplements that exceed the RDA.

BOX 6-14	Signs of Riboflavin Deficiency

Lips become swollen and cracked, and characteristic cracks develop at the corners of the mouth, a deficiency sign called cheilosis.

Nasal angles develop cracks and irritation.

Tongue becomes swollen and reddened (glossitis; see Figure 6-8).

Extra blood vessels develop in the cornea (corneal vascularization).

Eyes burn, itch, and tear.

Skin becomes greasy and scaly (seborrheic dermatitis), especially in skinfolds.

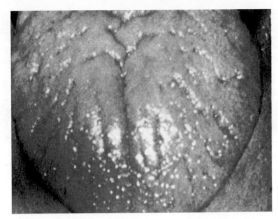

FIGURE 6-8   Glossitis. *(From McLaren DS:* A colour atlas and text of diet-related disorders, *ed 2, London, 1992, Mosby-Year Book Europe Limited.)*

Risk Groups

Certain populations may require additional riboflavin. Patients on hemodialysis are likely to require extra riboflavin to replace losses in the dialysate fluids.[54] Pregnant and lactating women and infants and children are at risk of riboflavin deficiency based on their rapid growth and high energy and protein metabolism.[59] People who engage in regular physical activity seem to have a greater need for riboflavin, likely related to increased energy expenditure and muscle maintenance and repair.[59]

Food Sources of Riboflavin

A major source of riboflavin is milk. One quart of milk contains 2 mg of riboflavin, more than the daily requirement, but the replacement of milk with soft drinks or juice drinks by children and youth reduces intake. Individuals who are lactose intolerant may not reach optimum intakes. Other good sources of riboflavin are meat, whole or enriched grains and ready-to-eat cereals, and vegetables. Because riboflavin is destroyed by exposure to light, milk is usually packaged in cardboard or opaque plastic containers. Nursing mothers who store their breast milk need to be reminded of potential riboflavin losses from glass containers. Riboflavin is stable to heat and not easily destroyed with proper cooking. Box 6-15 lists some food sources of riboflavin.

NIACIN

The age-old disease related to niacin is pellagra. It is characterized by a typical dermatitis and eventually has fatal effects on the nervous system.[60] Pellagra was first observed in eighteenth-century Europe and was common in the southern region of the United States in the early 1900s among families whose diet was largely based on corn. The American physician Goldberger noticed that children who did not have pellagra had higher intakes of meat and milk. His investigation established that pellagra was related to a certain food factor, not an infectious organism, but it was not until 1937 that a researcher at the University of Wisconsin associated niacin with pellagra by using it to cure a related disease—black tongue—in dogs.

Chemical and Physical Nature

Two forms of niacin have been identified: nicotinic acid and nicotinamide. Niacin (nicotinic acid) is easily converted to its amide form nicotinamide, which is water soluble, stable to acid and heat, and forms a white powder when crystallized.

Niacin also bears a close connection to the essential amino acid tryptophan, as described below:

- *Precursor role of tryptophan:* Curious observations by early researchers raised puzzling questions. Why was pellagra rare in some populations whose diets were low in niacin, but common in others whose diets were higher in niacin? Why did milk, which is low in niacin, cure or prevent pellagra? And why was pellagra so common in families subsisting on diets high in corn? In 1945 came the key discovery—tryptophan can be used by the body to make niacin; in

ariboflavinosis Group of clinical manifestations of riboflavin deficiency.

cheilosis Cracks and scaly lesions on the lips and mouth resulting from riboflavin deficiency.

glossitis Swollen, reddened tongue; symptom of riboflavin deficiency.

seborrheic dermatitis Greasy scales and crusts that appear on the skin in riboflavin deficiency; they are most likely to occur in the moist folds of the body.

BOX 6-15 | Food Sources of Riboflavin

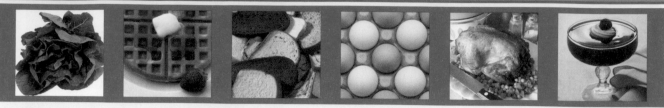

Food Source	Amount	Riboflavin (mg)
Grains Group		
Ready-to-eat cereals		
Product 19	1 cup	1.70
Wheaties	1 cup	0.85
Rice Krispies	1¼ cup	0.78
Corn flakes	1 cup	0.74
Instant oatmeal	1 packet	0.34
Waffle	1	0.26
Bagel	3½ in	0.20
Rice, parboiled, cooked	1 cup	0.13
Bread, enriched	1 slice	0.10
Vegetable Group		
Spinach, frozen, cooked	½ cup	0.17
Broccoli, frozen, cooked	½ cup	0.10
Meat, Beans, Eggs, and Nuts Group		
Pork, braised	3 oz	0.30
Egg	1	0.27
Turkey dark meat, roasted	1 cup	0.25
Kidney beans, cooked	1 cup	0.23
Baked beans, canned	1 cup	0.15
Milk Group		
Yogurt, flavored	1 cup	0.49
Milk, whole, skim, low fat	1 cup	0.45
Pudding	½ cup	0.25
Cottage cheese	½ cup	0.21

Images copyright 2006 JupiterImages Corporation.
Recommended Dietary Allowances for adults: women, 1.1 mg; men, 1.3 mg.

other words, tryptophan is a precursor of niacin. Milk prevents pellagra because it is high in tryptophan. A corn-based diet leads to pellagra because it is low in both tryptophan and niacin, but this depends on how the corn is prepared. In the American South, where corn was eaten as a vegetable or made into corn bread or corn meal, the bound niacin present in corn was not available for absorption. In Mexican families who soaked corn in lime (alkali) when preparing tortillas, pellagra was rare because the lime treatment released the bound niacin and made it available to be absorbed.[60] Others with diets low in niacin escaped pellagra because they had adequate amounts of tryptophan from animal protein.

- *Niacin equivalent:* The tryptophan-niacin relation led to the development of the unit of measure called a niacin equivalent (NE). In general, 60 mg of tryptophan can produce 1 mg of niacin, the amount designated as the NE. This unit is used in the DRI for niacin.[54]

Functions of Niacin

Coenzyme Role

Niacin has two coenzyme forms: nicotinamide-adenine dinucleotide (NAD) and nicotinamide-adenine dinucleotide phosphate (NADP). In these forms niacin partners with riboflavin in the cellular enzyme systems that convert amino acids and glycerol to glucose and then oxidize the glucose to release energy. (Recall that glycerol is obtained from the hydrolysis of triglycerides.)

Use as a Drug

Pharmacologic dosages of nicotinic acid have been prescribed for cardiovascular patients in an effort to raise blood high-density lipoprotein (HDL) cholesterol levels and reduce low-density lipoprotein (LDL) cholesterol and triglyceride levels. However, at intake levels of 1000 mg to 2000 mg (the RDA is 14 to 16 mg) nicotinic acid acts as a vasodilator and causes skin flushing and itching.

Harmful side effects can include gastrointestinal upset, hyperglycemia, and liver damage, so patients treated with these dosages require constant medical supervision[61] (see Chapter 20).

Niacin Deficiency and Clinical Applications

Niacin deficiency results in the disease pellagra with muscle weakness, anorexia, and indigestion. More specific symptoms involve the skin and nervous system. Skin areas exposed to sunlight develop a dark, scaly dermatitis (Figure 6-9). If the deficiency continues, deterioration of the central nervous system leads to confusion, disorientation, neuritis, and finally death.

Niacin Requirement

Dietary Reference Intake

The current RDAs for niacin are 16 mg NE/day for adolescent and adult men and 14 mg NE/day for adolescent and adult women.[54] These recommendations allow for differences in energy intake and body size and the availability and relative efficiency of converting tryptophan to niacin. Rapid growth, pregnancy, lactation, physical activity, or the need to replace tissues following surgery or trauma increases the need for niacin.

Food Sources of Niacin

Meat and dairy products are major sources of niacin and also high in tryptophan. Other foods include peanuts, dried beans and peas, and whole grain or enriched breads and cereals. Corn and rice are relatively poor sources because they are low in tryptophan. Box 6-16 lists some comparative food sources of niacin.

VITAMIN B_6 (PYRIDOXINE)

Chemical and Physical Nature

The chemical structure of vitamin B_6 is a pyridine ring, which accounts for its name. It is water soluble and heat stable but sensitive to light and alkaline solutions.

Forms

Vitamin B_6 is a generic term for a group of vitamins with a similar function. Three forms occur in nature: pyridoxine, pyridoxal, and pyridoxamine. All three forms are equally active in the body as precursors of the coenzyme pyridoxal phosphate (B_6-PO_4), or PLP.[54]

Absorption and Storage

Vitamin B_6 is well absorbed in the upper segment of the small intestine. It is stored in muscle but found in tissues

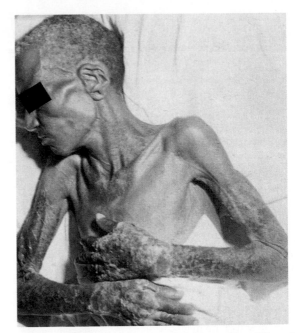

FIGURE 6-9 Pellagra results from a niacin deficiency. *(From McLaren DS: A colour atlas and text of diet-related disorders, ed 2, London, 1992, Mosby-Year Book Europe Limited.)*

throughout the body, evidence of its many metabolic activities involving protein.

Functions of Vitamin B_6

Coenzyme in Protein Metabolism

In its active phosphate form (PLP) vitamin B_6 is a coenzyme in more than 100 amino acid reactions involving the synthesis of important proteins. Key examples include:

- *Neurotransmitters:* Converts the essential amino acid tryptophan to serotonin, which carries messages across the cells in the brain; helps form gamma-aminobutyric acid (GABA) found in the gray matter of the brain
- *Amino group transfer:* Transfers nitrogen-containing amino groups from amino acids to form new amino acids and release carbon residues for energy
- *Sulfur transfer:* Moves sulfur from a sulfur-containing amino acid (methionine) to form other sulfur compounds
- *Niacin:* Controls formation of niacin from tryptophan
- *Hemoglobin:* Incorporates amino acids into heme, the nonprotein core of hemoglobin
- *Immune function:* Plays a role in the production and release of antibodies and immune cells

niacin equivalent (NE) A measure of the total dietary sources of niacin; 1 NE equals 1 mg of niacin or 60 mg of tryptophan.

BOX 6-16 | Food Sources of Niacin

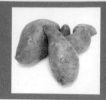 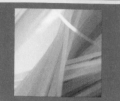 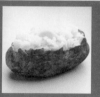 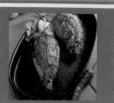 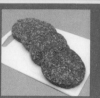 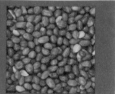

Food Source	Amount	Niacin (mg NE)*
Grains Group		
Ready-to-eat cereals		
Product 19	1 cup	20.0
Wheaties	1 cup	9.9
Rice Krispies	1¼ cup	7.1
Corn flakes	1 cup	6.8
Instant oatmeal	1 packet	3.6
Bagel	3½ in	2.4
Spaghetti	1 cup	2.3
Bread, enriched	1 slice	1.1
Vegetable Group		
Spaghetti sauce, no meat	1 cup	9.8
Potato, baked, with skin	1	2.1
Sweet potato, baked	1	2.1
Meat, Beans, Eggs, and Nuts Group		
Chicken breast	½	11.8
Tuna, canned in water	3 oz	11.2
Haddock, baked	3 oz	6.9
Beef, ground meat patty	3 oz	4.3
Peanuts, roasted	1 oz	3.9

Images copyright 2006 JupiterImages Corporation.
Recommended Dietary Allowances for adults: women, 14 mg NE; men, 16 mg NE.
*1 mg NE (Niacin Equivalent) = 1 mg niacin or 60 mg tryptophan.

Coenzyme in Carbohydrate and Fat Metabolism

PLP provides metabolites to be used for energy. It also converts the essential fatty acid linoleic acid to another fatty acid, arachidonic acid.

Vitamin B₆ Deficiency and Clinical Applications

Vitamin B₆ holds a key to a number of clinical situations, as follows:

- *Anemia:* A lack of vitamin B₆ interferes with heme formation, resulting in a hypochromic anemia. This can occur despite a ready supply of iron. The anemia is cured with restoration of vitamin B₆.
- *Central nervous system changes:* Through its role in the formation of the neurotransmitter serotonin and GABA, vitamin B₆ controls brain function. When a batch of commercial infant formula was mistakenly heated to a very high temperature, destroying the vitamin B₆, the babies fed this formula experienced increased irritability progressing to convulsions. Immediate supplementation with vitamin B₆ restored their normal function.

- *Physiologic demands in pregnancy:* Vitamin B₆ deficiency has been identified in mothers with preeclampsia (hypertension with edema and proteinuria) and eclampsia (convulsions).[54] Growth of the fetus along with rising metabolic needs of the mother increase the need for vitamin B₆. Vitamin B₆ supplements may relieve severe nausea and vomiting in some pregnant mothers.[62]
- *Blood homocysteine levels:* Vitamin B₆ may help to prevent a rise in blood homocysteine levels that accelerate arterial disease and increase cardiovascular risk.[63] (For a more detailed discussion, see the section on folate later in this chapter.)
- *Drug therapy:* The drug isoniazid (isonicotinic acid hydrazide or INH) used to treat tuberculosis is a vitamin B₆ antagonist; vitamin B₆ intakes of 50 to 100 mg/day are needed to overcome this effect. Levodopa, a medication for Parkinson's disease, lowers blood PLP levels.[54]

Vitamin B₆ Requirement

Dietary Reference Intakes

The RDA is intended to maintain optimum blood PLP levels.[54] The relatively high protein intakes in the general population increase the need for vitamin B₆. Men and

BOX 6-17 | Food Sources of Vitamin B₆ (Pyridoxine)

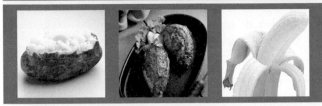

Vitamin B₆ (pyridoxine) is found in both plant and animal foods, although the milk group is low in this nutrient. Ready-to-eat cereals, potatoes, and poultry are especially good sources.

Food Source	Amount	Vitamin B₆ (mg)
Grains Group		
Corn flakes	1 cup	0.96
Instant oatmeal	1 packet	0.42
Vegetable Group		
Potato, baked, with skin	1	0.63
Spaghetti sauce, tomato	1 cup	0.43
Fruit Group		
Banana	1	0.43
Meat, Beans, Eggs, and Nuts Group		
Chicken breast	½	0.52
Tuna, canned, packed in water	3 oz	0.39

Images copyright 2006 JupiterImages Corporation.

Recommended Dietary Allowances for adults: men and women, ages 19-50, 1.3 mg; women, ages ≥51, 1.5 mg; men, ages ≥51, 1.7 mg.

women ages 19 to 50 years need 1.3 mg/day. Older adults require higher amounts of vitamin B₆ to maintain optimum blood levels, and older men need more than older women. The RDA for men over age 50 is 1.7 mg/day, and the RDA for women of this age is 1.5 mg/day.

Vitamin B₆ Toxicity

Vitamin B₆ toxicity occurred in women taking supplements 1000-fold higher than the RDA in the belief that such a dose would alleviate premenstrual syndrome. Such intakes interfere with muscle coordination and over time damage the nervous system.[54] Luckily for most of those women their symptoms gradually disappeared after they discontinued the supplements. The UL for vitamin B₆ is 100 mg/day.

Food Sources of Pyridoxine

Many foods contain vitamin B₆ but usually in rather small amounts. Good sources include grains, legumes, meat, poultry, bananas, and potatoes. The highest contributor of vitamin B₆ to the diets of U.S. adults is ready-to-eat cereals.[64] Box 6-17 displays some food sources of vitamin B₆.

PANTOTHENIC ACID

Discovery

Pantothenic acid was first isolated from yeast by researchers looking for a growth factor that prevented dermatitis.[54] Because it occurs in all living things and is an acid, it was named pantothenic acid. True to its name, it is widespread in nature and participates in many body functions. Intestinal bacteria synthesize considerable amounts. This source, along with its occurrence in a wide variety of foods, makes pantothenic acid deficiency unlikely.

Chemical and Physical Nature

Pantothenic acid is a white crystalline compound. It is readily absorbed in the intestine and combines with phosphorus to make the active molecule acetyl coenzyme A (CoA). In this form pantothenic acid has broad metabolic presence and use throughout the body. There is no known toxicity or natural deficiency.

Functions of Pantothenic Acid

As an essential constituent of CoA, pantothenic acid controls metabolic reactions involving carbohydrate, fat, and protein.[54]

Pantothenic Acid Requirements

The AI of 5 mg/day for all adults will replace the pantothenic acid lost daily in the urine. There is no UL for this nutrient.[54]

Food Sources of Pantothenic Acid

Pantothenic acid is found in both plant and animal foods. Good sources include egg yolk, milk, and broccoli.

BIOTIN

General Nature of Biotin

Biotin is a sulfur-containing vitamin. The minute traces of biotin in the body perform multiple metabolic tasks. Natural deficiency is unknown; however, induced deficiencies have occurred in patients on long-term parenteral nutrition that did not include biotin. Raw egg whites contain the protein avidin that binds biotin and, if eaten regularly, induces biotin deficiency. Cooking denatures this protein and destroys its ability to bind biotin. (Raw eggs also carry the risk of foodborne illness that can be fatal to young children, older adults, or those with compromised immune function.) There is no known toxicity for biotin.

Functions of Biotin

Biotin functions as a partner with CoA in reactions that transfer carbon dioxide from one compound to another. Examples of these cofactors at work include (1) the initial steps in the synthesis of some fatty acids, (2) the synthesis of some amino acids, and (3) carbon dioxide fixation to form purines needed for making genetic material.

Biotin Requirement

Because the amount of biotin needed is so small, the AI for this nutrient is 30 μg/day for all adults.[54] Intestinal bacterial synthesis also adds to the body's supply.

Food Sources of Biotin

Biotin is found in many foods, but its bioavailability varies greatly. The biotin in corn and soy is well absorbed, whereas that in wheat is almost completely unavailable. Excellent food sources include egg yolk, liver, tomatoes, and yeast.

FOLATE

Discovery

Folate is the generic name for a group of substances with similar nutritional properties and chemical structures. Early studies investigating an anemia occurring among poor pregnant Indian women led to the discovery of this vitamin group.[55] One folate compound was first extracted from dark green leafy vegetables and given the name folic acid from the Latin word for "leaf."

Chemical and Physical Nature

Folic acid is a yellow crystal made up of three parts: (1) pteroic acid, (2) *para*-aminobenzoic acid (PABA), and (3) glutamic acid (an amino acid). The chemical name for folic acid taken from its structure is pteroylmonoglutamic acid. Folic acid is seldom found naturally in food but is the form used in vitamin supplements and fortified foods. Naturally occurring folate or food folate is the compound pteroylpolyglutamate, which contains additional glutamic acid molecules.[54] Both forms of folate are well utilized by the body.

Functions of Folate

Coenzyme Role

Folate is the coenzyme with the important task of attaching single carbons to metabolic compounds. Several key molecules provide examples, as follows:

- *Purines:* Nitrogen-containing compounds in genetic material that participate in cell division and the transmission of inherited traits

- *Thymine:* A component of DNA, the material in the cell nucleus that controls and transmits genetic characteristics
- *Hemoglobin:* Heme is the iron-containing nonprotein portion of hemoglobin that transports oxygen and carbon dioxide in the blood

Folate Deficiency and Clinical Applications

Anemia

A nutritional megaloblastic anemia often occurs in simple folate deficiency. Because folate needs are high during periods of rapid growth, folate deficiency anemia is most likely to occur in pregnant women, growing infants, and young children. Adolescent girls who severely limit their food intake are also at risk.

Presence of Gastric Acid

An acid environment is required to release folate from its food source and enable its absorption. Low hydrochloric acid secretion in the stomach, a common problem in older people, or use of medications that raise the pH in the gastrointestinal tract can adversely affect folate status.[65]

Chemotherapy

The drug amethopterin (methotrexate) used in cancer treatment is a folate antagonist and prevents the synthesis of DNA and purines, thereby preventing the growth of the cancer.

Anticonvulsant Medications

High intakes of folate interfere with the action of phenobarbital used to control epilepsy.[54]

Folate Requirement

Clinical Factors

Folate and Birth Defects. Folate has an essential role in the formation and closure of the neural tube in the early weeks of fetal development. The neural tube eventually develops into the brain and spinal cord as fetal growth and maturation continue. Mothers with poor folate status *before* conception are more likely to give birth to an infant with a neural tube defect (NTD) and the accompanying physical and developmental disabilities (Figure 6-10)[66,67] (see the *Perspectives in Practice* box, "Folate Intake and Neural Tube Defects).

Folate and Chronic Disease. When folate is in short supply, the conversion of methionine to cysteine cannot be completed and homocysteine (the intermediate product) accumulates in the blood. High blood homocysteine levels increase the severity of atherosclerotic damage to the major arteries, adding to cardiovascular risk and stroke.[68] Folate intakes meeting the recommended level appear to offer some protection against peripheral artery disease.[69] Raising intake by even 100 μg/day helps lower elevated

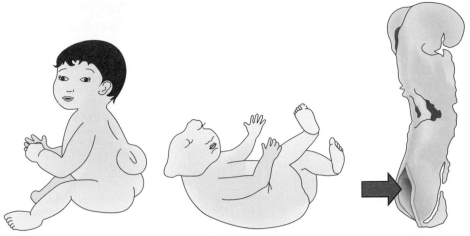

FIGURE 6-10 Neural tube defects include spina bifida and anencephaly. They result from a lack of folate needed to close the neural tube that becomes the spinal cord in the developing fetus. *(Redrawn from* www.cdc.gov/ncbddd/folicacid/excite, *Centers for Disease Control and Prevention, Atlanta, GA.)*

PERSPECTIVES IN PRACTICE
Folate Intake and Neural Tube Defects

A goal of health professionals worldwide is to prevent the incidence of neural tube defects (NTDs). NTDs are congenital abnormalities that occur when the spinal cord and its coverings fail to develop normally. When part of the brain fails to develop (anencephaly), the infant is likely to die shortly after birth. A more common NTD is spina bifida, in which the neural tube fails to close during embryonic development and the spinal cord remains on the outside of the body (see Figure 6-10). In less severe cases a child may be otherwise normal and live a productive life if surgical and medical intervention is effective. For many, however, a normal life cannot be achieved.

Researchers have focused on two possible causes of NTDs. First, it appears that some individuals have a genetic trait that alters their metabolism of folate and may increase their folate requirement, and this contributes to some NTD-affected births.[1] Poor nutritional status before conception is also related to NTD-affected births. Women with daily folate intakes below 400 μg are more likely to give birth to an infant with an NTD. Among 1136 mothers giving birth to infants with major congenital malformations, estimated daily folate intake was only 130 μg.[2] Since the mandatory folate fortification of grain products was initiated, the incidence of NTDs in the United States, previously about 0.5:1000 births, has dropped by 19%.[3]

There were several reasons for choosing food fortification rather than supplements as a way of improving folate nutrition in women of childbearing age. First, it is both difficult and expensive to provide supplements to all who may be at risk. Second, providing folate supplements to women following confirmation of their pregnancy would be too late. Development of the fetal nervous system occurs early, between day 21 and day 28 of gestation, before a woman is even aware that she might be pregnant. So it is critical that a mother be in good folate status at the time of conception.

Current fortification standards require the addition of 1.4 mg of folic acid per kilogram of grain. In practical terms one slice of fortified bread and one serving of fortified pasta provides 136 μg, or about one third of the RDA. Five servings from the grains group, depending on the portion size, could come close to meeting the target intake of 400 μg. Mexican American, Vietnamese American, and East Indian American women, for whom rice is the major grain in the diet pattern, should be urged to use rice fortified with folic acid.

Although health professionals recognize the importance of folic acid for a healthy pregnancy, a recent survey of women of childbearing age indicated that most had heard of folate, but only 25% knew it could help prevent certain birth defects or what foods could provide it.[4] Most had obtained their information from magazines or newspapers, radio or television, or their doctor. The folic acid content of grain products underscores the need to encourage women to eat the recommended servings from this food group.

References

1. Food and Nutrition Board, Institute of Medicine, *Dietary Reference Intakes for thiamin, riboflavin, niacin, vitamin B₆, folate, vitamin B₁₂, pantothenic acid, biotin, and choline,* Washington, DC, 1998, National Academies Press.
2. Olson BH et al: Effectiveness and safety of folic acid fortification, *Nutr Today* 39(4):169, 2004.
3. Oakley GP: Oral synthetic folic acid and vitamin B₁₂ supplements work—if one consumes them, *Nutr Reviews* 62(6):S22, 2004.
4. French MR, Barr SI, Levy-Milne R: Folate intakes and awareness of folate to prevent neural tube defects: a survey of women living in Vancouver, Canada, *J Am Diet Assoc* 103(2):181, 2003.

blood homocysteine levels.[70] Inappropriately high blood homocysteine levels also increase bone mineral loss and risk of bone fracture.[71] Folate intakes barely two thirds the recommended level[72] may contribute to the worsening bone health of older women in the United States.

megaloblastic anemia Anemia resulting from faulty production of abnormally large immature red blood cells; caused by vitamin B₁₂ or folate deficiency.

Folate Absorption

The absorption of folate depends on its source. Approximately 50% of the folate occurring naturally in plant foods (food folate) is absorbed, compared with 85% of the folic acid added to fortified foods. Conversion factors developed by the Food and Nutrition Board are helpful for calculating folate intakes (Box 6-18).[73]

Dietary Reference Intakes

The RDA for adolescents and adults of all ages is 400 μg/day; this increases to 600 μg/day in pregnancy to support fetal and maternal tissue growth.[54] To better ensure that women of childbearing age consume at least 400 μg of folate daily, mandatory fortification of flour, grain, and cereal foods was enacted in 1998. This has resulted in an average increase of more than 200 μg of folic acid a day in the diet of the U.S. population and is credited with the decrease in NTD-affected births.[66] We will learn more about food fortification in Chapter 9.

Folate Toxicity

The UL for folate is 1000 μg/day,[54] and supplements exceeding the recommended intake are best avoided. The basis for concern is the relationship between folate and vitamin B_{12}. If vitamin B_{12} levels are very low but folate levels are very high, folate can substitute for vitamin B_{12} and prevent the development of a megaloblastic anemia. This is a dangerous situation because, as we will learn in the next section, vitamin B_{12} also plays a critical role in maintaining nerve tissues, and folate does not meet that need. The appearance of a megaloblastic anemia is often the first sign alerting the health professional to the vitamin B_{12} deficiency. If high intakes of folate "mask" this effect, damage to the nervous system will continue unabated.

Food Sources of Folate

Folate is widely distributed in plant foods. Good sources include dark green leafy vegetables, citrus fruits, tomatoes, cantaloupe, and legumes. All grain products produced in the United States, including flour, bread, cereals, and baked products and mixes, are fortified with folic acid. Ready-to-eat cereal is the major contributor of folic acid in the U.S. diet.[64] Box 6-19 summarizes food sources of folate.

VITAMIN B_{12} (COBALAMIN)

Discovery

The discovery of vitamin B_{12} coincided with the search for a cure for pernicious anemia.[74] At first this disease was thought to be related to a deficiency of folate, but, although folate helped to initiate the regeneration of red blood cells, it did not alleviate the nerve damage associated with the disease. In 1948 workers crystallized a red

---

BOX 6-18	Calculating Dietary Folate Equivalents (DFEs)

1 μg of food folate (folate occurring naturally in a food) = 1 DFE
    1 μg folic acid (added in food fortification) = 1.7 μg DFE
(Folic acid added to foods is absorbed more efficiently than naturally occurring food folate.)
To estimate the DFEs in foods such as fortified breakfast cereals in which most or all of the folate is added folic acid, use the percent Daily Value on the food label:
% Daily Value $\times$ 400 μg (the Daily Value for folic acid) $\times$ 1.7 = DFEs per serving

Data from Suitor CW, Bailey LB: Dietary folate equivalents: interpretation and application, *J Am Diet Assoc* 100:88, 2000.

---

compound from liver that they numbered B_{12}. This new vitamin controlled both the blood-forming defect and the nerve involvement in pernicious anemia. The scientists named their vitamin discovery cobalamin because of its unique structure with a single red atom of the trace element cobalt at its center.

Chemical and Physical Nature

Vitamin B_{12} is a complex red crystal of high molecular weight with a single cobalt atom at its core. It occurs as a protein complex in foods of animal origin only. The ultimate source is the synthesizing bacteria in the intestinal tract of herbivorous animals. Some synthesis also takes place in the human intestine by local bacteria.

Absorption, Transport, and Storage
Absorption

Intestinal absorption occurs in the ileum. Vitamin B_{12} is first split from its protein complex by the hydrochloric acid in the stomach and then bound to a specific glycoprotein called intrinsic factor, secreted by the mucosal cells lining the stomach. This vitamin B_{12}–intrinsic factor complex then moves into the intestine, where it is absorbed by special receptors in the ileal wall.

Storage

Approximately 50% of body vitamin B_{12} is stored in the liver, with the remainder distributed among active tissues. These amounts are minute but held tenaciously and only slowly depleted. Vitamin B_{12} deficiency does not become apparent for 3 to 5 years after a gastrectomy with removal of the organ and loss of its secretions.

Functions of Vitamin B_{12}
Basic Coenzyme Role

Vitamin B_{12} participates in amino acid metabolism and the formation of the heme portion of hemoglobin. It is also involved in the synthesis of important lipids and

BOX 6-19	Food Sources of Folate

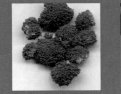 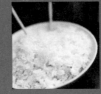 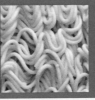 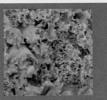 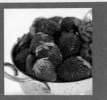

Food Source	Amount	Folate (µg DFE)*
Grains Group		
Fortified ready-to-eat cereals		
Product 19	1 cup	676
Wheaties	1 cup	336
Corn flakes	1 cup	222
Instant oatmeal	1 packet	138
Rice, parboiled, cooked	1 cup	222
Spaghetti, cooked	1 cup	172
Hamburger roll	1	73
Bread, white, enriched	1 slice	43
Vegetable Group		
Spinach, frozen, cooked	½ cup	115
Broccoli, frozen, cooked	½ cup	84
Lettuce, dark green (romaine or similar)	1 cup	76
Tomato juice	1 cup	49
Fruit Group		
Orange juice	1 cup	74
Strawberries	1 cup	40
Meat, Beans, Eggs, and Nuts Group		
Kidney beans, canned	1 cup	131

Images copyright 2006 JupiterImages Corporation.
  Recommended Dietary Allowances for adults: 400 µg.
  *1 µg DFE (Dietary Folate Equivalent) = 1 µg food folate.

proteins that form the myelin sheath that covers the nerves of the brain and spinal cord.

Vitamin B_{12} Deficiency and Clinical Applications

Vitamin B_{12} deficiency disrupts blood formation and affects cognitive function, as follows:

- *Pernicious anemia:* The megaloblastic anemia arising from vitamin B_{12} deficiency took on the name pernicious anemia because of its fatal consequences if left untreated. When vitamin B_{12} is not available, the production of red blood cells is halted because (1) the heme portion of the hemoglobin molecule cannot be synthesized and (2) the activated form of folate needed to assist in the process cannot be formed. The root cause of pernicious anemia is the lack of intrinsic factor required for the absorption of vitamin B_{12}, so another way must be found to supply this vitamin. A person with defective vitamin B_{12} absorption can be adequately maintained with monthly intramuscular injections of 1000 µg.[55] This treatment controls both the blood-forming disorder and prevents the degenerative effects on the nervous system.

- *Cognitive function:* A lack of vitamin B_{12} causes fatigue, lassitude, and a decline in cognitive function as the deficiency continues to damage the nervous system. Changes in gastric acid secretion adversely affect vitamin B_{12} absorption despite the availability of intrinsic factor because acid is needed to break the vitamin away from the protein complex in which it is found. As many as 30% of people over the age of 50 have low gastric acid levels[75]; those ages 75 and over[76] and Latino older adults[77] are at greatest risk. Crystalline vitamin B_{12} used to fortify foods is not dependent on the presence of gastric acid and is highly available for absorption. (See also the *Perspectives in Practice* box in Chapter 8, "Not Enough Stomach Acid: Is This a Problem?")

> pernicious anemia A macrocytic anemia caused by the absence of intrinsic factor necessary for the absorption of vitamin B_{12} (cobalamin); this condition is fatal unless treated with intramuscular injections of vitamin B_{12}.

TABLE 6-3	Summary of B-Complex Vitamins

Vitamin	Coenzyme: Physiologic Functions	Clinical Applications	Dietary Reference Intake	Food Sources
Thiamin	Carbohydrate metabolism Thiamin pyrophosphate (TPP): oxidative decarboxylation	Beriberi (deficiency) Neuropathy Wernicke-Korsakoff syndrome (alcoholism) Depressed muscular and secretory symptoms	Adults Males ages ≥19: 1.2 mg Females ages ≥19: 1.1 mg Pregnancy All ages: 1.4 mg Lactation All ages: 1.4 mg	Pork, beef, organ meats Whole or enriched grains and cereals Legumes
Riboflavin	General metabolism Flavin adenine dinucleotide (FAD) Flavin mononucleotide (FMN)	Cheilosis, glossitis, seborrheic dermatitis	Adults Males ages ≥19: 1.3 mg Females ages ≥19: 1.1 mg Pregnancy All ages: 1.4 mg Lactation All ages: 1.6 mg	Milk products, organ meats Enriched grains and cereals
Niacin (nicotinic acid, nicotinamide)	General metabolism Nicotinamide adenine dinucleotide (NAD) Nicotinamide adenine dinucleotide phosphate (NADP)	Pellagra (deficiency) Weakness, anorexia Scaly dermatitis Neuritis	Adults Males ages ≥19: 16 NE Females ages ≥19: 14 NE Pregnancy All ages: 18 NE Lactation All ages: 17 NE	Meat, protein foods containing tryptophan Peanuts Enriched grains and cereals
Vitamin B_6 (pyridoxine, pyridoxal, pyridoxamine)	General metabolism Pyridoxal phosphate (PLP): transamination and decarboxylation	Reduced serum levels associated with pregnancy and the use of certain oral contraceptives Antagonized by isoniazid, penicillamine, and other drugs	Adult males Ages 19-50: 1.3 mg Ages ≥51: 1.7 mg Adult females Ages 19-50: 1.3 mg Ages ≥51: 1.5 mg Pregnancy All ages: 1.9 mg Lactation All ages: 2.0 mg	Meat, organ meats Whole grains and cereals Legumes Bananas
Pantothenic acid	General metabolism Coenzyme A (CoA): acetylation	Many roles through acyl transfer reactions (e.g., lipogenesis, amino acid activation, and formation of cholesterol, steroid hormones, heme)	Adults Males/females ages ≥19: 5 mg Pregnancy All ages: 6 mg Lactation All ages: 7 mg	Egg, milk, liver
Biotin	General metabolism N-Carboxybiotinyl lysine: CO_2 transfer reactions	Deficiency induced by avidin (a protein in raw egg white) and by antibiotics	Adults Males/females ages ≥19: 30 μg Pregnancy All ages: 30 μg Lactation All ages: 35 μg	Egg yolk, liver Synthesized by intestinal microorganisms
Folate (folic acid, folacin)	General metabolism Single carbon transfer reactions (e.g., purine nucleotide, thymine, heme synthesis)	Megaloblastic anemia Elevated blood homocysteine levels	Adults Males/females ages ≥19: 400 μg Pregnancy All ages: 600 μg Lactation All ages: 500 μg	Green leafy vegetables Oranges, orange juice, tomatoes Liver and organ meats Fortified breads and cereals

NE, Niacin equivalent.

TABLE 6-3	Summary of B-Complex Vitamins—cont'd			
Vitamin	**Coenzyme: Physiologic Functions**	**Clinical Applications**	**Dietary Reference Intake**	**Food Sources**
Vitamin B$_{12}$ (cobalamin)	General metabolism Methylcobalamin: methylation reactions (e.g., synthesis of amino acids, heme)	Pernicious anemia induced by lack of intrinsic factor Megaloblastic anemia Methylmalonic aciduria Homocystinuria Peripheral neuropathy (vegan diet lacking B$_{12}$ supplements or fortified foods)	Adults Males/females ages ≥19: 2.4 μg Pregnancy All ages: 2.6 μg Lactation All ages: 2.8 μg	Meat, milk, cheese, egg, liver (all animal foods) Fortified cereals

BOX 6-20	Food Sources of Vitamin B$_{12}$ (Cobalamin)

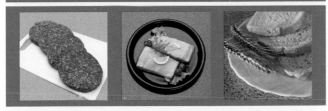

Vitamin B$_{12}$ (cobalamin) is found naturally in animal foods only, but various grain foods and juices are fortified with this vitamin. Vegans who consume no animal foods and older persons with reduced gastric acid levels should check the Nutrition Label to identify products with added vitamin B$_{12}$.

Naturally Occurring Sources of Vitamin B$_{12}$
Meat patty
Chicken leg
Fish serving
Milk

Examples of Nonanimal Foods Fortified With Vitamin B$_{12}$
Ready-to-eat cereal
Bread
Orange juice

Images copyright 2006 JupiterImages Corporation.
    Recommended Dietary Allowances for adults: 2.4 μg

Vitamin B$_{12}$ Requirement

The amount of vitamin B$_{12}$ needed for normal human metabolism is minute. The RDA for vitamin B$_{12}$ is 2.4 μg for both younger and older adults.[54]

Food Sources of Vitamin B$_{12}$

In nature vitamin B$_{12}$ is found only in animal foods; rich sources include lean meat, fish, poultry, milk, eggs, and cheese. For individuals consuming any ani-

mal foods, the recommended intake is easily obtained. Vegans who consume no animal foods or individuals with low gastric acid levels can obtain the amount needed from fortified cereal and grain products or vitamin B$_{12}$ supplements. Box 6-20 lists some sources of vitamin B$_{12}$.

A summary of the water-soluble B vitamins is presented in Table 6-3.

TO SUM UP

A vitamin is an organic, non–energy-yielding substance found in food that is (1) required in very small amounts; (2) participates in certain metabolic functions, often as a coenzyme; and (3) cannot be manufactured by the body. Vitamins may be fat soluble or water soluble, and their solubility affects their absorption and transport to target tissues.

The fat-soluble vitamins are A, D, E, and K. Their metabolic tasks focus on the synthesis of important proteins, the development and differentiation of cells and tissues, and the protection of structural membranes. They are absorbed and transported in the body associated with lipids. The possibility of toxicity is increased for fat-soluble vitamins because the body has a high storage capacity for these nutrients. Toxicity has occurred from abuse of high potency supplements.

The water-soluble vitamins include vitamin C (ascorbic acid) and the B complex. These vitamins share three characteristics: (1) they are synthesized by plants and (with the exception of vitamin B$_{12}$) are supplied in the diet by both plant and animal foods; (2) body stores are limited so they must be consumed regularly; and (3) they function as coenzymes in cell metabolism and the synthesis of vital molecules. Toxicity is uncommon with water-soluble vitamins because excess intake is excreted in the urine. However, two vitamins have shown toxic effects when taken in excessive amounts: pyridoxine (vitamin B_6) caused severe damage to the nerves, and ascorbic acid (vitamin C) was associated with gastrointestinal disturbances, renal calculi, and lowered resistance to infection. Folate if consumed in levels above what is recommended can mask a serious deficiency of vitamin B_{12}. Water-soluble vitamins, especially vitamin C and folate, are easily oxidized, and appropriate cooking and storage practices are required.

QUESTIONS FOR REVIEW

1. How do the absorption and storage of a vitamin affect the risk of deficiency or toxicity? Provide several examples to illustrate this concept.

2. List and describe three health problems caused by a vitamin A deficiency. Give three possible causes of a vitamin A deficiency.

3. Describe the formation and function of the vitamin D hormone calcitriol. Who is at risk for vitamin D deficiency? Why?

4. Vitamin E has an important role as an antioxidant. What is an antioxidant? How does it protect body tissues? A woman tells you that she is taking 1000 mg of vitamin E to prevent signs of aging—how would you advise her?

5. You have a client who is taking a prescription anticoagulant. What do you need to tell her about (1) food choices and (2) use of other supplements?

6. You are working with a child who has cystic fibrosis. What should you be telling her caregivers about her vitamin needs? Does she require a vitamin supplement? Why?

7. What three characteristics are shared by most water-soluble vitamins? Identify an exception to each and explain the reason.

8. Define the term *coenzyme* as applied to the role of the water-soluble vitamins. Give several examples.

9. Which water-soluble vitamins have an Upper Tolerable Intake level (UL)? What signs of toxicity have been observed for each?

10. Name the B vitamins involved in blood formation. Describe their roles and interactions.

11. You have been asked to speak at a senior citizens center on the topic of phytochemicals. Outline your presentation describing (1) what a phytochemical is, (2) why phytochemicals are important, and (3) good food sources to include in your diet. The senior center director has given you some money for groceries to provide taste treats to serve with your program. What foods or recipes will you prepare?

12. Visit a nearby grocery store, and from the food label record the folate content of (1) three different breads, (2) three different ready-to-eat cereals, (3) three types of rice or rice-containing dishes, and (4) three types of pasta or pasta-containing dishes. Rice and pasta dishes may be dry mixes or frozen entrees. Develop menus for 3 days that include a daily minimum of six servings from the grains group and provide at least 400 μg of folate.

REFERENCES

1. Marsh MN, Riley SA: Digestion and absorption of nutrients and vitamins. In Feldman M, Scharschmidt BF, Sleisenger MH, eds: *Gastrointestinal and liver disease,* ed 6, vol 2, Philadelphia, 1998, WB Saunders.

2. Carpenter KJ, Harper AE: Evolution of knowledge of essential nutrients. In Shils ME et al, eds: *Modern nutrition in health and disease,* ed 10, Baltimore, 2006, Lippincott Williams & Wilkins.

3. Krinsky NI: Human requirements for fat-soluble vitamins, and other things concerning these nutrients, *Mol Aspects Med* 24:317, 2003.

4. Food and Nutrition Board, Institute of Medicine: *Dietary Reference Intakes for vitamin A, vitamin K, arsenic, boron, chromium, copper, iodine, iron, manganese, molybdenum, nickel, silicon, vanadium, and zinc,* Washington, DC, 2001, National Academies Press.

5. West CE et al: Consequences of revised estimates of carotenoid bioefficacy for dietary control of vitamin A deficiency in developing countries, *J Nutr* 132:2920S, 2002.

6. Olson JA et al: Fat-soluble vitamins. In Garrow GS, James WPT, Ralph A, eds: *Human nutrition and dietetics,* ed 10, Edinburgh, 2000, Churchill Livingstone.

7. Ross DA: Recommendations for vitamin A supplementation, *J Nutr* 131:2902S, 2002.

8. Feskanich D et al: Vitamin A intake and hip fractures among postmenopausal women, *JAMA* 287:47, 2002.

9. Johanning GL, Piyathilake CJ: Retinoids and epigenetic silencing in cancer, *Nutr Reviews* 61(8):284, 2003.

10. Ross AC: Vitamin A and carotenoids. In Shils ME et al, eds: *Modern nutrition in health and disease,* ed 10, Baltimore, 2006, Lippincott Williams & Wilkins.

11. Paeratakul S et al: Fast-food consumption among U.S. adults and children: dietary and nutrient intake profile, *J Am Diet Assoc* 103(10):1332, 2003.

12. Thorsdottir I et al: Association of fish and fish liver oil intake in pregnancy with infant size at birth among women of normal weight before pregnancy in a fishing community, *Am J Epidemiol* 160:460, 2004.

13. Allen LH, Haskell M: Estimating the potential for vitamin A toxicity in women and young children, *J Nutr* 132:2907S, 2002.

14. Penniston KL, Tanumihardjo SA: Vitamin A in dietary supplements and fortified foods: too much of a good thing, *J Am Diet Assoc* 103:1185, 2003.

15. Holick MF: Vitamin D: importance in the prevention of cancers, type 1 diabetes, heart disease, and osteoporosis, *Am J Clin Nutr* 79:362, 2004.

16. Holick MF: Vitamin D. In Shils ME et al, eds: *Modern nutrition in health and disease,* ed 10, Baltimore, 2006, Lippincott Williams & Wilkins.

17. Gordon GM et al: Prevalence of vitamin D deficiency among healthy adolescents, *Arch Pediatr Adolesc Med* 158:531, 2004.

18. Bischoff-Ferrari HA et al: Effect of vitamin D on falls: a meta-analysis, *JAMA* 291:1999, 2004.

19. Zittermann A: Vitamin D in preventive health: are we ignoring the evidence, *Brit J Nutr* 89:552, 2003.

20. Stokstad E: The vitamin D deficit, *Science* 302:1886 (Dec 12), 2003.

21. Hollis BW, Wagner CL: Assessment of vitamin D requirements during pregnancy and lactation, *Am J Clin Nutr* 79:717, 2004.

22. Food and Nutrition Board, Institute of Medicine: *Dietary Reference Intakes for calcium, phosphorus, magnesium, vitamin D, and fluoride,* Washington, DC, 1997, National Academies Press.

23. Mascarenhas R, Mobarhan S: Hypovitaminosis D-induced pain, *Nutr Reviews* 62(9):354, 2004.

24. Moore C et al: Vitamin D intake in the United States, *J Am Diet Assoc* 104:980, 2004.

25. Newmark HL et al: Should calcium and vitamin D be added to the current enrichment program for cereal-grain products, *Am J Clin Nutr* 80:264, 2004.

26. Food and Nutrition Board, Institute of Medicine: *Dietary Reference Intakes for vitamin C, vitamin E, selenium, and carotenoids,* Washington, DC, 2000, National Academies Press.

27. Shekelle PG et al: Effect of supplemental vitamin E for the prevention and treatment of cardiovascular disease, *J Gen Intern Med* 19:380, 2004.

28. Eidelman RS et al: Randomized trials of vitamin E in the treatment and prevention of cardiovascular disease, *Arch Intern Med* 164:1552, 2004.

29. Kinkey S et al: Long term effect of combined vitamins E and C on coronary and peripheral endothelial function, *J Am Coll Cardiol* 43:629, 2004.

30. Mares J: High-dose antioxidant supplementation and cataract risk, *Nutr Reviews* 62(1):28, 2004.

31. Taylor A, Siegal M: Nutritional influences on risk for cataract, *Nutr & the MD* 28(10):1, 2002.

32. Taylor A et al: Long term intake of vitamins and carotenoids and odds of early age-related cortical and posterior subcapsular lens opacities, *Am J Clin Nutr* 75:540, 2002.

33. Traber MG: Vitamin E. In Shils ME et al, eds: *Modern nutrition in health and disease,* ed 10, Baltimore, 2006, Lippincott Williams & Wilkins.

34. Back EI et al: Antioxidant deficiency in cystic fibrosis: when is the right time to take action? *Am J Clin Nutr* 80:374, 2004.

35. Maras JE et al: Intake of alpha-tocopherol is limited among U.S. adults, *J Am Diet Assoc* 104:567, 2004.

36. Leonard SW et al: Vitamin E bioavailability from fortified breakfast cereal is greater than that from encapsulated supplements, *Am J Clin Nutr* 29:86, 2004.

37. Suttie JW: Vitamin K. In Shils ME et al, eds: *Modern nutrition in health and disease,* ed 10, Baltimore, 2006, Lippincott Williams & Wilkins.

38. Kalkwarf HJ et al: Vitamin K, bone turnover, and bone mass in girls, *Am J Clin Nutr* 80:1075, 2004.

39. Booth SL et al: Associations between vitamin K biochemical measures and bone mineral density in men and women, *J Clin Endocrinol Metab* 89:4904, 2004.

40. Feskanich D et al: Vitamin K intake and hip fractures in women: a prospective study, *Am J Clin Nutr* 69:74, 1999.

41. Geleijnse JM et al: Dietary intake of menaquinone is associated with a reduced risk of coronary heart disease: the Rotterdam Study, *J Nutr* 134:3100, 2004.

42. Booth SL, Centurelli MA: Vitamin K: a practical guide to the dietary management of patients on warfarin, *Nutr Rev* 57:288, 1999.

43. Jacob RA, Sotoudeh G: Vitamin C function and status in chronic disease, *Nutr Clin Care* 5(2):47, 2002.

44. Guyton AC, Hall JE: *Textbook of medical physiology,* ed 10, Philadelphia, 2000, WB Saunders.

45. Houston DK, Johnson MA: Does vitamin C intake protect against lead toxicity? *Nutr Rev* 58:73, 2000.

46. Winkler MA, Manchester S: Medical nutrition therapy for metabolic stress, sepsis, trauma, burns, and surgery. In Mahan KL, Escott-Stump S, eds: *Krause's food, nutrition, & diet therapy,* ed 11, Philadelphia, 2004, Elsevier.

47. Cogswell ME et al: Cigarette smoking, alcohol use and adverse pregnancy outcomes: implications for micronutrient supplementation, *J Nutr* 133:1722S, 2003.

48. Beitz R et al: Blood pressure and vitamin C and fruit and vegetable intake, *Ann Nutr Metab* 47:214, 2003.

49. Frei B: Efficacy of dietary antioxidants to prevent oxidative damage and inhibit chronic disease, *J Nutr* 134:3196S, 2004.

50. Lee KW et al: Vitamin C and cancer chemoprevention: reappraisal, *Am J Clin Nutr* 78:1074, 2003.

51. Satia-Abouta J et al: Association of micronutrients with colon cancer risk in African Americans and whites: results from the North Carolina colon cancer study, *Cancer Epidemiol Biomarkers Prev* 12:747, 2003.

52. Cho E et al: Premenopausal intakes of vitamins A, C, and E, folate, and carotenoids, and risk of breast cancer, *Cancer Epidemiol Biomark Prev* 12:713, 2003.

53. Rock CL et al: Antioxidant supplement use in cancer survivors and the general population, *J Nutr* 134:3194S, 2004.

54. Food and Nutrition Board, Institute of Medicine: *Dietary Reference Intakes for thiamin, riboflavin, niacin, vitamin B_6, folate, vitamin B_{12}, pantothenic acid, biotin, and choline,* Washington, DC, 1998, National Academies Press.

55. Thurnham DI et al: Water-soluble vitamins. In Garrow GS, James WPT, Ralph A, eds: *Human nutrition and dietetics,* ed 10, Edinburgh, 2000, Churchill Livingstone.

56. Suter PM, Vetter W: Diuretics and vitamin B1: are diuretics a risk factor for thiamin malnutrition? *Nutr Rev* 58:319, 2000.

57. Nakamura K et al: Polyneuropathy following gastric bypass surgery, *Am J Med* 115:679, 2003.

58. McCormick DB: Riboflavin. In Shils ME et al, eds: *Modern nutrition in health and disease,* ed 10, Baltimore, 2006, Lippincott Williams & Wilkins.

59. Powers HJ: Riboflavin (vitamin B-2) and health, *Am J Clin Nutr* 77:1352, 2003.

60. Bourgeois C, Cervantes-Laurean D, Moss J: Niacin. In Shils ME et al, eds: *Modern nutrition in health and disease,* ed 10, Baltimore, 2006, Lippincott Williams & Wilkins.

61. Goldberg AC: A meta-analysis of randomized controlled studies on the effects of extended-release niacin in women, *Am J Cardiol* 94:121, 2004.

62. Koren G, Maltepe C: Pre-emptive therapy for severe nausea and vomiting of pregnancy and hyperemesis gravidarum, *J Obstet Gynaecol* 24:530, 2004.

63. Tool JF et al: Lowering homocysteine in patients with ischemic stroke to prevent recurrent stroke, myocardial infarction, and death: the Vitamin Intervention for Stroke Prevention (VISP) Randomized Trial, *JAMA* 291(5):565, 2004.

64. Cotton PA et al: Dietary sources of nutrients among U.S. adults, 1994-1996 (additional tables accessed at *www.eatright.org* on November 3, 2004), *J Am Diet Assoc* 104:921, 2004.

65. Gregory JF: Case study: folate bioavailability, *J Nutr* 131:1376S, 2001.

66. Quinlivan EP, Gregory JF: Effect of food fortification on folic acid intake in the United States, *Am J Clin Nutr* 77:221, 2003.

67. Shane B: Folate fortification: enough already, *Am J Clin Nutr* 77:8, 2003.

68. Homocysteine Studies Collaboration: Homocysteine and risk of ischemic heart disease and stroke: a meta-analysis, *JAMA* 288:2015, 2002.

69. Merchant AT et al: The use of B vitamin supplements and peripheral arterial disease risk in men are inversely related, *J Nutr* 133:2863, 2003.

70. Venn BJ et al: Assessment of three levels of folic acid on serum folate and plasma homocysteine: a randomised placebo-controlled double-blind dietary intervention trial, *Eur J Clin Nutr* 56:748, 2002.

71. van Meurs JBJ et al: Homocysteine levels and the risk of osteoporotic fractures, *N Eng J Med* 350:2033, 2004.

72. Ervin RB et al: *Dietary intake of selected vitamins for the United States population: 1999-2000, advance data, vital and health statistics,* No. 339, Washington, DC, 2004 (March 12), United States Department of Health and Human Services.

73. Suitor CD, Bailey LB: Dietary folate equivalents: interpretation and application, *J Am Diet Assoc* 100(1):81, 2000.

74. Carmel R: Cobalamin (Vitamin B_{12}). In Shils ME et al, eds: *Modern nutrition in health and disease,* ed 10, Baltimore, 2006, Lippincott Williams & Wilkins.

75. Bailey LB: Folate and vitamin B_{12} recommended intakes and status in the United States, *Nutr Reviews* 62(6):S14, 2004.

76. Clarke R et al: Screening for vitamin B_{12} and folate deficiency in older persons, *Am J Clin Nutr* 77:1241, 2003.

77. Campbell AK et al: Plasma vitamin B_{12} concentrations in an elderly Latino population are predicted by serum gastrin concentrations and crystalline vitamin B_{12} intake, *J Nutr* 133:2770, 2003.

FURTHER READINGS AND RESOURCES

Readings

Olson BH et al: Effectiveness and safety of folic acid fortification, *Nutr Today* 39(4):169, 2004.

This article provides insight as to the value and the concerns pertaining to folate fortification of grain foods.

The following three articles point to community nutrition practice and fruit and vegetable intake:

Nanney MS et al: Rationale for a consistent "powerhouse" approach to vegetable and fruit messages, *J Am Diet Assoc* 104(3):352, 2004.

These authors suggest how nutrition professionals can join forces with other groups such as the American Heart Association to provide effective nutrition education and increase use of fruits and vegetables.

Akobundu UO et al: Vitamins A and C, calcium, fruit, and dairy products are limited in food pantries, *J Am Diet Assoc* 104:811, 2004.

Food pantries are a source of emergency foods for many women, children, and families. We need to consider how we can improve the nutrient quality of foods available to them.

Cullen KW et al: Effect of a la carte and snack bar foods at school on children's lunchtime intake of fruits and vegetables, *J Am Diet Assoc* 100:1482, 2000.

Children who have access to a snack bar in their school may not consume as many fruits and vegetables at lunch. This article helps us think about school food service issues and their influence on nutrient intake.

Websites of Interest

- United States Department of Agriculture, United States Department of Health and Human Services, *Dietary Guidelines for Americans 2005, ed 6;* the *Dietary Guidelines for Americans 2005* provides important information on choosing fruits and vegetables for good health: *www.healthierus.gov/dietaryguidelines/.*

- National Institute of Health, National Heart, Lung and Blood Institute, the DASH Eating Plan; the DASH diet provides advice for selecting fruits and vegetables and helpful recipes for their preparation: *http://www.nhlbi.nih.gov/health/public/heart/hbp/dash/index.htm.*

- Produce for Better Health Foundation; this site provides nutrition education materials and recipes to help consumers eat the recommended five to nine fruits and vegetables each day: *http://www.5aday.com/.*

CHAPTER 7

Minerals

Eleanor D. Schlenker

We completed our review of the three macronutrients, carbohydrate, fat, and protein, and one of the classes of micronutrients, the vitamins. Now we turn to the remaining class of micronutrients, the minerals, as well as the last nutrient category—water. As individual elements minerals seem simple in comparison to the complex vitamins, but they fulfill equally important roles.

Minerals having a requirement greater than 100 mg/day are called major minerals, not because they are more important but because there is more of them in the body. Those needed in smaller amounts are called trace elements, and a few required in only minute amounts are referred to as ultratrace elements.

As with the vitamins we will focus on why we need them and how we obtain them.

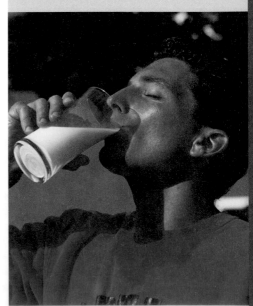

Copyright 1999-2006 Getty Images, Inc.

Probable Essential Trace Elements
Water-Electrolyte Balance
Water Balance
Overall Water Balance: Intake and Output
Water Requirements
Forces Controlling Water Distribution
Influence of Electrolytes on Water Balance
Influence of Plasma Protein on Water
    Balance
Influence of Hormones on Water Balance

MINERALS IN HUMAN NUTRITION

COMPARISON OF VITAMINS AND MINERALS

The two micronutrient classes, the vitamins and minerals, have both similarities and differences (Table 7-1). Vitamins are complex organic molecules that serve primarily as coenzymes or regulators of body metabolism, especially energy metabolism. Minerals, on the other hand, are simple elements with important roles in both structure and function. As is true for the vitamins, an excess of one mineral cannot remedy an existing deficit of another, emphasizing our need to eat a variety of foods.

CYCLE OF MINERALS

On Earth we live within a vast slow-motion cycle of minerals essential to life. Elements present in water find their way into rocks and soil and through plants, to animals and humans.[1] Until recent times our access to these elements depended on luck—where we happened to live—because most people obtained all of their food from nearby farms. But with expanding knowledge of how these elements are incorporated into foods, plus the fact that much of the food we eat is grown outside of our immediate community, people living in all parts of the country or world can be supplied with adequate mineral nutrition.

METABOLIC ROLES

Differing Functions

Minerals have roles in the body as varied as the elements themselves. They carry out an impressive array of structural and metabolic activities, as follows:

- *Structural:* Calcium and phosphorus give strength to the bones and body frame. Iron provides the core for the *heme* in hemoglobin that delivers oxygen to the tissues. Red cobalt is the atom at the center of the vitamin B_{12} molecule.
- *Metabolic:* Ionized sodium and potassium exercise control over body water. Iodine is a necessary constituent of the thyroid hormone that sets the rate of metabolism in the cells. Iron is a coenzyme in the mitochondrial oxidase system that provides our body with energy fuel.

Some minerals such as iron contribute to both structure and function. Far from being static and inert, minerals are active participants in many systems and activities that support life.

TABLE 7-1	Mineral and Vitamin Comparison	
Characteristic	**Minerals**	**Vitamins**
Similarities		
Essentiality	Must be obtained in food	Must be obtained in food
Unique role	One cannot take the place of another	One cannot take the place of another
Interactions	Can interfere with another if present in inappropriate amounts	Can interfere with another if present in inappropriate amounts
Impact on chronic disease	May have a role in prevention of chronic disease	May have a role in prevention of chronic disease
Differences		
Structure	Simple organic elements	Complex organic structures
Absorption	Problems in absorption from interfering or binding substances	More easily absorbed
Classification	Based on amount needed by the body	Based on solubility in water or lipid
Roles in the body	Structural and metabolic	Only metabolic
Amount needed	Varies based on the mineral	Needed in very minute amounts
Stability	Seldom lost in cooking	Easily lost in cooking

Differing Amounts

Minerals differ from vitamins in the amounts needed to complete their tasks. All vitamins are required in very small amounts; minerals, however, vary in the quantities needed from the larger amounts of the major minerals to the exceedingly small amounts of the trace elements. The major mineral calcium contributes a relatively large proportion of body weight—approximately 2%, and most of this calcium is in the skeleton. A man weighing 150 lb has about 3 lb of calcium in his body. This same adult contains only about 3 g ($\frac{1}{10}$ oz) of iron, mostly in the hemoglobin of red blood cells.

Concept of Bioavailability

In general the absorption of minerals is less efficient than the absorption of vitamins and macronutrients. The amount of mineral present in a food as determined by laboratory analysis may not be the amount that is actually available and absorbed by the body. The term bioavailability refers to the proportion of a nutrient that is absorbed and can be used in carrying out body functions.[2] Bioavailability depends on many factors relating to both the food source and the receiver, as follows:

- *Binding substances in plants:* In some plant foods minerals are bound to other substances and not easily released. Oxalates in some green leafy vegetables and phytates in grains bind minerals and prevent their absorption.
- *Gastric acidity:* Hydrochloric acid levels in the stomach affect bioavailability because many minerals are better absorbed in an acid environment.
- *Chemical form of the mineral:* Iron in the ferric form cannot be absorbed; it must first be reduced to ferrous iron for absorption to take place.
- *Other foods in the same meal:* Some foods such as tea contain substances that interfere with the absorption of particular minerals.
- *Body need:* Certain minerals are absorbed at higher rates in periods of active growth, pregnancy, and lactation.

Issues of bioavailability make it difficult to set dietary recommendations for minerals.

CLASSIFICATION

The minerals are organized into three general groups: major minerals, trace elements that are known to be essential, and trace elements that are probably essential. These divisions are based on (1) how much of the mineral is required and (2) how much we know about its essentiality.

Major Minerals

The seven minerals present in the body in large amounts are referred to as major minerals; these include calcium, phosphorus, magnesium, sodium, potassium, sulfur, and chloride.

Trace Elements

The remaining minerals are found in smaller amounts and termed the trace elements. Ten of these are known to be essential to body function. As for the remaining eight, their precise role in the body is not clear.

The minerals in each group are listed in Box 7-1. We will review (1) regulation of absorption, (2) physiologic function, (3) clinical applications, (4) daily requirement, and (5) food sources.

MAJOR MINERALS

CALCIUM

Of all the minerals in the body, calcium is by far present in the largest amount. Total body calcium is in constant

BOX 7-1	Major Minerals and Trace Elements

Major Minerals (Required Intake ≥100 mg/day)

Calcium (Ca)	Potassium (K)
Phosphorus (P)	Chloride (Cl)
Magnesium (Mg)	Sulfur (S)
Sodium (Na)	

Trace Elements

Essential (Required Intake <100 mg/day)

Iron (Fe)	Chromium (Cr)
Iodine (I)	Cobalt (Co)
Zinc (Zn)	Selenium (Se)
Copper (Cu)	Molybdenum (Mo)
Manganese (Mn)	Fluoride (F)

Essentiality Unclear

Silicon (Si)	Cadmium (Cd)
Vanadium (V)	Arsenic (As)
Nickel (Ni)	Aluminum (Al)
Tin (Sn)	Boron (B)

hemoglobin Oxygen-carrying pigment in red blood cells; a conjugated protein containing four heme groups combined with iron and four long polypeptide chains forming the protein globin, named for its ball-like form; made by the developing red blood cells in bone marrow, hemoglobin carries oxygen to body cells.

bioavailability Amount of a nutrient ingested in food that is absorbed and thus available to the body for metabolic use.

balance between food sources from the outside and body stores in the skeleton. Various mechanisms work to maintain body levels within normal ranges. Calcium balance is applied at three levels: (1) the intake-absorption-excretion balance, (2) the bone-blood balance, and (3) the calcium-phosphorus blood serum balance.

Intake-Absorption-Excretion Balance

Calcium Intake

Young adult women in the United States take in about 685 mg of calcium/day, and young adult men about 850 mg.[3] Milk, cheese, and bread with added nonfat milk powder contribute the most calcium to the typical U.S. diet.[4] Skeletal growth in childhood and adolescence creates a tremendous demand for calcium,[5-8] because one fourth of the adult skeleton is laid down in about 2 years during the adolescent growth spurt.[6] Boys have a greater need for calcium during this period based on their larger body size and appear to be more efficient in calcium absorption and retention.[5] If calcium intake is low or if the primary sources of dietary calcium have low bioavailability, skeletal demands are not met and bone growth is compromised. This has long-term effects; women reporting low milk intake as children and adolescents were twice as likely to experience a hip fracture in later life.[9]

Absorption of Calcium

Calcium absorption ranges from 20% to 60% of intake but decreases with age.[10] Most food calcium occurs in complexes with other dietary components. These complexes must be broken down and the calcium released in a soluble form before it can be absorbed. Absorption takes place in the small intestine, chiefly the duodenum. Here the gastric acidity is still effective, but, as the food mass continues to move along the intestine, it is buffered by pancreatic juices and becomes more alkaline.

Factors Increasing Calcium Absorption

The following factors promote calcium absorption:

- *Vitamin D hormone:* Vitamin D is necessary for calcium absorption. Calcitriol, the active form of vitamin D, controls the synthesis of a calcium-binding protein carrier in the duodenum that transports the mineral across the mucosal cell and into the blood.[1]
- *Body need:* Physiologic conditions over the life cycle—growth, pregnancy, lactation, and older age—strongly influence the rate of absorption. Absorption is higher in times of greatest need, such as the adolescent growth spurt or lactation. In all older persons but particularly in postmenopausal women, calcium absorption is greatly reduced.[1,10]
- *Dietary protein and carbohydrate:* A greater percentage of dietary calcium is absorbed when the diet is high

in protein,[11-13] but protein intakes in excess of the Recommended Dietary Allowance (RDA) also increase calcium excretion in the urine.[14] In short, higher intakes of calcium are needed to maintain calcium balance when the diet is high in protein. Soy protein, on the other hand, has a favorable effect on calcium balance through the action of its isoflavone genistein, which has estrogen-like activity.[15] Lactose, the major carbohydrate in milk, enhances calcium absorption through the action of the intestinal bacteria lactobacilli, which produce lactic acid and lower intestinal pH.

- *Acid environment:* Lower pH or a more acid environment favors the solubility of calcium and enhances absorption.

Factors Decreasing Calcium Absorption

The following factors lower calcium absorption:

- *Vitamin D deficiency:* A lack of vitamin D or inability to form the active vitamin D hormone calcitriol depresses calcium absorption.
- *Dietary fat:* Fat malabsorption or high fat intake creates an excess of fat in the intestine. These fatty acids released in digestion combine with calcium to form insoluble soaps that cannot be absorbed and are lost in the feces.
- *Fiber and other binding agents:* Dietary fiber can bind calcium and hinder its absorption. Other binding agents include *oxalic acid,* combining with calcium to produce calcium oxalate, and *phytic acid,* which forms calcium phytate. Oxalic acid is found in green leafy vegetables in varying amounts, making some vegetables better sources of calcium than others. The outer hull of many cereal grains, especially wheat, contains phytates.
- *Alkaline environment:* Calcium is insoluble at a high pH (alkaline medium) and poorly absorbed.

Calcium Output

Calcium balance is controlled primarily at the point of absorption. A large proportion of dietary calcium—50% to 90% of total intake, depending on body need—remains unabsorbed and is eliminated in the feces. A small amount of calcium is also excreted in the urine, about 200 mg/day, to maintain normal levels in body fluids.

Bone-Blood Balance

Calcium in the Bones

The skeleton is the major site of calcium storage. Bones and teeth contain about 99% of total body calcium. However, these tissues are not static. Bone is constantly being built and reshaped according to body needs and hormonal influences (Figure 7-1). As much as 700 mg of

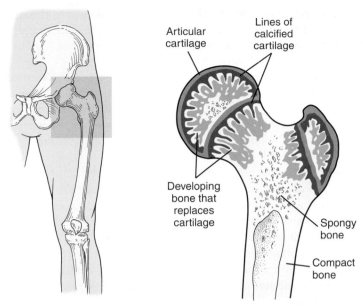

Articular
cartilage

Lines of
calcified
cartilage

Developing
bone that
replaces
cartilage

Spongy
bone

Compact
bone

FIGURE 7-1   Bone and cartilage development.

calcium enter and leave the bones each day. Under certain conditions withdrawals exceed deposits, causing an imbalance and calcium loss. Immobility from a body cast or the bone disease osteoporosis results in excess calcium withdrawal from bone. In periods of growth there is a net gain in bone calcium.

Calcium in the Blood

The small amount of body calcium that is not in bone—approximately 1%—circulates in the blood and other body fluids. Blood calcium exists in the following two forms:

1. *Bound calcium:* About 40% of the calcium in the blood is bound to plasma proteins and is not free or *diffusible,* that is, able to move into cells or enter into other activities.
2. *Free ionized calcium:* Free calcium, in an active ionized form and carrying an electrical charge, moves about unhindered and diffuses through membranes to control body functions. Free calcium accomplishes a great deal of metabolic work because it is in an activated form.

Calcium-Phosphorus Serum Balance

The final level of calcium balance is the calcium-phosphorus balance in the blood. These two minerals maintain a definite relationship based on their relative solubility. The calcium-phosphorus serum balance is the solubility product of calcium and phosphorus expressed in milligrams per deciliter (mg/dl). Normal calcium serum levels are 10 mg/dl in both children and adults. For phosphorus normal levels are 4 mg/dl in adults and 5 mg/dl in children. Thus the normal serum calcium-phosphorus solubility

products are $10 \times 4 = 40$ in adults and $10 \times 5 = 50$ in children. Any situation that increases the serum phosphorus level will bring about a decrease in the serum calcium level to keep the calcium-phosphorus solubility product constant. A drop in serum calcium interferes with important functions such as muscle contraction.

Control of Calcium Balance

The three control agents that work together to maintain calcium balance are parathyroid hormone, the vitamin D hormone calcitriol, and the hormone calcitonin. The cooperative action of these three hormones, as follows, is a good example of the synergism and interdependent relationship of metabolic control agents.

1. *Parathyroid hormone (PTH):* The parathyroid glands lie adjacent to the thyroid glands. They are particularly sensitive to changes in the blood level of free ionized calcium. When ionized calcium levels begin to fall,

osteoporosis Abnormal loss of bone mineral and matrix leading to porous, fragile bone tissue with enlarged spaces that is prone to fracture or deformity; common disease of aging in both men and women.

calcitonin A polypeptide hormone secreted by the C cells in the thyroid gland in response to hypercalcemia, which acts to lower both calcium and phosphate in the blood.

synergism The joint action of separate agents in which the total effect of their combined action is greater than the sum of their separate actions (adjective: synergistic).

PTH is released and restores levels to normal. PTH accomplishes this by the following different actions:

1. It stimulates the intestinal mucosa to absorb more calcium.
2. It rapidly withdraws calcium from bone.
3. It causes the kidneys to reabsorb more calcium and excrete more phosphorus.

These combined activities restore calcium and phosphorus to their correct balance in the blood.

2. *Vitamin D hormone (calcitriol):* Calcitriol cooperates with PTH to control the absorption of calcium in the small intestine and regulate the deposit of calcium and phosphorus in bone. Calcitriol exerts more control on calcium absorption and its deposit in bone, and PTH exerts more control on calcium withdrawal from bone and kidney excretion of phosphorus.

3. *Calcitonin:* Calcitonin is produced by special C cells in the thyroid gland. It prevents an abnormal rise in serum calcium by modulating the release of bone calcium. Thus its action counterbalances that of PTH to keep serum calcium at normal levels. The overall relationship of the factors involved in calcium balance and regulation is illustrated in Figure 7-2.

Physiologic Functions of Calcium

Bone Formation

Calcium, along with phosphorus, provides strength and rigidity to the skeleton. Building and maintaining bone mass is accomplished through the action of specialized cells that handle the deposit and withdrawal of bone calcium.

Tooth Formation

Special organs in the gums deposit calcium to form teeth, and this mineral exchange continues as in bone. Calcium deposit and withdrawal occur mainly in the dentin and cementum. Very little exchange occurs in the enamel once the tooth is formed.

General Metabolic Functions

A relatively small amount of body calcium (approximately 1%) carries out an amazing number of physiologic functions, as described below:

- *Blood clotting:* Serum calcium ions are required for the cross-linking of fibrin, giving stability to the fibrin threads.
- *Nerve transmission:* A current of calcium ions triggers the flow of signals from one nerve cell to another and on to the waiting target muscle.
- *Muscle contraction and relaxation:* Ionized serum calcium initiates the contraction of muscle fibers and controls their return to steady state after contraction. This action of calcium is particularly critical to the constant contraction-relaxation cycle of the heart muscle.
- *Cell membrane permeability:* Ionized calcium controls the passage of fluids and solutes across cell membranes by

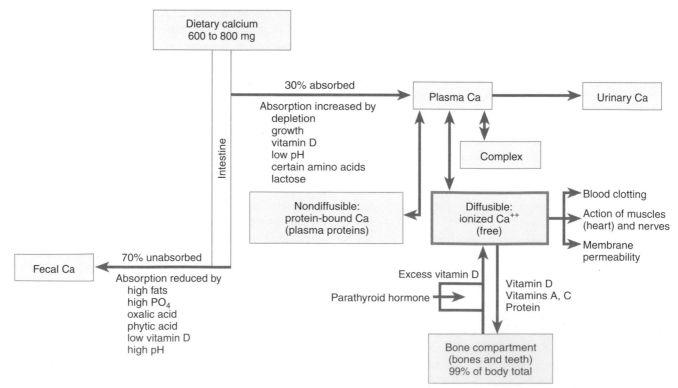

FIGURE 7-2 Calcium metabolism. Note the relative distribution of calcium in the body.

its effect on the integrity of the intercellular membrane cement.

- *Enzyme activation:* Calcium ions activate certain cell enzymes, especially those that release energy for muscle contraction. They have a similar role with protein-splitting enzymes and the lipase enzyme that digests fat.

Clinical Applications

Disruption of the physiologic and metabolic functions of calcium leads to various clinical problems.

Tetany

A decrease in serum ionized calcium causes *tetany,* marked by severe, intermittent spastic muscle contractions and muscular pain. Seizures and convulsions ensue if the situation is not corrected.

Rickets and Osteomalacia

A deficiency of vitamin D hormone causes *rickets* in growing children and *osteomalacia* in adults. When exposure to sunlight is inadequate and dietary intake of vitamin D is poor, calcium absorption and appropriate bone development do not take place.

Osteoporosis

Osteoporosis, which is characterized by a loss of bone mineral mass and disrupted bone architecture, occurs in older adults and carries with it increased risk of bone fracture and physical disability. It is associated with the loss of estrogen in postmenopausal women and the gradual decrease in testosterone in older men and the subsequent alterations in calcium balance. Once a large amount of bone has been lost, treatment with drug regimens is required to lower the risk of bone fracture.[16] Nutrition education promoting adequate calcium and vitamin D intakes and lifestyle practices that support bone health need to begin early in life.[17]

Resorptive Hypercalciuria and Renal Calculi

Resorption of calcium from bone and its excretion in the urine are accelerated in prolonged immobilization. A full body cast made necessary by orthopedic surgery or spinal cord injury or a body brace after a back injury decreases the normal muscle tension on bone. The risk of renal stones increases with the rise in urinary calcium.

Increased Risk of Chronic Disease

Low calcium intake may increase the risk of chronic problems unrelated to bone health, including obesity, hypertension, and certain types of cancer, as follows:

- *Obesity:* Dietary calcium has a role in energy metabolism in cells.[18] When calcium is in short supply, adipose cells store fat at an accelerated rate.[19] Weight

gain in midlife is proportionately higher for women consuming less than half the Adequate Intake (AI) for calcium as compared to those taking in the suggested amount.
- *Hypertension:* The hypertension intervention program Dietary Approaches to Stop Hypertension (DASH) advocates a diet rich in calcium and potassium. DASH participants were able to reduce their antihypertensive medications by as much as 35% and still control their blood pressure levels with higher intakes of these nutrients.[20] The DASH regimen also contains many servings of fruits and vegetables, adding a variety of phytochemicals to the diet.
- *Colon cancer:* A calcium intake reaching recommended levels, whether from food or supplements, may reduce the risk of colon cancer.[21,22]

Each of these interventions will be discussed in more detail in succeeding chapters.

Calcium Requirement

Dietary Reference Intake

Increasing concern about the amount of calcium required for lifetime maintenance of healthy bones led to a new Dietary Reference Intake (DRI).[10] For youth ages 9 through 18 the AI of 1300 mg/day ensures maximum deposition of bone calcium. Men and women ages 19 to 50 should take in 1000 mg/day to maintain positive calcium balance. After age 50, 1200 mg of calcium/day is needed to support bone health and prevent bone loss. Persons should not exceed the Tolerable Upper Intake Level (UL) of 2500 mg/day.

Food Sources of Calcium

Dairy products are ideal sources because the calcium is present in a highly available form. One quart of milk contains approximately 1200 mg of calcium along with 5 μg of vitamin D. Cheese and yogurt are good sources of calcium, and yogurt is sometimes fortified with vitamin D (Box 7-2). Green leafy vegetables, broccoli, legumes, nuts, and grains contribute calcium, but oxalic acid or phytates can compromise bioavailability. For those who are lactose intolerant, calcium-fortified soy milk, calcium-fortified juices, and calcium-fortified cereals can meet calcium needs. Some aged cheeses such as cheddar or Swiss are low in lactose and tolerated by those

---

solutes Particles of a substance in solution; a solution consists of a substance and a dissolving medium (solvent), usually a liquid.

| **Comparison of Calcium Sources**

Each of the foods listed below supplies approximately 300 mg of calcium. Those who are lactose intolerant can obtain their calcium from sources other than milk or dairy foods.

Foods Containing Approximately 300 mg Calcium

8-oz glass of milk
8-oz container of yogurt
1½-oz chunk of cheddar cheese
8-oz glass of calcium-fortified soy milk
8-oz container of calcium-fortified orange juice
1 cup of frozen cooked spinach
1½ cups cooked white beans
5 oz tofu

with lactase deficiency. It is important to emphasize dairy foods and other calcium sources low in fat and kilocalories (kcalories or kcal), because fear of gaining weight is a major concern for girls and women.[23] Box 7-3 lists many more food sources of calcium.

Calcium Supplements

Many persons cannot or will not consume enough calcium-rich food to meet their calcium needs and require supplements. Nevertheless, individuals should be encouraged to obtain at least half of their daily calcium from food sources that supply other important nutrients and support overall diet quality. Table 7-2 defines a number of criteria to be considered in the selection of a calcium supplement.

BOX 7-3 | **Food Sources of Calcium**

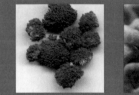 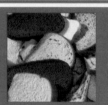 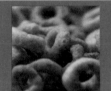 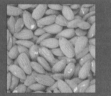

Food Source	Quantity	Calcium (mg)
Grains Group		
Fortified ready-to-eat cereals		
Total	¾ cup	1100
All Bran	½ cup	102
Cheerios	1 cup	100
Bread, whole wheat or white	1 slice	24
Vegetable Group		
Vegetable juice (fortified)	8 fl oz	300
Collards (boiled)	1 cup	148
Potato (baked, with skin)	1 med	115
Broccoli (raw)	½ cup	21
Fruit Group		
Orange juice (fortified)	8 fl oz	300
Figs (dried)	10 figs	269
Meat, Beans, Eggs, and Nuts Group		
Soybeans (boiled)	1 cup	175
Almonds (roasted)	1 oz	148
Milk Group		
Yogurt, whole-milk	8 fl oz	355
Milk, skim, low-fat, whole	8 fl oz	302
Soy milk fortified with calcium	8 fl oz	300
Fats, Oils, and Sugar		
These foods are not important sources of calcium		

Images copyright 2006 JupiterImages Corporation.
  Adequate Intakes for adults: ages 19 to 50, 1000 mg; ages ≥51, 1200 mg.

PHOSPHORUS

Phosphorus is closely associated with body calcium, although it has some unique characteristics and functions of its own. Phosphorus makes up about 1% of total body weight.

Absorption-Excretion Balance

Absorption

Free phosphate is absorbed along the entire length of the small intestine. Absorption is regulated by the vitamin D hormone calcitriol and phosphate carrier proteins.[24] Phosphorus occurs in food as a phosphate compound joined with calcium and before its absorption must be split off as a free mineral. When that is completed, absorption goes forward. An excess of other minerals such as aluminum or iron or calcium depresses phosphorus absorption. The phytates in whole grains prevent its absorption.

Excretion

The kidneys are the main excretion route for phosphorus and regulate serum phosphorus levels. Usually 85% to 95% of the plasma phosphate filtered by the renal glomeruli is reabsorbed in the renal tubules along with calcium under the influence of vitamin D hormone. But when phosphate must be excreted to preserve the normal serum calcium-phosphorus balance, PTH overrides vitamin D hormone and raises excretion levels.

Bone-Blood-Cell Balance

Bone

Approximately 80% to 90% of the body's phosphorus is in the skeleton and teeth combined with calcium. Bone phosphorus is in constant interchange with the phosphorus in blood and other body fluids.

Blood

The normal range for serum phosphorus in adults is 3.0 to 4.5 mg/dl; levels below 2.5 or above 5.0 mg/dl demand immediate medical attention.[24] High phosphorus intakes leading to elevated serum levels stimulate PTH release and mobilization of bone calcium to restore the serum calcium-phosphorus balance to normal. Continued use of phosphorus-binding antacids such as those containing aluminum lower serum levels.[24] Serum phosphorus levels

---

TABLE 7-2	Choosing a Calcium Supplement

Characteristic	Recommendation
Amount of elemental calcium present	Calcium compounds contain different amounts of elemental calcium by weight; calcium carbonate is 40% calcium, but calcium citrate is only 21% calcium; you would need twice as many tablets of calcium citrate to get the same amount of calcium.
Absorption	Calcium carbonate, calcium citrate, and calcium citrate malate (the form found in fortified juices) are all well absorbed; calcium citrate is better absorbed than calcium carbonate when gastric acid is low.
Purity	Do not use supplements made from bone meal or oyster shell or dolomite because they may contain lead or other toxic elements; coral calcium also may contain lead and mercury; look for either a well-known brand of pharmaceuticals or check for the USP (United States Pharmacopeia) symbol or the word "purified."
Dose	Calcium is absorbed best when taken in doses of 500 mg or less; depending on need, take divided doses of 500 mg each rather than one dose of 1000 mg.
When best taken	Calcium carbonate is best absorbed with food; calcium citrate can be taken anytime.
Combination products	Some calcium supplements are combined with other nutrients such as phosphorus, magnesium, or vitamin D; phosphorus is readily available in the U.S. diet; unless vitamin D is already provided in another supplement, it could be included here.
Potential interactions	Calcium can decrease the absorption of various medications, including digoxin, phenytoin, and tetracycline, or interact with thiazide and similar diuretics; medications to be taken on an empty stomach should not be taken with a calcium supplement; persons on prescription or over-the-counter medications should check with their physician or pharmacist before adding a supplement.
Form	Calcium supplements are available in tablets, gel capsules, liquids, and chewables; chewables and liquids might be helpful for those with difficulty in swallowing.
Ability to dissolve in the stomach	Chewables and liquids dissolve well because they are broken down before they enter the stomach; for tablets: place one in warm water for 30 minutes, and stir occasionally; if it has not dissolved in this time, it will likely not dissolve in your stomach.

Data from National Institute of Arthritis and Musculoskeletal and Skin Diseases: *Calcium supplements: what to look for,* Washington, DC, 2005, National Institutes of Health, U.S. Department of Health and Human Services. Retrieved September 18, 2005, from *www.niams.nih.gov/bone/hi/calcium_supp.htm;* Office of Dietary Supplements: *Dietary supplement fact sheet: calcium,* Washington, DC, 2005, National Institutes of Health, U.S. Department of Health and Human Services. Retrieved September 18, 2005 from *http://dietary-supplements.info.nih.gov/factsheets/Calcium_pf.asp;* and Blumberg S: Is coral calcium a safe and effective supplement? *J Am Diet Assoc* 104:1335, 2004.

are somewhat higher in children, ranging from 4 to 7 mg/dl, a significant clue to its active role in cell metabolism in the growth years.

Cells

In its active phosphate form, phosphorus participates in the structure and function of all living cells. Here it works with proteins, lipids, and carbohydrates to produce energy, build and repair tissues, and act as a buffer to maintain appropriate pH levels.

Hormonal Controls

Because calcium and phosphorus work closely together, phosphorus balance is under the control of two hormones that also control calcium—vitamin D hormone and PTH. Phosphate deficiency or depletion results from (1) low intake, (2) diminished absorption, usually caused by an interfering substance such as phytate or aluminum, or (3) excessive wasting by the kidney.

Physiologic Functions

Phosphorus has important functions both inside and outside of cells and enters practically every cellular metabolic pathway.

Bone and Tooth Formation

Phosphorus helps build bones and teeth. As a component of calcium phosphate it is constantly being deposited and resorbed in the continuing process of bone formation and remodeling.

General Metabolic Activities

Phosphorus is present in every living cell, where it participates in overall metabolism. Several of these activities are as follows:

- *Absorption of glucose and glycerol:* Phosphorus combines with glucose and glycerol to assist in their absorption from the intestine. Phosphorus also promotes the reabsorption of glucose in the renal tubules, preventing its loss in the urine.
- *Transport of fatty acids:* Phospholipids transport fats in the blood.
- *Energy metabolism:* Phosphorus-containing compounds such as adenosine triphosphate (ATP) are high-energy storage molecules that meet instant demands for energy.
- *Buffer system:* The phosphate buffer system of phosphoric acid and phosphate helps maintain blood acid-base balance.

Clinical Applications

Changes in the normal serum phosphorus level occur under various clinical and physiologic circumstances, as follows:

- *Recovery from diabetic acidosis:* Active carbohydrate absorption and metabolism place a high demand on serum phosphorus, causing temporary hypophosphatemia. (Phosphate is combined with glucose in the formation of glycogen.)
- *Growth:* Children have higher serum phosphate levels related to their high levels of growth hormone.
- *Hypophosphatemia:* Low serum phosphorus occurs in intestinal diseases such as sprue and celiac disease that hinder phosphorus absorption. Excessive secretion of PTH (primary hyperparathyroidism) causes inappropriate excretion of phosphorus and hypophosphatemia. Low serum phosphorus may accompany the refeeding syndrome sometimes seen in the first days of nutritional repletion of a severely wasted patient. As noted earlier, phosphorus is required for the storage of glycogen which follows refeeding, and this demand lowers blood levels. One symptom of hypophosphatemia is muscle weakness because cells are deprived of the phosphorus needed for energy metabolism. If left untreated, hypophosphatemia leads to metabolic acidosis, heart failure, and sudden death.[25]
- *Hyperphosphatemia:* In renal failure and hypoparathyroidism excess phosphate accumulates in the serum. This makes the serum calcium level drop, causing tetany.

Phosphorus Requirement

Dietary Reference Intake

The RDA for phosphorus is 1250 mg/day for those ages 9 to 18 years and 700 mg/day for all adults over age 18. At one time the relative intake of calcium to phosphorus was considered important in building and remodeling bone. Higher intakes of phosphorus than calcium were believed to be detrimental to bone mineral deposition. New studies indicate that having sufficient amounts of each nutrient is more important than their ratio to each other.[10] Because these two minerals are found in many of the same foods, meeting calcium needs will likely provide adequate phosphorus.

Food Sources of Phosphorus

Milk and milk products contain significant amounts of phosphorus, along with calcium. Because phosphorus is important in cell and muscle metabolism, lean meats are a good source. Phosphorus-containing additives in processed food and the high phosphorus content of soft drinks add this mineral to the American diet.

SODIUM

Sodium, the major cation in the extracellular fluids, is one of the most plentiful minerals in the body. The average adult contains approximately 120 g (4 oz), and nearly 95% is found in the extracellular fluid as free ionized sodium.

Absorption-Excretion Balance

Absorption

Sodium is easily absorbed in the small intestine; usually no more than 2% remains to be excreted in the feces.

Excretion

The major route of excretion is through the kidney under the control of aldosterone, the sodium-conserving hormone produced in the adrenal cortex. For individuals in a temperate climate with a steady state of fluid and sodium balance, urinary sodium excretion is about equal to intake. Sodium is lost in sweat as related to exercise or a hot environment.

Physiologic Functions of Sodium

Water Balance

Ionized sodium is the major guardian of the body water outside of the cells. Differences in the sodium concentrations of body fluids largely determine the distribution of water via osmosis from one area to another.

Acid-Base Balance

In cooperation with chloride and bicarbonate ions, ionized sodium helps regulate acid-base balance.

Cell Permeability

The sodium pump located in all cell membranes controls the passage of materials in and out of the cell. Potassium is moved into the cell, and sodium is moved out of the cell. Glucose also moves into cells via this active transport system.

Muscle Action

Sodium ions help to transmit electrochemical impulses along nerve and muscle membranes and maintain normal muscle action. Potassium and sodium ions work together to balance the response of nerves to stimulation, and control the flow of nerve impulses to muscles and the contraction of the muscle fibers.

Sodium Requirement

Dietary Reference Intake

The body can adjust to a wide range of sodium intakes. When intake is very low, the body conserves sodium by reducing output in urine and sweat. At high intakes excretion equals intake. The AI for sodium will cover sweat losses in individuals who are physically active or exposed to high environmental temperatures in the short term. Those with exceptionally high losses in sweat, such as endurance runners, will require greater amounts of sodium.[26] For young adults the AI is 1500 mg of sodium or 3800 mg of table salt. (Sodium chloride or table salt is 40% sodium by weight.) The suggested intake drops to 1300 mg sodium (approximately 3300 mg table salt) for those ages 51 to 70 years, and to 1200 mg (approximately 3000 mg table salt) for those ages 71 and over based on their lower energy intakes. Excessive amounts of sodium can raise blood pressure in sensitive people, so the goal for this nutrient is to limit rather than increase daily intake. The UL is 2300 mg sodium or 5800 mg of table salt.

Health Promotion

Sodium and Blood Pressure

High sodium intakes exert an effect on blood pressure and contribute to the growing prevalence of hypertension in the United States. Reducing dietary sodium is especially effective in helping to lower systolic blood pressure in blacks and people over age 45[26] (see the *Focus on Culture* box, "Low Mineral Intake: Does It Have an Effect on Blood Pressure Among Blacks?").

The DASH studies mentioned earlier took a broad view of diet and hypertension, looking beyond sodium intake, and encouraged volunteers to eat at least nine servings of fruits and vegetables and three servings of low-fat dairy products each day. This diet is high in fiber, calcium, magnesium, potassium, vitamins, and phytochemicals[27] and brought about a significant decline in systolic blood pressure.[28] When adults following the DASH diet also limited their sodium intake to 2300 mg per day (the current UL for sodium), systolic blood pressures fell even more than with the DASH diet alone.[29] Approximately 25% of adults in the United States have hypertension. A 5-mm Hg decrease in systolic blood pressure could reduce mortality from stroke by 14% and mortality from coronary heart disease by 9%.[26]

Dietary Intake of Sodium

Most adults consume more sodium than the current UL. The median sodium intake for young men is 4329 mg but drops to 3447 mg after age 59. Women consume less sodium with intakes of 2871 mg at younger ages and 2333 mg at older ages.[3] Compare these intakes with the UL of 2300 mg. Sodium intakes are highest in the southern region of the United States—which also has the highest average systolic blood pressure—and lowest in the western region, which has the lowest average systolic blood pressure.[30]

---

aldosterone Potent hormone of the cortex of the adrenal glands, which acts on the distal renal tubule to cause reabsorption of sodium in an ion exchange with potassium. The aldosterone mechanism is essentially a sodium-conserving mechanism but indirectly also conserves water because water absorption follows the sodium reabsorption.

◆ FOCUS ON CULTURE

Low Mineral Intake: Does It Have an Effect on Blood Pressure Among Blacks?

Blacks are especially at risk for hypertension, and in some cases this may be related to salt sensitivity.[1] But research evidence suggests that not only sodium, but other minerals—calcium, potassium, and magnesium—also play a role in regulating blood pressure. The DASH program (Dietary Approaches to Stop Hypertension) was successful in lowering blood pressure using an eating plan including foods rich in potassium, calcium, and magnesium. The DASH food plan provides the following calculated intakes[2]:

Potassium: 4706 mg (DRI = 4700 mg for those ages 51 and over)
Magnesium: 500 mg (DRI = 310 mg for those ages 51 and over)
Calcium: 1619 mg (DRI = 1200 mg for those ages 51 and over)

At the same time the DASH diet does not exceed the UL for sodium set at 2300 mg.

Among the individuals who participated in a recent National Health and Nutrition Examination Survey (NHANES) study, low potassium and calcium intakes were more predictive of elevated systolic blood pressure than were high intakes of sodium.[3] For many blacks calcium and potassium intakes fall well below recommended levels. Average intake of potassium is 2408 mg, and average intake of calcium is 612 mg, barely half of the recommended amount. Magnesium intake is 230 mg, or about two thirds of the suggested amount.[4]

Why are intakes of calcium and potassium so low in this group, and what can we do to improve them? Many blacks avoid dairy products because of lactose intolerance, resulting in low calcium intakes. Other foods that could provide calcium include fortified cereals or orange juice. We might also encourage the use of aged cheese, which is lower in lactose than milk and may be tolerable. Various vegetables, including broccoli, collard greens, cabbage, and kale, are good sources of calcium as well as potassium. Legumes add both calcium and potassium to the daily intake. Encouraging more use of fruits and vegetables will also supply potassium to the diet. (Refer to Boxes 7-2, 7-3, 7-5, and 7-6 to find good sources of these nutrients.)

All population groups will benefit from lowering their intakes of sodium. Cutting down on the use of processed luncheon meats and salty snacks and using frozen rather than canned vegetables removes sodium from the diet. Avoiding frozen dinners and canned soups that are not labeled low sodium will reduce sodium intakes (see Box 7-4).

Preventing or reducing elevated blood pressure must be two pronged. Lowering sodium intake to the extent possible is one step, but equally important is the need to help blacks raise their intakes of calcium, potassium, and magnesium.

References

1. U.S. Department of Health and Human Services: *The seventh report of the Joint National Committee on Prevention, Detection, Evaluation, and Treatment of High Blood Pressure,* NIH Publication No. 03-5230, Washington, DC, 2003 (May), U.S. Government Printing Office.
2. U.S. Departments of Health and Human Services, U.S. Department of Agriculture: *Dietary Guidelines for Americans 2005,* ed 6, Washington, DC, 2005, Author. Available at *www.healthierus.gov/dietary guidelines.*
3. Townsend MS et al: Low mineral intake is associated with high systolic blood pressure in the third and fourth National Health and Nutrition Examination Surveys, *Am J Hypertens* 18:261, 2005.
4. Champagne CM et al: Dietary intake in the lower Mississippi delta region: results from the Foods of Our Delta Study, *J Am Diet Assoc* 104:199, 2004.

Sources of Dietary Sodium in the American Diet

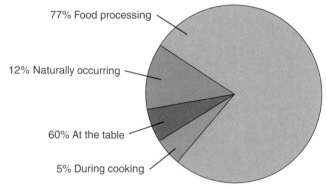

77% Food processing

12% Naturally occurring

60% At the table

5% During cooking

FIGURE 7-3   Sources of dietary sodium. Most of our dietary sodium comes from processed food. *(Redrawn from U.S. Department of Health and Human Services, U.S. Department of Agriculture:* Dietary Guidelines for Americans 2005, *ed 6, Washington, DC, 2005, Author.)*

Controlling Sodium Intake

The primary source of sodium for most people is processed food. As you can see in Figure 7-3, only 12% of the sodium in our diet comes from foods in their natural form, whereas 77% is added in food processing.[26] Varying amounts of sodium are added by individuals in cooking or at the table, but it is usually less than consumed in processed foods or when dining out. Food additives containing sodium serve a variety of functions in food products as flavorings, leavening agents, and preservatives (Table 7-3) and are responsible for the high sodium content of many processed items. A few vegetables, including spinach and celery, are fairly high in sodium. Compare the sodium in natural and processed foods in Box 7-4. Learn to use the Nutrition Label to check the sodium content of foods you buy.

POTASSIUM

Potassium is about twice as plentiful in the body as sodium. An adult body contains about 270 g or 4000 *milliequivalents (mEq).* Most body potassium is found inside cells, where it guards intracellular water; however, the relatively small amount of potassium in extracellular fluid is important for muscle activity, especially heart muscle. Plasma potassium levels are maintained within very narrow limits of 3.5 to 5.0 mg/dl.

Absorption-Excretion Balance

Absorption

Dietary potassium is readily absorbed in the small intestine. Potassium also circulates in the gastrointestinal secretions

TABLE 7-3	Sodium-Containing Additives Commonly Used in Food Processing	

Additive	Purpose	Where Used
Sodium chloride	Flavoring	Condiments (catsup, soy sauce, onion salt, bouillon cubes, Worcestershire sauce); food mixtures; heat-and-serve entrees, snack foods
	Dough conditioner	Yeast breads
	Preservative	Fermented products (pickles); luncheon meats and frankfurters; canned vegetables; smoked fish
Sodium citrate	Texture agent	Frozen foods
Sodium bicarbonate	Leavening agent	Muffins, biscuits, cakes
Sodium aluminum phosphate	Leavening agent	Muffins, biscuits, cakes
Sodium benzoate	Preservative	Many processed items
Sodium bisulfate	Preservative	Many processed items
Sodium nitrite	Preservative	Luncheon meats; frankfurters

and is reabsorbed in digestion. Prolonged vomiting or diarrhea results in serious losses.

Excretion

The principal route of potassium excretion is the urine. Because plasma potassium levels are critical to heart muscle action, the kidneys guard potassium carefully. At least 70% of the potassium filtered by the kidneys is reabsorbed. Aldosterone, the hormone that acts on the kidneys to conserve sodium also regulates plasma potassium, because potassium is lost in exchange for sodium in the renal tubule. Elevated plasma potassium levels stimulate the release of aldosterone. The normal obligatory potassium loss is about 160 mg/day. Certain diuretic drugs cause excessive loss of potassium.

Physiologic Functions of Potassium

Water Balance

The potassium inside the cells balances with sodium outside the cells to maintain normal osmotic pressures and protect cellular fluid.

Muscle Activity

Potassium is needed for the action of cardiac and skeletal muscles. Together with sodium and calcium, potassium regulates neuromuscular stimulation, transmission of electrochemical impulses, and contraction of muscle fibers. Low plasma potassium leads to muscle irritability and paralysis. This effect is particularly notable for the heart muscle, which develops a gallop rhythm ending in cardiac arrest. Even small variations in plasma potassium are reflected in electrocardiograms (ECGs).

Carbohydrate Metabolism

When glucose is converted to glycogen, 0.36 mmol of potassium is stored in each gram of glycogen. When a patient in diabetic acidosis is treated with insulin and glucose, the rapid glycogen production that ensues draws potassium from the plasma. Serious hypokalemia will result if adequate potassium replacement does not accompany treatment. Even moderate potassium deficiency without overt hypokalemia can aggravate existing glucose intolerance.

Protein Synthesis

Potassium is required for the storage of nitrogen as muscle protein or other cell protein. When tissue is broken down, potassium is lost along with nitrogen. Amino acid replacement in rehabilitation includes potassium to ensure nitrogen retention.

Control of Blood Pressure

Potassium has a role in controlling blood pressure.[26,28] Potassium appears to offset the pressor effect of sodium in raising blood pressure, such that persons with higher potassium intakes have lower pressures. Potassium also increases the excretion of sodium through the action of aldosterone.

Acid-Base Balance

Potassium, along with bicarbonate-yielding compounds in fruits and vegetables, helps to neutralize acids produced by the metabolism of meat and other animal protein foods. When potassium and bicarbonate buffers are not available in sufficient amounts, these acids act on bone, releasing bone calcium and reducing bone mass. Calcium-containing kidney stones can occur from such increases in bone turnover.[26]

Potassium Requirement

Dietary Reference Intake

The AI for potassium is set at 4700 mg/day for all adults.[26] This intake is expected to lower blood pressure and reduce risk of bone loss. Current potassium intakes fall far short of this goal. Men ages 40 and over have a median intake of about 3000 mg, and women of this age have median intakes of only 2900 mg.[3] In light of the age-related increase in blood pressure[31] and loss of bone[32]

BOX 7-4 | Sodium Content of Processed and Unprocessed Foods*

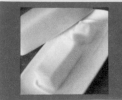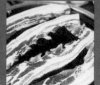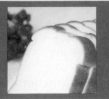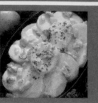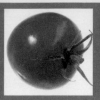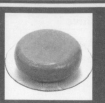

Food Source	Quantity	Sodium (mg)
Grains Group		
Ready-to-eat cereals		
Cheerios	1 cup	273
Total	¾ cup	192
All Bran	½ cup	80
Shredded Wheat, no salt added	2 biscuits	3
Bread, white	1 slice	135
Vegetable Group		
Potato salad, homemade	1 cup	1324
Stewed tomatoes (canned)	1 cup	564
Broccoli (frozen with cheese sauce)	½ cup	402
Potato (baked, with skin)	1 med	16
Broccoli (boiled with no salt)	½ cup	12
Tomato (raw)	1 med	10
Meat, Beans, Eggs, and Nuts Group		
Ham, canned (lean)	3½ oz	1255
Baked beans, canned	½ cup	510
Bacon (broiled/fried)	3 med pieces	303
Tuna, light, canned in water (with salt)	3 oz	303
Peanut butter, creamy (with salt)	1 tbsp	131
Ground beef, regular (broiled)	3½ oz	83
Beef top round, lean (broiled)	3½ oz	61
Halibut (baked)	3 oz	59
Black-eyed peas (boiled without salt)	1 cup	6
Peanut butter, creamy (unsalted)	1 tbsp	3
Milk Group		
Cottage cheese, creamed	1 cup	850
Cheddar cheese	1 oz	176
Milk, whole, low-fat, or skim	8 fl oz	124
Swiss cheese	1 oz	74
Fats, Oils, and Sugar		
Margarine, stick, corn oil (salted)	1 tbsp	132
Butter (salted)	1 tbsp	123
Butter (unsalted)	1 tbsp	2
Margarine, stick corn oil (unsalted)	1 tbsp	3

Images copyright 2006 JupiterImages Corporation.

Adequate intake for adults: ages 19-50, 1500 mg; ages 51-70, 1300 mg; ages ≥71, 1200 mg; Tolerable Upper Intake Level for adults: 2300 mg.

*Sodium is added to foods in home food preparation and in industry food processing.

commonly occurring in middle age and beyond, increased fruit and vegetable intakes could be a cost-effective intervention.

Clinical Implications of Excessive Intake

When kidney function is normal, excess potassium is easily excreted; thus the Food and Nutrition Board did not set a UL for this nutrient. Nevertheless, potassium supplements can be dangerous, regardless of kidney status. Hyperkalemia accompanied by serious cardiac arrhythmias has occurred in apparently healthy individuals who accidentally or intentionally took potassium supplements. Potassium-containing salt substitutes can be unrecognized sources of potassium. Individuals with diabetes, renal impairment, or heart failure are at increased risk of hyperkalemia. Certain medications impair potassium excretion.[26] These situations will be discussed in greater detail in Part 3.

BOX 7-5 | Food Sources of Potassium

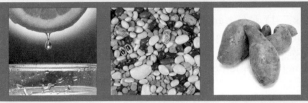

Food Source	Quantity	Potassium (mg)
Vegetable Group		
Potato, baked	1	610
Sweet potato	½ cup	397
Fruit Group		
Orange juice	1 cup	473
Banana	1	422
Meat, Beans, Eggs, and Nuts Group		
Lima beans	½ cup	484
Other		
Spaghetti sauce	½ cup	405

Images copyright 2006 JupiterImages Corporation.
Adequate intake for adults: 1700 mg.

BOX 7-6 | Food Sources of Magnesium

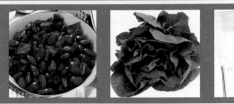

Food Source	Quantity	Magnesium (mg)
Grains Group		
Bite-Size Shredded Wheat cereal	1 cup	65
Vegetable Group		
Spinach	½ cup	81
Meat, Beans, Eggs, and Nuts Group		
Baked beans	1 cup	66
Peanuts	1 oz	50
Milk Group		
Soy milk	1 cup	61
Cow's milk	1 cup	34

Images copyright 2006 JupiterImages Corporation.
Recommended Dietary Allowance for adults: women ages 19-30, 310 mg; women ages ≥31, 320 mg; men ages 19-30, 400 mg; men ages ≥31, 420 mg.

Food Sources of Potassium

Potassium is found in many foods because it is an essential component of all living cells. Legumes, whole grains, fruits such as oranges and bananas, leafy green vegetables, broccoli, potatoes, meats, and milk supply considerable amounts (Box 7-5). Persons who eat many servings of fruits and vegetables have potassium intakes of about 8 to 11 g/day. It is important to note that potassium toxicity has not resulted from high intakes of potassium-containing foods, but rather from potassium supplements.

OTHER MAJOR MINERALS

Three additional minerals are assigned to the major minerals group based on their body content—magnesium, chloride, and sulfur.

MAGNESIUM

Magnesium is found in all body cells. An adult body contains approximately 25 g of magnesium, a little less than an ounce. Most is combined with calcium and phosphorus in bone and likely cooperates in bone health.[10] The remainder is distributed in muscle and other tissues and fluids. Magnesium activates enzymes for energy production and tissue building and has a role in normal muscle action. The magnesium found in whole grains may help to bring about the positive effect of these foods on insulin action.[33]

Magnesium Requirement

The RDA for magnesium is 400 mg for younger men and 310 mg for younger women. To compensate for age-related changes in the kidney that result in greater losses of magnesium, the RDA for persons above age 50 increases to 420 mg in men and 320 mg in women.[10]

Food Sources

Magnesium is widespread in nature and unprocessed foods. Whole grains are good sources, but more than 80% of the magnesium is lost when the germ and bran layers of the kernel are removed. Although milk contains only a modest amount of magnesium, it is a major source in the U.S. diet because it is consumed frequently.[4] Other sources include nuts, soybeans, cocoa, seafood, dried beans and peas, and green vegetables. Except for bananas, fruits are relatively poor sources, as are meat and fish. Diets rich in vegetables and unrefined grains are higher in magnesium than diets based on highly processed foods and meat. Box 7-6 lists some good sources of magnesium.

CHLORIDE

Chlorine appears in the body as the chloride ion (Cl^-). Chloride accounts for about 3% of the body's total mineral content and is found in the extracellular fluid, where it helps control water balance and acid-base balance. Spinal fluid has the highest concentration. A fair amount of ionized chloride is found in the gastrointestinal secretions as a component of gastric hydrochloric acid (HCl). Uncontrolled vomiting and diarrhea with continued loss of gastric fluids can result in chloride deficiency with muscle cramps and disturbed acid-base balance.

SULFUR

Sulfur is found in all body cells as a constituent of cell protein. Elemental sulfur forms sulfate compounds with sodium, potassium, and magnesium. Other forms of sulfur include (1) sulfur-containing amino acids such as methionine and cysteine; (2) glycoproteins in cartilage, tendons, and bone matrix; (3) detoxification products formed by intestinal bacteria; (4) organic molecules such as heparin, insulin, coenzyme A, thiamin, and biotin; and (5) keratin in hair and nails.

The major minerals are summarized in Table 7-4.

TRACE ELEMENTS: THE CONCEPT OF ESSENTIALITY

By the simplest definition an essential element is one required to sustain life and whose absence brings death. For major elements that occur in relatively large amounts in the body such a determination is fairly easy, based on the quantity available for study. It is much more difficult to establish the essentiality of the trace elements because we seem to need so little of them. Trace elements have a required intake of less than 100 mg/day, yet some of them exist in fairly large amounts in our diet and our environment.

Trace elements have two major functions: (1) to catalyze chemical reactions and (2) to serve as structural components of larger molecules.

ESSENTIAL TRACE ELEMENTS: DEFINITE AND PROBABLE

Based on current knowledge, the trace elements are separated into two groups: (1) those that are known to be essential and (2) those that are probably essential.

Essential Elements

Ten trace elements are considered essential in human nutrition based on defined function and need (see Box 7-1).

Probable Essential Elements

Eight other trace elements are thought to be essential for animals, but researchers have yet to demonstrate a role for them in *human* health.[34] As we develop better techniques

of tissue analysis and functional tests appropriate for human studies, we will learn more about their essentiality. For now they are categorized as probably essential (see Box 7-1). (Hair analysis is not recommended as a way to evaluate the body's need for trace minerals; see the *To Probe Further* box, "Hair Analysis: A Basis for Purchasing Mineral Supplements?")

ESSENTIAL TRACE ELEMENTS

IRON

Of all the micronutrients, iron has the longest history, and the body mechanisms regulating iron absorption and utilization are well understood.

Forms of Iron in the Body

The human body contains about 40 to 50 mg of iron per kilogram of body weight. This iron is distributed in the following four forms, each with a specific metabolic function:

1. *Transport iron:* A trace of iron, 0.05 to 0.18 mg/dl, is found in blood plasma bound to the transport carrier protein transferrin.
2. *Hemoglobin:* Most body iron, about 70%, resides in the red blood cells as part of the heme portion of hemoglobin. Another 5% helps form myoglobin, the molecule that carries oxygen to the muscles.
3. *Storage iron:* Approximately 20% is stored as the protein-iron compound ferritin in the liver, spleen, and bone marrow. Excess iron is held in the body as hemosiderin and interchanges with ferritin as needed.
4. *Cellular iron:* The remaining 5% is distributed across all body cells as an enzyme cofactor in oxidative enzyme systems that produce energy.

Absorption-Transport-Storage-Excretion Balance

Iron is regulated by a rather unique system as compared with most other nutrients. In most cases plasma and tissue levels are controlled by urinary excretion, which rids the body of any excess that has accumulated. For iron, control is exerted at the points of absorption, transport, and storage. There is no defined system for excreting iron.

---

ferritin Protein-iron compound in which iron is stored in tissues; the storage form of iron in the body.

hemosiderin Insoluble iron oxide–protein compound in which iron is stored in the liver if the amount of iron in the blood exceeds the storage capacity of ferritin.

TABLE 7-4	Summary of Major Minerals				
Mineral	**Metabolism**	**Physiologic Functions**	**Clinical Applications**	**Dietary Reference Intake**	**Food Sources**
Calcium (Ca)	Absorption according to body need; requires Ca-binding protein and regulated by vitamin D, parathyroid hormone, and calcitonin; absorption favored by protein and acidity Excretion chiefly in feces: 50%-90% of amount ingested Deposition-mobilization in bone tissue is regulated by vitamin D and parathyroid hormone	Constituent of bones and teeth Participates in blood clotting, nerve transmission, muscle action, cell membrane permeability, enzyme activation	Tetany (decrease in serum Ca) Rickets, osteomalacia Osteoporosis Hyperparathyroidism and hypoparathyroidism	Male/female adults 　Ages 19-50: 1000 mg 　Ages ≥51: 1200 mg Pregnancy 　Ages ≤18: 1300 mg 　Ages ≥19: 1000 mg Lactation 　Ages ≤18: 1300 mg 　Ages ≥19: 1000 mg	Milk, cheese, yogurt Green leafy vegetables Whole grains Legumes, nuts Fortified soy foods Fortified fruit juice
Phosphorus (P)	Absorption with Ca aided by vitamin D and parathyroid hormone as for calcium; hindered by binding agents Excretion chiefly by kidney according to serum level, regulated by parathyroid hormone Deposition-mobilization in bone compartment is constant	Constituent of bones and teeth, adenosine triphosphate (ATP), phosphorylated intermediary metabolites Participates in absorption of glucose and glycerol, transport of fatty acids, energy metabolism, and buffer system	Growth Recovery from diabetic acidosis Hypophosphatemia: bone disease, malabsorption syndromes, primary hyperparathyroidism Hyperphosphatemia: renal insufficiency, hypoparathyroidism, tetany	Male/female adults 　Ages ≥19: 700 mg Pregnancy 　Ages ≤18: 1250 mg 　Ages ≥19: 700 mg Lactation 　Ages ≤18: 1250 mg 　Ages ≥19: 700 mg	Milk, cheese Meat, egg yolk Whole grains Legumes, nuts Soft drinks
Magnesium (Mg)	Absorption according to intake load; hindered by excess fat, phosphate, calcium, protein Excretion (regulated by kidney)	Constituent of bones and teeth Coenzyme in general metabolism, smooth muscle action, neuromuscular irritability Cation in intracellular fluid	Low serum level following gastrointestinal losses Tremor, spasm in deficiency induced by malnutrition, alcoholism	Adults 　Males ages 19-30: 400 mg 　Males ages ≥31: 420 mg 　Females ages 19-30: 310 mg 　Females ages ≥31: 320 mg Pregnancy 　Ages ≤18: 400 mg 　Ages 19-30: 350 mg 　Ages 31-50: 360 mg Lactation 　Ages ≤18: 360 mg 　Ages 19-30: 310 mg 　Ages 31-50: 320 mg	Milk, cheese Meat, seafood Whole grains Legumes, nuts

Continued

TABLE 7-4	Summary of Major Minerals—cont'd				
Mineral	Metabolism	Physiologic Functions	Clinical Applications	Dietary Reference Intake	Food Sources
Sodium (Na)	Readily absorbed Excretion chiefly by kidney, controlled by aldosterone	Major cation in extracellular fluid, water balance, acid-base balance Cell membrane permeability, absorption of glucose Normal muscle irritability	Losses in gastrointestinal disorders, diarrhea Fluid-electrolyte and acid-base balance problems Muscle action	Male/female adults Ages 19-50: 1500 mg Ages 51-70: 1300 mg Ages >70: 1200 mg UL for all adults: 2300 mg Pregnancy All ages: 1500 mg Lactation All ages: 1500 mg	Salt (NaCl) Sodium compounds used in baking and food processing Milk, cheese Carrots, spinach, beets, celery
Potassium (K)	Readily absorbed Secreted and reabsorbed in gastrointestinal circulation Excretion chiefly by kidney, regulated by aldosterone	Major cation in intracellular fluid, water balance, acid-base balance Normal muscle irritability Glycogen formation Protein synthesis	Losses in gastrointestinal disorders, diarrhea Fluid-electrolyte, acid-base balance problems Muscle action, especially heart action Losses in tissue catabolism Treatment of diabetic acidosis: rapid glycogen production reduces serum potassium level Losses with diuretic therapy	Male/female adults All ages: 4700 mg Pregnancy All ages: 4700 mg Lactation All ages: 5100 mg	Fruits Vegetables Legumes, nuts Whole grains Meat
Chloride (Cl)	Readily absorbed Excretion controlled by kidney	Major anion in extracellular fluid, water balance, acid-base balance, chloride-bicarbonate shift Gastric hydrochloride—digestion	Losses in gastrointestinal disorders, vomiting, diarrhea, tube drainage Hypochloremic alkalosis	Male/female adults Ages 19-50: 2300 mg Ages 51-70: 2000 mg Ages >70: 1800 mg Pregnancy All ages: 2300 mg Lactation All ages: 2300 mg	Salt (NaCl)
Sulfur (S)	Elemental form absorbed as such; split from amino acid sources (methionine and cysteine) in digestion and absorbed into portal circulation Excreted by kidney in relation to protein intake and tissue catabolism	Essential constituent of protein structure Enzyme activity and energy metabolism through free sulfhydryl group (–SH) Detoxification reactions	Cystine renal calculi Cystinuria	Adults No specific recommendation: diets adequate in sulfur-containing amino acids are adequate in sulfur	Meat, eggs Milk, cheese Legumes, nuts

TO PROBE FURTHER

HAIR ANALYSIS: A BASIS FOR PURCHASING MINERAL SUPPLEMENTS?

With the growing attention to health and self-care, consumers are eager for food and nutrition information. This increases their vulnerability to health fraud, and older adults with health concerns are especially at risk.[1] Interest in nutrition and its benefits for preventing or improving chronic health problems makes people wonder about their personal nutritional status. One of the sales ploys used is the offer of a hair analysis to determine one's mineral status or need for dietary supplements.[2] For a few strands of hair and a sizable fee, a person can find out if his or her selenium levels are low, lead levels are high, or sodium levels are just right. Or can they?

Hair is formed of living cells containing the same vitamins and minerals as other body cells, but these cells die quickly. Dead cells are joined together by a sulfur-rich protein called keratin and, as more are added, the single strand of hair continues to grow longer. Vitamins disappear when cells die, so no vitamins are found in hair, but most of the inorganic minerals still remain. Yet, there are problems in hair analysis, as described below:

- Some minerals may be lost when hair cells die.
- The high sulfur level in keratin can mask the presence of some minerals and attract others at levels exceeding those found elsewhere in the body.
- Hair can be contaminated by hair care preparations and air pollution.
- Hair samples can be contaminated with other minerals in the process of preparing them for chemical analysis.

Hair analysis conducted by experts can provide valuable information in certain situations. Coroners use it to find out if a person has died from arsenic, lead, or other poisons. Public health researchers use it to study pollution levels and the potential for hazardous elements to find their way into the food supply and then into humans eating those foods. Hair analysis can help monitor occupational exposure to lead dust.[3] We have learned that women and children who eat certain fish more frequently have higher hair mercury levels than those who seldom eat fish,[4] and mothers with higher mercury levels transfer greater amounts to their newborns.[5] These reports by government researchers are useful for monitoring environmental hazards and developing food advisories.

But hair analysis cannot provide a valid determination of an individual's nutritional status. For most nutrients there are no standard laboratory values for normal hair content, and we do not know how hair levels and blood levels are related. A mineral found in very low levels in hair may be at normal levels in blood. Hair analysis requires highly specialized equipment and expertise that is generally available only in recognized university and government facilities. Companies that advertise hair analysis and request a hair sample by mail, often use this diagnosis as a sales technique. They report deficiencies and recommend purchasing dietary supplements to remedy the situation. Quality standards are also suspect with these groups. When researchers sent a split hair sample from a healthy volunteer to six different commercial laboratories for analysis, there was a tenfold difference between the highest value reported and the lowest value reported for more than half the minerals.[6] The reports on hair samples from two healthy teenagers advised supplements to remedy nutrient imbalances and prevent various chronic diseases.[2]

Persons should avoid any nutritional diagnosis from other than a health professional, especially when advice is being provided by mail and dietary supplements are recommended. When in doubt about the appropriateness of an organization, a good rule is to check with a physician or local hospital.

References

1. American Dietetic Association: Position of the American Dietetic Association: food and nutrition misinformation, *J Am Diet Assoc* 102:260, 2002.
2. Barrett S: Fads, frauds, and quackery. In Shils ME et al, eds: *Modern nutrition in health and disease,* ed 10, Baltimore, 2006, Lippincott Williams & Wilkins.
3. Strumylaite L, Ryselis S, Kregzdyte R: Content of lead in human hair from people with various exposure levels in Lithuania, *Int J Hyg Environ Health* 207:345, 2004.
4. McDowell MA et al: Hair mercury levels in U.S. children and women of child-bearing age: reference range data from NHANES 1999-2000, *Environ Health Perspect* 112:1165, 2004.
5. Morrissette J et al: Temporal variation of blood and hair mercury levels in pregnancy in relation to fish consumption history in a population living along the St. Lawrence River, *Environ Res* 95:363, 2004.
6. Steindel SJ, Howanitz PJ: The uncertainty of hair analysis for trace minerals, *JAMA* 285(1):67, 2001.

Absorption

Major control of iron balance takes place at the site of absorption in the small intestine. There are two forms of dietary iron—(1) heme iron and (2) nonheme iron (Table 7-5). The larger portion by far is nonheme iron, which includes all plant sources plus 60% of animal sources.[34] Nonheme iron is absorbed at a much slower rate than the smaller heme molecule because it is tightly bound to organic components in the form of ferric iron (Fe^{3+}). In the acid medium of the stomach, ferric iron must be separated and reduced to the more soluble ferrous form (Fe^{2+}) before it can be absorbed. If not enough gastric acid is available to convert the nonheme iron from the ferric to the ferrous form, it cannot be absorbed and is lost in the feces.

Iron distribution and transfer within the absorbing cells of the intestinal mucosa involve several carrier substances. Iron never travels unescorted. First, the ferrous iron is bound by a protein carrier in the mucosal cell. This protein carrier leaves behind a supply of iron to serve the needs of the energy-producing mitochondria of the absorbing cell and then delivers specific amounts to waiting

heme iron Form of dietary iron from animal sources, from the heme portion of hemoglobin in red blood cells. Heme iron is more easily absorbed and transported in the body than nonheme iron from plant sources, but it supplies the smaller portion of the body's total dietary iron intake.

nonheme iron The larger portion of dietary iron, including all the plant food sources and 60% of the animal food sources. This form of iron is not part of a heme complex and is less easily absorbed.

TABLE 7-5	Characteristics of Heme and Nonheme Dietary Iron	
	Dietary Iron	
	Heme (Smaller Portion)	Nonheme (Larger Portion)
Food sources	None in plant sources; 40% of iron in animal sources	All plant sources; 60% of iron in animal sources
Absorption rate	Rapid; transported and absorbed intact	Slow; tightly bound in organic molecules

carriers that control its destination. These compounds are (1) apoferritin, a protein receptor that combines with iron to form the iron-holding compound ferritin for storage in the cell and (2) apotransferrin, the protein receptor that combines with iron to form the iron-carrier compound serum transferrin, which circulates in the blood.

The proportion of dietary iron that is absorbed or rejected is determined by the amount of ferritin already present in the intestinal mucosal cells. When all available apoferritin has been bound to iron to form ferritin, any additional iron arriving at the binding site is rejected and returned to the lumen of the intestine for excretion in the feces. Approximately 1% to 15% of nonheme iron is absorbed compared to 15% to 45% of heme iron.[35] Most absorption takes place in the upper small intestine.

The following three factors favor absorption:

1. *Body need:* In iron deficiency or when body demands increase as in growth or pregnancy or weight training, more iron is absorbed.[34] When tissue reserves are ample or saturated, iron is rejected and excreted.
2. *Ascorbic acid (vitamin C) or other acids:* An acid environment increases iron absorption.[36] Acids act on ferric iron to reduce it to ferrous iron, the soluble form that is absorbed. Adding 50 mg of ascorbic acid to a meal by including orange juice or other food source can triple the absorption of nonheme iron.[34] Gastric hydrochloric acid provides the optimal acid medium to prepare iron for absorption.
3. *Animal tissues:* Meat, fish, and poultry improve iron absorption by providing some iron in the heme form. Heme iron is not only better absorbed than nonheme iron, but also improves the absorption of nonheme iron eaten at the same meal.[37] Peptides released from meat, fish, and poultry during digestion enhance the absorption of iron from other sources.[34]

The following five factors hinder iron absorption.

1. *Binding agents:* Phosphates, phytates, and oxalates bind iron and prevent its absorption. Certain vegetable proteins, including soy protein, decrease iron absorption independent of their phytate content. Substances in tea and coffee decrease absorption of nonheme iron.[38]
2. *Low gastric acid:* Surgical removal of stomach tissue (gastrectomy) reduces the number of cells available to secrete hydrochloric acid and can decrease iron absorption. Iron supplements may be required following bariatric surgery or stomach resection.[39] Persons who abuse antacids may have trouble absorbing nonheme iron.
3. *Infection:* Severe infection depresses iron absorption, as the body attempts to suppress the supply of iron to the infectious microorganisms.
4. *Gastrointestinal disease:* Malabsorption syndromes or diarrhea or steatorrhea hinder iron absorption.
5. *Calcium:* Large amounts of calcium may inhibit the absorption of both heme and nonheme iron consumed at the same meal. This interaction could affect the iron status of those taking calcium supplements with meals, although the addition of 300 mg of calcium (the equivalent of one glass of milk) at meals did not affect iron absorption over several days.[40] Adding calcium in the form of a food rather than a supplement is a better approach for supporting optimum absorption of all nutrients.

Transport

Following absorption, iron is bound with the protein transferrin for transport via the general circulation to storage sites or body cells. Normally only 20% to 35% of the iron-binding capacity of transferrin is filled. The remainder serves as a reserve for handling any emergency or variance in iron intake.

Storage

Bound to transferrin, iron is delivered to its storage sites in bone marrow and liver. Here it is recombined with apoferritin to form ferritin. Ferritin is a stable and exchangeable storage form that can release iron as needed. A second, less soluble storage form, hemosiderin, provides reserve storage in the liver. From these storage compounds iron is mobilized for hemoglobin synthesis and production of red blood cells or formation of other body cells. In the average adult 20 to 25 mg of iron/day is used for hemoglobin synthesis, but much of this represents iron that was conserved and recycled by the body when old red blood cells were destroyed. The average life span of a red blood cell is approximately 120 days. These interrelationships of body iron absorption-transport-storage are diagrammed in Figure 7-4.

Excretion

Because iron regulation occurs at the point of absorption, only minute amounts are lost through the kidneys. In

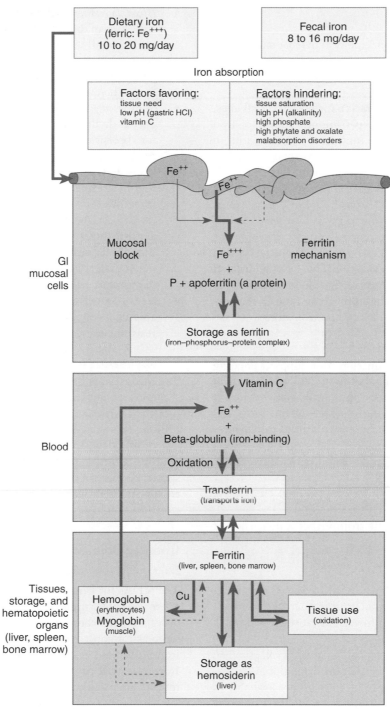

FIGURE 7-4 Summary of iron metabolism, showing its absorption, transport, use in hemoglobin formation, and storage forms (ferritin and hemosiderin).

this respect iron differs from other circulating minerals, which are excreted in the urine. Body iron is lost by the normal sloughing off of skin cells and gastrointestinal cells and through normal gastrointestinal and menstrual blood loss. Heavy menstrual flow, childbirth, surgery, acute and chronic hemorrhage, gastrointestinal disease, or parasitic infestation causes exceptional iron loss and depletes body stores.

Physiologic Functions of Iron

Oxygen Transport

Iron is "pocketed" within the heme molecule, the nonprotein portion of hemoglobin in the red blood cell. Iron carries oxygen to the cells for respiration and metabolism. Iron has a similar role in myoglobin, the compound that delivers oxygen to muscle.

Cellular Oxidation

Iron is a component of cell enzyme systems that oxidize glucose and other energy-yielding nutrients to produce energy.

Growth Needs

Positive iron balance is imperative for growth at all ages. At birth an infant has a 4- to 6-month supply of iron stored in the liver. Breast-fed infants obtain some iron in breast milk, and iron is added to commercial infant formulas. Supplementary iron-rich and iron-fortified foods are introduced to an infant's diet at 4 to 6 months of age to prevent milk anemia.[41] Throughout childhood iron is needed for continued growth and to build reserves for the physiologic stress of adolescence—muscle development in boys and the onset of menses in girls. The need for iron escalates during pregnancy for producing the additional red blood cells for the expanding blood volume and building iron reserves in the developing fetal liver. Normal blood loss in childbirth draws on iron stores.

Brain and Cognitive Function

Iron is important for brain function. Iron supports ongoing energy metabolism and the synthesis and breakdown of neurotransmitters. A sufficient amount of available iron is needed for infants and young children whose brain and nerve cells are growing rapidly. Iron status also influences cognitive function in children and adolescents with effects on memory, attention span, and the ability to concentrate.[42]

Iron Deficiency and Clinical Applications

Clinical abnormalities result from either a deficiency or an excess of iron.

Iron Deficiency Anemia

Iron deficiency occurs in both developed and developing countries and results in a hypochromic microcytic anemia. This deficiency may stem from various causes, as follows[34]:

- *Low iron intake:* Nutritional anemia develops when iron or other nutrients needed for hemoglobin synthesis and red blood cell production are not available in adequate amounts. The role of hemoglobin in carrying oxygen to the cells is important in understanding the symptoms of iron deficiency anemia (Box 7-7).

BOX 7-7	**Signs of Iron Deficiency**

Fatigue
Muscle weakness
Pale color
Decreased resistance to infection
Spoon nails
Angular stomatitis

- *Blood loss:* Hemorrhagic anemia results from excessive loss of blood and its associated iron. Aspirin causes small amounts of blood loss through the gastrointestinal tract, and its long-term use by older people for pain relief can lower body iron stores.[43] Severe hemorrhoids can lead to blood loss.
- *Gastrectomy:* Postgastrectomy anemia develops when gastric hydrochloric acid necessary to liberate iron for absorption is no longer available.
- *Malabsorption:* Iron deficiency anemia ensues when iron-binding agents prevent absorption or mucosal lesions damage the absorbing surface of the small intestine.
- *Chronic disease:* Anemia of chronic disease is related to abnormalities in the recycling of iron from old red blood cells and the production of new red blood cells, not iron deficiency. It is associated with infection, inflammatory disorders, heart disease, renal disease, and connective tissue diseases such as arthritis. This anemia is found mostly in older persons and is highly resistant to treatment.

Worldwide Problem of Iron Deficiency Anemia

Nutritional anemia, including iron deficiency anemia, is second only to protein-energy malnutrition as the most prevalent nutritional deficiency in the world. More than 2 billion persons across many nations are believed to be anemic or iron deficient, with women of childbearing age and children most likely affected.[44] Iron deficiency anemia respects neither social class nor geographic situation; iron balance is precarious based on low intakes of bioavailable iron and iron losses through parasitic infections.

Iron Requirement

Dietary Reference Intake

The RDAs for iron are set at 18 mg/day for women ages 19 to 50 and 8 mg/day for men ages 19 and over.[34] For older women whose menses have ceased the RDA is the same as for adult men, 8 mg/day. Pregnancy has a "high iron cost," and the daily allowance rises to 27 mg/day. Iron needs fall to 9 mg/day during lactation because the menses are usually absent during this period.[34]

Special Considerations for Vegetarians

Individuals eating only plant foods are at increased risk of iron deficiency. Not only is the bioavailability of iron lower in plant foods, but also heme iron is unavailable to enhance the absorption of nonheme iron. As a result, overall absorption from plant-only diets may be only 10% as compared to 18% for the typical American diet. With this in mind it is recommended that vegetarian men take in 14 mg of iron/day and vegetarian premenopausal women take in 33 mg/day. Vegetarian adolescent girls need 26 mg/day. Note that these recommendations are nearly twice the RDAs for persons of comparable age who consume a mixed diet containing meat, fish, or poultry.[34] (See Chapter 4 for a review of plant-based diets.)

Iron Toxicity

Hemochromatosis

Iron toxicity was first identified in a population in Southern Africa who cooked their food in iron vessels and also had a genetic tendency to absorb and store abnormally high amounts of iron.[34] In the United States accidental iron poisoning occurs in both children and adults who overuse iron supplements. But another cause of iron overload is the genetic disease hemochromatosis, in which iron continues to be absorbed at a high rate despite elevated liver stores. Excessive body iron contributes to cardiac arrhythmias, liver disease, and diabetes.[45] It is estimated that 1 of every 385 Americans has this genetic mutation, although not all develop hemochromatosis.[46]

Tolerable Upper Intake Level

Because iron becomes toxic at high levels, the Food and Nutrition Board has set a UL for this nutrient. Iron intake should not exceed 45 mg/day.[34] Although it would seem unlikely that a person could reach this level from food alone, current iron fortification practices developed to meet the iron needs of women in the childbearing years add significant amounts of iron to the diet. Individuals who eat more than one serving size of a cereal containing 15 to 18 mg of iron per serving along with other iron-containing foods and possibly an iron-containing multivitamin-mineral supplement can approach or exceed the UL. High iron stores were found in older men and women who ate large amounts of meat containing heme iron and took iron supplements[47,48] or used alcoholic beverages on a regular basis.[49] (Alcohol increases iron absorption.) Excessive iron stores may increase the risk of colorectal cancer.[46] Iron supplements should always be approved by a physician. (See the *Perspectives in Practice* box, "Do I Need a Vitamin-Mineral Supplement?" for important criteria to consider before using *any* mineral or vitamin supplement.)

Food Sources of Iron

The typical Western diet contains about 5 to 7 mg of iron per 1000 kcal.[44] Iron is found in highest amounts in meat, fish, poultry, eggs, dried peas and beans, and whole grain and fortified breads and cereals. Fortified grain products such as breakfast bars contain from 1 mg to 24 mg of iron per serving. Ready-to-eat cereals and bread make the highest contributions to the iron intake of adults.[4] Heme iron provides less than 10% of the iron intake of girls and women and less than 12% of the iron intake of boys and men.[34] Box 7-8 lists some comparative food sources of iron.

IODINE

Iodine has a long history of study based on the need to identify the cause of goiter and other disorders found to relate to iodine deficiency. Iodine is a component of the hormone thyroxine produced in the thyroid gland, which controls the rate of energy metabolism in cells. The body contains only 15 to 20 mg of iodine, and most of this (70% to 80%) is in the thyroid gland. The thyroid gland has a remarkable ability to concentrate iodine.

Absorption-Excretion Balance

Absorption

Iodine is absorbed in the small intestine in the form of iodides. Iodides are then loosely bound to proteins and carried by the blood to the thyroid gland, which takes up as much as it needs to continue appropriate hormone synthesis. About one third of the available iodide is used to produce active thyroid hormone, and the remainder is used to form hormone precursors that are held for later use.

Excretion

Absorbed iodide not needed by the thyroid gland is excreted in the urine. More than 90% of the iodine taken into the body appears in the urine.

Hormonal Control

Thyroid-stimulating hormone (TSH) from the anterior lobe of the pituitary gland directs the uptake of iodine by the thyroid cells in response to plasma thyroid hormone levels. When plasma levels are high, less thyroid hormone is produced. When plasma levels are low, the thyroid cells are stimulated to take up more iodine and produce more hormone. This feedback mechanism maintains a healthy circular balance between supply and demand and is the characteristic pattern for governing hormone production by the endocrine glands controlled by the master pituitary gland.

Physiologic Function of Iodine

Thyroid Hormone Synthesis

The major function of iodine is the synthesis of the thyroid hormone thyroxine. Thyroxine regulates cell oxidation and basal metabolic rate (BMR) by increasing oxygen uptake and the reaction rates of enzyme systems handling glucose. In this role iodine indirectly exerts tremendous control on the body's total metabolism. Thyroid hormone also regulates protein synthesis and controls maturation of the developing brain.[50]

Plasma Thyroxine

Free thyroxine is secreted into the bloodstream and bound to plasma protein for transport to the cells. After

PERSPECTIVES IN PRACTICE
Do I Need a Vitamin-Mineral Supplement?

We are constantly barraged by advertisements urging us to purchase a vitamin or mineral supplement to prevent or cure real or imagined nutrient deficiencies. Sales of dietary supplements now exceed $17.7 billion,[1] and the nutritional supplement market is one of the world's fastest growing industries.[2] The U.S. Food and Drug Administration estimates there are more than 29,000 supplements on the market including nutritional, herbal, botanical, and sports products.[3]

The best strategy for obtaining appropriate amounts of vitamins and minerals is to wisely choose a variety of foods.[3] All of the nutrients, fiber, and phytochemicals that we need for preserving good health and preventing chronic disease are available in the foods we eat. Many substances yet to be discovered that may be essential to health are found in food. Fortified foods such as breakfast cereals or juices can provide additional vitamins or minerals that are lacking in our usual diets. Vitamin or mineral supplements should be considered only in those situations when needs cannot be met with food alone.

Despite an emphasis on food, some individuals because of particular physiologic circumstances or cultural patterns may need supplements or certain fortified foods to meet their DRI for particular nutrients, as follows:

- Older adults with low levels of gastric acid are less able to absorb vitamin B_{12} from animal protein foods and need to find another source. Vitamin B_{12}–fortified breads, cereals, or juices or a supplement containing vitamin B_{12} could meet this need. Vegans who eat no animal foods require a vitamin B_{12} supplement or fortified plant food.
- Women of childbearing age who may become pregnant require 400 μg of folate daily to help prevent neural tube defects in a developing fetus. Mandatory folic acid fortification of grain products sold in the United States has raised the folate intakes of women who do not eat fruit and vegetable sources regularly. Still, the Surgeon General recommends that all women of childbearing age use a folate supplement to ensure an adequate intake.[4]
- Pregnant women, whose DRI for iron is 27 mg, are unlikely to obtain this amount from food, even including fortified foods. Physicians usually prescribe iron supplements in pregnancy and may include folate and calcium supplements as well.[3]
- Youth and adults who cannot tolerate milk or do not care for dairy products may find it difficult to meet their goals for calcium. Calcium-fortified juices and cereals can help but it may be necessary to include a supplement to add to the food total for the day.
- Older adults with low energy needs who eat very limited amounts of food and others who restrict their intake of kcalories may benefit from a multivitamin-mineral supplement. Energy intakes falling below 1500 to 1600 kcal are unlikely to contain all necessary vitamins and minerals in the required amounts.[3]
- Individuals who seldom spend time in the sun, vegans who do not use animal foods, and those whose skin pigment makes it difficult to synthesize vitamin D need to consider vitamin D–fortified foods or a supplement to ensure an adequate body supply.[3]

Although meeting the DRI for essential vitamins and minerals is important to health, we must help our audiences understand that there is no added benefit—and even a danger—to exceeding recommended levels through use of supplements[5] and it wastes money better spent for food. Dietary evaluations need to be individualized; no one piece of advice fits all. When reviewing a person's intake, consider the added nutrients in fortified foods. Some brands of ready-to-eat breakfast cereals approach the vitamin and mineral content of multivitamin-mineral supplements. In today's food market, combinations of nutrient-dense unprocessed foods and fortified foods plus a supplement containing 100% of the DRI can add up to potentially dangerous levels of certain nutrients. Intakes of preformed vitamin A exceeding the RDA are dangerous for pregnant women and can lead to congenital malformations (see Chapter 6). Men and postmenopausal women can be vulnerable to iron overload based on their genetic disposition. Because vitamin and mineral supplements interact with certain prescription and nonprescription medications, individuals taking medicines regularly need to check with their physician before using a supplement.

The following guidelines can help individuals make decisions about the need for a vitamin-mineral supplement:

- Use supplements in addition to, not in place of, real food. A poor diet with added supplements is still a poor diet. To the extent possible try to obtain needed nutrients with appropriate meal planning.
- Avoid multivitamin-mineral supplements or single nutrient supplements that exceed 100% of the RDA or AI for any nutrient. Individuals using highly fortified foods might aim for no more than 50% of the DRI in a supplement or reconsider whether a supplement is really necessary. Intake should not exceed the UL for any vitamin or mineral.
- Seek the advice of a physician before adding a supplement; this is especially important for individuals on prescription or nonprescription medications or who regularly eat a highly fortified cereal that supplies 100% of the recommended levels of most minerals and/or vitamins.
- Take the supplement with meals so that foods in the digestive tract will enhance nutrient absorption.

References

1. Marcason W: What are some resources that can help my clients sort through the conflicting information on dietary supplements? *J Am Diet Assoc* 103:712, 2003.
2. Foote JA et al: Factors associated with dietary supplement use among healthy adults of five ethnicities, *Am J Epidemiol* 157:888, 2003.
3. American Dietetic Association: Position of the American Dietetic Association: fortification and nutritional supplements, *J Am Diet Assoc* 105:1300, 2005.
4. U.S. Department of Health and Human Services: U.S. Surgeon General announces new folic acid recommendations (news release), Washington, DC, 2005 (January 24). Retrieved October 11, 2005, from *www.surgeongeneral.gov/pressreleases/sg01242005a.html/*.
5. Hunt JR: Tailoring advice on dietary supplements, *J Am Diet Assoc* 102:1754, 2002.

BOX 7-8 | Food Sources of Iron

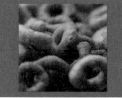 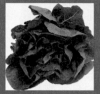 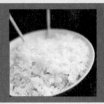 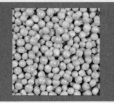 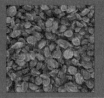 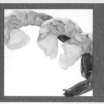

Food Source	Quantity	Iron (mg)
Grains Group		
Ready-to-eat cereals		
Total	¾ cup	18.00
Cheerios	1 cup	8.10
All Bran	½ cup	4.96
Rice, white, enriched (cooked)	1 cup	1.80
Bread, white	1 slice	0.76
Vegetable Group		
Spinach (boiled)	½ cup	3.21
Potato (baked, with skin)	1 med	2.75
Peas, green (boiled)	½ cup	1.24
Broccoli (boiled)	½ cup	0.89
Fruit Group		
Prune juice (canned)	8 fl oz	3.03
Raisins, seedless	⅔ cup	2.08
Meat, Beans, Eggs, and Nuts Group		
Lima beans (cooked)	1 cup	4.50
Shrimp (steamed)	3 oz (15 large)	2.62
Soybeans (cooked)	½ cup	2.30
Ground beef patty	3 oz	2.20
Refried beans	½ cup	2.10
Tuna, light, canned in water	3 oz	2.07
Chicken, dark (roasted, without skin)	3½ oz	1.33
Egg, whole	1 large	1.04
Ham, canned (lean)	3½ oz	0.94
Halibut (baked)	3 oz	0.91

Images copyright 2006 JupiterImages Corporation.

Recommended Dietary Allowances for adults: women ages 19-50, 18 mg; women ages ≥51, 8 mg; men, 8 mg.

completing its work the hormone is degraded in the liver and the iodine excreted in the bile.

Iodine Deficiency and Clinical Applications

Abnormal Thyroid Function

Both hyperthyroidism and hypothyroidism affect the rate of thyroxine production and the body's overall metabolic rate.

Iodine Deficiency Disorder: Goiter

Endemic goiter, visible as a great enlargement of the thyroid gland, is found in persons living where water and soil, and in turn locally grown foods, contain little iodine. Up to 2.2 billion people live in iodine-deficient areas in developing countries.[51] When iodine is not available, the thyroid gland cannot produce a normal quantity of thyroxine. Low plasma thyroxine levels sig-

nal the pituitary to release TSH, which attempts to stimulate the thyroid gland. In the absence of iodine the thyroid responds by making thyroglobulin (a colloid), which accumulates in the thyroid follicles. Over time the gland becomes increasingly engorged and may attain a size of 500 to 700 g (1 to 1½ lb) or more (Figure 7-5). In the West African goiter belt of New Guinea, Zaire, and the Sudan iodized rapeseed oil and iodine-treated drinking water have eradicated severe endemic goiter.[50,52] Goiter also results from eating foods that contain substances that inhibit important steps in the

goiter Enlargement of the thyroid gland caused by lack of sufficient available iodine to produce the thyroid hormone thyroxine.

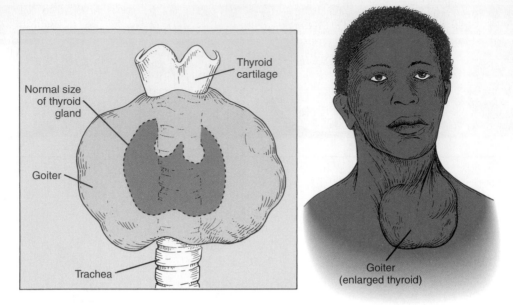

FIGURE 7-5 Goiter. The extreme enlargement shown here reflects an extended duration of iodine deficiency.

synthesis of thyroxine. Pearl millet, a cereal grain used in the Sudan region of Africa, has caused goiter in some preschool children.[50]

Iodine Deficiency Disorder: Cretinism

Iodine deficiency has been referred to as the leading cause of brain damage in the world,[53] and breast-fed infants of iodine-deficient mothers are especially at risk.[54] When iodine deficiency is severe in periods of critical brain development, the outcome is cretinism, with irreversible mental retardation and disability.

Iodine Requirement

Dietary Reference Intake

The iodine RDA for both men and women is 150 µg/day.[34] To meet the needs of both mother and developing fetus the RDA in pregnancy is 220 µg/day, and this rises to 290 µg/day in lactation. Because the iodine demand is great during periods of accelerated growth, the allowance for youth ages 14 to 18 is 150 µg/day, the same as for adults.

Iodine Overload

Food production and processing methods add to iodine intake. Dairy farms use iodophors, iodine-containing chemicals, for sanitizing milking machines and milk tanks. Other iodine-containing compounds that find their way into the human food supply are the iodates used as dough conditioners in breads, erythrosine used as food coloring, and derivatives of iodine supplements added to animal feeds. Case reports of iodine toxicity indicate that iodine-containing dietary supplements or topical medications, when added to the iodine contributed by food, result in intakes that exceed by many times the RDA.

Food Sources of Iodine

Seafood is rich in iodine. Other foods vary widely depending on the iodine content of the soil and the iodine compounds used in processing. Iodized table salt fortified at the level of 1 mg iodine per 10 g of salt is a major dietary source in the United States and elsewhere. Calcium iodate and potassium iodate are additives commonly found in commercially produced bread. Avoidance of salt for health reasons could contribute to an iodine deficiency.

OTHER ESSENTIAL TRACE ELEMENTS

ZINC

Zinc participates in many metabolic activities as a component of over 100 different enzymes and a factor in growth.[34] An adult's total body zinc ranges from 1.5 g in women to 2.5 g in men. It is present in minute quantities in all body organs, tissues, fluids, and secretions. Although zinc is vital throughout life, it is particularly important in growth periods such as pregnancy and lactation, infancy and childhood, and adolescence.[34,51,55] Zinc is closely involved with deoxyribonucleic acid (DNA) and ribonucleic acid (RNA) metabolism and protein synthesis and is necessary for tissue growth to progress at normal rates.

Zinc Deficiency and Clinical Applications

Several clinical problems stem from zinc deficiency, as follows:

- *Hypogonadism:* Dwarfism and arrested development and function of the gonads result from pronounced human zinc deficiency in childhood and adolescence.

- *Loss in taste and smell:* Hypogeusia (diminished taste) and hyposmia (diminished smell) are associated with severe zinc deficiency but may improve when zinc is restored.
- *Wound healing:* The healing of wounds or tissue injuries from trauma, surgery, or physiologic stress is retarded in zinc-deficient persons. Older people with pressure sores can sometimes benefit from zinc supplementation.
- *Growth, development, and life cycle needs:* Rapid growth in infants, children, and adolescents carries special needs for zinc. When zinc is inadequate, proteins necessary for the linear growth of the long bones are not produced and growth is stunted.[55] Sexual maturation is delayed in adolescent males deprived of zinc.[56] Poor zinc intake in pregnancy can result in congenital malformations and low infant birth weight.
- *Immune function:* Zinc is needed for optimum immune function.[57]
- *Malabsorption:* Malabsorption diseases such as Crohn's disease lead to zinc deficiency because the ulcerative lesions in the mucosal surface hinder absorption. Dietary restrictions imposed in the treatment of these conditions can limit zinc intake.

Zinc Requirement

Dietary Reference Intake

The RDAs for zinc are 11 mg for men and 8 mg for women.[34] The recommended intake for women is lower because of their generally smaller body mass. National surveys tell us that adolescent girls and persons over age 60 are most likely to have intakes below recommended levels.[58] In contrast, less than 1% of preschool children take in less than the DRI for their age group.[59] Milk, meat, and ready-to-eat cereals accounted for much of the children's intake. Beef is the major zinc source in the United States providing nearly 25% of total intake. Zinc can be a problem for vegetarians because phytates and other zinc-binding substances in plant foods interfere with absorption.[38]

Food Sources of Zinc

Good sources of dietary zinc are seafood (especially oysters), meat, and eggs. Less rich sources are legumes and whole grains. Bioavailability is a problem for those depending on plant foods for their zinc. Box 7-9 lists some comparative foods containing zinc.

COPPER

Copper and iron have many characteristics in common, as follows:

- Both are components of cell enzymes.
- Both are involved in energy production.
- Both participate in hemoglobin synthesis.

BOX 7-9	Food Sources of Zinc

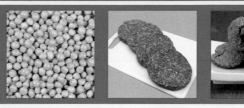

Food Source	Quantity	Zinc (mg)
Grains Group		
Bite-Size Shredded Wheat cereal	1 cup	1.50
Oat bran muffin	1	1.05
Vegetable Group		
Peas, green	1 cup	1.07
Meat, Beans, Eggs, and Nuts Group		
Oysters (steamed)	12	25.8
Ground-beef patty	3 oz	5.26
Baked beans	1 cup	4.24
Peanut butter	2 tbsp	0.94

Images copyright 2006 JupiterImages Corporation.
Recommended Dietary Allowance for adults: women, 8 mg; men, 11 mg.

Copper occurs naturally in many foods, so dietary deficiency is rare.[34] Copper deficiency has developed in patients on total parenteral nutrition (TPN) that excluded copper, persons using concentrated zinc supplements that interfered with copper absorption, and premature infants fed only cow's milk, which is low in copper.

The current RDA for copper is 900 μg/day (0.9 mg/day); however, it appears that many adults do not meet this level.[34] Copper like many trace elements is lost in food processing. The richest sources of copper are liver, seafood (particularly oysters), nuts, and seeds; smaller amounts are found in whole grains and legumes (see the *Focus on Food Safety* box, "Beware of Copper-Lined Utensils," for more information on copper).

MANGANESE

The adult body contains about 20 mg of manganese distributed in the liver, bones, pancreas, and pituitary gland.[34] Although a dietary essential, manganese is toxic at high levels. Like other trace elements, manganese is a part of important cell enzymes. Manganese deficiency has been reported in patients with pancreatic insufficiency

---

cretinism A congenital disease resulting from absence or deficiency of normal thyroid secretion, characterized by physical deformity, dwarfism, mental retardation, and often goiters.

FOCUS ON FOOD SAFETY
Beware of Copper-Lined Utensils

Some dishes and containers intended to be decorative are lined with copper. Copper is easily dissolved by acid—and this includes acids in food. It is dangerous to cook or serve foods in copper-lined containers because harmful amounts of copper can dissolve and enter your food. The body requires copper in very minute amounts, and high levels become toxic. The Food Code developed by the Food and Drug Administration to set standards for safe food handling in restaurants, institutions, and other food service operations forbids any use of copper-lined containers for cooking or serving. Think about using your copper-lined dish for a centerpiece rather than a serving dish.

Data from U.S. Food and Drug Administration: *Food Code: 2005,* Washington, DC, 2005, U.S. Government Printing Office.

and protein-energy malnutrition. Manganese toxicity is associated with industrial situations in which miners or other workers had prolonged exposure to manganese dust. Excess manganese accumulates in the liver and central nervous system, producing psychiatric disturbances and neuromuscular symptoms resembling those of Parkinson's disease. The AI for manganese is 2.3 mg/day for men and 1.8 mg/day for women.[34] The typical American diet supplies manganese at a level of 1.6 mg/1000 kcal. The best sources are plant foods—grains, legumes, seeds, nuts, leafy vegetables, tea, and coffee.

CHROMIUM

The precise amount of chromium in the body is not known, although it is found in minute amounts in liver, soft tissues, and bone. Chromium is part of a low-molecular-weight protein complex that potentiates insulin activity and assists in moving glucose into cells. Through its role with insulin, chromium influences carbohydrate, protein, and fat metabolism. Chromium supplements have not been found to have therapeutic value in the treatment of type 2 diabetes.[60] Chromium picolinate is widely advertised as a body-building supplement, although we lack definite evidence as to its value (see Chapter 14).

The AI for chromium is 35 μg/day for men and 25 μg/day for women ages 19 to 50. Based on their lower energy intakes, the AIs for those over age 50 drop to 30 μg and 20 μg, respectively.[34] Information about the chromium content of common foods is sparse.[60] Brewer's yeast is a rich source. Other food sources include liver, cheddar cheese, and wheat germ. Most whole grains provide this nutrient.

COBALT

Cobalt is found in only minute traces in body tissues with storage in the liver. As part of vitamin B_{12} (cobalamin) the known functions of cobalt are associated with red blood cell formation and support of the myelin sheath surrounding nerve fibers in the central nervous system. Cobalt is provided in the human diet only in the form of vitamin B_{12}.

SELENIUM

Selenium is deposited in all body tissues except fat. Concentrations are highest in liver, kidney, heart, and spleen. Selenium is an integral part of an antioxidant enzyme that protects cells and lipid membranes from oxidative damage. Selenium partners with vitamin E, each sparing the other.[61] Highly bioavailable selenium compounds are found in breast milk, suggesting an important role for this element in early life.[62] The RDA for all adults is 55 μg/day.[61] Foods vary in selenium based on the content of the soil in which they were grown. Generally good sources include seafood, legumes, whole grains, lean meats, and dairy products; vegetables contain the smallest amounts.

MOLYBDENUM

Molybdenum is an enzyme cofactor in hydroxylation reactions.[34] The RDA is set at 45 μg/day for men and women. The amount of molybdenum in foods varies depending on the soil content. The richest sources generally include legumes, whole grains, and nuts. Animal products, fruit, and most vegetables are poor sources.

FLUORIDE

Fluoride accumulates in the calcified tissues and protects bones and teeth from mineral loss. If fluoride is present when calcium-phosphorus crystals are being formed, a fluoride ion (F^-) replaces a hydroxyl ion (OH^-) in the crystal, resulting in a substance that is more resistant to resorption. (Resorption is the breaking down of bone crystals with release of the minerals into solution.) This effect is seen in bones and teeth. Microorganisms feeding on fermentable carbohydrates that adhere to the teeth after a meal form acids that dissolve tooth enamel and initiate tooth decay. Fluoride-containing crystals are more resistant to the erosive effect of bacterial acids.[63]

The AI for fluoride is expected to protect against dental caries. For men intake is set at 4 mg/day and for women, 3 mg/day.[10] Fish, fish products, and tea contain the highest amounts. Fluoridated dental products also contribute to fluoride intake. Adding fluoride to public water supplies in the amount of 1 part per million (ppm) leads to a decline in dental caries in those communities. Cooking with fluoridated water raises the level in many foods.

The roles of the trace elements are summarized in Table 7-6.

TABLE 7-6	Summary of Trace Elements			
Element	**Metabolism**	**Physiologic Functions**	**Clinical Applications**	**DRI**	**Food Sources**

Iron (Fe)	Absorption controls body supply; favored by body need, acidity, and reduction agents such as vitamin C; hindered by binding agents, reduced gastric HCl, infection, gastrointestinal losses
	Transported as transferrin, stored as ferritin or hemosiderin
	Excreted in sloughed cells, bleeding
		Hemoglobin synthesis, oxygen transport
		Cell oxidation, heme enzymes
			Anemia (hypochromic, microcytic)
			Excess: hemosiderosis, hemochromatosis
			Growth and pregnancy needs
				Adults
				  Males ages ≥19: 8 mg
				  Females ages 19-50: 18 mg
				  Females ages ≥51: 8 mg
				Pregnancy
				  All ages: 27 mg
				Lactation
				  Ages ≤18: 10 mg
				  Ages ≥19: 9 mg
					Meat, eggs, liver
					Whole grain and enriched breads and cereals
					Dark green vegetables
					Legumes, nuts
					Acid foods cooked in iron utensils

Iodine (I)	Absorbed as iodides, taken up by thyroid gland under control of thyroid-stimulating hormone (TSH)
	Excretion by kidney
		Synthesis of thyroxin, which regulates cell metabolism, basal metabolic rate (BMR)	Endemic colloid goiter, cretinism
			Hypothyroidism and hyperthyroidism
				Adults
				  Males/females ages ≥19: 150 µg
				Pregnancy
				  All ages: 220 µg
				Lactation
				  All ages: 290 µg
					Iodized salt
					Seafood

Zinc (Zn)	Absorbed in small intestine
	Transported in blood by albumin; stored in many sites
	Excretion largely intestinal
		Essential coenzyme constituent: carbonic anhydrase, carboxypeptidase, lactic dehydrogenase	Growth: hypogonadism
			Sensory impairment: taste and smell
			Wound healing
			Malabsorption disease
				Adults
				  Males ages ≥19: 11 mg
				  Females ages ≥19: 8 mg
				Pregnancy
				  Ages ≤18: 13 mg
				  Ages ≥19: 11 mg
				Lactation
				  Ages ≤18: 14 mg
				  Ages ≥19: 12 mg
					Beef and other meats; liver
					Oysters, seafood
					Milk, cheese, eggs
					Whole grains
					Widely distributed in food

Copper (Cu)	Absorbed in small intestine
	Transported in blood by histidine and albumin
	Stored in many tissues
		Associated with iron in enzyme systems, hemoglobin synthesis
		Metalloprotein enzyme constituent
			Hypocupremia: nephrosis and malabsorption
			Wilson's disease, excess copper storage
				Adults
				  Males/females ages ≥19: 900 µg
				Pregnancy
				  All ages: 1000 µg
				Lactation
				  All ages: 1300 mg
					Meat, liver, seafood
					Whole grains
					Legumes, nuts
					Widely distributed in food

Manganese (Mn)	Absorbed poorly
	Excretion mainly by intestine
		Enzyme component in general metabolism	Low serum levels in protein-energy malnutrition
			Inhalation toxicity
				Adults
				  Males ages ≥19: 2.3 mg
				  Females ages ≥19: 1.8 mg
				Pregnancy
				  All ages: 2.0 mg
				Lactation
				  All ages: 2.6 mg
					Whole grains and cereals
					Legumes, soybeans
					Green leafy vegetables

Continued

TABLE 7-6	Summary of Trace Elements—cont'd				
Element	Metabolism	Physiologic Functions	Clinical Applications	DRI	Food Sources
Chromium (Cr)	Absorbed in association with zinc Excretion mainly by kidney	Associated with glucose metabolism	Potentiates action of insulin	Adults Males ages 19-50: 35 μg Males ages ≥51: 30 μg Females ages 19-50: 25 μg Females ages ≥51: 20 μg Pregnancy Ages ≤18: 29 μg Ages ≥19: 30 μg Lactation Ages ≤18: 44 μg Ages ≥19: 45 μg	Whole grains and cereals Brewer's yeast Animal protein foods
Cobalt (Co)	Absorbed as component of food source, vitamin B₁₂ Stored in liver	Constituent of vitamin B₁₂, functions with vitamin	Deficiency associated only with deficiency of vitamin B₁₂	Unknown (usually consumed as part of the vitamin B₁₂ molecule)	Animal foods containing vitamin B₁₂
Selenium (Se)	Absorption depends on solubility of compound form Excreted mainly by kidney	Constituent of enzyme glutathione peroxidase Synergistic antioxidant with vitamin E	Marginal deficiency when soil content is low Deficiency secondary to total parenteral nutrition (TPN) or malnutrition Toxicity observed in livestock	Adults Males/females ages ≥19: 55 μg Pregnancy All ages: 60 μg Lactation All ages: 70 μg	Seafood Legumes Whole grains Vegetables Low-fat meats and dairy foods Varies with soil content
Molybdenum (Mo)	Readily absorbed Excreted rapidly by kidney Small amount excreted in bile	Constituent of oxidase enzymes, xanthine oxidase	Deficiency unknown in humans	Adults Males/females ages ≥19: 45 μg Pregnancy All ages 50 μg Lactation All ages: 50 μg	Legumes Whole grains Milk Organ meats Leafy vegetables
Fluoride (F)	Absorbed in small intestine; little known of bioavailability Excreted by kidney—80%	Accumulates in bones and teeth, increases hardness	Inhibits dental caries Osteoporosis: may reduce bone loss Excess: dental fluorosis	Adults Males ages ≥19: 4 mg Females ages ≥19: 3 mg Pregnancy All ages: 3 mg Lactation All ages: 3 mg	Fish and fish products Tea Drinking water (fluoridated) Foods cooked in fluoridated water

PROBABLE ESSENTIAL TRACE ELEMENTS

The metabolic functions of the remaining trace elements (see Box 7-1) are less well understood. Found to be essential in animal nutrition, they are probably essential for humans, acting as enzyme cofactors or adding to structure in special tissues. Such an example is the suggested role of boron in bone building. Based on the minute amounts needed, primary dietary deficiency is unlikely. However, induced deficiencies resulting when these elements are excluded from long-term TPN therapy reinforces their clinical importance.

WATER-ELECTROLYTE BALANCE

Several major minerals function as electrolytes in controlling body water balance. Fluid status is fundamental to health and a vital part of patient care. In this section we will look at the three interdependent factors that control fluid balance: (1) the water itself (the *solvent* base for solutions), (2) the various particles (*solutes*) in solution in the water, and (3) the separating membranes that control the flow.

WATER BALANCE

Body Water Distribution

If you are a woman, your body is about 50% to 55% water. If you are a man, your body is about 55% to 60% water. Men have higher water content because they have a greater proportion of muscle mass and a smaller proportion of fat. Muscle is higher in water than any other tissue except blood. Women have less muscle and a larger deposit of fat. Adipose tissue has a low water content compared to muscle.

Functions of Water

Body water has many important roles (Box 7-10). Much of our body form comes from the *turgor* water provides for tissues. Cell water furnishes the fluid environment for the vast array of chemical reactions that sustain life. Medications are dissolved in body fluids. The evaporation of water

BOX 7-10	Functions of Body Water

Form and structure
Fluid environment for chemical reactions
Fluid for dissolving important substances in tissues and cells
Fluid for transport of nutrients and waste
Control of body temperature
Fluid for dissolving medications

from the skin is an important means of controlling body temperature.

OVERALL WATER BALANCE: INTAKE AND OUTPUT

The average adult handles 2.5 to 3 L of water per day between intake and output. Water enters and leaves the body by various routes controlled by the mechanisms of thirst and regulatory hormones.

Water enters the body in the following three forms (Table 7-7):

1. As preformed water taken in as water or in other beverages
2. As preformed water in food
3. As metabolic water produced by cell oxidation

In general 81% of fluid intake comes from water and beverages and 19% comes from food.[26] Many common foods contain large amounts of water (Table 7-8). Metabolic water contributes less than beverages or food. All water entering the body, regardless of source, is of equal value in meeting fluid needs.

Water leaves the body through the kidneys, skin, and lungs and by fecal elimination (see Table 7-7). Vomiting and diarrhea result in abnormal losses of fluid and are serious clinical problems if prolonged. Extensive loss of body fluid is especially dangerous for infants and children, whose bodies contain a greater proportion of water than do adults and more of this water is outside the cells and easily lost. Water retention associated with cardiac failure or electrolyte disturbances is equally serious, requiring immediate medical attention. Intake and output must remain in balance to sustain normal hydration levels.

WATER REQUIREMENTS

For years we have been told to drink eight glasses of water a day, although it is difficult to find documentation on how this admonition came to be.[64-65] Recent concerns about hydration and encouragement of companies marketing bottled water have led to the practice of keeping a bottle of water close by. Nutrition experts have established guidelines for fluid intake but emphasize that for most individuals fluid needs are adequately met by thirst.[26]

Dietary Reference Intake

The AIs for fluids (Table 7-9) are based on the median water intake reported by participants in a recent national survey[26]; thus half of the persons in each age and sex category drank more and half drank less. Note, however, that these guidelines are intended for healthy individuals who are relatively sedentary and living in temperate cli-

TABLE 7-7	Approximate Daily Adult Intake and Output of Water		

	Intake (Replacement) (ml/Day)	Output (Loss) (ml/Day)	
		Obligatory (Insensible) (ml/Day)	Additional (According to Need) (ml/Day)
Preformed		Lungs 350	
Liquids	1200-1500	Skin	
In foods	700-1000	Diffusion 350	
Metabolism (oxidation of food)	200-300	Sweat 100	± 250
		Kidneys 900	± 500
		Feces 150	
		TOTAL 1850	750
TOTAL	2100-2800 (≈2600 ml/Day)	(≈2600 ml/Day)	

TABLE 7-8	Water Content of Selected Foods and Beverages

Food	Percent (%)
Coffee, milk, sports drinks, watermelon, broccoli, lettuce	91-100
Soda, fruit drinks, fruit juice, apples, oranges, grapes	80-90
Peas, frozen desserts, bananas, casseroles	70-79
Meat, fish, poultry	60-69
Bread, pasta	30-40
Cereals, nuts	<5

Data from Campbell S: Dietary Reference Intakes: water, potassium, sodium, chloride, and sulfate, *Nutr MD* 30(6):13, 2004.

TABLE 7-9	Adequate Intakes of Fluid*	

Age (Years)	Males	Females
1-3	4 cups	4 cups
4-8	5 cups	5 cups
9-13	8 cups	7 cups
14-18	11 cups	8 cups
≥19	13 cups	9 cups

Data from Food and Nutrition Board, Institute of Medicine: *Dietary Reference Intakes for water, potassium, sodium, chloride, and sulfate,* Washington, DC, 2004, National Academies Press.

*Expressed as cups of beverages/drinking water with additional fluid to be supplied in food.

mates. Athletes engaging in vigorous physical activity of long duration, the critically ill, or persons in very hot environments require special attention.

Over the years there have been conflicting opinions as to the value of caffeinated beverages in meeting fluid needs. It was common thought that the water in caffeine-containing fluids such as coffee or soft drinks was lost to the body. New studies indicate that people accustomed to drinking caffeinated beverages have no increase in urine output.[66] Alcohol does bring about water loss soon after it is consumed, but this effect is transient and does not result in appreciable losses over a 24-hour period.[26]

Special Clinical Applications

The following clinical situations influence water needs:

- *Uncontrolled diabetes mellitus:* Patients losing excessive amounts of water through the osmotic effect of large amounts of glucose excreted in the urine need additional fluid to replace body water.

- *Cystic fibrosis:* Children and adults with this disease have increased fluid needs.
- *High fiber intake:* As dietary fiber increases, so do fluid requirements. Adequate fluid intake is needed to replace the water absorbed by the fiber in the gastrointestinal tract.
- *High protein intake:* Protein metabolism produces urea and other nitrogenous wastes that must be excreted via the kidneys. Providing an appropriate level of fluid is important for patients given high-protein supplements.
- *Intense athletic activity:* Exercise of high intensity or duration such as marathon runs increase fluid requirements to replace water lost in sweat and allow this cooling mechanism to continue. A lack of fluid in such situations can lead to heat stroke and death (see Chapter 14).
- *Impaired thirst in older adults:* Many older persons, particularly frail older adults taking numerous medications or those in poor health, do not get thirsty when they should based on aging changes in the

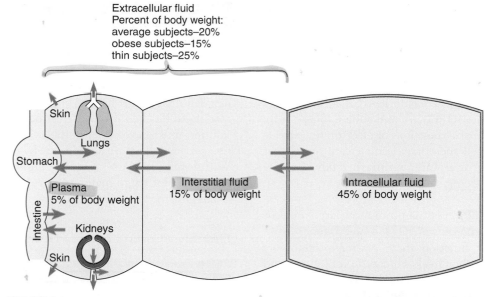

FIGURE 7-6 Body fluid compartments. Note the relative amounts of water in the intracellular compartment and extracellular compartment. *(Data from Gamble JL: Chemical anatomy, physiology, and pathology of extracellular fluid, Cambridge, Mass, 1964, Harvard University Press.)*

thirst center of the hypothalamus. In such cases it is prudent to monitor fluid intake.

- *Certain medications:* Diuretics increase fluid output, as do certain analgesics and decongestants.

Water Compartments

Body water is divided into two major compartments: (1) the water outside the cells—the *extracellular fluid compartment* and (2) the water inside the cells—the *intracellular fluid compartment* (Figure 7-6), as described below:

1. *Extracellular fluid (ECF):* The water outside the cells makes up approximately 20% of total body weight. It has four sections: (1) blood plasma, which accounts for about 25% of the ECF and 5% of body weight; (2) interstitial fluid, the water surrounding the cells; (3) secretory fluid, the water circulating in transit; and (4) dense tissue fluid, water in deep connective tissue, cartilage, and bone.
2. *Intracellular fluid (ICF):* The water inside the cells constitutes about 40% to 45% of total body weight. Because the body cells handle our vast metabolic activity, it would be expected that the total water inside the cells would be greater than the amount outside the cells (intracellular water is about twice the amount of extracellular water).

FORCES CONTROLLING WATER DISTRIBUTION

The forces that control the distribution of body water depend on two factors: (1) the amounts of solutes or particles in solution and (2) the membranes that separate water compartments. We will look at the important properties of each.

Solutes

A variety of particles are found in body water in varying concentrations. Two main types—(1) electrolytes and (2) plasma proteins—control water balance.

Electrolytes

Several minerals serve as major electrolytes in controlling body fluid compartments. In this role they are called electrolytes because they are free in solution and carry an electrical charge. Free, charged chemical forms are also called *ions,* a term that refers to atoms, elements, or

---

compartment The collective quantity of material of a given type in the body. The four body compartments are lean body mass (muscle and vital organs), bone, fat, and water.

interstitial fluid The fluid situated between parts or in the interspaces of a tissue.

electrolyte A chemical element or compound that in solution dissociates as ions carrying a positive or negative charge (e.g., H^+, Na^+, K^{++}, Ca^{2+}, and Mg^{+2+} and Cl^-, HCO_3^-, $HPO_4^{2-}-$, and SO_4^2). Electrolytes constitute a major force controlling fluid balances within the body through their concentrations and shifts from one place to another to restore and maintain balance—homeostasis.

groups of atoms that in solution carry either a positive or negative electrical charge. An ion carrying a positive charge is called a *cation:* examples are sodium (Na^+)—the major cation in extracellular water, potassium (K^+)—the major cation in intracellular water, calcium (Ca^{2+}), and magnesium (Mg^{2+}). An ion carrying a negative charge is called an *anion:* examples are chloride (Cl^-), bicarbonate (HCO_3^-), phosphate (HPO_4^{2-}), and sulfate (SO_4^{2-}). By virtue of their small size these ions or electrolytes can diffuse freely across cell membranes and create forces that control the movement of water within the body.

Plasma Proteins

Albumin and globulin, plasma proteins of large molecular size, influence the movement of water in and out of capillaries. In this function these plasma proteins are called *colloids* (from the Greek word *kolla* for "glue") and form colloidal solutions. Because of their large size, plasma proteins cannot pass through the capillary membrane into the interstitial fluid. Instead they remain in the blood vessels where they exert colloidal osmotic pressure (COP) to maintain vascular blood volume. We will learn more about this process a bit later.

Organic Compounds of Small Molecular Size

Other organic compounds small in size such as glucose, urea, and amino acids diffuse freely in and out of the various fluid compartments but do not influence shifts of water unless they are present in abnormally large concentrations. Such a situation occurs in patients with uncontrolled diabetes mellitus, when large amounts of glucose in the urine cause an abnormal osmotic diuresis or excess water output.

Water and solutes move across the separating membranes according to the physiologic mechanisms that handle fluid shifts. These mechanisms include osmosis, diffusion, filtration, active transport, and pinocytosis. We will learn more about these mechanisms in Chapter 8.

INFLUENCE OF ELECTROLYTES ON WATER BALANCE

Measurement of Electrolytes

The concentration of electrolytes or particles in a given solution determines the chemical activity of that solution. It is the *number* of particles, not the *size* of the particles, that determines chemical combining power, so electrolytes are measured according to the total number of particles in solution. Each particle contributes chemical combining power according to its valence, not its total weight. The unit of measure commonly used is the *equivalent.* Because small amounts are usually in question, most physiologic measurements are expressed in *milliequivalents (mEq),* or thousandths of an equivalent. This term refers to the number of ions—cations and anions—in solution in a given volume of body fluid and is expressed as the number of *milliequivalents per liter (mEq/L).*

Electrolyte Balance

Electrolytes are distributed in body water compartments in a definite pattern having physiologic significance. According to biochemical and electrochemical laws a stable solution must have equal numbers of positive and negative particles. This means it must be electrically neutral. When shifts or losses occur, compensating shifts and gains must follow to maintain this dynamic balance of *essential* electrochemical neutrality.

Electrolyte Control of Body Hydration

Ionized sodium is the chief cation of ECF, and ionized potassium is the chief cation of ICF. These two electrolytes control the amount of water retained in any given compartment. Shifts in water from one compartment to the other reflect changes in the ECF concentration of these electrolytes. The terms *hypertonic* and *hypotonic* refer to the electrolyte concentration of the water outside the cell. When surrounded by a hypertonic solution, water flows out of the cell and the cell becomes dehydrated and shrinks in size. When the cell is surrounded by a hypotonic solution, water flows into the cell causing it to swell and eventually burst if the situation is not corrected.

INFLUENCE OF PLASMA PROTEIN ON WATER BALANCE

Capillary Fluid Shift Mechanism

Water constantly circulates throughout the body in the blood vessels. However, fluid must move out of the vessels to service the tissues and then be drawn back into the vessels to maintain the normal transport flow. Two opposing pressures—(1) the hydrostatic pressure (blood pressure) of the capillary blood flow and (2) the COP from plasma proteins (mainly albumin)—control the movement of water and solute across capillary membranes. The constant flow of water, nutrients, and waste to and from the cells occurs by the shifting balance of these two pressures. It works as a filtration process operating according to the differences in osmotic pressure on either side of the capillary membrane.

When blood first enters the capillary system, the existing blood pressure forces water and small solutes such as glucose out into the tissues to bathe and nourish the cells. The plasma protein particles, however, are too large to pass through the pores of the capillary membranes. Hence the protein remains in the capillary vessel and exerts the now greater COP that draws fluid and waste materials from the cells back into the capillary circulation.

This process is called the capillary fluid shift mechanism. It is one of the most important homeostatic mechanisms in the body for maintaining water balance, without which cells would die.

Cell Fluid Control

Just as plasma protein provides COP to maintain the volume of the ECF, cell protein provides the osmotic pressure that maintains the volume of the ICF. Electrolytes also have a role with ionized potassium guarding water within the cell and ionized sodium guarding water outside the cell. This balance supports the sustaining flow of water, nutrients, metabolites, and waste in and out of cells.

INFLUENCE OF HORMONES ON WATER BALANCE

Antidiuretic Hormone

The antidiuretic hormone (ADH), also called *vasopressin,* is secreted by the posterior lobe of the pituitary gland. It controls the reabsorption of water by the kidneys according to body need, acting as a water-conserving mechanism. In any stress situation with threatened or actual loss of body water, this hormone is released to retain precious fluid.

Aldosterone

Aldosterone is a sodium-conserving hormone related to the renin-angiotensin system, but it also exerts secondary control over body water. Renin, an enzyme secreted by the kidney, and angiotensin, a product of the liver, trigger the release of aldosterone from the adrenal cortex. The complete name of this system is the renin-angiotensin-aldosterone mechanism. Aldosterone acts on the kidney to reabsorb sodium, but in the process water is also reabsorbed. Both aldosterone and ADH are activated by injury, surgery, or other physiologic stress.

TO SUM UP

Minerals are inorganic substances widely distributed in nature. They build body tissues; activate, regulate, and control metabolic processes; and help transmit messages across nerve fibers. Minerals are classified as (1) major minerals and (2) trace elements. Major minerals are required in larger amounts and make up 60% to 80% of all the inorganic material in the body. Trace elements, measured in amounts as small as a microgram (μg), make up less than 1% of the body's inorganic matter. Seven major minerals and 10 trace minerals are known to be essential in human nutrition; another 8 trace ele-

ments are probably essential, but their roles remain to be defined. The major minerals include calcium and phosphorus, with roles in bone health, energy metabolism, and nerve transmission, and magnesium, a participant in many metabolic reactions. The trace mineral iron as a part of hemoglobin transports oxygen to the cells and along with iodine and zinc regulates growth and body metabolism. Other trace minerals regulate day-to-day metabolic activities as partners with enzymes that maintain body cells. Sodium, potassium, and chloride are the particles in body fluids that, along with plasma proteins, control water balance and the distribution of fluids inside (intracellular fluid) and outside (extracellular fluid) the cells.

QUESTIONS FOR REVIEW

1. List the seven major minerals and describe their (a) physiologic function, (b) problems related to deficiency or excess, and (c) dietary sources.
2. List the 10 trace elements with proven essentiality for humans. Why has it been difficult to establish DRIs for these nutrients?

---

colloidal osmotic pressure (COP) Pressure produced by the protein molecules in the plasma and in the cell. Because proteins are large molecules, they do not pass through the separating membranes of the capillary cells. Thus they remain in their respective compartments, exerting a constant osmotic pull that protects vital plasma and cell fluid volumes in these compartments.

capillary fluid shift mechanism Process that controls the movement of water and small molecules in solution (electrolytes, nutrients) between the blood in the capillary and the surrounding interstitial area. Filtration of water and solutes out of the capillary at the arteriole end and reabsorption at the venule end are accomplished by shifts in balance between the intracapillary hydrostatic blood pressure and the colloidal osmotic pressure exerted by the plasma proteins.

renin-angiotensin-aldosterone mechanism Three-stage system of sodium conservation, hence control of water loss, in response to diminished filtration pressure in the kidney nephrons: (1) pressure loss causes kidney to secrete the enzyme renin, which combines with and activates angiotensinogen from the liver; (2) active angiotensin stimulates the adjacent adrenal gland to release the hormone aldosterone; and (3) aldosterone causes reabsorption of sodium from the kidney nephrons and water follows.

3. The AI for calcium for persons over age 50 is 1200 mg/day. Develop a menu for a frail 83-year-old woman that will provide this level of calcium within an energy intake of 1500 kcal.

4. You are working with a teenager who eats no red meat or fish but likes chicken. She is concerned about her weight and follows the diet pattern of MyPyramid that provides an intake of 1600 kcal. List the foods with portion sizes that you would select to reach her RDA of 18 mg of iron. When making your selections, consider other factors in the diet that will enhance or impede the absorption of the iron you provide.

5. What causes the edema in protein-energy malnutrition?

6. Why does prolonged diarrhea lead to potassium depletion?

7. Go to a nearby grocery store or drug store that sells mineral supplements. Check five supplements marketed for children (use the DRI of the age-group noted on the label) and five supplements marketed for adults. Prepare a table that lists each brand and include (a) the percent of the DRI provided for each mineral and (b) the cost of a 1-day supply of the supplement. Did any of the supplements you examined exceed the UL for any nutrient, and, if so, what is the danger of toxicity? Based on cost and content, would an individual be better advised to spend that extra amount of money for food? What specific foods would you recommend?

8. You are working with a 37-year-old man who is beginning to experience a gradual increase in his blood pressure and has been advised to increase his intakes of potassium and calcium and lower his intake of sodium. When his work takes him on the road, he has lunch at a fast-food restaurant; on other days he takes a sandwich from home to eat at his desk. Develop a menu for a fast-food lunch and a packed lunch that will provide 33% of the DRI for potassium and calcium and no more than 33% of the UL for sodium.

REFERENCES

1. Weaver CM, Heaney RP: Calcium. In Shils ME et al, eds: *Modern nutrition in health and disease,* ed 10, Baltimore, 2006, Lippincott Williams & Wilkins.

2. Hurrell RF: Influence of vegetable protein sources on trace element and mineral bioavailability, *J Nutr* 133:2973S, 2003.

3. Ervin RB et al: *Dietary intake of selected minerals for the United States population: 1999-2000, advance data, vital and health statistics,* No. 341, Washington, DC, 2004 (April 27), U.S. Department of Health and Human Services.

4. Cotton PA et al: Dietary sources of nutrients among U.S. adults, 1994-1996 (additional tables accessed at *www.eatright.org* on November 3, 2004), *J Am Diet Assoc* 104:921, 2004.

5. Whiting SJ et al: Factors that affect bone mineral accrual in the adolescent growth spurt, *J Nutr* 134:696S, 2004.

6. Weaver CM: 2003 W.O. Atwater Memorial Lecture: Defining nutrient requirements from a perspective of bone-related nutrients, *J Nutr* 133:4063, 2003.

7. Heaney RP: Long-latency deficiency disease: insights from calcium and vitamin D, *Am J Clin Nutr* 78:912, 2003.

8. Rozen GS et al: Calcium supplementation provides an extended window of opportunity for bone mass accretion after menarche, *Am J Clin Nutr* 78:993, 2003.

9. Kalkwarf HJ, Khoury JC, Lanphear BP: Milk intake during childhood and adolescence, adult bone density, and osteoporotic fractures in U.S. women, *Am J Clin Nutr* 77:257, 2003.

10. Food and Nutrition Board, Institute of Medicine: *Dietary Reference Intakes for calcium, phosphorus, magnesium, vitamin D, and fluoride,* Washington, DC, 1997, National Academies Press.

11. Dawson-Hughes B: Interaction of dietary calcium and protein in bone health in humans, *J Nutr* 133:852S, 2003.

12. Dawson-Hughes B et al: Effect of dietary protein supplements on calcium excretion in healthy older men and women, *J Clin Endocrinol Metab* 89:1169, 2004,

13. Rapuri PB, Gallagher JC, Haynatzka V: Protein intake: effects on bone mineral density and the rate of bone loss in elderly women, *Am J Clin Nutr* 77:1517, 2003.

14. Ince AB, Anderson EJ, Neer RM: Lowering dietary protein to U.S. Recommended Dietary Allowance levels reduces urinary calcium excretion and bone resorption in young women, *J Clin Endocrinol Metab* 89:3801, 2004.

15. Cotter A, Cashman KD: Genistein appears to prevent early postmenopausal bone loss as effectively as hormone replacement therapy, *Nutr Rev* 61(10):346, 2003.

16. Dawson-Hughes B: Osteoporosis. In Shils ME et al, eds: *Modern nutrition in health and disease,* ed 10, Baltimore, 2006, Lippincott Williams & Wilkins.

17. Fleming R, Patrick K: Osteoporosis prevention: pediatricians' knowledge, attitudes, and counseling practices, *Prevent Med* 34:411, 2002.

18. Zemel MB, Miller SL: Dietary calcium and dairy modulation of adiposity and obesity risk, *Nutr Rev* 62(4):125, 2004.

19. Heaney RP: Normalizing calcium intake: projected population effects for body weight, *J Nutr* 133:268S, 2003.

20. McCarron DA, Heaney RP: Estimated healthcare savings associated with adequate dairy food intake, *Am J Hypertens* 17:88, 2004.

21. Chia V, Newcomb PA: Calcium and colorectal cancer: some questions remain, *Nutr Rev* 62(3):115, 2004.

22. Peters U et al: Calcium intake and colorectal adenoma in a U.S. colorectal cancer early detection program, *Am J Clin Nutr* 80:1358, 2004.

23. Lappe JM et al: Girls on a high calcium diet gain weight at the same rate as girls on a normal diet: a pilot study, *J Am Diet Assoc* 104:1361, 2004.

24. Knochel JP: Phosphorus. In Shils ME et al, eds: *Modern nutrition in health and disease,* ed 10, Baltimore, 2006, Lippincott Williams & Wilkins.

25. Marinella MA: The refeeding syndrome and hypophosphatemia, *Nutr Rev* 61(9):320, 2003.

26. Food and Nutrition Board, Institute of Medicine: *Dietary Reference Intakes for water, potassium, sodium, chloride, and sulfate,* Washington, DC, 2004, National Academies Press.

27. Most MM: Estimated phytochemical content of the Dietary Approaches to Stop Hypertension (DASH) diet is higher than in the control study diet, *J Am Diet Assoc* 104:1725, 2004.

28. Sacks FM et al: Effects on blood pressure of reduced dietary sodium and the Dietary Approaches to Stop Hypertension (DASH) diet, *N Engl J Med* 344:3, 2001.

29. Bray GA et al: A further subgroup analysis of the effects of the DASH diet and three dietary sodium levels on blood pressure: results of the DASH-Sodium Trial, *Am J Cardiol* 94:222, 2004.

30. Hajjar I, Kotchen T: Regional variations of blood pressure in the United States are associated with regional variations in dietary intakes: the NHANES-III data, *J Nutr* 133:211, 2003.

31. Whelton PK et al: Primary prevention of hypertension: clinical and public health advisory from the National High Blood Pressure Education Program, *JAMA* 288:1882, 2002.

32. Doyle L, Cashman KD: The DASH diet may have beneficial effects on bone health, *Nutr Rev* 62(5):215, 2004.

33. McKeown NM: Whole grain intake and insulin sensitivity: evidence from observational studies, *Nutr Rev* 62(7):286, 2004.

34. Food and Nutrition Board, Institute of Medicine: *Dietary Reference Intakes for vitamin A, vitamin K, arsenic, boron, chromium, copper, iodine, iron, manganese, molybdenum, nickel, silicon, vanadium, and zinc,* Washington, DC, 2001, National Academies Press.

35. Hunt JR, Roughead ZK: Adaptation of iron absorption in men consuming diets with high or low iron availability, *Am J Clin Nutr* 71:94, 2000.

36. Hunt JR: High-, but not low-bioavailability diets enable substantial control of women's iron absorption in relation to body iron stores, with minimal adaptation within several weeks, *Am J Clin Nutr* 78:1168, 2003.

37. Wells AM et al: Comparisons of vegetarian and beef-containing diets on hematological indexes and iron stores during a period of resistive training in older men, *J Am Diet Assoc* 103:594, 2003.

38. Hunt JR: Bioavailability of iron, zinc, and other trace minerals from vegetarian diets, *Am J Clin Nutr* 78(suppl):633S, 2003.

39. Furtado MM, Shikora SA, Saltzman E: Long-term outcomes and complications of obesity surgery: an overview, *Nutr Clin Care* 7:31, 2004.

40. Grinder-Pedersen L et al: Calcium from milk or calcium-fortified foods does not inhibit nonheme-iron absorption from a whole diet consumed over a 4-day period, *Am J Clin Nutr* 80:404, 2004.

41. Kleinman RE, ed: *Pediatric nutrition handbook,* ed 4, Elk Grove Village, Ill, 1998, American Academy of Pediatrics.

42. Murray-Kolb LE, Beard JL: Iron status and cognitive performance, *Nutr and the MD* 29(10):1, 2003.

43. Fleming DJ et al: Aspirin and the use of serum ferritin as a measure of iron status, *Am J Clin Nutr* 74:219, 2001.

44. Fairbanks VF: Iron in medicine and nutrition. In Shils ME et al, eds: *Modern nutrition in health and disease,* ed 9, Philadelphia, 1999, Lippincott Williams & Wilkins.

45. Neff LM: Current directions in hemochromatosis research: towards an understanding of the role of iron overload and the HFE gene mutations in the development of clinical disease, *Nutr Rev* 61(1):38, 2003.

46. Heath ALM, Fairweather-Tait SJ: Health implications of iron overload: the role of diet and genotype, *Nutr Rev* 61(2):45, 2003.

47. Fleming DJ et al: Dietary factors associated with the risk of high iron stores in the elderly Framingham Heart Study cohort, *Am J Clin Nutr* 76:1375, 2002.

48. Beard J: Dietary iron intakes and elevated iron stores in the elderly: is it time to abandon the set-point hypothesis of regulation of iron absorption? *Am J Clin Nutr* 76:1189, 2002.

49. Liu JM et al: Body iron stores and their determinants in healthy postmenopausal U.S. women, *Am J Clin Nutr* 78:1160, 2003.

50. Hetzel BS, Clugston GA: Iodine. In Shils ME et al, eds: *Modern nutrition in health and disease,* ed 9, Philadelphia, 1999, Lippincott Williams & Wilkins.

51. Bryan J et al: Nutrients for cognitive development in school-aged children, *Nutr Rev* 62(8):295, 2004.

52. Solomons NW: Slow-release iodine in local water supplies reverses iodine deficiency disorders: is it worth its salt? *Nutr Rev* 56:280, 1998.

53. Lyons GH, Stangoulis JC, Graham RD: Exploiting micronutrient interaction to optimize biofortification programs: the case for inclusion of selenium and iodine in the HarvestPlant program, *Nutr Rev* 62(6 pt 1):247, 2004.

54. Semba RD, Delange F: Iodine in human milk: perspectives for infant health, *Nutr Rev* 59(8):269, 2001.

55. Hotz C, Brown KH: Identifying populations at risk of zinc deficiency: the use of supplementation trials, *Nutr Rev* 59(3):80, 2001.

56. Caulfield LE: Maternal zinc deficiency and maternal and child health in Peru, *Nutr Today* 39:78, 2004.

57. Raqib R et al: Effect of zinc supplementation on immune and inflammatory responses in pediatric patients with shigellosis, *Am J Clin Nutr* 79:444, 2004.

58. Gibson RS et al: The risk of inadequate zinc intake in United States and New Zealand adults, *Nutr Today* 38:63, 2003.

59. Arsenault JE, Brown KH: Zinc intake of U.S. preschool children exceeds new Dietary Reference Intakes, *Am J Clin Nutr* 78:1011, 2003.

60. Dattilo AM, Miguel SG: Chromium in health and disease, *Nutr Today* 38:121, 2003.

61. Food and Nutrition Board, Institute of Medicine: *Dietary Reference Intakes for vitamin C, vitamin E, selenium, and carotenoids,* Washington, DC, 2000, National Academies Press.

62. Burk RF, Levander OA: Selenium. In Shils ME et al, eds: *Modern nutrition in health and disease,* ed 10, Baltimore, 2006, Lippincott, Williams & Wilkins.

63. Palmer CA, Anderson JJB: Position of the American Dietetic Association: the impact of fluoride on health, *J Am Diet Assoc* 101(1):126, 2001.

64. Valtin H: "Drink at least eight glasses of water a day." Really? Is there scientific evidence for "8 × 8"? *Am J Physiol Regul Integr Comp Physiol* 283(5):R993, 2002.

65. Grandjean AC et al: Hydration: issues for the 21st century, *Nutr Rev* 61(8):261, 2003.

66. Grandjean AC et al: The effect of caffeinated, non-caffeinated, caloric and non-caloric beverages on hydration, *J Am Coll Nutr* 19:591, 2000.

FURTHER READINGS AND RESOURCES

Readings

Grandjean AC et al: Hydration: issues for the 21st century, *Nutr Rev* 61(8):261, 2003.
This article explains the importance of proper fluid intake for individuals in various states of health and levels of physical activity.

Heaney RP, Rafferty K, Bierman J: Not all calcium-fortified beverages are equal, *Nutr Today* 40:39, 2005.

Bowman SA: Beverage choice of young females: changes and impact on nutrient intakes, *J Am Diet Assoc* 102:1234, 2002.
These articles point to the issues related to calcium intake and the need to suggest beverages that promote bone health.

Caulfield LE: Maternal zinc deficiency and maternal and child health in Peru, *Nutr Today* 39:78, 2004.
Dr. Caulfield describes interventions to improve maternal and child health in developing countries and the consequences when there is not enough zinc in the diet.

Websites of Interest

- National Institutes of Health, Office of Dietary Supplements, *Dietary Supplement Fact Sheets: http://dietary-supplements.info.nih.gov/factsheets/*.
- National Institutes of Health, information on calcium and bone health: *http://health.nih.gov/result.asp/1101*.
- National Institutes of Health, information on sodium and blood pressure: *http://health.nih.gov/result.asp/329/10*.

- U.S. Department of Health and Human Services, U.S. Department of Agriculture: *Dietary Guidelines for Americans 2005: http://www.healthierus.gov/dietaryguidelines/*.
- U.S. Department of Agriculture, Center for Nutrition Policy and Promotion, MyPyramid food guidance system: *http://www.mypyramid.gov/*.
- U.S. Food and Drug Administration, Center for Food Safety and Applied Nutrition, Office of Nutritional Products, Labeling, and Dietary Supplements: *http://www.cfsan.fda.gov/~dms/supplmnt.html*.

CHAPTER 8

Digestion, Absorption, and Metabolism

Eleanor D. Schlenker

In this chapter we continue our narrative of what happens to the foods we eat and their ultimate fate in the body. We will consider all the steps that must occur for the tuna sandwich we had at lunch to be broken down into glucose, amino acids, and fatty acids. We look first at the integrated body systems that receive the foods we take in and transform them for our use.

The physiologic and biochemical process that turns the food we eat into energy and body tissue has three parts: digestion, absorption, and metabolism. We begin with a review of the gastrointestinal tract and then follow the path of the nutrients to the cells where they nourish and protect us. We see how each part of the system contributes to the integrated whole.

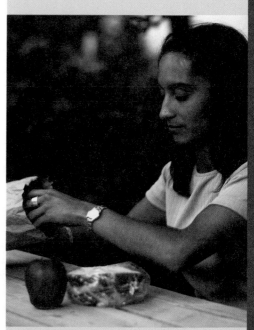

THE HUMAN BODY: ROLE OF NUTRITION

Food: Change and Transformation

The foods we eat contain the nutrients necessary for our survival, but these life-sustaining materials must first be released and transformed into units the body can use. Through a successive interrelated system, foods are broken down into simpler substances and then still simpler substances that can enter the metabolic pathways in the cell. Each section of the gastrointestinal tract has a unique function, but together they form a continuous *whole*. A problem in one organ has clinical consequences for the entire system.

Importance for Health and Nutrition

Nutritional status and gastrointestinal function are interdependent. *Food* as it occurs naturally and as we eat it is not a single substance but a mixture of chemical substances and nutrients. These substances must be separated into their respective components so the body can handle each as an individual unit. *Nutrients* released from food remain unavailable to the body until they cross the intestinal wall and are transported to tissues for storage or immediate use. Gastrointestinal health is a partner in nutritional well-being.[1] Diseases affecting the organs of the gastrointestinal tract or the absorbing surface of the intestinal wall have adverse effects on nutritional status because nutrients are not made available to the body in the amounts needed. Likewise, moderate to severe malnutrition brings changes in the secretion of digestive enzymes and a blunting of the absorbing structures, which limits nutrient passage. This vicious cycle adds to further deterioration of nutritional status.[1]

The gastrointestinal tract is one of the many body systems whose output is essential to the chemical work taking place in tissues and cells. The recognition of the human body as an integrated physiochemical organism is basic to an understanding of human nutrition in both health and in disease. The internal control that maintains a constant chemical environment and keeps the many functional systems operating in harmony with one another is referred to as homeostasis.[2]

THE GASTROINTESTINAL TRACT

Component Parts

The gastrointestinal tract, also called the alimentary canal, is a long hollow tube that begins at the mouth and ends at the anus. The specific parts that make up the tract are the mouth, esophagus, stomach, small intestine, large intestine or colon, and rectum. Other organs that lie outside the tract but support its work by their secretion of important enzymes and digestive fluids are the pancreas, gallbladder, and liver. Look at the respective components of the gastrointestinal tract and their relative position to one another as shown in Figure 8-1. These organs working as a team can break down and absorb several kilograms of carbohydrate, a half kilogram of fat, a half kilogram of protein, and 20 or more liters of water each day.[2] We will follow these food components as they travel *together* through the successive parts of the gastrointestinal tract and into body cells.

General Functions

The gastrointestinal tract has the following four major functions in digestion and absorption:

1. *Receives food:* The mouth is the entrance to the gastrointestinal tract. From here the food is moved on to the stomach and other organs for digestion and absorption.
2. *Releases nutrients from food:* Digestion and the separation of nutrients from other food components take place in the stomach and small intestine.
3. *Delivers nutrients into the blood:* Absorbing structures called microvilli located in the small intestine transfer the nutrients into the portal blood or lymph (fatty acids). Water is absorbed later in the colon.
4. *Excretes nondigestible waste:* The fecal mass moves from the colon into the rectum, where it is stored until excreted.

Both physical and chemical actions accomplish these tasks.

Sensory Stimulation and Gastrointestinal Function

Both physiologic and psychologic factors influence digestion. The physical presence of food in the mouth, stomach, or small intestine initiates a variety of responses that coordinate the muscular movements and chemical secretions necessary for digestion and absorption. However, sensory stimulation—sight, smell, or proximity to food—also brings about the secretion of digestive juices and muscle motility.[2] Smelling the aroma of cookies baking, hearing foods sizzle on an outdoor grill, or picking a fresh berry can evoke the physiologic process of digestion. Seeing a sign advertising your favorite food or thinking about food stimulates the gastrointestinal tract. On the other hand, dread of an unpleasant-tasting medication or recalling the nausea brought on by chemotherapy can repress the desire for food. Positive associations with food and mealtime promote efficient digestion and absorption of nutrients.

PRINCIPLES OF DIGESTION

Digestion is the first step in preparing food for use by the body. There are two types of actions involved—(1) muscular and (2) chemical.

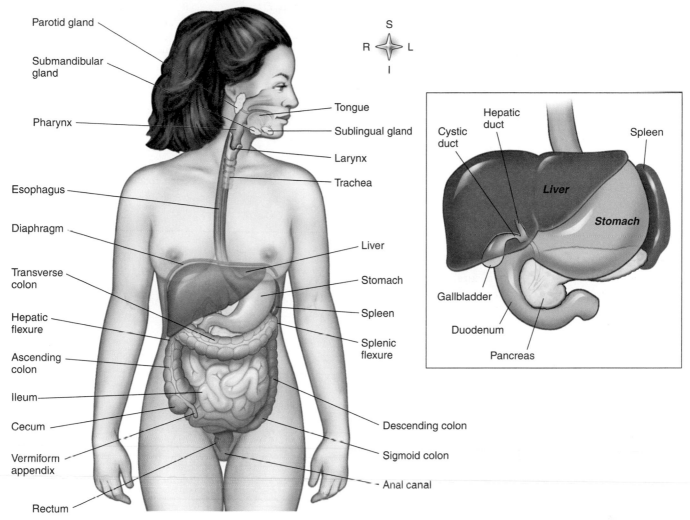

FIGURE 8-1   The gastrointestinal system. Through the successive parts of the gastrointestinal system, multiple activities of digestion liberate and reform food nutrients for our use. *(From Thibodeau GA, Patton KT:* Anatomy and physiology, *ed 5, St. Louis, 2003, Mosby/Elsevier.)*

Gastrointestinal Motility: Muscles and Movement

Digestion involves mechanical mixing and propulsive movements controlled by several neuromuscular, self-regulating systems. These actions work together to move the food mass along the alimentary tract at the best rate for digestion and absorption.

Types of Muscles

Organized muscle layers in the gastrointestinal wall provide the necessary motility for digestion (Figure 8-2). From the outer surface inward the layers are (1) the serosa, (2) a *longitudinal muscle layer*, (3) a *circular muscle layer*, (4) the *submucosa,* and (5) the mucosa. Embedded in the deeper layers of the mucosa are thin bundles of smooth muscle fibers called the *muscularis mucosae.* The coordinated interaction of the following four smooth

homeostasis State of dynamic equilibrium within the body's internal environment; a balance achieved through the operation of various interrelated physiologic mechanisms.

digestion The process of breaking down food to release its nutrients for absorption and transport to the cells for use in body functions.

serosa Outer surface layer of the intestines interfacing with the blood vessels of the portal system going to the liver.

mucosa The mucous membrane forming the inner surface layer of the gastrointestinal tract, with extensive nutrient absorption and transport functions.

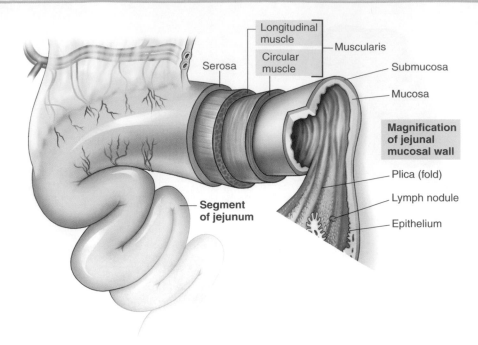

FIGURE 8-2   Muscle layers of the intestinal wall. Notice the five layers of muscle that produce the movements necessary for digestion. *(Modified from Thibodeau GA, Patton KT:* Anatomy & physiology, *ed 5, St. Louis, 2003, Mosby/Elsevier.)*

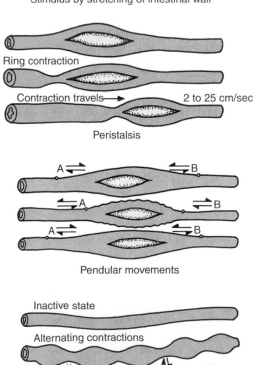

FIGURE 8-3   Types of movement produced by muscles of the intestine:
peristaltic waves from contraction of deep circular muscle, pendular movements from small local muscles, and segmentation rings formed by alternate
contraction and relaxation of circular muscle.

muscle layers makes possible four different types of
movement (Figure 8-3).

1. *Longitudinal muscles:* These long smooth muscles
   arranged in fiber bundles that extend lengthwise
   along the gastrointestinal tract help propel the food
   mass forward.
2. *Circular contractile muscles:* The circular smooth muscle fibers extend around the hollow tube forming the
   alimentary canal. These rhythmic contractile rings
   cause sweeping waves along the digestive tract push-
   ing forward the food mass. These regularly occurring
   propulsive movements are called peristalsis.
3. *Sphincter muscles:* More defined circular muscles at
   strategic points form muscle sphincters that act as
   valves—pyloric, ileocecal, and anal—to prevent reflux or backflow and keep the food mass moving in a
   forward direction.
4. *Mucosal muscles:* This thin embedded layer of smooth
   muscle produces *local constrictive contractions* every few
   centimeters. These contractions mix and chop the
   food mass, effectively churning and mixing it with
   secretions to form a semiliquid called chyme that is
   ready for digestion and absorption.

In summary, the muscles lining the gastrointestinal tract
produce the following two types of action:

1. General muscle tone or tonic contraction that ensures
   continuous passage of the food mass and valve control
2. Periodic rhythmic contractions that mix and propel
   the food mass forward

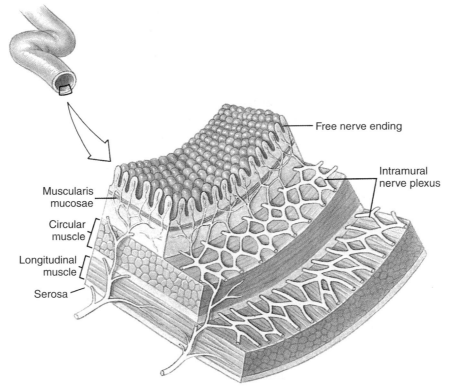

FIGURE 8-4   Innervation of the intestine by the intramural nerve plexus. A network of nerves controls and coordinates the movements of the intestinal muscles. *(Credit: Medical and Scientific Illustration.)*

Alternating contractions and relaxations of these muscles move the food contents along the tract and facilitate digestion and absorption.

Nervous System Control

Throughout the gastrointestinal tract specific nerves regulate muscle action. An interrelated network of nerves within the gastrointestinal wall called the intramural nerve plexus (Figure 8-4) extends from the esophagus to the anus. This network of about 100 million nerve fibers regulates the rate and intensity of muscle contractions, controls the speed at which the food mass moves along the tract, and coordinates the digestive process, including the secretion of enzymes and digestive juices.[3]

Gastrointestinal Secretions

Food is digested chemically through the combined action of a number of secretions. These secretions are of the following four types.

1. *Enzymes:* Specific enzymes attack designated chemical bonds within the structure of nutrient compounds, freeing their component parts.
2. *Hydrochloric acid and buffer ions:* These agents produce the pH necessary for the activity of certain enzymes.

3. *Mucus:* This sticky, slippery fluid lubricates and protects the lining of the inside wall of the gastrointestinal tract and eases the passage of the food mass.
4. *Water and electrolytes:* These agents provide an appropriate solution in the amounts needed to circulate the substances released in the digestive process.

Special cells in the mucosal lining of the gastrointestinal tract and in adjacent accessory organs, especially the pancreas, produce these secretions. The release of these secretions is stimulated by (1) the presence of food in the gastrointestinal tract, (2) the sensory nerve network activated by the sight, taste, or smell of food, and (3) hormones specific for certain nutrients.

---

peristalsis A wavelike progression of alternate contraction and relaxation of the muscle fibers of the gastrointestinal tract.

chyme Semifluid food mass in the gastrointestinal tract after gastric digestion.

intramural nerve plexus Network of nerves in the walls of the intestine that make up the intramural nervous system, controlling muscle action and secretions for digestion and absorption.

MOUTH AND ESOPHAGUS: PREPARATION AND DELIVERY

Up to this time we have looked at the integrated muscular-secretory functions that govern the overall operation of the gastrointestinal tract. Here we begin to follow this process through its successive stages to see what happens to the food we eat. Eating begins a physiologic process that uses muscle movement and specialized secretions to change food into a completely different form. The first step takes place in the mouth, which prepares food for digestion and then delivers it to the stomach by way of the esophagus.

Taste and Smell

Much of our enjoyment of food comes from its unique flavors and aromas. Taste buds located on the tongue, roof of the mouth, and throat contain chemical receptors that respond to food and produce the four sensations of taste: *salty, sweet, sour,* and *bitter.* Some individuals have a stronger perception of one taste over another, and this can influence food intake. Certain medications produce a bitter taste or loss of taste. Patients on chemotherapy often have distorted taste (dysgeusia). Zinc deficiency causes a loss of taste (hypogeusia). Some older people experience changes in taste as the number of taste buds decreases.[4]

Foods contain volatile components that move from the back of the mouth up into the nasal cavity, where they act on olfactory receptors to produce the pleasant odors we associate with particular foods. In fact, much of what we perceive as taste of a food may actually be its odor. Persons who have radiation therapy of the head or neck and patients with Parkinson's disease or senile dementia of the Alzheimer's type (SDAT) often have olfactory losses that lessen their enjoyment of eating.

Mastication

Initial biting and chewing begin to break food down into smaller particles. The incisors cut; the molars grind. The jaw muscles provide tremendous force: 55 lb of muscular pressure is applied through the incisors, and 200 lb is applied through the molars.[2] Because digestive enzymes act only on the surface of food particles, sufficient chewing to enlarge the surface area available for enzyme action is an important step in preparing food for digestion. Also, the fineness of the particles produced by chewing eases the passage of the food mass down the esophagus and into the stomach.

Ability to chew is necessary to prepare fiber-containing foods—fruits, vegetables, and whole grains—for digestion. Decayed teeth, loss of teeth, or poorly fitting dentures make eating difficult. Gingivitis and other diseases of the gums and supporting structures of the teeth leading to infection, mouth pain, or further loss of teeth restrict food intake and contribute to malnutrition.

Swallowing

Swallowing involves both the mouth and pharynx. It is intricately controlled by the swallowing center in the brain stem,[2] and damage to these nerves through radiation therapy, aging, or disease makes swallowing difficult. The tongue initiates a swallow by pressing the food upward and backward against the palate. From that point on, swallowing proceeds as an involuntary reflex and, once begun, cannot be interrupted. Swallowing occurs rapidly, taking less than 1 second, but in that time (1) the larynx must close to prevent food from entering the trachea and moving into the lungs and (2) the soft palate must rise to prevent food from entering the nasal cavity (Figure 8-5). Patients must never be fed in a supine position because it increases the risk of aspirating food into the lungs.

Esophagus

The esophagus is a muscular tube that connects the mouth and throat with the stomach and serves as a channel to carry the food mass into the body. Functionally, it has the following three parts[2]:

1. *Upper esophageal sphincter (UES):* The UES controls the entry of the food bolus into the esophagus. Between intakes the UES muscle is closed. Within 0.2 to 0.3 second after a swallow, nerve stimuli open the sphincter to receive the food mass.
2. *Esophageal body:* The mixed bolus of food passes immediately down the esophagus, moved along by peristaltic waves controlled by nerve reflexes. Changes in the muscles or nerves lower the intensity and frequency of the peristaltic waves, slowing passage down the channel. Diabetic neuropathy is one cause of esophageal problems.[5] Pain and discomfort associated with these changes can add to anorexia and weight loss in older persons. Gravity aids the passage of food down the esophagus when the person eats in an upright position.
3. *Lower esophageal sphincter (LES):* The LES controls the movement of the food bolus from the esophagus into the stomach. When the LES muscles maintain excessively high muscle tone, they fail to open following a swallow, preventing the passage of food into the stomach. This condition is called *achalasia,* meaning "unrelaxed muscle." (See Chapter 19 for a more detailed discussion of this condition.)

Entry Into the Stomach

At the point of entry into the stomach the gastro-esophageal constrictor muscle relaxes to allow the food to pass and then contracts quickly to prevent regurgitation or reflux of the acidic stomach contents back into the

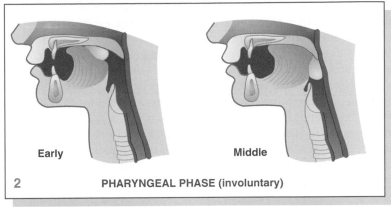

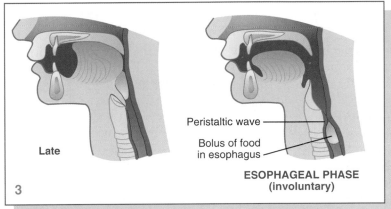

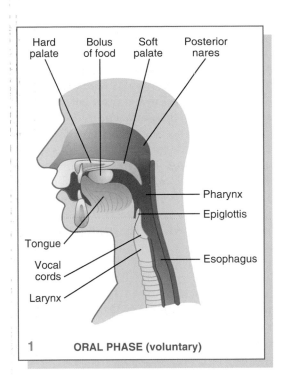

FIGURE 8-5   Swallowing is a highly coordinated task directed by a special nerve center in the hypothalamus. *(From Mahan KL, Escott-Stump S, eds: Krause's food, nutrition, and diet therapy, ed 11, Philadelphia, 2004, Saunders/Elsevier.)*

esophagus. When this mechanism fails and regurgitation happens, the person feels what is often referred to as "heartburn." The medical name for this condition is *gastroesophageal reflux disease (GERD),* and it is estimated that 30% of the population experience GERD on an occasional or chronic basis.[6] GERD causes damage to the tissues of the esophagus that are unprotected against the destructive effects of gastric acid. (Mucus secreted by cells in the stomach wall help to protect those tissues against the harsh effects of gastric acid.) Obesity, overeating, physical inactivity, and certain medications contribute to this condition.[6,7]

Two clinical problems hinder food passage into the stomach: (1) cardiospasm, caused by failure of the constrictor muscle to relax properly, and (2) hiatal hernia, the protrusion of the upper part of the stomach into the thorax through an abnormal opening in the diaphragm.

Chemical Digestion

In the mouth three pairs of salivary glands—(1) parotid, (2) submaxillary, and (3) sublingual—produce a watery fluid containing salivary amylase. This enzyme is specific for starch. The salivary glands also secrete mucus to lubricate and bind the food particles. Sensory stimuli—and even thoughts of favorite or disliked foods—influence these secretions. Saliva secretion ranges from 800 to 1500 ml a day with a pH range of 6.0 to 7.4 (approximately neutral) (Table 8-1). Food remains in the mouth for only a short time, so starch digestion here is brief. However, when salivary amylase binds to starch molecules, it is resistant to inactivation by gastric acid, and significant breakdown of starch continues in the stomach.[3] Smoking alters the composition of juices from the salivary glands. This effect may contribute to the loss of taste associated with smoking and the return of taste when smoking stops.[8]

Salivary secretions have other important functions, even though relatively little digestion takes place in the

---

gingivitis   Red, swollen, bleeding gums, most often caused by accumulation of bacterial plaque on the teeth.

bolus   Rounded mass of food formed in the mouth and ready to be swallowed.

mouth. These secretions (1) moisten the food particles so they bind together to form a bolus that moves easily down the esophagus and (2) they lubricate and cleanse the teeth and tissues of the mouth, destroying harmful bacteria and neutralizing toxic substances entering the mouth. Dry mouth or the more serious condition of xerostomia, the result of poor salivary secretion, creates swallowing problems because individual particles of food get separated in the esophagus. Infections and ulcers in the mouth along with tooth decay are serious outcomes of xerostomia. Medications can contribute to dry mouth.[9]

TABLE 8-1	Comparative pH Values and Approximate Daily Volumes of Gastrointestinal Secretions	
Secretion	**pH**	**Daily Volume (ml)**
Salivary	6.0-7.4	1000
Gastric	1.0-3.5	1500
Pancreatic	8.0-8.3	1000
Small intestinal	7.5-8.0	1800
Brunner's gland	8.0-8.9	200
Bile	7.5-7.8	1000
Large intestinal	7.5-8.0	200
TOTAL		6700

Modified from Guyton AC, Hall JE: *Textbook of medical physiology*, ed 10, Philadelphia, 2000, WB Saunders.

STOMACH: STORAGE AND INITIAL DIGESTION

Motility

The major parts of the stomach are shown in Figure 8-6. Muscles in the stomach wall have three motor functions: storage, mixing, and controlled emptying. As the food mass enters the stomach, it rests against the stomach walls, which stretch to store as much as 1 L of food and fluid. Local tonic muscle waves gradually increase their kneading and mixing action to move the mass of food and secretions toward the pyloric valve at the distal end of the stomach. Waves of peristaltic contractions reduce the food mass to a semifluid chyme. Finally, with each wave small amounts of chyme pass through the pyloric valve into the upper end of the small intestine. The pyloric sphincter muscle periodically constricts and relaxes to control the emptying of the stomach contents. The acid chyme is released slowly enough to allow it to be buffered by the alkaline secretions of the duodenum.

The energy (kcaloric) density of a meal, along with its volume and composition, influences the rate of stomach emptying. The speed at which food moves from the gastroesophageal sphincter to the distal end of the stomach and into the small intestine influences food intake, as messages to the brain signaling the arrival of food in the small intestine induce feelings of satiety.

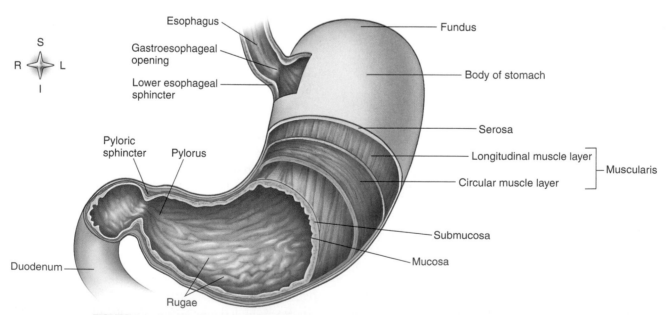

FIGURE 8-6 Stomach. The pyloric sphincter controls passage from the stomach into the duodenum, the upper section of the small intestine. See also the five layers of muscle found in the stomach wall. The mucosa lining the stomach forms folds called rugae. (*Modified from Thibodeau GA, Patton KT:* Anatomy & physiology, *ed 5, St. Louis, 2003, Mosby/Elsevier.*)

Chemical Digestion

Types of Secretions

Secretions produced in the stomach contain acid, mucus, and enzymes, as follows:

- *Acid:* Hydrochloric acid creates the acidic environment necessary for certain enzymes to work. For example, a pH of 1.8 to 3.5 is needed for the enzyme pepsin to act on protein; at a pH of 5.0 or above there is little or no pepsin activity. (See the *Perspectives in Practice* box, "Not Enough Stomach Acid: Is This a Problem?" to learn more about a clinical effect of low stomach acid levels.)
- *Mucus:* This viscous secretion protects the stomach lining from the eroding effect of the acid. Mucus also binds and mixes the food mass and helps move it along.
- *Enzymes:* The major enzyme in the stomach is pepsin, which begins the breakdown of protein. Pepsin is secreted in the form of pepsinogen and activated by hydrochloric acid. The stomach also produces a small amount of gastric lipase (tributyrase) that acts only on butterfat and has a relatively minor role in overall digestion. Children have a gastric enzyme called rennin (not to be confused with the renal enzyme renin) that aids in the coagulation of milk. Coagulation of the proteins in milk, changing them from a liquid to a semisolid (as occurs when egg white is heated), slows the rate of stomach emptying, ensuring a gradual passage of material to the small intestine. Rennin is absent in adults.

Control of Secretion

Stimuli for the release of gastric secretions come from the following two sources:

1. *Nerve stimulus* is produced in response to the visual and chemical senses, the presence of food in the gastrointestinal tract, and emotional distress. Anger and hostility increase gastric secretions; fear and depression lower secretions and inhibit both blood flow and gastric motility.
2. *Hormonal stimulus* is produced in response to food entering the stomach. Certain stimulants, especially caffeine, alcohol, and meat extracts, cause release of the local gastrointestinal hormone gastrin from the mucosal cells of the antrum. Gastrin, in turn, stimulates the secretion of more hydrochloric acid. When the pH falls below 3, a feedback mechanism halts the release of gastrin, preventing the accumulation of excess acid.[3] A second gastrointestinal hormone, enterogastrone, is produced in the mucosa of the duodenum. This hormone prevents excessive gastric activity by inhibiting hydrochloric acid secretion, pepsin secretion, and gastric motility.

SMALL INTESTINE: MAJOR DIGESTION, ABSORPTION, AND TRANSPORT

Motility

Intestinal Muscle Layers

The complex structural arrangement of the intestinal wall is shown in Figure 8-2. Coordination of intestinal motility is accomplished by three layers of muscle: (1) the thin layer of smooth muscle embedded in the mucosa (the muscularis mucosae) with fibers extending up into the villi, (2) the circular muscle layer, and (3) the longitudinal muscle lying next to the outer serosa.

Types of Intestinal Muscle Action

Under the control of the intramural nerve plexus of the intestinal nervous system, wall-stretch pressure from food or hormonal stimuli produces muscle action of the following two types:

1. *Propulsive movements:* Peristaltic waves from contractions of the deep circular muscles propel the food mass slowly forward. The intensity of the wave is increased by food or the presence of irritants that cause long sweeping waves over the entire intestine. A series of local segmental contractions also support the forward movement of the food bolus. Fiber and other indigestible materials from plant foods aid this process, providing bulk for the action of these muscles.
2. *Mixing movements:* Local constrictive contractions occurring every few centimeters mix and chop the food particles to form the semiliquid chyme.

The interaction of the muscles in the small intestine producing (1) general tonic contractions that ensure continuous passage and valve control and (2) periodic, rhythmic contractions that mix and propel the food mass forward facilitates ongoing digestion and future absorption.

---

distal Away from the point of origin.
duodenum The first section of the small intestine entered by food passing through the pyloric valve from the stomach.
viscous Sticky.
gastrin Hormone secreted by mucosal cells in the antrum of the stomach that stimulates the parietal cells to produce hydrochloric acid. Gastrin is released into the stomach in response to stimulants, especially coffee, alcohol, and meat extracts. When the gastric pH falls below 3, a feedback mechanism cuts off gastrin secretion and prevents excess acid formation.
antrum Lower section of the stomach.
enterogastrone A duodenal peptide hormone that inhibits gastric hydrochloric acid secretion and motility.

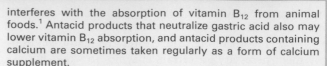

PERSPECTIVES IN PRACTICE
Not Enough Stomach Acid: Is This a Problem?

Nutrition surveys tell us that many younger and older adults have lower blood levels of vitamin B_{12} than they should. As we learned in Chapter 6, vitamin B_{12} is needed to form mature red blood cells and maintain nerves in the brain and spinal cord. In nature vitamin B_{12} is found only in animal foods, so vegans who eat no animal foods depend on vitamin B_{12} supplements or fortified plant foods. Persons who eat any animal foods are expected to get the vitamin B_{12} they need. A few individuals who lack the protein intrinsic factor needed to absorb vitamin B_{12} are given injections of the vitamin.

But now we know another reason why people may have trouble absorbing vitamin B_{12}. Some adults, especially older adults, have lower than normal levels of gastric acid because of changes in the acid-producing cells lining the stomach. The condition of low gastric acid is referred to as hypochlorhydria, and those who have no hydrochloric acid secretion are said to have achlorhydria. The vitamin B_{12} found in meats is strongly bound to protein fibers, and gastric acid is needed to activate pepsin, which breaks down the protein and releases the vitamin for absorption. Use of the widely advertised over-the-counter medications that suppress gastric acid secretion interferes with the absorption of vitamin B_{12} from animal foods.[1] Antacid products that neutralize gastric acid also may lower vitamin B_{12} absorption, and antacid products containing calcium are sometimes taken regularly as a form of calcium supplement.

There are food sources that do not require gastric acid for release of their vitamin B_{12}. The vitamin B_{12} added to fortified breads, cereals, or juices is easily freed from its food component and absorbed, even if gastric acid is limited.[2] Vitamin B_{12} also seems to be released more easily from dairy foods than muscle foods. Adults, especially older adults, should include a vitamin B_{12}-fortified food in their diet several times a week to ensure an adequate intake.

References

1. Dharmarajan TS, Adiga GU, Norkus EP: Vitamin B_{12} deficiency: recognizing subtle symptoms in older adults, *Geriatrics* 58:30, 2003.
2. Russell RM, Baik H, Kehayias JJ: Older men and women efficiently absorb vitamin B-12 from milk and fortified bread, *J Nutr* 131:291, 2001.

Chemical Digestion

Major Role of the Small Intestine

In comparison to other sections of the gastrointestinal tract, the small intestine carries the major burden of chemical digestion. It secretes many enzymes, each specific for one of the macronutrients—carbohydrate, fat, or protein. Other enzymes enter the small intestine from the pancreas to assist in digestion. The small intestine acts as a regulatory center that senses the nutrient content, pH, and osmolarity of its contents and controls enzyme secretion accordingly.[3]

Types of Secretions

The following four types of digestive secretions complete this final stage of chemical breakdown:

1. *Enzymes:* A number of specific enzymes (Table 8-2) act on specific macronutrients to bring about their final breakdown to forms the body can absorb and use.
2. *Mucus:* Glands located at the entrance to the duodenum secrete large amounts of mucus. As in the stomach, mucus protects the intestinal mucosa from irritation and digestion by the highly acid gastric juices in the chyme entering the duodenum. Other cells along the length of the intestinal surface secrete mucus when touched by the moving food mass, lubricating and protecting the mucosal tissues from abrasion.
3. *Hormones:* When signaled by the presence of acid in the food mass entering from the stomach, mucosal cells in the upper part of the small intestine produce the local gastrointestinal hormone secretin.[3] Secretin, in turn, stimulates the pancreas to send alkaline pancreatic

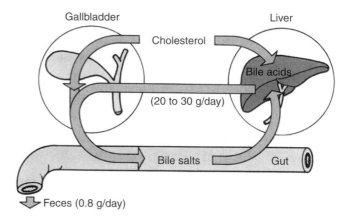

FIGURE 8-7   Enterohepatic circulation of bile salts. Bile salts are reabsorbed from the small intestine and returned to the liver and gallbladder to be used again and again.

juices into the duodenum to buffer the acidic chyme. The intestinal mucosa in the upper duodenum could not withstand the high acid of the entering chyme without the neutralizing action of the bicarbonate-containing pancreatic juice.

4. *Bile:* Bile emulsifies fats and facilitates their digestion. A large volume of bile is produced in the liver as a dilute, watery solution. It is then concentrated and stored by the gallbladder. When fat enters the duodenum, the local gastrointestinal hormone cholecystokinin (CCK) is secreted by glands in the intestinal mucosa and stimulates the gallbladder to contract and release bile. By means of the bile-conserving *enterohepatic circulation* (Figure 8-7), molecules of bile are returned to the liver and gallbladder and used over and over again. CCK also acts on the

TABLE 8-2	Summary of Digestive Processes		

Nutrient	Mouth	Stomach	Small Intestine
Carbohydrate	Starch $\xrightarrow{Alpha\text{-}amylase}$ Dextrins		Pancreas Starch $\xrightarrow{Amylase}$ Maltose and sucrose (Disaccharides) Intestine Lactose $\xrightarrow{Lactase}$ Glucose and galactose (Monosaccharides) Sucrose $\xrightarrow{Sucrase}$ Glucose and fructose Maltose $\xrightarrow{Maltase}$ Glucose and glucose
Protein		Protein $\xrightarrow{Pepsin\ HCl}$ Polypeptides	Pancreas Proteins, Polypeptides $\xrightarrow{Trypsin}$ Dipeptides Proteins, Polypeptides $\xrightarrow{Chymotrypsin}$ Dipeptides Polypeptides, Dipeptides $\xrightarrow{Carboxypeptidase}$ Amino acids Intestine Polypeptides, Dipeptides $\xrightarrow{Aminopeptidase}$ Amino acids Dipeptides $\xrightarrow{Dipeptidase}$ Amino acids
Fat		Tributyrin (butterfat) $\xrightarrow{Tributyrinase}$ Glycerol and Fatty Acids	Pancreas Fats $\xrightarrow{Lipase}$ Glycerol and Glycerides (di-, mono-) and Fatty acids Intestine Fats $\xrightarrow{Lipase}$ Glycerol and Glycerides (di-, mono-) and Fatty acids Liver and gallbladder Fats $\xrightarrow{Bile}$ Emulsified fat

TABLE 8-3	End Products of Digestion

Macronutrient	End Products of Digestion
Carbohydrate	Glucose, fructose, and galactose (monosaccharides)
Fat	Fatty acids, monoglycerides, diglycerides, and glycerol
Protein	Amino acids, dipeptides

pancreas to stimulate the release of enzymes to break down fats, proteins, and carbohydrates.[3]

Factors Influencing Secretion

Many factors influence the release of digestive secretions into the small intestine. Local gastrointestinal hormones and nerve systems are stimulated by physical contact with food materials and the senses and emotions. These factors are summarized in Figure 8-8.

Absorption

End Products of Digestion

When digestion of the macronutrients is complete, the simplified end products are ready for absorption. These end products are summarized in Table 8-3. At times incompletely digested nutrients remain in the small intes-

tine.[5] In persons who lack the digestive enzyme lactase the disaccharide lactose remaining in the intestine causes diarrhea and abdominal discomfort.[10] (See the *To Probe Further* box, "Lactose Intolerance: Common Problem Worldwide," and Box 8-1 to learn more about lactose

mucus Viscous fluid secreted by mucous membranes and glands, consisting mainly of mucin (a glycoprotein), inorganic salts, and water. Mucus lubricates and protects the gastrointestinal mucosa and helps move the food mass along the digestive tract.

secretin Hormone produced in the mucous membrane of the duodenum in response to the entrance of acid contents from the stomach into the duodenum. Secretin in turn stimulates the flow of pancreatic juices, providing needed enzymes and the proper alkalinity for their action.

cholecystokinin (CCK) A peptide hormone secreted by the mucosa of the duodenum in response to the presence of fat. Cholecystokinin causes the gallbladder to contract and propel bile into the duodenum, where it is needed to emulsify the fat. The fat is thus prepared for digestion and absorption.

absorption Transport of nutrients from the lumen of the intestine across the intestinal wall into the blood (carbohydrates and proteins) or the lymph (fats).

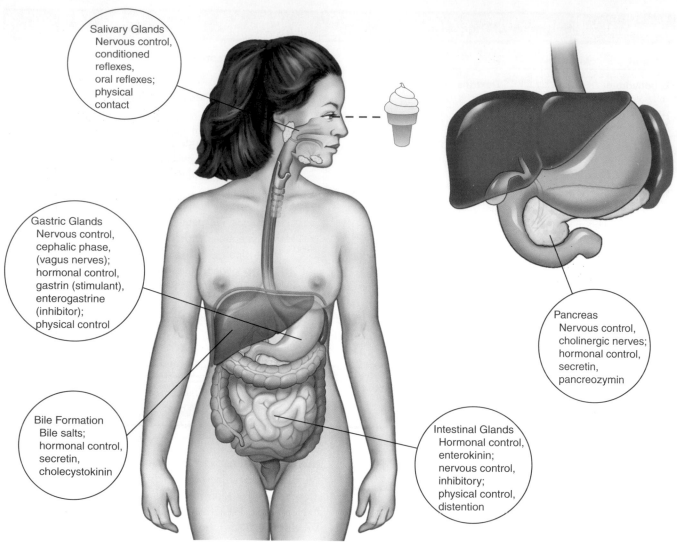

Salivary Glands
Nervous control,
conditioned
reflexes,
oral reflexes;
physical
contact

Gastric Glands
Nervous control,
cephalic phase,
(vagus nerves);
hormonal control,
gastrin (stimulant),
enterogastrine
(inhibitor);
physical control

Bile Formation
Bile salts;
hormonal control,
secretin,
cholecystokinin

Intestinal Glands
Hormonal control,
enterokinin;
nervous control,
inhibitory;
physical control,
distention

Pancreas
Nervous control,
cholinergic nerves;
hormonal control,
secretin,
pancreozymin

FIGURE 8-8   Summary of factors influencing secretions of the gastrointestinal tract. (*From Thibodeau GA, Patton KT: Anatomy and physiology, ed 5, St. Louis, 2003, Mosby/Elsevier.*)

BOX 8-1 | Food Sources of Lactose

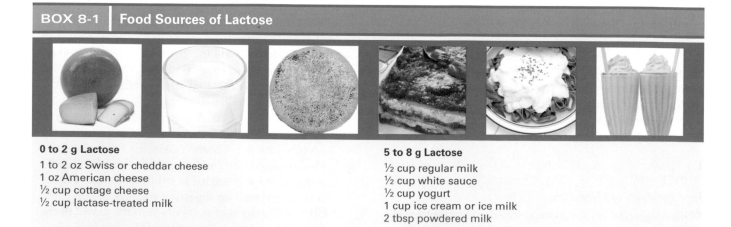

0 to 2 g Lactose
1 to 2 oz Swiss or cheddar cheese
1 oz American cheese
½ cup cottage cheese
½ cup lactase-treated milk

5 to 8 g Lactose
½ cup regular milk
½ cup white sauce
½ cup yogurt
1 cup ice cream or ice milk
2 tbsp powdered milk

Data from Bonci L: *American Dietetic Association guide to better digestion,* Hoboken, NJ, 2003, John Wiley & Sons.
Images copyright 2006 JupiterImages Corporation.

TO PROBE FURTHER

LACTOSE INTOLERANCE: COMMON PROBLEM WORLDWIDE

Lactose intolerance is a digestive problem facing 75% of the world's population—15% of whites, 80% of blacks and Latinos, and almost 100% of Asians.[1] Individuals with lactose intolerance may have symptoms after taking in 12 to 18 g of lactose (approximately 8 to 12 oz of milk).[1] This problem stems from a deficiency of lactase, the digestive enzyme in the microvilli of the small intestine that breaks lactose into its simple sugars—glucose and galactose. When undigested lactose remains in the small intestine and colon, it absorbs large amounts of water and is fermented by resident bacteria, producing diarrhea, bloating, and gas.

Infants produce enough lactase to digest the large amounts of lactose in mother's milk. But before man domesticated cows and goats, no one had lactose in their diet after weaning, so this enzyme was no longer needed. In some areas of the world milk-producing animals were rare. In those countries where cows became commonplace, the need to preserve milk led to fermented dairy foods such as cheese and yogurt that are lower in lactose than milk.[2] As a result, lactase activity drops to some extent in most people by the age of 20. Extreme intolerance to lactose is usually genetically related.

Conditions other than lactose intolerance can cause or worsen symptoms after eating dairy foods. Irritable bowel syndrome, celiac disease, cystic fibrosis, or any gastrointestinal disorder that damages the intestinal mucosa can interfere with the digestion of lactose, and medical diagnosis is often needed to confirm the problem.[1] Viral infections can cause temporary lactose malabsorption.

Having some degree of lactose intolerance does not mean that you are allergic to milk or dairy foods. A true milk allergy is caused by the *protein* in milk, not the *lactose*. Most people with problems digesting lactose do not need to follow a totally lactose-free diet, although milk may have to be limited in favor of other dairy foods[1] or they may need to relearn to tolerate lactose-containing foods.[3]

Persons with lactose malabsorption can begin to include dairy foods in their diet in several ways to increase intakes of calcium and vitamin D, such as the following[3]:

- *Add dairy foods gradually:* Begin with a small amount of one dairy food each day, a fourth cup of milk or half ounce of cheese; include only one lactose-containing food per meal. (See Box 8-1 for examples of food lactose content.)
- *Include lactose-containing foods with a meal or snack:* This slows the movement of lactose into the intestine and may reduce discomfort.
- *Choose dairy foods lower in lactose:* Use lactose-free or lactose-reduced milk. (*Acidophilus milk is not lactose-free.*) Add lactase enzyme drops (Lactaid or Dairy Ease) to milk to lower the lactose, but plan ahead because lactase drops need 24 hours to act. Lactase tablets taken right before eating dairy foods can reduce discomfort. In addition, aged cheeses such as cheddar or Swiss are lower in lactose than cheese spreads or other processed cheese.

Lactose is also found in nondairy foods that have milk as an ingredient. Breads and other baked products, some ready-to-eat breakfast cereals, pancake and cookie mixes, instant potatoes, cream soups, hot dogs, and luncheon meats may contain lactose. Read the Nutrition Label, and look for the word *milk* or *whey*. (Refer to Chapter 7 for food sources of calcium for those who cannot tolerate any dairy foods.)

References

1. Swagerty DL, Walling AD, Klein RM: Lactose intolerance, *Am Fam Physician* 65:1845, 2002.
2. Solomons NW: Fermentation, fermented foods and lactose intolerance, *Eur J Clin Nutr* 56(suppl 4):550, 2002.
3. Bonci L: *American Dietetic Association guide to better digestion,* Hoboken, NJ, 2003, John Wiley & Sons.

malabsorption and sources of lactose, respectively.) Some small peptides made up of several amino acids escape digestion. Vitamins and minerals have been liberated from their food source. With a water base for solution and transport, plus necessary electrolytes, the total fluid food mass is now ready for absorption, the next phase in the process (Table 8-4).

Surface Structures

Viewed from the outside the small intestine appears smooth, but the inner surface is quite different. Note in Figure 8-9 the following three types of convolutions and projections that greatly expand the area of the absorbing surface:

1. *Mucosal folds:* Large folds in the mucosa similar to hills and valleys in a mountain range can be easily seen with the naked eye.
2. *Villi:* Fingerlike projections on these folds called villi can be seen through a simple microscope.
3. *Microvilli:* These extremely small projections on each villus can be seen only with an electron microscope.

The array of microvilli covering the edge of each villus is called the *brush border* because it looks like bristles on a brush. Each villus has an ample network of blood capillaries for the absorption of monosaccharides and amino acids and a central lymph vessel called a *lacteal* for the absorption of fatty acids.

Absorbing Surface Area

The three structures lining the small intestine—(1) mucosal folds, (2) villi, and (3) microvilli—increase the inner absorbing surface area about 1000 times over that of

> villi Small protrusions from the surface of a membrane; fingerlike projections covering mucosal surfaces of the small intestine.
>
> microvilli Minute vascular structures protruding from the surface of villi covering the inner surface of the small intestine, forming a "brush border" that facilitates absorption of nutrients.

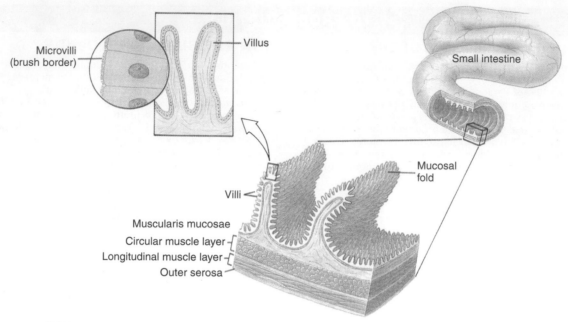

FIGURE 8-9 Intestinal wall. Note the arrangement of muscle layers and the structures of the mucosa that increase the surface area for absorption: mucosal folds, villi, and microvilli. *(Credit: Medical and Scientific Illustration.)*

TABLE 8-4	Daily Absorption Volume in Gastrointestinal System		
Substance	**Intake (L)**	**Intestinal Absorption (L)**	**Elimination (L)**
Food ingested	1.5		
Gastrointestinal secretions	8.5		
TOTAL	10.0		
Fluid absorbed in small intestine		9.5	
Fluid absorbed in large intestine		0.4	
TOTAL		9.9	
Feces			0.1

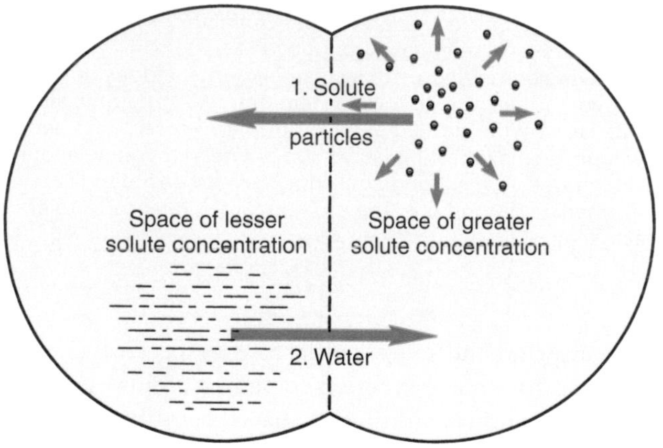

FIGURE 8-10 Movement of molecules, water, and solutes through osmosis and diffusion.

the outside serosa.[2] These special structures, plus the contracted length of the small intestine—630 to 660 cm (21 to 22 feet)—produce a tremendously large surface to capture and absorb nutrients. This absorbing surface, if stretched out flat, would be as large as a tennis or basketball court! All three of the mucosal structures serve as units for nutrient absorption. The small intestine is one of the most highly developed and specialized tissues in the body.

Mechanisms of Absorption

Absorption of the nutrients dispersed in this water-based solution involves several transport mechanisms. The par-

ticular transport used depends on the nutrient and the prevailing electrochemical fluid pressure gradient, as follows:

- *Passive diffusion and osmosis:* When there is no opposing fluid pressure, molecules small enough to pass through the capillary membranes diffuse easily into the villi (Figure 8-10). High concentrations of nutrients in the mucosal cells waiting to move into the capillaries where nutrient concentrations are low create an electrochemical gradient and osmotic pressure that promote absorption.[2]
- *Facilitated diffusion:* Even when the pressure gradient is favorable, flowing from a higher to a lower concentration, some molecules may be too large to pass easily

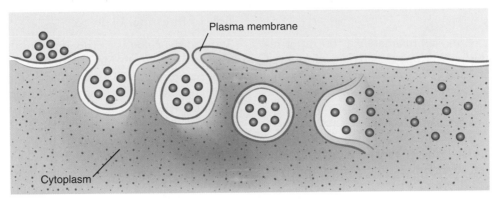

FIGURE 8-11   Pinocytosis, or engulfing of large molecules by the cell. *(From Nix S:* Williams' basic nutrition and diet therapy, *ed 12, St. Louis, 2005, Mosby/Elsevier.)*

through the membrane pores and need assistance. Specific proteins located in the membrane facilitate passage by carrying the nutrient across the membrane.

- *Energy-dependent active transport:* Nutrients must cross the intestinal membrane to reach hungry cells even when the fluid flow pressures are against them. Such active work requires extra energy along with a pumping mechanism. A special membrane protein carrier, coupled with the active transport of sodium, assists in the process. The energy-requiring, sodium-coupled transport of glucose is an example of this action. The enzyme *sodium- and potassium-dependent adenosine triphosphatase* (Na$^+$, K$^+$-ATPase), found in the cell membrane, supplies the energy for the pumping action.

- *Engulfing pinocytosis:* At times fluid and nutrient molecules are absorbed by pinocytosis. When the nutrient particle touches the absorbing cell membrane, the membrane dips inward around the nutrient, surrounds it to form a vacuole, and then engulfs it. The nutrient is then conveyed through the cell cytoplasm and discharged into the circulation. Smaller whole proteins and neutral fat droplets are sometimes absorbed through pinocytosis (Figure 8-11).

Routes of Absorption

Following their absorption by one of these mechanisms, the water-soluble monosaccharides and amino acids enter directly into the portal blood and travel to the liver and other tissues. Fat, which is not water soluble, is unique in its route. Fats packaged in a bile complex (the micelles described in Chapter 3) are carried into the cells of the intestinal wall, where they are processed into human lipid compounds and form a complex with protein as a carrier. These lipoproteins flow into the lymph, empty into the cisterna chyli, the central abdominal collecting vessel of the lymphatic system, travel upward into the chest through the thoracic duct, and finally flow into the venous blood at the left subclavian vein. These initial lipoproteins called chylomicrons are rapidly cleared from the blood by the special fat enzyme named lipoprotein lipase.

Exceptions to this route of fat absorption are the shorter-chain fatty acids with 10 or fewer carbons. Because these shorter-chain fatty acids are water soluble, they can be absorbed directly into the blood as are carbohydrate and protein breakdown products. However, most dietary fats are made of long-chain fatty acids that are not water soluble and must take the lymphatic route.

COLON (LARGE INTESTINE): FINAL ABSORPTION AND WASTE ELIMINATION

Role in Absorption

The absorption of water is the main task remaining for the colon. The capacity of the colon for water absorption is vast with a net daily maximum of 5 to 8 L.[2] Normally about 1 to 1.5 L is received from the ileum, and 95% of that is absorbed. Nutrients and other materials, including electrolytes, minerals, vitamins, intestinal bacteria, and nondigestible residue, remain in the chyme delivered to the large intestine.

---

cisterna chyli Cistern or receptacle of the chyle; a dilated sac at the origin of the thoracic duct, which is the common trunk that receives all the lymphatic vessels. The cisterna chyli lies in the abdomen between the second lumbar vertebra and the aorta. It receives the lymph from the intestinal trunk, the right and left lumbar lymphatic trunks, and two descending lymphatic trunks. The chyle, after passing through the cisterna chyli, is carried upward into the chest through the thoracic duct and empties into the venous blood at the point where the left subclavian vein joins the left internal jugular vein. This is the way absorbed fats enter the general circulation.

colon The large intestine extending from the cecum to the rectum.

Water Absorption

Within a 24-hour period approximately 1500 ml of remaining food mass leaves the *ileum,* the last section of the small intestine, and enters the *cecum,* the pouch at the entrance to the colon. Here the *ileocecal valve* controls the passage of the semiliquid chyme. Normally the valve remains closed, but each peristaltic wave relaxes the valve muscle, squirting a small amount of chyme into the cecum. This holds the food mass in the small intestine long enough to ensure maximum digestion and absorption of vital nutrients.

The watery chyme continues to move slowly through the colon, aided by muscle contractions and the mucus secreted by the mucosal glands along the passageway. Most of the water in the chyme (350 to 400 ml) is absorbed in the first half of the colon. Only approximately 100 to 150 ml remains to form the feces.[2] The absorption of water in the colon is important in the regulation of water balance and the elimination of fecal waste. When the chyme first enters the colon, it is a semiliquid, but water absorption during passage changes it to the semisolid nature of normal feces.

The amount of water absorbed in the colon depends on motility and rate of passage. Poor motility and a slow passage rate, often related to low dietary fiber and low fecal mass, allow greater absorption of water, resulting in hard stools difficult to pass and constipation. Excess motility and too rapid passage limit the absorption of water and important electrolytes, producing a high volume of loose, watery stool (diarrhea). Severe and extended diarrhea leads to dehydration and serious loss of electrolytes. Diarrhea is caused by disease, microbial infection or irritants as in foodborne illness, or large amounts of undigested sugar such as lactose that exert osmotic pressure and hold vast amounts of fluid.

Mineral Absorption

Sodium and other electrolytes are absorbed from the colon. Intestinal absorption exerts major control on body content of many minerals, and much of the dietary intake remains unabsorbed and is excreted in the feces. As we learned in Chapter 7, up to 90% of the calcium and iron in the food we eat is not absorbed. The bioavailability of nutrients, especially minerals, is reflected in their overall absorption from the gastrointestinal tract.[11] This is an important aspect of nutrient balance and dietary evaluation.

Vitamin Absorption

Conditions in the gastrointestinal tract influence the absorption of vitamins. When gastric acid is lower than normal, vitamin B_{12} is not easily released from its animal protein source and is lost in the feces. On the other hand, colon bacteria synthesize vitamin K and biotin, which are actively absorbed and serve as a major source of the body's supply.

Role of Intestinal Bacteria

At birth the colon is sterile, but intestinal bacteria soon become established. More than 500 different species of bacteria are found in the normal gastrointestinal tract, and intestinal contents may contain as many as 1 billion bacteria per gram.[12] The composition of the microflora differs according to diet and other factors. Intake of fiber or other nondigestible carbohydrates, immune responses favoring one group of bacteria over another, or the use of antibiotics influence the types and numbers of particular bacteria. Bacterial populations also differ along the gastrointestinal tract based on differences in structure and pH.[13] Many bacteria ingested with food do not survive the extreme acid environment in the stomach.

Intestinal bacteria make up about one third of fecal weight[2] and affect the color and odor of the stool. The customary brown color comes from bile pigments produced by colon bacteria from bilirubin. Thus when bile flow is hindered, the feces may become clay colored or white. The characteristic odor of the stool comes from amines, especially *indole* and *skatole* formed by the action of bacterial enzymes on amino acids.

Intestinal microflora have many different roles. Particular microflora produce bothersome gas or increase the risk of gastrointestinal disease. Other species make positive contributions to health (Box 8-2).

Excessive Gas Production

Fermentation of Complex Carbohydrates

Intestinal bacteria are the major contributors to gas production, including CO_2, H_2, methane, and sometimes hydrogen sulfide. Gas formation is a normal occurrence and, while harmless, is distressful when it causes pain or embarrassment. Intestinal gas or flatus can be exaggerated as a result of specific foods or physiologic circumstances in the person eating them. Foods associated with increased gas production are listed in Box 8-3.[14] Excessive gas also results from problems with intestinal motility.

For the most part gas is produced by the bacterial fermentation of undigested or incompletely absorbed carbohydrate. Humans lack the enzymes necessary to digest the oligosaccharides raffinose and stachyose in legumes that cause the intestinal gas associated with

---

BOX 8-2 | Healthful Effects of Intestinal Bacteria

Produce butyrate and other fatty acids that nourish the intestinal cells
Assist in absorbing and activating phytochemicals
Assist in excreting harmful bacteria
Prevent harmful bacteria from growing and forming colonies
Support immune cells that attack harmful body invaders

these foods. Certain starches in grains, fruits, and vegetables are resistant to pancreatic amylase and cannot be broken down and absorbed. When we encourage people to increase their intakes of foods high in resistant starch and fiber, we need to warn them that they may experience increased intestinal gas as they become accustomed to these new foods. Increasing fiber intake gradually allows a more comfortable adjustment with limited gastrointestinal distress.[15] (Benefits of dietary fiber and resistant starch are discussed later in this chapter.)

Excessive gas has social implications. Although CO_2, H_2, and methane are odorless, hydrogen sulfide carries a striking odor. Hydrogen sulfide is most often caused by cruciferous vegetables (cabbage, cauliflower, or broccoli) or large amounts of beer, all foods high in sulfur. Various over-the-counter products claim to reduce the formation of gas or eliminate gaseous odors, but all have limitations. Persons should check with their physicians before using such preparations.[14] (See the *Complementary and Alternative Medicine (CAM)* box, "Bismuth and Certain Herbs: A Dangerous Combination," for cautions on use of certain preparations.)

Fermentation of Sugars

Fructose can be a source of gas production and intestinal distress. Fructose absorption is limited in most people. The use of high fructose corn syrup (HFCS) in highly sweetened soft drinks and fruit drinks has increased the identification of fructose intolerance among users of these beverages.[16] Avoidance of fructose successfully reduces or eliminates symptoms. Certain sugar alcohols cause distress. Apple juice contains both fructose and sorbitol, another naturally occurring sugar that is not absorbed, and results in diarrhea and abdominal discomfort in some children.[17]

Some major aspects of nutrient absorption are summarized in Table 8-5.

Waste Elimination

Fully formed and ready for elimination, normal feces contain about 75% water and 25% solids.[2] The solids include fiber, bacteria, inorganic matter such as minerals, a small amount of fat and its derivatives, some mucus, and sloughed-off mucosal cells.

The mass of food residue now slows its passage. Approximately 4 hours after a meal is consumed, it enters the cecum, having traveled the entire length of the small intestine, 630 to 660 cm (21 to 22 feet). About 8 hours later it reaches the sigmoid colon, having traveled an additional 90 cm (3 feet) through the large intestine. In the sigmoid colon the residue descends still more slowly toward its final destination, the rectum.

The rectum begins at the end of the large intestine immediately following the descending colon and ends at the anus. Feces are usually stored in the descending colon; however, when it becomes full, feces pass into the rectum, leading to an urge to defecate. Anal sphincters under voluntary control regulate the elimination of feces from the body. As much as 25% of a meal may remain in the rectum for up to 72 hours.

Health Promotion

Dietary Fiber and Intestinal Health

Fiber helps maintain the health and function of the gastrointestinal tract, particularly the colon. Because humans are unable to break down this plant material, the fiber residue remains after nutrient digestion and absorption is complete. Fiber contributes important bulk

---

BOX 8-3	Foods Promoting Intestinal Gas

Dried beans
Cabbage-family foods (broccoli, brussels sprouts, cabbage, cauliflower)
Bran
Carbonated beverages
Corn
Fatty foods
Juices or foods high in sugar alcohols (apple juice, sugar-free products)

Data from Bonci L: *American Dietetic Association guide to better digestion,* Hoboken, NJ, 2003, John Wiley & Sons.

COMPLEMENTARY AND ALTERNATIVE MEDICINE (CAM)
Bismuth and Certain Herbs: A Dangerous Combination

Bismuth-containing medications such as Pepto-Bismol are sometimes used to ease gas and bloating. Bismuth also binds with the odor-causing sulfur compounds in intestinal gas and helps relieve embarrassment. However, bismuth when combined with various herbs can have serious side effects. When taken with ginger, garlic, or ginseng, bismuth can affect blood glucose levels, a real danger for diabetic patients. Bismuth and these herbs working together also act as anticoagulants.

Bonci L: *American Dietetic Association guide to better digestion,* Hoboken, NJ, 2003, John Wiley & Sons.

---

bilirubin A reddish bile pigment resulting from the degradation of heme by reticuloendothelial cells in the liver; a high level in the blood produces the yellow skin symptomatic of jaundice.

TABLE 8-5	**Absorption of Some Major Nutrients**

Nutrient	Form	Means of Absorption	Control Agent or Required Cofactor	Route
Carbohydrate	Monosaccharides (glucose and galactose)	Competitive	—	Blood
		Selective	—	
		Active transport via sodium pump	Sodium	
Protein	Amino acids	Selective	—	Blood
	Whole protein (rare)	Pinocytosis	—	Blood
	Some dipeptides	Carrier transport systems	Vitamin B_6 (pyridoxal phosphate)	Blood
Fat	Fatty acids	Fatty acid–bile complex (micelles)	Bile	
	Glycerides (mono-, di-)		—	Lymph
	Few triglycerides (neutral fat)	Pinocytosis	—	Lymph
Vitamins	B_{12}	Carrier transport	Intrinsic factor (IF)	Blood
	A	Bile complex	Bile	Blood
	K	Bile complex	Bile	From large intestine to blood
Minerals	Sodium	Active transport via sodium pump	—	Blood
	Calcium	Active transport	Vitamin D	Blood
	Iron	Active transport	Ferritin mechanism	Blood (as transferrin)
Water	Water	Osmosis	—	Blood, lymph, interstitial fluid

needed to form normal feces, increase stool weight, and promote efficient bowel emptying.[18,19] The continuing passage of the food residue through the colon is stimulated by the presence of a bulk mass. Fiber hastens the movement of the food residue, decreasing transit time and limiting exposure of surface cells to potentially toxic materials. Fiber residues also dilute the content of any toxic material and by these actions appear to reduce the risk of colon cancer.[11,20]

Lack of dietary fiber has been implicated in the development of diverticulosis and constipation, conditions involving the colon and lower bowel. When dietary fiber is limited or absent, the muscles in the colon contract with greater force and develop greater intraluminal pressure in an effort to move the small food mass forward. Over time this leads to the development of small pouchlike projections (diverticula) along the inner wall of the colon. Inflammation of the diverticula with bleeding and perforation, a condition referred to as diverticulitis, can have serious complications.

Constipation occurs in 20% of the U.S. population, who spend more than $400 million a year on laxatives.[21]

Although metabolic conditions such as diabetes mellitus or hypothyroidism, disorders of the nervous system, or certain medications including antidepressants and nonsteroidal antiinflammatory drugs (NSAIDs) contribute to constipation, dietary fiber will help prevent this condition. Adding fiber to the diet in the form of food is also a first step in intervention. Chronic constipation can have serious consequences with damage to the nerves or rectum or fecal impaction. Dietary fiber is also used to treat irritable bowel disease, a condition characterized by abdominal discomfort, pain, and changes in bowel habits. (Prevention and treatment of all of these conditions will be discussed further in Part 3.)

GASTROINTESTINAL FUNCTION AND CLINICAL APPLICATIONS

Chronic Gastrointestinal Distress

Most of the time the gastrointestinal tract is a smoothly working system that allows us to enjoy the food we eat while effectively handling digestion, absorption, and the

BOX 8-4	Factors Contributing to Chronic Dyspepsia

Delayed gastric emptying
Excess amount of gastric acid
Large amount of food at one meal
Sensitivity to stomach distention
Smoking
Use of nonsteroidal antiinflammatory drugs (NSAIDs)
Emotional distress
Psychologic distress

elimination of waste. But for some people abdominal pain, nausea, vomiting, or diarrhea is a regular occurrence and no specific biochemical or structural explanation can be found.[22,23] Many ideas have been put forth as possible causes of chronic dyspepsia (Box 8-4).[23-25] Medical researchers have identified a microorganism, *Helicobacter pylori,* that attacks the lining of the stomach and duodenum and is a major cause of ulcers. Current studies are trying to learn if this organism may also cause chronic dyspepsia.[26]

Mental and emotional stress, depression, certain prescription medications, and chronic disease all influence gastrointestinal function. Some populations appear to be particularly vulnerable to chronic gastrointestinal distress (see the *Focus on Culture* box, "Prevalence of Digestive Distress in Black and Hispanic Americans"). We need to listen carefully when people tell us about gastrointestinal difficulties that interfere with eating and their enjoyment of food.[27] Health education for self-care should point to the dangers of over-the-counter supplements such as food enzymes advertised to enhance digestion, inappropriate laxatives, or ill-advised procedures such as colonic irrigation. Chronic digestive problems demand medical assessment and intervention.

Prebiotics and Probiotics

Prebiotics and probiotics are new tools for clinical intervention to improve gastrointestinal function.

Prebiotics

Prebiotics are indigestible carbohydrates, mostly polysaccharides, that promote the growth of lactobacilli and bifidobacteria, types of bacteria with positive effects on health (see Box 8-2). Any dietary component that reaches the colon intact is a potential prebiotic. Prebiotics used clinically include (1) oligosaccharides (chains of 8 to 10 glucose units) isolated from soy; (2) oligosaccharides isolated from fruits and vegetables such as onions, bananas, garlic, and asparagus; (3) guar gum, a water-soluble fiber used as a food additive; and (4) lactulose, a synthetic disaccharide.[28-30]

✦ FOCUS ON CULTURE

Prevalence of Digestive Distress in Black and Hispanic Americans

Chronic digestive distress can influence food choices, nutrient intake, and general health. Black and Hispanic Americans may be at greater risk than other groups. When adults were asked to complete a questionnaire asking about abdominal pain and fullness, nausea, vomiting, or gastric reflux, almost one third indicated having at least one of these problems.[1] The majority with problems were blacks, and many were found to have previously undiagnosed gastric ulcers, duodenal ulcers, or damage to the mucosa of their esophagus. Blacks and Mexican Americans are more likely to be infected with *Helicobacter pylori,* the microorganism known to have a role in causing ulcers.[2] This burden of infection may contribute to dyspepsia or digestive disease in these groups.

References

1. Shaib Y, El-Serag HB: The prevalence and risk factors of functional dyspepsia in a multiethnic population in the United States, *Am J Gastroenterol* 99:2210, 2004.
2. Kruszon-Moran D, McQuillan GM: *Seroprevalence of six infectious diseases among adults in the United States by race/ethnicity: data from the third National Health and Nutrition Examination Survey, 1988-94, advance data, vital and health statistics,* No. 352, Hyattsville, Md, 2005 (March 9), U.S. Department of Health and Human Services.

Increases in lactobacilli and bifidobacteria have various favorable actions, as follows:

- *Increase in mineral absorption:* Although most minerals are absorbed in the small intestine, the lower pH in the colon resulting from bacterial fermentation stimulates the absorption of zinc, calcium, magnesium, and iron still remaining in the food residue.[28]
- *Promotion of normal laxation:* The fermenting action of bacteria on lactulose relieves constipation and helps avoid dependence on laxatives. Guar gum is effective in preventing the common problem of diarrhea in patients on tube feeding.[28,29]
- *Protection against colon cancer:* The fermentation products of healthful bacteria destroy cancer cells and toxic enzymes produced by harmful bacteria.[28]

Probiotics

Probiotics are nutritional supplements made up of living microorganisms having advantages to health. The benefits

---

constipation Difficult or infrequent passage of hard dry stools; fewer than three bowel movements a week.

dyspepsia Gastric distress or indigestion involving nausea, pain, burning sensations, or excessive gas.

of probiotics depend on the particular strain of bacteria and the active substances that it produces. Lactic acid–producing bacteria have been used over the centuries to acidify and preserve foods. Commonly used fermented foods include cultured milk and yogurt, cheese, distilled mash, cabbages, and meats.[31] Although probiotic cultures are available from pharmaceutical companies for clinical use, species of lactic acid–producing bacteria that survive the passage through the gastrointestinal tract and thrive in the colon can be obtained from commercially produced yogurt.[32]

The following list describes several clinical applications of probiotics:

- *Diarrhea:* Species of *Lactobacillus* are effective in treating infectious diarrhea in children and diarrhea induced by the use of antibiotics.[33] Loss of the normal microflora from antibiotics allows the growth of harmful bacteria and can cause serious diarrhea, adding an average of 8 days to the usual hospital stay.[28]
- *Infant allergies:* Poi, a probiotic made from the taro plant native to the Pacific Islands, has been used to feed babies allergic to cereals. When given in capsule form to expectant mothers with a family history of cereal allergy, only half of the infants showed signs of potential allergy.[33]
- *Inflammatory bowel disease:* Patients with ulcerative colitis and Crohn's disease have an abnormal pattern of intestinal bacteria that fosters these diseases. Probiotics may assist in prevention or treatment.[33]
- *Inhibition of H. pylori:* This pathogenic bacterium attaches to the gastric mucosa and is implicated in the development of peptic ulcer, gastric cancer, and chronic gastritis. Probiotics appear to inhibit its growth and prevent its burrowing into the stomach lining.[33]
- *Gastrointestinal immune response:* Probiotics support the immune cells living in the gastrointestinal tract that provide the first line of defense against pathogens entering the body.

Although lactic acid–producing bacteria have been used safely in food and therapeutic preparations, any new strain must be determined safe before being added to food. Yogurt continues to be a source of both important nutrients and probiotics and is a positive addition to the diet. At the same time persons should avoid supplements containing new strains of lactic acid–producing bacteria that have not been tested for safety.[32]

METABOLISM

Following absorption, the various nutrients are transported to the cells for use as energy or to produce the substances and tissues needed to sustain life. Cell metabolism encompasses the total complex of chemical changes that determine the final use of the individual nutrients.

Carbohydrate Metabolism

Glucose is an immediate energy source for all body cells, but the preferred energy source for cells of the brain and nervous system. Because glucose is so important to life, its level in the blood is carefully regulated.

Sources of Blood Glucose

Both carbohydrate and noncarbohydrate molecules are sources of blood glucose, as follows:

- *Carbohydrate sources:* Three carbohydrate substances can be converted to glucose: (1) dietary starches and sugars, (2) glycogen stored in liver and muscle, and (3) products of carbohydrate metabolism such as lactic acid and pyruvic acid.
- *Noncarbohydrate sources:* Both protein and fat provide indirect sources of glucose. Certain amino acids are called *glucogenic amino acids* because they can form glucose after their amino ($NH_2{}^+$) group is removed. Approximately 58% of the protein in a mixed diet is made of glucogenic amino acids. Thus more than half of dietary protein could ultimately be used for energy if sufficient carbohydrate and fat were not available. After fats are broken down into fatty acids and *glycerol,* the glycerol portion (about 10% of the fat) can be converted to glycogen in the liver and made available for glucose formation. The formation of glucose from protein, glycerol, and carbohydrate metabolites is called **gluconeogenesis.**

Uses of Blood Glucose

Blood glucose is maintained within a normal range of 70 to 140 mg/dl (3.9 to 7.8 mmol/L) but is in constant flux as absorbed glucose is transported to cells for immediate use or removed from the circulation and stored as glycogen or fat. When blood glucose levels begin to fall, stored glucose is released into the blood for use as needed. Blood glucose is used in three different ways as follow:

- *Energy production:* The primary function of glucose is to supply energy to meet the body's constant demand. A vast array of metabolic pathways using many specific and successive enzymes accomplish this task.
- *Energy storage:* There are two storage forms for glucose: (1) glycogen, into which glucose is converted and stored in limited amounts in the liver and muscle, and (2) fat, into which any excess glucose is converted and stored as adipose tissue after energy demands have been met. Only a small supply of glycogen exists at any one time, and it turns over rapidly. Adipose tissue can store unlimited amounts of fat and provides long-term energy stores.
- *Glucose products:* Small amounts of glucose are used to produce various carbohydrate compounds with important roles in body metabolism. Examples include deoxyribonucleic acid (DNA) and ribonucleic acid (RNA), galactose, and certain amino acids.

These sources and uses of glucose act as checks and balances to maintain normal blood glucose levels, adding glucose or removing it as needed.

Hormonal Controls

A number of hormones directly and indirectly influence glucose metabolism and regulate blood glucose levels.

Blood Glucose–Lowering Hormone. Only one hormone—insulin—lowers blood glucose. Insulin is produced by the beta cells in the pancreas. These cells are scattered in clusters forming "islands" in the pancreas—giving rise to the name *islets of Langerhans* after the German scientist Paul Langerhans (1847-1888), who first discovered them. Insulin lowers blood glucose by the following actions:

- *Glycogenesis* stimulates the conversion of glucose to glycogen in the liver for constant energy reserve
- *Lipogenesis* stimulates the conversion of glucose to fat for storage in adipose tissue
- *Cell permeability* to glucose increases, allowing it to enter the cells to be oxidized for energy.

Blood Glucose–Raising Hormones. The following hormones effectively raise blood glucose levels:

- *Glucagon,* produced by the alpha cells in the pancreas, acts in opposition to insulin, increasing the breakdown of liver glycogen to glucose and maintaining blood glucose levels during fasting or sleep hours. (The hydrolysis of liver glycogen to yield glucose is called glycogenolysis.)
- *Somatostatin,* produced in the delta cells of the pancreas and the hypothalamus, suppresses insulin and glucagon and acts as a general modulator of related metabolic activities.
- *Steroid hormones* secreted by the adrenal cortex release glucose-forming carbon units from protein and oppose the actions of insulin.
- *Epinephrine,* originating from the adrenal medulla, stimulates the breakdown of liver glycogen and quick release of glucose.
- *Growth hormone (GH)* and *adrenocorticotropic hormone (ACTH),* released from the anterior pituitary gland, oppose the actions of insulin.
- *Thyroxine,* originating in the thyroid gland, increases the rate of insulin breakdown, increases glucose absorption from the small intestine, and liberates epinephrine.

Lipid Metabolism

Lipid Synthesis and Breakdown

Two organ tissues—(1) liver and (2) adipose tissue—form a balanced axis of lipid metabolism. Both participate in lipid synthesis and breakdown. The fatty acids released from lipids are used by body cells as concentrated fuel for energy.

Lipoproteins

Lipid-protein complexes are the transport forms of lipids in the blood. An excess of blood lipoproteins produces a clinical condition called *hyperlipoproteinemia.* Lipoproteins are produced (1) in the intestinal wall after the initial absorption of dietary lipids and (2) in the liver for constant recirculation to and from cells.

Hormonal Controls

Because lipid and carbohydrate metabolism are interrelated, the same hormones are involved, as follows:

- *GH, ACTH,* and *thyroid-stimulating hormone (TSH),* all from the pituitary gland, increase the release of free fatty acids from stored lipids when energy demands are imposed.
- *Cortisol* and *corticosterone,* from the adrenal gland, release free fatty acids.
- *Epinephrine* and *norepinephrine* stimulate the breakdown of lipids and release of free fatty acids.
- *Insulin* from the pancreas promotes lipid synthesis and storage, whereas glucagon has the opposite effect of breaking down lipid stores to release free fatty acids.
- *Thyroxine* from the thyroid gland stimulates lipid release of free fatty acids and also lowers blood cholesterol levels.

Protein Metabolism

Anabolism (Tissue Building)

Protein metabolism centers on the critical balance between anabolism (tissue building) and catabolism (tissue breakdown). The process of anabolism builds tissue through the synthesis of new protein. The making of new protein is governed by a definite pattern or "blueprint" provided by DNA in the cell nucleus that calls for specific amino acids. Specific enzymes and coenzymes along with certain hormones—GH, gonadotropins, and thyroxine—control and stimulate the building of tissue protein.

Catabolism (Tissue Breakdown)

Amino acids released by tissue breakdown, if not reused for making new proteins, are further broken down and

---

gluconeogenesis Production of glucose from keto acid carbon skeletons from deaminated amino acids and the glycerol portion of fatty acids.

glycogenolysis Specific term for conversion of glycogen into glucose in the liver; chemical process of enzymatic hydrolysis or breakdown by which this conversion is accomplished.

used for other purposes. The breakdown of these amino acids yields two parts: (1) the nitrogen-containing group and (2) the remaining nonnitrogen residue, as follows:

1. *Nitrogen group:* The nitrogen portion is split off first, a process called deamination. This nitrogen can be converted to ammonia and excreted in the urine or retained for use in making other nitrogen compounds.
2. *Nonnitrogen residue:* The nonnitrogen residues are called keto acids. They can be used to form either carbohydrates or fats. With the addition of a nitrogen group they can form a new amino acid.

Cell enzymes and coenzymes along with hormones control tissue breakdown. In health there is a dynamic equilibrium between anabolism and catabolism to sustain growth and maintain sound tissue.

Metabolic Interrelationships

Each of the chemical reactions in body metabolism is purposeful, and all are interdependent. They are designed to fill two essential needs: produce energy and support growth and maintenance of healthy tissue. The controlling agents necessary for these reactions to proceed in an orderly manner are the cell enzymes, their coenzymes (that often include vitamins and minerals), and special hormones. Overall, human metabolism is an exciting biochemical process designed to develop, sustain, and protect our most precious possession—life itself.

TO SUM UP

The process of digestion and absorption breaks down food to release and convert the nutrients to simple forms that the body can use. Metabolism refers to the many chemical reactions in which the body uses these nutrients to produce energy, build and replace body tissues, and maintain normal body functions. Digestion involves two types of activities: mechanical and chemical. Muscle action breaks down food through mixing and churning motions and moves the food mass along the gastrointestinal tract. The chemical activity of gastrointestinal enzymes breaks down food into smaller and smaller components for absorption. Nutrients move across the intestinal wall by the process of diffusion, facilitated diffusion, active transport, or pinocytosis. Monosaccharides and amino acids are water soluble and pass directly from the mucosal cells of the small intes-

tine into the portal blood circulation. Long-chain fatty acids are not water soluble and, packaged in lipid-protein complexes, must first enter the lymph and then pass through the thoracic duct into the blood. Water absorption is the main activity in the colon. The day-to-day function of the gastrointestinal tract, often taken for granted, is fundamental to health and well-being.

QUESTIONS FOR REVIEW

1. List the muscle types and their locations in the walls of the gastrointestinal tract. What types of motions or movements do they provide in each section of the tract? What is the role of the intramural nerve plexus in controlling gastrointestinal muscle function?
2. You are working with an older adult man who had a stroke resulting in damage to the nerves in the swallowing center of the hypothalamus. What are the implications for his food intake and nutritional well-being?
3. Make a chart describing the chemical actions of digestion that occur in each section of the gastrointestinal tract. List across the top of the page the mouth, esophagus, stomach, and small intestine. List along the side of the page (a) the enzymes or fluids that act on the food mass in that location, (b) the sources of those enzymes or fluids, (c) the factors that stimulate their release, and (d) the factors that inhibit their activity.
4. Describe what happens in absorption. Explain the four mechanisms by which nutrients are absorbed from the small intestine.
5. You have just eaten a lunch that included a hamburger on a whole wheat bun, a glass of low-fat milk, and a bunch of grapes. Trace the digestion and final use of each of the macronutrients present in your lunch. Indicate (a) the enzymes, locations, and breakdown products formed in the complete digestion of these foods; (b) the routes taken by the breakdown products after absorption; and (c) one possible use for each breakdown product.
6. Differentiate between probiotics and prebiotics. Indicate two clinical effects or applications for each.
7. Visit a local supermarket or drug store and examine three over-the-counter medications that claim to (a) reduce stomach acid or (b) alleviate intestinal gas. Make a table that includes each product and list the active ingredients on the product label. Using the *Physicians Desk Reference* or other drug index, identify the specific actions of the active ingredients. Explain the mechanism by which each active ingredient is believed to bring about the desired effect.
8. At your local drug store examine three fiber supplements advertised to relieve constipation or ensure "regularity." Compare these products according to (a) source of the fiber, (b) daily dose in grams, and (c) cost per day. Compare the cost of these supplements with the cost of a similar amount of fiber obtained from a serving of fruit, vegetable, or whole grain bread.

---

deamination Removal of an amino group (NH_2) from an amino acid.

keto acid Amino acid residue after deamination. The glycogenic keto acids are used to form carbohydrates.

REFERENCES

1. Mason JB: Nutrition and gastroenterology: a mutually supportive partnership, *Nutr Clin Care* 7(3):91, 2004.

2. Guyton AC, Hall JE: *Textbook of medical physiology,* ed 10, Philadelphia, 2000, WB Saunders.

3. Klein S, Cohn SM, Alpers DH: The alimentary tract in nutrition. In Shils MA et al, eds: *Modern nutrition in health and disease,* ed 10, Baltimore, 2006, Lippincott Williams & Wilkins.

4. Mattes RD: The chemical senses and nutrition in aging: challenging old assumptions, *J Am Diet Assoc* 102:192, 2002.

5. Avunduk C: *Manual of gastroenterology: diagnosis and therapy,* ed 3, Philadelphia, 2002, Lippincott Williams & Wilkins.

6. Modlin I, Kidd M: GERD 2004: issues from the past and a consensus for the future, *Best Pract Res Clin Gastroenterol* 18(suppl):55, 2004.

7. Pilotto A: Aging and upper gastrointestinal disorders, *Best Pract Res Clin Gastroenterol* 18(suppl):73, 2004.

8. Ma L et al: Cigarette smoke increases apoptosis in the gastric mucosa: role of epidermal growth factor, *Digestion* 60:461, 1999.

9. Ship JA, Pillemer SR, Baum BJ: Xerostomia and the geriatric patient, *J Am Geriatr Soc* 50:535, 2002.

10. Szilagyi A: Review article: lactose—a potential prebiotic, *Aliment Pharmacol Ther* 16:1591, 2002.

11. American Dietetic Association: Position of the American Dietetic Association: health implications of dietary fiber, *J Am Diet Assoc* 102:993, 2002.

12. Mai V: Dietary modification of the intestinal microbiota, *Nutr Rev* 62:235, 2004.

13. Turner NJ, Thomson BM, Shaw IC: Bioactive isoflavones in functional foods: the importance of gut microflora on bioavailability, *Nutr Rev* 61:204, 2003.

14. Bonci L: *American Dietetic Association guide to better digestion,* Hoboken, NJ, 2003, John Wiley & Sons.

15. McEligot AJ et al: High dietary fiber consumption is not associated with gastrointestinal discomfort in a diet intervention trial, *J Am Diet Assoc* 102:549, 2002.

16. Johlin FC, Panther M, Kraft N: Dietary fructose intolerance: diet modification can impact self-rated health and symptom control, *Nutr Clin Care* 7(3):92, 2004.

17. Kleinman RE, ed: *Pediatric nutrition handbook,* ed 5, Washington, DC, 2004, American Academy of Pediatrics.

18. Slavin J: Why whole grains are protective: biological mechanisms, *Proc Nutr Soc* 62:129, 2003.

19. Muir JG et al: Combining wheat bran with resistant starch has more beneficial effects on fecal indexes than does wheat bran alone, *Am J Clin Nutr* 79:1020, 2004.

20. Satia-Abouta et al: Associations of total energy and macronutrients with colon cancer risk in African Americans and whites: results from the North Carolina Colon Cancer Study, *Am J Epidemiol* 158:951, 2003.

21. Shiels A, ed: *The Washington manual gastroenterology subspecialty consult,* Philadelphia, 2004, Lippincott Williams & Wilkins.

22. Rabeneck L et al: Sociodemographics, general health, and psychologic health in uninvestigated dyspepsia: a comparison of public and private patients, *J Clin Gastroenterol* 34:516, 2002.

23. Locke GR et al: Psychosocial factors are linked to functional gastrointestinal disorders: a population based nested case-control study, *Am J Gastroenterol* 99:350, 2004.

24. Lee KJ et al: A pilot study on duodenal acid exposure and its relationship to symptoms in functional dyspepsia with prominent nausea, *Am J Gastroenterol* 99:1765, 2004.

25. Shaib Y, El-Serag HB: The prevalence and risk factors of functional dyspepsia in a multiethnic population in the United States, *Am J Gastroenterol* 99:2210, 2004.

26. Bode G et al: Dyspeptic symptoms in middle-aged to old adults: the role of *Helicobacter pylori* infection, and various demographic and lifestyle factors, *J Intern Med* 252:41, 2002.

27. Beyer PL: Gastrointestinal disorders: roles of nutrition and the dietetics practitioner, *J Am Diet Assoc* 98:272, 1998.

28. Broussard EK, Surawicz CM: Probiotics and prebiotics in clinical practice, *Nutr Clin Care* 7(3):104, 2004.

29. Slavin JL, Greenberg NA: Partially hydrolyzed guar gum: clinical nutrition uses, *Nutrition* 19:549, 2003.

30. Bouhnik Y et al: The capacity of nondigestible carbohydrates to stimulate fecal bifidobacteria in healthy humans: a double-blind, randomized, placebo-controlled, parallel-group, dose-response relation study, *Am J Clin Nutr* 80:1658, 2004.

31. Clemens R: Progress in probiotics, *Nutr and the MD* 30(8):1, 2004.

32. Adolfsson O, Meydani SN, Russell RN: Yogurt and gut function, *Am J Clin Nutr* 80:245, 2004.

33. Brown AC, Valiere A: Probiotics and medical nutrition therapy, *Nutr Clin Care* 7(2):56, 2004.

FURTHER READINGS AND RESOURCES

Readings

Mattes RD: The chemical senses and nutrition in aging: challenging old assumptions, *J Am Diet Assoc* 102:192, 2002.

This author tells us about the genetic factors that influence taste and their relationships to food preferences. Genetic differences in taste may influence one's preference for sweet, high-fat, or bitter foods.

Gerstein DE et al: Clarifying concepts about macronutrients' effects on satiation and satiety, *J Am Diet Assoc* 104:1151, 2004.

Melanson KJ: Food intake regulation in body weight management: a primer, *Nutr Today* 39:203, 2004.

The growing obesity crisis worldwide has brought new attention to the internal and environmental influences that control our desire to eat and how much we eat. These researchers tell us more about what regulates our food intake.

Brown AC, Valiere A: The medicinal uses of poi, *Nutr Clin Care* 7:69, 2004.

Poi is a tropical plant that is being used as a probiotic and provides an example of an alternative therapy in the treatment of medical conditions.

Websites of Interest

- National Institutes of Health, information on the digestive system; this site offers information on a host of digestive medical problems: *http://health.nih.gov/search.asp/5.*

- National Institutes of Health, National Institute of Diabetes and Digestive and Kidney Diseases; this site offers specific information on lactose intolerance: *http://health.nih.gov/result.asp/391/5.*

- National Institutes of Health, National Institute of Diabetes and Digestive and Kidney Diseases, National Digestive Diseases Information Clearinghouse; this site offers information on drugs that cause bleeding or damage the mucosa of the digestive tract: *http://digestive.niddk.nih.gov/ddiseases/pubs/bleeding/.*

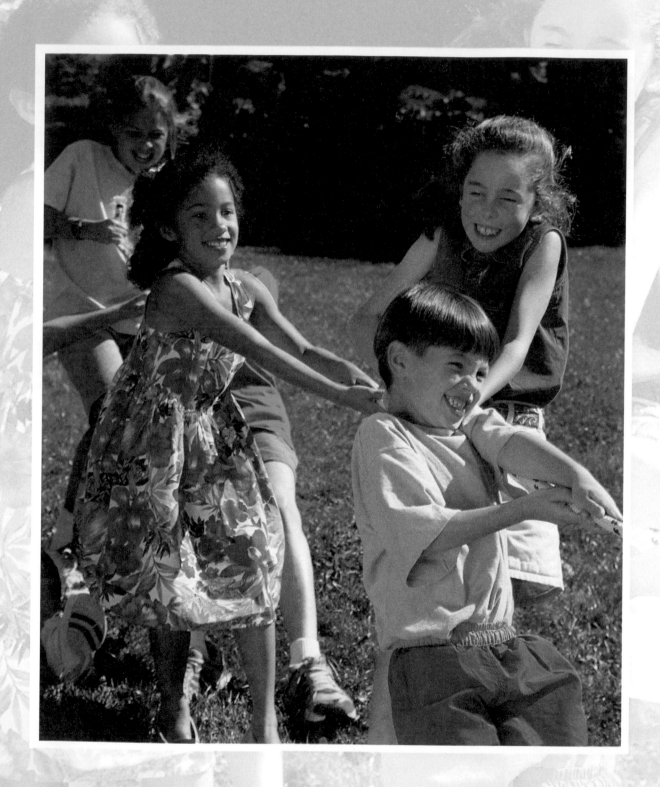

Community Nutrition: The Life Cycle

CHAPTER 9

The Food Environment and Food Habits

Eleanor D. Schlenker

Here we begin the second section of our study of nutrition with a two-chapter sequence on food habits and family nutrition counseling. In this section we apply the principles of nutrition science to the food needs of individuals and families.

The science of human nutrition comes alive when we focus on personal needs. Respect and concern for individual differences are as important as practical skills for applying knowledge in a useful and helpful way.

We look first at our changing food environment and the web of factors that influence personal food choices.

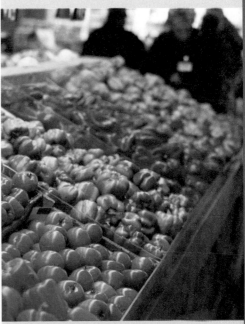

HOW OUR FOOD HABITS DEVELOP

Food habits like other human behaviors do not develop in a vacuum. They grow out of our personal, cultural, social, and psychologic environment. These factors interweave in each of us to develop a unique individual.

Cultural Influences

Cultural Identity

Culture is broadly defined as the values, beliefs, attitudes, and practices accepted by members of a group or community.[1] Often the most significant thing about a culture is what is taken for granted in daily living. Culture involves not only the more obvious aspects of life—language, religion, family structure, and historical heritage—but also the patterns of everyday living such as preparing and serving food and caring for children or elders. These facets of a culture are passed from generation to generation and learned gradually as a child grows up within the community. Socially acquired knowledge and habits we learn as part of our culture.[2]

Food in a Culture

Foodways (food customs or traditions) are among the oldest and most deeply rooted aspects of a culture. They determine what food shall be eaten, when and how it shall be eaten, and who shall prepare it.[1] What is a special treat for families in one part of the world may be viewed as an unacceptable food in another. The geography of the land, the agriculture practiced in that locality, experiences related to health and food safety, and local history and traditions influence food choices. Within every culture certain foods are deeply infused with symbolic meaning. From early times designated foods or meals have commemorated special events of religious significance or national heritage or rites of passage. Many of these customs remain today.[3]

Social Influences

Internal Factors

Food has various social roles. Food is a symbol of acceptance, warmth, and friendliness. People are more likely to accept food from those they view as friends or allies, and in many cultures the offering of food is an expected act of hospitality. Strong food patterns develop within the primary social unit of the family, and food habits associated with family sentiments are held tenaciously throughout life (Figure 9-1). Long into adulthood certain foods trigger a flood of childhood memories and are valued for reasons totally apart from their nutritional contribution. Nevertheless, family income, local availability, and market conditions ultimately influence food choices. Persons eat foods that are readily available and that they have the money to buy.

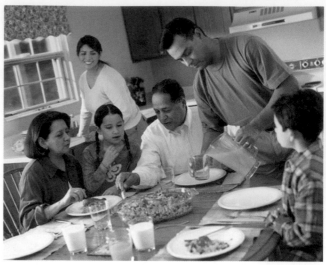

FIGURE 9-1   A family sharing food. Sharing food with guests is an established custom among many cultural and ethnic groups. *(From Food and Nutrition Service, U.S. Department of Agriculture and Food and Nutrition Information Center, National Agricultural Library: Food stamp nutrition collection: photo gallery, Beltsville, Md, 2005, Authors. Retrieved December 9, 2005, from* http://grande.nal.usda.gov/foodstamp_album.php?mode=mealtime.*)*

External Factors

Peer pressures influence food choices. Foods may be selected because they are high-prestige foods or rejected because they are associated with low economic status. Individuals immigrating to the United States may reject their traditional foods to adopt American foods perceived to be popular across the general population. Children may plead for a particular snack item if that is what their friends eat.

Psychologic Influences

Individual behaviors result from many interrelated psychosocial influences. Persons who enjoy a bountiful food supply think less about food because it is always available,[4] whereas those with chronic hunger think, talk, and dream about food. For most of us the concern for food is relatively abstract and associated with other needs. Maslow's classic hierarchy describes the five levels of human need, each building on the one before, as follows[5]:

1. *Basic physiologic needs:* Hunger and thirst
2. *Need for safety:* Physical comfort, security, and protection
3. *Need to belong:* Love; giving and receiving affection
4. *Need for recognition:* Self-esteem, sense of self-worth, self-confidence, and capability
5. *Need for self-actualization:* Self-fulfillment and creative growth

Although these levels of need vary with time and circumstance, we can use them to help understand the needs of our clients and to plan our care accordingly.

BOX 9-1	Factors Determining Food Choices

Physical Factors

Food availability
Food technology
Geography, agriculture, food distribution
Personal economics, income
Sanitation, housing
Season, climate
Storage and cooking facilities

Social Factors

Advertising
Culture
Education, food, and nutrition knowledge
Political and economic policies
Religion and social customs
Social class role
Social problems, poverty, or alcoholism

Physiologic Factors

Allergy
Physical disability
Health-disease status
Personal food acceptance
Energy or nutrient needs
Therapeutic diets

BOX 9-2	Five Top Global Food Trends

1. The Quick Fix—foods easy to prepare
2. Drive and Go—take-out foods, including meals from full-service restaurants
3. Inherently Healthy—foods that are fresh and less processed
4. Fancy That—foods that emphasize gourmet, ethnic, and upscale dining
5. Farm-Friendly—foods perceived to be natural and organic and to support sustainable agriculture

Data from Sloan AE: Top 10 global food trends, *Food Tech* 59:20, 2005.

TRENDS IN PERSONAL FOOD HABITS

Basic Determinants of Food Choices

Family, ethnic, and regional patterns are strong influences in our lives. At the same time new technology and mass media put old influences in conflict with new forces. As summarized in Box 9-1, a complex set of physical, social, and physiologic factors influence what a person eats.

All food patterns have several characteristics in common, although they differ in the actual foods they contain. When working with individuals with food patterns different from your own, this is one way to begin to look at their meal pattern and nutrient intake. Several common components are as follows[1]:

- *Core and complementary foods:* Core foods, usually complex carbohydrates, are eaten every day and provide the bulk of the energy intake. Complementary foods are those items added to improve palatability such as the vegetables or meat added to a rice meal.
- *Food flavors:* How foods are prepared and seasoned is distinctive to each cultural or ethnic group and is as important as the foods themselves.
- *Meal patterns:* The number of meals or snacks eaten each day, when they are eaten, and the items they contain define food intake among individuals and cultures.

Maintaining core foods, familiar flavors, and the meal sequence to the extent possible serves as a bridge to developing new patterns made necessary by health or other considerations.

Changing American Food Patterns

Changes in our society are bringing changes in traditional food patterns. Households are getting smaller with fewer children, and more families are single-parent families (see the *Case Study* box, "Planning the Family Dinner"). Working parents in both single- and two-parent families are putting in more hours on the job and have less time for meal preparation. As a result, almost one half of the family food dollar is spent for food away from home.[6] With the busy lifestyles of parents and children, families eat fewer meals together, and children prepare more of their own meals or snacks. Growing numbers of households are made up of unrelated persons or single people living alone. As the older population increases in age with growing disability,[7] the market for appropriate meals requiring little or no preparation will continue to expand.

Convenience Meals

According to a food industry survey, the leading consumer trend is the "Quick Fix" (Box 9-2).[8] Consumers want foods that can be heated quickly and served in minutes after they arrive home. Supermarkets, fast-food outlets, and upscale restaurants offer meals to take home that are hot and ready to eat. Fast foods meet the needs of many families because they are quick, reasonably priced, and readily available. Every day one fourth of the adult population of the United States eats at a fast-food restaurant; Americans spend more money on fast food than on higher education.[9]

Unfortunately, fast food and many heat-and-serve packaged entrees are often high in total fat, saturated fat, and sodium, and rather low in calcium and important vitamins. (Review Box 7-4 to compare the sodium content of processed foods and their fresh counterparts.) A reasonable compromise for a busy student or parent might be a combination of fast food or convenience items along with some fresh items that are easily prepared. A rotisserie chicken from the supermarket or chicken from a fast-food restaurant could be combined with a frozen

Planning the Family Dinner

Mrs. G is a single parent with two children. Her daughter is in third grade, and her son is in ninth grade. They ride different buses to school, but both get home about 3:30 PM. Mrs. G is a secretary in a real estate office and usually has to work until about 6:00 PM. She arrives home at approximately 6:45 PM. Usually by the time she gets home her children have already filled up on snacks and are not really hungry for a meal. Sometimes she calls ahead to tell them that she is stopping at a fast-food restaurant and they should wait to eat with her, but most of the time they get something to eat for themselves. Mrs. G's son has been gaining weight rapidly and has a body mass index (BMI) of 29. She also has been told that his blood pressure is above normal. The doctor recommended that he reduce his sodium intake to improve his long-term health.

Questions for Analysis

1. Is it important that the family eat together when Mrs. G returns home in the evening? How would you approach this with her?

2. What are some appropriate snack foods that the children might have when they get home from school that would hold them over until dinnertime?

3. What are important facts on the Nutrition Label that Mrs. G could use in selecting after-school snacks for her children?

4. MyPyramid recommends an energy intake of 2400 kcal for a 14-year-old moderately active boy. What should be the upper level of fat and sodium included in his food for the day? If one fourth of his daily energy intake is reserved for snacks, recommend some food combinations that would provide the appropriate amounts of kcalories, sodium, and fat.

5. What are some dinner alternatives to fast food? What might Mrs. G bring home, or what could the children begin to prepare before she arrives home?

6. Develop five rules for food safety that the children should practice when preparing and eating their after-school snacks.

vegetable and a fresh salad or fruit in place of french-fried potatoes. Washed, packaged salad greens can be served or a frozen vegetable cooked in the microwave in the time it takes to set the table and get the family seated. Helping people identify nutrient-rich accompaniments to fast-food meals can improve the nutrient intake of the entire family.

The Grazers

Another food trend that has contributed to the growing energy intake of both children and adults is the increase in the number of times that people eat each day. The traditional 3 meals has expanded to as many as 11 or 12 eating occasions over the course of a day with midmorning and midafternoon snack breaks and several periods of eating in the evening while watching television or surfing the Internet. Eating on the go is commonplace, and every day over 100 million people purchase food from a vending machine.[8] Several small meals and snacks (a grazing pattern) rather than 1 or 2 very large meals represent a positive shift in food intake if the energy and nutrient content of the foods eaten across the day is monitored wisely. Snacks of fruits, vegetables, low-fat dairy foods, and low-fat grain products add important nutrients with low to moderate amounts of kilocalories (kcalories, kcal)

and complement the meal pattern. But in most cases common snacks include chips, baked items, and sugar-sweetened beverages high in sugar and fat that escalate energy intake.

Eating as a Family

As both children and adults have become involved in more activities outside the home, family meals have become less frequent. Still, about two thirds of adolescents eat dinner with their family at least 3 to 4 times each week.[10] Eating together as a family influences both nutritional and emotional well-being. The more meals children eat with their parents, the greater their intakes of calcium-rich foods, fruits, and vegetables.[10] Also, youth eating at the family dinner table enjoy a higher degree of "family connectedness," do better in school, and are less likely to use tobacco, alcohol, and drugs.[11] Eating more meals with their family appears to be a protective strategy against disordered eating patterns in both girls and boys.[12]

Health Concerns

More Americans are concerned about their health, and this is demonstrated in various ways. First, there is greater attention to foods lower in fat and kcalories and higher in other nutrients. More than 60% of shoppers reported purchasing a food item because of a health-related claim they read on the label.[8] Whole grains and foods low in fat, saturated fat, and kcalories or high in calcium and vitamin C were of greatest interest. Salads are now the fourth most popular restaurant entree.[8] Fresh fruits and vegetables are becoming more popular. Consumers have an increased interest in the wholesomeness of the food supply and are seeking out plant foods that have been grown without the use of pesticides and animal foods produced without the use of antibiotics. Mothers report trying to restrict their children's intakes of candy, soda, and high-fructose corn syrup.[8]

Cutting Food Costs

Many consumers are finding it necessary to economize on food. Warehouse food markets that provide limited services but offer items in bulk at lower prices are growing in popularity with consumers stocking up on bargains. Brand loyalty has declined, and the purchase of generic products has increased. Consumers look more carefully at food labels to compare price and value. In Chapter 10 we will review the information on food labels that can help shoppers make good decisions when buying food in bulk.

Gourmet and Ethnic Cooking

Gourmet foods and specialty ethnic dishes are getting increasing attention. Food specialty shops and bookstores offer a wide variety of new cookbooks and television cooking shows and celebrity chefs are helping consumers learn about international foods. Gourmet cooking has become a popular hobby, and magazines are featuring recipes for unusual foods.[13] Supermarkets are establishing specialty shops that feature ingredients for preparing ethnic foods, fueled by the growing international population. Increasing interest in Asian food has led to large supermarket sections devoted to Asian vegetables and fruits.[14] This phenomenon of preparing more expensive items made from fresh ingredients parallels the general trend toward meals that are easy to prepare in little time.

The Problem of Food Misinformation

Concerns for a safe and wholesome food supply have existed across the centuries. Most cultural and ethnic groups had beliefs about the healing properties or dangers of particular foods, and certain religious food laws may be rooted in concerns for food safety. Some scientifically unsubstantiated beliefs about certain foods are harmless, but others have serious implications for health. Pursuing claims that megadoses of vitamins are necessary for vitality or using certain herbs that produce a dangerous interaction with a prescription drug carry both financial and physical costs. False information may come from folklore, be built on half-truths, or stem from intentional deception and fraud.

Types of False Food Claims

Exaggerated food claims are of the following four types:

1. Certain foods will cure specific diseases or conditions.
2. Certain foods are harmful and should be avoided.
3. Certain food combinations have special therapeutic effects.
4. Only "natural" foods can meet body needs and prevent disease.

Notice that each claim focuses on foods as such, not on the chemical components or nutrients that they contain. Certain foods contain certain nutrients—and it is the nutrients, not the specific foods—that have defined functions in the body. Moreover, each nutrient can be found in a number of different foods. Persons require specific nutrients, not specific foods.

Why should we be concerned about food misinformation and its influence on food habits? Several reasons are outlined below:

- *Danger to health:* Self-diagnosis and self-treatment can delay efforts to seek out appropriate medical treatment in an effective time frame. Patients with difficult-to-treat conditions such as cancer, diabetes, or arthritis can be especially vulnerable to fraudulent claims.
- *Money spent needlessly:* As much as $18.8 billion per year is spent on various dietary supplements,[15] and

many are unnecessary or inappropriate. If dollars are scarce, money spent on supplements may be at the expense of nutritious food.
- *Distrust of the food supply:* Changes in our food environment have led to erroneous teaching about dangerous chemicals and plants in the food supply, breeding public suspicion and distrust of agriculture and food technology. We will discuss some of these issues later in this chapter.

Groups Vulnerable to Food Misinformation

The following groups with particular needs and concerns are often the target of materials and products making false claims:

- *Older persons:* Progressing physical changes and chronic disease make older individuals vulnerable to products promising to restore youthful vigor. Older adults suffering pain and disability are easy prey for exaggerated health claims or cures.
- *Teenagers:* Figure-conscious adolescent girls and muscle-minded adolescent boys often respond to crash programs in hopes of attaining the perfect body and peer-group acceptance.
- *Obese persons:* Obese individuals desperate to lose large amounts of weight over a short period of time may respond to the bewildering barrage of advertisements advocating diets, pills, various devices, and special foods.
- *Athletes:* Always looking for something to give them the competitive edge, athletes can be lured by nutrition myths and false promises.

Although these groups are especially vulnerable to food misinformation and false claims, no segment of the population is completely free of the appeal of unscrupulous marketers of worthless or worse yet harmful products.

Answers

How do we respond to food habits or erroneous beliefs built on food misinformation or deception? Several approaches have merit, as follows:

- *Educate consumers:* Help consumers learn to evaluate advertisements about diets, food products, or dietary supplements. The U.S. Department of Health and Human Services has developed a checklist for spotting health scams that provides simple criteria for differentiating legitimate products and health advice from those that can be harmful and a waste of money (Box 9-3).
- *Stay current:* Be well informed about new products—both their content and reputed effects on the body. Search out studies by universities or government agencies using the scientific method to evaluate advertising claims and product safety. Review publications and website materials of responsible

✓ Promises a quick or painless cure
✓ Claims to be made from a special, secret, or ancient formula available from only one source
✓ Uses testimonials or undocumented case histories from satisfied patients
✓ Claims to be effective for a wide range of ailments
✓ Claims to cure a disease such as arthritis or cancer that is not fully understood by physicians and medical scientists
✓ Requires advance payment and claims limited availability of the product

Modified from National Institute on Aging, U.S. Department of Health and Human Services: *Health quackery: spotting health scams,* Bethesda, Md, 2002 (reprinted 2005), Author. Retrieved December 9, 2005, from *www.niapublications.org/engagepages/healthqy.asp.*

government, professional, and private organizations such as the American Dietetic Association, the American Medical Association, the U.S. Food and Drug Administration (FDA), and the International Food Information Council Foundation.

- *Think scientifically:* Use the problem-solving approach when working with both children and adults. In everyday situations look for research data to support your position and be able to answer the questions, "How do you know?" and "What is your evidence?"

BIOTECHNOLOGY AND FOOD: PROMISE AND CONTROVERSY

Throughout human history, scientific discoveries leading to new products and opportunities have created change and challenges for society. The discovery of antibiotics directed our attention from the control of infectious diseases to the challenge of chronic diseases. Biotechnology, the field of science involved with gene technology, allows us to manage deoxyribonucleic acid (DNA) material, adding or removing a gene from the DNA of a plant or animal species.[16] Biotechnology has the potential to improve the food supply, as in Chapter 4 we noted the development of new varieties of rice with improved amino acid patterns; nonetheless, these scientific advances have also raised questions about the safety of these new foods.

Two biotechnology applications that provide examples of the biosafety review process are growth hormone in dairy cows and genetic engineering in plants.

Bovine Growth Hormone

Growth hormone is secreted naturally in the pituitary glands of animals and humans and plays an essential role in growth, development, and health. Bovine growth hormone (BGH) extracted from the pituitary glands of cattle

was used for more than 60 years in the dairy industry to boost milk production. When it became possible in the 1980s to make large quantities of BGH using recombinant DNA methods, farmers petitioned the FDA for permission to use the rBGH in their dairy herds,[17,18] and in 1993 permission was granted. The assessment of potential benefit versus risk to humans conducted by an FDA expert panel considered the following factors:

- *Absorption of rBGH from milk:* Proteins such as rBGH are broken down into amino acids in the human digestive tract. They are not absorbed as proteins.
- *Antibody response:* The amount of rBGH that could bring about an antibody response in humans is several hundred–fold higher than could be consumed in milk. (Allergic reactions to milk proteins that occur in some individuals are not related to rBGH.)
- *Production of insulin-like growth factor (IGF):* IGF is a protein produced by humans and animals in response to growth hormone. IGF is a normal component of cow's milk and found in similar amounts in both rBGH-treated and untreated cows.

When assessing risk, answers are seldom clear cut; no action by either a government agency or an individual is ever completely risk free.[19] Risk must be evaluated in light of the potential benefits versus the potential harm and involves weighing numerous and often subtle variables. Available research evidence must form the basis for judgments that serve the public interest.

Genetically Modified Plants

Genetically modified (GM) organisms are plants or bacteria in which the natural genetic DNA material has been modified to produce a desired trait. Genetic modification can take place through plant breeding techniques or through genetic engineering, the process that allows us to transfer a gene from one organism to another.[20] Genetic engineering was first applied to the development of pharmaceuticals, and nearly 95 such therapeutic agents have been approved for human use. Genetically modified bacteria produce human insulin for managing diabetes and erythropoietin, the hormone that stimulates the production of red blood cells.[21]

Genetically Modified Food Plants

Genetically modified food crops were introduced in the early 1990s, and their use has increased dramatically. Six million farmers in 16 countries are planting genetically modified plant species representing 62% of the soybeans, 21% of the maize, and 5% of the rapeseed (canola oil) produced worldwide.[22] In the United States the sale and use of genetically modified seeds are regulated by the FDA, the Environmental Protection Agency (EPA), and the U.S. Department of Agriculture (USDA).[23,24]

Goals for Genetic Modification

Since humans first began to cultivate plants for food, various practices have been used to improve the yield or desirability of particular species. Selection and breeding using Mendel's principles of inheritance and the development of hybrid plants led to the green revolutions of the 1960s and 1970s and varieties of wheat and rice with double the yields of those grown previously. These transformations in crop production are credited with helping to reduce the food shortages in the developing world.[25]

The genetic modification of food plants has centered on the following three goals[16,25]:

1. *Resistance to disease and insects:* These plants can better tolerate weed-killing herbicides or carry a protein that acts as a built-in insecticide making pesticide sprays unnecessary. Such plants enable farmers to reduce their use of both pesticides and herbicides for protection of the environment.
2. *Increased tolerance to weather conditions:* New plant varieties are able to survive more extreme environmental conditions. A delayed-ripening tomato is less likely to be destroyed by a late frost.
3. *Increased nutritional value:* Genetic modification has increased the monounsaturated fatty acid content of soybean oil, and efforts are underway to produce a tomato with a greater lycopene content. Improved grains with increased protein and micronutrients could lessen the continuing nutrient deficiencies in developing countries.

Corn, soybeans, canola, potatoes, and tomatoes are among the 12 genetically altered food crops approved for sale in the United States.[20]

Safety of Genetically Modified Crops

Genetically modified crops and their sale and use remain controversial. Various public groups have questioned their safety for human health and their long-term effects on the environment. Following are the three major concerns:

1. *Risk of allergic reaction:* A concern of health professionals and allergic consumers is the possible transfer of a known allergen into a new food. For example, adding a peanut allergen to a corn plant would make those corn products unsafe for a person allergic to peanuts. Industry and government agencies worldwide have joined together to develop a vigorous assessment process for all genetically modified foods before they may enter the marketplace. To date, no genetically modified food has been shown to be allergenic.[26]
2. *Potential toxicity to humans:* The presence of new DNA in a food carries no inherent risk to human health because all foods contain DNA.[27] People eating a normal diet already consume as much as 1 g of DNA

a day. All genetically engineered foods undergo toxicity testing before being approved for sale.[28]
3. *Potential danger to the environment:* Plants with specific genes that resist the effects of insects or herbicides may be harmful to helpful insects such as butterflies[29] or pass those genes along to weeds or invasive plants. Farmers are urged to confine these plants to specific growing areas.

Currently, it is not required that food labels identify food ingredients from a genetically modified plant *unless* the modification has increased the allergenicity or reduced the nutrient content of the food as compared to the conventional product.[20]

Biotechnology and Animal Foods

New techniques have identified genes in cattle that lead to higher milk production, more tender meat, and more favorable nutrient composition. Conventional breeding methods have produced eggs with a lower cholesterol content and beef with reduced fat. Marker-assisted breeding, which combines the skills of classic breeders and molecular geneticists, offers even greater potential for the development of healthy animal foods. In marker-assisted breeding, molecular geneticists identify existing DNA patterns in living animals that influence important traits such as muscle amount or composition, enabling breeders to better select for positive characteristics.

ENSURING A SAFE AND WHOLESOME FOOD SUPPLY

The sources of our food have changed dramatically over the years. No longer do families produce their own food or purchase food from their neighbors. Food from all over the world is available at the local grocery market, and fresh produce picked on a farm on one continent can be served on a dinner table on another continent the next day. Farmers and food processors have at their disposal a wide variety of technologies to expand and preserve our food supply and create new products in response to consumer demand. This flow of food from across the nation and the world has implications for food safety and the need to monitor the overall food environment.

Government Agencies Monitoring Food Safety

A Shared Regulatory System: USDA and FDA

The current system for ensuring a safe food supply began in 1906 when Congress charged the USDA with the responsibility of monitoring the safety of the nation's food. Early on USDA began the continuous on-site inspection of meatpacking plants and poultry-processing plants, an enormous job that is still being carried out by thousands

PERSPECTIVES IN PRACTICE
Mad Cow Disease: A Continuing Prevention Effort

Meredith Catherine Williams

Mad cow disease first gained international attention in the mid-1990s when several people in the United Kingdom died from a new form of a rare brain disease. Researchers discovered that this new human disease was apparently connected with eating beef from cattle afflicted with the so-called mad cow disease that had been seen in British cattle since 1986. Since then more than 170,000 cattle in the United Kingdom and Western Europe have been slaughtered in an attempt to prevent infected meat from reaching the public. Despite the efforts of government officials to prevent the spread of this disease to the United States, an infected cow was found in Washington State in 2003, causing Food and Drug Administration (FDA) investigators to act quickly to ensure that our national food supply was not contaminated. That incident led to a reassessment of the safety of U.S. beef and the development of new methods of testing and screening.

Mad cow disease is the name given by the press to bovine spongiform encephalopathy (BSE). It is a rare neurologic disorder in cattle that causes afflicted animals to be disorientated, stare at imaginary objects, and kick and paw at the ground. This disease is unique in that it is not caused by a bacterium or virus, or even a genetic connection, but rather by a malformed protein called a *prion*. Normal prions are present in lymph and brain tissue and their three-dimensional coiled helix shape helps maintain the integrity of nerve cells. Diseased prions uncoil to form straight protein sheets that destroy surrounding brain tissue. Diseased prions proliferate by inducing healthy prion proteins to change their shape. Deformed prions can incubate in the lymph for as long as 10 years before moving to the brain. Once in the brain, a buildup of these diseased proteins will lead to harmful changes in the neural tissue.[1]

Cattle contract the abnormal prions causing BSE from their feed. In a process known as *rendering,* scrap pieces of meat and bone, glands, and spinal cord from sheep and cattle not used in human food were ground and prepared for cattle feed. Rendering did not destroy the malformed prions because the more virulent strains are not destroyed by heat or by enzymes in the stomach. It is suspected that cows contracted BSE from eating processed feed infected with scrapie, a sheep version of the fatal brain disorder. Rendering, now outlawed in both Europe and the United States, continued for years until whole cattle populations became infected with mad cow disease.[2]

The same prions that caused BSE in cows may have produced a variant of Creutzfeldt-Jakob disease (vCJD) in humans. The original and extremely rare form of CJD strikes persons in their 50s or older, causing dementia, uncoordinated movements, sleep disorders, and death within several months. However, the variant form that surfaced in the United Kingdom in the mid-1990s affected people in their 20s, and death usually occurred within about 14 months. Although there is no conclusive evidence to prove that the infection stemmed from eating beef, researchers are working on a diagnostic test that would scan for mutant prions in the blood and allow an earlier diagnosis of this condition.[3]

Since 1986 more than 95% of all BSE-infected cattle have been in Great Britain, although mad cow disease has spread to cattle populations in other European countries. In the late 1980s the United States imposed a ban on all beef imports, including live cattle and all bovine products such as beef tallow and bone meal from Great Britain and other European countries where BSE had been detected. In 1997 the United States instituted a countrywide ban on the manufacture and use of cattle feed that contains rendered parts from other cattle and sheep.

Despite these efforts, in December 2003 a U.S. Department of Agriculture (USDA) surveillance program identified a case of BSE in the United States.[4] The infected dairy cow in Washington State had been purchased from a farm in Canada and imported to the United States. The cow had already been slaughtered and its parts sent to different processing plants with the potential of being incorporated in small amounts in edible meats, feeds, and fat for soap products. The FDA and the USDA promptly activated their BSE Emergency Response Plan, and all the meat was officially recalled. Teams worked to trace quickly all parts of the cow and ensure their destruction. Local stores and plants worked with officials, in some cases discarding their entire meat stock to prevent the possibility of contamination. By the end of the search, approximately 2000 tons of cattle products had been procured and destroyed. The response to the incident was labeled a success in that the protective institutions and field agents were able to prevent any further contamination or infection of the local cattle population. In addition, there was no public panic with the persons involved remaining calm and rational.

The beef supply in the United States is considered very safe. The critical control point (see the discussion of Hazard Analysis and Critical Control Points (HACCP) on p. 217) is the ban on cattle feed containing rendered parts from other cattle. A recent study by a university expert panel concluded that "the U.S. appears very resistant to a BSE challenge, primarily because of the FDA feed ban which greatly reduces the chance that an infected animal would infect other animals."[5] This prohibition breaks the cycle by which BSE is spread among cattle and possibly passed on to humans eating this meat. However, the FDA and the USDA are continuing to expand and strengthen their inspection and enforcement of cattle feed regulations.[6] New kits have been developed that allow easier testing for the presence of animal proteins in feed.[7] These kits will allow ranchers to inspect any cattle feed they purchase, thereby acting as a second check against infection.

Both BSE in cattle and vCJD in humans are dramatic and frightening diseases. The FDA and the USDA are working hard to establish and enforce safety precautions across national, state, and local levels to prevent BSE in U.S. cattle herds and uphold public confidence in the safety of the food supply.

References

1. Yam P: Mad cow's human toll, *Sci Am* 284(5):12, 2001.
2. Animal and Plant Health Inspection Service, U.S. Department of Agriculture: Bovine spongiform encephalopathy (BSE), Riverdale, Md, 2005, Author. Available at *www.aphis.usda.gov/lpa/issues/bse/bse.html.*
3. Caughey B: A sane look at mad cows, *Discover* 22(3):16, 2001.
4. Brem L: FDA investigators respond to mad cow emergency, *FDA Consumer,* p 38, May-June 2004. Retrieved December 12, 2005, from *www.fda.gov/fdac/features/2004/304_bse.html.*
5. Harvard Center for Risk Analysis, Harvard School of Public Health: Risk analysis of transmissible spongiform encephalopathies in cattle and the potential for entry of the etiologic agent(s) into the U.S. food supply, Cambridge, Mass, November 2001 (revised October 2003), Author. Retrieved March 21, 2006 from http://www.hcra.harvard.edu/peer_reviewed_analysis.html.
6. Newman L: Risk of BSE in USA is low, *Lancet* 358(9298):2053, 2001.
7. Center for Veterinary Medicine, U.S. Food and Drug Administration: *FDA evaluates test kits to detect animal proteins in animal feed,* Rockville, Md, 2004 (November), Author. Retrieved December 12, 2005, from *www.fda.gov/cvm/BSEkitup.htm.*

of inspectors nationwide. Today the FDA has responsibility for ensuring the safety of all foods except meat and poultry. These two agencies work with the EPA to ensure that pesticide residues in food do not exceed tolerance standards. Interagency cooperation is essential for mounting an effective response to new food-related threats to health. The USDA and the Centers for Disease Control and Prevention (CDC) work closely together to prevent the introduction and spread of such hazards as mad cow disease or avian flu from other countries to the United States (see the *Perspectives in Practice* box, "Mad Cow Disease: A Continuing Prevention Effort").

Food and Drug Administration

The FDA is a law enforcement agency charged by Congress to ensure that our food supply is safe, pure, and wholesome. The FDA enforces federal food safety regulations pertaining to many aspects of the food supply (Box 9-4).[30] The most common means of enforcement is the recall or seizure of contaminated food. Because it is impossible to inspect all food products before they are sold, the FDA has put in place surveillance and risk assessment procedures in food manufacturing facilities to prevent food contamination. These procedures referred to as HACCP (Hazard Analysis and Critical Control Points) identify potential sources of food contamination and help plant managers set up ways to control them during the production process. HACCP also requires systematic testing for the presence of dangerous microbes at production points where they might enter the system. The joint efforts of the FDA and the USDA to implement HACCP procedures in poultry processing are credited with reducing by 50% the number of chickens contaminated with *Salmonella*. A new responsibility of FDA is to effectively monitor today's global food economy and the threat of food bioterrorism (see the *To Probe Further* box, "The Threat of Bioterrorism to the Food Supply: Risk Assessment and Policy Responses").

The FDA Division of Consumer Education conducts an active program of public education through its website, electronic newsletters, and publications. Combating food and nutrition misinformation and encouraging safe food storage and preparation practices in the home and in food service facilities receive special attention. Consumer specialists work through FDA district offices and are available to speak to consumer groups.

Food Safety Laws: Drugs, Foods, Additives, and Supplements

Approval Process for Drugs

The FDA's control over food and drug ingredients began in 1938 with the passage of the Federal Food, Drug, and Cosmetic Act (FFDCA). Pharmaceutical drugs are the most highly regulated based on the great dangers they carry if poorly formulated or misused. When in development a new drug must undergo intensive testing, often extending over a period of years. The manufacturer must present to the FDA convincing scientific evidence that the drug meets the legal standard of "safe and effective," and formal approval must be obtained before the drug can be sold.

Regulation of Food Ingredients and Food Additives

The makers of all foods and food additives are legally obligated to assure the public that their products are safe. For conventional foods the FFDCA requires that the food and all ingredients not be "ordinarily injurious." Safety is assumed for ingredients with a long history of use, and such food products may be marketed without prior FDA approval. Cookies with the ingredients of flour, brown sugar, eggs, butter, and baking soda would meet this standard.

In 1960 the FFDCA was expanded to create two legal classes of food additives. The first group included all food additives and ingredients that had been marketed before 1958. These were placed in a category called Generally Recognized as Safe (GRAS). There are thousands of additives on the GRAS list. One example is the yellow coloring added to margarine that has been in use since the 1930s. The safety standard under the FFDCA is that a food is unsafe if the additive "may render injurious" the food product. Food processors are not required to obtain FDA approval to use additives on the GRAS list. The presumed safety of GRAS additives was based on their wide prior use; most have not been tested to determine their safety. But in 1977 Congress directed the FDA to begin testing the thousands of additives on the GRAS list, and this testing is ongoing.

The second legal category of food additives includes any additive developed since 1958. These additives are not on the GRAS list. The same legal standard of "may render injurious" applies, but these newer additives must undergo rigid testing for safety under FDA scrutiny, and FDA approval must be obtained before any food product containing the new additive may be legally sold. Aspartame, the nonnutritive sweetener marketed under the brand name NutraSweet, is an example of a new additive that received FDA approval after extensive testing; it has enjoyed wide use as a sweetener in many sugar-free soft drinks, baked products, and snacks.

BOX 9-4	**Food-Related Activities of the Food and Drug Administration**

- Ensure that processed foods are free of pathogens and contaminants
- Inspect food processing facilities (other than meat and poultry plants)
- Approve food additives
- Monitor the content of infant formulas and medical foods
- Regulate the movement of food across state lines
- Oversee nutrition labeling
- Check shipments of imported foods for purity
- Approve drugs and supplements added to animal feeds

TO PROBE FURTHER

THE THREAT OF BIOTERRORISM TO THE FOOD SUPPLY: RISK ASSESSMENT AND POLICY RESPONSES

Meredith Catherine Williams

Food poisoning and foodborne illness are natural dangers that public health agencies combat continuously; however, in most cases the contamination of food with disease-causing bacteria is accidental, based on the carelessness of a food service worker or an infection from an animal source. But in recent years the threat of bioterrorism—attacks against people or agriculture using deadly biological organisms—has received increasing attention from government agencies charged with overseeing the safety of our food.

Agriculture is considered to be vulnerable to a bioterrorist attack for a number of reasons as follows:

- Many animal and crop pathogens are relatively easy to obtain and do not require sophisticated equipment or expertise to use.
- Only small amounts of a pathogen are needed to start a contamination.
- Growing crops are openly exposed, and poultry and livestock are often raised in large numbers on farms and feedlots.
- Animals and animal foods are shipped over wide areas in short periods of time, which increases the potential of spreading a communicable disease quickly.

The Centers for Disease Control and Prevention (CDC) has assessed the vulnerability of the U.S. food supply to widespread contamination. The most important factor is the availability of disease agents and how medically dangerous they are. The CDC has classified biological agents into the following three categories of danger:

1. *Category A:* This category includes diseases with a high degree of morbidity and mortality that are easily spread throughout a population and such pathogens as *Clostridium botulinum* (botulism), neurotoxins, and anthrax.
2. *Category B:* These agents are easily disseminated but have significantly lower morbidity and mortality rates. *Salmonella, Shigella,* and *Escherichia coli* O157:H7 fall into this group.
3. *Category C:* Weaker agents such as hepatitis A and the *Cryptosporidium paramecium* are included here. Many of these agents are available in the wild or can be purchased under the guise of legitimate research.

Another important component in assessing vulnerability is the increasing centralization of the production, packaging, and distribution of food products. The extent of damage in a bioterrorist attack would depend upon the point of contamination in the supply chain and how quickly it is contained. In addition, more food is being imported from other countries, increasing the potential sources for external tampering.

Up to now, detection methods for monitoring the safety of food have been designed to protect against negligence, poor handling, and spoilage, not direct and intentional contamination. Increased surveillance and coordination is now the key to providing national and local officials with the information needed to respond quickly and contain any spread of foodborne illness. The Public Health Security and Bioterrorism Preparedness and Response Plan requires all groups and organizations involved in food safety and food handling—state and local regulatory and safety agencies and food manufacturers and sellers—to develop response, crisis communication, and public awareness strategies. Increased surveillance and faster detection methods will become part of the normal cycle of food

production and shipment. The U.S. Department of Agriculture (USDA) has offices in almost every county in the nation, and many USDA employees are first responders in their communities. The USDA in cooperation with the Food and Drug Administration (FDA) has expanded food security training for all personnel involved with the U.S. food supply.

The threat of bioterrorism is a legitimate concern for the American public. Food contamination incidents in the United States and other countries have shown that a deliberate attack on the food supply could lead to significant illness and death with implications for agriculture, the healthcare system, and the economy. Tighter security in all stages of food production and distribution, improved screening and detection of possible food contamination, increased coordination among all levels of government leading to faster and more effective responses to biological incidents, and heightened public awareness all help to mitigate the risks of bioterrorism. Although accidental and naturally occurring food-related illnesses will still occur, the chances of a successful intentional event have been greatly reduced through effective planning and concerted public effort.

References

Bruemmer B: Food biosecurity, *J Am Diet Assoc* 103(6):687, 2003.

Center for Food Safety and Applied Nutrition, U.S. Food and Drug Administration: *Public Health Security and Bioterrorism Preparedness and Response Act of 2002 (PL107-188),* Rockville, Md, 2002, Author. Retrieved December 9, 2005, from *www.cfsan.fda.gov/~dms/sec-ltr.html.*

Center for Food Safety and Applied Nutrition, U.S. Food and Drug Administration: *Risk assessment for food terrorism and other food safety concerns,* Rockville, Md, 2003, Author. Retrieved December 9, 2005, from *www.cfsan.fda.gov/~dms/rabtact.html.*

Center for Infectious Disease Research and Policy, University of Minnesota: *Agricultural biosecurity,* Minneapolis, 2005, Regents of the University of Minnesota. Available at *www.cidrap.umn.edu/cidrap/content/biosecurity/ag-biosec/index.html.* Accessed December 9, 2005.

Food Safety and Inspection Service, U.S. Department of Agriculture: *Protecting the food supply from intentional adulteration: an introductory training session to raise awareness,* Washington, DC, 2005, Author. Retrieved December 9, 2005, from *www.fsis.usda.gov/news_&_events/food_security_awareness_training/index.asp.*

Peregrin T: Bioterrorism and food safety: what nutrition professionals need to know to educate the American public, *J Am Diet Assoc* 102(1):614, 2002.

Sobel J et al: Threat of biological terrorist attack on the U.S. food supply: the CDC perspective, *Lancet* 359:874, 2002.

Sorvillo F et al: Bioterrorism. In Detels R et al, eds: *Oxford textbook of public health,* ed 4, Oxford, England, 2004, Oxford University Press.

U.S. Department of Agriculture: *Statement by Agriculture Secretary Ann M. Veneman regarding the completion of the National Response Plan,* Washington, DC, 2005 (January 6), Author. Retrieved December 9, 2005, from *www.usda.gov/wps/portal/usdahome?contentidonly=true&contentid=2005/01/0006.xml.*

U.S. Department of Homeland Security: *Department of Homeland Security Secretary Tom Ridge announces completion of the National Response Plan,* Washington, DC, 2005 (January 6), Author. Retrieved December 9, 2005, from *www.dhs.gov/dhspublic/interapp/press_release/press_release_0582.xml.*

See *Websites of Interest* on pp. 234 and 235 for further information on food safety and food bioterrorism.

FOCUS ON CULTURE

Cultural and Ethnic Differences in Health Practices

Many health beliefs and practices spring from our cultural and ethnic backgrounds. The word *health* was derived from an Anglo-Saxon word meaning wholeness, or the interaction of the mind and body in reaching a state of well-being.[1] Most cultures emphasize the melding of our physical and spiritual beings in harmony with nature as the basis of health. In contrast, healthcare in mainstream America rests on biomedicine, applying the sciences of biology, biochemistry, and physiology to the study and treatment of human diseases. Although traditional healthcare focuses on the present, biomedicine focuses on the future, relating the treatment of today to physical well-being in years to come.

The unity between physical, emotional, and psychological health is the cornerstone of traditional healthcare, often referred to as alternative medicine. These healing therapies use botanical remedies and interventions such as massage or acupuncture to rectify imbalances in physical and spiritual systems. Mind-body therapies, including prayer, relaxation, or meditation, along with plant remedies are still used to prevent or cure disease by groups favoring alternative medicine.[2] The use of these alternative methods to improve health or relieve problem conditions continues to grow as individuals assert greater responsibility over their own health.

East Asian traditional medicine is based on Ayurvedic medicine developed in ancient times. *Ayur* means "longevity," and *veda* means "knowledge of." This system of medicine uses diet, herbal remedies, and meditation to realign the mind, body, and soul. Over time Ayurvedic botanical remedies have been used to treat digestive disorders, heart problems, diabetes, and urinary tract disorders,[1] and along with other traditional plant medicines provided the foundation for many of the prescription and over-the-counter drugs commonly used today.

Many traditional home remedies making use of herbs and plants remain popular today. Teas made from the yellowroot shrub or sassafras are used to relieve stomach distress, and many families use lemon-flavored water with honey to ease the symptoms of a cold.[1] Herbal teas prepared from peppermint, chamomile, parsley, and wormwood are commonly used for diarrhea or other illnesses. Tonics made from eggnog or malt are used to stimulate the appetite or build strength in pale children or pregnant and postpartum women. Certain alternative medicines, however, can be hazardous. Medicines that contain mercury or lead and are highly toxic are sometimes brought into the United States from Mexico, and individuals need to be warned of their danger. In some cultures infants may be given honey (a source of infant botulism) to relieve digestive upset.

It is important to know not only what health strategies your patients are following, but also the basis of their attitudes and beliefs. Those individuals with the greatest risk of health problems are often less likely to use biomedical preventive measures.[3] Low-income women who could benefit from added iron or folate are not typical supplement users. Asian and Latino Americans at risk of low bone density are not encouraged to use calcium supplements. We need to develop effective approaches to working with individuals from various backgrounds, combining the strengths of both alternative medicine and biomedicine.

References

1. Kittler PG, Sucher KP: *Food and culture*, ed 4, Belmont, Calif, 2004, Brooks/Cole, a division of Thomson Learning.
2. Barnes PM et al: *Complementary and alternative medicine use among adults: United States, 2002, advance data, vital and health statistics*, No. 343, Hyattsville, Md, 2004, National Center for Health Statistics.
3. Jacti S, Siega-Riz AM, Bentley ME: Dietary supplement use in the context of health disparities: cultural, ethnic and demographic determinants of use, *J Nutr* 133:2010S, 2003.

Overview of Dietary Supplements

Dietary supplements enjoy a very favorable legal status. In 1994 Congress passed the Dietary Supplement Health and Education Act (DSHEA) which effectively deregulated the dietary supplement industry. All ingredients marketed as supplements before 1994 were assumed to be safe, as was the case for the GRAS food additives, whether or not research evidence existed to support this decision. The dietary supplement industry markets thousands of products containing vitamins, minerals, herbs, botanical compounds, Asian medicinal herbals, and related substances. Under this law supplements are legally classified as neither foods nor drugs. No scientific testing by the manufacturer to demonstrate either product safety or effectiveness of claims is required. For newer supplement ingredients developed after 1994 the safety standard is simply that there be no "unreasonable risk." The manufacturer must notify the FDA before marketing the product, but no prior FDA approval is required.

The DSHEA has been a controversial law. Dietary supplements have become a major industry with large advertising budgets and a wide range of products, from single vitamins to complex mixtures of compounds. Under the law a dietary supplement cannot claim to cure a disease; however, statements about how the human body will respond to the supplement, such as a claim that it will make you burn fat faster, are completely unregulated and require no proof. Supplements containing growth hormone and other potentially dangerous substances expected to restore youthful vitality are often marketed to older adult audiences. Steps to ensure consumer safety along with honest claims describing appropriate uses, expected effects, recommended dosage, and potential drug-herb interactions are very much needed. (See the *Focus on Culture* box, "Cultural and Ethnic Differences in Health Practices," for more information about cultural and ethnic differences in the use of supplements and alternative medicines.)

Food Safety Laws: Agricultural Practices

Agricultural Chemicals

American farmers have come to depend on various agricultural chemicals to increase crop production. Such chemicals help control destructive insects and weeds, improve seed sprouting to increase yield, prevent plant diseases, and improve market quality. But the overuse of pesticides increases residues on food and adds to the exposure of farm

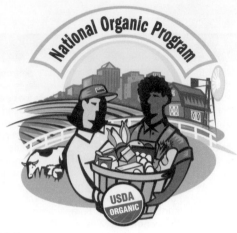

FIGURE 9-2   Seal of the National Organic Program. The U.S. Department of Agriculture has developed a certification program to enable organic farmers to label their produce as organically grown. *(From National Organic Program, Agricultural Marketing Service, U.S. Department of Agriculture: The organic seal, Washington, DC, 2002, Author. Available at* www.ams.usda.gov/nop.*)*

workers to powerful chemicals. Many universities are helping farmers reduce their use of chemical pesticides through programs called Integrated Pest Management. These programs help the environment by making use of the natural enemies of certain insect pests to reduce their population and their destruction of farm crops. The FDA has the difficult task of assessing health risks and establishing guidelines for the thousands of agricultural chemicals in development and in use.

Organic farming—which excludes the use of chemical pesticides and herbicides—is receiving increasing attention. Organic farming includes both organically grown plant foods and organically raised beef and poultry. Organic farmers, with help from soil scientists, are developing systems of sustainable agriculture that do not rely on pesticide use. Growing numbers of consumers are seeking out organically produced food. In 2002 the USDA established national standards for producers who wish to label their food as "organic." These standards govern both growing procedures and the handling of produce after it is picked, and a farmer must be certified by the USDA before a food can display the seal of the National Organic Program (Figure 9-2).[31]

Despite the trend toward food globalization, consumers are showing a growing willingness to support local farmers. A diet based on locally produced food has many advantages, both for the environment and for health: local farmland is retained, the environmental damage from food production and transport is minimized, the food supply becomes more sustainable, and exposure to foodborne contamination and illness is reduced.[32]

Food Safety Laws: Pollution and Waste

Contamination of Lakes and Oceans

The dumping of waste into rivers, lakes, and oceans by industries and local governments has raised concentrations of polychlorinated biphenyls (PCBs) and heavy metals such as

mercury in these bodies of water. In some cases these pollutants have been concentrated in fish, shellfish, or other wildlife living in or drinking these waters. State and local health departments often offer advisories to local fishermen regarding the safety or potential hazards associated with fish caught in lakes or streams within their boundaries. The FDA monitors the mercury content of ocean and farm-raised fish sold in the United States. Although fish is a valued food for the protein and n-3 fatty acids that it contains, current advisories recommend that women who are pregnant or nursing or may become pregnant limit their fish intake and choose fish low in mercury to prevent harm to their unborn child or infant (Box 9-5).[33] This advisory also applies to young children because mercury can damage the developing nervous system.

The Food Label

If people are to choose their food wisely, they must have an understanding of the nutrients they need for good health, the amounts they need, and the nutrient content of the various foods in the marketplace. Over the past 30 years the FDA, with the advice of panels of experts representing agriculture, food, nutrition, and health, has developed a framework of food labeling to help consumers understand and monitor their nutrient intake.

Early Efforts at Food Labeling

In the mid 1970s new regulations added to the FFDCA and the Fair Packaging and Labeling Act set requirements for the food label. All cans and packages had to provide general nutrition information about the food,

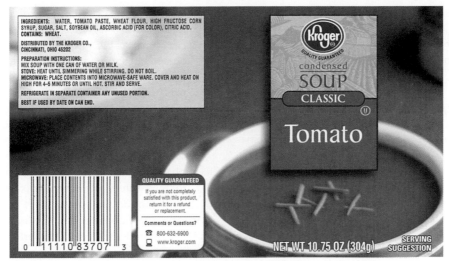

FIGURE 9-3   Example of a food label. The label on a package or container of processed food must describe the food contents, list the ingredients in descending order by weight, and provide the name and address of the producer. Notice that this label also informs the consumer that the product contains wheat—one of eight food allergens that must be clearly stated on a food label to protect individuals having this allergy. (*Courtesy of The Kroger Company, Cincinnati, OH.*)

including package weight, a list of ingredients, and the name and address of the manufacturer (Figure 9-3). Some producers voluntarily added other nutrition information to their label in response to increasing consumer demand. The goal of the label at that time was to protect consumers from *economic* risk—providing true information about food weight and ingredients—not *health* risk. But surveys indicated that consumer groups wanted access to more nutrition information including the amounts of the macronutrients (carbohydrates, fats, and protein), the total energy value (kcalories), key micronutrients (vitamins and minerals), and sodium, cholesterol, and saturated fat.

Current Food Labeling Regulations

The Nutrition Label that appears on food products is mandated by the Nutrition Labeling and Education Act of 1990 (NLEA). This law made major changes to the nutrition information available to consumers. The NLEA requires nutrition labels on all processed foods subject to enforcement by the FDA. Labeling is voluntary for fresh fruits, vegetables, and seafood, although guidelines are being developed.[34] The USDA is responsible for standards and consumer information on fresh meat, poultry, and dairy products. The label format was designed to provide descriptive information about the amount and nutrient content of the food contained, along with guidance as to the relative adequacy or suggested upper intake of those nutrients. Health claims included on the food label with the approval of FDA help consumers make choices related to health promotion and disease prevention.

Health Promotion: The Nutrition Label

The Nutrition Label has been used on food products since 1994 (Figure 9-4). The common format allows consumers to compare the nutritional value of one product with

Nutrition Facts

Serving Size: 1/2 cup (114 g)
Servings Per Container: 4

Amount per Serving	
Calories 260	
Calories from Fat 120	

	% Daily Value*
Total Fat 13 g	20%
Saturated Fat 5 g	25%
Cholesterol 30 mg	10%
Sodium 660 mg	28%
Total Carbohydrate 31 g	11%
Dietary Fiber 0 g	0%
Sugars 5 g	
Protein 5 g	

Vitamin A 4%	•	Vitamin C 1%	
Calcium 15%	•	Iron 4%	

*Percents (%) of a Daily Value are based on a 2,000 calorie diet. Your Daily Values may vary higher or lower depending on your calorie needs.

Nutrient	2,000 calories	2,500 calories
Total Fat	<65 g	<80 g
Saturated Fat	<20 g	<25 g
Cholesterol	<300 mg	<300 mg
Sodium	<2,400 mg	<2,400 mg
Total Carbohydrate	300 g	375 g
Dietary Fiber	25 g	30 g

1 g Fat = 9 calories
1 g Carbohydrate = 4 calories
1 g Protein = 4 calories

FIGURE 9-4   Example of a Nutrition Label. The Nutrition Label is designed to assist consumers in choosing a healthy diet. (*From U.S. Food and Drug Administration, Rockville, Md.*)

another. The legal definitions assigned to the terms *light* or *reduced* protect the public from inappropriate or misleading labels describing kcalorie, fat, sodium, or cholesterol content.[35] At the same time confusion about serving sizes[36] and differences between the Daily Reference Values used to describe the vitamin and mineral content on the food label and the Dietary Reference Intakes for various age-groups create problems for users.

The major components of the Nutrition Label are as follows:

- *Food amount and energy content:* The amount of food in the container is described by weight, serving size, and number of servings expected. As noted in Chapter 1, the general public does not equate standard serving sizes with the amount of food they are accustomed to eating. A food package perceived to contain two or three portions of one cup each may be labeled to contain five to six servings of one half cup each, so the actual energy intake of the consumer is double what was expected. Food manufacturers sometimes present serving sizes in a way that makes their food item appear lower in kcalories. A supersized muffin that consumers would expect to represent an individual portion may actually be labeled as containing two servings or more.

- *Macronutrient content:* Protein, carbohydrate, and fat content are listed in grams. The specific amounts of saturated fat and cholesterol must be indicated, and some processors voluntarily add the amounts of monounsaturated and polyunsaturated fats. Effective in 2006, the Nutrition Label must list the gram content of *trans* fatty acids. Total carbohydrates are also broken down into dietary fiber and sugars.

- *Vitamin and mineral content:* Sodium and four leader nutrients—vitamin A, vitamin C, calcium, and iron—are required on the Nutrition Label. For sodium the label lists the content in milligrams and as a percentage of the upper limit recommended for good health. The vitamins and minerals are given as percentages of the Daily Reference Values. Fortified foods such as cereals list the vitamins and minerals added as ingredients in the manufacturing process. The Daily Reference Values were derived from the Dietary Reference Intakes for specific use on food labels. The Daily Reference Value for each vitamin and mineral represents the highest Dietary Reference Intake among the various age and sex groups.

- *Daily Reference Values:* For most people the number of grams of fat, carbohydrate, protein, or fiber holds little meaning. To help consumers compare the per-serving content of these nutrients to current health recommendations, suggested daily intakes are related to reference diets containing 2000 or 2500 kcalories.

- *Health claims:* Health claims describe a relationship between a food or food component and a chronic disease or health-related problem.[37] Based on the scientific evidence presented for review, FDA has approved 13 health claims that may be printed on the nutrition label.[38] These approved health claims address such relationships as calcium and bone health,

fiber and heart health, and folate and neural tube defects (Table 9-1).

- *Labels for special needs:* Additional information is included on some nutrition labels to meet the needs of particular populations. Products that have been processed and packaged under the overview of a rabbi and meet Jewish dietary standards are labeled as kosher for the benefit of individuals who adhere to those standards. Beverages or other foods with added aspartame, the nonnutritive sweetener containing phenylalanine, must include a warning on the label for the safety of individuals with phenylketonuria who cannot metabolize this amino acid. The Food Allergen Labeling and Consumer Protection Act to become effective in 2006 will require food labels to indicate any content of eight major allergens known to cause life-threatening reactions, including anaphylactic shock, in allergic individuals. These include milk (casein), peanuts, tree nuts, fish, shellfish, wheat, eggs, and soybeans (see Figure 9-3 and note the presence of wheat in this product).

New products that are blurring the distinction between foods and supplements are beverages or foods to which herbs or other botanicals such as ginseng are being added. Manufacturers adding botanicals or other novel ingredients to their foods must show proof that these substances are on the GRAS list or present evidence that the intended use is safe.[39] These products claim to increase energy level and fitness, and often contain added vitamins, minerals, and amino acids.

FOOD SAFETY AND FOOD PROCESSING

Foodborne Illness

Prevalence and Causes

Foodborne illness is a serious public health problem. Many disease-bearing microorganisms inhabit our environment and can contaminate our food and water. New

---

allergens Substances that can produce a hypersensitivity reaction in the body; proteins present in milk, eggs, fish, wheat, tree nuts, peanuts, soybeans, and shellfish can result in serious and sometimes fatal reactions in allergic individuals, and the presence of any of these foods must be noted on the food label beginning in 2006.

anaphylactic shock A serious and sometimes fatal hypersensitivity reaction to a drug, food, toxin, chemical, or other allergen; the patient can experience weakness, sweating, and shortness of breath or such life-threatening responses as loss of blood pressure and shock, respiratory congestion, or cardiac arrest.

TABLE 9-1	Health Claims Approved by the FDA for Nutrition Labels*

Claim	Food Requirement	Model Statement
Calcium and osteoporosis	High in calcium	Regular exercise and a healthy diet with enough calcium helps teens and young adult white and Asian women maintain good bone health and may reduce their high risk of osteoporosis later in life.
Sodium and hypertension	Low in sodium	Diets low in sodium may reduce the risk of high blood pressure, a disease associated with many factors.
Dietary fat and cancer	Low fat	Development of cancer depends on many factors. A diet low in total fat may reduce the risk of some cancers.
Dietary saturated fat and cholesterol and risk of coronary heart disease	Low saturated fat Low cholesterol Low fat	Although many factors affect heart disease, diets low in saturated fat and cholesterol may reduce the risk of this disease.
Fiber-containing grain products, fruits, and vegetables and cancer	A grain product, fruit, or vegetable that contains dietary fiber Low fat Good source of dietary fiber without fortification	Low-fat diets rich in fiber-containing grain products, fruits, and vegetables may reduce the risk of some types of cancer, a disease associated with many factors.
Fruits, vegetables, and grain products that contain fiber, particularly soluble fiber, and risk of coronary heart disease	A fruit, vegetable, or grain product that contains fiber Low saturated fat Low cholesterol Low fat At least 0.6 g soluble fiber per serving (without fortification) Soluble fiber content provided on label	Diets low in saturated fat and cholesterol and rich in fruits, vegetables, and grain products that contain some types of dietary fiber, particularly soluble fiber, may reduce the risk of heart disease, a disease associated with many factors.
Fruits and vegetables and cancer	A fruit or vegetable Low fat Food source (without fortification) of at least one of the following: Vitamin A Vitamin C Dietary fiber	Low-fat diets rich in fruits and vegetables (foods that are low in fat and may contain dietary fiber, vitamin A, or vitamin C) may reduce the risk of some types of cancer, a disease associated with many factors. *Example:* Broccoli is high in vitamins A and C and is a good source of dietary fiber.
Folate and neural tube defects	Good source of folate (at least 40 μg per serving)	Healthful diets with adequate folate may reduce a woman's risk of having a child with a brain or spinal cord defect.
Dietary sugar alcohols and dental caries	Sugar-free Sugar alcohol must be xylitol, sorbitol, mannitol, maltitol, isomalt, lactitol, hydrogenated starch hydrolysates, hydrogenated glucose syrups, erythritol, or a combination Food must not lower plaque pH below 5.7	Frequent between-meal consumption of foods high in sugars and starches promotes tooth decay. The sugar alcohols in this food do not promote tooth decay.
Soy protein and risk of coronary heart disease	At least 6.25 g soy protein per serving Low saturated fat Low cholesterol Low fat	25 g of soy protein a day, as part of a diet low in saturated fat and cholesterol, may reduce the risk of heart disease. The grams of soy protein that can be derived from a serving varies with food.†

Modified from U.S. Food and Drug Administration: *A food labeling guide—Appendix C: Health claims,* Rockville, Md, 1994 (rev 1999, 2004), Author. Retrieved December 9, 2005, from *http://vm.cfsan.fda.gov/~dms/flg-6c.html.*

EPA, Eicosapentaenoic acid; *DHA,* docosahexaenoic acid.

*Food contains without fortification at least 10% of the Daily Value for the named vitamin, mineral, or fiber, and less than 13 g fat, 4 g saturated fat, 60 mg cholesterol, and 480 mg sodium per serving.

†Label will list the amount found in that particular food serving.

Continued

TABLE 9-1	Health Claims Approved by the FDA for Nutrition Labels*—cont'd

Claim	Food Requirement	Model Statement
Plant sterol/stanol esters and risk of coronary heart disease	At least 0.65 g plant sterol esters per serving of spreads and salad dressings *or* At least 1.7 g plant stanol esters per serving of spreads or salad dressings Low saturated fat Low cholesterol	Foods containing at least 0.65 g per serving of vegetable oil sterol esters, eaten twice a day with meals for a daily total intake of at least 1.3 g, as part of a diet low in saturated fat and cholesterol, may reduce the risk of heart disease. The grams of vegetable oil sterol esters that can be derived from a serving varies with food.†
Monounsaturated fat from olive oil and coronary heart disease	Must contain monounsaturated fat	Eating about 2 tablespoons of olive oil daily may reduce the risk of coronary heart disease due to the monounsaturated fat in olive oil. To achieve this benefit, olive oil should replace a similar amount of saturated fat and not increase the total number of calories eaten in a day. The grams of olive oil that can be derived varies with food.†
Omega-3 (n-3) fatty acids and coronary heart disease	Must contain both EPA and DHA omega-3 (n-3) fatty acids	Eating EPA and DHA omega-3 (n-3) fatty acids may reduce the risk of coronary heart disease. The grams of EPA and DHA fatty acids that can be derived from 1 serving varies with food.†
Whole grain foods and risk of heart disease and certain cancers	Contains 51% or more whole grain ingredients by weight per serving Good fiber source Low fat	Diets rich in whole grain foods and other plant foods and low in total fat, saturated fat, and cholesterol may reduce the risk of heart disease and some cancers.
Potassium and the risk of high blood pressure and stroke	Good source of potassium Low sodium Low total fat Low saturated fat Low cholesterol	Diets containing foods that are a good source of potassium and low in sodium may reduce the risk of high blood pressure and stroke.

technologies ranging from refrigerated trucks to freeze-drying to food irradiation have brought major improvements in food handling and food safety, yet Americans are still vulnerable to foodborne pathogens. According to the CDC, 76 million persons get sick, 300,000 are hospitalized, and 5000 die of foodborne illness each year.[40]

New trends in how our food is produced and how we consume it give foodborne pathogens new opportunities to enter the food chain. The worldwide distribution of fresh and processed food by large food corporations can spread foodborne illness both regionally and globally. Contemporary eating habits hold potential for food contamination. Fruits and vegetables are often eaten raw or unpeeled, and people may not take the time to wash them thoroughly. In today's fast-paced life, families eat more precooked foods, seafood salads, deli meats, and food kept warm for extended periods, as compared to cooked meals eaten immediately after being prepared.

Individuals who eat at their desk or eat in their cars while traveling may not take time to wash their hands or use a hand sanitizer, increasing their risk of infection.

Costs of Foodborne Illness

Foodborne illness has both economic and health consequences. The USDA estimates that $5.6 to $9.4 billion dollars a year are spent on medical intervention and lost productivity associated with foodborne illness.[41] Microbial foodborne illness results in acute but self-limiting symptoms—diarrhea, vomiting, and abdominal pain—and most people do not seek medical attention or require only general supportive care.[42] But for young children, older adults, and immunocompromised patients such as those with cancer, recent organ or bone marrow transplants, or autoimmune deficiency disease, foodborne pathogens can result in serious illness, septicemia, acute renal failure, or death. In pregnant women, foodborne illness can result in

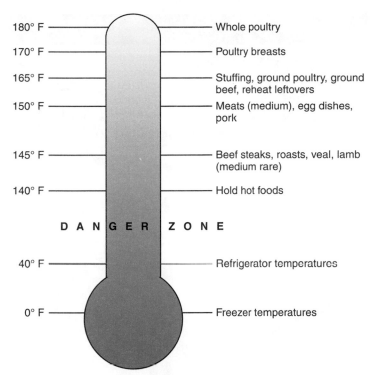

180° F —————— Whole poultry

170° F —————— Poultry breasts

165° F —————— Stuffing, ground poultry, ground beef, reheat leftovers

150° F —————— Meats (medium), egg dishes, pork

145° F —————— Beef steaks, roasts, veal, lamb (medium rare)

140° F —————— Hold hot foods

D A N G E R   Z O N E

40° F —————— Refrigerator temperatures

0° F —————— Freezer temperatures

FIGURE 9-5 Chart of food temperatures. Foods should be held at temperatures below 45° F or above 140° F to prevent microbial growth. Microorganisms grow rapidly between 45° F and 140° F. Meat and poultry products should be cooked to the internal temperature indicated above. *(From U.S. Department of Health and Human Services and U.S. Department of Agriculture:* Dietary Guidelines for Americans 2005, *ed 6, Washington, DC, 2005, Authors. Retrieved December 9, 2005, from http://www.healthierus.gov/dietaryguidelines/dga2005/document/html/chapter10.htm.)*

miscarriage. One in four Americans is likely to experience some form of foodborne illness each year,[49] although stomach distress is often attributed to other causes. Bottled water has been a cause of foodborne illness.[44]

Prevention

Sanitation Procedures

Strict sanitation practices and rigid personal hygiene are essential to prevent foodborne illness. Food and everything it touches must be scrupulously clean. Attention to final cooking temperatures and holding temperatures are particularly important in food preparation facilities serving schools, meal programs for older adults, healthcare facilities, and all programs in which food is prepared at one location and transported to other buildings or other areas in the city. Leftover food must be cooled and stored within a specific period of time (Figure 9-5) and reheated to the recommended temperature before serving. Dishwashing equipment should meet public health standards for water and drying temperatures and be used to sanitize both cooking and serving utensils. Garbage or discarded food must be removed from the food preparation area immediately. Although these guidelines are well known, they are not always practiced. Frequent hand washing and use of gloves should be required of all food handlers in public food service operations, food processing and packaging plants, public markets, or delicatessen shops. Persons with any infectious disease or hand injury, however small, should not work with food. Figure 9-6 illustrates and provides directions for proper hand washing.

Food Irradiation

Food irradiation is a technology that can extend the shelf life and increase the safety of many foods.[45] By this process food is irradiated using energy sources such as gamma rays, similar to microwaves, that pass through the food and safely kill harmful bacteria. Food does not become radioactive, and there is almost no loss of nutrients. Irradiation is used to sterilize rations for astronauts in space travel, and hospitals irradiate food for patients needing completely germ-free food, such as those with bone marrow transplants. Most of the cooking spices, herbs, and seasonings sold in the United States are irradiated. Irradiation destroys more than 99% of any *Escherichia coli* in ground meat and more than 99% of any *Salmonella* bacteria in fresh eggs and poultry.[45]

Although this technology has been proven to be both safe and effective, less than one tenth of 1% of the fruits, vegetables, meat, and poultry sold in the United States is

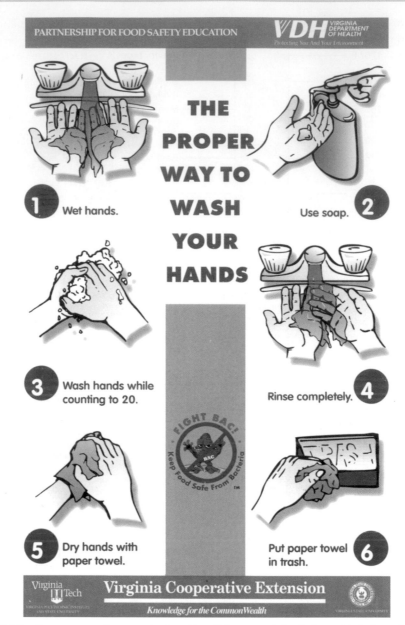

FIGURE 9-6   Six-step process for proper hand washing. Failure to wash hands thoroughly before and after food preparation and before eating is a common cause of foodborne illness. *(Courtesy Virginia Cooperative Extension, College of Agriculture and Life Sciences, Virginia Polytechnic Institute and State University, Blacksburg, Va, and Virginia Department of Health, Richmond, Va.)*

irradiated. Healthcare facilities and food service programs serving at-risk populations are the primary users of irradiated foods. Unfortunately, the sale of irradiated food has been opposed by those who erroneously believe that the food becomes radioactive and by others who are concerned that irradiation will be used to mask unsanitary processing practices.[45] Irradiation has been endorsed as safe by the American Medical Association, the American Dietetic Association, the World Health Organization, and the United Nations Food and Agriculture Organization, among others.

Forms of Foodborne Illness

Bacterial Food Infection

Bacterial food infections occur when individuals eat food contaminated with large colonies of bacteria. Specific bacteria cause specific diseases. The CDC has established an active surveillance system called *FoodNet* to monitor the incidence of foodborne illness. The FoodNet system includes 10 state and local health departments with a population base of 38 million persons.[43] Data collected from clinical laboratories and physicians document the illnesses and related complications caused by seven bacteria and two parasites of importance in food safety.

Following are descriptions of five common bacteria causing foodborne illness:

1. *Escherichia coli O157:H7:* This microorganism inhabits the intestines of animals and humans. Most types of *E. coli* are benign, and some even do nutritionally important work such as fermenting resistant starch. However, other strains such as *E. coli* O157:H7 produce toxins that cause serious disease. *E. coli* O157:H7 has emerged as a major cause of individual cases and large outbreaks of inflammatory diarrhea associated with bloody stool and fever.[40] Serious infections can result in kidney impairment or death.[41]

   E. coli O157:H7 is destroyed by heat, and most outbreaks occur from unpasteurized or undercooked foods. Cases have been reported in persons who drank unpasteurized cider made from apples that had fallen to the ground, been contaminated with animal droppings, and not thoroughly washed. A major outbreak resulted from beef that was contaminated in processing and then undercooked at a fast-food restaurant. The latter incident demonstrates that all parties across the food chain are responsible for food safety, those who process foods and those who prepare food for immediate consumption. Ground beef must be cooked to a temperature of 165° F to ensure safety against *E. coli.*

2. *Salmonella:* These bacteria were first isolated and identified by Daniel Salmon (1850-1914) and are a common cause of human foodborne infections. *Salmonella* bacteria grow quickly in high-protein foods such as milk, custard, egg dishes, and sandwich filling. Seafood, especially shellfish such as oysters and clams from polluted waters, can be a source of infection. The contamination of eggs with *Salmonella enteritidis* is a worldwide problem. Persons of all ages should avoid eating raw cookie dough, drinking unpasteurized beverages containing milk or egg, or eating poorly cooked eggs, but this is particularly important for older adults. According to the CDC 40% of deaths from *Salmonella* occur in people over the age of 65.[43] Symptoms develop slowly, usually 12 to 24 hours after ingestion, and range from mild to bloody diarrhea with fever.

3. *Campylobacter: Campylobacter* is a common cause of bacteria-related acute diarrhea in America and around the world. *Campylobacter* bacteria are found in raw and undercooked beef, poultry, and seafood; raw milk; and untreated water; they are destroyed by heating food to 160° F and appropriate water treatment. Cross-contamination of foods is a significant danger with this bacterium. One outbreak of *Campylobacter*-related illness occurred when a cutting board used for raw poultry was then used to chop lettuce without appropriate cleaning.[43] *Campylobacter* infection is also associated with the development of Guillain-Barré syndrome.

4. *Shigella:* The bacterium *Shigella* was first discovered as the cause of a dysentery epidemic in Japan in 1898. Foodborne illness arising from *Shigella* infection is usually confined to the large intestine and varies from simple cramps and diarrhea to fatal dysentery. Treatment with antibiotics may be required. Young children are at particular risk of fatal complications. *Shigella* bacteria are found in contaminated water and the intestinal tract of animals and are spread by insects and unsanitary food-handling practices. They grow rapidly in moist or protein foods such as milk, beans, tuna, and turkey. Apple cider or raw fruits and vegetables contaminated by animal droppings are sources of *Shigella* bacteria. Foods need to be washed and cooked thoroughly and chilled quickly to prevent infection.

5. *Listeria:* The bacterium *Listeria* has long been known as a major cause of infection after surgery, but only recently was *Listeria monocytogenes* linked with foodborne illness. In older adults, pregnant women, infants, or those with suppressed immune systems, the organism produces diarrhea and flulike fever and headache. Related complications such as pneumonia, sepsis, meningitis, endocarditis, and miscarriage require medical intervention. Outbreaks of *Listeria*-related illness have been traced to unpasteurized dairy products, particularly soft Mexican cheeses made with unpasteurized milk. Undercooked poultry and deli foods have been implicated in *Listeria* infections.[41] Thorough cooking and careful washing of raw fruits and vegetables are preventive measures (see the *Focus on Food Safety* box, "Do I Really Need to Wash That Melon?").

---

dysentery A general term given to a number of disorders marked by inflammation of the intestines, especially the colon, and accompanied by abdominal pain and frequent stools containing blood and mucus. The cause may be chemical irritants, bacteria, protozoa, or parasites.

sepsis Presence in the blood or other tissues of pathogenic microorganisms or their toxins; conditions associated with such pathogens.

meningitis Inflammation of the meninges, the three membranes that envelop the brain and spinal cord; the cause is a bacterial or viral infection leading to high fever, severe headache, and stiff neck or back muscles.

endocarditis Inflammation of the endocardium, the serous membrane that lines the cavities of the heart.

Bacterial Food Poisoning

Some types of foodborne illness are caused not by the ingestion of the bacteria, but by toxins produced by the bacteria before the food was eaten. These powerful toxins are ingested directly, and symptoms develop rapidly, within 1 to 6 hours after eating. The two most common types of bacterial food poisoning are staphylococcal and clostridial, as follows:

1. *Staphylococcal food poisoning: Staphylococcus aureus* is responsible for the most common form of bacterial poisoning in the United States. Symptoms come on suddenly and include severe cramping and abdominal pain with vomiting and diarrhea, accompanied by sweating, headache, and fever. In some cases there may be shock and prostration. Recovery is fairly rapid but depends on the amount of toxin ingested. A common source of contamination is an infection on the hand of a food worker, often minor or unnoticed. This bacterium grows rapidly in custard- and cream-filled bakery goods, chicken and ham salads, egg products, processed meats, cheese, and sauces, all moist foods. The toxin produces no change in the normal odor, taste, or appearance of the food, so the person eating it has no warning.

2. *Clostridial food poisoning: Clostridium perfringens* spores are in soil, water, dust, and refuse-virtually everywhere. The organism multiplies in cooked meat and meat dishes and develops its toxin in foods held for extended periods at warming or room temperatures.

As a result outbreaks can occur in food service facilities where foods are held for long periods of time following cooking. Prevention rests with thorough cooking of meat, prompt serving after cooking, and immediate refrigeration.

The toxins produced by another *Clostridium* bacterium, *Clostridium botulinum*, cause far more serious food poisoning that is often fatal. Depending on the amount of toxin consumed and the individual response, death can ensue within 24 hours. Vomiting, weakness, and dizziness are initial complaints. Progressively, the toxin irritates motor nerve cells and blocks transmission of neural impulses, causing gradual paralysis. Sudden respiratory paralysis with airway obstruction is the major cause of death. *C. botulinum* spores are found in soils throughout the world and can be carried on harvested food to the canning process. Like all clostridia, this species is anaerobic (develops in the absence of air). A relatively air-free environment can provide ideal conditions for toxin production if spores are not destroyed in the canning process. The commercial canning industry follows processing standards that eliminate the risk of botulism, but cases still result from eating foods canned at home using inappropriate methods. Boiling for 10 minutes destroys the toxin (although not the spore), so all home-canned food, no matter how well preserved, should be boiled at least 10 minutes before eating. Cases of botulism have occurred in Alaska from native food practices involving uncooked or partially cooked meats.[46]

Table 9-2 summarizes these bacterial sources of food contamination.

Viruses

Viruses from the Caliciviridae family are the leading cause of gastrointestinal upset in the United States. Although these viruses can be spread by the fecal-oral route, the CDC reports that 39% of outbreaks arise from contaminated food. Nursing homes are subject to outbreaks if healthcare workers disposing of vomitus or feces or bed linens or water glasses used by ill persons touch food or serving dishes without thoroughly washing their hands. In food service facilities illness can spread from worker to worker and on to the food. Vomiting and diarrhea resulting from calicivirus contamination usually last no more than 5 days, but the diarrhea has been known to continue for as long as 28 days.[43]

Food Safety Education

Government agencies, food industry representatives, and health organizations have joined forces to develop food safety education programs and certifications to meet the needs of consumers, food service professionals and entrepreneurs, and food processors. The FightBAC! program, an initiative of the Partnership for Food Safety Education,

---

FOCUS ON FOOD SAFETY
Do I Really Need to Wash That Melon?

We often associate foodborne illness with improperly cooked ground meat or poultry or deli foods left to stand at room temperature, but 25% of reported cases of foodborne illness are caused by vegetables and fruits. Produce can become contaminated with *Escherichia coli* O157:H7, *Salmonella*, or *Cyclospora* through contact with animals, fertilizers containing animal waste, contaminated irrigation water, or poor sanitation practices of workers who pick or sort fresh produce.

Following are safety tips for washing fresh fruits and vegetables:

- *Rinse raw produce under running water*, even if you are not going to eat the skin or rind. Any bacteria on the outer surface that are not removed will be transferred to your hands or to the knife as you peel or cut, and then to the food itself. Rub firm-skinned fruits and vegetables or scrub with a small vegetable brush to remove surface dirt.
- *Remove and discard the outermost leaves* of a head of lettuce or cabbage. Wash each lettuce leaf under running water. Scrub melons thoroughly. Do not clean by dipping the entire head of lettuce or melon in water. You may just be rinsing the item in contaminated water.
- *Store fruits and vegetables in the refrigerator within 2 hours of peeling or cutting.* Be especially careful with cut melon. Melons are low in acid as compared to oranges, apples, or pineapple, and this allows more rapid growth of bacteria on cut surfaces when the melon stands at room temperature.

TABLE 9-2	Selected Examples of Bacterial Foodborne Disease

Foodborne Disease	Causative Organisms (Genus and Species)	Food Source	Symptoms and Course
Bacterial Food Infections			
Salmonellosis	*Salmonella* *S. typhi* *S. paratyphi*	Milk, custards, egg dishes, salad dressings, sandwich fillings, polluted shellfish	Mild to severe diarrhea, cramps, vomiting; appears ≥12-24 hr after eating; lasts 1-7 days
Shigellosis	*Shigella* *S. dysenteriae*	Milk and milk products, seafood, salads	Mild diarrhea to fatal dysentery (especially in young children); appears 7-36 hr after eating; lasts 3-14 days
Listeriosis	*Listeria* *L. monocytogenes*	Soft cheese, poultry, seafood, raw milk, meat products (pâté)	Severe diarrhea, fever, headache, pneumonia, meningitis, endocarditis; can cause miscarriage in pregnant women; symptoms begin after 3-21 days
Bacterial Food Poisoning			
Enterotoxins			
Staphylococcal	*Staphylococcus* *S. aureus*	Custards, cream fillings, processed meats, ham, cheese, ice cream, potato salad, sauces, casseroles	Severe abdominal pain, cramps, vomiting, diarrhea, perspiration, headache, fever, prostration; appears suddenly 1-6 hr after eating; symptoms subside generally within 24 hr

Clostridial
  Perfringens enteritis
  Botulism
	Clostridium
	C. perfringens
	C. botulinum
		Cooked meats, meat dishes held at warm or room temperature
		Improperly home-canned foods; smoked and salted fish, ham, sausage, shellfish
			Mild diarrhea, vomiting; appears 8-24 hr after eating; lasts ≤1 day
			Symptoms range from mild discomfort to death within 24 hr; initial nausea, vomiting, weakness, dizziness, progressing to motor and sometimes fatal breathing paralysis

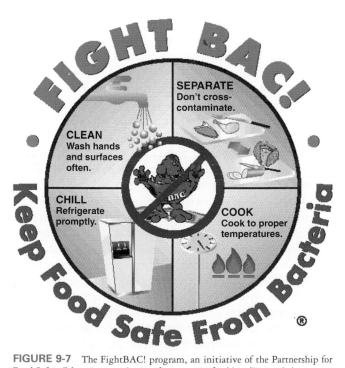

FIGURE 9-7   The FightBAC! program, an initiative of the Partnership for Food Safety Education, emphasizes four steps in food handling to help prevent foodborne illness: (1) clean, (2) separate, (3) cook, and (4) chill. (*Courtesy Partnership for Food Safety Education, Washington, DC. Available at www.fightbac.org/graphics.cfm.*)

offers lessons and publicity materials on their website for both consumers and professionals (Figure 9-7). Fight-BAC! contains food safety messages useful to teachers, nutritionists, nurses, or food service managers working with children or adults. The National Restaurant Association Foundation offers a 16-hour national certification program called *ServSafe* designed for restaurant managers, school food service managers, day care operators, and food managers in healthcare facilities such as hospitals, nursing homes, and rehabilitation centers. Many state public health departments require all food service managers to have the ServSafe certification or equivalent. Training and certification in the HAACP program mentioned earlier is available to food processors through government and university training programs.

Commercial Food Processing

Processing Methods

As consumers continue to expect fast and convenient foods to feed their families, food processors have sought

prostration Extreme exhaustion.

new methods of food preservation and packaging to meet this demand. Several of the methods that commercial processors use are similar to those that consumers use to keep their food safe. At the same time food scientists are always looking for new ways of packaging and controlling the environment of foods to maintain freshness and flavor and prohibit microbial growth. Following is a list of some common methods used to preserve and process food:

- *Application of heat:* Cooking procedures used routinely in the home soften food for chewing, increase food palatability, and prepare food for digestion. Heat is also an important means of ensuring food safety in both home and industry processing. Most bacteria are killed at temperatures of 180° to 200° F, although high-acid foods require less heat.[47] Heat also inactivates enzymes that promote the deterioration of foods such as fruits and vegetables. This is why vegetables are first blanched in boiling water to prevent further enzyme activity before being frozen.

- *Maintaining a cold temperature:* Microbial activity slows at temperatures below 50° F; thus refrigeration at 45° F or lower will preserve food for a limited period of time.[47] Freezing also protects against microbial growth and destroys some but not all microorganisms. Because certain bacteria remain alive although dormant, it is important not to refreeze food that has been thawed for some time, allowing microorganisms to begin to multiply. Cold temperatures will decrease but not eliminate enzyme activity in food.

- *Removal of moisture:* Drying reduces the water activity in a food. Foods dried at high temperatures, such as ready-to-eat cereals, and foods that are frozen and then dried retain more flavor and color. Drying a food removes the water from any microorganisms that are present and prevents their growth. The removal of water from a food also slows or prevents enzyme activity.

- *Addition of acid, sugar, salt, or chemical additives:* Foods that contain more acid and are lower in pH are more resistant to the growth of bacteria and require a shorter period of heat treatment to destroy any microorganisms present. Before the era of refrigeration, people used fermentation and the production of acid to turn highly perishable milk into yogurt or cheese that could be safely stored for a longer period. The addition of salt or sugar to a food controls the growth of bacteria by removing the water from any microorganisms that may be present. For example, the high sugar content of jams prevents spoilage. Chemical additives such as sodium benzoate or calcium propionate are added to bread to retard the growth of bacteria and mold and increase its shelf life. All of these substances also slow any enzyme activity.

- *Change in atmosphere:* A newer method of food preservation involves changing the atmosphere—that is, removing the oxygen needed for bacterial growth and enzyme activity and replacing it with carbon dioxide or nitrogen to slow these activities. Modified atmosphere packaging is used for ready-to-eat chicken pieces and other highly perishable protein foods.

Use of Chemical Additives

The use of chemical additives continues to expand as consumers demand new flavors, increased shelf life, and improved textures as part of their food. Additives enrich food with nutrients, provide color, standardize functional factors such as thickening, and improve flavor and texture. Table 9-3 lists some examples of food additives. Various micronutrients and antioxidants are being added to processed foods, not to increase their nutrient content, but to enhance shelf life by preventing undesirable oxidation reactions or similar changes.

Nutritional Aspects of Food Processing

An ongoing concern of health professionals is the effect of food processing on nutrient content. In general carbohydrates, fats, proteins, and minerals are the least affected by food processing; vitamins are the most likely to be destroyed or lost. However, the characteristics of the food and the methods used to preserve or process it greatly influence the stability or loss of important nutrients. Effects on various nutrients are detailed in the following list:

- *Macronutrients:* The major nutritional consequence of food processing for carbohydrates and proteins is the Maillard reaction or browning reaction that takes place between sugars and amino acids at high temperatures. The browning reaction occurs in normal baking, forming new sugar–amino acid compounds that cannot be digested or absorbed. The indispensable amino acid lysine enters into the browning reaction, resulting in some loss of this important amino acid. However, cereals and baked products are not important sources of this nutrient. Hydrogenation of liquid oils to produce solid table fats forms *trans* fatty acids that have negative effects on health. (See Chapter 3 to review fat hydrogenation.)

- *Minerals:* The major loss of minerals occurs in the refining of cereal grains. When the germ and bran portion of wheat and other grains is removed to produce a finer-textured flour or cereal, iron along with other trace minerals, including zinc, chromium, and manganese, is lost. Under current food enrichment regulations, iron is added back to refined cereals, although these other important minerals are not. In general mineral content and bioavailability is retained by most other processing methods.

- *Vitamins:* No vitamin is completely stable to food processing, although losses vary from one vitamin to another. Niacin is generally resistant to loss, whereas

TABLE 9-3	Examples of International Food Additives

Function	Chemical Compounds	Common Food Uses
Acids, alkalis, buffers	Sodium bicarbonate	Baking powder
	Tartaric acid	Fruit sherbets
		Cheese spreads
Antibiotics	Chlortetracycline	Dip for dressed poultry
Anticaking agents	Aluminum calcium silicate	Table salt
Antimycotics	Calcium propionate	Bread
	Sodium propionate	Bread
	Sorbic acid	Cheese
Antioxidants	Butylated hydroxyanisole (BHA)	Fats
	Butylated hydroxytoluene (BHT)	Fats
Bleaching agents	Benzoyl peroxide	Wheat flour
	Chlorine dioxide	
	Oxides of nitrogen	
Color preservative	Sodium benzoate	Green peas
		Maraschino cherries
Coloring agents	Annatto	Butter, margarine
	Carotene	
Emulsifiers	Lecithin	Bakery goods
	Monoglycerides, diglycerides	Dairy products
	Propylene glycol alginate	Confections
Flavoring agents	Amyl acetate	Soft drinks
	Benzaldehyde	Bakery goods
	Methyl salicylate	Candy, ice cream
	Essential oils, natural extracts	
	Monosodium glutamate	Canned meats
Nonnutritive sweeteners	Saccharin	Diet-packed canned fruit
	Aspartame	Low-kcalorie soft drinks and other beverages
	Sucralose	Baked goods and other sweets
Nutrient supplements	Potassium iodide	Iodized salt
	Vitamin C	Fruit juices and fruit drinks
	Vitamin D	Fruit juices, fruit drinks, and milk
	Vitamin A	Milk and margarine
	B vitamins and folate	Bread and cereal
	Iron	Bread and cereal
	Calcium	Bread, cereal, fruit juices and fruit drinks
Sequestrants	Sodium citrate	Dairy products
	Calcium pyrophosphoric acid	
Stabilizers and thickeners	Pectin	Jelly
	Vegetable gums (carob bean, carrageenan, guar)	Dairy desserts and chocolate milk
	Gelatin	Confections
	Agar-agar	Low-kcalorie salad dressings
Yeast foods and dough conditioners	Ammonium chloride	Bread and rolls
	Calcium sulfate	
	Calcium phosphate	

vitamin B_{12} is rather unstable. Various factors influence vitamin losses (Box 9-6). Vitamins are lost naturally during the storage of fruits and vegetables, and heat processing adds to losses in some foods. Certain synthetic forms of vitamins are more stable than the naturally occurring form, as is the case for vitamin E, but in general, factors affecting vitamin losses influence all forms of a particular vitamin.[48]

• *Fat-soluble vitamins:* Vitamin A is relatively stable to heat. Rather small amounts of vitamin A are lost in

BOX 9-6	Factors Affecting Vitamin Losses in Food Processing

- Temperature (losses increase at very high and very low temperatures)
- Moisture (low moisture content increases losses)
- Oxygen (presence of oxygen increases losses)
- Light (increases losses of photosensitive vitamins)
- pH (certain vitamins are more stable in acid)
- Presence of certain minerals (iron and copper increase oxidation of vitamins)

Data from Henry CJK, Chapman C, eds: *The nutrition handbook for food processors,* Boca Raton, Fla, 2002, CRC Press.

milk pasteurization, but holding milk at high temperatures for long periods increases losses. Beta carotene is more likely to be lost in normal cooking of fruits and vegetables than some other carotenoids. Vitamin E in oils is not usually lost in heat treatment or frying, but is rapidly destroyed at freezing temperatures. Naturally occurring vitamin D is not harmed by heat, but must be protected from light and atmospheric oxygen.[48]

- *Water-soluble vitamins:* Thiamin is destroyed by heat, and losses occur in baking and in foods cooked in an alkaline medium. Light is extremely destructive to riboflavin, although it withstands the heat treatment and pasteurization of milk. It is important that riboflavin-containing foods be stored in opaque containers. Niacin and pantothenic acid are generally stable in all foods. Folate is lost through exposure to light, and heating vegetables to high temperatures in large amounts of water result in serious losses. Pyridoxine is sensitive to light, and losses occur in both cooking and canning of vegetables. Long exposure to heat or hot storage causes the destruction of ascorbic acid. It is best that vitamin C–containing beverages and foods be packaged with no head space, because the presence of oxygen leads to serious losses over time.[48]

Food processing, whether general cooking procedures in the home or large-scale commercial food manufacturing, often leads to some degree of nutrient loss. As foods are refined, with removal of the bran or germ or peel, both nutrients and fiber are left behind. Extended cooking times, elevated temperatures, and the reduction of a natural food into smaller and smaller pieces, increasing surface area, exert a toll on nutritional quality. Choosing whole grains and fresh or frozen fruits and vegetables more of the time and avoiding items processed with the addition of large amounts of sodium and other additives improves nutrient intake and health.

TO SUM UP

Food habits evolve from a social perspective. As our society changes, so do our food patterns. More women are employed outside the home, more persons are living alone, and more meals are eaten away from home. We also are more conscious of nutrition and health. At the same time, however, fast food and convenience meals have become the norm in many families. As more of our food comes from farmers and processors around the world, the risk of food contamination and threat of foodborne illness grow in importance. In the United States two government agencies, the FDA (Food and Drug Administration) and the USDA (U.S. Department of Agriculture), carry major responsibility for maintaining a safe and wholesome food supply. Although the USDA oversees meat, poultry, and dairy processing, the FDA regulates the processing, labeling, and formulation of other foods, including genetically modified foods. Food labels including the nutrition label help consumers select food to maximize their nutrient intake but limit kcalories, sodium, and fat. The CDC (Center for Disease Control and Prevention) monitors the incidence of foodborne illness and provides public education to promote safe food-handling practices. Health professionals need to monitor not only the food preservation methods used in commercial food processing, but also their effects on food nutrient content.

QUESTIONS FOR REVIEW

1. What are some social and psychologic factors that influence our food habits? Using your own experience, give an example of a family custom or special observance that involves food.
2. What influences the acceptance of food misinformation? Name several groups that are highly vulnerable to nutrition or health fraud and explain why.
3. You have been asked to prepare a 15-minute lesson on how to evaluate dietary supplements for a group of senior citizens. Visit the Dietary Supplement Education section on the website of the Food and Drug Administration and the Center for Food Safety and Applied Nutrition (*www.cfsan. fda.gov/~dms/supplmnt.html* [perform a search on "supplements" on the home page of the FDA]). Select appropriate information, and develop an outline for your talk. Review the brochures available on the website, and choose one that would be suitable for the senior audience.
4. A pregnant mother who is trying to eat more fish to obtain a good supply of n-3 fatty acids read a newspaper article indicating that all ocean fish are contaminated with mercury. She is concerned about the safety of her baby and asks your advice. Review the current advisory of the Food and Drug Administration (*www.fda.gov*) regarding the consumption of fish by pregnant women. What would you tell her? Develop some practical menu suggestions that might be helpful.

5. You are working with a day care provider to develop a food safety program for her facility. Develop a list of 10 guidelines for the staff that will help to reduce the risk of foodborne illness among the children and the staff. (Visit the FightBAC! website at *http://www.fightbac.org/main.cfm* for some good ideas.)

6. Select a type of frozen entree, and review the nutrition labels for five examples of that product. Make a table that lists the number of servings; kcalories per serving; grams of protein, fat, and fiber; milligrams of sodium; and Daily Value for calcium, iron, vitamin A, and vitamin C. Compare the relative merits and disadvantages of each. Which is the best choice based on its contribution of protein, fiber, and vitamins and minerals? Which is the poorest choice in terms of fat, kcalories, and sodium?

7. Name five different methods of food preservation used in food processing. Which methods destroy harmful bacteria, and which methods merely retard their growth? What are the appropriate storage conditions for food preserved by each of these methods?

8. What is the difference between a bacterial infection and illness arising from a bacterial toxin? Give an example of each type of foodborne illness and the microorganism involved. Name the population groups that are the most vulnerable to foodborne illness. What types of food are most subject to the growth of bacteria?

REFERENCES

1. Kittler PG, Sucher KP: *Food and culture,* ed 4, Belmont, Calif, 2004, Brooks/Cole, a division of Thomson Learning.

2. Kittler PG, Sucher KP: *Food and culture in America,* ed 2, New York, 1998, The West Group.

3. Counihan C, Van Esterik P: *Food and culture: a reader,* New York, 1997, Routledge.

4. Belasco W, Scranton P: *Food nations: selling taste in consumer societies,* New York, 2002, Routledge.

5. Maslow AH: *Motivation and personality,* New York, 1954, Harper & Row.

6. Economic Research Service, U.S. Department of Agriculture: *Briefing room: Food cpi, prices, and expenditures—food and alcoholic beverages: total expenditures,* Washington, DC, 2005, Authors. Retrieved December 9, 2005, from *www.ers.usda.gov/Briefing/CPI-FoodAndExpenditures/Data/table1.htm.*

7. Federal Interagency Forum on Aging-Related Statistics: *Older Americans 2004: key indicators of well-being,* Washington, DC, 2004 (November), Author.

8. Sloan AE: Top 10 global food trends, *Food Technol* 59(4):20, 2005.

9. Schlosser E: *Fast food nation: the dark side of the all-American meal,* New York, 2002, Perennial (Imprint of HarperCollins Publisher).

10. Neumark-Sztainer D et al: Family meal patterns: associations with sociodemographic characteristics and improved dietary intake among adolescents, *J Am Diet Assoc* 103:317, 2003.

11. Eisenberg ME et al: Correlations between family meals and psychosocial well-being among adolescents, *Arch Pediatr Adolesc Med* 158(8):792, 2004.

12. Neumark-Sztainer D et al: Are family meal patterns associated with disordered eating behaviors among adolescents, *J Adolesc Health* 35:350, 2004.

13. Lewandowski J: Grocery goes gourmet, *Grocery Headquarters* 70(8):18, 2004.

14. Heller A: Ethnic allure, *Supermarket News* 53(61):16, 2005.

15. Radimer K et al: Dietary supplement use by U.S. adults: data from the National Health and Nutrition Examination Survey, 1999-2000, *Am J Epidemiol* 160:339, 2004.

16. Fogg-Johnson N, Merolli A: Food biotechnology: nutritional considerations. In Bowman BA, Russell RM, eds: *Present knowledge in nutrition,* ed 8, Washington, DC, 2001, ILSI Press.

17. Barbano D: *BST fact sheet,* Rockville, Md/Ithaca, NY, FDA Prime Connection, Center for Food Safety and Applied Nutrition, U.S. Food and Drug Administration/Cornell University Department of Food Science. Retrieved December 9, 2005, from *www.cfsan.fda.gov/~ear/CORBST.html.*

18. Center for Veterinary Medicine, U.S. Food and Drug Administration, U.S. Department of Health and Human Services: *Report on the Food and Drug Administration's review of the safety of recombinant bovine somatotropin,* Rockville, Md, 1993, Authors. Retrieved December 9, 2005, from *www.fda.gov/cvm/RBRPTFNL.htm.*

19. International Food Information Council Foundation: The myth of zero: the elusive goals of absolute safety and guaranteed benefits, *Food Insight,* p 1, Nov/Dec 2004.

20. Wilkins J: Fact or fishberry? Answering consumer questions about genetically engineered foods, *ADA Times* 2(4):5, 2005.

21. Goldstein DA, Thomas JA: Biopharmaceuticals derived from genetically modified plants, *QJM* 97:705, 2004.

22. Azevedo JL, Araujo WL: Genetically modified crops: environmental and human health concerns, *Mutat Res* 544:223, 2003.

23. Maryanski JH: *Safety assurance of foods derived by modern biotechnology in the United States,* Rockville, Md, 1996, Center for Food Safety and Applied Nutrition, U.S. Food and Drug Administration, U.S. Department of Health and Human Services. Retrieved December 9, 2005, from *www.cfsan.fda.gov/~lrd/biojap96.html.*

24. Formanek R Jr: Proposed rules issued for bioengineered foods, *FDA Consumer,* p 1, Mar/Apr 2001. Retrieved December 9, 2005, from *www.fda.gov/fdac/features/2001/201_food.html.*

25. Davies WP: An historical perspective from the green revolution to the gene revolution, *Nutr Rev* 61(suppl 6):S124, 2003.

26. Lehrer SB, Bannon GA: Risks of allergic reactions to biotech proteins in foods: perception and reality, *Allergy* 60:559, 2005.

27. Malarkey T: Human health concerns with GM crops, *Mutat Res* 544:217, 2003.

28. Board on Agriculture and Natural Resources: *Safety of genetically engineered foods: approaches to assessing unintended health effects,* Washington, DC, 2004, National Academies Press.

29. Hampton T: Prevent genetically modified organisms from escaping into nature, report urges, *JAMA* 291(9):1055, 2004.

30. U.S. Food and Drug Administration, U.S. Department of Health and Human Services: *FDA's growing responsibilities for the year 2001 and beyond,* Rockville, Md, 2001, Author. Retrieved December 9, 2005, from *www.fda.gov/oc/opacom/budgetbro/budgetbro.html.*

31. U.S. Department of Agriculture: *The National Organic Program,* Washington, DC, Author. Available at *www.ams.usda.gov/nop.* Accessed December 9, 2005.

32. American Dietetic Association: Position of the American Dietetic Association: dietetics professionals can implement practices to conserve natural resources and protect the environment, *J Am Diet Assoc* 101:1221, 2001.

33. U.S. Department of Health and Human Services and U.S. Environmental Protection Agency: Backgrounder for the 2004 FDA/EPA consumer advisory: *What you need to know about mercury in fish and shellfish,* Washington, DC, 2004, Authors. Retrieved December 9, 2005, from *www.cfsan.fda.gov/~dms/admehg3b.html.*

34. U.S. Food and Drug Administration: Food labeling: guidelines for voluntary nutrition labeling of raw fruits, vegetables, and fish—identification of the 20 most frequently consumed raw fruits, vegetables, and fish: reopening of the comment period, *Fed Reg* 70(63):16995, 2005.

35. Center for Food Safety and Applied Nutrition, U.S. Food and Drug Administration: *A food labeling guide*—Appendix A: Definitions of nutrient content claims, Rockville, Md, 1994 (rev 1999, 2004), Author. Retrieved December 9, 2005, from *www.cfsan.fda.gov/~dms/flg-6a.html.*

36. Seligson FH: Serving size standards: can they be harmonized, *Nutr Today* 38(6):247, 2003.

37. Center for Food Safety and Applied Nutrition, U.S. Food and Drug Administration: *Claims that can be made for conventional foods and dietary supplements,* Rockville, Md, 2001 (rev 2003), Author. Retrieved December 9, 2005, from *http://www.cfsan.fda.gov/~dms/hclaims.html.*

38. Center for Food Safety and Applied Nutrition, U.S. Food and Drug Administration: *A food labeling guide*—Appendix C: Health claims, Rockville, Md, 1994 (rev 1999, 2004), Author. Retrieved December 9, 2005, from *www.cfsan.fda.gov/~dms/flg-6c.html.*

39. U.S. Food and Drug Administration: FDA issues letter to industry on foods containing botanical and other novel ingredients, *FDA Talk Paper,* p 1, Feb 5, 2001. Retrieved December 9, 2005, from *www.cfsan.fda.gov/~lrd/tpnovel.html.*

40. Foodborne Illness Primer Work Group: Foodborne illness primer for physicians and other health care professionals, *Nutr Clin Care* 7:134, 2004.

41. Hemminger J: *Food safety: a guide to what you really need to know,* Ames, 2000, Iowa State University Press.

42. Walls I: Microbial food-borne diseases, *Nutr Clin Care* 7:131, 2004.

43. McCabe-Sellers BJ, Beattie SE: Food safety: emerging trends in foodborne illness surveillance and prevention, *J Am Diet Assoc* 104:1708, 2004.

44. American Dietetic Association: Position of the American Dietetic Association: food and water safety, *J Am Diet Assoc* 103:1203, 2003.

45. Parnes RB, Lichtenstein AH: Food irradiation: a safe and useful technology, *Nutr Clin Care* 7:149, 2004.

46. Cody MM, Kunkel ME: *Food safety for professionals,* ed 2, Chicago, 2002, American Dietetic Association.

47. Parker R: *Introduction to food science,* Albany, NY, 2003, Delmar/Thomson Learning.

48. Henry CK, Chapman C, eds: *The nutrition handbook for food processors,* Boca Raton, Fla, 2002, CRC Press.

FURTHER READINGS AND RESOURCES

Readings

American Dietetic Association: Position of the American Dietetic Association: food and water safety, *J Am Diet Assoc* 103:1203, 2003.
This article describes how all healthcare professionals must work together to ensure a safe food and water supply. A current list of food safety education resources for professionals is also provided.

Foodborne Illness Primer Work Group: Foodborne illness primer for physicians and other health care professionals, *Nutr Clin Care* 7:134, 2004.
This work group has prepared an overview of foodborne illness as it relates to the health and well-being of patients. It alerts us to the symptoms and causes of foodborne illness that should be included in food safety education with individuals and community groups.

Neumark-Sztainer D et al: Family meal patterns: associations with sociodemographic characteristics and improved dietary intake among adolescents, *J Am Diet Assoc* 103:317, 2003.

Eisenberg ME et al: Correlations between family meals and psychosocial well-being among adolescents, *Arch Pediatr Adolesc Med* 158(8):792, 2004.

Neumark-Sztainer D et al: Are family meal patterns associated with disordered eating behaviors among adolescents, *J Adolesc Health* 35:350, 2004.
This series of articles by Dr. Neumark-Sztainer and her co-workers point to the importance of family meals in supporting nutrient intake, the development of appropriate eating patterns, and psychological and physical well-being among children and adolescents. These findings can help us reinforce with parents and caregivers why their families should plan meals together.

Seligson FH: Serving size standards: can they be harmonized? *Nutr Today* 38(6):247, 2003.
This author points out some of the problems associated with serving sizes on labels and how we can help consumers resolve this confusion.

Websites of Interest

Food Product Labeling, Food Advertising, and Genetically Engineered Foods

- The Public Issues Education Project of Cornell University Cooperative Extension; this website contains consumer information about genetically engineered organisms and their regulation and safety: *www.geo-pie.cornell.edu.*

- Center for Food Safety and Applied Nutrition, U.S. Food and Drug Administration; this website is an excellent source of information on food labeling, food safety, and harmful foods or drugs being removed from the market: *www.cfsan.fda.gov/list.htm.*

- National Institutes of Health, U.S. Department of Health and Human Services; this website provides guidelines to assist consumers in evaluating advertisements for food and health products and selecting reputable websites and other sources of health information: *http://health.nih.gov/result.asp?disease_id=1107&terms=health.*

- International Food Information Council; this website provides information on food labeling, food additives, and food ingredients of interest to the consumer: *http://ific.org/.*

- FightBAC!, Partnership for Food Safety Education; many consumer food safety materials for adults, children, and food service workers are available on this website: *www.fightbac.org/main.cfm.*

Food Safety and Bioterrorism

- EDEN-Extension Disaster Education Network; the EDEN website links USDA Extension educators from across the United States and various disciplines, enabling them to use and share resources to reduce the impact of disasters. The site is managed by Louisiana State University and funded by the USDA: *www.agctr.lsu.edu/eden/.*

- U.S. Department of Agriculture—Homeland Security Home Page; this site is the starting place for news and information about numerous USDA programs and activities, with links to detailed websites related to food and agriculture security: *www.usda.gov/homelandsecurity/.*

- Food Safety and Inspection Service of the U.S. Department of Agriculture—Food Security and Emergency Preparedness; this site presents what the Department of Agriculture is doing to keep the public food supply safe and offers information on how families can be prepared and protected in the event of either a natural disaster or an intentional attack: *www.fsis.usda.gov/food_security_&_emergency_preparedness/index.asp.*
- Center for Food Safety and Applied Nutrition (CFSAN) of the U.S. Food and Drug Administration; this website is the FDA's main portal for news, information, and links to all programs, regulations, and documents relating to food and food safety and is an excellent starting point for learning in depth about food safety: *www.cfsan.fda.gov/.*
- FoodSafety.gov—Gateway to Government Food Safety Information for all aspects of food safety, including how consumers can report contaminated food and foodborne illnesses to local health officials: *www.foodsafety.gov/.*

CHAPTER 10

Family Nutrition Counseling: Food Needs and Costs

Eleanor D. Schlenker

This chapter continues our sequence on food habits and family nutrition counseling that introduced our study of Community Nutrition and the Life Cycle. In Chapter 9 we looked at the food environment that influences and shapes our food habits. Here we continue with family counseling and educational approaches to nutrition problems, often in the face of economic difficulties. Knowledge of the ecology of the food environment and the malnutrition that exists in many settings provides a context for sensitive counseling.

In our clinics and communities we must interpret complex information to assist families in meeting their health and nutritional needs. In this chapter we seek approaches and resources to help make this possible.

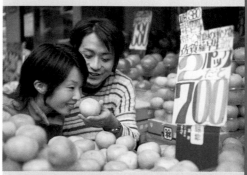

Copyright 2006 JupiterImages Corporation.

FAMILY NUTRITION COUNSELING

Community health and nutrition professionals apply the principles of health education in family nutrition counseling. Health and nutrition are inseparable, and the term *counseling* is appropriate. The skilled nutrition counselor helps family members explore their situation, express their needs, and meet those needs in ways that are best suited to their particular circumstances and goals. Societies shape their own patterns of disease, and economic and demographic factors largely influence health at all ages.[1,2] Nutrition counselors must come to understand the diet patterns of people from many different ethnic and national backgrounds and recognize the difficulties they may face in acculturation to a new environment.[3] Our job is to help families explore their options and make decisions based on appropriate information and personal support.

Person-Centered Goals

Family counseling must be person-centered. It involves close attention to personal and family needs, nutrition and health problems, and food choices and costs. The nutrition counselor has the following three main goals:

1. To obtain information about the individual or family as related to nutritional and health needs
2. To provide the knowledge and practical skills to help meet those needs
3. To support the individual or family with encouragement, caring, reinforcement, and referral

The Dietary Interview

All healthcare professionals should develop the ability to put clients at ease and discuss their problems in a helpful manner. In some situations the dietary interview is a formal or structured history taking, but a more common application is a purposeful, planned conversation in the hospital, clinic, community center, or home. It may be a simple telephone call to determine ongoing needs or progress. The following are four general principles that guide the interview:

1. The purpose or goal for the interview
2. What is needed to achieve the goal
3. How these actions will be accomplished
4. How outcomes or success will be measured

Purpose or Goal

The focus of all healthcare is the individual client and his or her personal health needs. This need may be a short-term or intermediate goal relating to some aspect of overall care or a long-term goal. An example of an intermediate goal might be learning to choose foods lower in sodium.

The long-term goal could include overall diet planning and weight management to control blood pressure. Our purpose is to help evaluate needs, set goals, and suggest practical ways to meet those goals.

Building a Foundation

The personal qualities of the interviewer and the social environment that she or he creates are critical to success or failure. Early in the process the nutrition counselor must provide a foundation for future communication by building a helping relationship, creating a comfortable climate, and developing positive attitudes, as follows:

1. *Building a relationship:* Counseling is a dynamic and person-centered process rooted in a helping relationship. The first step in offering help is establishing a relationship of mutual trust and respect. Within such a relationship, true healing can take place. The most significant tool we have for helping others is ourselves. Our role is that of a helping vehicle.
2. *Creating a climate:* The counseling climate is influenced by both the approach of the counselor and the physical setting. The physical setting should be as comfortable as possible as to space, ventilation, heating, lighting, and physical position. It is important to allow sufficient time for the interview in a quiet setting free from interruption and with the privacy needed to ensure confidentiality. In an office setting the desk should be to the side, not between the counselor and client (Figure 10-1).
3. *Developing positive attitudes:* The word *attitude* refers to that aspect of personality leading to a consistent behavior toward persons, situations, or objects. Our attitudes are learned and develop from life experiences and influences. Because they are learned, they can be examined, and we can become more aware of them.

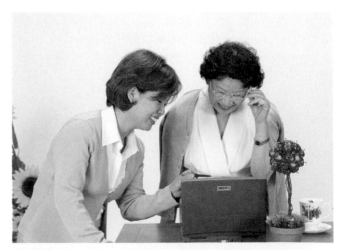

FIGURE 10-1 Sitting at a table with your client in a quiet place provides a friendly setting for communication. Online nutrition education materials can be helpful in nutrition counseling. *(Copyright 2006 JupiterImages Corporation.)*

We can strengthen those attitudes that are desirable and constructive and try to change or modify those attitudes that are less desirable or more destructive. For a healthcare professional, certain attitudes are essential, as follows:

- *Warmth:* A genuine concern displayed by interest, friendliness, and kindness; we convey warmth by being thoughtful.
- *Acceptance:* Meeting people as they are and where they are. Acceptance does not mean approval of behavior. It does carry the realization that individuals usually regard their behavior as purposeful and meaningful or act in a certain manner as a way of handling stress. An attitude of acceptance conveys that a person's thoughts, ideas, and actions are important and worth attention simply because he or she has the right to be treated as having personal worth and dignity.
- *Objectivity:* To be objective is to be nonjudgmental and free of bias. Although complete objectivity may not be possible, reasonable objectivity is an attainable goal. We must be aware of our own feelings and biases and attempt to control them. Our evaluation of a situation must be based on what is actually happening, that is, the facts as we perceive them, not on opinions, assumptions, or inferences.
- *Compassion:* Compassion enables us to feel with and for another person. It means accepting the impact of an emotion, holding it long enough to absorb its meaning, and entering into a kind of fellowship of feeling with the person who expressed it. It is not easy to develop compassion; it requires emotional maturity.

Steps in the Counseling Process

Nutrition counseling can have many different goals or purposes depending upon the audience. In a clinical setting it may be helping a newly diagnosed diabetic choose foods that will assist in maintaining appropriate blood glucose levels. In a school setting the goal of individual or group counseling could be helping children learn to choose lower-fat snacks to support a healthy weight. In a community center counseling of a mother may focus on meal planning to improve the nutrient intake of her family. Regardless of the audience and goal, the counseling process includes several basic steps.

The following sequence of questions summarizes the ongoing counseling process:

- *Need:* What is wrong? What is the need or health problem of this individual?
- *Goal:* What does the individual want to do about it? What is his or her immediate goal? What is the long-range goal?

- *Information:* What information do I need to help this person? What information does he or she need for personal decision making? What knowledge and skills are necessary to solve the health problem or achieve the goal?
- *Action:* What has to happen to reach the goal set by the client? What plan of action is best for solving the health problem and meeting the client's personal needs?
- *Result:* What happened? What was the result of the action that was planned and carried out? Did it solve the problem or meet the need? If not, why not? What changes or additions to the plan are indicated?

Important Actions of the Interview

All interviews, regardless of their specific health or nutrition purpose, include certain important steps: observing, listening, responding, terminating the interview, and recording. As you begin to develop interviewing skills, give attention to each of these actions in the process.

1. Observing

Ordinarily we do not deliberately look at all the persons we meet; however, when caring for persons with health needs, our role requires such behavior. Our purpose is to gather information that will guide us in understanding our clients and their environment. Valid observation is a skill developed through concentration, study, and practice. Important areas of observation include the following:

- *Physiologic function and features:* Refer to Table 1-1, and review the clinical signs of nutritional status. These characteristics provide a basis for detailed observations of physical well-being and can help you develop greater accuracy and objectivity.
- *Behavior patterns:* The behavior of the client or patient provides clues relating to self-concept and attitudes toward healthcare. Individuals with poor self-esteem may be uneasy about asking questions about their illness or treatment. Others may appear distracted or show disinterest in nutrition or the process. Persons giving careful attention to the interview may be demonstrating a stronger intent to initiate new behaviors.

---

demographic Relating to statistical data describing a population according to age, income, gender, household size, ethnic or cultural group, education, births or deaths.

acculturation The process by which newcomers to a country or region begin to adopt the practices of their neighbors; this term is often used to refer to the adoption of new foods or food patterns by individuals moving to the United States.

2. Listening

Hearing and listening are not the same thing. *Hearing* is a physiologic function—only the first step in the listening process. The function of *listening* is to hear, to identify the sound, to understand its meaning, and to learn by it. Although much of our communication involves listening, the average person without special training hears only about 25% of what is actually said.

The nutrition counselor must develop the art of creative listening. First, we must learn to be comfortable as listeners. Usually our lives are so filled with activity that to sit and listen quietly is difficult. We practice listening by staying close by, assuming a comfortable position, and giving our full attention to the person speaking. We show genuine interest by indicating agreement or understanding with a nod of the head or making such responses as "Uh-huh" or "I see" at appropriate times in the conversation. We must learn to remain silent when the other person's comment jogs a personal memory or parallel experience of our own. We learn to listen not only for the words a person uses but also for the repetition of key words, the hesitant or aggressive expression of words or ideas, and the softness or harshness of tone. We listen to the overall content of what is being said, to the main ideas expressed, and to the topics chosen. We listen for the feelings, needs, and goals being stated. We learn to listen to the silences and to be comfortable with them, giving the person time to frame thoughts and express them.

3. Responding

The responses we give can be verbal or nonverbal. Nonverbal responses include gestures and movements, silences, facial expressions, nods of the head, and touch. Verbal responses make use of language—words and meanings (Table 10-1). But we give our own meanings to the words we use. Thus we must give attention to our choice of words in creating a supportive and nonthreatening environment for responses. Sometimes a verbal response can be a simple restatement of what the individual has said. This gives you an opportunity to hear the statement again, think about it, and thus reinforce, expand, or correct it. At other times your response may be a reflection of what the expressed feelings seem to be. This enables the client to verify or correct what was meant. We should never act on an assumption about a client's feelings without verifying them first. (See the *Focus on Culture* box, "Counseling and Culture: What Do We Need to Know?," to learn more about beliefs and actions.)

4. Terminating the Interview

The close of the interview should have several components. This is a good time to summarize the main points covered or to reinforce learning. If contact is to continue, plans for follow-up visits or activities need to be set. The client should be left with the sense that the counselor has a sincere concern for his or her welfare and the door is always open for further communication.

5. Recording

The important points of the interview need to be recorded. This should be as unobtrusive as possible with little note taking, if any, during the interview itself. Members of the healthcare team compile information about the patient and the health problem in the patient's chart, a legal document admissible in court. The health professional has a legal obligation to respect confidentiality, and most healthcare facilities have guidelines that indicate what and how much information can be shared and with whom. At the same time healthcare professionals have a responsibility to relay to other members of the healthcare team pertinent information important to the total plan of care.

TABLE 10-1	Verbal Responses Used by the Helping Professions	
Purpose of Response	**Type of Response**	**Description**
Clarification	Content	Counselor summarizes content of the conversation up to that point
	Affective	Counselor paraphrases or defines a concern that the client has implied but not actually stated
Leading	Closed question	Question that can be answered with "yes" or "no" or with very few words
	Open question	Question that cannot be answered briefly; often triggers discussion or a flow of information
	Advice	Suggestion of an alternative type of behavior for the client; may be an activity or thought
	Teaching	Information presented with the intention of helping the client acquire the knowledge and skills to perform appropriate nutrition-related behaviors
Self-revealing	Self-involving	Response made to client's statements that reflects the personal feelings of the counselor
	Self-disclosing	Response made to client's statements that reflects factual information about the counselor
	Aside	Statement counselor makes to self

Two pieces of information from the health or nutrition interview need to be documented, as follows:

- A description of the individual's general physical and emotional status along with his or her immediate and long-term needs for care
- A description of whatever care and teaching were provided

Any plans for follow-up with the patient and family or notes concerning referrals to other agencies might be shared in oral team reports or case conferences.

Nutrition History and Analysis

Life Situation and Food Patterns

In both hospital and community settings the health or nutrition interview often includes a general nutrition history. A nutrition history provides an overview of the individual's past and present food intake and gives insight as to past or current nutrition problems. Such a record also includes a description of living situation and general accessibility to food. Several methods are used—either separately or in combination—as follows to collect the information needed.

- *24-Hour recall:* By this method the person is asked to recall all food and beverages consumed during the previous 24 hours, noting the nature and amount of each item.[4] Individuals whose memory may be limited, such as young children or elderly adults, may not be able to recall the types and amounts of all foods eaten. A second disadvantage of this method is that it does not reveal long-term food habits. Plastic food models or pictures representing food servings can help quantify the reported food intake.
- *Food records:* Persons may record their food intake for a brief period, usually no more than 3 days. Individuals are taught how to describe food items used singly or in combination and how to measure amounts consumed. A 3-day record is sometimes used periodically after an initial diet history to monitor food intake.

◆ FOCUS ON CULTURE

Counseling and Culture: What Do We Need to Know?

Culture has sometimes been compared to an iceberg. An iceberg has a section above the water line that is clearly visible and a section below the water line that is not visible. So does culture. All societies have underlying assumptions and values—invisible to others—that guide a person's observed behavior. As we work with families to help them improve their nutrition and health, we must consider those invisible beliefs that bring about the behaviors that we see.

We must be sensitive to both what people do and why they do it.

Individual or Group Orientation

Some cultures emphasize the "I" and others the "we." Individuals who tend to be group oriented are more likely to share whatever food or other resources they have with neighbors or their extended family. In a counseling situation, group-oriented individuals may also try to save face for their family and not admit if there is a lack of food or inappropriate living conditions.

Locus of Control

Cultures differ in their view of people's ability to control the forces around them and shape their own destiny. Persons who have an internal locus of control believe there are very few limits to what they can do or become as long as they set their mind to it. Such an individual with a family history of heart disease may be very receptive to lifestyle changes that will lower his or her risk of a heart attack. A person with an external locus of control assumes that life is predetermined—what will be will be—and there is not much that one can do about it. This individual may be less receptive to dietary changes believed to be ineffectual in altering a health outcome.

Patterns of Communication

Messages between members of different cultures can be easily misinterpreted or misunderstood. Some cultures are very direct in their communication with explicit and to-the-point words and phrases. Other cultures have an indirect style, with an emphasis on understatement and nonverbal cues. In these groups what is not said may be the true message. Body language, eye contact, and tone of voice are important aspects of indirect communication. Mannerisms that are distracting or inappropriate, interpreted as rude or condescending, or considered to indicate lack of interest in what is being said will quickly disrupt any rapport that has developed and end true communication between counselor and client. Following are just a few examples:

- *Personal space:* Americans like a lot of room. Try sitting next to the only passenger on a city bus and note the level of anxiety you create. In many other cultures closeness is considered acceptable behavior. Our distance from a client may affect his or her comfort level.
- *Eye contact:* Americans show respect by looking each other straight in the eye. Asians indicate respect by looking downward. Interchanging these behaviors is often interpreted as being rude.
- *Speech inflection:* The tone of voice and its loudness and inflection may be viewed as threatening or comforting depending on the cultural expectations of the listener.

You cannot always be aware of your clients' attitudes toward body language ahead of time. However, you can take note of any signs of uneasiness and invite them to discuss anything about the interview that is making them uncomfortable.

References

Holli BB, Calabrese RJ, O'Sullivan-Maillet J: *Communication and education skills for dietetics professionals,* ed 4, Philadelphia, 2003, Lippincott, Williams & Wilkins.

Peace Corps Information Collection and Exchange: *Culture matters: the Peace Corps cross-cultural workbook,* Washington, DC, 1997, U.S. Government Printing Office.

- *Food frequency:* This is a structured questionnaire that lists common food items or food groups and obtains information about the quantity and frequency of use. This tool is helpful in determining particular disease risk because it describes the use of specific groups of foods over an extended period.

- *Nutrition history:* At the initial interview with an individual or family a nutrition history collects the information needed to plan continuing care. Nutrition professionals use this comprehensive approach in both clinical and community settings and evaluate their findings by computer-assisted nutrient analysis. Other healthcare team members can contribute helpful nutrition information using a tool such as the activity-associated daily food pattern given in Figure 10-2. Most people structure their eating around their schedule of work or activity, where they are, what they are doing, and whom they are with. An activity-associated guide gives both interviewer and client a framework for data collection and provides a series of memory jogs to help flesh out information and permit constructive counseling. Questions refer to general habits—the nature of foods eaten and their frequency, preparation, portion size, and seasoning. Another practical method is a brief household food inventory such as a short checklist of high-fat foods combined with an assessment of how often each item is eaten.[5] See Box 10-1 for open-ended questions useful in obtaining dietary information. If you are interested and nonjudgmental, the information received should be valid and straightforward. Conversely, if you are critical and authoritarian, people will probably tell you only what they think you want to hear.

Food intake records are a helpful tool as a starting point for nutrition counseling; however, the underreporting of food intake is a pervasive problem. Some individuals underreport their food intake by as much as 45%.[6] Underreporting occurs most frequently among children, women, and obese persons. In some cases people may forget what or how much they ate, especially if they were eating and doing something else at the same time, such as watching television or surfing the Internet. Others may find it embarrassing to admit how much they con-

---

Name _____ Date _____

Height (in) _____ Weight (lb) _____ (kg) _____ Age _____

Referral   BMI _____

Diagnosis

Nutrition intervention

Members of household

Occupation

Recreation, physical activity

Present food intake	Place	Hour	Frequency, form, and amount checklist
Morning			Milk
			Cheese
			Meat
			Fish
			Poultry
Noon/afternoon			Eggs
			Nuts
			Soy foods
			Butter, margarine
			Other fats
Evening			Vegetables, green
			Vegetables, other
			Fruits (citrus)
			Legumes
			Potato
			Bread–kind
			Sugar
			Desserts
			Beverages
Summary			Alcohol
			Vitamin/mineral supplements
			Candy

FIGURE 10-2   Nutrition history and associated physical activity. When helping individuals evaluate their food intake it is useful to also review their associated physical activity to see how this corresponds with both the timing and content of their meals and snacks. BMI, body mass index.

sumed of a certain food. Establishing a relationship of trust so persons feel at ease reporting their true food intake and helping individuals develop an awareness of how much food they actually consume at an eating session are important goals for nutrition counseling.

Plan of Care

A careful review of the diet history along with current health status and health problems provides the foundation for the nutrition care plan and follow-up care. This may take the form of return clinic visits, telephone calls to share progress, home visits, consultation and referral with other members of the healthcare team, or use of community resources. Ongoing guidance and support with reinforcement of prior learning, introduction of new learning as needs develop, and/or adjustment of the care plan will keep the individual or family focused. Client follow-up requires patience, recognizing that there are various ways of reaching a goal.

THE TEACHING-LEARNING PROCESS

Learning and Behavior

Despite our knowledge of learning theory and the need to motivate individuals to use the information they have learned, the myth still prevails that if health information is provided, negative health practices will automatically improve. Unfortunately, there is a vast difference between a person who has learned and a person who has only been informed. Learning is ultimately measured by a change in behavior. Education must focus on the learner, not on the teacher or the content. The health educator's task is to create situations in which clients and their families can successfully develop motivation and direction for self-care. The application of learning to self-care is especially important when working with adults. Children are accustomed to learning ideas or facts because they are expected to. Adults will learn only those new concepts for which they believe they have an immediate need.[7]

Human Personality and Learning

The teaching-learning experience involves three aspects of the human personality—thinking, feeling, and the will to act.

Thinking

We each grasp information through our personal thought process. Some of us learn better by hearing information, and others learn better by looking at visuals. We take in information selectively and then process and shape it according to our needs. Our total thought process provides the background knowledge that forms the basis for reasoning and analysis. The learner senses the contribution of this thinking to the learning process as "I know how to do it."

Feeling

In each of us, specific feelings and responses are associated with given items of knowledge. These emotions reflect desires and needs that are aroused by what we hear or read. Emotions provide impetus, creating the tensions that spur us to act. The learner senses the contribution of emotion to the learning process as "I want to do it."

Will to Act

The will to act arises from the conviction that this new knowledge can fulfill a felt need and relieve the symptoms of tension. The will causes us to act on the knowledge received so that an attitude, value, thought, or pattern of behavior can be changed. The learner senses the contribution of the will to the learning process as "I will do it."

Principles of Learning

Learning follows three basic laws: (1) learning is *personal* and occurs in connection with a perceived individual need, (2) learning is *developmental* and builds on prior knowledge and experience, and (3) learning brings *change* and results in a change in behavior.

Individuality

Learning is an individual response. We all learn according to our own needs, in our own way and time, and for our own purpose. The teacher must discover who the learner is by asking questions that clarify the learner's relationship to the problem. As nutrition educators we must devise new teaching strategies to meet the differing needs of learners and learning situations.

Need Fulfillment

An initial force in learning is personal motivation. Persons learn only what they believe will be useful to them, and they retain only what they think they will need. The sooner a person can put new learning to use, the more readily he or she will grasp it. The more it satisfies his or her immediate goals, the more effective the learning will be.

Point of Contact

Learning starts from a point of contact between prior experience and knowledge and the new information being presented, an overlap of the new with the familiar. Find out what the individual already knows and to what past experiences the new knowledge can be related, and start the process of learning at this point. Search for areas of association, and relate your teaching to that point of contact.

> motivation Forces that affect individual goal-directed behavior toward satisfying needs or achieving personal goals.

PERSPECTIVES IN PRACTICE
A Person-Centered Model Applied to Diabetes Education

A paradigm for nutrition education referred to as *holistic education* can be effective in teaching good self-care practices to persons with chronic diseases such as diabetes. This approach draws on both sound management and sound medicine: (1) varying its style to meet the needs of the particular situation and (2) focusing on the wellness of the whole person—mind, body, and spirit. Holistic education views clients and patients as active partners in caring for their health, and further, it teaches persons to use both their "boxes and their bubbles" as part of a thinking model. Our "box" is our rational left side of the brain. Our "bubbles" emerge from our intuitive right side of the brain, and both are important. We need to combine our rational processes and our intuitive capacity to build creative thinking skills. Providing information alone does not help individuals build creative solutions to health problems or learn how to implement new behaviors in everyday situations.

To achieve long-term success, health education programs must incorporate learning theories in the design of the program. Learning theories are based on the psychosocial as well as the educational needs of individuals. Nutrition educators must assess learner attitudes and look for ways to change those attitudes that will modify behavior. Diabetes education can serve as a model for nutrition education and counseling across the continuum of healthcare. Persons with diabetes must manage their disease on a day-to-day basis to maintain positive health and avoid debilitating complications. This involves the adoption of attitudes and lifestyle behaviors needed to meet the nutritional and medical requirements of the disease.

When designing any nutrition education program, ask yourself the following questions:
- **Is the teaching process effective?**
  Does the teaching process take the following into account:
  - How do people learn?
  - What is worth learning?
  - Who is most responsible for a person's health?
  - What responsibilities lie with the learner versus the counselor?
- **Is the learning process effective?**
  Does the learning process consider the following:
  - How significant is this condition at this point in the life of the learner?

- Does the learner have a sense of psychologic safety—that is, does he or she have the security to discuss any problems openly and honestly?
- How will the instructor know if the learner's attitude has changed after receiving or using new information?

These questions are important reminders of those issues that influence learning behavior. Self-care for any chronic disease lies primarily in the hands of the person with the disease. No matter how much information is provided, it is ultimately up to that individual to decide what foods are selected, how much is eaten, and when it is consumed. Nutrition educators must keep in mind the major aspects of the learner's personal life that influence these decisions, such as family finances, work situation, or social activities. They also must recognize the effect of these circumstances on the individual's sense of personal responsibility for his or her health.

Dietitians and other healthcare professionals can benefit from the systematic methods of assessment developed in the field of clinical psychology. Therapists have identified five stages of disease acceptance and responsibility, with intervention strategies for each stage (see Table 10-2). Such a system for assessing client attitudes can guide education for effective self-care not only in diabetics but also in any individual diagnosed with a chronic condition such as hypertension, obesity, or heart disease.

There are various benefits to use of this method, as follows:
- It recognizes and reinforces that the client is ultimately responsible for his or her health.
- It gives the instructor an objective, measurable way of assessing client attitudes that can be used to evaluate progress.
- It serves as a basis for selecting appropriate teaching methods and counseling techniques that match the client's current stage of responsibility.

References

Leontos C et al: National Diabetes Education Program: opportunities and challenges, *J Am Diet Assoc* 98(1):73, 1998.

Saylor C: Health redefined: a foundation for teaching nursing strategies, *Nurse Educ* 28(6):261, 2003.

BOX 10-1	Examples of Open-Ended Questions for a Dietary Interview

- What is your first meal of the day, and what foods do you usually eat?
- Who plans and prepares the meals in your home?
- Are you currently restricting your food choices in any way for health reasons?
- You mentioned that you eat lunch away from home. Where do you usually eat? What types of food do you eat?
- Describe for me your general physical activity, starting when you get up in the morning and continuing through the day.
- Tell me about any dietary supplements that you take regularly.
- Where do you usually shop for groceries? Is this a satisfactory arrangement for you?
- What is your favorite grain food? How many servings do you eat over the course of a day?

Active Participation

Because learning is an active process, learners must become personally involved. Indeed, effective teaching strategies require the active participation of learners to bring about desired changes in attitudes and behaviors. One means of securing participation is through planned feedback. Feedback may take several forms, as follows:

- Ask questions that require more than a "yes" or "no" answer and reveal the learner's degree of understanding and motivation.

- Provide opportunities within the session to practice new skills or procedures. Such guided practice develops ability, self-confidence, and security. It enables the learner to clarify the principles that form the basis for decision making in particular situations and actions.

TABLE 10-2   Levels of Personal Responsibility and Intervention Methods: A Diabetes Example

Level of Personal Responsibility	Client Characteristics	Intervention Method
1. Being diabetic is a disaster	Feels hopeless, helpless, defeated; self-care may be difficult	Educate family member or other caregivers
2. Being diabetic is a burden	Blames problem on others; expects others to feel sorry for him or her; feels angry, threatened	Provide emotional support; help client accept anger to move on
3. Being diabetic is a problem	Blames self as often as others; personal growth is possible	Reinforce attitudes that reflect sense of responsibility; examine irresponsible attitudes in a nonjudgmental way
4. Being diabetic is a challenge	Rarely blames others for problem; recognizes responsibility, but does not always act on it; good self-care expected	Point out discrepancies between stated need and actual behavior
5. Being diabetic is an opportunity	Takes total responsibility for the problem; acts positively on decisions; optimal self-care is expected	Provide tools required for good self-care

- Have the learner try out the new activities in situations outside the teacher-directed location. Alternate such trials with return visits to review these experiences. Answer, or help the person to answer, any questions that arise and continue to provide support and reinforcement.

Appraisal

At appropriate intervals take stock of the changes that your clients have made in outlook, attitude, and actions toward their health or nutrition goals. Careful, sympathetic questions may reveal any blocks to learning and show if you are communicating clearly, making contact, or choosing the best method of teaching. It also may remind you of principles that you glossed over. In the final analysis the measure of success in teaching lies not in the number of facts transferred but rather in the changes for the better that were initiated in your client's life.

The nutrition educator who builds on clients' needs and goals, imparts strong knowledge and interest in the subject, shows respect and concern for each individual, and projects self-confidence has the greatest chance for success. In the long run, clients who follow a personal goal-setting approach will have more opportunity to develop responsibility for self-care and personal choice than will those who follow a prescriptive approach. Personal goal setting may require more time initially but achieves far greater results over the long-term.

The American Dietetic Association advocates the following four nutrition principles for helping persons improve their diets[8]:

1. It is the total diet rather than one meal or one food that is important.
2. All foods can fit into a healthy diet if used in appropriate amounts and combined with physical activity.
3. Balance, variety, and moderation are the keys to a healthy diet.
4. Take a positive approach to food.

Nutrition educators following these nutrition principles can help clients avoid confusion in the face of the many and often conflicting media reports about health and nutrition. Nutrition education is most effective when it builds on easy-to-understand principles such as MyPyramid: choose a variety of fruits, vegetables, and grains; limit fats, sugars, and salt; and exercise regularly.[9] (See the *Perspectives in Practice* box, "A Person-Centered Model Applied to Diabetes Education," and Table 10-2 for more about individual learning.)

THE ECOLOGY OF MALNUTRITION

As a health professional you will be counseling individuals from all social and economic groups and varying levels of resources. Although malnutrition occurs at all income levels, it is especially prevalent in lower-income families who lack the funds to purchase appropriate and adequate amounts of food. These individuals are also likely to have inferior housing, a limited education that constrains their job opportunities, and low self-confidence. All of these factors combine to negatively influence nutrition and health. In this section we explore the common elements of these problems as found in the United States and around the world and consider our role as health professionals in addressing these needs.

> paradigm A pattern or model serving as an example; a standard or ideal practice or behavior based on a fundamental value or theme.

TO PROBE FURTHER

INCOME, FOOD INSECURITY, AND WELL-BEING: HOW ARE THEY RELATED?

A family's income influences not only how much money is available for food, but also the level of healthcare that is accessible to its members. Both have implications for long-term physical and emotional well-being. The appropriate types and quantities of food are critical for optimal growth and health and resisting infection and degenerative disease. Ongoing healthcare—to treat acute conditions, monitor growth, and detect any developing chronic disease—supports personal productivity at work and school and quality of life. Unfortunately, a stable supply of nutritious food and routine healthcare are out of reach for many low-income families.

Food insecurity is a persistent national problem with implications for both the physical and emotional well-being of children in low-income families. Income level is influenced by race and ethnic group, and black and Hispanic families have a disproportionately higher burden of poverty. Ten percent of white households have incomes that fall below the poverty line, but 24% of black households and 22% of Hispanic households live in poverty.[1] These differences in income influence the amount of money that families can spend on food. Black households spend on average 25% less per person per year on food than white households similar in size.[2] The Third National Health and Nutrition Examination Survey reported that black women had lower intakes of folate, vitamin B_6, and vitamin B_{12} than white or Hispanic women.[3] Fruits, vegetables, and animal proteins, foods that tend to be higher in cost, are major contributors of these nutrients. Hispanic families with children are also at higher risk of food insufficiency than comparable white families. Hispanic families are five times more likely to run out of food, two times more likely to cut the meal size of adults in the family to save food, and five times more likely to cut the meal size of children in the family to save food.[4]

Children who experience food insecurity express worry, sadness, and anxiety about their family's food situation.[5] They eat more food and eat fast when food is available, which may contribute to problems of overweight among low-income children. Families who are food insecure have limited food choices, and their diet often lacks variety, consisting of a few kinds of low-cost foods. A study that traced the development of children from kindergarten through third grade revealed that children from food-insecure families made lower progress in reading and social skills but gained weight more rapidly.[6]

For optimal nutrition and health, families need both the resources to obtain food and the knowledge and skills to select appropriate foods in the marketplace. Access to nutrition intervention and counseling is often influenced by an individual's health insurance coverage. Sessions with a healthcare provider to establish a positive diet and exercise pattern are less accessible to those with chronic conditions who do not have health insurance. Nearly one third of Hispanic households, 19% of black households, and 11% of white households are without health insurance.[1] Thus individuals whose food resources are most limited may also find it difficult to obtain help in solving their food problems. Referral of food-insufficient households to available food assistance programs and appropriate educational resources is an important responsibility of health professionals who assist in their care.

References

1. DeNavas-Walt C, Proctor BD, Mills RJ: *Income, poverty, and health insurance coverage in the United States: 2003, current population reports P60-226,* Washington, DC, 2004, U.S. Census Bureau.
2. Blisard N: Food spending by U.S. households grew steadily in the 1990s, *Food Rev* 23(3):18, 2000.
3. Arab L et al: Ethnic differences in the nutrient intake adequacy of premenopausal U.S. women: results from the Third National Health Examination Survey, *J Am Diet Assoc* 103:1008, 2003.
4. Mazur RE, Marquis GS, Jensen HH: Diet and food insufficiency among Hispanic youths: acculturation and socioeconomic factors in the Third National Health and Nutrition Examination Survey, *Am J Clin Nutr* 78:1120, 2003.
5. Connell CL et al: Children's experiences of food insecurity can assist in understanding its effect on their well-being, *J Nutr* 135:1683, 2005.
6. Jyoti DF, Frongillo EA, Jones SJ: Food insecurity affects school children's academic performance, weight gain, and social skills, *J Nutr* 135:2831, 2005.

The Food Environment and Malnutrition

Out of necessity our food habits are linked to our environment. Today's rapidly changing environment and growing problems of pollution and malnutrition often threaten health. The word *ecology* comes from the Greek word *oikos,* which means "house," and refers to the relationship between individuals and their environment. Just as many forces within a family interact to influence its members, so even greater forces in our physical and social environment can interact to produce disease.

Worldwide Prevalence of Malnutrition

Malnutrition as a public health problem worldwide continues to grow. Globally, the unequal distribution of food leaves a fifth of the world's population chronically undernourished.[10] Over half of the child deaths occurring worldwide are associated with malnutrition, and about one third of the children under age 5 who survive have stunted growth.[11] Micronutrient deficiencies are common in the developing world, as more than 20% of the population is deficient in iodine and vitamin A and 40% of women are anemic. Issues of food and income distribution rather than a lack of available food are often the causes of malnutrition. Close to 80% of the malnourished children around the world live in countries that report food surpluses.

Even in the midst of plenty in America, malnutrition exists.[12-15] Approximately 11% of U.S. households are food insecure, meaning they have limited or uncertain availability of nutritionally safe and adequate food (Box 10-2).[13] More than one third of families with incomes below the poverty level experience food shortages, and such shortages influence health[13,14] (see the *To Probe Further* box, "Income, Food Insecurity, and Well-Being: How Are They Related?"). Malnutrition in pregnancy can result in low birth weight, putting an infant at risk.

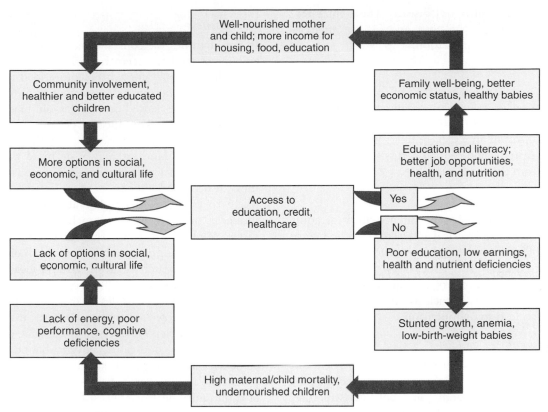

FIGURE 10-3   Breaking out of the cycle of despair. Access to education, healthcare, and credit enable mothers to adequately care for themselves and their children. *(Redrawn from American Dietetic Association: Position of the American Dietetic Association: addressing world hunger, malnutrition, and food insecurity, J Am Diet Assoc 103:1046, 2003, with permission from the American Dietetic Association.)*

BOX 10-2	Questions to Identify Food Insecurity

- In the last 12 months did you ever run out of food and have no money to purchase food?
- In the last 12 months did you or your children ever skip a meal because you had run out of food and had no money to purchase food?
- In the last 12 months were you or your children ever hungry but didn't eat because you didn't have enough food and had no money to purchase additional food?
- In the last 12 months did you ever cut the size of your children's meals because there wasn't enough food in the house and you had no money to purchase additional food?

Data from Hampl JS, Hall R: Dietetic approaches to U.S. hunger and food insecurity, *J Am Diet Assoc* 102:921, 2002.

Malnutrition occurs in older adults adding to weakness and disability. Alcoholism and drug addition can lead to poor food intake. Food insecurity is associated with homelessness. In the developed world, malnutrition is partner to a distorted obsession with thinness. Human misery and human waste of life from malnutrition occur in both hemispheres. Worldwide, it is estimated that hunger and malnutrition have a cost equal to 46 million years of productive life.[11]

At the biologic level malnutrition results from an inadequate supply of nutrients to maintain cell growth and function. Within communities malnutrition in mothers and their children result from interconnecting circumstances: physical, social, cultural, economic, political, and educational (Figure 10-3). Each is more or less important at a given time and place for a given individual. If the adverse circumstances are only temporary, the malnutrition will be short term and rapidly alleviated with no long-standing harm to life. But chronic malnutrition with no relief carries irreparable harm, and in severe conditions death ensues. For the epidemiologist a triad of

> poverty line   The minimum amount of income required to provide food, clothing, shelter, and other basic necessities for a family of a given size and composition; this index is calculated by government economists and used to determine eligibility for various government programs such as food stamps or free or reduced-cost school lunches.
>
> food insecurity   Limited or uncertain availability of food and the inability to obtain a sufficient supply of nutritionally safe, adequate, and acceptable food through socially acceptable means.

variables influences health and disease. These three factors—(1) the agent, (2) the host, and (3) the environment—also influence malnutrition.

The Agent

The agent in malnutrition is a lack of food. As a result, nutrients essential to maintaining cell activity are missing and physiologic changes begin to occur. Many circumstances can result in a lack of food: famine, poverty, war, unequal distribution of food across a region, or unwise choices from the foods available.

The Host

The host is the individual—the infant, child, or adult who is malnourished. Physical characteristics influence the severity of the problem: the presence of other diseases; increased needs during times of growth, pregnancy, lactation, or heavy labor; or congenital defects or premature birth. Personal factors such as emotional problems and poverty can lead to malnutrition.

The Environment

Environmental factors influence malnutrition. These can include lack of clean water, poor sanitation, social problems, cultural beliefs, economic and political structure, and agricultural production. This debilitating group of factors, in one combination or another, still occurs every day in numerous places around the world.

Economic and Political Environment

Food Availability and Use

In all societies both financial and government policies influence food availability and use. Money is a necessity for obtaining adequate food. Sometimes the role of government in setting programs and policies is less evident. Nonetheless, both are intertwined in securing adequate nutrients.

Government Programs

Food and agricultural programs at all levels of government influence food availability and distribution. Agricultural policies relating to land management and erosion practices, water distribution, or pesticide use influence food production. Food assistance programs for persons in need may support adequate nutrition among low-income and vulnerable population groups.

The Problem of Poverty

Daily news reports from around the world remind us that malnutrition leading to starvation and death exists in many countries ravaged by war or overwhelmed by social conditions of desperate poverty. But even in the United States, one of the wealthiest nations, reports document hunger and malnutrition, especially among minority groups.[13]

Hopelessness

In poor families the constant need to acquire a sufficient amount of food can seem to be almost insurmountable. Individuals may be forced to acquire food that has been discarded by others and carries the risk of foodborne illness or purchase dented cans or day-old foods being sold at a cheaper price. Low-income persons may fish in polluted streams or lakes despite the health risk if food is in short supply.[16] Mothers may visit more than one food pantry to obtain a sufficient amount of food for their families. When food money is very limited, families are likely to purchase foods that are high in kilocalories (kcalories or kcal), rather than high in micronutrients. Figure 10-4 tells us that fresh fruits and vegetables that are high in vitamins may be out of reach of low-income persons. Staples such as bread, ground meat, and cereals provide more kcalories and satiety for a hungry family.[17]

The values and attitudes of other groups within our society can set low-income families apart even more than do physical barriers. As a result of extreme pressures and difficult living conditions, poverty-bound persons become victims of negative stereotypes and feel isolated, powerless, and insecure—feelings that influence their use of community health services. Based on their day-to-day struggle to exist, poor persons may see little value in long-range preventive health measures. Hazards to health inherent in poor housing and poor nutrition are often compounded by distance from sources of healthcare. An inadequate supply of food, with its deep psychologic and emotional impact, adds to both mental and physical risk.

Isolation

Feelings of alienation from mainstream society are common among the poor. In many communities few, if any, channels of communication exist between the lowest-income groups and the other segments of the community. A poor person responds to such alienation with further withdrawal and feelings of isolation, concluding that no one is concerned.

Role of the Health Professional

How can concerned health professionals help individuals and families crushed by years of poverty? In the face of overpowering feelings of isolation, helplessness, and insecurity, how can we best reach these individuals and serve their needs? Some guidelines are provided below.

Self-Awareness

First, we must explore our own feelings about the poor. We must be aware of any distorted vision based on our own values and attitudes. If we are to be agents of constructive change, we must first understand an individual's situation and its broad social setting. We must also understand ourselves and confront any cultural conditioning or biases that we may have.

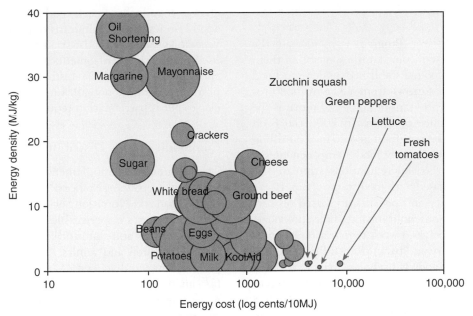

FIGURE 10-4   Relationship between energy density (megajoules/kg) and food costs (cents/10 megajoules) for foods in the USDA Thrifty Food Plan. The size of the bubble indicates the amount of energy that each food contributes to the diet of a family of four over 1 week. Fresh fruits and vegetables that are high in price and contain many important vitamins and minerals make a very small contribution to energy intake. *(Redrawn from Drewnowski A, Barratt-Fornell A: Do healthier diets cost more,* Nutr Today *39(4):165, 2004.)*

Rapport

Genuine warmth, interest, friendliness, and kindness grow from within. *Rapport* is that sense of relationship between persons that is born of mutual respect, regard, and trust. This relationship gives the helper and the helped a strong feeling of working together. Its most basic ingredient is a concern for people and the desire to improve their situation. It is born of the knowledge of what it means to be human.

Client Focus

We need to begin where the client is in relation to his or her needs and concerns. What we may see as an overriding health problem may not be viewed by the individual as the most critical life factor needing attention. We must work with other team members—the social worker, psychologist, and nurse—to cut through the maze of factors that hinder an individual from implementing the health or dietary advice given. It may be necessary to provide actual food resources before practical diet intervention can begin.

FAMILY ECONOMIC NEEDS: FOOD ASSISTANCE PROGRAMS

Many families under economic stress need financial help to meet their food needs. Food assistance programs funded by local communities or the U.S. government can supply food directly or increase food buying power to provide additional nutrients. Federally funded assistance programs often target particular population groups, whereas most local food banks serve all age or gender groups with food needs. As a health professional working in the community it is important for you to be aware of available food assistance programs and make appropriate referrals.

U.S. Department of Agriculture Food Assistance Programs

The U.S. Department of Agriculture (USDA) oversees food assistance programs designed to provide a food "safety net" for low-income Americans. The goals of these programs are to provide (1) access to food, (2) a healthy diet, and (3) nutrition education. It is estimated that one in six Americans participates in a food assistance program.[18] Some of these programs are entitlement programs, which means there are specific income guidelines that determine eligibility. The Food Stamp program is an entitlement program. The School Lunch Program serves all children regardless of family income; however, children from low-income households are eligible for free or reduced-cost meals.

---

entitlement program   A government program for which a person is eligible or "entitled" based on income; all persons falling below a certain income level are eligible to receive food stamps.

Food Stamp Program

The goal of the Food Stamp Program is to increase the food-buying power of low-income families, enabling them to purchase additional food. Established under the Food Stamp Act of 1964, it has grown from a $13 million program to a $20.7 billion program in 2002 and remains the largest U.S. food assistance program. In 2002 the Food Stamp Program served 19.8 million people in 8.2 million households. The average monthly food stamp benefit per household was $173.[19] Federal regulations stipulate the items that may be purchased with food stamps (Box 10-3).

Food stamp eligibility and benefits are based on several factors, including household income, household size, housing costs, total assets, and work registration requirements. Income eligibility and benefits are adjusted annually. The individuals and households receiving food stamps have incomes at or below the federal poverty level, which limits their ability to purchase adequate and appropriate food. Food stamps increase the amount of money they have to spend for food. The average income of food stamp households is $633 per month (average household size is 2.3 persons), and the average benefit is $80 per person. More than 51% of Food Stamp Program participants are children, and 9% are older adults. Of the households with children, more than one third are headed by a single parent (mostly women).[20] Although food stamps make a significant contribution to the food resources of low-income families, many recipients still run out of food before the end of the month and are forced to rely on local food pantries for assistance.

Historically, participants were issued coupons (food stamps) that could be used to purchase food at participating food stores. In recent years states have converted to electronic benefit transfer cards (EBT) with funds transferred from the client's food stamp account to the retailer's account.[20] Although food stamps are intended to improve the nutrient intake of low-income families, this goal is not always achieved. Families can purchase whatever foods they wish, so nutrient intake will vary according to the choices they make. Snack foods or high-sugar beverages add kcalories but not vitamins or minerals as would fruit, vegetables, or dairy foods. Food Stamp Act funds are also used to provide nutrition education to food stamp recipients.[21] Although all 50 states have approved nutrition education programs, not all families are reached by these classes nor is participation required.

Commodity Foods Distribution Programs

The Commodities Supplemental Food Program and The Emergency Food Assistance Program (TEFAP) managed by the Food and Nutrition Service of the USDA distribute market surpluses of perishable foods to eligible individuals and families and state and local programs serving low-income children and adults. These foods include meat, poultry, fruits and vegetables, eggs, dried beans and peas, fats, and cheese. Some items are distributed through local government and social service agencies to persons with incomes below the federal poverty guidelines or who qualify for food stamps. Commodity foods are also made available to (1) schools for use in the National School Lunch and School Breakfast Programs, (2) congregate and home-delivered meals programs serving older adults, (3) Head Start and other child care programs, and (4) food pantries or soup kitchens serving homeless and indigent families.

Child Nutrition Programs

National School Lunch Program

The National School Lunch Program was initiated in 1946 and since that time has served over 187 billion meals. This program provides nutritionally balanced lunches to children in public schools, nonprofit private schools, and residential child care programs. Schools receive either commodity foods or cash reimbursement based on the number of students eating the school lunch. Meals are offered at no cost or reduced cost to children from low-income families meeting the federal income guidelines. Each meal is required to provide one third of the Dietary Reference Intake (DRI) for the following nutrients—protein, vitamin A, vitamin C, iron, calcium, and kcalories. It is also recommended that no more than 30% of kcalories come from fat and less than 10% from saturated fat. In 2003 the National School Lunch Program served 28.4 million children in more than 99,800 schools. More than 26 million children received free or reduced-cost lunches.[22]

School meal programs offer unique opportunities for nutrition education. The school lunch can provide a good example of a well-balanced meal including foods from the protein, fruit, vegetable, grain, and dairy groups. Teachers and school health and nutrition professionals can join together to provide educational experiences that connect the school meal with science and biology, social studies, and health (Table 10-3). In-school nutrition education can help to address the growing problem of child obesity. A comprehensive program called Team Nutrition makes

---

| BOX 10-3 | Items That Can Be Purchased With Food Stamps |

Allowable Items
Most foods (see exceptions below)
Garden plants for raising food
Seeds for raising food

Nonallowable Items
Hot, ready-to-eat foods
Foods that will be eaten in the store
Vitamin or mineral supplements
Pet foods
Cleaning supplies
Tobacco items
Alcohol

educational materials available and suggests activities for use in the school classroom, lunchroom, and after-school setting that encourage good food choices, portion control, and physical activity.

National School Breakfast Program

In 1966 it was apparent that many children were coming to school without breakfast, which seriously impeded their ability to learn, and the National School Breakfast Program was launched. Children eligible for free or reduced-cost lunches are also able to receive a school breakfast at the same level of payment. Under current regulations the school breakfast must contain one fourth of the DRI for protein, calcium, iron, vitamin A, vitamin C, and kcalories. As required for the school lunch, the breakfast meal must limit total fat to no more than 30% of total kcalories and saturated fat to less than 10% of total kcalories. More than 78,000 schools offer the School Breakfast Program. In 2003 8.4 million children had a school breakfast every day, and 6.9 million of these received their breakfast free or at a reduced price.[23]

The suggested meal pattern for school breakfast and school lunch is described in Table 10-4.

Summer Food Service Program

The Summer Food Service Program provides a noon meal for low-income children during summer vacation periods. Meals must meet the same nutritional guidelines as those offered through the school year. This program usually accompanies a summer school or camp experience

---

TABLE 10-3	Nutrition Education Ideas for the School Classroom

Subject	Activities for Different Grade Levels
Language arts	Read a story about food; keep a food diary for 3 days; write an article on nutrition for the school newspaper; write a food history of your family.
Mathematics	Using food pictures, count out the servings you need from each food group; calculate the kcalories, fat, protein, and carbohydrate in your lunch meal; look at the nutrition label on your favorite candy bar, and, using the 2000-kcalorie diet, calculate how much fat you have left for the rest of the day.
Science	Learn about the nutrients that plants need to grow; trace the paths by which the body breaks down food to release protein, carbohydrate, and fat; do some simple microbiological tests before and after you wash your hands.
Social studies	Learn about the different types of breads that are eaten in various countries around the world and how they are prepared; learn what nutrients must be listed on the nutrition label and how the Food and Drug Administration enforces food labeling; work with the school lunch manager to have an international food day and learn about the culture of each country.
Art	Draw pictures of foods that we should eat every day; prepare posters advertising healthy foods offered in the school lunch program or telling students why they should eat breakfast; invent a healthy food, and prepare a package and food label.
Health	Draw a picture of a healthy meal that includes all of the food groups; set up a plan of activities that will give you 60 minutes of physical activity every day; evaluate your food diary according to the food portions suggested in MyPyramid.

Ideas from Shepherd SK, Whitehead CS: *Team Nutrition's teacher handbook: tips, tools and jewels for busy educators*, Washington, DC, 1997, U.S. Department of Agriculture.

TABLE 10-4	USDA School Breakfast and Lunch Patterns*

Food Group	School Breakfast	School Lunch
Grains/Bread (includes whole grain or enriched bread, rolls, muffins, cereal, rice, macaroni, or noodles)	1 slice bread or 1 muffin or ¾ cup cereal	1 slice bread or 1 muffin or 1 roll, and/or ½ cup rice, pasta, or macaroni for total of 2 servings
Juice/Fruit/Vegetables (includes fruit, vegetables, fruit or vegetable juice)	½ cup	½ cup fruit and ½ cup vegetable (minimum)
Milk	1 cup	1 cup
Meat or meat alternate (includes meat, poultry, fish, soy, cheese, egg, peanut butter, peas and beans, yogurt)	1 oz meat, soy, or cheese or ½ egg or 2 tbsp peanut butter or ½ cup yogurt	2 oz of lean meat, poultry, fish, soy or cheese or 1 egg or ½ cup peas or beans or 4 tbsp peanut butter or 1 cup yogurt

USDA, U.S. Department of Agriculture.
*Amounts recommended for children in grades 7 to 12; portions vary for younger children.

sponsored by the local school district, recreation department, or other government or nonprofit community group.[24] Such a program is especially important for children who depend on the school breakfast and lunch programs for a significant portion of their nutrient intake.

School Milk Program

To encourage the use of milk among all children, schools or child care facilities that do not participate in the School Lunch or Breakfast Programs can receive cash reimbursement for milk. All children are eligible to participate regardless of their income level. More than 116 million half-pints of milk were served in 2001.

Child and Adult Care Food Program

The Child and Adult Care Food Program provides cash equivalents or commodity foods for child care programs serving children up to 12 years of age, adult day care programs serving persons age 60 and over, or programs caring for younger adults with disabilities. Such settings include day care centers, recreation centers, settlement houses, homeless shelters, and some Head Start programs. Children or adults are eligible to receive two meals and one snack per day with an additional meal or snack if care exceeds 8 hours.

Special Supplemental Nutrition Program for Women, Infants, and Children

The Special Supplemental Nutrition Program for Women, Infants, and Children (commonly called *WIC*) was approved by the U.S. Congress in 1974 and is administered by the Food and Nutrition Service of USDA through state health departments. This program provides nutritious food to low-income women who are pregnant, postpartum, or breast-feeding and at nutritional risk. Postpartum mothers can receive supplementary food for 6 months, and breast-feeding mothers can receive supplementary food for 12 months. Infants at nutritional or medical risk can receive formula and cereal up to the age of 1 year, and children are eligible for supplemental foods up to the age of 5.[25] In general, participants receive vouchers to purchase designated foods that are rich sources of protein, calcium, iron, vitamin A, and vitamin C, although some states deliver packages of food. Different food packages or vouchers are provided for different categories of participants. Box 10-4 provides a list of WIC-approved foods. WIC also includes nutrition education and counseling by public health nutritionists and serves as a source of referral to medical or social service providers.

Eligibility for WIC must be determined by a health professional based on federal guidelines. The following two types of nutritional risk carry WIC eligibility[25]:

1. *Medically-based risk:* anemia, underweight, overweight, prior poor pregnancy outcomes, or history of pregnancy complications

---

BOX 10-4 | WIC-Approved Foods

- Iron-fortified formula
- Iron-fortified infant cereal
- Iron-fortified adult cereal
- Vitamin C–rich fruit juice
- Vitamin C–rich vegetable juice
- Eggs
- Milk
- Cheese
- Peanut butter
- Dried beans and peas
- Canned tuna fish
- Carrots

WIC, Special Supplemental Nutrition Program for Women, Infants, and Children.

---

2. *Dietary risk:* nutrient deficiencies or inappropriate nutrition practices

Over the years the WIC program has been cost effective, bringing about improved birth outcomes and savings in healthcare costs. Research with WIC mothers and children indicates that WIC participation (1) reduces the number of premature and low-birth-weight infants, (2) results in a savings of more than $3 in healthcare costs within the first 60 days after birth for every $1 paid out in benefits, and (3) lowers the number of children with anemia.[26] The WIC program allows participants to use their food vouchers to purchase fresh fruits and vegetables at farmers' markets, supporting the national goals for increasing intakes of fruits and vegetables.

Although the WIC program is directed toward low-income women and children, it is not an entitlement program. Income eligibility does not automatically entitle one to benefits. There is a ceiling each year on total funding and therefore on the number of participants, so only those judged to be at the highest medical or nutritional risk can be served. Nevertheless, 7.6 million persons received benefits each month in 2003. Of this group 3.8 million were children, 1.9 million were infants, and 1.9 million were women.[25]

Nutrition Program for Older Adults

The Older Americans Act established the Elderly Nutrition Program in 1972, and it continues to benefit our growing numbers of older adults. The Elderly Nutrition Program was developed to provide one meal a day for older people who do not have an adequate diet. For those who are able to leave their homes, congregate meals offered at noon in community centers, churches, high-rise apartment buildings for older persons, or similar facilities provide nourishing food in a social setting. Meals are served Monday through Friday, and social events and nutrition education accompany the meals. Each meal is required to provide one third of the DRI for people age 60 and older.

When older people are unable to leave their homes because of illness or disability or the need to care for a dependent spouse, home-delivered meals, sometimes called Meals-on-Wheels, help to maintain nutritional adequacy. Programs provide one hot meal at noon on weekdays and may include a cold lunch for the evening meal or extra lunches for the weekend. As the costs of daily home delivery continue to rise, programs have experimented with weekly delivery of several frozen meals that can be defrosted and reheated as needed. Unfortunately, the occasional delivery of several frozen meals takes away the social aspect of a daily visitor that can be important to a homebound and isolated senior.

The Elderly Nutrition Program, managed by the U.S. Administration on Aging, serves all persons ages 60 and older regardless of income, although the program does target frail older adults and those at risk. Recipients are not required to pay for their meal, although they are encouraged to make a donation. More than 3 million older adults participate in this program on a regular basis.[27]

Expanded Food and Nutrition Education Program

The Expanded Food and Nutrition Education Program (EFNEP) funded by USDA does not provide actual food but supports limited-resource families by helping them obtain the knowledge and skills necessary for making healthy food choices. Serving both adults and youth, EFNEP is delivered to families by Cooperative Extension agents, paraprofessionals, and volunteers. Most of the paraprofessionals are indigenous to the communities they serve. An experiential series of lessons offers hands-on opportunities to develop skills in food preparation, food safety, food budgeting, and wise shopping. Individuals are recruited through neighborhood contacts, food stamp offices, and WIC. Group classes, media methods, one-on-one instruction, and educational mailings are used to reach different audiences. More than 380,000 youth and 158,000 adults are reached by EFNEP each year. The EFNEP reporting system indicates that 84% of adults improved their food management practices (e.g., planning meals and shopping more wisely) and 74% of youth improved their food preparation and food safety skills.[28]

The food assistance programs described above are intended to provide some degree of food security for low-income individuals and families; however, food shortages continue to exist, especially among the working poor. Those most at risk for hunger include children, single-parent families, and older adults.

FOOD-BUYING GUIDES

The amount of money spent for food is influenced by the size and composition of the household, the total household income, and personal preferences. As household size increases so do food costs, and the ages of the members of

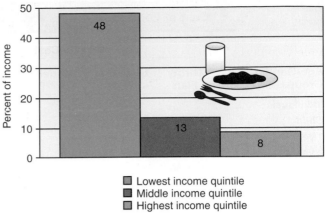

FIGURE 10-5 The percentage of income spent for food decreases as income rises. Low-income families must spend almost half of their income on food as compared with high-income families, which spend only 8% of their income on food. (*Data from Blisard N: Food spending by U.S. households grew steadily in the 1990s,* Food Rev 23(3):18, 2000.)

the household influence the amount of money spent. The weekly average food cost of a preschooler is about half that of an adult, and women consume less food than men.[29] As household income rises, the total amount of money spent for food also rises—but not proportionately—low-income households are forced to spend almost half of their income for food (48%) as compared to higher-income households, which spend only 8% (Figure 10-5).[30] Those with higher incomes do not necessarily eat greater amounts of food, but they select more expensive foods, buy more convenience items, and eat in restaurants more often.

USDA Food Plans

The USDA developed several food plans to serve as guides for food assistance programs. They are referred to as liberal, moderate, low, and thrifty food plans, based on the money spent per person of a given age or gender, but in reality they are all fairly low-cost plans and are tied to the poverty index. The thrifty plan is used to calculate the dollar value of food stamps granted to an individual or family. These food plans are developed by nutritionists, economists, and computer experts at USDA and are based on a predetermined level of spending. For each food plan there is a market basket list of the grocery items that will together meet the DRIs and the Dietary Guidelines for Americans for various age and gender groups (Tables 10-5 and 10-6).[29,31]

Developing a Family Food Plan

Many factors influence how much money a family can spend for food and how they divide their food dollars. When working with families a first step is to identify their food resources as well as their values and preferences about food, because these traits will enter into their household food plan.

TABLE 10-5	Cost of Food at Home for the Four USDA Food Plans*†‡

Age-Gender Groups	Weekly Cost				Monthly Cost			
	Thrifty Plan	Low-Cost Plan	Moderate-Cost Plan	Liberal Plan	Thrifty Plan	Low-Cost Plan	Moderate-Cost Plan	Liberal Plan
Individuals								
Child								
1 year	17.90	22.60	26.40	31.70	77.70	97.90	114.30	137.20
2 years	18.00	22.30	26.60	32.10	77.80	96.70	115.20	139.10
3-5 years	19.80	24.60	30.40	36.50	86.00	106.60	131.60	158.20
6-8 years	25.00	33.20	41.00	47.90	108.30	143.80	177.50	207.50
9-11 years	29.30	37.40	47.80	55.60	127.00	162.00	207.10	240.70
Male								
12-14 years	30.60	42.30	52.40	61.70	132.50	183.20	226.90	267.40
15-19 years	31.70	43.60	54.40	63.20	137.20	189.00	235.80	273.90
20-50 years	33.80	43.50	54.20	66.20	146.40	188.40	234.70	286.70
51 years and over	30.70	41.30	51.00	61.30	132.90	179.10	221.00	265.40
Female								
12-19 years	30.50	36.50	44.40	53.50	132.20	158.20	192.20	231.70
20-50 years	30.50	37.80	46.30	59.60	132.30	163.90	200.50	258.10
51 years and over	30.00	36.80	45.80	54.90	129.80	159.30	198.60	238.00
Families								
Family of 2								
20-50 years	70.80	89.50	110.50	138.30	306.60	387.60	478.70	599.20
51 years and over	66.70	85.90	106.50	127.80	289.00	372.20	461.50	553.80
Family of 4								
Couple, 20-50 years and children—								
2 and 3-5 years	102.10	128.20	157.40	194.30	442.50	555.60	682.00	842.10
6-8 and 9-11 years	118.60	151.90	189.20	229.20	514.00	658.20	819.70	993.00

From Center for Nutrition Policy and Promotion, U.S. Department of Agriculture: *Official USDA food plans: cost of food at home at four levels, U.S. average,* Alexandria, Va, 2005, Author. Available at *www.cnpp.usda.gov.*

USDA, U.S. Department of Agriculture.

*Average across the United States, October 2005.

†Expects that all meals and snacks are purchased at stores and prepared at home; see Table 10-6 for a list of specific food items to be purchased.

‡The costs given for individuals of certain ages expect that they live in four-person families; costs for children and adults living in smaller households or for adults living alone are somewhat higher.

Food Resources and Skills

Food resources can include money to purchase the appropriate amounts and types of food; however, food handling skills that enable a person to "cook a meal from scratch" is also a food resource. See the comprehensive list of food resources and skills that follows:

- *Family income in dollars*
- *Food produced or preserved in the home:* Some families have a vegetable garden and freeze or can that food for later use; those in rural areas may raise animals for meat or eggs.
- *Access to food assistance programs:* Food stamps, the Special Supplemental Nutrition Program for Women, Infants, and Children, commodity foods, free or reduced-cost

lunches for school-age children, meal programs for older adults, or accessible food pantries may be sources of food.

- *Access to a well-stocked grocery store with competitive prices:* As supermarkets move to suburban areas where profit margins are greater, persons living in the inner city that lack transportation are forced to food shop at convenience stores with limited selection and higher prices. Older people who no longer drive may have to shop at the store to which they can get a ride with a neighbor or friend. Families in rural areas may need to drive considerable distances to a supermarket with a good selection.
- *Time for food shopping:* Working single parents or working students with limited time may have to rush with shopping and not take time to read labels

TABLE 10-6	Weekly Food Market Basket on the Various USDA Food Plans*†		
Food Category	**Low-Cost**	**Moderate-Cost**	**Liberal**
	Pounds per week		
Grains			
Breads, yeast and quick	1.25	1.48	1.61
Breakfast cereals, cooked and ready to eat	.44	.42	.39
Rice and pasta	1.33	1.33	1.62
Flours	.47	.53	.58
Grain-based snacks and cookies	.17	.22	.18
TOTAL GRAINS	**3.66**	**3.98**	**4.38**
Vegetables			
Potato products	2.39	2.27	2.59
Dark-green and deep-yellow vegetables	.56	.77	.94
Other vegetables	2.73	3.29	3.57
TOTAL VEGETABLES	**5.68**	**6.33**	**7.10**
Fruits			
Citrus fruits, melons, berries, and juices	2.48	2.61	1.68
Noncitrus fruits and juices	1.84	2.46	4.78
TOTAL FRUITS	**4.32**	**5.07**	**6.46**
Milk Products			
Whole milk, yogurt, and cream	1.69	1.86	1.87
Lower fat and skim milk and lowfat yogurt	5.03	5.33	6.27
Cheese	.30	.34	.29
Milk drinks and milk desserts	.34	.39	.44
TOTAL MILK PRODUCTS	**7.36**	**7.92**	**8.87**
Meat/Meat Alternates			
Beef, pork, veal, lamb, and game	1.50	1.68	2.55
Chicken, turkey, and game birds	1.60	2.02	1.87
Fish and fish products	.48	.80	1.10
Bacon, sausages, and luncheon meats	.31	.33	.37
Eggs and egg mixtures	.41	.42	.44
Dry beans, lentils, peas, and nuts	.47	.44	.39
TOTAL MEAT/MEAT ALTERNATES	**4.77**	**5.69**	**6.72**
Other Foods			
Table fats, oils, and salad dressings	.39	.45	.47
Gravies, sauces, condiments, spices, and salt	.23	.27	.29
Fruit drinks, soft drinks, and ades	4.84	3.82	4.64
Sugars, sweets, and candies	.39	.17	.44
Coffee and tea	.19	.17	.12
TOTAL OTHER FOODS	**6.04**	**4.88**	**5.96**
TOTAL POUNDS	**31.83**	**33.87**	**39.49**

From Center for Nutrition Policy and Promotion, U.S. Department of Agriculture: *The low-cost, moderate-cost, and liberal food plans, 2003, administrative report, CNPP-13,* Alexandria, Va, 2003 (March), Author. Available at *www.cnpp.usda.gov.*

USDA, U.S. Department of Agriculture.

*Average pounds per person per week.

†Food as purchased includes uncooked grains; raw, canned, and frozen vegetables; fruit juice concentrates; dry beans and legumes; and meat and poultry with bones. Coffee and tea are included in small amounts. Fruit drinks, soft drinks, and ades equal less than one 16-oz bottle per day.

or look for the most economical choice. A retired older person or full-time homemaker may see food activities as an enjoyable way to pass the time.

- *Skills and experience in food management—planning, buying, preparation:* Many younger people never learned to cook and rely on convenience foods regardless of their nutritive content or cost. Those with limited food knowledge need help with reading food labels and understanding freshness codes. Older homemakers may have extensive knowledge about food but find it difficult to move about the kitchen based on physical limitations.

- *Facilities to store and cook food:* Most people have access to a cooking appliance and refrigerator, but homeless persons or older people living in single rooms may not have cold storage or food preparation facilities.

Family Food Needs and Preferences

Families have their own goals for use of food as a meaningful part of their relationships with each other, neighbors, and friends. Work and school patterns influence when and where family members eat. Characteristics that will be important in developing a family food plan follow:

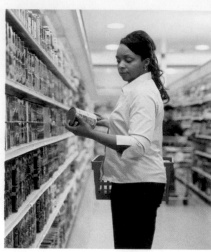

FIGURE 10-6 Shoppers are faced with a dazzling array of food choices. *(From Food and Nutrition Service, U.S. Department of Agriculture and Food and Nutrition Information Center, National Agricultural Library:* Food stamp nutrition collection: photo gallery, *Beltsville, Md, 2005, Authors. Retrieved December 12, 2005, from http://grande.nal.usda.gov/viewer.php?file=fs_recipes/imgs/shopping/shopping_vertical.jpg&file_loc=shopping_vertical.jpg.)*

- *Family traditions and food likes and dislikes:* Cultural, ethnic, and national groups often have specific food patterns that they wish to continue. It may be difficult to obtain certain foods or ingredients common to their food pattern, or, if available, they could be high in price.
- *Special dietary needs:* Individuals following a sodium-restricted diet may need certain foods.
- *Amount and kind of food entertaining:* Families may enjoy sharing meals or participating in potluck socials with their neighbors, community organizations, or religious groups.
- *Meals eaten away from home:* Family work or school schedules may demand that persons eat some meals away from home, either taking a packed lunch or purchasing food at that location. People may enjoy eating out and consider this part of their social framework.
- *Value placed on food and eating:* Food and mealtime may be an important part of family structure and interaction.

An extended discussion with family members about their food resources and preferences will provide the framework for helping them develop and implement a successful food plan.

Food Shopping Practices

Learning to Shop Wisely

Many American families spend more time shopping for food than preparing it once they arrive home. Food marketing is a big business, and buying food for a family is more complex than it may seem. The typical American supermarket offers over 40,000 different food

Before shopping, I:	Hardly ever	Sometimes	Most of the time
Check to see what foods I have on hand	☐	☐	☐
Plan meals to include a variety of foods from each of the major food groups	☐	☐	☐
Plan food purchases to keep amounts of fat, sugars, and sodium limit	☐	☐	☐
Consider how much money I have to spend on food	☐	☐	☐
Make a shopping list	☐	☐	☐
While shopping, I:			
Read ingredient labels, watching for ingredients that provide fat, sugars, and sodium	☐	☐	☐
Use nutrition labels to help select food products	☐	☐	☐
Use open dating information to ensure quality and freshness	☐	☐	☐
Use unit pricing (when available) to compare prices	☐	☐	☐
After shopping, I:			
Store foods promptly and properly to maintain their nutritive value and quality	☐	☐	☐
Place newer foods in the back of refrigerator, freezer, and cabinet shelves, so older foods will be used first	☐	☐	☐
Use perishable foods promptly to avoid food waste	☐	☐	☐

FIGURE 10-7 The Super Shopper Checklist. Most people have a general routine when they shop for food. Check the boxes above that best describe what you do before, during, and after each trip to the supermarket. Small changes in your shopping habits may make it easier to prepare meals at home that meet the Dietary Guidelines. If "most of the time" is your answer, you are a super shopper! *(From U.S. Department of Agriculture:* Shopping for food and making meals in minutes using The Dietary Guidelines, *Home and Garden Bulletin No. 232-10, Hyattsville, Md, {no date available}, Author.)*

items,[32] and a single food item may be marketed in many different ways, all with different prices, presenting many choices for the shopper (Figure 10-6). The food stamps nutrition education program noted earlier helps families develop food shopping skills. Supermarket tours can be an informative tool in helping families develop good shopping skills. Wise meal planning and food shopping practices will not only improve the nutrient content of meals but also increase the food value obtained from the money spent (Figure 10-7).

TABLE 10-7	Cost Comparisons of Home-Prepared Foods and Preprepared Foods		
Food*	**Ingredients**	**Preprepared**	**Added Preparation**
Carrots	Unpeeled and uncut	Small baby carrots peeled and washed	Shredded carrots
	3-oz serving (raw)	3-oz serving (raw)	3-oz serving (raw)
	15 cents	37 cents	94 cents
Broccoli	Frozen flowerets in family-size bag	Frozen spears in 10-oz package	Frozen spears with butter sauce
	3-oz serving	3-oz serving	3-oz serving
	18 cents	30 cents	57 cents
Potato	Fresh potatoes (purchased in 10-lb bag)	Instant mashed potatoes	Refrigerated mashed potatoes ready to heat
	½ cup (cooked/mashed)	½ cup (reconstituted/heated)	½ cup
	14 cents	34 cents	49 cents
Chicken	Raw chicken breasts	Refrigerated roasted chicken breasts, ready-to-eat	Cooked chicken breast cut in strips for salads (no bones)
	$1.49 per pound	$7.98 per pound	$9.57 per pound
Ground beef	Ground chuck hamburger	Ground chuck hamburger preshaped into patties	Meat loaf refrigerated and ready to heat
	3-oz serving (cooked)	3-oz serving (cooked)	3-oz serving (heated)
	$0.67 cents	$0.99 cents	$1.23
Oatmeal	Old-fashioned oats	Quick 1-minute oats	Instant oatmeal, regular flavor
	¾-cup serving	¾-cup serving	¾-cup serving (one packet)
	16 cents	16 cents	37 cents

NOTE: The more preparation that has been completed for you, the higher will be the purchase price.

*Costs based on market prices at The Kroger Company, Blacksburg, Va, April 2005, and Network Grocers, accessed April 28, 2005, at *www.netgrocer.com/*. Ground meat costs calculated on the basis of cooked weight.

Planning Ahead

To ensure that family members eat a variety of foods and obtain the number of food servings recommended in MyPyramid (see Chapter 1), it is best to plan meals for the week and then develop a shopping list. When planning meals consider the food on hand and how perishable items can be used to avoid waste. Checking local newspapers or store flyers for specials can target those items that the family enjoys. Fresh fruits and vegetables that are in season are lower in price. Preparing a market list ahead of time helps avoid impulse buying and extra trips to the store. Grocery lists should be organized in the same order as the supermarket aisles to save time. Shopping when you are not hungry or rushed means you are less tempted to buy items that you do not need or cannot afford.

Buying Wisely

Food product labels provide important information about food quality, quantity, and safety. Purchasing sale items in quantity saves money only if the food can be adequately stored or used before it spoils, and food labels indicate when a food will no longer be safe to eat. Shoppers should be cautious in selecting convenience foods, because the time saved may not be worth the added cost (Table 10-7).

Supplying recipes that are both convenient and nutritious can help busy homemakers make better use of their food dollars, especially if recipes are simple and easily remembered.[33] Comparing one food product with another helps consumers get the best value for their food dollar. The following pieces of information on the food label and store shelf are helpful in evaluating food purchases.

Unit Pricing. Large packages are sometimes cheaper per unit weight than small packages, but any savings depend on how much of the product you need and whether it can be used within the appropriate time. If an item has an extended shelf life or is something that you use regularly, one large box rather than two smaller boxes is a wise choice. Use the unit pricing label to determine the true food price per unit weight when comparing different brands or packages of different sizes (Box 10-5). Unit pricing can help you decide if a store brand is less expensive than a national brand for which you also pay the cost of television or magazine advertising.

Open Dating. These dates tell you about the freshness of the item or how soon it must be used. Box 10-6 describes the types of dating information used on food labels.

BOX 10-5 | Unit Pricing

The unit price is the price per pound, ounce, quart, or other unit. Unit price labels can be found on the display shelves or below canned and packaged foods. Comparison of unit prices can help consumers find the brand of food and the specific container that cost the least amount per unit.

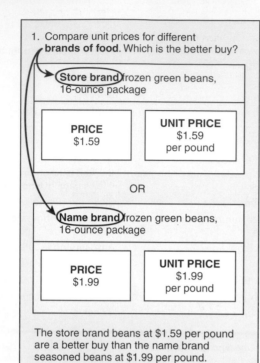

1. Compare unit prices for different **brands of food.** Which is the better buy?

(Store brand) frozen green beans, 16-ounce package

| PRICE $1.59 | UNIT PRICE $1.59 per pound |

OR

(Name brand) frozen green beans, 16-ounce package

| PRICE $1.99 | UNIT PRICE $1.99 per pound |

The store brand beans at $1.59 per pound are a better buy than the name brand seasoned beans at $1.99 per pound.

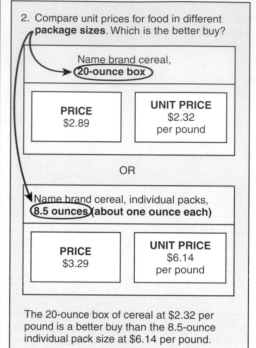

2. Compare unit prices for food in different **package sizes.** Which is the better buy?

Name brand cereal, (20-ounce box)

| PRICE $2.89 | UNIT PRICE $2.32 per pound |

OR

Name brand cereal, individual packs, (8.5 ounces)(about one ounce each)

| PRICE $3.29 | UNIT PRICE $6.14 per pound |

The 20-ounce box of cereal at $2.32 per pound is a better buy than the 8.5-ounce individual pack size at $6.14 per pound.

BOX 10-6 | Types of Open Dating Used on Food Packages

Sell by	The last date the item should be sold by the store
Best if used by	The date that indicates maximum freshness; after this date check for signs of spoilage and expect a reduced price
Expiration date or use by	The last date when active ingredients will be good (commonly used with yeast for baking); do not purchase foods after their expiration date because spoilage may have occurred even if not immediately visible
Pack date	The date when the food was packed; commonly found on canned foods; look for a recent pack date

Package Weight or Volume. Check the label to determine the actual contents of a package by weight or volume and the number of servings it contains. Deceptive packaging can suggest that the food content is greater than it really is.

CASE STUDY

Helping With Family Shopping

You are working with a family that includes three adults—two men ages 27 and 69 and a woman age 26—and two boys ages 5 and 2. The children are receiving foods from the Special Supplemental Nutrition Program for Women, Infants, and Children (WIC). The family was referred to you by the nurse at WIC, who is concerned about the children's nutrition as well as the food shopping and preparation practices in the family. To save money the homemaker buys foods reduced for quick sale and tries to use it all regardless of the length of time. She seldom buys fresh fruits and vegetables because they seem to be more expensive, but she often uses fruit drinks.

Questions for Analysis

1. Based on the various food plans developed by the U.S Department of Agriculture (USDA), what is the minimum amount of money that this family must spend on food to meet their nutritional requirements?
2. What questions would you ask this homemaker about her shopping practices?
3. What advice would you give her about food-buying practices to ensure food safety for her family? Which family members are most vulnerable to foodborne illness?
4. What are some suggestions that you would give her about purchase of fruits and vegetables (see Box 10-7 and Table 10-6)? Are fruit drinks a good use of her food dollars?
5. Prepare a 1-day menu for the children meeting the MyPyramid recommendations using the WIC foods available.

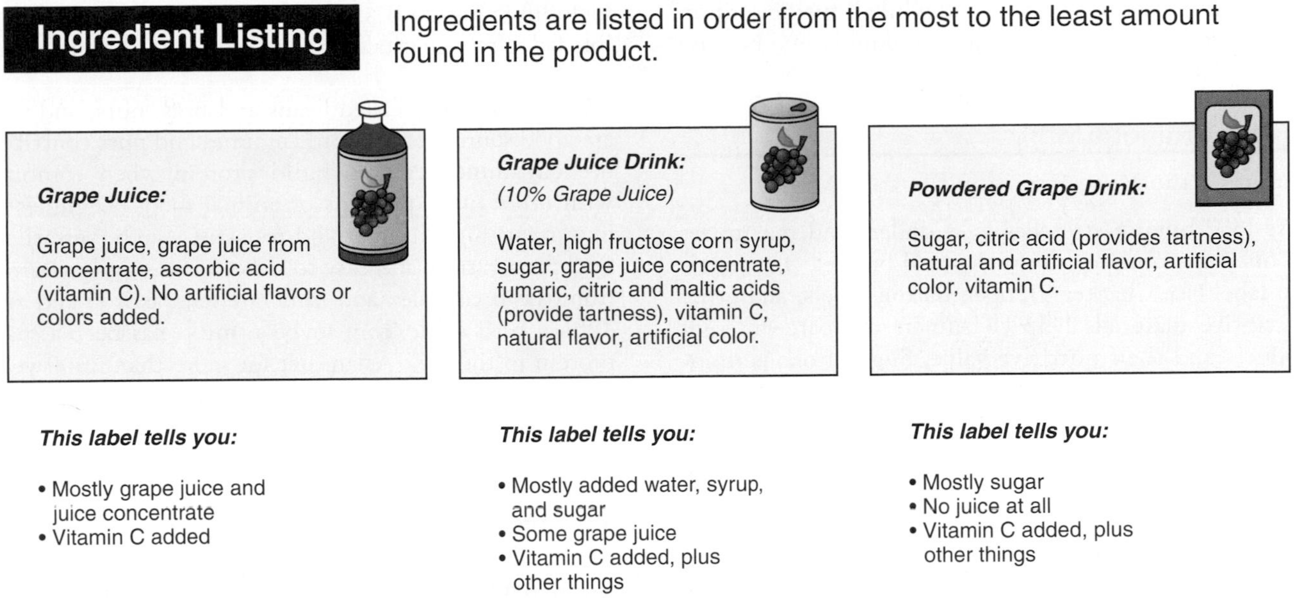

Ingredient Listing

Ingredients are listed in order from the most to the least amount found in the product.

Grape Juice:

Grape juice, grape juice from concentrate, ascorbic acid (vitamin C). No artificial flavors or colors added.

Grape Juice Drink:

(10% Grape Juice)

Water, high fructose corn syrup, sugar, grape juice concentrate, fumaric, citric and maltic acids (provide tartness), vitamin C, natural flavor, artificial color.

Powdered Grape Drink:

Sugar, citric acid (provides tartness), natural and artificial flavor, artificial color, vitamin C.

This label tells you:

- Mostly grape juice and juice concentrate
- Vitamin C added

This label tells you:

- Mostly added water, syrup, and sugar
- Some grape juice
- Vitamin C added, plus other things

This label tells you:

- Mostly sugar
- No juice at all
- Vitamin C added, plus other things

FIGURE 10-8   Products with similar names can have very different ingredients and nutrient content. It is important to read labels carefully to know what you are paying for. *(From U.S. Department of Agriculture:* Do you use unit prices to find the best buys? Make your food dollars count, *Program Aid No 1345, Washington, DC, 1984, Author.)*

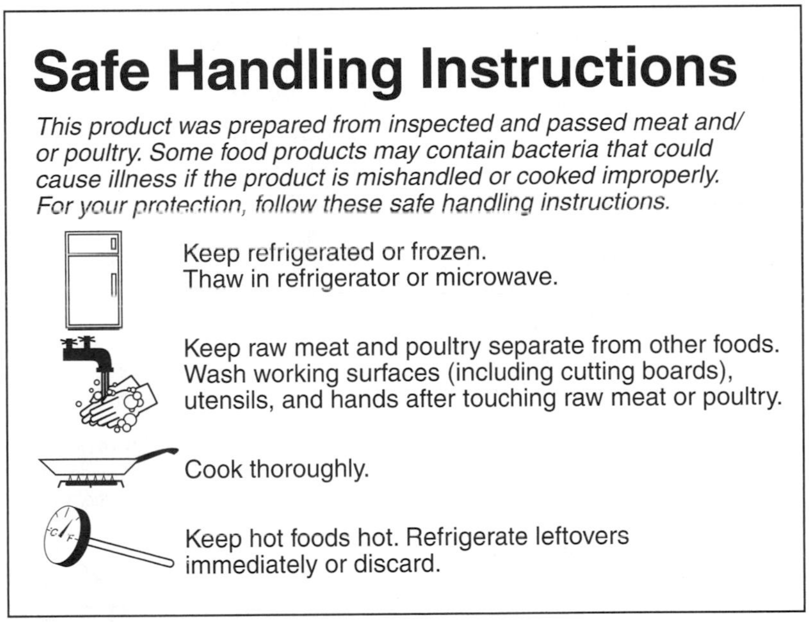

Safe Handling Instructions

This product was prepared from inspected and passed meat and/or poultry. Some food products may contain bacteria that could cause illness if the product is mishandled or cooked improperly. For your protection, follow these safe handling instructions.

 Keep refrigerated or frozen.
Thaw in refrigerator or microwave.

 Keep raw meat and poultry separate from other foods. Wash working surfaces (including cutting boards), utensils, and hands after touching raw meat or poultry.

 Cook thoroughly.

 Keep hot foods hot. Refrigerate leftovers immediately or discard.

FIGURE 10-9   Food safety instructions on the food label. The food label provides important information about the safe storage and cooking of perishable foods. The food label on fresh and frozen meat, fish, and poultry advises consumers to store, thaw, and cook these foods to avoid foodborne illness. *(From U.S. Department of Agriculture:* Safe handling label, *Washington, DC, {no date available}, Author.)*

List of Ingredients.   Ingredients are listed in order by weight, from the highest to the lowest amount found in the product. By reviewing this list you can see what you are paying for. As we see in Figure 10-8, fruit drinks may contain sugar, water, and flavoring, but little or no juice. (See the *Case Study* box, "Helping With Family Shopping," to apply these principles.)

Storing Food Safely

Controlling kitchen waste resulting from food spoilage helps protect the family food dollar. Conserve food using covered containers for dry storage, refrigeration, or freezing. Opened and partly used food packages are best kept at the front of the shelf where they will remain visible and be used first. Labels found on highly perishable foods such as meat, poultry, and fish give directions for preventing spoilage and contamination (Figure 10-9).

Cooking Food Well

Nutrition education for meal preparers should focus on how to retain maximum food value when preparing or cooking fruits and vegetables (see Chapter 6). A variety of seasonings can give zest to food while limiting sodium and fat. Persons eat because they are hungry and because the food looks and tastes good.

Health Promotion

Obtaining the Most Nutrition for Your Money

Wise food buying stretches food dollars and maximizes the nutrients obtained from the food budget. The nutrition label (see Chapter 9), open dating labels, and other descriptive materials help consumers compare different products and their nutritive value. Suggestions pertaining to the purchase of foods from the various food groups are given below.

Vegetables and Fruits

Vegetables and fruits supply important nutrients, phytochemicals, and fiber. They are major sources of vitamins A, C, and B_6, folate, potassium, and trace minerals. MyPyramid suggests the amounts of fruits and of each category of vegetables to be included in the weekly food pattern. Home gardening is a way to increase availability and encourage use of vegetables. In some urban areas community agencies sponsor gardening programs using vacant lots, offering opportunities for youth- and family-oriented activities. Box 10-7 provides suggestions on purchasing vegetables, fruits, and juices.

Breads, Cereals, and Grains

Enriched and whole grain breads, cereals, and other grains are well liked, relatively inexpensive, and fit easily into meal plans. They provide complex carbohydrates and important vitamins and minerals. Under federal law all grain foods produced in the United States must be enriched with folate to prevent the occurrence of neural tube defects. Some enriched cereals and grains have added vitamin B_{12} and help prevent deficiency among older people with low gastric acid. Whole grain foods are rich in dietary fiber and especially high in certain trace minerals. The fiber, vitamins, and trace minerals occurring naturally in grain foods are found in the bran and kernel, which are removed when whole grains are refined (Figure 10-10). MyPyramid recommends that at least three of our daily servings of grains be whole grains.

Protein Foods: Meat, Poultry, Fish, Eggs, Legumes, and Nuts

Animal Proteins.   Meat, fish, poultry, and eggs provide complete protein, the B complex vitamins, and trace minerals. Eggs are relatively inexpensive sources of high-quality protein and are lower in cholesterol than had been believed. For most persons four eggs per week is acceptable. Fish is a healthy choice for both children and adults and adds polyunsaturated fatty acids, especially n-3 fatty acids, to the diet. Red meats are good sources of well-absorbed forms of iron and zinc and the B vitamins,

including vitamin B_{12}. Choose lean cuts, and trim all visible fat to reduce intakes of cholesterol and saturated fat.

Plant Proteins.   Dried beans and peas, nuts, and seeds are good sources of protein. Legumes and nuts contribute needed amino acids to build protein when combined with other plant proteins or animal foods. Legumes are low in fat, high in fiber and resistant starch, versatile in food preparation, and easy to store. They supply vitamins from the B complex and minerals such as iron and zinc. Tofu, a curd made from soybean milk, has been a major protein in the East Asian diet for more than 2000 years. Soy protein and soybeans are common ingredients in chips, pasta, trail mix, and other prepared foods.

Dairy Foods

Milk products, including fluid or nonfat dried milk, cheese, and yogurt, are important sources of protein, calcium, magnesium, vitamin B_{12}, and riboflavin. Most fluid and nonfat dried milk and yogurt are fortified with vitamin D, adding to their nutritional value and facilitating the absorption of calcium. Dairy products naturally contain both saturated fat and cholesterol; low-fat varieties are lower in kcalories and total and saturated fat.

Fats and Oils

Fats and oils contain the essential fatty acids and provide a concentrated source of kcalories for those with high

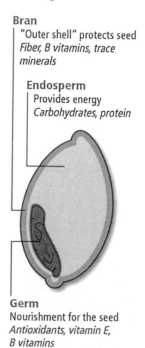

Whole grain kernel

Bran
"Outer shell" protects seed
Fiber, B vitamins, trace minerals

Endosperm
Provides energy
Carbohydrates, protein

Germ
Nourishment for the seed
Antioxidants, vitamin E, B vitamins

FIGURE 10-10   The nutrients in the bran and the germ of whole grains are lost when these grains are refined and the bran and germ are removed. *(From U.S. Department of Agriculture:* Get on the grain train: putting the guidelines into practice, *Home and Garden Bulletin No. 267-2, Washington, DC, 2002 {May}, Author.)*

BOX 10-7 | Getting the Most for Your Food Dollar

Fruits and Vegetables

- Buy fresh fruits and vegetables in season when they are less expensive. Visit a farmers' market or a pick-your-own outlet, which provides cost savings along with a fun family activity.
- Choose fresh produce that is firm, crisp, and free of brown or soft spots.
- Compare costs of fresh fruits and vegetables sold by weight or count. Look for the number of items in bags sold by weight.
- Check the cost of store brands versus national brands when buying canned vegetables and fruits. Avoid fancy grades that are priced higher. Grading is based on shape, size, and perfection of pieces; lower grades are equal in food value and taste.
- Compare the cost of family-size bags versus individual packages of frozen vegetables. It may be more economical to buy the family-size bags and pour out what you need, saving the remainder for later. Replace the unused portion in the freezer immediately to prevent thawing and loss of quality. Avoid frozen vegetables with special sauces that add both cost and additional fat and sodium.
- If possible, select juice- or water-packed canned fruits rather than syrup-packed with added sugar. If using syrup-packed fruit, rinse before serving.
- If possible, select low-sodium canned vegetables rather than the usual variety, or rinse the higher-sodium product before using.

Breads and Cereals

- Check the weight of bread loaves when doing price comparisons, because a large loaf may not weigh more than a small loaf; higher-priced breads advertised as having fewer kcalories per slice may be similar to other breads, just cut into thinner slices.
- Look for whole grain breads or cereals; check the label for the words *whole grain*. The word *whole* should appear first on the ingredient list; breads darker in color may have added molasses and may not be whole grain. Choose products made from whole wheat, whole oats, oatmeal, whole rye, or whole grain corn or corn meal. (Popped corn is an easy, whole grain snack!)
- Avoid bread or cereal products in which some form of sugar is the first or second ingredient. It is more economical to add your own sugar to cereal and be in control of the amount added. Learn to recognize the names of different types of sugars, such as sucrose, fructose, molasses, honey, corn syrup, and high-fructose corn syrup (HFCS), that appear on food labels.
- Cereals providing 100% of the Dietary Reference Intake (DRI) for many vitamins and minerals are more expensive; if you eat a good diet, these additional nutrients may be unnecessary. Look for those nutrients that you really need; if you eat more than one serving of these cereals along with other foods you may take in inappropriately high levels of certain nutrients.
- Use a variety of whole grains. Bulgur, buckwheat, barley, and millet can be used in place of rice or potatoes or added to soup or salads; bulgur is cooked like rice and has a toast-like color and wheat flavor.
- Emphasize less-processed grains. Highly processed grains not only lose nutrients and fiber but are also higher in sodium and more expensive.

Meat, Fish, Poultry, and Eggs

- Eggs are sold according to grade and size, which do not affect food value; extra large eggs are not worth the additional cost. Shell color varies according to the breed of chicken but does not influence nutrient content.
- Check the expiration date on fresh poultry because it has a relatively short shelf life; boneless chicken pieces are more expensive because you are paying for convenience.
- Fresh or frozen fish is expensive in some geographic locations, and this is also true for shellfish. Fresh fish has a short shelf life and should not have a "fishy" odor because this indicates it is several days old; if fresh fish will not be used in 1 or 2 days, it is best to freeze it. Canned fish, especially tuna, is a good buy; water-packed tuna will be lower in kcalories than oil-packed.
- Lower grades of beef are less expensive and also lower in fat. Beef roasts will keep safely in the refrigerator for several days, but ground meat with a greater area of exposure to the air and potential pathogens should be held for no more than 1 to 2 days.
- Trim all visible fat from beef, pork, or ham before cooking.
- When choosing meat, poultry, or fish for family meals, consider the number of portions and number of meals it will provide.

Milk, Cheese, and Other Dairy Foods

- Fluid milk can contain varying levels of fat: nonfat, 1%, 2%, or 3.3% (whole milk); for persons above 2 years of age, nonfat or low-fat milk is a better choice. Canned evaporated milk with a long shelf life is available in regular and nonfat forms.
- Nonfat dry milk is a very economical form of milk and can be added to casseroles, mashed potatoes, or soups to increase their nutrient content; reconstituted nonfat dry milk can be mixed 1:1 with fluid milk to provide a low-cost and palatable milk for drinking.
- Families using large amounts of milk will find it economical to buy gallon containers; be sure to check the sell by date when buying fluid milk (see Box 10-6).
- Natural cheeses such as cheddar or Swiss provide more calcium and vitamins and are lower in fat and sodium than processed cheeses; cheeses prepackaged in individual slices are more expensive than block cheeses that you slice yourself. Packages of shredded cheese cost more than the same weight of the same cheese in wedges or blocks.
- Cottage cheese contains less calcium than an equal weight of milk or yogurt. Cottage cheese is also fairly high in sodium. Be sure to check the expiration date before purchase.

Fats and Oils

- Liquid oils such as canola or soybean oil are high in polyunsaturated fats and can become rancid; they must be stored tightly closed in a cool dry place.
- Partially hydrogenated fats (soft-tub fats) are good choices as table fats, but check the label and select those with few or no *trans* fatty acids. Some margarines have added plant sterols to reduce the absorption of dietary cholesterol, but they are much higher in price.

energy needs. Polyunsaturated and monounsaturated oils are the best sources of the essential n-6 and n-3 fatty acids and vitamin E. Hydrogenated fats such as margarine may contain *trans* fatty acids harmful to health (see Chapter 3), and consumers should read nutrition labels to avoid *trans* fats. Butter, an animal fat high in saturated fatty acids, is best used in only limited amounts.

Sources of Groceries

Retail Grocery Stores

Most people have access to at least one supermarket or grocery store that carries a wide variety of fresh and processed foods at reasonable prices. When several food outlets are close by, individuals can select where they want to shop or vary their location depending on the particular specials for the week. With supermarket chains moving out of the inner city where crime and low profit margins make business less desirable, these residents are becoming more dependent on convenience stores that carry limited amounts of fresh foods, offer little choice of package size, and charge higher prices. Neighborhood groups are working with city governments to improve access to food supplies.[34] Individuals in rural areas may be dependent on small general stores that cater to travelers and tourists and offer limited options for weekly food shopping.

Farmers' Markets

Farmers' markets make local produce directly available to consumers at prices that are often lower than those at supermarkets. The public considers local fruits and vegetables to be fresher and look and taste better. Buying local produce also supports a sustainable local agricultural economy.[35]

Consumer Cooperatives

Consumer cooperatives strive to offer high-quality foods at the lowest possible price. Food cooperatives usually deal in bulk sales of whole or minimally processed foods. Many food cooperatives emphasize locally grown foods, thus supporting local farmers while providing very fresh foods for consumers. They usually require a certain number of hours of volunteer time from each member in addition to or in lieu of a membership fee.

Food Discount Stores

Food stores that stock fresh and processed foods, paper goods, and cleaning supplies at discount prices are growing in popularity. These stores offer few services, and furnishings are sparse, but in exchange, food and other supplies are usually lower in price than at traditional supermarkets. Processed foods sold at food discount stores may be closeouts or excess stock from large food manufacturers that is nearing the date of expiration or best use. The units sold often include several cans or packages, so consumers must decide if the quantity being purchased is actually needed and can be used within the appropriate time period.

Food Banks

Food banks are warehouses that collect and store donations of food from supermarkets, food processors, food distributors, growers, and the general public. These foods are made available to nonprofit programs such as soup kitchens serving limited-resource families or to food pantries that distribute groceries to those in need. The food banks across the United States distribute more than a billion pounds of food each year.[36] For many families food pantries are a source of emergency assistance when their food supplies are depleted and they have no money or food stamps to purchase food. Food banks usually have more plentiful supplies of foods from the grains and meat groups. Fruit and dairy products are often limited, decreasing the vitamin A, vitamin C, and calcium available to those receiving food.[37]

TO SUM UP

Nutrition counselors translate food and nutrition information into simple ideas and suggestions that will help individuals and families make appropriate diet-related decisions. Important concepts must be presented in ways that are easily understood, retained, applied, and evaluated to determine their effectiveness. Health and nutrition education must focus on the needs of the learner, and both goals and strategies must be developed jointly by the health professional and the individual or family if they are to be successful. Many families are in economic stress and need help in obtaining appropriate amounts of food. Various food assistance programs can add to a family's food resources, and referrals to appropriate agencies are an important part of nutrition intervention. Support in developing good shopping and food handling practices—planning ahead, buying wisely, storing safely, and cooking appropriately to preserve nutrient values—will lead to positive changes in nutrient intake.

QUESTIONS FOR REVIEW

1. Identify and describe the skills necessary for effective nutrition counseling.
2. List the basic principles of learning. Apply these principles to one of the following situations:
   - A low-income Hispanic mother with limited English skills and a 2-year-old son who is underweight for his age
   - A 71-year-old woman with hypertension who has been told to lower her sodium intake
3. What is meant by food insecurity, and how is it determined? Describe the government-funded food assistance programs available to help limited-resource families obtain sufficient amounts of food. Using your local telephone

directory, prepare a list of organizations in your community that provide food resources for individuals or families in need. Working with other students in the class, prepare a pamphlet for distribution that lists the organization, contact information, type of assistance provided, and any requirements or qualifications for receiving assistance.

4. Describe the types of information provided under the "open dating" legislation. Develop a handout with visuals that could be used to teach these concepts to a low-literacy audience.

5. Using unit pricing, compare the cost per serving of eight different ready-to-eat cereals: two sugar-coated cereals, two granola cereals, two whole grain cereals, and two cereals advertised as meeting 100% of the DRIs. Which is the most expensive per serving, and which is the least expensive per serving? Which cereal seems to provide the best nutritional value for the money?

6. Obtain a map of your city or county, and, using the telephone directory, identify supermarkets or food stores offering a good selection of fresh and processed foods. Mark their location on your map. Does each general neighborhood or community have access to a supermarket, or are there areas that lack food access? Visit the web site of The Food Trust (*www.thefoodtrust.org*), which is based in Philadelphia and helps inner-city communities keep or attract appropriate food markets.

REFERENCES

1. Hayes DK et al: Racial/ethnic and socioeconomic disparities in multiple risk factors for heart disease and stroke—United States, 2003, *MMWR Morb Mortal Wkly Rep* 54(5):113, 2005.

2. Centers for Disease Control and Prevention: *The burden of chronic diseases and their risk factors: national and state perspectives,* Atlanta, 2004 (February), U.S. Department of Health and Human Services.

3. Kittler PG, Sucher KP: *Food and culture,* ed 4, Belmont, Calif, 2004, Brooks/Cole, a division of Thomson Learning.

4. Holli BB, Calabrese RJ, O'Sullivan-Maillet J: *Communication and education skills for dietetics professionals,* ed 4, Philadelphia, 2003, Lippincott, Williams & Wilkins.

5. Patterson RE et al: Using a brief household inventory as an environmental indicator of individual dietary practices, *Am J Public Health* 87(2):272, 1997.

6. Novotny JA et al: Personality characteristics as predictors of underreporting of energy intake on 24-hour dietary recall interviews, *J Am Diet Assoc* 103:1146, 2003.

7. Kicklighter JR: Characteristics of older adult learners: a guide for dietetics practitioners, *J Am Diet Assoc* 91(11):1418, 1991.

8. American Dietetic Association: Position of the American Dietetic Association: total diet approach to communicating food and nutrition information, *J Am Diet Assoc* 102:100, 2002.

9. U.S. Department of Agriculture: *MyPyramid food guidance system,* Washington, DC, 2005, Author. Available at *www.mypyramid.gov.*

10. Mackey M, Montgomery J: Plant biotechnology can enhance food security and nutrition in the developing world, part 1, *Nutr Today* 39:52, 2004.

11. American Dietetic Association: Position of the American Dietetic Association: addressing world hunger, malnutrition, and food insecurity, *J Am Diet Assoc* 103:1046, 2003.

12. Champagne CM et al: Dietary intake in the Lower Mississippi Delta Region: results from the Foods of Our Delta Study, *J Am Diet Assoc* 104:199, 2004.

13. Stuff JE et al: Household food insecurity is associated with adult health status, *J Nutr* 134:2330, 2004.

14. Cook JT et al: Food insecurity is associated with adverse health outcomes among human infants and toddlers, *J Nutr* 134:1432, 2004.

15. Sharkey JR: Risk and presence of food insufficiency are associated with low nutrient intakes and multimorbidity among homebound older women who receive home-delivered meals, *J Nutr* 133:3485, 2003.

16. Kempson KM et al: Educators' reports of food acquisition practices used by limited-resource individuals to maintain food sufficiency, *Fam Econ Nutr Rev* 14(2):44, 2002.

17. Drewnowski A, Barratt-Fornell A: Do healthier diets cost more, *Nutr Today* 39(4):161, 2004.

18. Boyle MA: *Community nutrition in action: an entrepreneurial approach,* Belmont, Calif, 2003, Wadsworth/Thomson Learning.

19. U.S. Department of Agriculture: Food stamp households: 2002, *Fam Econ Nutr Rev* 16(1):56, 2004.

20. Food and Nutrition Service, U.S. Department of Agriculture: *Food stamp program: frequently asked questions,* Washington, DC, 2005, Author. Retrieved December 12, 2005, from *www.fns.usda.gov/fsp/faqs.htm.*

21. Food and Nutrition Service, U.S. Department of Agriculture: *Nutrition program facts: food stamp nutrition education,* Washington, DC, 2005, Author. Retrieved December 12, 2005, from *www.fns.usda.gov/fsp/nutrition_education/factsheet.htm.*

22. Food and Nutrition Service, U.S. Department of Agriculture: *Nutrition program facts: National School Lunch Program,* Washington, DC, 2005, Author. Retrieved December 12, 2005, from *www.fns.usda.gov/cnd/lunch/AboutLunch/NSLPFactSheet.pdf.*

23. Food and Nutrition Service, U.S. Department of Agriculture: *Nutrition program facts: the school breakfast program,* Washington, DC, 2005, Author. Retrieved December 12, 2005, from *www.fns.usda.gov/cnd/breakfast/AboutBFast/FactSheet.pdf.*

24. Food and Nutrition Service, U.S. Department of Agriculture: *Summer Food Service Program: frequently asked questions,* Washington, DC, 2005, Author. Retrieved December 12, 2005, from *www.fns.usda.gov/cnd/summer/about/faq.html.*

25. Food and Nutrition Service, U.S. Department of Agriculture: *Nutrition program facts: WIC, the Special Supplemental Nutrition Program for Women, Infants and Children,* Washington, DC, 2005, Author. Retrieved December 12, 2005, from *www.fns.usda.gov/wic/factsheets.htm.*

26. Food and Nutrition Service, U.S. Department of Agriculture: *About WIC: how WIC helps,* Washington, DC, 2005, Author. Retrieved December 12, 2005, from *www.fns.usda.gov/wic/aboutwic/howwichelps.htm.*

27. Administration on Aging, U.S. Department of Health and Human Services: *Elderly Nutrition Program,* Washington, DC, 2005, Author. Retrieved December 12, 2005, from *www.aoa.gov/press/fact/fact.asp#quantitys.*

28. Cooperative State Research, Education, and Extension Service, U.S. Department of Agriculture: *About EFNEP,* Washington, DC, 2005, Author. Retrieved December 12, 2005, from *www.csrees.usda.gov/nea/food/efnep/about.html.*

29. Center for Nutrition Policy and Promotion, U.S. Department of Agriculture: *Official USDA food plans: cost of food at home at four levels, U.S. average,* Alexandria, Va, 2005 (March), Author. Available at *www.cnpp.usda.gov.*

30. Blisard N: Food spending by U.S. households grew steadily in the 1990s, *Food Rev* 23(3):18, 2000.

31. Lino M: The thrifty food plan, 1999: revisions of the market baskets, *Fam Econ Nutr Rev* 13(1):50, 2001.

32. Tillotson JE: Who's filling your grocery bag, part 1, *Nutr Today* 39:176, 2004.

33. Harper R: Easy does it, *Supermarket News,* p 57, Jan 17, 2005.

34. The Food Trust: *www.thefoodtrust.org,* Philadelphia, 2004, Author.

35. Storper B: Moving toward healthful sustainable diets, *Nutr Today* 38:57, 2003.

36. Cotugna N, Beebe PD: Food banking in the 21st century: much more than a canned handout, *J Am Diet Assoc* 102:1386, 2002.

37. Akobundu UO et al: Vitamins A and C, calcium, fruit, and dairy products are limited in food pantries, *J Am Diet Assoc* 104:811, 2004.

FURTHER READINGS AND RESOURCES

Readings

Jonnalagadda SS: Dietary counseling is an important component of cardiac rehabilitation, *J Am Diet Assoc* 105(10):1529, 2005.

Nutrition counseling can help individuals with chronic disease lower their risk and establish more healthy lifestyles. Dr. Jonnalagadda applies the principles of nutrition assessment and counseling to patients with cardiovascular disease.

Lockeretz W, Merrigan KA: Selling to the eco-conscious food shopper, *Nutr Today* 40(1):45, 2005.

Storper B: Moving toward healthful sustainable diets, *Nutr Today* 38(2):57, 2003.

These articles discuss our social responsibility as food shoppers for maintaining the environment and sustaining plant and agricultural systems.

Cotugna N, Beebe PD: Food banking in the 21st Century: much more than a canned handout, *J Am Diet Assoc* 102(10):1386, 2002.

McCullum C et al: Evidence-based strategies to build community food security, *J Am Diet Assoc* 105(2):278, 2005.

An important source of food for many limited-resource families is the local food pantry. Dr. Cotugna and Dr. Beebe tell us how these programs got started in local communities and provide examples of some very successful programs. Dr. McCullum and co-workers provide us with ideas on how communities can work together to ensure that all families have enough food.

Scheier LM: What is the hunger-obesity paradox, *J Am Diet Assoc* 105(6):883, 2005.

Overweight and obesity are prevalent among limited-resource individuals and families. Dr. Scheier discusses how hunger and obesity may be related.

Websites of Interest

- Food and Nutrition Service, U.S. Department of Agriculture; this website offers links to many different food assistance programs, including the National School Breakfast Program, the Food Stamp Program, and the Special Supplemental Nutrition Program for Women, Infants, and Children: *www.fns.usda.gov/fns/.*

- Center for Nutrition Policy and Promotion, U.S. Department of Agriculture; this website contains a series of short reports entitled Nutrition Insights that tell us about food and nutrition problems of various population groups in the United States: *www.cnpp. usda.gov/insights.html.*

- The World Bank Group; this website describes programs to improve the health and nutrition of women and children around the world: *www.worldbank.org/html/extdr/hnp/hnp.htm.*

- U.S. Agency for International Development (USAID); this agency sponsors nutrition programs in many developing countries. Its website describes programs for vitamin A fortification of foods, infant and child feeding, and community programs to ensure safe water and sanitation practices: *www.usaid.gov/our_work/global_health/nut/index.html.*

- The Food Trust; the website of this Philadelphia-based organization describes efforts to bring both nutrition education programs and appropriate food resources including supermarkets to inner-city neighborhoods: *www.thefoodtrust.org/.*

CHAPTER 11

Nutrition During Pregnancy and Lactation

Sharon M. Nickols-Richardson

In this chapter we begin a three-chapter sequence on nutrition in health care throughout the life cycle. In each chapter, we will relate principles of nutrition to the remarkable process of human growth and development.

As we focus first on the beginning of new life, we examine the prenatal nutritional demands of the pregnant woman and her developing fetus, as well as maternal nutritional needs during lactation. Mother and offspring possess great adaptive abilities to meet nutritional demands during these life cycle stages.

Here, we explore the tremendous physiologic changes during pregnancy and lactation and some possible complications. You will see how vital optimal nutrition is for a successful course and outcome.

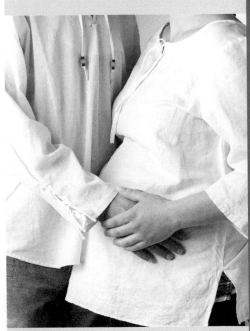

MATERNAL NUTRITION AND THE OUTCOME OF PREGNANCY

Early Medical Practice

For centuries, in all cultures, a great body of folklore has surrounded pregnancy. Various traditional practices and diets have been followed, many of which have had little factual basis, and much clinical advice has been based only on supposition. For example, early obstetricians even held the notion that semistarvation of the pregnant woman was really a blessing in disguise because it produced a small baby of light weight who would be easier to deliver. To this end, they used diets restricted in kilocalories (kcalories or kcal), protein, water, and salt. Despite the lack of any scientific evidence to support such ideas, two assumptions, now known to be false, governed practice: (1) the *parasite theory:* whatever the fetus needs, it draws from maternal stores despite the maternal diet and (2) the *maternal instinct theory:* whatever the fetus needs, the pregnant woman instinctively craves and consumes.

Healthy Pregnancy

It is clear now that until recently much of the counsel given to pregnant women over the past few decades has been based more on tradition than on scientific fact. Increasing evidence indicates that positive nutritional support of pregnancy, rather than past negative restrictions born of limited knowledge and false assumptions, promotes a successful outcome with increased health and vigor of mothers and infants alike. This struggle over the past few decades, particularly to define the "healthy pregnancy," has not been easy. A healthy pregnancy has often been defined by the birth weight of the newborn, because infant mortality, or death, is low for infants with birth weights of 3500 to 4500 g.[1] The two key factors that predict infant birth weight are maternal preconception weight and weight gain during pregnancy.[2] Nutrition and other lifestyle factors affect maternal weight and weight gain; many of these factors, particularly nutrition, are modifiable or may be controlled by the pregnant woman. Healthy pregnancy may also be described in broader terms of mother, infant, and family. We are beginning to understand more about what this really means, especially as we see around us fetal damages from malnutrition, drug abuse, and other factors. We know that we must assess and support more fully the quality of life of each mother and her family if we are to achieve the healthy pregnancy we desire for all women.

Directions for Current Practice

Clinical observations and developing science in both nutrition and medicine have provided directions for healthier pregnancies. They have long refuted previous false ideas and laid a sound base for our current practice. A classic report of the National Research Council (NRC) first reflected this applied scientific base and led the way. This report, *Maternal Nutrition and the Course of Human Pregnancy,* was a clear turning point and provided undeniable direction for a new positive approach to the management of pregnancy.[3] Indeed, continuing research has reinforced this positive direction. On the basis of the significant NRC findings, guidelines for the nutritional care of pregnant women were then issued by the American College of Obstetrics and Gynecology and the American Dietetic Association.[4,5] These reports continue to provide useful guidelines for physicians, nutritionists, dietitians, and nurses in their prenatal care. Nutritional guidelines for pregnancy and lactation for all nutrients are also included in the Dietary Reference Intake (DRI) recommendations published by the Food and Nutrition Board of the Institute of Medicine.[6-10] We are reminded by these guides that an infant is nutritionally 9 months old at birth, even older when we consider the significance of the mother's preconception status.

The *fetal origins hypothesis* supports the notion that nutrition during gestation, or the lack thereof, sets the course for chronic disease in adulthood.[11] Development of cardiovascular disease, hypertension, obesity, type 2 diabetes, metabolic syndrome, and gestational diabetes, among other chronic diseases, have been shown in the offspring of animals for which maternal dietary intakes of macronutrients and micronutrients were manipulated, as well as in human epidemiologic studies of the relationship between infant anthropometric measurements and adult disease incidence.[12,13] In these epidemiologic studies, infant body size, shape, and weight measurements served as indicators of maternal nutrition. Changes in maternal nutrition during pregnancy require that the fetus adapt. These adaptations to nutrient supplies may lead to programming, or the mechanism(s) through which permanent changes in organ system structures and functions occur, leading to risk of chronic disease. This hypothesis presumes that nutritional insults that occur during critical stages of embryonic and fetal development are most harmful, leading to future disease risk. The merits of the fetal origins hypothesis have been debated, and much remains to be discovered.[14] Although research regarding the influence of nutrition on fetal growth and development has unique ethical and moral considerations, outcomes-based research is essential for appropriate evidence-based practice for healthy pregnancies.

Factors Determining Nutritional Needs

It is evident from an expanding body of research and the wide experience of many clinicians that maternal nutrition is critically important to both the mother and newborn (Figure 11-1). It lays the fundamental foundation for the successful outcome of pregnancy—a healthy mother and infant.[15] Several vital factors that determine

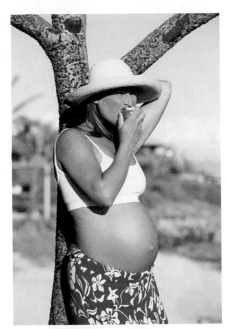

FIGURE 11-1   Adequate intake of fruits and vegetables is essential during pregnancy. *(Copyright 2006 JupiterImages Corporation.)*

nutritional requirements of the woman during her pregnancy are well-recognized.

Age, Gravida, and Parity

Age plays a major role in pregnancy; the teenage girl adds her own growth and maturation needs to those imposed by pregnancy. Also, the number of pregnancies (gravida) and the number of viable offspring (parity), as well as the time intervals between them, greatly influence the woman's nutrient reserves, her increased nutritional needs, and the outcome of the pregnancy.

Complex Physiologic Interactions of Gestation

Three distinct biologic entities are involved during gestation: the woman, the fetus, and the placenta, which nourishes fetal growth. Together they form a unique biologic whole. Constant metabolic interactions occur among them. Their functions, although unique, are at the same time interdependent. It is this unique biologic synergism that nourishes and sustains the pregnancy.

Basic Concepts Involved

As a result of our increased knowledge of pregnancy and nutrition, we can provide better nutritional guidance. Three basic concepts form a fundamental framework for assessing maternal nutritional needs and for planning supportive prenatal care for the woman.

Perinatal Concept

The prefix *peri-* comes from the Greek root meaning "around, about, or surrounding." Thus the word *perinatal* refers more broadly to the scope of factors that surround a

birth than merely the 9 months of the physical gestation. Certainly, as nutrition knowledge and understanding have increased, health professionals realize that all of a woman's life experiences surrounding her pregnancy must be considered. Her nutritional status and food patterns, which have developed over a number of years, and the degree to which she has established and maintained nutritional reserves are all important factors. Cultural and social influences have shaped beliefs and values of the woman about pregnancy. All of these influences come to bear on any pregnancy.

Synergism Concept

The word *synergism* is a term used to describe biologic systems in which the cooperative action of two or more factors produces a total effect greater than and different from the mere sum of the parts. In short, a new whole is created by the unified, joint effort of blending the parts in which each part makes more powerful the action of the others. Of the many biologic and physiologic examples of synergism, pregnancy is a prime case in point. Maternal organism, fetus, and placenta combine to produce a new whole, a system not existing before and producing a total effect greater than and different from the sum of the parts, all for the sole purpose of sustaining and nurturing the pregnancy and its offspring. Physiologic measures change. Blood volume and cardiac output increase, ventilation rate and tidal volume of breathing increase, and basal metabolic rate increases. The physiologic norms of the nonpregnant woman do not apply.

Thus the normal physiologic adjustments of pregnancy cannot be viewed as pathologic with application of treatment procedures for that same type of response in

---

programming The mechanism(s) through which adaptations to nutrient supplies during gestation result in permanent changes in organ and body system structures and functions, potentially leading to chronic disease risk.

gravida A pregnant woman.

parity The condition of a woman with respect to having borne viable offspring.

gestation The period of embryonic and fetal development from fertilization to birth; pregnancy.

fetus The unborn offspring in the postembryonic period, after major structures have been outlined; in humans, the growing offspring from 7 to 8 weeks after fertilization until birth.

placenta Special organ developed in early pregnancy that provides nutrients to the fetus and removes metabolic waste.

synergism The joint action of separate agents in which the total effect of their combined action is greater than the sum of their separate actions.

the nonpregnant state. For example, a normal physiologic generalized edema of pregnancy is a protective response. It reflects the normal increase in total body water necessary to support the increased metabolic work of pregnancy and is associated with enhanced reproductive performance.

Life Continuum Concept

In a real sense, throughout her life a woman is providing for the ongoing continuum of life through food that she eats. Each offspring obviously becomes a part of this continuing process during the pregnancy when the mother's diet directly sustains growth and development. But in the broader sense, the mother transfers her nutritional heritage, practices, and beliefs to her growing children, who in the next generation pass on this heritage both genetically and culturally. Other family members also play important roles in this generational sustenance of the life continuum.

Health Promotion

Preconception Nutrition

A woman brings to each pregnancy all of her previous life experiences, including her diet and eating habits. Her general health and fitness and her state of nutrition at the time of conception are products of her lifelong dietary habits and her genetic heritage. The importance of preconception nutrition is increasingly recognized. The Maternal, Infant and Child Health Goal included in *Healthy People 2010: Understanding and Improving Health* (see the *Further Readings and Resources* section at the end of this chapter) addresses the need for improvements in preconception nutrition and health in women in the United States.[16] Preconception counseling is an avenue to such improvements. Related to nutrition, preconception counseling may include screening for medical conditions such as iron deficiency anemia, eating disorders, drug-nutrient interactions, and genetic disorders, as well as assessment of current body weight, recent and previous weight changes, body mass index (BMI), fitness and exercise status, folate status, and specific nutrient intakes, eating patterns, and dietary and botanical supplement use. Evaluation of existing medical conditions such as hypertension, diabetes, thyroid disease, celiac disease, phenylketonuria (PKU), and others, is important. Inquiry about the home and family environment, including income, education, safety, lead exposure, abuse, etc., should also be conducted during preconception counseling so that guidance, recommendations, and referrals may be thoroughly provided. Each of these nutrition and health-related factors has documented effects on pregnancy outcome, many of which are adverse. However, preconception counseling and optimal preconception nutrition may increase the odds for a healthy pregnancy and desirable infant outcome.

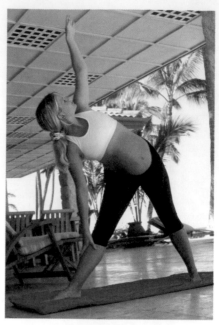

FIGURE 11-2 Excercise during pregnancy benefits both the pregnant woman and the fetus. *(Copyright 2006 JupiterImages Corporation.)*

Exercise

Women who exercise before pregnancy should continue a reasonable exercise regimen during pregnancy. In fact, women who engage in prenatal exercise have been shown to have health benefits compared to nonexercising women.[17] Moderate exercise programs may also be beneficial to the woman and fetus, even if the woman was sedentary before conception. As the woman's body size and shape change throughout the course of pregnancy, exercise type, duration, and intensity should be adjusted to promote safety for the woman and her fetus (Figure 11-2). Exercises that are not recommended during pregnancy include scuba diving and those with risk of trauma to the abdominal area.[18]

The energy cost of exercise impacts kcalorie needs of the pregnant woman. Kcalories must be consumed to meet the energy cost of exercise and to promote appropriate maternal weight gain and fetal growth and development. Adequate hydration is also vital, and the woman should increase fluid intake during exercise.

NUTRITIONAL DEMANDS OF PREGNANCY

Basic Nutrient Allowances and Individual Variation

Gestation is characterized by exceedingly rapid growth and development. During this 40-week period, a single fertilized egg cell (ovum) grows into a fully developed infant weighing about 3500 g, on average. What nutrients must the woman supply to support this intense period of

| TABLE 11-1 | Dietary Reference Intakes per Day of Some Selected Nutrients for Pregnancy and Lactation |

| Nutrients | Nonpregnant Girl | | Nonpregnant Woman | During Pregnancy | Lactation | |
	9-13 yr 46 kg 101 lb	14-18 yr 55 kg 120 lb	19-50 yr 63 kg 138 lb	19-50 yr	(600 ml/day) First 6 mo	(750 ml/day) Second 6 mo
Kilocalories	2000-2100	2300-2400	2400	No change in first trimester; + 340 kcal/day for second trimester and + 450 kcal/day for third trimester	+ 500 kcal/day (170 kcal/day from maternal stores)	+ 400 kcal/day
Protein (g)	34	46	46	71	71	71
Calcium (mg)	1300	1300	1000	1000 mg throughout	1000 mg throughout	
Iron (mg)	8	15	18	27 mg throughout	9 mg throughout	
Vitamin A (μg RAE)*	600	700	700	770 μg RAE throughout	1300 μg throughout	
Thiamin (mg)	0.9	1.0	1.1	1.4 mg throughout	1.4 mg throughout	
Riboflavin (mg)	0.9	1.0	1.1	1.4 mg throughout	1.6 mg throughout	
Niacin (mg NE)†	12	14	14	18 mg NE throughout	17 mg NE throughout	
Vitamin C (mg)	45	65	75	85 mg throughout	120 mg throughout	
Vitamin D (μg)	5	5	5	5 μg throughout	5 μg throughout	
Folic acid (μg)‡	300	400	400	600 μg throughout	500 μg	

Data from Food and Nutrition Board, Institute of Medicine: *Dietary Reference Intakes for calcium, phosphorus, magnesium, vitamin D, and fluoride,* Washington, DC, 1997, National Academies Press; Food and Nutrition Board, Institute of Medicine: *Dietary Reference Intakes for thiamin, riboflavin, niacin, vitamin B$_6$, folate, vitamin B$_{12}$, pantothenic acid, biotin, and choline,* Washington, DC, 1998, National Academies Press; Food and Nutrition Board, Institute of Medicine: *Dietary Reference Intakes for vitamin C, vitamin E, selenium, and carotenoids,* Washington, DC, 2000, National Academies Press; Food and Nutrition Board, Institute of Medicine: *Dietary Reference Intakes for vitamin A, vitamin K, arsenic, boron, chromium, copper, iodine, iron, manganese, molybdenum, nickel, silicon, vanadium, and zinc,* Washington, DC, 2000, National Academies Press; Food and Nutrition Board, Institute of Medicine: *Dietary Reference Intakes for energy, carbohydrate, fiber, fat, fatty acids, cholesterol, protein, and amino acids (macronutrients),* Washington, DC, 2005, National Academies Press.

*As retinal activity equivalents (RAEs). One RAE is equal to 1 μg all-*trans* retinal or 12 μg beta-carotene.

†As niacin equivalents (NE). One NE is equal to 1 milligram of niacin or 60 milligrams of tryptophan.

‡As dietary folate equivalents (DFEs). One DFE is equal to 1 μg food folate or 0.6 μg of folic acid from fortified food or as a supplement consumed with food or 0.5 μg of a supplement taken on an empty stomach.

fetal growth and development? What must her diet provide to meet fetal nutritional demands and her own needs during this critical period?

Throughout the pregnancy there is an increased need for most of the basic nutrients, as indicated by the DRI guidelines from the Food and Nutrition Board of the Institute of Medicine[6-10] (Table 11-1). However, it is important to remember that these are guidelines; individual variances in nutrient needs must be examined for each pregnancy. Individual variations such as BMI, physical activity, and health status must be considered. Also, the quantitative need for nourishment of pregnant adolescents and multifetal pregnancies must be noted. Individual counseling and correct use of nutritional guidelines is imperative.[19] In considering the nutritional needs of the *healthy* pregnant woman, we will review here the macronutrients and selected micronutrients with increased needs, rationale for increased needs, and how such nutrients may be obtained from foods.

Energy Needs

The kcalories must be sufficient to perform the following two functions:

1. Supply the increased energy and nutrient demands created by the increased metabolic workload, including some maternal fat storage and fetal fat storage to ensure an optimal newborn size for survival
2. Spare protein for tissue building

The DRI standard recommends an additional amount of energy of approximately 340 kcal/day during the second trimester and approximately 450 kcal/day during the third trimester of pregnancy to supply needs during this time of rapid growth.[10] Total daily kcalorie intake during mid- and late-pregnancy should be based on the woman's nonpregnant estimated energy requirement plus the additional energy need and will typically increase by about 15% to 20% over the woman's general prepregnancy need.

This primary emphasis on sufficient kcalories is critical to ensure nutrient and energy needs to positively support the pregnancy. Appropriate weight gain during pregnancy indicates whether sufficient kcalories are being provided.

Much of our knowledge regarding the importance of sufficient energy intake during pregnancy arose from records of pregnancy and infant statistics through periods of famine during World War II. Insufficient kcalorie intake during the first trimester of pregnancy was associated with infertility and increased incidence of neural tube defects and other metabolic changes, whereas inadequate kcalorie consumption in the second and third trimesters of pregnancy was associated with increased numbers of congenital abnormalities, infants of low birth weight, and infant mortality. Current famine and food insecurity in various locations around the world continue to support these earlier findings regarding the essential need for adequate kcalories during pregnancy to support an optimal infant outcome. Energy needs of pregnancy may be met through a balanced intake of macronutrients.

Protein, Fat, and Carbohydrate Needs

The total amount of protein recommended for a pregnant woman is 71 g/day, an increase of 25 g/day.[10] Protein, with its essential nitrogen, is the nutrient basic to tissue growth. Nitrogen balance studies suggest that a large amount of nitrogen is used by the woman and fetus during pregnancy and emphasize the importance of preconception maternal reserves to meet initial pregnancy needs. More protein is necessary for demands posed by the following:

- Rapid fetal growth
- Enlargement of the uterus, mammary glands, and placenta
- Increase in maternal circulating blood volume and subsequent demand for increased plasma proteins to maintain colloidal osmotic pressure and circulation of tissue fluids to nourish cells
- Formation of amniotic fluid
- Storage reserves for labor, delivery, and lactation

Milk, egg, cheese, and meat are complete protein foods of high biologic value. Protein-rich foods also contribute other nutrients, such as calcium, iron, and B vitamins. Additional protein may be obtained from legumes and whole grains, with lesser amounts in other plant sources.

An adequate supply of essential fatty acids is also vital throughout pregnancy. Tissue growth, especially the proper development of cell membranes in nerve and brain tissue, and development of organ function, notably cognition and visual acuity, require that essential fatty acids and their converted forms reach the developing fetus in sufficient amounts. Depending on individual needs, supplementation of the mother's essential fatty acid intake may be useful to maintain adequate levels.[20,21] However, most pregnant women may consume adequate amounts of linoleic (13 g/day) and alpha-linolenic (1.4 g/day) acids through consumption of canola, soybean, and walnut oils, in addition to other dietary fat sources.[10] Docosahexaenoic acid (DHA), important for visual and cognitive development, is found in salmon, mackerel, striped bass, and other fish products.

Carbohydrate intake of at least 175 g/day during pregnancy is important for an adequate supply of glucose and nonprotein energy.[10] Whole grain breads and cereals and fresh fruits and vegetables should be consumed to meet maternal and fetal glucose needs, as well as provide fiber for satiety and bowel regulation. Currently popular low-carbohydrate "diets" are not recommended during pregnancy because various phases of these diets do not provide the minimum glucose load required by the maternal and fetal bodies. In general, total daily dietary kcalorie intake should comprise 15% protein, 30% fat, and 55% carbohydrate, keeping in mind the individual needs of the pregnant woman.

Mineral Needs

All the major and trace minerals play roles in maternal health. Four that have special functions in relation to pregnancy—calcium, iodine, iron, and zinc—deserve particular attention.

Calcium

The pregnant woman's DRI recommendation is 1000 mg of calcium per day, the same as the general recommendation for all women ages 19 to 50.[6] Calcium is the essential element for the construction and maintenance of bones and teeth. It is also an important factor in the blood-clotting mechanism and is used in normal muscle action and other essential metabolic activities. Improved absorption of calcium supplies the needs arising from the accelerated fetal mineralization of skeletal tissue during the final period of rapid growth. Dairy products are a primary source of calcium. Consumption of milk or equivalent milk foods (cheese or nonfat milk powder used in cooking) is recommended. Additional calcium is obtained in whole or fortified cereal grains and in green leafy vegetables.

Iodine

The recommendation for iodine increases by 70 μg/day during pregnancy.[9] Iodine is vital for thyroid hormone synthesis and prevention of goiter. The need increases during gestation to support changes in maternal thyroid economy, increased maternal renal clearance, and fetal uptake of iodine. An inadequate supply of iodine to the fetus may lead to hypothyroidism in the newborn and is often associated with poor and abnormal growth, deficits in cognitive development, and poor motor function. Although infrequently encountered in the United States, infant hypothyroidism continues to be found in many developing countries. Iodine consumption is critical in the first half of pregnancy, and programs designed to provide oil- and water-based iodine supplements to women in preconception and prenatal periods in developing countries have been successful in reducing the incidence of infant hypothyroidism. Iodized salt is the primary dietary source for women in developed countries. Seafood is also a noted source of iodine.

Iron

The pregnant woman needs 27 mg of iron per day, a substantial increase over her general needs.[9] Some pregnant women may need supplementary iron in addition to increased dietary sources to meet the additional requirement of pregnancy. The iron cost of pregnancy is high. With increased demands for iron, often insufficient maternal stores, and inadequate provision through the usual diet, a daily supplement of 30 to 60 mg of iron may be prescribed. If a woman has iron deficiency anemia at conception, a larger therapeutic amount of 120 to 200 mg/day of iron may be necessary to reduce the risk of a preterm delivery and/or low-birth-weight baby.

During normal pregnancy the maternal circulating blood volume expands by 40% to 50% and may increase more with multiple fetuses. This adaptation reduces the strain on the maternal heart, minimizes hemoglobin losses at delivery, and enhances nutrient flow to the fetus. Although red blood cell mass also increases during gestation, this change does not parallel blood volume expansion, resulting in hemodilution of red blood cell mass. Thus specific guidelines are used to determine iron deficiency anemia during pregnancy (see the discussion under the heading "Anemia" later in this chapter). Maternal iron is needed to supply iron to the developing placenta and fetal liver. Adequate maternal iron stores also help protect the woman against iron losses related to blood loss at delivery.

To obtain the needed amount of iron, check the percentage of elemental iron in the iron preparation being used. For example, the commonly used compound ferrous sulfate is a hydrated salt ($FeSO_4$ $7H_2O$), which contains 20% iron. It is usually dispensed in tablets containing 195, 300, or 325 mg of the ferrous sulfate compound. Each tablet, then, would contain 39, 60, or 65 mg of iron, respectively. Thus to supply a regular daily supplement of 60 mg of iron, one 300-mg tablet of ferrous sulfate is required, and for a therapeutic dose of 120 mg iron, two 300-mg tablets are required.

Problems with routine iron supplementation for pregnant women include unpleasant gastrointestinal side effects (see the discussion under the heading "Effects of Iron Supplements" later in this chapter) and less motivation to maintain a good diet. Of major concern are imbalances with other trace elements, such as zinc, that compete with iron for absorption. Excess iron intake, when not needed,

may actually mask inadequate pregnancy-induced hemodilution. Thus some prenatal clinics follow protocols that prescribe regular prenatal vitamins with iron at the first clinic visit, adding additional iron supplementation only if hemoglobin falls to 10.5 g/dl or less at any time during the pregnancy.

The major food source of iron is liver; however, liver intake is often avoided during pregnancy. Other food sources include meat, legumes, dried fruit, green leafy vegetables, eggs, and enriched bread and cereals (see list of iron-containing foods in Chapter 7).

Zinc

During pregnancy the DRI recommendation for zinc increases from 8 to 11 mg/day.[9] Zinc is vital for enzymatic reactions and is essential to growth and development due to its role in deoxyribonucleic acid (DNA) and ribonucleic acid (RNA) synthesis and protein production. Inadequate zinc consumption during gestation has been associated with low birth weight and congenital malformations. Iron supplementation may inhibit zinc absorption; thus additional dietary sources of zinc are critical when maternal iron supplementation is prescribed. Seafood, eggs, and meat are primary sources of zinc.

Vitamin Needs

Increased amounts of vitamins A, B complex, and C are needed during pregnancy. If these needs are met, sufficient amounts of vitamins E and K are also available. The recommended amount of vitamin D does not increase during pregnancy but is important to fetal skeletal development.

Vitamin A

The daily amount of vitamin A recommended for pregnancy is 770 μg of retinol activity equivalents (RAE), a slight increase over the woman's regular need.[9] For most women in the United States, no extra amount is needed. However, malnourished, underweight women and those with multiple pregnancies need more. Vitamin A is an essential factor in cell differentiation, organ formation, maintenance of strong epithelial tissue, tooth formation, and normal bone growth. Liver, egg yolk, butter and fortified margarine, dark green and yellow vegetables, and fruits are good food sources.

Excessive consumption of retinol and retinoic acid, two forms of vitamin A, has been associated with fetal

---

amniotic fluid The watery fluid within the membrane enveloping the fetus, in which the fetus is suspended.

PERSPECTIVES IN PRACTICE
Preventing Spina Bifida: The Importance of Folate

Meredith Catherine Williams

The Centers for Disease Control and Prevention estimates that in the United States about 3000 infants are born every year with a neural tube defect (NTD), with the most common defects being anencephaly and spina bifida. Babies with anencephaly do not develop any brain tissue, and most are stillborn or die soon after birth. Spina bifida is caused by a defect in the development of the spinal column in which the vertebrae surrounding the spinal cord do not close properly in early development. In the mild form, *spina bifida occulta*, there is only a small gap between two vertebrae of the spine. This usually produces no symptoms, and the only sign may be a small dimple in the skin covering the gap. The severe form is *spina bifida aperta*, where a larger space develops in the spine. There is a visible sac, called a meningocele, on the infant's back where spinal fluid bulges out, most commonly in the lower back. This causes little to no muscle paralysis once repaired by surgery, but in the majority of cases of spina bifida aperta, part of the undeveloped spinal cord sticks through the gap and into the protruding sac on the baby's back. This undeveloped or damaged spinal cord that extends beyond the vertebrae, called a *myelocele* or *meningomyelocele*, causes the most acute cases of paralysis, bladder or bowel incontinence, scoliosis (a sideways bending of the spine), and mental retardation. Again, surgery can help reduce these symptoms, and 85% to 90% of infants with spina bifida are able to survive into adulthood.

However, a woman can reduce the risk of her baby being born with an NTD by increasing her consumption of folate. Folate is often consumed in the form of folic acid from a fortified food or from a food supplement. Folic acid helps to ensure normal embryonic tissue growth and to prevent malformation of the neural tube. Folic acid is the synthetic version of the B vitamin folate and slightly easier for the body to absorb. Recommended intakes are expressed in units of dietary folate equivalents (DFE). One DFE equals 1 μg of food folate or 0.6

μg of folic acid from fortified foods or from a supplement consumed with food or 0.5 μg of a supplement taken on an empty stomach.

Folic acid is also recommended for women who are not pregnant because the beneficial effect of folic acid must be present in the first 2 weeks of pregnancy, a time when the woman typically does not know she is pregnant. Neurulation, or the creation of the neural tube, crest, and covering, and the possibility for defects, occurs in humans from approximately day 21 through day 28 of development. More than half of all pregnancies are unexpected; therefore the U.S. Public Health Service recommends that all women capable of becoming pregnant consume 400 μg of folate per day, to ensure an adequate supply for the fetus.

To achieve the recommended 400 μg DFE/day, women can take a vitamin supplement that contains folic acid; eat a variety of folate-rich foods, such as dark green leafy vegetables, fruits, and dried beans and peas; or eat folic acid–fortified enriched products. As part of the public health effort to increase folic acid consumption, the Food and Drug Administration has mandated that all manufacturers of grain products, including cereals, breads, flours, corn meals, and pastas, include 0.43 to 1.4 mg of folic acid in each pound of product. This addition will not harm males and nonpregnant women and is a benefit for women who are pregnant. The goal in fortifying food for an entire population is to increase general intake levels of folic acid while remaining below the upper limit of 1 mg/day so as to be safe for everyone. Although the effects of high folic acid consumption are not generally well known, there is evidence to suggest that high intake can interfere with the diagnosis of a vitamin B_{12} deficiency. It is recommended that women consume 600 μg of folate/day when pregnant to ensure that the fetus is completely supplied. During lactation the recommended folate intake daily is 500 μg.

Data from Food and Nutrition Board, Institute of Medicine: *Dietary Reference Intakes for thiamin, riboflavin, niacin, vitamin B_6, folate, vitamin B_{12}, pantothenic acid, biotin, and choline,* Washington, DC, 1998, National Academies Press.

malformations such as heart, facial, and ear defects. Overconsumption is generally due to use of supplements or medications such as Accutane. Harmful effects are most damaging during the first few months of pregnancy, again emphasizing the need for prenatal counseling and appropriate preconception nutrition.

B Vitamins

There is a special need for various B vitamins, including thiamin, riboflavin, niacin, pyridoxine, cobalamin, pantothenic acid, and folate, during pregnancy. The B vitamins are important as coenzyme factors in a number of metabolic activities related to energy production, tissue protein synthesis, and function of muscle and nerve tissue; therefore they play key roles in the increased metabolic work of pregnancy.[22] These B vitamins are usually supplied by a well-balanced diet that is increased in quantity and quality to supply needed energy and nutrients.

There is a special increased metabolic need for the B vitamin folate during pregnancy. Folate deficiency usually occurs in conjunction with general malnutrition, making the pregnant woman in low-socioeconomic conditions especially vulnerable. A specific megaloblastic anemia caused by maternal folate deficiency sometimes occurs and warrants supplementation of the diet with folic acid. This added amount is particularly needed where such demands are greater, as in a multiple pregnancy.

Preconception folic acid supplementation has been shown in randomized clinical trials to greatly reduce a woman's risk of bearing an infant with a neural tube defect, which is the source of the serious defects of spina bifida and anencephaly. These congenital defects in the formation of the spine develop in the first few weeks of pregnancy, when the neural tube, which forms the spinal cord, does not close completely, leaving part of one or more vertebrae of the spinal cord exposed at birth (see Chapter 26). Each year in the United States approximately 3000 infants are born with spina bifida and anencephaly, and an estimated 1500 affected fetuses are spontaneously aborted.[23] Since 1992 the U.S. Public Health Service has recommended that all women of childbearing age who are capable of becoming pregnant consume from food or supplementation 400 μg of folic acid per day to prevent such deficiencies. This recommendation continues in the latest DRI guidelines, which recommend 400 μg/day for nonpregnant women, rising to 600 μg/day during pregnancy and 500 μg/day during lactation.[7] The Food and Drug Administration, acting to increase folic acid consumption nationally, began requiring in 1996 that enriched cereal grain products be fortified with folic acid.[24-26] These fortified foods are good sources of folic acid in addition to orange and pineapple juices, oranges, and dried beans (see the *Perspectives in Practice* box, "Preventing Spina Bifida: The Importance of Folate").

Vitamin C

Special emphasis must be given to the pregnant woman's need for ascorbic acid. Vitamin C is essential to the formation of intercellular cement substance in developing connective tissues and vascular systems. It also increases the absorption of iron, which is needed for the increasing quantities of hemoglobin. The DRI standard recommends 85 mg/day for the pregnant women, an increase of 10 mg/day over the regular adult female need of 75 mg/day.[8] Additional food sources such as citrus fruit and other vegetables and fruits should be included in the woman's diet.

Vitamin D

Women who have adequate exposure to sunlight probably need little additional vitamin D. During pregnancy, because of the need for calcium and phosphorus presented by the developing fetal skeletal tissue, vitamin D is used to promote the absorption and utilization of these minerals. The daily recommended amount for pregnancy is 5 μg cholecalciferol (200 IU/day), which is the same as for the nonpregnant woman.[6] Food sources include fortified milk, liver, egg yolk, and fortified margarine.

Dietary Patterns: General and Alternative

General Daily Food Pattern

Two useful general principles concerning eating habits for all persons also apply during pregnancy, as follows:

1. Eat an appropriate quantity of food.
2. Eat regularly, avoiding fasting or skipping meals, especially breakfast.

During pregnancy a variety of familiar foods usually supply the woman's need for added nutrients and make eating a pleasure. The increased quantities of essential nutrients needed during pregnancy may be met in many ways by planning around a daily food pattern and using key types of suggested core foods. A general daily food pattern that meets basic nutrient needs is suggested in Table 11-2. Compare the increases in each food group suggested for the pregnant or lactating adolescent or woman during the reproductive cycle with the basic amounts for the nonpregnant woman. The comparison indicates the need for increased amounts of basic foods during pregnancy to meet increased key nutrient needs. It may be used as a guide, with additional foods added according to individual energy needs and personal desires. This pattern represents the "orthodox middle-class American diet." It has been labeled the "biomedically recommended prenatal diet," which is generally used worldwide by most health professionals in industrialized, affluent countries.

Alternative Food Patterns

With the increasing ethnic diversity in the United States, it is especially important to use the woman's personal cultural food patterns in dietary counseling. We are ethnocentric if we rigidly adhere to the orthodox pattern previously discussed as the pattern for all pregnant women, because it is but one diet pattern among many others from different cultures, belief systems, and lifestyles. We must always remember that specific nutrients, not specific foods, are required for a successful pregnancy and that these nutrients are found in a wide variety of food choices. If we are wise, we will encourage our clients to use foods that serve their nutritional needs, whatever those foods might be (see the *Case Study* box, "A Baby for the Delgados"). A number of resources are available as guides for cultural, religious, and vegetarian food patterns. Suggestions for improving transcultural nutrition counseling skills are also available.[27-29]

Dietary Supplements

Often, "prenatal vitamins" are prescribed for pregnant women. These supplements include a variety of vitamins and minerals and are intended to add to nutrient intake from foods rather than replace food and nutrient consumption. Iron and folate are generally the two nutrients that require supplementation during pregnancy. Some women may need additional nutrients, however. For example, pregnant women who follow vegan diets, have one or more nutritional deficiencies, smoke cigarettes, or use or abuse drugs and/or alcohol, or have multiple fetuses need prenatal vitamin and mineral supplements that include additional nutrients.

Herbal and botanical supplement use during pregnancy is discouraged due to the potentially harmful or unknown effects to the woman and fetus. However, based on cultural and traditional medicine practices and emerging trends, pregnant women may include such products in their daily routines (see the *Case Study* box, "Nutrition Counseling in Pregnancy"). Several reference materials are available regarding the risks associated with use of specific herbals and botanicals during pregnancy (see the *Further Readings and Resources* section at the end of this chapter).[30-32]

WEIGHT GAIN DURING PREGNANCY

General Amount of Weight Gain

Healthy women produce healthy babies over a wide range of total weight gain. During pregnancy therefore the nutri-

---

TABLE 11-2   Daily Food Guide for Women

Food Group	One Serving Equals	Recommended Servings		
		Nonpregnant		Pregnant/ Lactating
		11-24 yr	25+ yr	
Protein Foods Provide protein, iron, zinc, and B vitamins for growth of muscles, bone, blood, and nerves; vegetable protein provides fiber to prevent constipation	***Animal Protein*** 1 oz cooked chicken or turkey 1 oz cooked lean beef, lamb, or pork 1 oz or ¼ cup fish or other seafood 1 egg 2 fish sticks or hot dogs 2 slices luncheon meat ***Vegetable Protein*** ¼ cup cooked dry beans, lentils, or split peas ¼ cup tofu ½ oz nuts 1 tbsp peanut butter	5 1 serving of vegetable protein daily	5 1 serving of vegetable protein daily	7 1 serving of vegetable protein daily
Milk Products Provide protein, calcium, and vitamin D to build strong bones, teeth, and healthy nerves and muscles and to promote normal blood clotting	8 oz milk 8 oz yogurt 1 cup milkshake ½ cup cream soup (made with milk) 2 oz low-fat processed cheese 1½ -2 slices presliced American cheese 2 cups cottage cheese 1 cup pudding 1 cup custard or flan 1½ cups ice milk, ice cream, or frozen yogurt	3	3	3
Breads, Cereals, Grains Provide carbohydrates and B vitamins for energy and healthy nerves; also provide iron for healthy blood; whole grains provide fiber to prevent constipation	1 slice bread 1 dinner roll ½ bun or bagel ½ English muffin or pita 1 small tortilla 1 cup dry cereal ½ cup granola ½ cup cooked cereal ½ cup rice ½ cup noodles or spaghetti ¼ cup wheat germ 1 4-in pancake or waffle 1 small muffin	7*	6*	9*

Data from U.S. Department of Health and Human Services, U.S. Department of Agriculture: *Dietary Guidelines for Americans 2005,* ed 6, Washington, DC, 2005, U.S. Government Printing Office.

NOTE: The Food Guide may not provide the kcalories you require. The best way to balance your intake is to include more or less than the servings recommended.

*4 servings of whole grain products daily.

TABLE 11-2	Daily Food Guide for Women—cont'd

Food Group	One Serving Equals	Recommended Servings		
		Nonpregnant		Pregnant/ Lactating
		11-24 yr	25+ yr	
Breads, Cereals, Grains—cont'd	8 medium crackers			
	4 graham cracker squares			
	3 cups popcorn			
Vitamin C–Rich Fruits and Vegetables Provide vitamin C to prevent infection and to promote healing and iron absorption; also provide fiber to prevent constipation	4 oz orange, grapefruit, or fruit juice enriched with vitamin C	1-2	1-2	1-2
	4 oz tomato juice or vegetable juice cocktail			
	1 orange, kiwi, or mango			
	½ grapefruit or cantaloupe			
	½ cup papaya			
	2 tangerines			
	½ cup strawberries			
	½ cup cooked or 1 cup raw cabbage			
	½ cup broccoli, brussels sprouts, or cauliflower			
	½ cup snow peas, sweet peppers, or tomato puree			
	2 tomatoes			
Vitamin A–Rich Fruits and Vegetables Provide beta-carotene and vitamin A to prevent infection and to promote wound healing and night vision; also provide fiber to prevent constipation	4 oz apricot nectar or vegetable juice cocktail	1-2	1-2	1-2
	3 raw or ¼ cup dried apricots			
	¼ cantaloupe or mango			
	1 small or ½ cup sliced carrots			
	2 tomatoes			
	½ cup cooked or 1 cup raw spinach			
	½ cup cooked greens (beet, chard, collards, dandelion, kale, mustard)			
	½ cup pumpkin, sweet potato, winter squash, or yams			
Other Fruits and Vegetables Provide carbohydrates for energy and fiber to prevent constipation	4 oz fruit juice (if not listed previously)	3-4	3-4	3-4
	1 medium or ½ cup sliced fruit (apple, banana, peach, pear)			
	½ cup berries (other than strawberries)			
	½ cup cherries or grapes			
	½ cup pineapple			
	½ cup watermelon			
	½ cup dried fruit			
	½ cup sliced vegetable (asparagus, beets, green beans, celery, corn, eggplant, mushrooms, onion, peas, potato, summer squash, zucchini)			
	½ artichoke			
	1 cup lettuce			
Unsaturated Fats Provide vitamin E to protect tissue and essential fatty acids	⅛ medium avocado	3	3	3
	1 tbsp low-fat mayonnaise			
	2 tbsp light salad dressing			
	1 tsp margarine			
	1 tsp mayonnaise			
	1 tsp vegetable oil			

CASE STUDY

A Baby for the Delgados

Mrs. Delgado is a 19-year-old married primigravida who tested positive for urinary human chorionic gonadotropin (hCG) 2 weeks earlier. Mrs. Delgado is 160 cm (5 ft 3 in) tall with an average pregravid weight of 57 kg (125 lb). Her current gestational age is 6 weeks. Her history for chronic disorders and other serious health problems is negative.

During her initial nutrition interview Mrs. Delgado indicated that the pregnancy was unplanned. She seemed especially worried about the effects of her irregular diet on the baby. As college students, she and her 21-year-old husband had erratic meals, dominated by junk food. Mrs. Delgado's 24-hour diet history revealed an inadequate intake of dark green or yellow vegetables and milk products, as well as meat or eggs and citrus fruits. The couple realized that these types of foods were an important part of a nutritious diet but felt inexperienced as cooks and lacked the time and money to prepare healthful meals every day.

At the end of the initial counseling session the nutritionist told the couple about a series of prenatal group discussions conducted by members of the clinic's perinatal health team, including sessions on pregnancy, labor and delivery, and the care and feeding of the infant. These are attended primarily by a mixture of experienced parents and young, first-time parents-to-be and are offered as a means of introducing practical aspects of pregnancy and parenting.

The Delgados attended every prenatal group meeting and kept all consequent diet-counseling sessions. Their food choices improved in time, and Mrs.

Delgado's weight gain progressed normally, to a total of 13 kg (28 lb) by the time of delivery. The Delgados had a healthy 4 kg (8 lb 13 oz) baby girl.

Questions for Analysis

1. What health professionals ideally should be included on the health care team caring for Mrs. Delgado? Describe the significance of each role to the outcome of her pregnancy. What are the roles of Mr. and Mrs. Delgado?
2. What nutritional deficiencies would you expect in Mrs. Delgado's diet? What practical problems would you expect her to encounter in attempting to improve her diet?
3. Write a 1-day meal plan for Mrs. Delgado, taking into account her lifestyle and schedule, as well as the amounts of nutrients considered adequate for pregnancy.
4. Write a lesson plan for a group session on nutrition during pregnancy. Include a general description, behavioral objectives, content outline, teaching methods and materials, and evaluation tool(s) you would use.
5. Would you encourage Mrs. Delgado to breast-feed? If so, why? What factors would you expect might discourage her from trying? How would you discuss these factors?
6. Write a lesson plan for an infant feeding session, addressing breast-feeding and bottle-feeding methods. Include the components listed in Questions 3 and 4.

CASE STUDY

Nutrition Counseling in Pregnancy

Ms. McLane is a 33-year-old white woman who is in her twenty-ninth week of pregnancy. This is her second pregnancy. During her first pregnancy (at age 29), she gained 24 lb during a normal pregnancy and had a delivery without complications. She is presently 165.1 cm (5 ft 5 in) tall and weighs 81.8 kg (180 lb). Her prepregnancy weight was 72.7 kg (160 lb). Ms. McLane visited her obstetrician (OB) before her second pregnancy for prepregnancy planning. She has been consuming a healthy diet and a prenatal vitamin supplement every day. After her first visit to the OB during the current pregnancy (at week 10), Ms. McLane did not return for any further appointments, because of her prior positive experience with pregnancy and belief that she "didn't need anything because the first pregnancy went so well."

Ms. McLane has a positive family history for diabetes, and her mother had gestational diabetes. Ms. McLane should have been screened for gestational diabetes between the twenty-fourth and twenty-eighth weeks of her current pregnancy; however, this was not done. She experienced frequent urination and fatigue that she reported as "different" from her first pregnancy. This prompted her to return to her OB. The OB completed a full examination and administered an oral glucose tolerance test. One hour after consuming a 100-g solution of glucose, Ms. McLane's blood glucose concentration was 218 mg/dl. She was scheduled for follow-up testing, and gestational diabetes was confirmed. A 2200-kcal/day diabetic diet was prescribed to allow Ms. McLane to control this condition through diet.

Ms. McLane has been referred to you for nutrition counseling. This is now the thirty-first week of her pregnancy, and she shares with you that a friend suggested that she "use some natural products to help her high blood sugar." In addition to consuming her prenatal supplement on a daily basis, she takes 500 mg of burdock root and 1 tbsp of flaxseed and drinks 3 cups of

hot fenugreek tea per day. Her prenatal supplement contains 400 μg of folate, 250 mg of calcium, 40 mg of iron, 100 mg of vitamin C, 5 μg of vitamin D, 3 mg of thiamin, 3 mg of riboflavin, 4 mg of pyridoxine, 40 mg of niacin, 10 mg of vitamin E, 5 μg of cobalamin, 30 mg of zinc, and 10 mg of copper. Completion of a dietary intake analysis shows that Ms. McLane's kcaloric intake is 1750 per day. She reported that she has been nauseated for about 2 weeks, so she also added 300 mg of powdered ginger to each cup of the fenugreek tea. She reported some diarrhea and Braxton Hicks contractions during the last week, as well a lack of desire to be physically active.

Questions for Analysis

1. What is Ms. McLane's body mass index based on her prepregnancy weight?
2. What is the recommended amount of weight gain for Ms. McLane based on prepregnancy weight and/or her body mass index? Has she experienced an appropriate weight gain so far?
3. Is the current level of kcalories appropriate based on her condition of gestational diabetes, body mass index, and weight gain?
4. What additional information would you collect from Ms. McLane to complete a nutritional assessment?
5. How would you approach a nutritional intake plan for Ms. McLane?
6. Why would Ms. McLane's friend have recommended burdock root, flaxseed, and fenugreek? Be specific for each botanical. Are burdock root, flaxseed, fenugreek, and/or ginger recommended for use during pregnancy?
7. Identify at least five points that you would make during a nutrition counseling session with Ms. McLane. Discuss the priority for the first counseling session with Ms. McLane.

TABLE 11-3	Approximate Weight of Products of Normal Pregnancy

Products	Weight
Fetus	3500 g (7.5 lb)
Placenta	450 g (1 lb)
Amniotic fluid	900 g (2 lb)
Uterus (weight increase)	1100 g (2.5 lb)
Breast tissue (weight increase)	1400 g (3 lb)
Blood volume (weight increase)	1800 g (4 lb) (1500 ml)
Maternal stores	1800-3600 g (4-8 lb)
TOTAL	10,850-12,650 g (10.9-12.7 kg; 24-28 lb)

tional focus should always be on an individualized assessment of need and the quality of the weight gain. An average weight gain during normal pregnancy is about 11 to 16 kg (25 to 35 lb).[33] Around this average many individual variations occur. There is no specific rigid norm or restriction to which all women should be held regardless of individual needs; such a course is obviously unwise and unscientific. Current recommendations are therefore usually stated in terms of ranges to accommodate variances in needs. An initial base for evaluation, however, may be the average weight of the products of pregnancy as shown in Table 11-3. In addition to the components of growth and development usually attributed to a pregnancy, an important part is maternal stores. This laying down of extra adipose fat tissue is necessary for maternal energy reserves to sustain rapid fetal growth during the latter half of pregnancy and for labor and delivery and maintaining lactation after birth. Approximately 1.8 to 3.6 kg (4 to 8 lb) of adipose tissue is commonly deposited for these needs. A report of the Food and Nutrition Board of the Institute of Medicine, *Nutrition During Pregnancy*, recommends setting weight gain goals together with the pregnant woman according to her prepregnancy nutritional status and BMI, as follows[33]:

- Normal weight women with BMI of 19.8 to 26.0: 11.5 to 16 kg (25 to 35 lb)
- Underweight women with BMI of less than 19.8: 13 to 18 kg (28 to 40 lb)
- Overweight women with BMI of greater than 26.0 to 29.0: 7 to 11.5 kg (15 to 25 lb)
- Obese women with BMI of greater than 29.0: minimum of 7 kg (15 lb)

The recommendation for adolescent girls is that they should strive for the upper end of the targeted range. The recommendation for a woman carrying twins is a weight gain range of 16 to 20.5 kg (35 to 45 lb).[33] Compared with single-birth infants, twin-birth infants are 5 times more likely to be born premature (less than 37 weeks'

gestation), 9.5 times more likely to be very low birth weight (less than 1500 g), and 8.5 times more likely to be low birth weight (less than 2500 g).[34]

Quality of Weight Gain

The important consideration, as indicated, lies in the nutritional quality of the gain. Specifically, the foods consumed should be nutrient dense, not full of empty kcalories, to meet the nutrient requirements. Also, there has been failure in some cases to distinguish between weight gained as a result of edema and that as a result of deposition of fat—maternal stores for energy to sustain rapid fetal growth during the latter part of pregnancy and energy for lactation to follow.[35] Analysis of the total tissue gained in an average pregnancy shows that the largest component, 62%, is water. Fat accounts for 31% and protein for 7%. Water is also the most variable component of the tissue gained, accounting for a range of 8 kg (18 lb) to as much as 11 kg (24 lb). Of the 8 kg of water usually gained, about 5.5 kg (12 lb) is associated with fetal tissue and other tissues gained in pregnancy. The remaining 2.5 kg (6 lb) accumulates in the maternal interstitial tissues.[33] Gravity causes the maternal tissue fluids to pool more in the lower extremities, leading to general swelling of the ankles, which is seen routinely in pregnant women. This fluid retention is a normal adaptive phenomenon designed to support the pregnancy and to exert a positive effect on fetal growth. Connective tissue becomes more hygroscopic as a result of the estrogen-induced changes in the ground substance and thus becomes softer and more easily distended. This facilitates delivery of the infant through the cervix and vaginal canal. Also, the increased tissue fluid during pregnancy provides a means for handling the increased metabolic work and circulation of numerous metabolites necessary for fetal growth.

Clearly, severe kcalorie restriction is harmful to the developing fetus and the woman. It is inevitably accompanied by restriction of the vitally needed nutrients essential to the growth process.[35] Moreover, *weight reduction should never be undertaken during pregnancy*. Sufficient weight gain should be encouraged with the use of a nourishing diet.

Rate of Weight Gain

On the whole, about 1 to 2.3 kg (2 to 5 lb) is an average weight gain during the first trimester. Thereafter, an average weight gain of about 0.5 kg (1 lb)/week during the remainder of the pregnancy is usual, although some women may need to gain more. There is no scientific justification for routinely limiting weight gain to lesser amounts. Moreover, an individual woman who needs to gain more should not have unrealistic patterns imposed

---

hygroscopic Taking up and retaining moisture readily.

on her. It is only unusual patterns of gain, such as a sudden sharp increase in weight after the twentieth week of pregnancy that may signal abnormal water retention, which should be monitored closely, especially if it occurs in conjunction with blood pressure elevation and proteinuria. Conversely, an insufficient or low maternal weight gain during the second or third trimester increases the risk for intrauterine growth retardation.[35,36]

Weight Gain and Sodium Intake

In relation to weight gain, questions are sometimes raised about the use of salt during pregnancy. A moderate amount of dietary sodium is needed for the following two essential reasons:

1. It is the major mineral required to control the extracellular fluid compartment.
2. This vital body water is increased during pregnancy to support its successful outcome.

Current practice usually follows a regular diet with moderate sodium intake, 1.5 to 2.3 g/day, with light use of salt to taste.[37] Limiting sodium beyond this general use is contrary to physiologic need in pregnancy and is unfounded. The NRC and professional obstetric guidelines have labeled routine salt-free diets and diuretics as potentially dangerous.[3-5] Maintaining the needed increase in circulating blood volume during pregnancy requires adequate amounts of sodium and protein, as well as adequate fluid intake to prevent dehydration and possible premature contractions.

GENERAL DIETARY PROBLEMS

Functional Gastrointestinal Problems

Nausea and Vomiting

Some general dietary problems temporarily interfere with food and nutrient intake. Most are easily resolved through dietary counseling and with medical attention and have no long-term adverse effect on the quality of maternal weight gain. Symptoms of nausea and vomiting are usually mild and short term, the so-called "morning sickness" of early pregnancy because it occurs more often on arising than later in the day. At least 50% of all pregnant women, most of them in their first pregnancy, experience this condition, beginning during the fifth or sixth week of the pregnancy and usually ending about the fourteenth to sixteenth week. A number of factors may contribute to the situation. Some are physiologic, with causal factors based on hormonal changes that occur early in pregnancy or on low blood sugar, which can be relieved by carbohydrate foods but *which will* return within 2 to 3 hours after a meal. Others may be psychologic, based on situational tensions or anxieties about the pregnancy itself. Still others may be dietary problems, based

on poor food habits. Simple treatment generally improves food tolerance. Frequent small low-fat meals and snacks, which are fairly dry and consisting chiefly of easily digested energy-yielding foods such as carbohydrates (mainly starches), are usually more readily tolerated. Also, it may help to avoid cooking odors as much as possible. Liquids are best taken between meals instead of with meals.

Hyperemesis

In a small number of pregnant women, about 3.5:1000 pregnancies, a severe form of persistent nausea and vomiting occurs that does not respond to usual treatment. This condition, *hyperemesis,* begins early in the pregnancy and may last throughout. It may develop into the more serious pernicious form of hyperemesis gravidarum. This persistent condition causes severe alterations in fluids and electrolytes, weight loss, and nutritional deficits, sometimes requiring hospitalization and alternative feeding by enteral or parenteral methods to sustain the pregnancy (see Chapter 18). Continued personal support and reassurance are important.

Constipation

The complaint of constipation is seldom more than minor, but it contributes to discomfort and concern. Placental hormones relax the gastrointestinal muscles, and the pressure of the enlarging uterus on the lower portion of the intestine may make elimination somewhat difficult. Increased fluid intake and the use of naturally laxative foods containing dietary fiber, such as whole grains, fruits and vegetables, dried fruits (especially prunes and figs), and other fruits and juices, generally promote regularity. Laxatives should be avoided. Appropriate daily exercise is essential for overall health during pregnancy.

Hemorrhoids

A fairly common complaint during the latter part of pregnancy is that of hemorrhoids. These are enlarged veins in the anus, often protruding through the anal sphincter. This vein enlargement is usually caused by the increased weight of the fetus and its downward pressure. The hemorrhoids may cause considerable discomfort, burning, and itching. Occasionally, they may rupture and bleed under pressure of a bowel movement, causing anxiety. The problem is usually controlled by the dietary suggestions given for constipation. Also, sufficient rest during the latter part of the day may help relieve some of the downward pressure of the uterus on the lower intestine.

Heartburn or Gastric Pressure

The related complaints of heartburn or a full feeling are sometimes voiced by pregnant women. These discomforts occur especially after meals and are usually caused by the pressure of the enlarging uterus crowding the stomach. Gastric reflux of some of the food mass, now a liquid chyme mixed with stomach acid, may occur in the lower esophagus, causing an irritation and a burning sensation. Obviously this common complaint has nothing to do with heart action but is so called because of the close proximity of the lower esophagus to the heart. The full feeling comes from general gastric pressure, lack of normal space in the area, a large meal, or gas formation. These complaints are usually remedied by dividing the day's food into a series of small meals, avoiding eating large meals at any time, and not lying down after a meal. Comfort is also improved by wearing loose-fitting clothing.

Effects of Iron Supplements

The effects of an iron supplement may include gray or black stools and sometimes nausea, constipation, or diarrhea. To help avoid food-related effects, the iron supplement should be taken 1 hour before a meal or 2 hours after with liquid such as water or orange juice but not with milk or tea. The absorption of iron is increased with vitamin C and decreased with milk, other dairy foods, eggs, whole grain bread and cereal, and tea.

HIGH-RISK PREGNANCIES

Identify Risk Factors Involved

To avoid the consequences of sustained poor nutrition during pregnancy, a first procedure is to identify women at risk. In a joint report, the American College of Obstetrics and Gynecology and the American Dietetic Association issued a set of risk factors, as shown in Box 11-1, that identify women with special nutritional needs during pregnancy.[5] These nutrition-related factors are based on clinical evidence of inadequate nutrition. However,

rather than waiting for clinical symptoms of poor nutrition to appear, a better approach would be to identify poor food patterns that will induce nutritional problems and to prevent these problems from developing. On this basis, three types of dietary patterns predict failure to support optimal maternal and fetal nutrition: (1) insufficient food intake, (2) poor food selection, and (3) poor food distribution throughout the day. These patterns, added to the list of risk factors in Box 11-1, are much more sensitive for nutritional risk.

Plan Personal Care

Once early assessment identifies risk factors, practitioners can then give more careful attention to these women. By working closely with each woman and her personal food pattern and living situation, a food plan can be developed with her to ensure an optimal intake of energy and nutrients to support her pregnancy and its successful outcome.

Recognize Special Counseling Needs

Several special needs require sensitive counseling. These areas of need include the age and parity of the woman; any use of harmful agents such as alcohol, cigarettes, drugs, or pica; and socioeconomic problems.

Age and Parity

Pregnancies at either age extreme of the reproductive cycle pose special problems. The adolescent pregnancy carries many social and nutrition-related risks associated with higher incidence of low birth weight and perinatal mortality, among other poor outcomes. The obstetric history of a woman is expressed in terms of number and order of pregnancies, or her gravida status. A nulligravida (no prior pregnancy) who is 15 years of age or younger is especially at risk because her own growth is incomplete; therefore sufficient weight gain and the quality of her diet are particularly important.[33] Sensitive counseling provides both information and emotional support; it should involve family members or other persons significant to the adolescent. On the other hand, the older primigravida (first pregnancy), older than 35 years, also requires special attention. She may be more at risk for hypertension, either preexisting or pregnancy induced, and may need more attention to the rate of weight gain and amount of sodium used, as well as any drug therapy

---

BOX 11-1	**Nutritional Risk Factors in Pregnancy**

Risk Factors Present at the Onset of Pregnancy

- Age: ≤15 yr or ≥35 yr
- Frequent pregnancies: 3 or more during a 2-year period
- Poor obstetric history or poor fetal performance
- Poverty
- Bizarre or faddist food habits
- Abuse of nicotine, alcohol, or drugs
- Therapeutic diet required for a chronic disorder
- Weight: <85% or >120% of standard weight

Risk Factors Occurring During Pregnancy

- Low hemoglobin or hematocrit: Hgb <12 g/dl; Hct <35%
- Inadequate weight gain: Any weight loss *or* weight gain of <1 kg (2 lb)/month after the first trimester
- Excessive weight gain: >1 kg (2 lb)/week after the first trimester

From American College of Obstetrics and Gynecology and American Dietetic Association Task Force on Nutrition: *Assessment of maternal nutrition*, Chicago, 1978, Authors.

---

hyperemesis gravidarum Severe vomiting during pregnancy, which is potentially fatal.
nulligravida A woman who has never been pregnant.
primigravida A woman who is pregnant for the first time.

prescribed. In addition, several pregnancies within a limited number of years leave a mother drained of nutritional resources and entering each successive pregnancy at a higher risk.

Social Habits: Alcohol, Cigarettes, and Drugs

These three personal habits may cause fetal damage and are contraindicated during pregnancy. No safe level of alcohol consumption has yet been found for pregnant women. Extensive or habitual alcohol use may lead to one of the fetal alcohol spectrum disorders known as *fetal alcohol syndrome (FAS),* which is currently a leading cause of mental retardation.[38] FAS is characterized by growth retardation, malformed facial features, joint and limb abnormalities, cardiac defects, mental retardation, and in serious cases, death. FAS signs have been seen in tests with rats as early as the human equivalent of the third week of gestation, when most women are unaware of their pregnancies. Thus moderate-to-heavy drinking among sexually active women of childbearing age may carry potential danger. Even moderate prenatal alcohol exposure has been associated with low birth weight and has effects on a child's psychomotor and cognitive development in the absence of malformations, known as *fetal alcohol effects (FAE).*[39]

Cigarette smoking during pregnancy is also contraindicated.[40] Harmful substances in tobacco and impaired oxygen transport cause fetal damage and special problems of placental abnormalities, leading to greater risk of spontaneous abortion (miscarriage), prematurity, low birth weight, impairment of mental and physical growth, and increased potential mortality.[40,41] Counseling with women and families who smoke should stress the importance of quitting for pregnancy and beyond.

Drug use, both recreational and medicinal, also poses numerous problems.[41] Self-medication with over-the-counter drugs carries potential adverse effects. The use of illicit drugs is especially hazardous, exposing the developing fetus to the risks of addiction and possibly acquired immunodeficiency syndrome (AIDS) from the woman's use of contaminated needles during drug injections. Dangers come not only from the drug itself or contaminated needles but also from impurities contained in illicit drugs. Evaluation of the effects of street drugs (marijuana, cocaine, heroin, methadone) on nutritional status is difficult because of multiple drug use, uncertain purity, unknown dosage and timing, and inadequate nutritional status of many drug users. A high incidence of meconium staining (which could relate to fetal damage), poor prenatal weight gain, very short (less than 3 hours) or prolonged labor, operative delivery (cesarean, forceps), and other perinatal problems among marijuana users has been reported. Such outcomes indicate that abstinence of marijuana use during pregnancy is prudent.

Abuse from megadosing with basic nutrients such as vitamin A or use of prescription medications such as

Accutane during pregnancy may cause fetal damage as previously described (see the *Further Readings and Resources* section at the end of this chapter). A number of drugs are often prescribed for female patients to treat a variety of psychologic and mental health disorders. However, if taken during pregnancy, they exhibit teratogenic effects. If any of these drugs are taken on a long-term basis for the treatment of serious conditions, such as clinical depression, bipolar disorder, or schizophrenia, comprehensive medical and psychologic assessment and follow-up is needed throughout the pregnancy. Lithium has been associated with an increased risk for Epstein's anomaly (a rare cardiovascular abnormality), goiter, and diabetes insipidus, as well as neonatal toxic disturbances such as cyanosis, hypothermia, and bradycardia. A diminished suck reflex will impede attempts to nourish the infant exposed to lithium in utero. Diazepam (Valium) is associated with an abnormal fetal heart rate. The neonate risks delivery by cesarean section, with oral-facial malformations, a depressed Apgar score, and a reluctance to feed. Rats exposed to diazepam in utero have exhibited abnormal motor skills and arousal processes. *Tricyclic antidepressants* (e.g., imipramine) have led to morphologic and behavioral abnormalities in rats.

Hydantoin (Dilantin, Phenytoin) is prescribed to control seizures caused by epilepsy and other conditions. Even though this drug has caused malformations in the offspring of rats, physicians are reluctant to discontinue it for their patients with epilepsy during pregnancy. Because only 7% of children born to mothers using the drug develop malformations, and significantly more develop malformations and developmental disabilities when the mother's epilepsy is untreated, this may be one case in which prenatal drug use is more beneficial than not using it. Thus, with the exception of drugs used to treat individuals with seizure disorders or natural replacement therapy (e.g., insulin for persons with type 1 diabetes), drugs should be avoided at all costs during pregnancy to ensure the health of the woman and a safe and healthy outcome of the pregnancy. The nutrition counselor is well advised to keep up with the most recent findings regarding medications (prescribed, over-the-counter, and street drugs) to evaluate the nutritional status of the woman using them and to allow the practitioner and woman to design a plan of action to safely eliminate the drug, preferably before conception. In addition, evaluation of herbal and botanical supplements, which are not regulated in the same manner as prescription and over-the-counter drugs, is necessary to inform the woman of potential safety issues and to counsel her appropriately.

Caffeine

Although milder in its effect (depending on the extent of use) than the agents just discussed, caffeine remains a

FOCUS ON CULTURE

Pica During Pregnancy: Cultural Norm of Concern

Pica is the ingestion of nonfood substances or food components including but not limited to clay, dirt, chalk, cornstarch, laundry starch, baking powder, baking soda, ice, and freezer frost. These substances are often craved with subsequent consumption. Approximately 20% of pregnant women engage in pica, and the prevalence of this psychobehavioral disorder is higher in rural compared to urban areas and in certain cultures.

Normal Cultural Behavior or Pregnancy-Induced Disorder

In a group of women living in Kenya from a variety of ethnic and religious backgrounds, more than 80% reported consumption of approximately 1 cup of soil on a daily basis. Soil intake was more common in the latter part of pregnancy. In these cultures, pica represents a cultural norm that may increase in prevalence during pregnancy.

Nearly 45% of women born and living in western Mexico engaged in pica during pregnancy, whereas only about 30% of Mexican-born women currently residing in California practiced pica during pregnancy. Although pica may be a culturally accepted norm, changes in prevalence may be induced with acculturation into a society where this behavior is less common.

Consequences of Pica and Need for Counseling

A pregnant woman who engages in pica, regardless of cultural background, should be informed about the health consequences of pica. Although it is unclear if nutrient deficiencies precipitate pica behaviors or vice versa, many pica substances are capable of binding nutrients to render them unavailable for absorption. Nutritional anemias may occur, having adverse effects on both mother and baby. Exposure to toxins and teratogens from nonfood substances such as battery acid or

ashes is also possible. Gastrointestinal perforation, constipation, and microbial infections are additional potential outcomes of pica.

An understanding by the health care practitioner regarding factors leading to pica is vital to affecting behavior change. For example, the pregnant woman who believes that a nonfood substance has an essential role in the body's balance or harmony with her environment may be less willing to avoid consumption of that nonfood substance. On the other hand, a pregnant woman who consumes eggshells because of the sensory cravings associated with the texture may be amenable to substituting a crunchy food substance for this nonfood product. Inquiry regarding the history of pica in the pregnant woman is important to identify sources of pica substances and to involve other family members or cultural leaders who may support such behavior and need counseling to facilitate appropriate behavior changes. Such nutrition counseling must be delivered in a culturally sensitive and appropriate manner, with emphasis on the importance of behavior changes for an optimal outcome for the infant.

References

Corbett RW et al: Pica in pregnancy: does it affect pregnancy outcomes? *MCN Am J Matern Child Nurs* 28(3):183, 2003.

Geissler PW et al: Perceptions of soil-eating and anaemia among pregnant women on the Kenyan coast, *Soc Sci Med* 48(8):1069, 1999.

Horner RD et al: Pica practices of pregnant women, *J Am Diet Assoc* 91(1):34, 1991.

Rainville AJ: Pica practices of pregnant women are associated with lower maternal hemoglobin level at delivery, *J Am Diet Assoc* 98(3):293, 1998.

Simpson E et al: Pica during pregnancy in low-income women born in Mexico, *West J Med* 173(1):20, 2000.

---

widely used drug that can cross the placenta and enter fetal circulation.[42] Its use at levels of 500 mg/day or greater has been associated with an increased risk of first-trimester spontaneous abortion.[43,44] Most health agencies have recommended that pregnant women limit caffeine consumption from foods, beverages (coffee, tea, cocoa, cola), and medications to less than 300 mg/day because of the many uncertainties regarding the fetal effects of maternal caffeine consumption.[45]

Pica

Pica is the craving and consumption of unusual nonfood substances such as laundry starch, clay, dirt, or ice. This practice during pregnancy is more widespread than health care workers have believed, particularly in southern regions of the United States and among specific ethnic and cultural groups. Some pica practices have been associated with iron deficiency anemia, although the direction of causality is unknown.[46,47] Where these unusual practices exist, they must be appreciated as cultural patterns that require a respectful approach and understanding by health workers who seek to negotiate appropriate behavior changes (see the *Focus on Culture* box, "Pica During Pregnancy: Cultural Norm of Concern").[48]

Socioeconomic Challenges

Special counseling is required for women and young girls facing economic challenges. Numerous studies and clinical observations indicate that lack of prenatal care, often associated with racial prejudices and fears, as well as a lack of adequate financial resources, places the expectant mother in grave difficulty. Special counseling that is sensitive to personal needs is required to help plan resources for care and financial assistance. Resources include programs such as the federally funded Special Supplemental Nutrition Program for Women, Infants, and Children (WIC), described in Chapter 10, as well as numerous state and local programs. An example of a community partnership program promoting prenatal care is Stork's Nest, sponsored by the March of Dimes in affiliation with a national women's organization and local community service agencies. Another successful program targeted for low-income women is BabyCare, administered by the Virginia Department of Health. The BabyCal program, now a web-based educational site sponsored by the California Department of Health Services, provides another approach to increasing prenatal care and decreasing adverse infant outcomes (see the *Further Readings and Resources* section at the end of this chapter).

COMPLICATIONS OF PREGNANCY

Anemia

Anemia is common during pregnancy. It is often associated with the normal maternal blood volume increase of 40% to 50% and a disproportionate increase in red cell mass of about 20%. Of all women in large prenatal clinics in the United States, about 10% have hemoglobin concentrations of less than 10 g/dl and a hematocrit reading below 32%. Anemia is far more prevalent among the poor, many of whom live on diets barely adequate for subsistence. However, anemia is by no means restricted to lower economic groups.

Iron Deficiency Anemia

A deficiency of iron is by far the most common cause of anemia in pregnancy. The total cost of a single normal pregnancy in iron stores is large—approximately 500 to 800 mg. Of this amount nearly 300 mg is used by the fetus. The remainder is used in the expanded maternal blood volume and its increased red blood cells and hemoglobin mass. This iron requirement typically exceeds the available reserves in the average woman. Thus, in addition to including iron-rich foods in the diet, a daily supplement or higher therapeutic dose may be required as previously described.

Folate Deficiency Anemia

A less common megaloblastic anemia of pregnancy results from folate deficiency. During pregnancy, the fetus is sensitive to folate inhibitors and therefore has increased metabolic requirements for folate. To prevent this anemia the DRI standard recommends 600 µg of folate per day during pregnancy. Women with poor diets will need supplementation to reach this intake goal.

Hemorrhagic Anemia

Anemia caused by blood loss is more likely to occur during labor and delivery than during pregnancy. Blood loss may occur earlier, as a result of abortion or ruptured tubular pregnancy. Most women undergoing these physiologic problems receive blood via transfusion, and iron therapy may be indicated for adequate replacement for hemoglobin formation.

Pregnancy-Induced Hypertension

Relation to Nutrition

A number of clinicians have presented clinical and laboratory evidence that *pregnancy-induced hypertension* (PIH) is a disease that principally affects young women with their first pregnancy. Although the genetic and immune-related causes of PIH are becoming clearer, diet plays a role in the risk of preeclampsia. For example, diets poor in kcalories, protein, calcium, magnesium, potassium, and dietary fiber have been associated with risk of PIH. Regardless of the underlying causes and multiorgan effects, nutritional support of the pregnancy is, as always, a primary concern. Certainly, as many practitioners have observed, PIH is classically associated with poverty, inadequate diet, and little or no prenatal care. Much of the PIH problem, which seems to develop early from the time of implantation of the fertilized ovum into the uterine lining, may be reduced by good prenatal care from the beginning of the pregnancy, which inherently includes attention to sound nutrition. It is this sound nutritional status, which a woman brings to her pregnancy and maintains throughout, that provides her with optimal resources for adapting to the physiologic stress of gestation. Her fitness during pregnancy is a direct function of her past state of nutrition and her optimal nutrition throughout pregnancy.

Clinical Symptoms

PIH is defined according to its manifestations, which generally occur in the third trimester toward term. These symptoms are hypertension, abnormal and excessive edema, albuminuria, and, in severe cases, convulsions or coma, a state called eclampsia.

Treatment

Specific treatment varies according to the individual patient's symptoms and needs. Optimal nutrition is a fundamental aspect of therapy in any case. Emphasis is given to a regular diet with adequate dietary protein and calcium and one that is rich in fruits and vegetables, providing magnesium, potassium, and dietary fiber. Correction of plasma protein deficits stimulates the capillary fluid shift mechanism and increases circulation of tissue fluids, with subsequent correction of the hypovolemia. In addition, adequate salt and sources of vitamins and minerals are needed for correction and maintenance of metabolic balance.

Multiple Fetuses

The incidence of multifetal pregnancies has increased in recent decades and presents unique concerns. Infants born from a multifetal pregnancy are more likely to have lower-than-average birth weights and are at risk for preterm delivery.[34] Thus nutritional needs of these women must be given special attention. Energy intake must be increased beyond the needs of a singleton pregnancy such that the recommended weight gain for multiple fetuses is achieved. This increase in energy intake often provides for the additional nutrient demands that exist. Attention to adequate folate intake is critical to reduce risks of low birth weights and preterm delivery. Supplemental iron may be necessary to reduce the incidence of anemia, more commonly found in women with multiple fetuses. Additional calcium and vitamin D are needed with multiple fetuses to promote adequate calcium absorption for optimal bone mineralization *in utero*. Zinc, copper, and pyridoxine supplementation may also be required to support multifetal growth and development.

Maternal Disease Conditions

Preexisting clinical conditions in the woman further complicate pregnancy. In each case, management of these conditions is based on general principles of care related to both pregnancy and the particular disease involved. Examples of such maternal conditions are reviewed here; they are hypertension, diabetes mellitus, PKU, AIDS, and eating disorders.

Hypertension

Preexisting hypertension in the pregnant woman can cause considerable maternal and fetal consequences. Many of these problems can be prevented by initial screening and continued monitoring by the prenatal nurse, with referral to the clinical nutritionist for a plan of care. The hypertensive disease process begins long before signs and symptoms appear, and later symptoms are inconsistent. Risk factors for hypertension before and during pregnancy are listed in Box 11-2. Nutritional therapy centers on the following three principles:

1. Prevention of weight extremes, underweight or obesity
2. Correction of any dietary deficiencies and maintenance of optimal nutritional status during pregnancy
3. Management of any related coexisting disease such as diabetes mellitus or hyperlipidemia

---

BOX 11-2 | **Risk Factors for Pregnancy-Induced Hypertension**

Before Pregnancy

- Nulligravida
- Diabetes
- Preexisting condition (hypertension, renal or vascular disease)
- Family history of hypertension or vascular disease
- Diagnosis of pregnancy-induced hypertension in a previous pregnancy
- Dietary deficiencies
- Age extremes
  ≤20 years
  ≥35 years

During Pregnancy

- Primigravida
- Large fetus
- Glomerulonephritis
- Fetal hydrops
- Hydramnios
- Multiple gestation
- Hydatidiform mole

Sodium intake may be moderate but should not be unduly restricted because of its relation to fluid and electrolyte balances during pregnancy and its controversial therapy in hypertension in general. Initial and continuing client education and a close relationship with the nurse-nutritionist care team contribute to successful management of the hypertension and prevent problems that may occur. (For a more detailed discussion of vascular disease, see Chapter 20.)

Diabetes Mellitus and Gestational Diabetes Mellitus

The management of preexisting diabetes in pregnancy presents special problems. Today, however, improved expectations for the diabetic woman's pregnancy constitute one of the success stories of modern medicine.[49] Contributing factors to this improved outlook include advances in technology for monitoring fetal development, increased knowledge of nutrition and diabetes, and management refinements in tight blood glucose control through self-monitoring.[50,51] Chapter 21 details care of persons with types 1 and 2 diabetes mellitus.

During pregnancy, glycosuria is not uncommon because of the increased circulating blood volume and its load of metabolites. Routine screening protocols, typically conducted between the twenty-fourth and twenty-eighth week of gestation, are used during pregnancy to detect gestational diabetes mellitus (GDM). GDM is an intolerance of carbohydrate such that blood glucose concentration increases during pregnancy. In 95% of cases this carbohydrate or glucose intolerance resolves after delivery. Treatment during pregnancy is important because of the higher risk these women carry for fetal damage during this gestational period.[52] The most common outcome for an infant born to a mother with GDM is macrosomia, a larger than normal body size. Other infant complications include hypoglycemia, jaundice, and trauma at birth. Although GDM occurs in 2% to 13% of the pregnant population, up to 50% of women with pregnancy-induced abnormal glucose tolerance subsequently develop overt diabetes. Team management is required for adequate care of gestational and preexisting types 1 and 2 diabetes mellitus.[53,54] (See Chapter 21 for a detailed discussion of diabetes care.)

Maternal Phenylketonuria

The successful detection and management of infants with PKU through newborn screening programs in all states have ensured their normal growth and development to adulthood. PKU is a genetic metabolic disease caused by

---

eclampsia Advanced pregnancy-induced hypertension (PIH), manifested by convulsions.

hypovolemia Abnormally decreased volume of circulating blood in the body.

a missing enzyme for the metabolism of the essential amino acid phenylalanine. It is controlled by a special low-phenylalanine diet initiated at birth. Now a new generation of young women with PKU since birth are beginning to have children of their own. However, maternal PKU presents potential fetal hazards. Experience has shown how crucial it is for the woman to follow a strict low-phenylalanine diet before conception, whenever possible, to minimize risks of fetal damage in the early cell differentiation weeks of pregnancy.

Acquired Immunodeficiency Syndrome

Carefully monitored care throughout pregnancy and after birth is essential for pregnant women who are infected by the human immunodeficiency virus (HIV). Two goals are most important: (1) to reduce the rate of the disease progression in the woman through nutritional support and (2) to minimize the chance of HIV vertical transmission from mother to infant either in the womb or after birth via breast-feeding. Nutrient deficiencies are often found in HIV-positive patients. Although specific nutrient requirements for HIV-infected pregnant women have not been established, these patients may need up to 150% of normal pregnancy intakes of both macronutrients and micronutrients. Continual individual monitoring and adjustment are essential. Infants can be infected by HIV during labor and delivery and through breast milk. Where safe alternatives to breast milk are available, such as commercial formula or banked human milk, a decision on breast-feeding depends on the HIV status of the newborn infant. In the United States, both the Centers for Disease Control and Prevention (CDC) and the American Academy of Pediatrics recommend HIV-positive mothers do not breast-feed when the infant is not infected.[55,56]

Eating Disorders

Eating disorders, specifically anorexia nervosa (AN) and bulimia nervosa (BN), have been previously described (see Chapter 5). Diagnosis and treatment of these disorders in the nonpregnant state require multidisciplinary approaches, and even greater consideration with further specialized care is required for a pregnant woman with AN or BN. AN is uncommon during pregnancy, because amenorrhea is a diagnostic criteria for the disorder; however, ovulation and subsequent conception has been reported.[57] Compared to AN, pregnancy in a woman with BN is more likely, due to more typical menstrual patterns, weight status, and less restrictive eating. BN has been linked to spontaneous abortion, poor weight gain, low infant birth weight, premature deliveries, and congenital malformations.[58] A team approach that emphasizes nutritional needs of the growing fetus, anticipated maternal body size and shape changes, and postpartum care is critical to a successful course and outcome.[58,59]

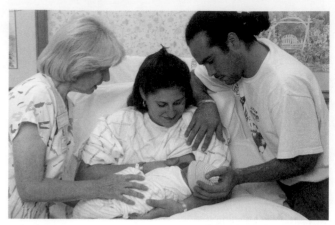

FIGURE 11-3 By teaching about the newborn and family, the nurse helps parents develop confidence in their ability to provide care for the infant. *(From McKinney ES et al: Maternal-child nursing, Philadelphia, 2000, WB Saunders.)*

NUTRITION DURING LACTATION

Current Breast-Feeding Trends

Data from the National Immunization Survey show that approximately 71% of mothers initiate breast-feeding.[60] Several factors contribute to this rate of breast-feeding initiation, as follows:

- More mothers are informed about the benefits of breast-feeding[61,62] (Figure 11-3).
- Practitioners recognize the ability of human milk to meet infant needs (Table 11-4) and promote immune function.[63-65]
- Maternity wards and alternative birth centers have been modified to facilitate successful lactation.
- Community support is increasingly available, even in workplaces.[66,67]
- Programs that promote breast-feeding are increasingly responsive to a wider range of maternal socioeconomic conditions and cultural backgrounds.[68-75]

Exclusive breast-feeding by well-nourished mothers can be adequate for periods ranging from 2 to 15 months.[76-79] Unfortunately, exclusive breast-feeding declines to less than 43% and less than 14% of mothers by 3 months and 6 months, respectively.[60] Solid foods are usually added to the baby's diet at about 6 months of age; the American Dietetic Association's position is that breast-feeding should continue for at least the first 12 months of the infant's life.[79]

Nutritional Needs

The physiologic needs of lactation are different from those of pregnancy, and they demand adequate nutritional support (see Tables 11-1 and 11-2). The basic nutritional needs for lactation include the following additions to the mother's prepregnancy needs.

TABLE 11-4	Selected Nutritional Components of Human Milk (per 100 ml)			
Milk Component	**Colostrum**	**Transitional**	**Mature**	**Cow's Milk**
Kilocalories	57.0	63.0	65.0	65.0
Vitamins, fat-soluble				
A (μg)	151.0	88.0	75.0	41.0
D (IU)	—	—	5.0	2.5
E (mg)	1.5	0.9	0.25	0.07
K (μg)	—	—	1.5	6.0
Vitamins, water-soluble				
Thiamin (μg)	1.9	5.9	14.0	43.0
Riboflavin (μg)	30.0	37.0	40.0	145.0
Niacin (μg)	75.0	175.0	160.0	82.0
Pantothenic acid (μg)	183.0	288.0	246.0	340.0
Biotin (μg)	0.06	0.35	0.6	2.8
Vitamin B_{12} (μg)	0.05	0.04	0.1	1.1
Vitamin C (mg)	5.9	7.1	5.0	1.1

Energy

The recommended caloric increase is 330 kcal/day (plus 170 kcal/day from maternal stores) in the first 6 months and 400 kcal/day in the second 6 months of breast-feeding more than the usual adult allowance. This makes a daily total of about 2700 to 2800 kcal.[10] This additional energy need for the overall total lactation process is based on the following four factors:

1. *Milk content:* An average daily milk production for lactating women is 780 ml (26 oz). The energy content of human milk averages 0.67 to 0.74 kcalories/g. Thus 26 oz of milk has a value of about 525 kcalories.
2. *Milk production:* The metabolic work involved in producing this amount of milk is about 80% efficient and requires from 400 to 450 kcalories. During pregnancy the breast is developed for this purpose, stimulated by hormones from the placenta, and forms special milk-producing cells called *lobules* (Figure 11-4). After birth the mother's production of the hormone *prolactin* continues this milk-production process, which the suckling infant stimulates. Thus milk production depends on the demand of the infant. The suckling infant stimulates the brain's release of the hormone *oxytocin* from the pituitary gland to initiate the letdown reflex for the release of the milk from storage cells to travel down to the nipple. This reflex is easily inhibited by the mother's fatigue, tension, or lack of confidence, a particular source of anxiety in the new mother. She may be reassured that a comfortable and satisfying feeding routine is usually established in 2 to 3 weeks (Figure 11-5).

3. *Maternal adipose tissue storage:* A component of the energy need for lactation (170 kcal/day in the first 6 months) is drawn from maternal adipose tissue stores deposited during pregnancy in normal preparation for lactation to follow in the maternal cycle. Depending on the adequacy of these stores, additional energy input may be needed in the lactating woman's daily diet.
4. *Exercise:* Lactating women generally balance energy expenditure from exercise with increased energy intake and alterations in prolactin to maintain an adequate milk supply.[80,81] In some women, the weight gained during pregnancy may be largely retained and contribute to obesity. Some overweight women who are breast-feeding have concerns regarding whether a weight loss program might endanger the growth of their infants. Research with overweight women who were exclusively breast-feeding has shown that a diet and exercise program that led to a weight loss of around 0.5 kg/week (approximately 1 lb/week) from 4 to 14 weeks postpartum did not affect infant growth.[82] However, the mother who is involved in any specific weight loss program during lactation should be monitored closely as should her infant.[82,83]

Protein

The recommendation for protein needs during lactation is 71 g/day during both the first 6 months and second 6 months.[10] This is an increase of about 25 g/day from the regular needs of the adult woman.

Minerals

The DRI standard for calcium during lactation is 1000 mg/day, the same as for the nonpregnant or pregnant

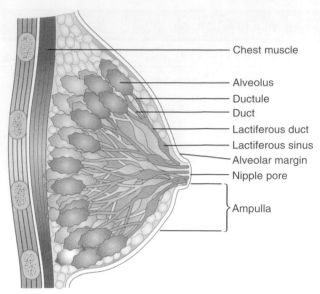

FIGURE 11-4   Structural features of the human mammary gland. *(From Mahan LK, Escott-Stump S, eds:* Krause's food, nutrition, and diet therapy, *ed 11, Philadelphia, 2004, WB Saunders/Elsevier.)*

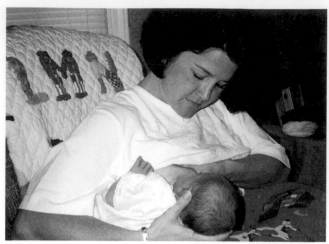

FIGURE 11-5   Breast-feeding infant and mother. *(From Lowdermilk DL, Perry SE, Bobak IM:* Maternity and women's health care, *ed 7, St Louis, 2000, Mosby.)*

adult woman.[6] The amount of calcium that was required during gestation for the mineralization of the fetal skeleton is now diverted into the mother's milk production. Iron, because it is not a major mineral component of milk and because of lactational amenorrhea, need not be increased during lactation.

Vitamins

The DRI standard for vitamin C during lactation is 120 mg/day.[8] This is a considerable increase from the regular 75 mg/day for adult women. Increases over the mother's prenatal intake are also recommended for vitamin A because it is a constituent of milk[9] and for the B-complex vitamins because they are involved as coenzyme factors in energy metabolism.[7] The quantities of vitamins needed, therefore, invariably increase as the kcalorie intake increases.

Fluids

Ample fluid intake is needed and should be based on the mother's urine color. A pale yellow color of the urine suggests adequate fluid intake. Beverages such as juices and milk contribute both fluid and kcalories.[37]

Dietary Supplements

Many health practitioners recommend that women continue their prenatal nutrient supplements during lactation. Specifically, women with certain health conditions or nutrient needs may require supplements while breast-feeding.[84] For example, mothers who consume vegan diets will need cobalamin supplementation.[85] Individual recommendations for nutrient supplementation during lactation should be based on a full assessment of the

mother's nutritional status and other environmental factors.

Women may desire to use herbal or botanical products as *galactogogues* (agents that stimulate breast milk production), relaxants, or analgesics. The safety for mother and infant and efficacy of such products during lactation have not been adequately evaluated in randomized, placebo-controlled trials. In general, women should not use herbals and botanical during lactation; however, some may be appropriate for use within defined quantities.[32]

Rest and Relaxation

In addition to the increased diet, the nursing mother requires rest, moderate exercise, and relaxation. Both parents may benefit from counseling focused on reducing the stresses of their new family situation, as well as meeting their own personal needs. Postpartum depression is increasingly recognized as a specific, and sometimes very serious, condition in mothers. Ranging from "baby blues" to postpartum psychosis, the relationship of this condition with nutritional status and impact on breast-feeding duration requires further investigation.[86,87]

Maternal Medical Conditions

Breast-feeding should be encouraged in most mothers (see the *To Probe Further* box, "Breast-Feeding: The Dynamic Nature of Human Milk"). However, some conditions exist for which it is recommended that women in the United States not breast-feed, including HIV-positive status, active untreated tuberculosis, human T-lymphocytic virus, illicit drug use, and with specific chemotherapeutic agents. Other conditions or medications should be discussed with health practitioners.[79]

BREAST-FEEDING: THE DYNAMIC NATURE OF HUMAN MILK

There is no question that human milk is the ideal first food for human infants. Its dynamic nature changes to match growth needs. The mother's choice to breast-feed her infant depends on a number of factors, however, especially for new mothers, who often need information and counseling from early pregnancy.

Even premature infants can thrive on human milk. Mothers and physicians have sometimes been reluctant to consider breast-feeding for babies born prematurely or delivered by cesarean section, fearing that there may be some negative effect on the quantity or quality of human milk. This uncertainty about the nutritional quality of mother's milk has also led them to encourage adding formula and/or solid foods to the diet to make sure the baby is well fed. These practices are usually unnecessary. They often contribute to allergies, obesity, and digestive problems because of the extra stress placed on an immature gut.

Breast Milk for the Preterm Infant
Levels of nutrients in mother's milk shift according to the gestational age of the infant at birth. The preterm infant is often denied its mother's milk by some hospital workers because they think of it as mature milk having too little protein and too much lactose to meet the child's needs. An analysis of the nutritional quality of preterm milk, however, reveals energy and fat concentrations that are 20% to 30% higher, protein levels 15% to 20% higher, and lactose levels 10% lower than those found in mature milk. Premature milk can meet the preterm infant's needs.

Breast Milk During Weaning
Nutrient levels continue to change with time to match changing growth patterns and developing digestive abilities. Mother's milk does provide sufficient kcalories and nutrients to keep babies well fed without supplemental formula or food. Even when the infant is being weaned, the nature of human milk ensures adequate nutrients, just in case the new, solid-food diet cannot meet the child's needs. Human milk collected during gradual weaning has been found to have higher concentrations of protein, sodium, and iron. Lactose levels are lower, possibly so that higher amounts of kcalories can be supplied by fats, a more concentrated source.

Breast Milk and the Cesarean Section Infant
The quality of human milk is not influenced by the way the baby comes into the world. Many women fear that a baby born by cesarean section cannot be nursed because they think that this method of delivery delays or prevents the production of mature milk. Milk production is stimulated by the release of the placenta, which occurs whether the delivery is vaginal or not. Studies confirm that there is no significant difference in the length of time it takes for mature milk to come in after vaginal or cesarean deliveries.

Thus premature or cesarean deliveries should not discourage women from breast-feeding. Mothers should not underestimate the nutritive quality of their milk simply because it does not appear as rich and thick as cow's milk. After all, cow's milk is made for young calves, who are up and running around after birth and have a much shorter, faster growth period. For the human infant, in both nutritional and immunologic terms, breast milk remains the best milk.

Mothers' Fact and Fancy About Breast-Feeding
In early counseling, mothers express a variety of concerns about breast-feeding. Following are a few such statements:
"My breasts aren't big enough." When it comes to breast-feeding, all women are created equal. The only parts of the breast that participate in milk production are the glandular and nervous tissue and the nipple; these are basically the same in healthy women. The only difference between a size 32A and a size 42DD is the amount of fat the breast contains.

"Breast-feeding causes cancer." Actually, investigators have been looking to breast-feeding as a possible means of preventing breast and ovarian cancer. Epidemiologic studies suggest a decreased risk for these cancers in women who breast-feed.

"Breast-feeding will ruin my figure." Breast-feeding might actually help a woman regain her figure more quickly. Because the caloric demand of breast-feeding exceeds that of the nonpregnant woman by about 400 to 500 kcal, a slightly faster rate of weight loss may be expected, although hormonal adaptations may limit the extent to which weight loss is experienced during lactation. Oxytocin, the hormone manufactured to stimulate the letdown reflex, also stimulates uterine contractions, helping reduce the uterus to its prepregnancy size more rapidly.

"Breast-feeding is painful." It may be painful in the first few days or even weeks as mother and baby establish a pattern of feeding and proper latch and release techniques. Milk should not be allowed to collect in the breast to the point of engorgement, the nipples should be kept clean and dry, and a variety of feeding positions may be used while nursing to decrease the chances of having a painful experience. *Mastitis* is a painful infection of the breast(s) that requires medical attention and often antibiotic treatment.

"Breast milk isn't nutritious." The thin, bluish appearance of breast milk has some women convinced that it is no more nourishing than water. Let them look at Table 11-4; they will be pleasantly surprised at how well breast milk meets the nutritional needs of the infant.

"I will have to change my diet to breast-feed." Foods that were eaten during pregnancy may be consumed during lactation. Some women report that after they eat onions, cauliflower, cabbage, or other foods that their infants do not like the taste of their breast milk. Other women say that eating chocolate or drinking coffee, for example, "makes their babies fussy" when breast-feeding. Scientific evidence does not exist to discourage moderate intake of these foods or drinks. A well-balanced diet that includes a variety of colorful foods and fluids is encouraged during breast-feeding.

"I can't go to work or school if I breast-feed." Breast milk can be stored for 24 hours in the refrigerator or several months in the freezer. Many working mothers take advantage of this by expressing their milk and storing it for use by care providers. In fact, women often express milk on their breaks at school or work. (Some places of employment even have lactation rooms and provide breast pumps at the workplace.) Not only does this relieve the pressure of buildup, but it also allows the milk to be stored for later use at home.

Other women would like to breast-feed but are worried about special "what if" situations, such as the following:
"What if I need a cesarean section?" The method of delivery does not affect the quality or quantity of milk produced. The baby can be held in such a way (the "football hold") that he or she does not rest on the mother's abdominal stitches.

"What if the baby is premature?" Mother's milk changes to meet the infant's needs at all stages of development.

"What if the baby has Down syndrome?" This baby can be nursed; however, it does require time, patience, and the use of slightly different nursing techniques. The mother should be told about the special nursing needs of this

Continued

TO PROBE FURTHER—cont'd

BREAST-FEEDING: THE DYNAMIC NATURE OF HUMAN MILK

infant to avoid disappointment or a feeling of failure in case breast-feeding becomes impractical for her particular living situation.

"What if I have twins?" Believe it or not, it has been done. It takes time, patience, and good coordination, but it can be done. Triplets, however, are another matter altogether. Women have successfully nursed triplets, but often they did very little else until the babies were weaned. This mother will need emotional support whether she attempts to nurse or, finding the amount of time and patience required overwhelming, prefers to bottle-feed.

"What if I have pierced nipples or have had breast surgery?" Nipple jewelry appears to interfere with breast-feeding; however, retainers may be used by a mother who wishes to maintain her piercing and breast-feed. Women should be made aware that serious complications due to nipple piercing, requiring pharmaceutical or surgical treatments that have required up to 12 months for resolution, have been reported. Very little is known about later breast-feeding successes or complications after earlier removal of a nipple piercing. Breast augmentation and reduction surgeries have shown mixed results related to successful breast-feeding; however, this issue has not been adequately investigated. At least one retrospective study shows that previous breast reduction did not impair the ability to breast-feed. Women should be informed about the current lack of knowledge surrounding these issues but presented with guidance for decision making.

"What if I become pregnant?" Some women may purposefully choose to breast-feed to avoid pregnancy, but this is not a dependable contraception method. Well-nourished women of the world tend to be more fertile and may find themselves pregnant and breast-feeding at the same time. Women who breast-feed must understand that the lack of a menstrual period during lactation *(lactational amenorrhea)* does not mean they cannot become pregnant. Contraceptives may be required if another pregnancy is not desired at that time. If pregnancy occurs, the woman should discuss appropriate infant feeding solutions with her healthcare team.

Advantages and Barriers to Breast-Feeding

These factors need to be reviewed with each individual mother in her particular situation. Only on this basis can she make the informed decision that is best for the baby and for herself.

There are many nutritional, physiologic, psychologic, and practical advantages to breast-feeding; six are identified as follows:

1. *Human milk changes* to meet changing nutrient and energy needs of both the newborn and the maturing infant during the first months of life. It is always there in the correct form to meet the growing infant's needs.
2. Infants experience *fewer infections* because the mother transfers certain antibodies and immune properties in human milk to her nursing infant. Also, there is no exposure of the infant to infectious organisms in the environment that can contaminate preparation and equipment for bottle-feeding, especially in poorer living situations.
3. *Fewer allergies and intolerances* occur, especially in allergy-prone infants, because cow's milk contains a number of potentially allergy-causing proteins that human milk does not have.
4. *Ease of digestion* is greater with breast milk because human milk forms a softer curd in the gastrointestinal tract that is easier for the infant to digest.

5. The *convenience and economy* of breast milk are greater because the mother is free from the time and expense involved in buying and preparing formula, and her breast milk is always ready and sterile.
6. Breast-feeding provides *psychologic bonding* because the mother and infant relate to one another during feeding, regular times of rest and enjoyment, cuddling and fulfillment.

Despite the advantages of breast-feeding, some women do have to deal with perceived barriers associated with misinformation, personal feelings of modesty, family pressures, or outside employment, among other factors. Addressing these barriers, such as the following, before delivery rather than after will increase the likelihood that the mother breast-feeds her infant:

- *Misinformation,* a major barrier, creates negative impressions and ideas. Women in today's world often lack positive role models in extended families or experienced friends with whom they can discuss their feelings and obtain much practical guidance. Experienced breast-feeding mothers or lactation consultants can fill this need, especially for young first-time mothers.
- *Personal modesty and anxiety,* or a fear of appearing immodest in breast exposure, may hinder some mothers from breast-feeding. Sensitive counseling, especially with a positive role model as described, can help to allay some of these personal fears. Most of women's breast-feeding is done in the privacy of the home rather than around others; therefore early support during initial experiences would be helpful.
- *Family pressures,* especially from the husband, not to breast-feed have strong influences on the mother, even though she may want to do so. Initial counseling and education about breast-feeding should include both parents whenever possible. Reasons for negative attitudes can be explored and misinformation clarified with sound education.
- *Outside employment,* with a limited maternity leave and job loss if the mother does not return to work at that time, can complicate the mother's decision, even though she may want to breast-feed her baby. However, if the mother does have the will, there are ways to do both. After breast-feeding is well established, she can regularly express milk by hand or with a breast pump into sterile disposable nursing bags to use with disposable holder, cap, and nipple ensemble. Rapid chilling and strict sanitation are required, but it can be planned, given the commitment. Some companies provide child care facilities for their employees, recognizing this modern need as good business. The mother can plan occasional formula feeds to fill in with the sustained breast-feeding.

All of these approaches to breast-feeding have real rewards for the infant. In addition, they can strengthen the mother's confidence in her maternal capabilities. The importance even of these intangible benefits should not be underestimated.

References

American Academy of Pediatrics Work Group on Breast-Feeding: Policy statement on breast-feeding, *Pediatrics* 100:1035, 1997.

Armotrading DC et al: Impact of WIC utilization rate on breast-feeding among international students at a large university, *J Am Diet Assoc* 92(3):352, 1992.

Cruz-Korchin N, Korchin L: Breast-feeding after vertical mammaplasty with medial pedicle, *Plast Reconstr Surg* 114(4):890, 2004.

Ghaemi-Ahmadi S: Attitudes toward breast-feeding among Iranian, Afghan, and Southeast Asian immigrant women in the United States: implications for health and nutrition education, *J Am Diet Assoc* 92(3):354, 1992.

TO PROBE FURTHER—cont'd

BREAST-FEEDING: THE DYNAMIC NATURE OF HUMAN MILK

Jernstrom H et al: Breast-feeding and the risk of breast cancer in BRCA1 and BRCA2 mutation carriers, *J Natl Cancer Inst* 96(14):1094, 2004.

Lewis CG et al: *Mycobacterium fortuitum* breast infection following nipple-piercing, mimicking carcinoma, *Breast J* 10(4):363, 2004.

Martin J: Is nipple piercing compatible with breastfeeding? *J Hum Lact* 20(3):319, 2004.

Pisacane A et al: Down syndrome and breastfeeding, *Acta Paediatr* 92(12):1479, 2003.

Position of the American Dietetic Association: Breaking the barriers to breastfeeding, *J Am Diet Assoc* 101(10):1213, 2001.

Position of the American Dietetic Association: Promotion of breast-feeding, *J Am Diet Assoc* 97(6):662, 1997.

Siskind V et al: Breastfeeding, menopause, and epithelial ovarian cancer, *Epidemiology* 8(2):188, 1997.

TO SUM UP

Pregnancy involves synergistic interactions among three distinct biologic entities: the fetus, the placenta, and the woman. Maternal needs reflect the increasing nutritional needs of the fetus and the placenta, as well as the need to meet maternal needs and to prepare for lactation. An optimal weight gain of about 11 kg (25 lb), or more as needed, is recommended during pregnancy to accommodate rapid growth. Even more significant than the actual weight gain is the quality of the diet.

Common problems occurring during pregnancy include nausea and vomiting, heartburn, and constipation. In most cases they are easily relieved without medication by simple, often temporary, changes in the diet. Serious problems with pregnancy may be associated with preexisting chronic maternal conditions, such as diabetes mellitus, or conditions arising as a result of the physical or metabolic demands of pregnancy, such as iron deficiency anemia and PIH. Unusual or erratic eating habits, age, parity, prepartum weight status, and low income are among the many related factors that also place the woman at risk for complications.

The American Dietetic Association strongly encourages public health and clinical efforts that promote breast-feeding to optimize the indisputable nutritional, immunologic, psychologic, and economic benefits. The ultimate goal of prenatal care is a healthy infant and a mother physically capable of breast-feeding her child, should she choose to do so. Human milk provides essential nutrients in quantities required for optimal infant growth and development. It also supplies immunologic factors that offer protection against infection. Lactation requires an increase in kcalories beyond the needs of pregnancy. Adequate fluid intake is guided by the mother's natural thirst.

QUESTIONS FOR REVIEW

1. List and discuss five factors that influence the nutritional needs of the woman during pregnancy. Which factors would place a woman in a high-risk category? Why?

2. List six nutrients that are required in larger amounts during pregnancy. Describe their special role during this period. Identify four food sources of each.

3. Identify two common problems associated with pregnancy, and describe the dietary management of each.

4. List and describe the screening indicators and risk factors for hypertension and diabetes mellitus during pregnancy.

5. List and discuss five major nutritional factors of lactation.

REFERENCES

1. Mathews TJ et al: Infant mortality statistics from the 2002 period: linked birth/infant death data set, *Natl Vital Stat Rep* 53(10):1, 2004.

2. Nahum GG et al: Accurate prediction of term birth weight from prospectively measurable maternal characteristics, *Prim Care Update Ob Gyns* 5(4):193, 1998.

3. Food and Nutrition Board Committee on Maternal Nutrition, National Research Council National Academy of Sciences: *Maternal nutrition and the course of human pregnancy*, Washington, DC, 1970, National Academies Press.

4. American College of Obstetricians and Gynecologists, Committee on Nutrition: *Nutrition in maternal health care*, Chicago, 1974, Author.

5. American College of Obstetrics and Gynecology and American Dietetic Association Task Force on Nutrition: *Assessment of maternal nutrition*, Chicago, 1978, Authors.

6. Food and Nutrition Board, Institute of Medicine: *Dietary Reference Intakes for calcium, phosphorus, magnesium, vitamin D, and fluoride*, Washington, DC, 1997, National Academies Press.

7. Food and Nutrition Board, Institute of Medicine: *Dietary Reference Intakes for thiamin, riboflavin, niacin, vitamin B_6, folate, vitamin B_{12}, pantothenic acid, biotin, and choline*, Washington, DC, 1998, National Academies Press.

8. Food and Nutrition Board, Institute of Medicine: *Dietary Reference Intakes for vitamin C, vitamin E, selenium, and carotenoids*, Washington, DC, 2000, National Academies Press.

9. Food and Nutrition Board, Institute of Medicine: *Dietary Reference Intakes for vitamin A, vitamin K, arsenic, boron, chromium, copper, iodine, iron, manganese, molybdenum, nickel, silicon, vanadium, and zinc*, Washington, DC, 2000, National Academies Press.

10. Food and Nutrition Board, Institute of Medicine: *Dietary Reference Intakes for energy, carbohydrate, fiber, fat, fatty acids, cholesterol, protein, and amino acids (macronutrients)*, Washington, DC, 2005, National Academies Press.

11. Barker DJ: Fetal origins of coronary heart disease, *BMJ* 311(6998):171, 1995.
12. Barker DJ: In utero programming of cardiovascular disease, *Theriogenology* 53(2):555, 2000.
13. Hindmarsh PC et al: Intrauterine growth and its relationship to size and shape at birth, *Pediatr Res* 52(2):263, 2002.
14. Rasmussen KM: The "fetal origins" hypothesis: challenges and opportunities for maternal and child nutrition, *Annu Rev Nutr* 21:73, 2001.
15. Nutrition-Cognition National Advisory Committee: *Statement on the link between nutrition and cognitive development in children,* Medford, Mass, 1998, Center on Hunger, Poverty, and Nutrition Policy, Tufts University.
16. U.S. Department of Health and Human Services: *Healthy people 2010: understanding and improving health,* ed 2, Washington, DC, 2000, U.S. Government Printing Office.
17. De Ver Dye T et al: Recent studies in the epidemiologic assessment of physical activity, fetal growth, and preterm delivery: a narrative review, *Clin Obstet Gynecol* 46(2):415, 2003.
18. Committee on Obstetric Practice: ACOG committee opinion: exercise during pregnancy and the postpartum period, *Int J Gynaecol Obstet* 77(1):79, 2002.
19. Food and Nutrition Board, Institute of Medicine: *Dietary Reference Intakes: applications in dietary assessment,* Washington, DC, 2000, National Academies Press.
20. Al MDM et al: Long-chain polyunsaturated fatty acids, pregnancy, and pregnancy outcome, *Am J Clin Nutr* 71(suppl 1):285S, 2000.
21. Uauy R, Hoffman DR: Essential fat requirements of preterm infants, *Am J Clin Nutr* 71(suppl 1):245S, 2000.
22. Reynolds RD: Perinatal vitamin B_6 deficiency and poverty: is there a link? *Nutr Today* 35(6):222, 2000.
23. Centers for Disease Control and Prevention: Use of vitamins containing folic acid among women of childbearing age: United States, 2004, *MMWR Morb Mortal Wkly Rep* 53(36):847, 2004.
24. Mills JL: Fortification of foods with folic acid: how much is enough? *N Engl J Med* 342(19):1442, 2000.
25. Kloeblen AS: Folate knowledge, intake from fortified grain products, and periconceptional supplementation patterns of a sample of low-income pregnant women according to the Health Belief Model, *J Am Diet Assoc* 99(1):33, 1999.
26. Mackey AD, Picciano MF: Maternal folate status during extended lactation and the effect of supplemental folic acid, *Am J Clin Nutr* 69(2):285, 1999.
27. O'Hagan K: *Cultural competence in the caring professions,* London, 2001, Jessica Kingsley Publishers.
28. Hogan-Garcia M: *Four skills of cultural diversity competence: a process for understanding and practice,* Belmont, Calif, 1999, Brooks/Cole.
29. Bronner Y: Cultural sensitivity and nutrition counseling, *Top Clin Nutr* 9(2):13, 1994.
30. Blumenthal M et al: *Herbal medicine: expanded commission E monographs,* Boston, 2000, Integrative Medicine Communications.
31. Foster S, Tyler VE: *Tyler's honest herbal,* ed 8, Binghamton, NY, 1999, The Haworth Herbal Press, Inc.
32. *Physician's desk reference (PDR) for herbal medicine,* ed 2, Montvale, NJ, 2000, Medical Economics Co.
33. Food and Nutrition Board, Institute of Medicine: *Nutrition during pregnancy,* Washington, DC, 1990, National Academies Press.
34. Luke B, Leurgans S: Maternal weight gains in ideal twin outcomes, *J Am Diet Assoc* 96(2):178, 1996.
35. Strauss RS, Dietz WH: Low maternal weight gain in the second or third trimester increases the risk for intrauterine growth retardation, *J Nutr* 129(5):988, 1999.
36. Butte NF et al: Adjustments in energy expenditure and substrate utilization during late pregnancy and lactation, *Am J Clin Nutr* 69(2):299, 1999.
37. Food and Nutrition Board, Institute of Medicine: *Dietary Reference Intakes for water, potassium, sodium, chloride, and sulfate,* Washington, DC, 2004, National Academies Press.
38. Ikonomidou C et al: Ethanol-induced apoptotic neurodegeneration and fetal alcohol syndrome, *Science* 287(5455):1056, 2000.
39. Barinaga M: Neurobiology: a new clue to how alcohol damages brains, *Science* 287(5455):947, 2000.
40. Kirchengast S, Hartmann B: Nicotine consumption before and during pregnancy affects not only newborn size but also birth modus, *J Biosoc Sci* 35(2):175, 2003.
41. Ness RB et al: Cocaine and tobacco use and the risk of spontaneous abortion. *N Engl J Med* 304(5):333, 1999.
42. Eskenazi B: Caffeine: filtering the facts, *N Engl J Med* 341(22):1688, 1999.
43. Danish Epidemiology Science Centre at the Institute of Preventive Medicine: Does caffeine and alcohol intake before pregnancy predict the occurrence of spontaneous abortion? *Hum Reprod* 18(12):2704, 2003.
44. Signorello LB, McLaughlin JK: Maternal caffeine consumption and spontaneous abortion: a review of the epidemiologic evidence, *Epidemiology* 15(2):229, 2004.
45. Position of the American Dietetic Association: Nutrition and lifestyle for a healthy pregnancy outcome, *J Am Diet Assoc* 102(10):1479, 2002.
46. Lopez LB et al: Pica during pregnancy: a frequently underestimated problem, *Arch Latinoam Nutr* 54(1):17, 2004.
47. Rainville AJ: Pica practices of pregnant women are associated with lower maternal hemoglobin level at delivery, *J Am Diet Assoc* 98(3):293, 1998.
48. Boyle JS, Mackey MC: Pica: sorting it out, *J Transcult Nurs* 10(1):65, 1999.
49. American Diabetes Association: Gestational diabetes mellitus, *Diabetes Care* 9(4):430, 1986.
50. Langer O et al: A comparison of glyburide and insulin in women with gestational diabetes mellitus, *N Engl J Med* 343(16):1134, 2000.
51. Slocum J et al: Preconception to postpartum: management of pregnancy complicated by diabetes, *Diabetes Educ* 30(5):740, 2004.
52. Alberico S et al: Gestational diabetes: universal or selective screening? *J Matern Fetal Neonatal Med* 16(6):331, 2004.
53. Gabbe SG, Graves CR: Management of diabetes mellitus complicating pregnancy, *Obstet Gynecol* 102(4):857, 2003.
54. Mensing C et al: National standards for diabetes self-management education, *Diabetes Care* 28(1, suppl):S72, 2005.
55. Wunderlich SM: Nutritional assessment and support of HIV-positive pregnant women and their children: perspective from an industrialized country, *Nutr Today* 35(3):107, 2000.
56. Taren DL: The infant feeding and HIV transmission controversy impacts public health services, *Nutr Today* 35(3):103, 2000.
57. James D: Eating disorders, fertility, and pregnancy: relationships and complications, *J Perinatal Neonatal Nurs* 15(2):36, 2001.
58. Morrill ES, Nickols-Richardson SM: Bulimia nervosa during pregnancy: a review, *J Am Diet Assoc* 101(4):448, 2001.
59. Position of the American Dietetic Association: nutrition intervention in the treatment of anorexia nervosa, bulimia nervosa, and eating disorders not otherwise specified (EDNOS), *J Am Diet Assoc* 101(7):810, 2001.

60. Li R et al: Breastfeeding rates in the United States by characteristics of the child, mother, or family: the 2002 national immunization survey, *Pediatrics* 115(1):E31, 2005.

61. Ryan AS: The resurgence of breastfeeding in the United States, *Pediatrics* 99(4):E12, 1997.

62. World Health Organization: WHO advises: ten steps to successful breast-feeding, *World Health* 2:28, 1997.

63. Schanler RJ et al: Pediatricians' practices and attitudes regarding breastfeeding promotion, *Pediatrics* 103(3):E35, 1999.

64. Lawrence RA, Lawrence RM: *Breastfeeding: a guide for the medical profession,* St Louis, 1998, Mosby.

65. Emmett PM, Rogers IS: Properties of human milk and their relationship with maternal nutrition, *Early Hum Dev* 49(suppl 1):S7, 1997.

66. Chezem J, Friesen C: Attendance at breast-feeding support meetings: relationship to demographic characteristics and duration of lactation in women planning postpartum employment, *J Am Diet Assoc* 99(1):83, 1999.

67. Wright AL et al: Increasing breast-feeding rates to reduce infant illness at the community level, *Pediatrics* 101(5):837, 1998.

68. Carmichael SL et al: Breast-feeding practices among WIC participants in Hawaii, *J Am Diet Assoc* 101(1):57, 2001.

69. Chapman DJ et al: Effectiveness of breastfeeding peer counseling in a low-income, predominantly Latina population: a randomized controlled trial, *Arch Pediatr Adolesc Med* 158(9):897, 2004.

70. Philipp BL, Merewood A: The baby-friendly way: the best breast-feeding start, *Pediatr Clin North Am* 51(3):761, 2004.

71. Misra R, James DCS: Breast-feeding practices among adolescent and adult mothers in the Missouri WIC population, *J Am Diet Assoc* 100(9):1071, 2000.

72. Pobocik RS et al: Effect of a breastfeeding education and support program on breastfeeding initiation and duration in a culturally diverse group of adolescents, *J Nutr Educ* 32(3):139, 2000.

73. Schmidt MM, Sigman-Grant M: Perspectives of low-income fathers' support of breastfeeding: an exploratory study, *J Nutr Educ* 32(1):31, 2000.

74. Sharma M, Petosa R: Impact of expectant fathers in breast-feeding decisions, *J Am Diet Assoc* 97(11):1311, 1997.

75. Kannan S et al: Cultural influences on infant feeding beliefs of mothers, *J Am Diet Assoc* 99(1):88, 1999.

76. Kramer MS, Kakuma R: Optimal duration of exclusive breast-feeding, *Cochrane Database Syst Rev,* 2002.

77. Murtaugh M: Optimal breast-feeding duration, *J Am Diet Assoc* 97(11):1252, 1997.

78. American Academy of Pediatrics: Breastfeeding and the use of human milk. American Academy of Pediatrics, work group on breastfeeding, *Breastfeed Rev* 6(1):31, 1998.

79. Position of the American Dietetic Association: Breaking the barriers to breastfeeding, *J Am Diet Assoc* 101(10):1213, 2001.

80. Lederman SA: Influence of lactation on body weight regulation, *Nutr Rev* 62(7, part 2):S112, 2004.

81. Dewey KG: Effects of maternal caloric restriction and exercise during lactation, *J Nutr* 128(suppl 2):386S, 1998.

82. Lovelady CA et al: The effect of weight loss in overweight, lactating women on the growth of their infants, *N Engl J Med* 342(7):449, 2000.

83. Butte NF: Dieting and exercise in overweight, lactating women, *N Engl J Med* 342(7):502, 2000.

84. Picciano MF: Pregnancy and lactation: physiological adjustments, nutritional requirements and the role of dietary supplements, *J Nutr* 133(suppl 1):1997S, 2003.

85. Weiss R et al: Severe vitamin B_{12} deficiency in an infant associated with a maternal deficiency and a strict vegetarian diet, *J Pediatr Hematol Oncol* 26(4):270, 2004.

86. Brockington I: Postpartum psychiatric disorders, *Lancet* 363(9405):303, 2004.

87. Falceto OG et al: Influence of parental mental health on early termination of breast-feeding: a case-control study, *J Am Board Fam Pract* 17(3):173, 2004.

FURTHER READINGS AND RESOURCES

Readings

Office of Nutrition Policy and Promotion: Nutrition for a healthy pregnancy: National guidelines for the childbearing years, Ottawa, Ontario, Canada, 1999, Health Canada. Retrieved November 28, 2005, from www.hc-sc.gc.ca/fn-an/nutrition/prenatal/national_guidelines_cp-lignes_directrices_nationales_pc_e.html.
This excellent resource provides helpful guidance for healthy pregnancies, as well as important information for identifying women at nutritional risk.

Rasmussen KM: The "fetal origins" hypothesis: challenges and opportunities for maternal and child nutrition, *Annu Rev Nutr* 21:73, 2001.
Does chronic disease begin in utero? A critical evaluation of epidemiologic and experimental evidence to support and refute this hypothesis is provided. Implications and limitations are addressed.

Vozenilek GP: What they don't know could hurt them: increasing public awareness of folic acid and neural tube defects, *J Am Diet Assoc* 99(1):20, 1999.
This informative article draws a clear picture of the cloud of ignorance that still hangs over the general population about the devastating results of neural tube defects in an affected child from birth because of the mother's folic acid deficiency early in pregnancy.

Websites of Interest

- U.S. Department of Health and Human Services, Office of Disease Prevention and Health Promotion: *Healthy People 2010:* www.healthypeople.gov.
- U.S. Department of Health and Human Services, National Institutes of Health, National Center for Complementary and Alternative Medicine: http://nccam.nih.gov.
- U.S. Department of Health and Human Services, Food and Drug Administration, Center for Food Safety and Applied Nutrition: www.cfsan.fda.gov.
- March of Dimes Birth Defects Foundation: www.marchofdimes.com.
- Virginia Department of Health, Office of Family Health Services, BabyCare: www.vahealth.org/babycare.
- California Department of Health Services, BabyCal: www.dhs.ca.gov/babycal/default.htm.

CHAPTER 12

Nutrition for Normal Growth and Development

Sharon M. Nickols-Richardson

In this second chapter in our life cycle series, we look at growing infants, children, and adolescents. We consider their physical growth and their inseparable psychosocial development at each progressive stage. This unified growth and development nurture the integrated progression of the child into the adult.

Within this dual framework of physical and psychosocial development, we consider food and feeding and their vital roles in the development of the whole child. In each age-group we relate nutritional needs and the food that supplies them to the normal physical maturation and psychosocial development achieved in each stage.

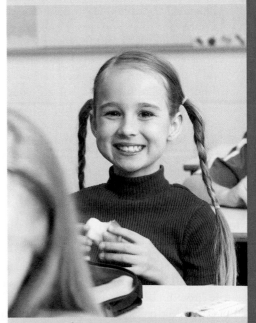

HUMAN GROWTH AND DEVELOPMENT

Individual Needs of Children

Growth may be defined as an increase in body size. Biologic growth of an organism occurs through cell multiplication (*hyperplasia*) and cell enlargement (*hypertrophy*). *Development* is the associated process by which growing tissues and organs take on a more complex function. Both of these processes are part of one whole, forming a unified and inseparable sequence of growth and development. Through these changes a small dependent newborn is transformed into a fully functioning independent adult. However, each child is a unique entity with individual needs. This is a paramount principle in working with children. Thus we must always seek to discover these individual human needs if we are to help each child reach his or her greatest growth and development potential.[1]

Normal Life Cycle Growth Pattern

The normal human life cycle includes the following four general stages of overall growth and development: (1) infancy, (2) childhood, (3) adolescence, and (4) adulthood:

1. *Infancy:* Growth velocity is rapid during the first year of life, with the rate tapering off in the latter half of the year. At 6 months of age an infant has typically doubled its birth weight, and at 1 year he or she will likely have tripled it.
2. *Childhood:* During the latent period of childhood after infancy and before adolescence, the growth rate slows and becomes erratic. During some periods there are plateaus. At other times, small spurts of growth occur. This overall growth deceleration affects appetite accordingly. At times, children will have little or no appetite; at other times, they will eat voraciously. Parents who know that this is a normal pattern can relax and avoid making eating a battleground with their children.
3. *Adolescence:* With the beginning of puberty, the second period of growth acceleration occurs. Because of hormonal influences involved, enormous physical changes take place, including growth and maturation of long bones, development of the sex characteristics, and gains in fat and muscle mass.
4. *Adulthood:* In the final stage of a normal life cycle, growth levels off on the adult plateau. Then it gradually declines during old age—the period of senescence.

Measuring Childhood Physical Growth

Growth Charts

Children grow at widely varying individual rates. In clinical practice a child's pattern of growth is compared with percentile growth curves derived from measurements of large numbers of children throughout the growth years. Contemporary growth chart grids, developed by the National Center for Health Statistics (NCHS), were recently revised to reflect the growth patterns of both breast-fed and formula-fed infants and to provide a broad baseline for evaluating growth patterns in children today.[2] These charts are based on data from nationally representative samples of children that include various racial and ethnic groups (see the *Further Readings and Resources* section at the end of this chapter). Two age intervals are presented: birth to 3 years and 2 to 20 years, with separate curves for boys and girls. A variety of grids are available to monitor growth based on weight and age, length (or stature) and age, weight-for-length (or body mass index [BMI]), and head circumference and age (see Appendix C, CDC Growth Charts: United States). Directions for use of these growth charts for infants and children with special growth patterns are also available.

Anthropometry

Practitioners use anthropometry to monitor a child's growth, with growth charts and other clinical standards as points of reference. A number of methods and measures may be used, as follows:

- *Body weight and height:* These are common general measures of physical growth. They provide a basic measure of change in body size but give only a crude index of growth without the finer details of individual variations in body fat or muscle or bone. They are used mainly to monitor patterns of growth over time, as the individual child's pattern is plotted on the growth chart for a given age. The recumbent length of infants and small children is measured initially, and then standing height (stature) is measured as they grow older.
- *Body circumferences and skinfolds:* The head circumference is a valuable measure in infants, but it is seldom measured routinely after 3 years of age. Circumference measures of abdomen, chest, and leg at its maximal girth of the calf are usually included at periodic intervals. Other measures for monitoring muscle mass growth and body composition include the midarm circumference and the triceps skinfold taken at the same point. Using these two measures, the midarm muscle circumference can be calculated easily (see Chapter 16). Skinfold measures, taken at a number of body sites, are performed with special calipers and require skill and practice for accuracy. Longitudinal growth studies in research centers use many measures of development in addition to these basic ones to monitor growth in general practice. Because national statistics inform us of the growing prevalence of fatness among children of all ages,[3] the use of skinfold thicknesses or other measures to monitor the relative increase in muscle versus fat should be incorporated into regular physical examinations.

Clinical Signs

Various clinical signs of optimal growth can be observed as indicators of a child's nutrition status. These include such indicators as general vitality; sense of well-being; good posture; healthy gums, teeth, skin, hair, and eyes; appropriate muscle development; and nervous control. (See Table 1-1 for a review of these general signs and observations.)

Laboratory Tests

Other measures of growth can be obtained with various laboratory tests, including studies of blood and urine to determine levels of hemoglobin, vitamins, and similar substances (see Appendix F, Normal Constituents of Blood and Urine in Adults). Radiographs of the hand and wrist are useful for assessment of skeletal development.

Nutritional Analysis

A nutritional analysis of general eating habits (see Chapter 10) provides helpful information for assessing the adequacy of the diet for meeting growth needs. A diet history form (see Figure 10-2) and food value tables (see the nutrient analysis program on the CD-ROM that accompanied your textbook) may be used. In clinical practice, diet evaluations and nutrient intake calculations are usually completed using computer analysis. The dietitian evaluates information obtained from a variety of methods to complete a food and nutrient intake analysis to use in diet counseling with the parent(s) and child.

Motor, Mental, and Psychosocial Development

Motor Growth and Development

Gross motor skills, such as sitting, standing, walking, and running, develop within the first 18 months of life. Fine motor skills gradually develop over a longer period of time. Such control over and coordination of voluntary muscle develops in conjunction with mental, emotional, social, and cultural growth as the child interacts and reacts to sensory stimulants in the environment. Motor skills greatly influence feeding skills and energy needs of the child.

Mental Growth and Development

Measures of mental growth usually involve abilities in speech and other forms of communication, as well as the ability to handle abstract and symbolic material in thinking. Young children think in very literal terms. As they develop in mental capacity, they can handle more than single ideas, and they can form constructive concepts.

Emotional Growth and Development

Emotional growth is measured in the capacity for love and affection, as well as the ability to handle frustration and anxieties. It also involves the child's ability to control aggressive impulses and to channel hostility from destructive to constructive activities.

Social and Cultural Growth and Development

The social development of a child is measured as the ability to relate to others and to participate in group living and cultural activities. These social and cultural behaviors are first learned through relationships with parent(s) and family, and these relationships greatly influence food habits and feeding patterns. As the child's horizon broadens, relationships are developed with those outside the family, with friends, and with others in the community at school or at religious or other social gatherings. For this reason, a child's play during the early years is a highly purposeful activity.

NUTRITIONAL REQUIREMENTS FOR GROWTH

Energy Needs

During childhood, the demand for kilocalories (kcalories or kcal) is relatively great. However, there is much variation in need with age and condition. For example, the total daily energy intake of a 5-year-old child is spent in the following way:

- Approximately 50% supplies basal metabolic requirements (BMR).
- Approximately 5% is used in the thermic effect of food (TEF).
- Approximately 25% goes toward daily physical activity.
- Approximately 12% is needed for tissue growth.
- Approximately 8% is lost in the feces.

Protein Needs

Protein provides amino acids, the essential building materials for tissue growth. As a child grows, the protein requirements per unit of body weight gradually decrease. For

> growth velocity Rapidity of motion or movement; rate of childhood growth over normal periods of development compared with a population standard.
> growth deceleration Period of decreased speed of growth at different points of childhood development.
> growth acceleration Period of increased speed of growth at different points of childhood development.
> percentile One of 100 equal parts of measured series of values; rate or proportion per hundred.
> growth chart grids Grids comparing stature (length), weight, and age of children by percentile; used for nutritional assessment to determine how their growth is progressing. The most commonly used grids are those of the National Center for Health Statistics (NCHS).
> anthropometry The science of measuring the size, weight, and proportions of the human body.
> body composition The relative sizes of the four basic body compartments that make up the total body: lean body mass (muscle and vital organs), fat, water, and bone.

example, during the first 6 months of life an infant requires 1.52 g of protein/kg/day.[4] This amount gradually decreases throughout childhood until adulthood, when protein needs are only about 0.8 g/kg/day.[4] Usually, the healthy, active, growing child will consume the necessary amounts of kcalories and protein if a variety of food is provided.

Essential Fatty Acid Needs

Fat kcalories are important as backup energy sources but are particularly needed to supply the essential fatty acids—linoleic and alpha-linolenic acids. Linoleic acid is required for the synthesis of brain and nerve tissue and normal mental development. However, an excess of fat, especially from animal sources, should be avoided.[4]

Carbohydrate Needs

Carbohydrates are the primary energy source and are important in sparing protein for its vital role in tissue formation. Most importantly, carbohydrates provide glucose for essential brain function.[4]

Fiber

Many complex-carbohydrate foods also provide dietary fiber. Fiber is important to satiety and bowel regulation and affects blood lipid and glucose concentrations as well as the vascular system. Fiber may also provide protection against some types of cancer and overweight.[4]

Water Requirements

The infant's relative need for water is greater than that of the adult. The infant's body content of water is approximately 70% to 75% of total body weight, whereas in the adult, water contributes only 60% to 65% of total body weight. Also, a large amount of the infant's total body water is outside of cells and more easily lost. Thus, prolonged water loss because of diarrhea, as occurs among infants in developing countries given formula prepared from contaminated water, is a serious threat to life and requires immediate oral hydration therapy.[5] The child's water need is related to energy intake and urine concentration. Generally, an infant drinks a daily amount of water equivalent to 10% to 15% of body weight, whereas the adult's daily water intake equals 2% to 4% of body weight. A summary of approximate daily fluid needs during the growth years is given in Table 12-1.[6]

Mineral and Vitamin Needs

Minerals and vitamins play essential roles in tissue growth and maintenance and in overall energy metabolism. Positive childhood growth and development depend on an adequate amount of these essential substances. For example, rapidly growing young bones require calcium and phosphorus. A

TABLE 12-1	Approximate Daily Fluid Needs During Growth Years
Age	**ml/kg**
0-3 months	120
3-6 months	117
6-12 months	89
1-3 years	108
4-8 years	85
9-13 years	67 (boys)
	57 (girls)
14-18 years	54 (boys)
	43 (girls)

From Food and Nutrition Board, Institute of Medicine: *Dietary References Intakes for water, potassium, sodium, chloride, and sulfate,* Washington, DC, 2004, National Academies Press.

radiograph of a newborn's body would reveal a skeleton appearing as a collection of disconnected, separate bones requiring mineralization. Calcium is also needed for tooth development, muscle contraction, nerve excitation, blood coagulation, and heart muscle action. Another mineral of concern is iron, essential for hemoglobin formation and mental and psychomotor development.[7,8] The infant's fetal iron stores are depleted in 4 to 6 months after birth. Thus solid food additions at that time help supply needed iron. Such foods as iron-fortified cereals, and later meat, accomplish this. The use of iron-fortified formulas and other foods by high-risk children enrolled in the Special Supplemental Nutrition Program for Women, Infants, and Children (WIC) assists in reducing the incidence of iron deficiency anemia among infants and young children from limited-resource families, including the homeless.[9]

Excess amounts of particular micronutrients are also of concern in feeding children. Excess intake is usually the result of inappropriate use of vitamin or mineral supplements and may occur because of misunderstanding, illiteracy, or carelessness. When supplements are indicated because of a specific and defined medical or nutrition condition, parents must be carefully instructed to use only the amount directed and no more. The following two nutrients pose particular hazards when consumed in excessive amounts:

1. *Vitamin A:* Symptoms of toxicity from excess vitamin A include lack of appetite, slow growth, drying and cracking of the skin, enlargement of the liver and spleen, swelling and pain in the long bones, and bone fragility.
2. *Vitamin D:* Symptoms of toxicity from excess vitamin D include nausea, diarrhea, weight loss, excess urination (especially at night), and eventual calcification of soft tissues, including the renal tubules, blood vessels, bronchi, stomach, and heart.

Summaries of the Dietary Reference Intakes (DRIs) for overall nutritional needs and growth, developed by the Food and Nutrition Board of the Institute of Medicine, are provided in Tables 12-2, 12-3, and 12-4.

TABLE 12-2	Dietary Reference Intakes for Energy and Protein

| | Age | Weight | | Height | | Energy* (kcalories) | Protein (g) |
		kg	lb	cm	in		
Infants	0-0.5	6	13	62	24	438-645	9.1
	0.5-1	9	20	71	28	608-844	13.5
Children	1-3	12	27	86	34	768-1683	13
	4-8	20	44	115	45	1133-2225	19
Males	9-13	36	79	144	57	1530-3038	34
	14-18	61	134	174	68	2090-3804	52
Females	9-13	37	81	144	57	1415-2762	34
	14-18	54	119	163	64	1718-2858	46

From Food and Nutrition Board, Institute of Medicine: *Dietary Reference Intakes for energy, carbohydrate, fiber, fat, fatty acids, cholesterol, protein, and amino acids (macronutrients),* Washington, DC, 2002, National Academies Press.
   *Varies according to sex, body size, age, and level of physical activity.

TABLE 12-3	Dietary Reference Intakes for Vitamins

Age (yr)	Vitamin A (µg RAE)	Vitamin D (µg)	Vitamin E (mg TE)	Vitamin K (µg)	Vitamin C (mg)	Thiamin (mg)	Riboflavin (mg)	Niacin (mg NE)	Vitamin B_6 (mg)	Folate (µg)	Vitamin B_{12} (µg)
Infants 0-0.5	400	5	4	2	40	0.2	0.3	2	0.1	65	0.4
Infants 0.6-1.0	500	5	5	2.5	50	0.3	0.4	4	0.3	80	0.5
Children 1-3	300	5	6	30	15	0.5	0.5	6	0.5	150	0.9
Children 4-8	400	5	7	55	25	0.6	0.6	8	0.6	200	1.2
Boys 9-13	600	5	11	60	45	0.9	0.9	12	1	300	1.8
Boys 14-18	900	5	15	75	75	1.2	1.3	16	1.3	400	2.4
Girls 9-13	600	5	11	60	45	0.9	0.9	12	1	300	1.8
Girls 14-18	700	5	15	75	65	1.0	1.0	14	1.2	400	2.4

From Food and Nutrition Board, Institute of Medicine: *Dietary Reference Intakes for calcium, phosphorus, magnesium, vitamin D, and fluoride,* Washington, DC, 1997, National Academies Press; Food and Nutrition Board, Institute of Medicine: *Dietary Reference Intakes for thiamin, riboflavin, niacin, vitamin B_6, folate, vitamin B_{12}, pantothenic acid, biotin, and choline,* Washington, DC, 1998, National Academies Press; Food and Nutrition Board, Institute of Medicine: *Dietary Reference Intakes for vitamin C, vitamin E, selenium, and carotenoids,* Washington, DC, 2000, National Academies Press; Food and Nutrition Board, Institute of Medicine: *Dietary Reference Intakes for vitamin A, vitamin K, arsenic, boron, chromium, copper, iodine, iron, manganese, molybdenum, nickel, silicon, vanadium, and zinc,* Washington, DC, 2001, National Academies Press.
   RAE, Retinal activity equivalents; *TE,* tocopherol equivalents; *NE,* niacin equivalents.

TABLE 12-4	Dietary Reference Intakes for Minerals

Age (yr)	Calcium (mg)	Phosphorus (mg)	Magnesium (mg)	Iron (mg)	Zinc (mg)	Iodine (µg)	Selenium (µg)	Fluoride (mg)
Infants 0-0.5	210	100	30	0.27	2	110	5	0.01
Infants 0.6-1.0	270	275	75	11	3	130	20	0.5
Children 1-3	500	460	80	7	3	90	20	0.7
Children 4-8	800	500	130	10	5	90	30	1
Boys 9-13	1300	1250	240	8	8	120	40	2
Boys 14-18	1300	1250	410	11	11	150	55	3
Girls 9-13	1300	1250	240	8	8	120	40	2
Girls 14-18	1300	1250	360	15	9	150	55	3

From Food and Nutrition Board, Institute of Medicine: *Dietary Reference Intakes for calcium, phosphorus, magnesium, vitamin D, and fluoride,* Washington, DC, 1997, National Academies Press; Food and Nutrition Board, Institute of Medicine: *Dietary Reference Intakes for vitamin C, vitamin E, selenium, and carotenoids,* Washington, DC, 2000, National Academies Press; Food and Nutrition Board, Institute of Medicine: *Dietary Reference Intakes for vitamin A, vitamin K, arsenic, boron, chromium, copper, iodine, iron, manganese, molybdenum, nickel, silicon, vanadium, and zinc,* Washington, DC, 2001, National Academies Press.

STAGES OF GROWTH AND DEVELOPMENT: AGE-GROUP NEEDS

The Stages of Human Life

Throughout the human life cycle, food and feeding not only supply nutrients for physical and motor growth but also play a role in personal and psychosocial development. The nutritional age-group needs of children cannot be understood apart from the child's overall maturation as a unique person. A leading American psychoanalyst, Erik Erikson,[10] has contributed to our understanding of human personality and growth throughout critical periods of development. His theory of human development has come to play a significant role in our view of the human life cycle.

Psychosocial Development

Erikson identified eight stages in human growth and a basic psychosocial developmental problem with which the individual struggles at each stage.[10] The developmental problem at each stage has a positive ego value and a conflicting negative counterpart, as follows:

1. *Infancy:* trust versus distrust
2. *Toddler:* autonomy versus shame and doubt
3. *Preschooler:* initiative versus guilt
4. *School-age child:* industry versus inferiority
5. *Adolescent:* identity versus role confusion
6. *Young adult:* intimacy versus isolation
7. *Adult:* generativity versus stagnation
8. *Older adult:* ego integrity versus despair

Given favorable circumstances, a growing child develops positive ego strength at each life stage and builds increasing inner resources and strengths to meet the next life crisis. The struggle at any age, however, is not forever won at this point. A residue of the negative remains, and in periods of stress, such as an illness, some regression is likely to occur. But as the child gains mastery at each stage of development, assisted by significant positive and supportive relationships, integration of self-controls takes place. Changes occurring at each stage influence both food intake and the interaction of the child with family members, peers, and counselors, as follows[11]:

- *Infant:* Infants require appropriate stimulation to thrive; they enjoy seeing different colors, engaging in verbal interactions, and being physically held. Activities such as holding objects, looking at pictures, or hearing nursery rhymes support motor and cognitive development. The attention span is short, which can create problems at feeding time.
- *Toddler:* Toddlers grow rapidly and begin to demonstrate autonomy with display of temper tantrums or other negative behaviors. They begin to develop language skills and can recall past experiences. Play is

an important medium for self-expression and allows the child to express some control over his or her environment.
- *Preschooler:* The preschool years are a time for increasing social experiences, and children begin to interact more with other children. Preschoolers have an increased ability to express themselves and may try to exert control through demands for or refusal of certain foods.
- *School-age child:* The school-age child enters a formal learning environment, and attention span increases. At this age, children are more selective in choosing friends, and the influence of peers becomes more obvious. As the environment becomes more structured, physical activity may decline, despite the need for play and further coordination of motor skills.
- *Adolescent:* Adolescents become more autonomous in their actions and attempt to exert independence from parental control. Teens perceive themselves to be invulnerable to illness or injury, and risk-taking behaviors involving drugs or alcohol may begin. Obsession with body image may result in inappropriate nutrition practices.

Various related developmental tasks surround each of these stages. These learnings, when accomplished, contribute to successful resolution of the core problem.

Physical Growth

The developmental tasks of choosing and consuming food do not develop in a vacuum. They flow as an integral part of physical, motor, and psychosocial development. In this section we discuss food and feeding practices at each of the stages of childhood and their relationship to normal physical and psychosocial maturation. Developing neuromuscular motor skills enable the child to accomplish related physical activities involved with food. Psychosocial development influences food attitudes, behavior, patterns, and habits.

Infant (Birth to 1 Year)

Physical Characteristics of a Full-Term Infant

The full-term infant is born after successful growth and development during a normal gestation period of about 40 weeks (280 days). During the first year of life the infant generally triples in weight, growing rapidly from an average birth weight of about 3.5 kg (7.5 lb) to a 1-year-old child ready to walk and weighing about 10 kg (22 lb). Thus energy requirements during this first year of tremendous growth are high.

Full-term infants have the ability to digest and absorb protein, a moderate amount of fat, and simple carbohydrates. They have some difficulty with starch because amylase, the starch-splitting enzyme, is not being produced at birth. However, as starch is introduced, this enzyme begins to function. The renal system functions well in infancy, but more water relative to body size is needed than in the adult to manage the renal solute load in urinary excretion. The first baby teeth do not erupt until about the fourth month; therefore food must initially be liquid and later semiliquid.

Nutrition for the Full-Term Infant

The first food for infants, breast milk or infant formula, generally provides all the nutrients required by a healthy infant for the first 6 months of life. Exclusive breast-feeding can, in fact, be adequate for the first 12 months of life; however, most mothers choose to supplement their infants' diets with complementary foods around the sixth month.[12] Nearly all infants born in a hospital receive an injection of vitamin K shortly after birth to ensure an adequate level of this nutrient, and it is important that infants born at home also receive supplemental vitamin K. It may be necessary to provide vitamin D supplements to breast-fed infants, because breast milk may not supply adequate vitamin D to prevent deficiency and the development of rickets. This is especially critical in the case of black mothers, who are less able to initiate the synthesis of vitamin D in their skin, or for mothers who wear special clothing for religious reasons that limits their skin exposure to the sun (see the *Focus on Culture* box, "Nutritional Rickets: Role of Culture").[13] Fomon, a noted pediatrician specializing in infant nutrition, recommends that breast-fed infants who receive no feedings of iron-fortified formula be supplemented with iron to the level of 5 mg/day, to make up for the limited amount of iron in breast milk.[14] It has been suggested that fluoride supplements be provided for breast-fed infants or formula-fed infants above 6 months of age in geographic regions where the water is low in fluoride, but not all nutritionists agree on this matter.[5,15] It is important that breast-feeding mothers be well nourished to supply optimal levels of nutrients in their milk.

Infants have limited nutritional stores from gestation, and this is especially true for iron. By the age of 6 months, semisolid foods such as iron-fortified cereals may be added to the diet to help meet increasing nutritional needs.

Psychosocial and Motor Development

The core psychosocial developmental task during infancy is the establishment of trust in others. Much of the infant's early psychosocial development is tactile in nature from touching and holding, especially with feeding. Feeding is the infant's primary means of establishing human relationships. The close mother-infant or caregiver-infant bonding in the feeding process fills the basic need to build trust. The need for sucking and the development of the oral organs, the lips and mouth, as sensory organs represent adaptations that ensure an adequate early food intake for survival. As a result, food becomes the infant's general means of exploring the environment and is one of the early means of communication. The infant has an additional "nonnutritive" sucking need that is satisfied, especially with the extra effort required in sucking while breast-feeding. As muscular coordination involving the tongue and the swallowing reflex develops, infants gradually learn to eat a variety of semisolid foods, beginning about 6 months of age. As physical and motor maturation proceed, infants begin to show a desire for self-feeding. When these stages of development occur, the exploration of new motor skills and autonomy should be encouraged. If their needs for food and love are fulfilled in this early relationship with the mother, father, other caregivers, and family members, trust is developed. Infants evidence this trust by an increasing capacity to wait a few minutes for feedings until they are prepared.

Breast-Feeding

The ideal food for the human infant is human milk. It has specific characteristics that match the infant's nutritional requirements during the first year of life. The process of breast-feeding today, as in the past, is successfully initiated and maintained by most mothers who try. However, sometimes there are problems when getting started, as well as a high degree of variability among nursing mothers as to frequency of feedings, intake per feeding, and infant growth (see Chapter 11). Thus, in providing support for mothers who want to breast-feed their babies, experienced nutritionists and nurses, many of whom are certified professional lactation consultants, advise flexibility rather than a rigid approach (see the *Further Readings and Resources* section at the end of this chapter). The World Health Organization and the United Nations Children's Fund created The Baby Friendly Hospital Initiative (BFHI)[16,17]; this program has increased the breast-feeding initiation rate of mothers in participating hospitals.[18] Box 12-1 lists the actions that hospitals must carry out to earn BFHI status. Many hospitals employ lactation consultants to oversee compliance with the actions and to promote breast-feeding practices that are optimal, yet realistic, for mother and infant.

The mother's breasts, or mammary glands, are highly specialized secretory organs, as indicated in Chapter 11 and illustrated in Figure 11-4. They are composed of

---

autonomy The state of functioning independently, without extraneous influence.

renal solute load Collective number and concentration of solute particles in a solution carried by the blood to the kidney nephrons for excretion in the urine. The particles are usually nitrogenous products from protein metabolism and the electrolyte sodium.

tactile Pertaining to the touch.

glandular tissue, fat, and connective tissue. The secreting glandular tissue has 15 to 24 lobes, each containing many smaller units called *lobules.* In the lobules, secretory cells called *alveoli* form milk from the nutrient material supplied to them via a rich capillary system. During

pregnancy the breasts are prepared for lactation. The alveoli enlarge and multiply, and toward the end of the prenatal period they secrete a thin, yellowish fluid called colostrum, which contains important antibodies and proteins. Hormonal components in breast milk also enhance the maturation of the gastrointestinal tract. Typically by the end of the second week, mature milk is produced; as the infant grows, the breast milk develops, adapting in composition to meet growth needs.

Breast milk is produced under the stimulating influence of the hormone *prolactin* from the anterior pituitary gland. After the milk is formed in the mammary lobules by alveoli, it is carried through converging branches of the lactiferous ducts to reservoir spaces called ampullae or the lactiferous sinus located under the areola, the pigmented area of skin surrounding the nipple. Another pituitary hormone, *oxytocin,* stimulates the ejection of the milk from the alveoli to the ducts, releasing it to the baby. This is commonly called the *let-down reflex.* It causes a tingling sensation in the breast and the flow of milk. The initial sucking of the baby stimulates this reflex. The newborn rooting reflex, oral need for sucking, and basic hunger drive usually induce and maintain breast-feeding by the healthy mother.

BOX 12-1	Prioritizing Breast-Feeding: The Baby Friendly Hospital Initiative (BFHI)

Actions to Earning BFHI Status
- Write and implement a breast-feeding policy
- Train health care personnel to support the policy
- Tell pregnant women how to breast-feed and of its benefits
- Assist mothers with breast-feeding their newborns in the first 30 minutes after delivery
- Demonstrate to mothers how to breast-feed and express breast milk
- Provide only breast milk to infants, unless contraindicated
- Allow infant to be with mother at all times
- Educate mothers about on-demand feeding
- Avoid pacifiers or other synthetic nipples
- Educate mothers about breast-feeding issues and finding support after leaving the hospital

 FOCUS ON CULTURE

Nutritional Rickets: Role of Culture

The eradication of nutritional rickets, or the vitamin D deficiency of childhood, is one of the greatest public health success stories in the United States. Fortification of cow's milk and supplementation of infant formula with vitamin D ensured the virtual disappearance of this nutritional disease by 1970. The understanding of the importance of sunlight exposure in the initiation of the conversion of inactive to active vitamin D, in addition to adequate dietary intake, was monumental. Unfortunately, rickets is on the rise due to a variety of cultural and related behavioral factors.

Factors Linked to Rickets
Several case series and studies describe causes of nutritional rickets. Two common factors among these reports include exclusive and prolonged breast-feeding and inadequate sunlight exposure in infants. Although most women do not continue to breast-feed their infants beyond 6 months, certain women, primarily white of high educational and economic backgrounds, have extended periods of breast-feeding. In many cases, vitamin D supplementation is not provided to the infant; thus, with an average human milk content of 68 IU/L in white women, the vitamin D source is inadequate to meet the skeletal demands for this nutrient.

Inadequate sunlight exposure of infants with darkly pigmented skin is another primary cause of rickets. For example, several case studies have shown a rise in rickets incidence in black infants, even those infants residing in southern climates with an abundance of sunlight. Other reports have documented rickets in infants required to be fully covered by clothing due to religious or cultural demands.

Rickets has also been documented in infants of lactating mothers who consume vegan diets. Children who are raised

on vegan diets or macrobiotic diets may also have vitamin D deficiency disorders. Often these diets are practiced to support cultural or religious beliefs.

Prevention and Treatment of Rickets
Rickets can be easily prevented, but health care practitioners must be able to recognize the clinical signs and symptoms of rickets once developed (see Chapter 6). Dietary intake assessment is often the first indicator of underlying biochemical and clinical indicators of nutritional deficiency diseases. Screening for special diets, infant feeding method and duration, supplementation, and behaviors related to sunlight exposure of both mother and child is necessary. Vitamin D supplementation of mother and/or child is typically decided on a case-by-case basis. Increased sunlight exposure is another avenue to increasing vitamin D concentration in the blood. Culturally sensitive counseling is required for prevention and treatment of nutritional rickets. Targeted public health and community interventions may also help to diminish rickets once again.

References

Greer FR: Do breastfed infants need supplemental vitamins? *Pediatr Clin North Am* 48(2):415, 2001.
Kreiter SR et al: Nutritional rickets in African American breast-fed infants, *J Pediatr* 137(2):153, 2000.
McCaffree J: Rickets on the rise, *J Am Diet Assoc* 101(1):16, 2001.
Tomashek KM et al: Nutritional rickets in Georgia, *Pediatrics* 107(4):E45, 2001.

The author would like to thank Melissa K. Zack for her assistance in creating this box.

The mother should follow the baby's lead with an on-demand schedule. The baby's continuing rhythm of need establishes feedings, usually about every 2 to 3 hours in the first few weeks after birth.[5,15] The newborn's rooting reflex and somewhat recessed lower jaw are natural adaptations for feeding at the breast. The mother can feed the baby for about 5 to 10 minutes on each breast, burping the baby gently between each period of sucking to expel swallowed air. When the baby is satisfied, he or she can be released from the breast. The nipple should air dry to prevent irritation and soreness (see the *Focus on Food Safety* box, "Ensuring the Safety of Breast Milk and Infant Formula").

The mother's diet and rest are important factors in establishing lactation and breast-feeding. Table 11-2 suggests a balanced diet to support ample milk production, including food choices from various food groups for meals and snacks (see Chapter 11). Natural thirst guides adequate fluid intake. Sufficient rest and relaxation for the mother are essential. An adequate energy intake is especially important in the early weeks to establish regular milk production. A gradual weight loss occurs as maternal fat stores are slowly depleted, but the mother should not expect a rapid return to her prepregnancy weight. Overweight mothers with a body mass index between 25 and 30 kg/m^2 lost about 1 lb/week while successfully breast-feeding their infants.[19] These infants were fed on demand and grew normally; however, rigorous dieting should not be undertaken by breast-feeding mothers.

Breast-feeding may influence feeding behavior and taste preferences into childhood.[20-24] One study suggests that breast-fed infants are less likely to become overweight as children compared to infants who are formula-fed, although more studies are needed to affirm this finding.[25] Infants who develop a pattern of eating in moderation are less likely to become overweight, and breast-fed infants have more control over the amount of milk they consume than do formula-fed infants.[14] Formula-fed infants may be urged to empty their bottle, even though they may turn away when they are satisfied. Force-feeding is less likely to occur in the breast-fed infant but should be avoided in all infants. Feeding should be discontinued at the first sign that the infant has had enough. Children who gain weight more rapidly during the first 4 months of life are more likely to be overweight at age 7.[26] A breast-feeding mother needs to be aware that her infant will likely gain weight more slowly than bottle-fed infants, but this should not be a concern.[27] Acceptance of a wide variety of tastes and preferences for foods may occur if the infant is breast-fed. Odorous compounds transfer into breast milk[22]; such flavor exposure during breast-feeding often impacts acceptance of same-flavored foods in childhood.[23,24]

A growing public health issue in the United States and worldwide is the advisability of breast-feeding by human immunodeficiency virus (HIV)-positive mothers, because breast-feeding can be a route of HIV transmission to an infant.[28] In some countries where formula is

---

FOCUS ON FOOD SAFETY
Ensuring the Safety of Breast Milk and Infant Formula

Breast milk or formula can be a source of food-related illnesses in an infant if these fluids are not properly used and stored. All equipment used in the expression or pumping of breast milk, including pump components and containers, and in the preparation of formula, including scoops and containers, should be sterilized. Most equipment and bottle parts, including synthetic nipples, are dishwasher safe and may be sterilized in this manner. Alternatively, such components may be sterilized in boiling water for 10 to 12 minutes.

Breast milk may stand at room temperature (77° F or less) for up to 6 hours. Breast milk may be stored for no more than 8 days in a 32° to 38° F refrigerator or in a self-defrosting freezer for up to 3 months. If not used within these time frames, breast milk should be discarded and not used to feed the infant.

Mixed or reconstituted infant formula may be stored for up to 24 hours in a 32° to 38° F refrigerator. Formula should not be left to stand at room temperature and cannot be frozen. If mixed formula has been in the refrigerator for more than 24 hours or left at room temperature, it should be thrown away and not used to feed the infant.

Data from Ogundele MO: Techniques for the storage of human breast milk: implications for anti-microbial functions and safety of stored milk, *Eur J Pediatr* 159(11):793, 2000.

---

colostrum Thin yellow fluid first secreted by the mammary gland a few days before and after childbirth, preceding the mature breast milk. It contains up to 20% protein, including a large amount of lactalbumin, more minerals and less lactose and fat than in mature milk, and immunoglobulins representing the antibodies found in maternal blood.

lactiferous ducts Branching channels in the mammary gland that carry breast milk to holding spaces near the nipple ready for the infant's feeding.

ampullae A general term for a flasklike wider portion of a tubular structure; spaces under the nipple of the breast for storing milk.

areola A defined space; a circular area of different color surrounding a central point, such as the darkened pigmented ring surrounding the nipple of the breast.

rooting reflex A reflex in a newborn in which stimulation of the side of the cheek or the upper or lower lip causes the infant to turn its mouth and face to the stimulus.

very expensive and clean water is not readily available, the risks of bottle feeding may still outweigh the risk of HIV transmission for breast-fed infants. For the premature and low-birth-weight baby, feeding through the first year of life poses additional problems.

Bottle-Feeding

Formula feeding by bottle may be preferred by some mothers, due to a variety of reasons. If the mother does not choose to breast-feed or stops breast-feeding before her infant reaches the age of 1 year, bottle-feeding of an appropriate formula is an acceptable alternative. A variety of commercial formulas that attempt to approximate the composition of human milk are available. Some of the cow's milk-based formulas are adjusted with whey protein to more nearly approximate the protein ratio in human milk.

A topic of current interest is the nutritional benefit of substantial amounts of the long-chain fatty acids *arachidonic acid* (ARA) and *docosahexaenoic acid* (DHA) provided in breast milk.[29] These fatty acids appear to play a special role in development of the brain and tissue of the retina,[30] and it has been suggested that the addition of these fatty acids to formula would be beneficial to formula-fed infants. In fact, based on the presence of ARA and DHA in human breast milk and the normal metabolic conversion of linoleic acid to ARA and alpha-linolenic acid to DHA along with evidence linking ARA and DHA to visual acuity and cognitive development,

the Food and Drug Administration approved the addition of these long-chain polyunsaturated fatty acids to infant formula.[31-34]

Special formulas have been developed for infants with allergies, lactose intolerance, diarrhea, fat malabsorption, or other problems,[35] and several types of constituent proteins and carbohydrates are used. These include cow's milk protein, soy protein, casein hydrolysate, or elemental formulas (Table 12-5). Hypoallergenic formulas have been developed for infants who are allergic to cow's milk or commercial formulas based on cow's milk and have existing symptoms of that allergy.[35] Even partially hydrolyzed proteins can provoke an allergic response in infants with hypersensitivity to cow's milk. In the preparation of hypoallergenic formulas, all proteins are completely hydrolyzed to free amino acids. Although soy formulas are tolerated by some infants allergic to cow's milk, they are not hypoallergenic.

In recent years, there has been growing use of soy protein–based infant formulas, and it is estimated that by 6 months of age, 16% of formula-fed infants in the United States are on this type of formula.[36] At one time, soy protein–based formula was used primarily to feed infants who could not tolerate the protein from cow's milk or the lactose found in standard formulas, but the use of soy protein–based formulas has been growing among parents who wish to feed their infants vegetarian diets. Also, soy protein–based formulas have been effective in the management of babies with acute diarrhea. To ensure

TABLE 12-5	**A Comparison of Types of Formulas Manufactured for Full-Term Infants**			
Type of Formula Used		**Protein Content**	**Fat Content**	**Carbohydrate Content**
Milk-based routine	Source:	Nonfat cow's milk	Vegetable oils	Lactose
	g/100 kcal:	2.2-2.3	5.4-5.5	10.5-10.8
	% kcalories:	9	48-50	41-43
Whey-adjusted routine	Source:	Nonfat cow's milk plus demineralized whey	Vegetable and oleo oils	Lactose
	g/100 kcal:	2.2	5.4	10.8
	% kcalories:	9	48	43
Soy isolate (cow's milk sensitivity)	Source:	Soy isolate	Vegetable oils	Corn syrup solids and/or sucrose
	g/100 kcal:	2.5	5.3-5.5	10.3-10.6
	% kcalories:	10	47-50	41-42
Casein hydrolysate (protein sensitivity, galactosemia)	Source:	Casein hydrolysate	Corn oil, other vegetable oils, and MCT	Tapioca starch and glucose, sucrose, or corn syrup solids
	g/100 kcal:	2.8	5.0-5.6	10.2-11.0
	% kcalories:	11	45-50	41-44
Meat-based (cow's milk sensitivity, galactosemia)	Source:	Beef hearts	Sesame oil and beef heart fat	Tapioca starch and sucrose
	g/100 kcal:	4.0	4.8	9
	% kcalories:	16	47	37

MCT, Medium-chain triglycerides.

an appropriate complement of amino acids, soy protein–based formulas are supplemented with methionine, one of the sulfur-containing essential amino acids.

Standards for the levels of nutrients required in infant formulas are based on recommendations from the American Academy of Pediatrics. Minimum levels have been established for protein, fat, and 27 micronutrients. Maximum levels have been set for 9 nutrients, including vitamins A and D and iron.[37]

When feeding formula, the baby should be cradled in the arm, as in breast-feeding, keeping the baby's head upright as much as possible to avoid milk running into the ear canals and resulting in an ear infection. The close human touch and warmth are important. When the infant is obviously satisfied, extra milk should not be forced, regardless of the amount remaining in the bottle. Any remaining formula should be thrown away and not refrigerated for reuse (see the *Focus on Food Safety* box, "Ensuring the Safety of Breast Milk and Infant Formula"). Infants usually take the amount of formula they need. Today most infants are fed on demand versus scheduled, which works out to be about every 2 to 3 hours. Healthy infants soon establish their individual feeding patterns according to their individual growth requirements. Only infant formula and water are appropriate for bottle-feeding; other fluids such as juice, flavored drinks, and carbonated beverages should not be provided through bottles.

Breast-Feeding and Formula-Feeding Combination

Some women may desire the flexibility of both breast-feeding and formula-feeding their infants. For example, a mother working outside of the home may choose to breast-feed her infant in the morning before work and in the evening after work and use formula during the day. This combination is possible but is recommended only after an adequate supply of breast milk and infant feeding pattern have been established. Factors to consider include infant's acceptance of a synthetic nipple and formula's taste, mother's ability or need to express breast milk during the day, and growth of the infant.

Cow's Milk

Regular unmodified cow's milk is not suitable for infants for several reasons, as follows:

- It causes gastrointestinal bleeding.
- Its renal solute load is too concentrated for the infant's renal system to handle; this leaves too small a margin of safety for maintaining water balance, especially during illness, diarrhea, or hot weather.
- Early exposure to cow's milk increases the risk of developing allergies to milk proteins.
- It adversely affects nutrition status.[14,15] Not only is cow's milk low in iron, but also iron status in the infant is lowered even further by the associated gastroin-

testinal bleeding and blood loss caused by this milk. In addition, cow's milk is a poor source of vitamins C and E and essential fatty acids. Infants have need for fat; thus they should not be fed reduced-fat milks such as nonfat or 2% fat. Low-fat or nonfat milks do not provide (1) sufficient energy to support growth requirements, leading the infant to consume increased volumes of milk and excessive protein, and (2) sufficient linoleic acid, the essential fatty acid needed for growth and development of body tissues, found in the fat portion of milk.[15] A specific form of eczema has been observed in infants deficient in linoleic acid, and a low-fat diet in infancy may impair physical and intellectual development.

To meet the special needs of infants, the American Academy of Pediatrics recommends breast milk or formula as the major food source up to 1 year of age, with a gradual addition of appropriate foods beginning at 4 to 6 months.[5,14] There is no need for special formulas for older infants; such formulas also present an added expense to the family.

Premature and Small-for-Gestational-Age Infants

Infants born too early or too small have many food-related difficulties to overcome and present a special challenge in feeding. A poor sucking reflex, difficulty in swallowing, small gastric capacity, reduced intestinal motility, tiring easily from eating and being handled, and increased nutrient requirements for catch-up growth all need to be considered. The health team involved in the care of premature and small-for-gestational-age infants is faced with a myriad of decisions to overcome these feeding difficulties. Whenever possible, these infants should be fed breast milk, usually fortified with additional protein, vitamins, and minerals to the levels found in special formulas developed to meet the particular needs of premature infants. Delivery of breast milk or formula using tube feeding (enteral feeding) carries less risk of complications than the delivery of nutrients through the veins (parenteral feeding).

---

casein hydrolysate formula Infant formula composed of hydrolyzed casein, a major milk protein, produced by partially breaking down the casein into smaller peptide fragments, making a product that is more easily digested.

elemental formula A nutrition support formula composed of single elemental nutrient components that require no further digestive breakdown and thus are readily absorbed. Infant formula produced with elemental, ready-to-be-absorbed components of free amino acids and carbohydrate as simple sugars.

A comparison of the nutrient content of breast milk and special formulas for the premature infant is presented in Table 12-6. Formulas developed for the premature infant may have as much as 30% more protein per fluid volume than those developed for the normal infant, as well as higher amounts of calcium, zinc, and the B-complex vitamins. This enriched formula also supports catch-up growth in term infants who are small for gestational age.[38] Nutrition support of the high-risk infant requires a team approach that includes the pediatrician, nurse, dietitian, and a lactation consultant who can assist the mother and family in developing a routine for expressing and safely storing her breast milk to feed her infant.

Beikost: Solid Food Additions

Beikost feeding begins the transition from a predominantly liquid diet to a predominantly solid food diet.[39] Nutritional and medical authorities agree that for the first 4 to 6 months of life the optimal single food for the infant is human breast milk or an appropriate formula. There is no nutritional basis for introducing solid foods to an infant earlier than 4 to 6 months of age; before this age, it may contribute to overfeeding.[14] Until then, the infant does not need any additional food and is not able to adequately handle other foods. In addition to nutritional reasons, there are developmental reasons for delaying the addition of solid foods until the age of 4 to 6 months. The

following developmental tasks must have been mastered before the infant is prepared to receive solid foods:

- The infant can communicate desire and interest in food by opening his or her mouth and leaning forward or, conversely, leaning back or turning away, participating in the feeding process.
- The infant can sit up with support and has good control of the trunk and neck.
- The infant has developed the ability to move food to the back of the mouth for swallowing.

Developmental abilities to use the hands and fingers are required before self-feeding can be initiated. Self-feeding efforts begin first with a whole hand (palmar) grasp and then move to a more refined finger (pincer) grasp by the end of the first year. The first item for self-feeding may be a piece of Melba toast that can be grasped with the whole hand. As solid food is gradually added, the amount of breast milk or formula consumed is reduced accordingly.

Both cultural patterns and the age and educational level of the mother influence infant-feeding practices. Some of these practices, such as adding cereal to the infant's bottle to help the baby sleep through the night, are related more to the convenience of the mother than to the benefit of the infant.[40,41] It may not be in the infant's best interests to sleep through the night at a very early age or to adapt as early as possible to three meals a day. Smaller

---

TABLE 12-6 | **Nutritional Value of Special Formulas and Human Milk for the Preterm Infant**

| Nutritional Component | Advisable Intake for Birth Weight | | Human Milk Content | | Standard Formulas | | Special Premature Formulas | |
	1.0 kg (2.2 lb)	1.5 kg (3.3 lb)	Preterm	Mature	Enfamil®* Similac®† SMA®‡	Enfamil® Premature LIPIL®*	Similac® Special Care®†	"Preemie" SMA®‡
Kcal/dl			73.0	73.0	67.0	81.0	81.0	81.0
Protein (g/200 kcal)	3.1	2.7	2.6§	1.5	2.2	6.0	2.7	2.5
Vitamins, Fat-Soluble								
D (IU/120 kcal/kg/day)	600.0	600.0	—	4.0	70.0-75.0	288.0	180.0	76.0
E (IU/120 kcal/kg/day)	30.0	30.0	—	0.3	2.0-3.0	7.6	5.0	2.0
Vitamins, Water-Soluble								
Folic acid (µg/120 kcal /kg/day)	60.0	60.0	—	8.0	9.0-19.0	48.0	45.0	14.0
C (mg/120 kcal /kg/day)	60.0	60.0	—	7.0	10.0-14.0	24.0	45.0	10.0
Minerals								
Calcium (mg/100 kcal)	160.0	140.0	40.0	43.0	63.0-78.0	197.0	180.0	92.0
Phosphorus (mg/100 kcal)	108.0	95.0	18.0	20.0	42.0-53.0	99.0	100.0	49.0
Sodium (mEq/100 kcal)	2.7	2.3	1.5¶	0.8	1.0-1.8	1.8	1.9	1.7

*Mead Johnson Nutritional Division, Evansville, Ind.
†Ross Laboratories, Columbus, Ohio.
‡Wyeth Laboratories, Philadelphia.
§Range: 1.9-2.8 g/100 kcal.
¶Range: 0.9-2.3 mEq/100 kcal.

amounts of food, eaten on a more frequent basis, may contribute to the pattern of eating in moderation.[14]

The traditional transition food is fortified infant cereal—specifically, infant rice cereal mixed with a little milk or formula—because rice cereal has the least potential for allergic reaction. Vegetables, fruits, potato, egg yolk, and finally meat can be added to the diet in a gradual sequence. No one sequence of food additions must be followed. A general guide is given in Table 12-7. Single foods are given first, one at a time in small amounts, about 5 to 7 days apart; in this way, adverse reactions can be identified. These foods are usually offered before the milk feeding. Individual responses and needs can be a basis for choice, as food becomes a source of enjoyment and a new means of building warm family relationships. A basic goal during this time is to have the infant learn to enjoy many different foods. This is the perfect time to introduce a wide variety of foods, because infants appear to be more willing to taste new foods than are toddlers; in fact, the greater the variety of foods presented when the addition of solid food is begun, the greater the number of foods the infant will accept when first presented.[42] Breast-fed infants seem to be more receptive to new foods with new flavors, and it has been suggested that exposure to a variety of flavors in breast milk, the result of the mother's varied diet, helps prepare an infant to accept new flavors and foods.[43]

Many commercial baby foods are available and are prepared without the formerly used ingredients of sugar, salt, or monosodium glutamate. Some mothers prefer preparing their own baby food. This can be done by cooking and straining vegetables and fruits and forming a puree using a blender, food processor, or Foley mill. These foods can be frozen in ice cube trays or in 1-tbsp amounts on a cookie sheet. The cubes or individual portions are easily stored in plastic bags in the freezer. Then a single portion can be reheated conveniently for use at a feeding. When working with mothers, it is important to stress the need for a clean environment when preparing infant foods to avoid the danger of foodborne illness.

Two foods that require special attention in infant feeding are honey and fruit juices. Honey should never be given to an infant who is younger than 1 year, because it can lead to botulism, a fatal condition in infants. Some fruit juices, including apple, pear, and prune, contain sorbitol, which can lead to diarrhea in infants and toddlers. If given, fruit juice should be limited to no more than 4 oz per day.

Summary Principles

The following two basic principles should guide the feeding process:

1. Nutrients are needed, not specific foods.
2. Food is a main basis of early learning

Food not only provides for physical sustenance but also fulfills other personal development and cultural needs.

TABLE 12-7	Guideline for Adding Solid Foods to Infant's Diet During the First Year*

When to Start	Foods Added	Feeding
Months 5-6	Infant cereal	10 AM and 6 PM
	Pureed baby foods such as cooked vegetable or fruit	2 PM
	Zwieback or hard toast that easily dissolves	At any feeding
Months 7-9	Potato: baked or boiled and mashed or sieved	10 AM and 6 PM
	Egg yolk (at first, hard cooked and sieved or scrambled, soft boiled or poached later)	

Suggested Meal Plan for 8 Months to 1 Year or Older

7 AM	Milk	240 ml (8 oz)
	Infant cereal	2-3 tbsp
	Strained fruit	2-3 tbsp
	Zwieback or dry toast	
Noon	Milk	240 ml (8 oz)
	Strained vegetables	2-3 tbsp
	Chopped meat or one whole egg	
	Puddings or cooked fruit	2-3 tbsp
3 PM	Milk	120 ml (4 oz)
	Toast, zwieback, or crackers	
6 PM	Milk	240 ml (8 oz)
	Whole egg or chopped meat	
	Potato: baked or mashed	2 tbsp
	Pudding or cooked fruit	2-3 tbsp
	Zwieback or toast	

*Semisolid foods should be given immediately before milk feeding. One or 2 tsp should be given first. If food is accepted and tolerated well, the amount should be increased to 1 to 2 tbsp per feeding.
NOTE: Banana or cottage cheese may be used as substitution for any meal.

palmar grasp Early grasp of the young infant, clasping an object in the palm and wrapping the whole hand around it.
pincer grasp Later digital grasp of the older infant, usually picking up smaller objects with a precise grip between thumb and forefinger.

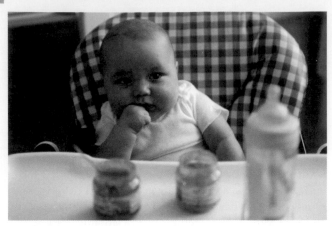

FIGURE 12-1   This child is taking a variety of solid food additions and developing wide tastes. Here, feeding serves as a source not only of physical growth but also of psychosocial development. Optimal physical development and security are evident, the result of sound nutrition and loving care. *(Credit: PhotoDisc.)*

Good food habits are formed early in life and continue to develop as a child grows older. By the time infants are about 8 or 9 months old, they should be able to eat many family foods that are cooked, chopped, or mashed and simply seasoned, without the need for special infant foods. Throughout the first year of life the infant's needs for physical growth and psychosocial development will be met by breast milk or formula, a variety of solid food additions, and a loving, trusting relationship between parents and child (Figure 12-1).

Toddler (1 to 3 Years)

Physical Characteristics and Growth

After the rapid growth of the first year the growth rate of children slows. But although the rate of gain is less, the pattern of growth produces significant changes in body form. The legs become longer, and the child begins losing "baby fat." There is less total body water, and more of the remaining water is inside cells. The young child begins to look and feel less like a baby and more like a child. Energy demands are lower because of the decelerated growth rate. However, important muscle development is taking place. In fact, muscle mass development accounts for about one half of the total weight gain during this period. As the child begins to walk and stand erect, more muscle is needed to strengthen the body and support these movements. For example, there is special need for big muscles in the back, the buttocks, and the thighs. The overall rate of skeletal growth slows, with greater deposits of mineral in existing bone rather than a lengthening of bones. The increased mineralization strengthens bones to support the increasing body weight. The child has six to eight teeth at the beginning of the toddler period. By 3 years of age, the remaining deciduous teeth have erupted.

Psychosocial and Motor Development

The psychosocial development of the toddler is pronounced. The core developmental problem they struggle with is the desire for autonomy. Each child has a profound increasing sense of self—of being a distinct and individual person apart from the parents, not just an extension of them. As physical mobility increases with increased gross and fine motor skill development, the sense of autonomy and independence grows. An expanding curiosity leads to much exploration of the environment, and increasingly the mouth is used as a means of exploring. Touch is important, providing the means of learning what objects are like. The constant use of "no" reflects the significant struggle with newly emerging ego needs in conflict with the caregiver's control efforts. The child wants to do more and more, but the attention span is fairly short and interest shifts quickly from one thing to another.

Food and Feeding

Physical growth and psychosocial development during the toddler period influence nutrient needs (see Tables 12-2, 12-3, and 12-4) and food patterns (see the *Perspectives in Practice* box, "Feeding Toddlers and Preschoolers: Eating Is a Family Affair"), as follows:

- *Energy:* The energy requirement now increases very slowly in small spurts. At about 1 year of age, children need approximately 850 kcal/day; this rises to a range of 1160 to 1680 kcal/day for boys and 1080 to 1650 kcal/day for girls by age 3.[4] The variation in energy need for toddlers is due to the wide range of physical activity. More active toddlers require more energy, whereas sedentary toddlers do not. From age 1 to 2, some children do not eat as much as they did in the second half of infancy. Caregivers will avoid conflict with their toddler about eating if they remember this decrease in need for kcalories is normal, resulting from a slowing in the growth rate and the child's necessary struggle for autonomy and selfhood, which often involves refusal of food. Appetite varies in the toddler; therefore food intake may be irregular with periods of good appetite and periods of disinterest in food. Encouragement is needed from caregivers, but constant conflict with the child about eating serves no useful purpose. A small plate of snacks, including finger-food pieces of raw fruit and cheese kept in the refrigerator or a few crackers on a special colorful plate, can give the child a measure of positive control when hungry. Toddlers will eat when they are hungry. Positive early experiences help develop appropriate food acceptance patterns.[1]

- *Protein:* In relation to energy needs, protein needs are relatively increased during this stage of life. The toddler requires about 13 g of protein per day.[4] Muscle

PERSPECTIVES IN PRACTICE
Feeding Toddlers and Preschoolers: Eating Is a Family Affair

No matter what their age, children need the same nutrients as adults but in different amounts. The challenge for parents and caregivers is to make available appropriate and appealing foods and to set the time and place for eating. Young children must learn how to make food choices and to decide how much food they need to consume.

We can help parents and caregivers develop child-feeding strategies based on the developmental needs of their young children. First, we must remind them that their children are not growing as fast as they did during the first year of life; it follows that they need less food. Also, a child's energy needs are sporadic; therefore periods of greater food intake will vary with periods of smaller intake. Forcing food during periods of low intake may encourage overeating or food aversion, leading to food intake problems later in life.

Amount of Food

Children are not ready for adult-sized portions and may be overwhelmed by large amounts of food on their plate. It is better to serve less food than they are likely to eat and to have them ask for more. In planning portion sizes, a good rule of thumb is 1 tbsp of food for every year of age. When the child begins to play with the food on the plate or seems to lose interest in eating, remove the plate and provide another activity.

Feeding Frequency

Children do best with a regular feeding schedule; try to keep meals and snacks at regular times. Young children have small stomachs, and it is difficult for them to consume enough food at one meal to last them until the next meal. They may need to eat 5 or 6 times a day. Try to allow at least 1½ or 2 hours between snacks and meals. When choosing between-meal snacks, look to foods that will provide not only additional kcalories but also protein and important vitamins and minerals. Fruit, crackers, raw vegetables (as appropriate), cheese, milk, and cereal are good snacks. It is best if children are not overtired at mealtime; if possible, plan a short rest period immediately before a meal.

What Foods

Over time, it is important for the young child to learn to eat a variety of foods, although it may be necessary to offer a new food 8 to 10 times, each including at least a taste, before it will be accepted. The child should learn to eat what other family members are eating and not be provided with special foods. But when planning meals, be sure to have one item that the child likes and will eat. Also, children are more willing to try a new food if it is accompanied by a favorite food; try to pair such foods at the same meal. Serve dessert, if any, with the main meal rather than later; it should not assume special importance in relation to other foods. Do allow your toddler or preschooler to make some choices about foods for meals or snacks just as older children are able to do. This develops skills in making food choices.

Avoid Forbidding Certain Foods

All foods, including sweets, can be included in a healthy diet for young children if limited in frequency and amount. It is important that children learn how to moderate their intakes of such foods. Excluding certain foods makes them more attractive and may ultimately lead to increased intake when they do become available.

Food Safety

Two major safety considerations in feeding children are avoidance of foodborne illness and the possibility of choking. Young children are very vulnerable to foodborne illness resulting from (1) foods that are not fully cooked, such as hamburger or eggs, (2) foods that became contaminated by contact with an unwholesome food or other source of bacteria, or (3) improperly stored food with bacterial growth. Eating such foods can lead to serious illness or even death in the young child, as occurred when preschoolers ate improperly cooked hamburger at a fast-food restaurant. Children must be taught at a young age to wash their hands thoroughly after they use the bathroom and before they touch a food. Parents should ask about food handling and other sanitary practices when evaluating the suitability of a caregiver or a care facility.

Children younger than 4 years are at greatest risk for choking and death by asphyxiation. Foods most likely to cause choking are those that are round and hard and do not dissolve in saliva. Typical items that cause choking are hot dogs, grapes, peanut butter in globs, hard pieces of raw fruits and vegetables, hard candy, or popcorn. Young children should always be supervised when eating and should eat sitting down.

Social Environment at Meal Time

Try to keep mealtime as pleasant as possible. Allow enough time for the young child to eat. Having to hurry adds stress to mealtime and takes away the pleasure of eating, especially for the child who is still learning to self feed. Be patient about spills or accidents; it takes time to develop feeding skills. Choose appropriate utensils that are unbreakable and easy for the child to grasp. Children are less likely to accept a food that was first introduced in a negative meal situation; therefore make mealtime an enjoyable family time that reinforces positive eating behaviors. Parental modeling is an important influence in encouraging children to try new foods. Toddlers are more likely to taste a new food if they see an adult, especially a familiar adult or parent, eating it. Children model the eating behavior of parents and caregivers; be sure that others at the table are eating vegetables and drinking milk. Parental modeling is as important in the choice of snacks as it is at mealtime.

References

Duyff RL: *The American Dietetic Association complete food and nutrition guide,* ed 2, Indianapolis, Ind, 2002, Wiley.

Fisher JO, Birch LL: Restricting access to palatable foods affects children's behavioral response, food selection, and intake, *Am J Clin Nutr* 69(6):1264, 1999.

Kleinman RE, ed: *Pediatric nutrition handbook,* ed 4, Elk Grove Village, Ill, 1998, American Academy of Pediatrics.

Nicklas TA et al: Family and child-care provider influences on preschool children's fruit, juice, and vegetable consumption, *Nutr Rev* 59(7):224, 2001.

Thorpe M: Parents as role models: nutrition is a family affair, *J Am Diet Assoc* 102(1):64, 2002.

Tibbs T et al: The relationship between parental modeling, eating patterns, and dietary intake among African-American parents, *J Am Diet Assoc* 101(5):535, 2001.

and other body tissues are growing rapidly. At least half of this protein should be of animal origin, because animal protein has high biologic value. However, toddlers who follow a balanced and well-planned ovolactovegetarian diet grow just as well and attain similar heights as their nonvegetarian counterparts.[5] Diets planned for vegan children will need to incorporate soy and legume protein and build on the complementarity of plant proteins (see Chapter 4).

- *Minerals:* Calcium and phosphorus are needed for bone mineralization. The bones are strengthening to keep pace with muscle development and increasing activity. Iron is needed to maintain adequate hemoglobin levels because the increase in body size requires an increasing blood volume. Adequate levels of zinc are necessary to support protein synthesis and cell division. The principle of increasing iron absorption from nonheme sources such as vegetables by including a small amount of heme iron from meat at the same meal, as discussed in Chapter 7, holds true for feeding the toddler.
- *Vitamins:* The fat-soluble and water-soluble vitamins are critical to macronutrient utilization and growth and development. A variety of food intake eaten in proportion to energy needs should provide adequate vitamins to the toddler.
- *Fiber:* Because solid foods make up a greater portion of the diet of toddlers than that of infants, constipation often become more prevalent. Adequate fiber of 19 g/day is recommended for children ages 1 to 3 years.[4]
- *Food choices:* About 2 to 3 cups of milk daily is sufficient for the young child's needs. Sometimes excessive milk intake, a habit carried over from infancy, excludes many solid foods from the diet. As a result, the child may lack iron and develop a so-called milk anemia. On the other hand, if a child dislikes milk as a beverage, replacement can be made with cheese, creamed soups, puddings, or custards, or nonfat dry milk can be used in cooked cereals, mashed potatoes, meatloaf, and casseroles. Calcium-fortified foods can assist in adding calcium to the diet. Offering the child an increasing variety of foods will help to develop good food habits; food habits are learned, and there is little opportunity for learning if a child is not exposed to a wide variety of foods. Refined sweets are best avoided, reserving them for special occasions, not for habitual use or to bribe a child to eat.

Another important consideration when selecting food for the toddler is the risk of choking and death by asphyxiation. Foods that are round, hard, and not easily dissolved can cause choking. Such food items include hot dogs, grapes, peanut butter in globs, hard pieces of raw fruits and vegetables, hard candy, and popcorn. Young children should always be supervised when eating and should eat sitting down. Running when eating can lead to choking.

It is best that children not eat in a moving car unless a second adult, in addition to the driver, is available to assist if needed.

Summary Principles

The following two important principles should be emphasized when working with caregivers to guide feeding practices during this period:

1. The child needs fewer kcalories but relatively more protein and minerals for physical growth; therefore a variety of foods should be offered in appropriate portion sizes to provide key nutrients. It is important that day care providers and parents work cooperatively to support the development of good food patterns.[44]
2. The child is struggling for selfhood as part of normal psychosocial development. This struggle is expressed in refusing food and the desire to do things for self before being fully able to do them efficiently. If caregivers are patient, offer a variety of foods in small amounts, and encourage some degree of food choice and self-feeding in the child's own ceremonial manner, eating can be a happy, positive means of development.

If we are to achieve the goal of establishing good food patterns for life, it is especially important to introduce a variety of fruits and vegetables along with grains and meats during this stage of development (Figure 12-2). A study of 72 children from 2 to 5 years of age found that they ate rather few fruits and vegetables and that their food choices changed very little over the 3 years.[45] Only three fruits (apples, bananas, and grapes) and four vegetables (carrots, green beans, corn, and french fries) were included among their list of 19 favorite foods given by both mothers and children. Macaroni and cheese, pizza, chicken, and cereal were their four top foods, and fruit drinks, carbonated beverages, milk, and apple juice were the most commonly used beverages.[45]

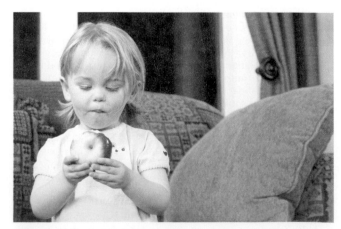

FIGURE 12-2 Grains are an important part of the toddler's diet. *(Copyright 2006 JupiterImages Corporation.)*

Preschooler (3 to 6 Years)

Physical Characteristics and Growth

As shown in normal childhood growth charts (see Appendix C), CDC Growth Charts: United States), each child tends to settle into a regular genetic growth channel as physical growth continues in spurts. On occasion the child bounds with energy. Play is hard play—running, jumping, and testing new physical resources. At other times, the child will sit for increasing periods of time engrossed in passive types of activities. Mental capacities are developing, and there is more thinking and exploring of the environment. Energy needs and specific nutrients are shown in Tables 12-2, 12-3, and 12-4. Protein requirements continue to increase as the child grows older. Preschool children need about 13 to 19 g/day of good-quality protein,[4] as found in milk, egg, meat, cheese, legumes, and soy. They continue to need calcium and iron to support growth and to build body stores. Because vitamins A and C and folate are often lacking in the diets of preschool children, a variety of fruits and vegetables should be provided. Vitamin D, important for calcium absorption, can be obtained in fortified milk or soy products or by spending time playing outdoors in the sun.

Psychosocial and Motor Development

Each stage of development builds on the previous one. The psychosocial developmental stage for preschool children involves increased socialization and initiative. They are beginning to develop their superego—the conscience. As powers of active movement increase, they have a growing imagination and curiosity. This is a period of increasing imitation. Boys and girls may imitate adults who serve as role models. Much of this becomes evident in their play by the use of grown-up clothes and role-playing in a variety of situations. Self-feeding skills increase, and eating takes on greater social aspects. The family mealtime is an important event for socialization, because children imitate their parents and others at the table.[46] Role-modeling may have long-term implications in respect to nutrient intake and health. For example, in nearly 200 girls of kindergarten age, the best predictor of their milk intakes was the milk intakes of their mothers. If the mother drank soft drinks rather than milk, so did her daughter.[47]

Food and Feeding

The preschool child is beginning to form definite responses to various types of foods, as follows:

- *Vegetables and fruits:* Fruits are usually well liked. However, of all the food groups, vegetables usually are the least well liked by children, yet these foods contain many vitamins and minerals needed for growth. Where there is space or opportunity, involving the young child in planting and growing vegetables in a small garden or in containers is an excellent way to draw the child's interest to vegetables to be tasted. Trips to the market or learning activities in the day care setting can help a child see a variety of shapes and colors in vegetables and discover new ones that can be prepared in a variety of ways. It is important to remember that children have a keen sense of taste; therefore flavor and texture are important. Children usually dislike strong vegetables such as cabbage and onions but do like crisp raw vegetables or fruits cut in small pieces to eat as finger foods. Mixed vegetables and fruits are often less tolerated than individual ones. Children also react to consistency of vegetables, disliking them overcooked. Tough strings and hard pieces are difficult to chew and swallow and should be removed.

- *Milk, cheese, egg, meat, and legumes:* It is helpful if children can set their own goals of quantities of food. Portions need to be relatively small (see the *Perspectives in Practice* box, "Feeding Toddlers and Preschoolers: Eating Is a Family Affair"). If children can pour their own milk from a small pitcher into a small glass, they will drink more. Smaller children like their milk more at room temperature, not icy cold. Also, they prefer it in small glasses that hold about 4 to 6 oz rather than in large, adult-sized glasses. Cheese is a favorite finger food or snack; however, the major source of calcium in this age-group is milk. Egg is usually well liked if hard-cooked or scrambled. Meat should be tender and easy to cut and chew; hence, ground meat is popular. Ground meat also must be well cooked to make it safe. (To avoid the risk of foodborne illness that can be fatal in the young child, ground meat should be cooked to a temperature of 160° F, the meat should have a gray-white color, and juices should be clear.)

- *Grains:* The wide variety in which grains can be eaten adds to their appeal to children who enjoy breads, cereals, and crackers. Whole grains provide important fiber. To avoid unwanted kcalories, presweetened cereals should be used infrequently if at all.

- *Temperature:* Because children prefer their foods lukewarm and not hot, some foods may remain on their plates and become dry and gummy such that the child refuses to eat it. Thus very small portions should be served at a time.

---

growth channel The progressive regular growth pattern of children, guided along individual genetically controlled channels, influenced by nutritional and health status.

- *Single foods:* Children usually prefer single foods to combination dishes such as casseroles or stews. Preschool is also a period of language learning. Children like to learn names of foods and to be able to recognize and name them on the basis of their shape, color, texture, and taste; these identifiable characteristics need to be retained as much as possible.
- *Finger foods:* Children like to eat food they can pick up with their fingers. Often, a variety of raw fruits and vegetables cut into finger-sized pieces and offered to children for their own selection provide a source of needed nutrition.
- *Food jags:* Because of developing social and emotional needs, preschool children commonly have food jags, refusing to eat all except one particular food. This may last for several days, but it is usually short lived and of no major consequence.

Summary Principles

The preschool period is one of important growth for the young child. Lifetime food habits are forming. Food continues to play an important part in the developing personality, and group eating becomes significant as a means of socialization. The following two principles should be considered when interacting with preschoolers:

1. The social and emotional environment and companionship at mealtime with family, other caregivers, or other children greatly influence the young child's food intake and diet quality. The child learns food patterns at the family table and follows the examples of food eaten by parents or older siblings.[48] The child may attend a day care or preschool in which group eating occurs. Food habits of preschoolers are greatly affected by peer modeling, and food preferences develop according to what the group is eating. Children in this stage of development may begin to respond to environmental cues encouraging them to consume more food than they need. In a day care setting, it was found that 5-year-old children ate more food when presented with larger portions, whereas 3½-year-old children were not affected by portion size.[49] In light of the growing numbers of overweight children, we need to encourage parents to be alert to portion size when serving their children's food.

2. Many food preferences and tolerances are established during this period. Exposure to a wide variety of foods in appropriate portion sizes may set the stage for lifetime food habits and associated patterns of health. This stage of growth is also a time for the young child to develop appropriate physical exercise habits, and games including activities such as skipping or jumping should be encouraged in a safe environment. Physical fitness established at an early age can lower the risk of overweight and obesity in childhood and adulthood, respectively.[50] Encouraging young children to participate in active games rather

than sedentary pastimes such as watching videos or television may support appropriate food patterns as well (see the *Further Readings and Resources* section at the end of this chapter). Even a 30-second commercial for a snack food has been shown to influence the food choices of preschool-age children.[51]

The School-Age Child (6 to 12 Years)

Physical Characteristics and Growth

The school-age period preceding adolescence has been called the latent time of growth. During this stage, the rate of growth slows and body changes occur very gradually. However, resources are being laid down for the rapid adolescent growth that lies ahead; sometimes this has been called the lull before the storm. By now the body type has been established, and growth rates vary widely. Girls usually outdistance boys in the latter part of this period.

Psychosocial and Motor Development

Psychosocial development during these early school years centers on the formal learning environment and its expectations. Children have widening horizons, new school experiences, and challenging learning opportunities. They develop increased cognitive capacity and the ability to problem solve. They learn to cooperate in group activities and begin to experience a sense of adequacy and accomplishment and sometimes the realities of competition. The child begins to move from a dependence on parental standards to those of peers (Figure 12-3). Pressures are generated for self-control of a growing body, and inappropriate concepts of body image that lead to chronic dieting or eating disorders likely take root during this period. Negative attitudes sometimes expressed and changes in temperament are evidence of these struggles for growing independence. It is a diffuse period of gangs, cliques, hero worship, pensive daydreaming, emotional stress, and learning to get along with other children. This is also a period during which nutrition and health concepts can be learned.

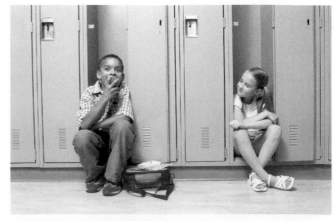

FIGURE 12-3 The nutrition habits of school-age children are influenced by their peers. *(Copyright 2006 JupiterImages Corporation.)*

Food and Feeding

The slowed rate of growth during this period results in a gradual decline in the food requirement per unit of body weight. This decline continues up to the period just before approaching adolescence. Likes and dislikes are a product of earlier years. Family food attitudes are imitated, but increasing outside activities compete with family mealtimes, and family conflicts may arise.

School and the Learning Environment

Research has firmly established the close relationship between sound nutrition and childhood learning.[50] Breakfast is particularly important for the school-age child. It breaks the fast of the sleep hours and prepares the child for problem solving and memory in the learning hours at school.[52] The School Breakfast and Lunch Programs provide nourishing school meals that many children would not otherwise have (see Chapter 10). Studies have documented the positive relationship between breakfast intake and school performance,[52,53] and innovative programs to increase school breakfast participation have been developed.[54,55] School programs implemented by the U.S. Department of Agriculture help to maintain sound nutrition by implementing the *Dietary Guidelines for Americans* (see the *Further Readings and Resources* section at the end of this chapter) into child breakfast and lunch programs,[56,57] developing recipes that lower the fat in school lunch entrees and desserts,[58] and preventing the initiation of snack bars that sell soft drinks and snack foods as an alternative to the cafeteria school lunch.[59] Schools should also take a premier role in promoting lifelong physical activity patterns in children. Health professionals must take leadership roles in their communities to ensure that school meal programs provide positive examples of nutritionally appropriate meal patterns and introduce children to new foods that they may not have tasted previously.

The *MyPyramid Food Guidance System* was released by the U.S. Department of Agriculture in September 2005. These program materials are designed to assist individuals in identifying energy needs, setting goals for food and nutrient intakes, and developing food intakes based on food groups. The *MyPyramid for Kids* (Figure 12-4) was developed for 6- to 11-year-olds to build knowledge related to food and nutrient intake along with energy intake and energy expenditure through physical activity. Classroom-based activities are available on the website of the U.S. Department of Agriculture (*http://teamnutrition. usda.gov/resources/mypyramidclassroom.html*) for implementation in schools.

The school-age child has increasing exposure to both positive and negative influences on food habits. Television becomes a powerful source of food information. At the same time, positive learning opportunities can occur in the classroom when nutrition education is integrated with other activities and parents provide support and reinforcement at home. An important learning experience can be the preparation of simple meals; in an urban community, 35% of the children in third grade ate at least one meal a day that they prepared themselves or a brother or sister prepared.[60]

Although declines in physical activity no doubt have contributed to the growing number of overweight children, some researchers have also pointed to changes in snacking habits. A comparison of diet surveys during the past 25 years indicated that today's children do not select snacks that are higher in kcalories than children in past years but they eat more snacks more often, which has added to their energy intakes.[61] An important message to children should be to snack only when they are hungry; snacking should not be a pastime, and the best snacks are those that are relatively low in kcalories but rich in protein, vitamins, and minerals.

Sound nutrition is especially critical for the child athlete. Children ages 6 to 12 years engaged in athletic competition need appropriate nutritional advice from parents, coaches, and trained professionals to meet their energy, protein, and fluid needs for training and competition.[62]

Summary Principles

Growth slows during the school-age years, yet development rapidly continues. Individual and group learning experiences greatly influence the individual. The following two principles should be considered when working with school-age children:

1. Energy needs decline; however, the quality of the diet is essential to provide the minerals and vitamins essential to school performance and physical demands.
2. The school and home environments must be conducive to assisting 6- to 12-year-olds with making appropriate food and activity choices. These choices should be based on sound evidence related to nutritional needs of the school-age individual.

The Adolescent

Physical Characteristics and Growth

During the adolescent period, with the onset of puberty, the final growth spurt of childhood occurs. Maturation during this time varies so widely that chronologic age as a reference point for discussing growth ceases to be useful. **Physiologic age** becomes more important in dealing with individual boys and girls. Adolescent growth accounts for wide fluctuations in physical size, metabolic

> **physiologic age** Rate of biologic maturation in individual adolescents that varies widely and accounts more for wide and changing differences in their metabolic rates, nutritional needs, and food requirements than does chronologic age.

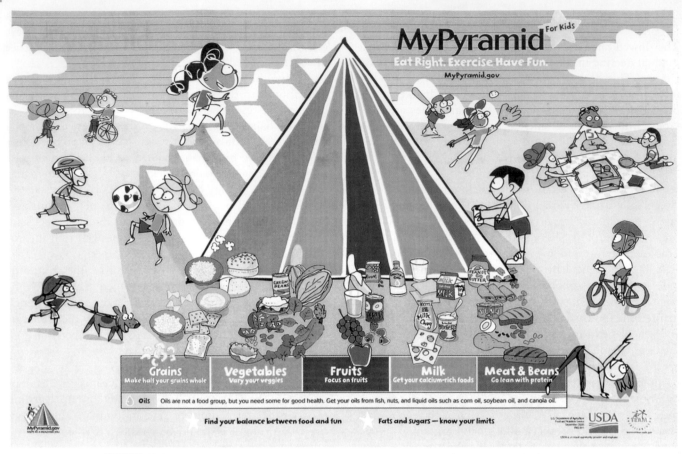

FIGURE 12-4 MyPyramid for Kids for younger children. *(From U.S. Department of Agriculture, Food and Nutrition Service: MyPyramid for Kids, FNS-381, Washington, DC, 2005, U.S. Government Printing Office.)*

rate, food needs, and even illness. These capacities can be more realistically viewed only in terms of physiologic growth.

The profound body changes occurring in the adolescent result from the release of estrogen and testosterone, the sex steroid hormones that regulate the development of the sex characteristics. The rate at which these body changes occur varies widely and is particularly distinct in the growth patterns that emerge between the sexes. In girls, the amount of subcutaneous fat increases, and the hip breadth widens in preparation for childbearing. This fat accumulation and change in body shape are often sources of anxiety to many figure-conscious young girls. In adolescent boys, physical growth is manifested by an increased muscle mass and long bone growth. The growth spurt in boys is slower than that in girls, but he soon passes her in weight and height.

Psychosocial and Motor Development

Adolescence is an ambivalent period marked by stresses and strains. On the one hand, teenagers look back to the securities of childhood; on the other hand, they reach for the maturity of adulthood. Emergence of a self-identity is

the major psychosocial developmental task of the adolescent years. The search for self, begun in early childhood, reaches its peak. The profound body changes associated with sexual development and the capability of reproduction also result in changes in body image and resulting tensions in maturing girls and boys. Motor development and skilled coordination is complete.

The identity crisis of the adolescent years, largely revolving around sexual development and preparation for an adult role in a complex society, produces many psychologic, emotional, and social pressures. Although the period of most rapid physical growth is relatively short, only 2 or 3 years, the attendant psychosocial development continues over a much longer period. The pressure for peer group acceptance is strong, and fads in dress and food habits play out this theme. Also, in a technologically developed society such as the United States, high values are placed on education and achievement. Social tensions and family conflicts are often created. These conflicts may have nutritional consequences as teenagers eat away from home more often and develop snacking patterns reflective of personal and peer-group choices.

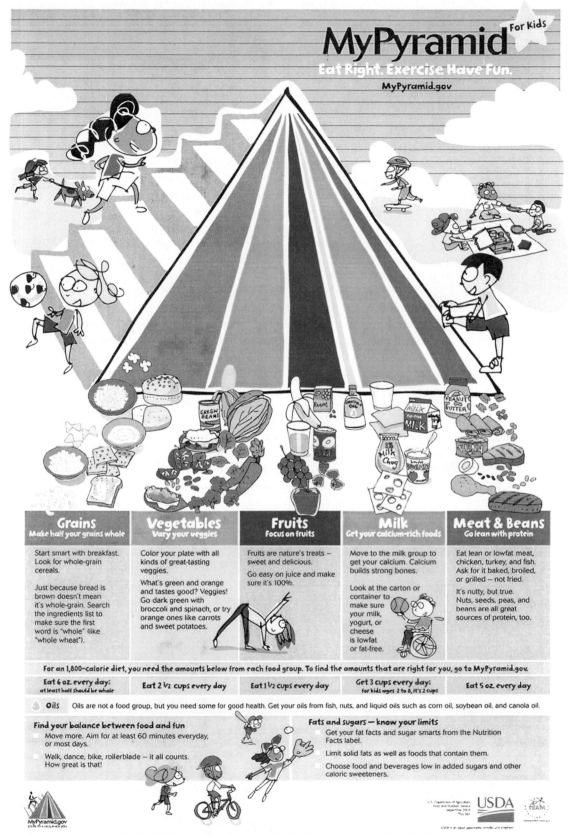

FIGURE 12-4, cont'd MyPyramid for Kids, a detailed image for older children.

Food and Feeding

With the rapid growth of adolescence comes increased demands for energy, protein, vitamins, and minerals, as follows:

- *Energy:* The kcalorie needs increase with the metabolic demands of growth and energy expenditure. Although individual needs may vary, girls require fewer kcalories than boys, based on their smaller body size and body composition.[4] Sometimes the large appetite, characteristic of this rapid growth period, leads adolescents to satisfy their hunger with snack foods that are high in sugar and fat and low in essential protein, vitamins, and minerals.

- *Protein:* Adolescent growth needs for protein increase to support the pubertal changes in both sexes and the developing muscle mass in boys. Girls require 46 g/day, and boys require 52 g/day to sustain daily needs and to maintain nitrogen reserves.[4]

- *Minerals:* The calcium requirement for all adolescents rises to 1300 mg/day to meet the demands of bone growth. In fact, adolescence is a critical time for the development of bone mass under the influence of the increasing levels of the sex hormones, especially estrogen. Poor bone mineralization in adolescence increases vulnerability to bone fracture at later ages.[63] Menses and consequent iron losses in the adolescent girl predispose her to simple iron deficiency anemia. Young female athletes who begin training before menarche and develop secondary amenorrhea may in turn have reduced bone mineral density resulting from low estrogen levels.[64] For all young athletes, fluid replacement in any exercise or performance period is essential.[62]

- *Vitamins:* The B vitamins are needed in increased amounts to meet the extra demands of energy metabolism and tissue development. Intakes of vitamins C and A may be low because of erratic food intake and low intake of vegetables and fruits. A high prevalence of folate deficiency exists among adolescent girls, increasing the risk of neural tube defects in babies born to teenage mothers. (For a review of neural tube defects see Chapter 6.)

In the development of nutrition intervention programs for teens, it is important to consider their cultural and ethnic backgrounds, recognizing that food habits and problems may differ (see the *Case Study* box, "Nutrition Program for Adolescents"). A study of more than 2800 adolescents that included Vietnamese, Hispanic, black, and white students showed clearly that intakes of fruits, vegetables, and dairy products differed according to group.[65] The Vietnamese adolescents were the least likely to meet the recommended three servings of dairy products each day compared with the black, Hispanic, or white adolescents. Conversely, the Vietnamese students were the most likely to meet the goal of five fruits and vegetables a day. We also need to consider cost when making nutritional recommendations to students or parents. Among limited-resource mothers, fruits and some vegetables were perceived as being less filling, and one mother noted it was more important to have her son's hunger satisfied than to provide particular fruits or vegetables.[66] Nutrition counseling must be individualized, taking into consideration both cultural food preferences and other circumstances existing within the family.

Eating Habits

Physical and psychosocial pressures influence adolescent eating behavior (see the *To Probe Further* box, "Food

---

CASE STUDY

Nutrition Program for Adolescents

Amanda is a graduate student of clinical nutrition assigned to the "Save Our Senior High" project in a metropolitan community of 300,000 located in northwestern United States. A representative of the city's educational advisory board approached her institution for assistance in developing a program that addresses three major problems faced by the majority of high school students: (1) popularity of fad diets among athletes, (2) overweight, and (3) iron deficiency anemia.

Amanda and other members of her class met with students who were learning other health professions (medicine, dentistry, nutrition, nursing, social work), as well as several student representatives from the high school, to plan the program. After they developed goals and objectives, they decided that the nutrition topics would be addressed in a series of workshops entitled "Nutrition and Physical Fitness," "Food for the Teen Years," and "Snack Facts."

The program was introduced to the students through an advance bulletin distributed at the largest high school in the city, where the project was to begin. The bulletin included an article written by Amanda: "Teenage Nutrition: A Seeming Paradox." This article responded to a common concern expressed by adolescents: the apparent preoccupation of school officials with the students' food habits when they, as a group, looked and usually felt very healthy.

Amanda's article stirred a tremendous interest in the student population. Attendance at each session was high, and the discussions were lively. The evaluation results were positive. In reviewing the evaluative data and low cost of the project, the city council asked Amanda and her classmates to repeat the program at two other high schools where these problems were also prevalent. The council approached the school board about the possibility of including the project in the citywide high school curriculum for the coming year.

Questions for Analysis

1. Outline the content of Amanda's article to reflect major points that you would have included.

2. Write a class outline for each workshop, including objectives, major topics, and questions you would expect from the students. What teaching methods and materials would you expect to be most effective in each workshop?

3. What outside influences on eating habits would you expect in this student population? How effective would you expect this educational program to be in influencing a change of behavior in eating habits?

4. Aside from in-school nutrition education programs, describe possible tactics for influencing the eating habits of teenagers.

Habits of Adolescents: Where Do We Begin?"). By and large, boys fare better than girls. Their large appetites and the sheer volumes of food they consume usually ensure generally adequate nutrient intakes, but the adolescent girl may be less fortunate. The following two factors combine to increase issues surrounding nutrition and food intake in adolescent girls:

1. *Physiologic sex difference:* Because sexual maturation in girls brings about increased fat deposition during the adolescent growth period and because many teenage girls are relatively inactive, it is easy for them to gain weight.
2. *Social and personal tensions:* Social pressures dictating thinness sometimes cause adolescent girls to follow unwise and self-imposed diets for weight loss. In some cases actual self-starvation regimens lead to complex and far-reaching eating disorders such as anorexia nervosa and bulimia nervosa (see Chapter 5). These problems, which can assume severe proportions, usually involve a distorted self-image and an irrational pursuit of thinness, even when actual body weight is normal or even below age norms. In the absence of described eating disorders, constant dieting can still result in varying degrees of poor nutrition in the teenage girl at the very time in life when her body needs to be building reserves for potential reproduction. The harmful effects that bad eating habits can have on the future course of a pregnancy are clearly indicated in many studies relating preconception nutrition status to the outcome of gestation (see Chapter 11).

Summary Principles

The following two principles should be considered when intervening with food habits during adolescence:

1. Nutrient demands are high for final growth and development. The quality of the diet is vital (Figure 12-5).

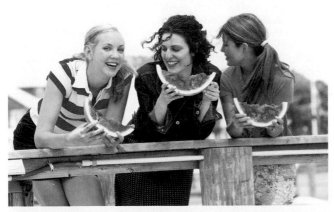

FIGURE 12-5 Fruits and vegetables help meet the high nutrient demands during adolescence. *(Copyright 2006 JupiterImages Corporation.)*

2. Food choices and eating patterns may be less than optimal due to the many influential factors that impact choices during adolescence.

Health Promotion

Children and Adolescents: Seeking Fitness

The *Dietary Guidelines for Americans 2005* provides direction for the development of a healthy diet and lifestyle for all persons aged 2 years and older.[67] The 2005 edition set goals for not only food patterns in all age-groups but also appropriate physical activity. Many chronic diseases that influence well-being in later life actually begin in childhood. Thus lifestyle practices that promote healthy behaviors related to diet and physical activity must be introduced at an early age when patterns are being developed that will continue for a lifetime.

Weight Management

Body weight and physical activity are intrinsically related. A regular pattern of exercise beginning in childhood will promote lifelong heart health and prevent the accumulation of excess body fat. Large numbers of U.S. children are overweight, and the numbers continue to climb. Among 5000 children between the ages of 9 and 11, the proportion classified as overweight increased by 11% during a 2 year period.[68] There also appear to be racial, ethnic, and regional differences in overweight among children. Boys, blacks, Hispanics, and those living in the southern states are more likely to be overweight.[68] High-energy diets coupled with inactivity patterns leading to increased body fat are associated with the growing incidence of type 2 diabetes in children of school age.

Body fat increases rapidly during the first year of life and then slows until about age 6, when again there is a normal increase in both the size and number of body fat cells. For some children, an inappropriate accumulation of body fat begins about this time or even earlier. This addition of body fat can be accelerated by a high energy intake in relation to energy needs or a sedentary life pattern with low energy expenditure. Although there are differences in opinion on this matter, several experts suggest that children who are overweight do not consume more kcalories than normal-weight children but rather are less physically active. The best insurance to prevent inappropriate accumulation of body fat in a child of any age is regular physical activity. The goal is to promote body weight gain within healthy ranges to support normal growth and development.[67] In overweight children and adolescents the goal is to slow gains in body weight while promoting optimal growth and development.[5]

TO PROBE FURTHER

FOOD HABITS OF ADOLESCENTS: WHERE DO WE BEGIN?

Adolescents who have entered their growth spurt seem to eat all the time. The questions for health professionals are "What are they eating?" and "How do we go about making it better?" Both quantity and quality of food are important during this period of rapid growth. Lean body mass increases by about 35 kg in boys and 19 kg in girls over these years, and 45% of total bone mass is accrued. Generous supplies of iron, zinc, calcium, and essential vitamins are needed to support these changes in body size and development.

Food Intake in the Teen Years

Despite the critical nutrient needs in this life stage, national dietary surveys indicate that of all age-groups, teens have the poorest diets. Their intakes of calcium, iron, zinc, vitamin A, and folate often fall below recommended levels. Although on the average teens eat 3 or 4 servings of vegetables each day, 1 or 2 of these servings are potatoes, most likely french fries; dark green and deep yellow vegetables are eaten infrequently. Boys and girls between the ages of 12 and 19 years eat about 1½ servings of fruit each day, and about half comes from citrus sources. From the dairy group boys have only 2½ servings and girls only 1½ servings each day, which will not meet a teen's need for calcium (1 dairy serving = 300 mg calcium). At the same time, most adolescents are exceeding their need for protein. Foods such as hamburgers, pizza with cheese, tacos, and milkshakes, popular among teens, are good sources of protein. Foods high in sugar such as soft drinks and candy and items high in fat, including pastries, fatty meats, and fried foods, are eaten regularly by many teens. Both boys and girls obtain 20% of their kcalories from added sugars, 33% from fat, and 13% from saturated fat. Twenty-one percent of adolescents use vitamin-mineral supplements, but the supplement users have better diets and obtain higher intakes of nutrients from food. Teens also indulge in risk-taking behaviors: about one third smoke, and 28% of girls and 35% of boys report at least one episode of binge drinking per month.

Lifestyle and Nutritional Behavior

Lifestyle choices in the teen years are influenced by peer pressure and teens' growing need to express their independence and make their own decisions. Teens also lead busy lives with school, sports, and jobs. Focus-group interviews with teens in Minnesota indicated that (1) food taste and appeal, (2) time, and (3) convenience were the three most important factors influencing their food choices. They liked foods that looked good and chose the same foods over and over because they knew how they were going to taste. Foods such as pastries and other high-sugar or high-fat items were perceived as tasting better than more healthy foods such as fruits, vegetables, or dairy products. Fast-food restaurants are popular because the food is served quickly. Teens often skip breakfast. Individuals in this age-group do not want to spend time preparing food or cleaning up afterward. Food items must be easy to prepare or ready-to-eat, easy to eat on the go or carry in a backpack, or delivered to the house.

Unfortunately, health is often not an important personal issue at this life stage. A feeling of invulnerability and the idea that they have plenty of time in future years to worry about their health are common in teens. At the same time, body weight and appearance are major concerns for 49% of girls and 43% of boys. The need to be thin causes some adolescent girls to adopt nutritionally inadequate diets or, worse, develop anorexia or bulimia nervosa (see Chapter 5). Adolescent boys trying to increase their muscle mass or "bulk up" may resort to unproven and potentially dangerous supplements or eat high-fat foods in an effort to obtain more kcalories. When working with teens who claim to be dieting, it is necessary to talk with them individually about what kind of diet they are following. For some teens dieting means drastically reducing their food intake or choosing foods erroneously believed to have special effects on appearance; for others, dieting refers to healthful practices like increasing their intakes of fruits and vegetables or cutting down on fats and sweets.

How Do We Help Teens Improve Their Food Choices?

Improving the food choices of this age-group will require the combined efforts of parents, health professionals, food manufacturers, restaurant personnel, and food retailers. An important message to teens is that appropriate food choices along with regular physical activity can help to achieve and maintain (1) a healthy weight and positive level of fitness, (2) a high energy level for school and work, and (3) an overall sense of well-being. Physical education and health teachers, nutrition educators, athletic coaches, school nurses, and parents must work together to develop programs that will reach teens at school and on the playing field.

Teens want information that they can use now, not 10 years from now. One topic of immediate use would be selecting a lower-fat or lower-kcalorie meal at a fast-food restaurant or choosing a more healthy pizza for home delivery. Snacks such as bananas, oranges, or apples; plastic containers of juice; or individual packages of ready-to-eat cereal travel well in a backpack, as do new ultrapasteurized milk drinks that do not require refrigeration. Simple-to-prepare or carry-along breakfasts such as ready-to-eat cereal or bread or a bagel with peanut butter could be encouraged. Among junior high school students, ready-to-eat cereals provided a breakfast that was lower in cost, lower in fat, and higher in important nutrients including calcium, iron, vitamins A and D, and folate than fast-food breakfast meals, granola, or toaster pastries.

Because taste is the most important factor in food selection for teens, it is important that healthy foods taste good. School cafeteria managers need to produce good-tasting and satisfying food that is attractively served. This means that the school meal must be viewed as an extension of the school's educational mission and supported by both teachers and parents. Salad bars have become popular among some teens, and salads to go might meet the need of both taste and convenience. Recipes that are reduced in fat and sugar but pleasing in taste and texture need to be developed for quantity food programs.

Food manufacturers must be urged to improve the nutrient quality of ready-to-eat main dishes as well as snack foods. Taste-testing parties with teens that compare lower-fat or reduced-sugar items with the less-nutritious product may help to dispel the myth that healthy foods do not taste good. Many popular foods among teens such as pizza or tacos can be exceedingly healthy foods with attention to reducing the levels of ingredients high in fat and saturated fat.

Finally, food retailers who cater to the teen audience must be urged to both sell and advertise healthy foods. Some fast-food restaurants include orange juice or low-fat milk as drink options in combination meals, as an alternative to soft drinks. Salads are an option at many fast-food outlets, and baked potatoes may be available as an alternative to french-fried potatoes. Advertisements for soft drinks or less-healthy food items often carry the endorsements of popular sports stars. Such endorsements have been applied to foods such as milk that are important to health and well-being. Community coalitions involving health professionals, educators, and parents con-

TO PROBE FURTHER—cont'd

FOOD HABITS OF ADOLESCENTS: WHERE DO WE BEGIN?

cerned about adolescents and their future health will be necessary to bring about needed changes.

References

Dixon LB et al: Let the pyramid guide your food choices: capturing the total diet concept, *J Nutr* 131(suppl 2):461S, 2001.

Dwyer JT et al: Do adolescent vitamin-mineral supplement users have better nutrient intakes than nonusers? Observations from the CATCH tracking study, *J Am Diet Assoc* 101(11):1340, 2001.

Hampl JS, Betts NM: Cigarette use during adolescence: effects on nutritional status, *Nutr Rev* 57(7):215, 1999.

Kleinman RE, ed: *Pediatric nutrition handbook,* ed 4, Elk Grove Village, Ill, 1998, American Academy of Pediatrics.

Neumark-Sztainer D et al: Are family meal patterns associated with disordered eating behaviors among adolescents? *J Adolesc Health* 35(5):350, 2004.

Neumark-Sztainer D et al: Factors influencing food choices of adolescents: findings from focus-group discussions with adolescents, *J Am Diet Assoc* 99(8):929, 1999.

Nicklas TA et al: Efficiency of breakfast consumption patterns of ninth graders: nutrient-to-cost comparisons, *J Am Diet Assoc* 102(2):226, 2002.

O'Dea JA: Children and adolescents identify food concerns, forbidden foods, and food-related beliefs, *J Am Diet Assoc* 99(8):970, 1999.

Physical Activity

Although children and adolescents are more active than most adults, many of our youth appear to be settling into a sedentary lifestyle that is common among adults.[69] We know that 48% of girls and 26% of boys do not exercise vigorously on a regular basis.[69] Schools now offer fewer physical education opportunities to students, and over the past decade, daily participation in physical education dropped to 29%, although about half of all youth have such classes at least once each week.[69] Television, computer games, the Internet, and similar sedentary pastimes are growing in popularity. Watching television for more than 2 hours per day during childhood is related to overweight and the presence of other risk factors for chronic diseases.[70] The goal is to have children and adolescents engage in a minimum of 1 hour of exercise, every day. This exercise need only be of moderate intensity.

Helping Children Develop an Active Lifestyle

Parents and caregivers, schools, and communities need to work together to increase physical activity among children.[71] Children are more likely to develop an active lifestyle if parents and role models also demonstrate such behavior. Taking your teddy bear for a walk can be a meaningful activity for a preschooler who belongs to a family that walks together regularly. School games and physical education programs should focus on activities such as walking or running that allow all students to participate, rather than on games in which several students are active but the majority sit and watch. Moving away from competitive games that discourage participation by overweight or less skilled players to such activities as kick ball or dancing or aerobics that can be done alone to music or in groups after school are worthwhile objectives for physical education. Bike riding and jumping rope are good forms of vigorous exercise. Making school facilities such as a gymnasium or walking track available to families and students after school hours might encourage a higher level of physical activity. Figure 12-6 illustrates guidelines regarding activity levels for children of all ages.

TO SUM UP

Normal growth and development depend on nutrition to support heightened physiologic and metabolic processes. Nutrition, in turn, depends on a multitude of social, psychosocial, cultural, and environmental influences that affect individual growth potential throughout the life cycle.

Four types of growth interact during each phase of development: (1) physical, (2) mental, (3) emotional, and (4) sociocultural. Each type of growth must be evaluated when assessing the child's nutrition status and planning an effective counseling approach. Nutritional needs change with each growth period and must be individualized according to the unique growth pattern of every child.

Infants experience rapid growth. They have immature digestive systems and limited ability to absorb and excrete metabolites efficiently. Breast-feeding is preferred during the first year of life. Solid foods are not needed, nor can they be adequately tolerated, until 4 to 6 months of age.

Toddlers (ages 1 to 3 years), preschoolers (ages 3 to 6 years), and school-age children (ages 6 to 12 years) experience the slowed and erratic latent growth of childhood. Their energy requirements per unit of body weight are not as great as those of infants. Their nutritional needs center on protein for growth with attendant minerals and vitamins. Social and cultural factors influence the development of food habits in these age-groups. Appropriate food behavior by parents and caregivers that can be modeled by children of these ages strongly influences the adoption of good eating habits during these periods of development.

Adolescents (ages 12 to 18 years) experience the second large growth spurt before reaching adulthood. This rapid growth involves both sexual maturation and

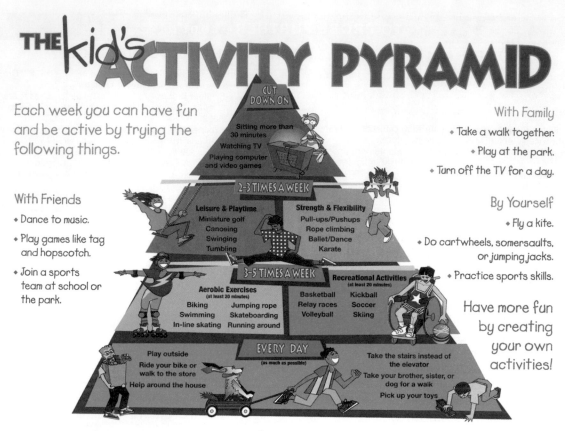

FIGURE 12-6   The Activity Pyramid. *(Copyright © 2003 Park Nicollet HealthSource, Minneapolis, U.S.A., 1-888-637-2675. Reprinted with permission.)*

physical growth. During this period girls increase their body proportion of fat, whereas boys increase their body proportion of muscle. Reaching peak bone mass is an important milestone for both sexes during this period of development. In general, the increased kcaloric and nutrient needs of adolescence are more easily achieved by boys, who consume larger amounts of food. In contrast, girls, who may feel social and peer pressure to restrict food intake to avoid weight gain, are less likely to meet their optimal nutrient requirements for growth. This pressure may also inhibit their ability to acquire the nutritional reserves necessary for later reproduction.

QUESTIONS FOR REVIEW

1. How is physical growth measured? What are the NCHS growth charts, and how are they used? What are the limitations of these charts? What are some clinical, biochemical, and dietary measures that are helpful in assessing the nutritional status of infants and children?
2. Describe the physical and psychosocial characteristics of the newborn. What are the capabilities of the newborn's digestive and renal systems, and how do they relate to infant feeding?
3. Why is breast-feeding the preferred method for feeding infants (discuss both nutritional and psychosocial factors)?

Describe the anatomic and hormonal components that participate in the delivery of breast milk to the nursing infant.
4. You are planning a nutrition education class to prepare pregnant mothers for breast-feeding. Outline the material that you would present, including (a) dietary needs for the new breast-feeding mother, (b) techniques for holding and feeding the baby, and (c) nipple care.
5. You are counseling a pregnant mother who has decided not to breast-feed. Describe some types of commercial formulas that would provide an appropriate alternative feeding for her infant. Describe the feeding techniques that will be important in meeting the psychosocial needs of her infant.
6. You are working with a mother whose newborn has been found to be allergic to milk proteins. What might be an appropriate food source for this infant?
7. You are working with a low-income mother who has chosen not to breast-feed. She is concerned about the high cost of infant formula and would like to feed her infant cow's milk because it is cheaper. What would you tell her?
8. Outline a general schedule for a new mother to use as a guide for adding solid foods to her infant's diet during the first year of life; indicate both the time of addition and the items to be offered.
9. What changes in physical growth and psychosocial development influence eating habits in the (a) toddler, (b) preschool

child, and (c) school-age child? How do these factors influence the nutritional needs of each age-group?

10. What factors influence the changing nutritional needs of adolescents? Who is usually at greater nutritional risk during this stage—boys or girls? Why? What nutritional deficiencies may be associated with this vulnerable age?

11. You are the director of a school food service program in an elementary school and want to start a nutrition education program. You are working with a science teacher, a social studies teacher, and the school nurse to develop lessons that will connect learning in the classroom with good nutrition in the lunchroom. Visit the U.S. Department of Agriculture's Food and Nutrition Information Center website for Team Nutrition at *www.fns.usda.gov/tn* to find some ideas and materials that will assist you in this project. Develop a lesson plan for presentation in the science or social studies class that focuses on nutrition or food patterns, and indicate how you will connect this lesson with the lunch program.

REFERENCES

1. Chumlea WC, Guo SS: Physical growth and development. In Samour PQ et al, eds: *Handbook of pediatric nutrition,* ed 2, Gaithersburg, Md, 1999, Aspen Publishers.
2. Kuczmarski RJ et al: *CDC growth charts: United States, advance data, vital and health statistics,* No. 314, Hyattsville, Md, 2000, Centers for Disease Control and Prevention.
3. Strauss RS, Pollack HA: Epidemic increase in childhood overweight, 1986-1998, *JAMA* 286(22):2845, 2001.
4. Food and Nutrition Board, Institute of Medicine: *Dietary Reference Intakes for energy, carbohydrate, fiber, fat, fatty acids, cholesterol, protein, and amino acids (macronutrients),* Washington, DC, 2002, National Academies Press.
5. Kleinman RE, ed: *Pediatric nutrition handbook,* ed 4, Elk Grove Village, Ill, 1998, American Academy of Pediatrics.
6. Food and Nutrition Board, Institute of Medicine: *Dietary References Intakes for water, potassium, sodium, chloride, and sulfate,* Washington, DC, 2004, National Academies Press.
7. Holst M-C: Developmental and behavioral effects of iron deficiency anemia in infants, *Nutr Today* 33(1):27, 1998.
8. Hurtado EK et al: Early childhood anemia and mild or moderate mental retardation, *Am J Clin Nutr* 69(1):115, 1999.
9. Partington S et al: The prevalence of anemia in a WIC population: a comparison by homeless experience, *J Am Diet Assoc* 100(4):469, 2000.
10. Erikson E: *Childhood and society,* New York, 1963, WW Norton.
11. Klawitter BM: Nutrition counseling. In Samour PQ et al, eds: *Handbook of pediatric nutrition,* ed 2, Gaithersburg, Md, 1999, Aspen Publishers.
12. Position of the American Dietetic Association: Breaking the barriers to breastfeeding, *J Am Diet Assoc* 101(10):1213, 2001.
13. Pettifor JM: Nutritional rickets: deficiency of vitamin D, calcium, or both? *Am J Clin Nutr* 80(6, suppl):1725S, 2004.
14. Fomon SJ: Feeding normal infants: rationale for recommendations, *J Am Diet Assoc* 101(9):1002, 2001.
15. Akers SM, Groh-Wargo SL: Normal nutrition during infancy. In Samour PQ et al, eds: *Handbook of pediatric nutrition,* ed 2, Gaithersburg, Md, 1999, Aspen Publishers.
16. Philipp BL, Merewood A: The baby-friendly way: the best breastfeeding start, *Pediatr Clin North Am* 51(3):761, 2004.
17. Chalmers B: The Baby Friendly Hospital Initiative: where next? *BJOG,* 111(3):198, 2004.
18. Philipp BL et al: Sustained breastfeeding rates at a U.S. baby-friendly hospital, *Pediatrics* 112:234, 2003.
19. McCrory MA: Does dieting during lactation put infant growth at risk? *Nutr Rev* 59(1, part 1):18, 2001.
20. Fisher JO et al: Breast-feeding through the first year predicts maternal control in feeding and subsequent toddler energy intakes, *J Am Diet Assoc* 100(6):641, 2000.
21. Hediger ML et al: Early infant feeding and growth status of U.S.-born infants and children aged 4-71 mo: analyses from the third National Health and Nutrition Examination Survey, 1988-1994, *Am J Clin Nutr* 72(1):159, 2000.
22. Desage M et al: Gas chromatographic-mass spectrometric method to characterize the transfer of dietary odorous compounds into plasma and milk, *J Chromatogr B Biomed Appl* 678(2):205, 1996.
23. Mennella JA, Beauchamp GK: Experience with a flavor in mother's milk modifies the infant's acceptance of flavored cereal, *Dev Psychobiol* 35(3):197, 1999.
24. Mennella JA et al: Flavor programming during infancy, *Pediatrics* 113(4):840, 2004.
25. Hediger ML et al: Association between infant breastfeeding and overweight in young children, *JAMA* 285(19):2453, 2001.
26. Stettler N et al: Infant weight gain and childhood overweight status in a multicenter, cohort study, *Pediatrics* 109(2):194, 2002.
27. Butte NF et al: Infant feeding mode affects early growth and body composition, *Pediatrics* 106(6):1355, 2000.
28. Humphrey J, Iliff P: Is breast not best? Feeding babies born to HIV-positive mothers: bringing balance to a complex issue, *Nutr Rev* 59(4):119, 2001.
29. Koo WW: Efficacy and safety of docosahexaenoic acid and arachidonic acid addition to infant formulas: can one buy better vision and intelligence? *J Am Coll Nutr* 22(2):101, 2003.
30. Williams C et al: Stereoacuity at age 3.5 y in children born full-term is associated with prenatal and postnatal dietary factors: a report from a population-based cohort study, *Am J Clin Nutr* 73(2):316, 2001.
31. Uauy R et al: Term infant studies of DHA and ARA supplementation on neurodevelopment: results of randomized controlled trials, *J Pediatr* 143(suppl 4l):S17, 2003.
32. Auestad N et al: Visual, cognitive, and language assessments at 39 months: a follow-up study of children fed formulas containing long-chain polyunsaturated fatty acids to 1 year of age, *Pediatrics* 112(3, part 1):E177, 2003.
33. Hoffman DR et al: Visual function in breast-fed term infants weaned to formula with or without long-chain polyunsaturates at 4 to 6 months: a randomized clinical trial, *J Pediatr* 142(6):669, 2003.
34. Innis SM et al: Docosahexaenoic acid and arachidonic acid enhance growth with no adverse effects in preterm infants fed formula, *J Pediatr* 140(5):547, 2002.
35. American Academy of Pediatrics, Committee on Nutrition: Hypoallergenic infant formulas, *Pediatrics* 106(2, part 1):346, 2000.
36. American Academy of Pediatrics, Committee on Nutrition: Soy protein–based formulas: recommendations for use in infant feeding, *Pediatrics* 101(1, part 1):148, 1998.
37. Sharpless KE et al: Certification of nutrients in Standard Reference Material 1846: infant formula, *J AOAC Int* 80(3):611, 1997.

38. Fewtrell MS et al: Catch-up growth in small-for-gestational-age term infants: a randomized trial, *Am J Clin Nutr* 74(4):516, 2001.

39. Fomon SJ: Infant feeding in the 20th century: formula and beikost, *J Nutr* 131(2):409S, 2001.

40. Kannan S et al: Cultural influences on infant feeding beliefs of mothers, *J Am Diet Assoc* 99(1):88, 1999.

41. Bronner YL et al: Early introduction of solid foods among urban African-American participants in WIC, *J Am Diet Assoc* 99(4):457, 1999.

42. Birch LL: Development of food preferences, *Annu Rev Nutr* 19:41, 1999.

43. Gerrish CJ, Mennella JA: Flavor variety enhances food acceptance in formula-fed infants, *Am J Clin Nutr* 73(6):1080, 2001.

44. Briley ME et al: Dietary intake at child-care centers and away: are parents and care providers working as partners or at cross-purposes? *J Am Diet Assoc* 99(8):950, 1999.

45. Skinner JD et al: Longitudinal study of nutrient and food intakes of white preschool children aged 24 to 60 months, *J Am Diet Assoc* 99(12):1514, 1999.

46. Nicklas TA et al: Family and child-care provider influences on preschool children's fruit, juice, and vegetable consumption, *Nutr Rev* 59(7):224, 2001.

47. Fisher JO et al: Maternal milk consumption predicts the tradeoff between milk and soft drinks in young girls' diets, *J Nutr* 131(2):246, 2001.

48. Tibbs T et al: The relationship between parental modeling, eating patterns, and dietary intake among African-American parents, *J Am Diet Assoc* 101(5):535, 2001.

49. Rolls BJ et al: Serving portion size influences 5-year-old but not 3-year-old children's food intakes, *J Am Diet Assoc* 100(2):232, 2000.

50. Position of the American Dietetic Association: Dietary guidance for healthy children aged 2 to 11 years, *J Am Diet Assoc* 104(4):660, 2004.

51. Borzekowski DLG, Robinson TN: The 30-second effect: an experiment revealing the impact of television commercials on food preferences of preschoolers, *J Am Diet Assoc* 101(1):42, 2001.

52. Kleinman RE et al: Diet, breakfast, and academic performance in children, *Annu Nutr Metab* 46(suppl 1):24, 2002.

53. Pollitt E, Mathews R: Breakfast and cognition: an integrative summary, *Am J Clin Nutr* 67(4):804S, 1998.

54. Gross SM, Cinelli B: Coordinated school health program and dietetics professionals: partners in promoting healthful eating, *J Am Diet Assoc* 104(5):793, 2004.

55. Kennedy E, Davis C: U.S. Department of Agriculture school breakfast program, *Am J Clin Nutr* 67(4):798S, 1998.

56. Friedman BJ et al: Texas school menu compliance with U.S. Dietary Guidelines for Americans, *J Am Diet Assoc* 98(11):1325, 1998.

57. Friedman BJ, Hurd-Crixell SL: Nutrient intake of children eating school breakfast, *J Am Diet Assoc* 99(2):219, 1999.

58. Rankin LL, Bingham M: Acceptability of oatmeal chocolate chip cookies prepared using pureed white beans as a fat ingredient substitute, *J Am Diet Assoc* 100(7):831, 2000.

59. Cullen KW et al: Effect of a la carte and snack bar foods at school on children's lunchtime intake of fruits and vegetables, *J Am Diet Assoc* 100(12):1482, 2000.

60. Melnick TA et al: Food consumption patterns of elementary school-children in New York City, *J Am Diet Assoc* 98(2):159, 1998.

61. Jahns L et al: The increasing prevalence of snacking among U.S. children from 1977 to 1996, *J Pediatr* 138(4):493, 2001.

62. Position of Dietitians of Canada, the American Dietetic Association, and the American College of Sports Medicine: Nutrition and athletic performance, *Can J Diet Pract Res* 61(4):176, 2000.

63. Wosje KS, Specker BL: Role of calcium in bone health during childhood, *Nutr Rev* 58(9):253, 2000.

64. Beals KA, Manore MM: Nutritional status of female athletes with subclinical eating disorders, *J Am Diet Assoc* 98(4):419, 1998.

65. Wiecha JM et al: Differences in dietary patterns of Vietnamese, white, African-American, and Hispanic adolescents in Worcester, Mass, *J Am Diet Assoc* 101(2):248, 2001.

66. Hampl JS, Sass S: Focus groups indicate that vegetable and fruit consumption by food stamp–eligible Hispanics is affected by children and unfamiliarity with non-traditional foods, *J Am Diet Assoc* 101(6):685, 2001.

67. U.S. Department of Health and Human Services, U.S. Department of Agriculture: *Dietary Guidelines for Americans 2005,* ed 6, Washington, DC, 2005, U.S. Government Printing Office. Available at *www.healthierus.gov/dietaryguidelines.*

68. Dwyer JT et al: Prevalence of marked overweight and obesity in a multiethnic pediatric population: findings from the Child and Adolescent Trial for Cardiovascular Health (CATCH) study, *J Am Diet Assoc* 100(10):1149, 2000.

69. Troiano RP et al: Be physically active each day: how can we know? *J Nutr* 131(2, suppl1):451S, 2001.

70. Hancox RJ et al: Association between child and adolescent television viewing and adult health: a longitudinal birth cohort study, *Lancet* 364(9430):257, 2004.

71. Veugelers PJ, Fitzgerald AL: Effectiveness of school programs in preventing childhood obesity: a multilevel comparison, *Am J Public Health* 95(3):432, 2005.

FURTHER READINGS AND RESOURCES

Readings

Auestad N et al: Visual, cognitive, and language assessments at 39 months: a follow-up study of children fed formulas containing long-chain polyunsaturated fatty acids to 1 year of age, *Pediatrics* 112(3, part 1):E177, 2003.

Hoffman DR et al: Visual function in breast-fed term infants weaned to formula with or without long-chain polyunsaturates at 4 to 6 months: a randomized clinical trial, *J Pediatr* 142(6):669, 2003.

Koo WW: Efficacy and safety of docosahexaenoic acid and arachidonic acid addition to infant formulas: can one buy better vision and intelligence? *J Am Coll Nutr* 22(2):101, 2003.

Uauy R et al: Term infant studies of DHA and ARA supplementation on neurodevelopment: results of randomized controlled trials, *J Pediatr* 143(suppl 4):S17, 2003.

Is it possible that the addition of docosahexaenoic acid (DHA) and arachidonic acid (ARA) to infant formula increases neurodevelopment, visual acuity, and language skills? Evidence from randomized clinical trials prompted the Food and Drug Administration to approve the inclusion of these long-chain polyunsaturated fatty acids into infant formula.

Dwyer J: Should dietary fat recommendations for children be changed? *J Am Diet Assoc* 100(1):36, 2000.

Krebs NF, Johnson SL: Guidelines for healthy children: promoting eating, moving, and common sense, *J Am Diet Assoc* 100(1):37, 2000.

Satter E: A moderate view on fat restriction for young children, *J Am Diet Assoc* 100(1):32, 2000.

The increasing incidence of overweight in children and concern for the prevention of chronic diseases later in life have led to a discussion about the optimum level of dietary fat for children. These articles discuss this controversy.

Briley ME et al: Dietary intake at child-care centers and away: are parents and care providers working as partners or at cross-purposes? *J Am Diet Assoc* 99(8):950, 1999.

Florencio CA: Developments and variations in school-based feeding programs around the world, *Nutr Today* 36(1):29, 2001.

Gable S, Lutz S: Nutrition socialization experiences of children in the Head Start program, *J Am Diet Assoc* 101(5):572, 2001.

Position of the American Dietetic Association: Local support for nutrition integrity in schools, *J Am Diet Assoc* 100(1):108, 2000.

Children attending day care or Head Start or schools with a breakfast and lunch program receive a major proportion of their meals for the day at that location. These articles provide some insight into the role of day care centers and schools in supporting the development of good food habits in children and the role of community health professionals in supporting school food programs, both in the United States and in developing countries.

Bronner YL et al: Early introduction of solid foods among urban African-American participants in WIC, *J Am Diet Assoc* 99(4):457, 1999.

Fomon SJ: Feeding normal infants: rationale for recommendations, *J Am Diet Assoc* 101(9):1002, 2001.

Mennella JA, Beauchamp GK: Early flavor experiences: research update, *Nutr Rev* 56(7):205, 1998.

Position of the American Dietetic Association: Breaking the barriers to breastfeeding, *J Am Diet Assoc* 101(10):1213, 2001.

Sills IN: Nutritional rickets: a preventable disease, *Topics Clin Nutr* 17(1):36, 2001.

These articles provide some insight into early feeding experiences and nutrition issues in feeding infants.

O'Dea J: Body basics: a nutrition education program for adolescents about food, nutrition, growth, body image, and weight control, *J Am Diet Assoc* 102(suppl 3):S68, 2002.

Reed DB et al: Clueless in the mall: a web site on calcium for teens, *J Am Diet Assoc* 102(3, suppl):S73, 2002.

Sigman-Grant M: Strategies for counseling adolescents, *J Am Diet Assoc* 102(suppl 3):S32, 2002.

Story M et al: Individual and environmental influences on adolescent eating behaviors, *J Am Diet Assoc* 102(suppl 3):S40, 2002.

Adolescents are an important target group for nutrition education. We need to learn more about the food-related beliefs and practices of this group and strategies to improve their nutrition and health behaviors. A supplement entitled Adolescent Nutrition: A Springboard to Health, Volume 102, March 2002, Journal of the American Dietetic Association, is devoted to issues and programs relevant to adolescent nutrition. The articles listed here offer practical ideas for intervention.

Websites of Interest

- Centers for Disease Control and Prevention (CDC), National Center for Health Statistics, 2000 CDC Growth Charts: United States: *www.cdc.gov/growthcharts.*
- La Leche League International: *www.lalecheleague.org.*
- International Lactation Consultant Association: *www.ilca.org.*
- Centers for Disease Control and Prevention, National Center for Chronic Disease Prevention and Health Promotion, Division of Nutrition and Physical Activity: *www.cdc.gov/nccdphp/dnpa.*
- *Dietary Guidelines for Americans 2005: www.healthierus.gov/dietaryguidelines.*
- U.S. Department of Agriculture, Center for Nutrition Policy and Promotion: *MyPyramid food guidance system: www.mypyramid.gov.*
- U.S. Department of Agriculture, *MyPyramid food guidance system for kids: www.mypyramid.gov/kids/.*
- U.S. Department of Agriculture, Food and Nutrition Service, Team Nutrition: *www.fns.usda.gov/tn/.*

CHAPTER 13

Nutrition for Adults: Early, Middle, and Later Years

Eleanor D. Schlenker

This chapter completes our three-chapter sequence on nutrition through the life cycle. Following the tumultuous adolescent years come the challenges, opportunities, and concerns of maturity and adulthood.

When adolescents come of age they have three quarters of their potential years of life still remaining. They face a changing world of accelerated pace, complexity, and global perspective. A part of this changing world is an aging and increasingly diverse population.

Here we review adulthood—the early, middle, and later years. We will look at individual needs in each stage and the role of nutrition in optimal health.

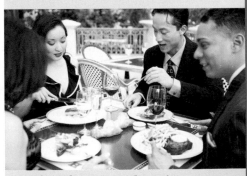

ADULTHOOD: CONTINUING GROWTH AND DEVELOPMENT

Aging Across the Life Cycle

Aging begins at the moment of conception and continues until death. It encompasses the whole of life as we grow and mature, not simply the latter years. All periods of life have their unique potential and fulfillment, and the stages of adulthood—young, middle, and later—are no exceptions.

The adult years should be a positive period of life.[1] They are distinguished by the attainment of optimal function in all body systems. A lifetime of personality and experience is available to be used and enjoyed.[2] The following two important considerations govern the physiologic, psychosocial, and nutritional needs across the adult years:

1. *The individual:* Although gradual aging as occurs throughout adulthood has implications for society, this sequence of change is an individual process.
2. *The total life:* Although specific changes occur during each stage of the life span, aging is a total life process. Experiences in one stage of life hold importance for well-being in later stages.

Both genetics and the environment play a role in the rate and magnitude of age-related changes.

Aging in America

Changes in population and available technology are affecting the personal and working lives of adults in the United States and around the world. The large group of baby boomers born after World War II are reaching their 50s and facing a world of computers, high-tech medical care, and increasing financial responsibilities. The so-called sandwich generation must cope with the costs of educating their children while caring for their aging parents, and in some cases, aging grandparents, and preparing for their own retirement. Medical life support systems present difficult decisions for professionals and families caring for older adult patients. As the life span continues to lengthen and the older population grows in size, their personal, social, and healthcare needs will be felt in all our lives.

Following are listed some of these changes and their impact on health and nutrition services:

*   *Growth in numbers:* The number of older adults in the United States has almost tripled in the past 50 years and now totals 35 million (Figure 13-1). The fastest-growing age cohort is the group age 85 and older, which now totals over 4 million.[3] By 2030 these numbers will have doubled again. As persons continue to age, they are more likely to develop some

degree of physical disability, be in poorer health, and require more health and community services than their younger counterparts (Figure 13-2). Individuals who are unable to stoop, reach over their head, or lift 10 lb will have difficulty shopping for groceries and preparing meals.

*   *Ethnic and racial diversity:* Currently 83% of all persons age 65 and older are white. But by 2050 nearly 40% of the older U.S. population will belong to other racial or ethnic groups[3] (Figure 13-3). Health professionals must respect the differences in food habits, attitudes toward health, and family roles in various cultural and ethnic groups and develop educational programs and materials that are appropriate.
*   *Education:* In 1950 only 17% of older adults had completed high school; currently 72% have a high school diploma, and nearly 17% of older adults hold

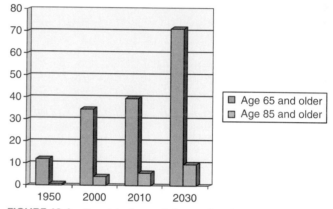

FIGURE 13-1   Growth in the population age 65 and older (in millions). By the year 2030 nearly 72 million persons will be at least 65 years of age and nearly 10 million persons will be at least 85 years of age. (*Redrawn from Federal Interagency Forum on Aging-Related Statistics: Older Americans 2004: key indicators of well-being, Washington, DC, 2004, U.S. Government Printing Office.*)

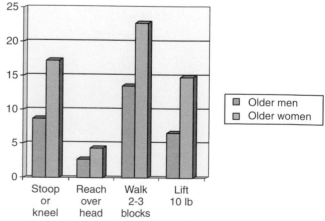

FIGURE 13-2   Percent of persons age 65 and older who are unable to perform these tasks without help. These tasks are important for an older person to remain independent. (*Redrawn from Federal Interagency Forum on Aging-Related Statistics: Older Americans 2004: key indicators of well-being, Washington, DC, 2004, U.S. Government Printing Office.*)

bachelor's degrees.[3] But older racial and ethnic groups differ widely in their levels of education. Only one third of Hispanic older adults and one half of black older adults have high school diplomas compared with three fourths of white older adults.[3] Individuals with more education can take more responsibility for their own health and self care. The older person who cannot read labels on food or medications is less able to implement sound health practices.

- *Income:* Approximately 10% of persons age 65 and over have incomes below the poverty line; however, certain groups are more likely to be poor. Black and Hispanic older adults and older persons living alone have higher poverty rates (Figure 13-4).[3,4] When food money is limited, protein foods, fruits, and vegetables

may not be available in adequate amounts. (Review the discussion of poverty and food in Chapter 10.)

- *Living arrangements:* Because women live longer, more older women are widowed and more older men still live with a spouse. About half of all women above age 74 live alone, whereas three fourths of the men of this age are married. Widowed Asian and Hispanic women are more likely to live with other family members, whereas widowed white and black women often live alone.[3] Older men and women living alone tend to have less money to spend on food and less help with meal preparation.

Influences on Adult Growth and Development

Adults grow and develop in various ways. Physical, socioeconomic, psychosocial, and nutritional forces shape the path of adult development.

Physical Characteristics

Physical growth governed by genetic potential levels off in the late teens and early adult years. When we reach physical maturity, growth is no longer marked by increasing numbers of cells and changing body size; rather, we begin the process of replication, forming new cells to replace old ones and maintain body structure and function. At older ages physical growth gradually declines as cells are lost more rapidly than they can be replaced. Individual vigor reflects the lifestyle patterns of previous years. Poor food choices coupled with low physical activity accelerate normal aging and the progression of chronic disease with its toll on health.

Socioeconomic Status

We all live our lives in a social and cultural environment. A changing world brings major social shifts—new mores and expected behaviors, fears for personal safety, and unfamiliar languages in the marketplace. Many adults experience changes in resources as they move through early, middle, and later adulthood. Financial pressures at any

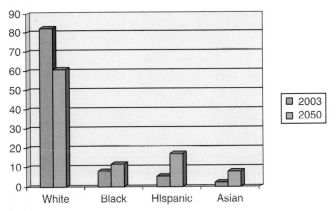

FIGURE 13-3   Percent of persons age 65 and older according to race and ethnic group. The older population will continue to become more diverse. *(Redrawn from Federal Interagency Forum on Aging-Related Statistics: Older Americans 2004: key indicators of well-being, Washington, DC, 2004, U.S. Government Printing Office.)*

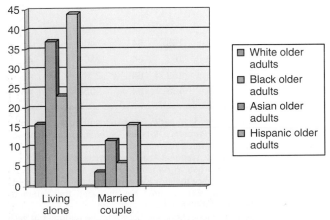

FIGURE 13-4   Percent of older groups living in poverty. Race, ethnicity, and marital status influence poverty risk. *(Redrawn from Federal Interagency Forum on Aging-Related Statistics: Older Americans 2004: key indicators of well-being, Washington, DC, 2004, U.S. Government Printing Office.)*

replication Making an exact copy; to repeat, duplicate, or reproduce. In genetics, replication is the process by which double-stranded deoxyribonucleic acid (DNA) makes copies of itself with each separating strand synthesizing a complementary strand. Cell replication is the process by which living cells under gene control divide to produce exact copies of themselves a programmed number of times during the life span of the organism. Cultured cell lines reproduced in the laboratory are used to study the aging process.

life stage influence food security and the availability of healthcare.

Psychosocial Development

Three developmental tasks of psychosocial growth characterize the adult years: (1) young adults develop intimacy and expand relationships outside of their parents and siblings; (2) middle adults pursue creative expression or explore new career directions; and (3) older adults seek fulfillment and strength of purpose. Each stage affects lifestyle and health.

Nutritional Needs

Nutrient needs remain important even after maturation and physical growth are complete. Each stage of adult life provides the foundation for the one that follows. Neglect of positive health behaviors in the teen and young adult years accelerates the physiologic changes leading to hypertension, cardiovascular disease, and diabetes in the middle years and the risk of premature disability or death. By the same token, lifestyle changes in middle age—beginning a walking program that reduces waist circumference or cutting down on dietary fat—slows metabolic and physical changes and may alleviate existing disease. Nutrient requirements remain dynamic throughout life according to age, physical activity, lifestyle, illness, chronic disease, or pregnancy and lactation.

ADULT STAGES: CHANGING NUTRIENT NEEDS

Young Adult: 19 to 45 Years

Physical Characteristics

Following the turbulent physical growth and sexual development of the adolescent years, the growth pattern levels off into adult homeostasis. Finely regulated genes control neural and hormonal activity and feedback, maintaining a stable internal environment. Body functions are fully developed with sexual maturation and reproductive capacity.

Socioeconomic Status

The early adult years contain the social and economic pressures of continuing education or professional development in preparation for adult responsibilities. Households are established, and individuals may take on the parenting role. Given the changing work environment, many face difficulty in meeting the life tasks of education, work, and family. Young adults ages 18 to 24 report more days of sadness or depression per month than any other adult group, and these feelings are associated with risky health behaviors and poorer self-rated health.[5] This is also the time when we establish lifestyle patterns that will influence our health in middle age and beyond.

Psychosocial Development

The core psychosocial task of the young adult is building relationships outside of the core family of which he or she is part (Figure 13-5). It is a time to become comfortable with the physical self and the demands of the adult role. If positive development is achieved, the individual can build on personal relationships leading to self-fulfillment.

Nutritional Needs

The differences in growth patterns that emerge between males and females in adolescence are strengthened in their adult bodies. Young men have larger muscle mass and long bone growth. In young women the wider hip breadth and pelvic girdle of subcutaneous fat, genetically developed to support reproduction, can prompt concerns and unwise dietary behavior in response to social pressures for thinness. Nutritional concerns for the young adult include energy, calcium, iron, and micronutrients, as follows:

- *Energy:* The Recommended Dietary Allowance (RDA) for active men ages 19 to 30 is about 3000 kcal/day, and for active women it is 2400 kcal/day (Table 13-1).[6] Resting energy expenditure (REE) is about 10% lower in females, reflecting their greater

TABLE 13-1	Dietary Reference Intakes for Energy and Protein*†					
	Weight		**Height**		**Energy (kcal)**	**Protein (g)**
Age (yr)	**kg**	**lb**	**cm**	**in**		
Males						
19-30	70	154	177	70	3000	56
31-50	70	154	177	70	2900	56
51-70	70	154	177	70	2700	56
≥71	70	154	177	70	2500	56
Females						
19-30	57	126	163	64	2400	46
31-50	57	126	163	64	2300	46
51-70	57	126	163	64	2100	46
≥71	57	126	163	64	2000	46

Data calculated from standards found in Food and Nutrition Board, Institute of Medicine: *Dietary Reference Intakes for energy, carbohydrate, fiber, fat, fatty acids, cholesterol, protein, and amino acids (macronutrients),* Washington, DC, 2002, National Academies Press.

* Because adults are urged to remain physically active throughout their lives, there is no evidence that body weight should change as adults continue to age; thus the Expert Panel has indicated that reference weights remain the same for all adult age categories.

†These energy recommendations are based on the midpoint of each age range: age 25, age 40, age 60, and age 80. Calculated values were rounded to the nearest 100. Energy needs in men decline by 10 kcal per year after the age of 19; energy needs in women decline by 7 kcal per year after the age of 19.

proportion of body fat.[6] The male's larger body size and greater amount of metabolically active muscle require more energy for maintenance and repair. Physical activity makes up a smaller proportion of the energy requirement in both sexes (Figure 13-6). Additional kcalories are needed to support pregnancy and lactation (see Chapter 11).

- *Protein:* The RDA is 56 g/day for young men and 46 g/day for young women.[6] These standards are based on a daily protein need of 0.8 g/kg body weight. An additional 25 g/day is required during pregnancy and lactation. Protein intakes among young adults are one and a half to two times the current RDA,[7] and discussion continues as to the relationship between excessive protein intake and development of chronic kidney disease.[6]

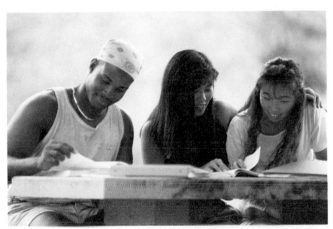

FIGURE 13-5   The early adult years center on the core problem of intimacy versus isolation. *(Credit: PhotoDisc.)*

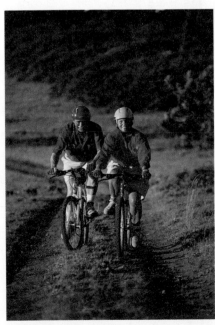

FIGURE 13-6   Energy needs vary according to level of physical activity. *(Credit: PhotoDisc.)*

- *Minerals:* The Dietary Reference Intakes (DRIs) for most minerals are met with a well-planned diet (Table 13-2); however, two minerals, calcium and iron, warrant special attention. Young adults need 1000 mg of calcium a day to ensure the development of peak bone mass.[8] Neither men nor women in this age-group take in enough calcium. More than half of the men fall below 85% of the Adequate Intake (AI), and more than half of the women fall below 65%.[9]

  Iron can be a problem for both young men and young women, but for different reasons. Women of childbearing age must offset the iron lost through the menses, making their RDA 18 mg/day.[10] National studies tell us that young women have a median iron intake less than 67% of their RDA. In contrast, men have an average intake more than two times their RDA.[9] Excessive intakes of iron over time could lead to iron overload. Iron intake is closely related to energy intake, which helps to explain the higher intakes of men. The iron requirement in pregnancy is 27 mg/day, which is usually met with a supplement. Iron needs in lactation are 9 mg daily based on the expectation that the menses have not resumed.

- *Vitamins:* Intakes of certain vitamins are less than optimal in many young adults. Dietary folate falls below 400 μg for many young women, who need to build body stores before conception. Young adults who spend little time in the sun and do not use vitamin D–fortified dairy products or take supplements are low in this vitamin and less able to absorb calcium. Vitamin D status is especially critical in Hispanic and black populations with greater skin pigmentation and a decreased ability to synthesize vitamin D.[11] (See Table 13-3 for the vitamin DRIs.)

Health Issues

Public health leaders are concerned about the health behaviors of young adults and their worsening health profiles. In a national study of risk behaviors smoking, low physical activity, and low intakes of fruits and vegetables were most prevalent among young adults.[12] New responsibilities of home and family along with pressures of the workplace allow less time for healthy behaviors such as physical activity. Also, the threat of chronic disease seems remote to an individual with youthful vigor. Various health risks are evident in this age-group.

Food Habits.   Restaurant meals, especially fast-food meals, are popular among busy young adults. The proportion of their daily kilocalories (kcalories or kcal) obtained at

> median In statistics the middle number in a sequence of numbers such that half are higher and half are lower.

TABLE 13-2 | Dietary Reference Intakes for Minerals, Electrolytes, and Water

Age (yr)	Calcium (mg)	Phosphorus (mg)	Magnesium (mg)	Iron (mg)	Zinc (mg)	Iodine (μg)	Selenium (μg)	Fluoride (mg)	Potassium (mg)	Sodium (mg)	Chloride (mg)	Water (L/day)
Males												
19-30	1000	700	400	8	11	150	55	4	4700	1500	2300	3.7
31-50	1000	700	420	8	11	150	55	4	4700	1500	2300	3.7
51-70	1200	700	420	8	11	150	55	4	4700	1300	2000	3.7
≥71	1200	700	420	8	11	150	55	4	4700	1200	1800	3.7
Females												
19-30	1000	700	310	18	8	150	55	3	4700	1500	2300	2.7
31-50	1000	700	320	18	8	150	55	3	4700	1500	2300	2.7
51-70	1200	700	320	8	8	150	55	3	4700	1300	2000	2.7
≥71	1200	700	320	8	8	150	55	3	4700	1200	1800	2.7

Data from Food and Nutrition Board, Institute of Medicine: *Dietary Reference Intakes for calcium, phosphorus, magnesium, vitamin D, and fluoride,* Washington, DC, 1997, National Academies Press; Food and Nutrition Board, Institute of Medicine: *Dietary Reference Intakes for thiamin, riboflavin, niacin, vitamin B$_6$, folate, vitamin B$_{12}$, pantothenic acid, biotin, and choline,* Washington, DC, 1998, National Academies Press; Food and Nutrition Board, Institute of Medicine: *Dietary Reference Intakes for vitamin C, vitamin E, selenium, and carotenoids,* Washington, DC, 2000, National Academies Press; Food and Nutrition Board, Institute of Medicine: *Dietary Reference Intakes for vitamin A, vitamin K, arsenic, boron, chromium, copper, iodine, iron, manganese, molybdenum, nickel, silicon, vanadium, and zinc,* Washington, DC, 2001, National Academies Press; Food and Nutrition Board, Institute of Medicine: *Dietary Reference Intakes for water, potassium, sodium, chloride, and sulfate,* Washington, DC, 2004, National Academies Press.

| TABLE 13-3 | Dietary Reference Intakes for Vitamins |

Age (yr)	Vitamin A (µg)	Vitamin D (µg)	Vitamin E (mg)	Vitamin C (mg)	Thiamin (mg)	Riboflavin (mg)	Niacin (mg NE)	Vitamin B₆ (mg)	Folate (µg)	Vitamin B₁₂ (µg)
Males										
19-30	900	5	15	90	1.2	1.3	16	1.3	400	2.4
31-50	900	5	15	90	1.2	1.3	16	1.3	400	2.4
51-70	900	10	15	90	1.2	1.3	16	1.7	400	2.4
≥71	900	15	15	90	1.2	1.3	16	1.7	400	2.4
Females										
19-30	700	5	15	75	1.1	1.1	14	1.3	400	2.4
31-50	700	5	15	75	1.1	1.1	14	1.3	400	2.4
51-70	700	10	15	75	1.1	1.1	14	1.5	400	2.4
≥71	700	15	15	75	1.1	1.1	14	1.5	400	2.4

Data from Food and Nutrition Board, Institute of Medicine: *Dietary Reference Intakes for calcium, phosphorus, magnesium, vitamin D, and fluoride,* Washington, DC, 1997, National Academies Press; Food and Nutrition Board, Institute of Medicine: *Dietary Reference Intakes for thiamin, riboflavin, niacin, vitamin B₆, folate, vitamin B₁₂, pantothenic acid, biotin, and choline,* Washington, DC, 1998, National Academies Press; Food and Nutrition Board, Institute of Medicine: *Dietary Reference Intakes for vitamin C, vitamin E, selenium, and carotenoids,* Washington, DC, 2000, National Academies Press; Food and Nutrition Board, Institute of Medicine: *Dietary Reference Intakes for vitamin A, vitamin K, arsenic, boron, chromium, copper, iodine, iron, manganese, molybdenum, nickel, silicon, vanadium, and zinc,* Washington, DC, 2001, National Academies Press.

NE, Niacin equivalent.

restaurants has doubled in recent years,[13] and the more meals eaten away from home, the higher the intakes of both energy and fat.[14] Young adults are drinking more sweetened beverages, and alcohol supplies nearly 4% of their total kcalories.[13] Young men are taking in more than three times the recommended level of sodium; young women are taking in more than twice the recommended amount.[9] More than one third of young adults do not meet the suggested standard of five fruits and vegetables a day,[12] limiting their intakes of fiber, potassium, and other important vitamins and minerals. High intakes of simple carbohydrates and low use of fiber foods adds to the risk of obesity and elevated blood glucose levels. Excessive sodium coupled with low potassium has an unfavorable effect on blood pressure in susceptible individuals.

Body Weight. Young adults are vulnerable to weight gain based on changes in living arrangements and lifestyle. Even adolescents who achieve the recommended level of daily physical activity fail to continue these patterns into adulthood.[15] Repeated follow-up evaluations of young adults between the ages of 18 and 25 revealed an average increase in body mass index (BMI) of 2.5 kg/m² in the men and 1.7 kg/m² in the women.[16] Many had established households over the 7-year interval, and living with a partner increased their likelihood of weight gain. New personal roles can influence eating and snacking patterns, as well as available time for exercise.

Disease Risk. The development of cardiovascular disease and diabetes are associated with such risk factors as an increase in BMI and waist circumference, elevated blood pressure, inappropriate blood lipid levels, and elevated blood glucose or insulin levels. As a group these factors are sometimes referred to as the metabolic syndrome.[17] Although we usually associate these risk factors with middle or older adults, they are beginning to appear in younger adults with poorly chosen diets and low physical activity. A survey of young adults ages 19 to 38 revealed that over 40% had at least one or two of these risk factors and more than 10% had three or more.[18] Low intakes of calcium and poor vitamin D status in the young adult years increase the risk of hip fracture, osteoporosis, and disability in the later adult years.

Middle Adult: 45 to 65 Years

Physical Characteristics

The homeostasis established in the young adult continues, although the cell replication rate begins to slow with gradual loss of body cells. From their 30s and 40s onward, both men and women begin to experience a decline in skeletal muscle mass and muscle strength, a condition called *sarcopenia,* meaning "vanishing flesh."[19] As muscle tissue is slowly lost, body fat begins to rise. Although most persons increase in body fat during this period, total fat accumulation is most rapid among those with sedentary lifestyles, leading to a growing obesity.[20,21] Regular physical and laboratory assessment to monitor body weight, blood pressure, and blood lipid levels can identify health risks that respond to early intervention.

Psychosocial Development

The middle-age adult has moved beyond the period of self-analysis and early career focus to the stage of active involvement with others—family, grandchildren, and community. Some experience the "empty nest" as their children, now adults, set up their own households, whereas others become caregivers to grandchildren or aging family members. Individuals with fewer responsibilities have opportunities to expand their personal horizons (Figure 13-7).

Socioeconomic Status

Increasing technology in business and manufacturing, company mergers and dissolutions, and shifts in the nature of employment can bring job loss for workers at all levels of responsibility. No longer can employees expect to remain with the same company all of their working lives, and reductions in salary or loss of retirement benefits can wreck havoc on both personal and financial well-being. Displaced workers may seek out new educational opportunities or workforce training for new careers.

Nutritional Needs

Nutrient needs change for both men and women in the middle-adult years. Energy needs decline based on loss of muscle mass and low physical activity. Waist circumference can increase by nearly 1 cm per year over this age range and beyond.[22] Calcium intake assumes special importance, particularly for women. Menopause and the loss of estrogen brings about a decrease in calcium absorption and an increase in bone turnover with a net loss of bone mass and increased risk of bone fracture.[23,24] At age 51 the DRIs for calcium and vitamin D increase for both men and women,[8] and optimum intakes of these nutrients promote bone health. With cessation of the menses, iron needs in women drop from 18 mg to 8 mg, the recommended intake for adult men[10] (see Tables 13-1 to 13-3).

Health Issues

The middle adult years hold the key to health both in this stage of life and beyond. Those who established positive health habits as young adults enter their middle years with a minimum of chronic disease. On the other hand, poor lifestyle choices in past years magnify the risk of overt disease, and intervention is essential to reverse the downhill slide.

Food Habits. Middle adults came to maturity during the early growth of the fast-food industry, and they continue to choose hamburgers, cheeseburgers, and french fries, although in lesser amounts than their younger counterparts.[13] Use of soft drinks declines over the adult years, but sweetened beverages still provide more than 5% of total energy. Alcohol supplied from 0% to nearly 15% of total kcalories in one group of this age.[22] Over the past 20 years middle adults have lowered their use of red meats and luncheon meats,[13] likely in response to health messages to eat less fat. Nevertheless, fat still provides 33% of total kcalories, and saturated fat more than 11%.[25] Salty snacks and desserts combined add up to almost 13% of energy intake.[13] Dietary folate is below recommended levels, increasing the risk of cardiovascular disease.[9] Fruits and vegetables, important sources of fiber and micronutrients, fall below MyPyramid goals.[12] Middle-age adults as compared to young adults are higher users of dietary supplements, especially vitamins E and C, the B complex vitamins, and calcium.[26]

Chronic Disease. Cardiovascular disease, diabetes, and cancer rise during this stage of life. Nearly half in this age-group have at least two modifiable risk factors for heart disease or stroke (Box 13-1), but more than one

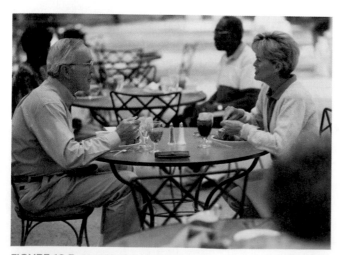

FIGURE 13-7 Middle adult years can be a time to expand personal growth. *(Credit: PhotoDisc.)*

BOX 13-1	Modifiable Risk Factors for Heart Disease and Stroke*

High blood pressure
High blood cholesterol levels
Diabetes (type 2)
Tobacco use
Obesity
Lack of exercise

From United States Department of Health and Human Services, Centers for Disease Control and Prevention: Racial/ethnic and socioeconomic disparities in multiple risk factors for heart disease and stroke—United States, 2003, *MMWR Morb Mortal Wkly Rep* 54(5, Feb 11), 2005.
  *These risk factors can be modified through prevention, early recognition, and treatment.

fourth do not have their blood cholesterol level checked regularly.[27] The prevalence of overweight and obesity has helped to fuel the rise in diabetes and younger age of diagnosis (46 versus 52 years).[28]

Food habits influence both weight gain and mortality in this age-group. Diets higher in alcohol, sweets, fast food, and processed meats result in greater increases in waist circumference[22] and risk of cardiovascular disease and diabetes. Mortality from all causes was lower in both men and women with a history of eating more fruits, vegetables, and whole grains.[29] The health implications of alcohol remain controversial.[30] Additional kcalories in the form of alcohol can stimulate unwanted weight gain, and at excessive levels alcohol is toxic to the liver. Even moderate amounts of alcohol appear to increase cancer risk in middle-age women and reduce bone mineral mass, adding to the risk of osteoporosis and bone fracture. At the same time, limited amounts of alcohol appear to offer some protection against cardiovascular disease.

Older Adult: 65 to 85 Years

Physical Characteristics

The later adult years bring a gradual waning of physical vigor, work capacity, and strength. Changes can be minimal immediately following retirement but become more pronounced as individuals move through their 70s and into their 80s. Chronic diseases such as osteoarthritis, heart disease, pulmonary disease, and diabetes may limit physical activity, adding to problems with energy balance. Advancing age also brings alterations in major tissues and organ systems that threaten homeostasis and the ability to respond to infection or disease. Physiologic changes that influence nutritional status in the aging adult are summarized in the following sections.

Body Composition.   Body water, bone mass, and muscle mass are lost, while fat mass increases in size. Even if body weight remains unchanged, the older adult has proportionately more fat.[31] The position of fat on the body also changes, moving from the extremities to the trunk, especially the abdomen. This too has implications for health because abdominal fat releases large amounts of fatty acids into the blood, raising both blood lipid and blood insulin levels.[32] Although some older adults experience weight gain, others undergo progressive weight loss, leading to frailty, disability, and diminished quality of life.[33]

Cardiovascular System.   Changes occur in both the heart and the vascular system, which carries nutrients and oxygen to the cells and removes waste. The heart weakens as a pump and is less able to respond to increased demands for oxygen as occurs in strenuous exercise, emotional stress, or acute disease. A fall in the amount of blood pumped with each beat of the heart lowers the blood supply to major organs such as the kidney and lungs. Major arteries, including those delivering vital nutrients to the heart muscle itself, become stiff and narrowed with atherosclerotic deposition. The stiffening of the major arteries, which limits their ability to stretch when blood is delivered from the heart, is responsible in part for the rise in blood pressure commonly seen in older adults.[1,34]

Renal System.   The older kidneys are less efficient and require more time to clear waste products from the blood. Urine can no longer be concentrated to the same extent, and greater amounts of water are required to excrete a given amount of waste. This is why older people receiving high-protein supplements that produce large amounts of nitrogen-containing waste need additional fluid. Fluid balance is poorly regulated at very high or very low intakes of fluid and sodium.[34]

Respiratory System.   The air sacs in the aging lung become less elastic, making it more difficult to move volumes of air in and out. Changes in the air sacs reduce the surface area for exchange of oxygen and carbon dioxide. Widening areas of the lungs do not participate in air exchange, and this "dead space" becomes vulnerable to the growth of bacteria and pathogens. Smoking and air pollution contribute to loss of lung function and reduce the supply of oxygen needed for normal activity as well as more strenuous exercise.[1,34]

Gastrointestinal System.   Changes in the gastrointestinal system can affect secretions, muscles, and nerves. Loss of gastric acid interferes with the absorption of vitamin B_{12}, thiamin, and folate.[35] Loss of nerve and muscle function add to constipation in frail older adults by increasing the time needed for food to pass through the lower digestive tract.

Psychosocial Development

Psychosocial development in the later adult years requires continuing adaptation to new challenges as physical abilities decline and emotional supports are lost. Depending on one's resources, a sense of wholeness or a sense of despair prevails. If life's experiences have been positive, the older individual enters this stage rich in the wisdom of the years and rewarding relationships. Nevertheless, problems with declining health, financial worries, or other circumstances over which the aging individual has no control can result in depression or failure to thrive.[36,37]

Socioeconomic Status

Older adults usually enter retirement on a fixed income. Some older adults have no stable source of income, and economic insecurity is a constant worry. Financial resources influence nutrient intake, and lower-income older people have poorer diets than higher-income older people.[38] Living alone and social isolation can lead to depression and a lack of incentive to prepare nourishing meals.[39-42] An older individual living alone with no neighbors or near relatives may have no one to call on for help in periods of illness or other emergency. Frail older adults confined to their homes may experience both economic and social deprivation.

Nutritional Needs

The DRIs have the following two age categories for persons above age 50[6]:

1. Ages 51 to 70
2. Ages 71 and older

These categories were established to recognize the physiologic changes and chronic diseases that continue to develop as we age and influence our nutritional needs, as follows (The DRIs for persons over age 50 are listed in Tables 13-1, 13-2, and 13-3.):

*   *Energy:* The energy allowance for older adults takes into consideration age-related changes in muscle and active tissue and expected levels of physical activity. A physically active 65-year-old man weighing 77 kg needs about 2600 kcal/day, and a physically active woman of this age weighing 57 kg needs about 2100 kcal/ day.[6] Beyond age 70 further declines in energy expenditure are more likely the result of decreasing physical activity than changes in lean body mass.[43,44] Physical activity to the extent possible helps maintain muscle mass and physical well-being. The sharp decline in energy expenditure seen in sedentary older adults is neither inevitable nor desirable.
*   *Protein:* The RDA for protein is the same for all adults ages 25 and older (see Table 13-1). A level of 0.8 g/kg body weight is recommended for both genders with reference intakes of 56 g/day for men and 46 g/day for women.[6] Health status influences protein needs. Physically impaired older adults with chronic disease use protein less efficiently and may lose body nitrogen on a protein intake of 0.8 g/kg body weight.[45,46]
*   *Minerals:* The DRI for calcium rises from 1000 mg to 1200 mg for persons over age 50 as a strategy to reduce bone loss, bone fracture, and the development of osteoporosis.[8] (Review the causes and consequences of bone mineral loss in Chapter 7.) The iron needs of postmenopausal women and older men are the same[10] (see Table 13-2).
*   *Vitamins:* Vitamin needs are unchanged from middle to older age, except for vitamin B_6 and vitamin D (see Table 13-3). Vitamin B_6 is used less efficiently by the older adult, so the RDA is higher.[47] Vitamin B_6 is stored and metabolized mainly in muscle, so muscle loss in older age may change the body's handling of

this nutrient. To ensure adequate vitamin D for calcium absorption and bone health, the AI rises from 10 μg (400 IU) for those ages 51 to 70 to 15 μg (600 IU) for persons over age 70.[8]

Health Issues

Food Intake.   In contrast to younger age-groups, who struggle with unwanted weight gain, the more likely problem in the older adult is unwanted weight loss with increasing frailty and disability (see the *Perspectives in Practice* box, "Involuntary Weight Loss: Danger Sign in Older Adults" and Boxes 13-2 and 13-3). Nevertheless, older adults who continue to consume the same number of kcalories despite a reduction in physical activity experience weight gain, making walking or other activities even more difficult. Although energy intake continues to decline, the proportions of kcalories from fat and saturated fat do not change from middle age.[25] Dietary sodium is lower in older adult men as compared to middle adult men. Sodium intakes are similar for middle and older adult women, but lower than in men.[9] Older men exceed the Tolerable Upper Intake Level (UL) for sodium by more than 1100 mg, likely adding to problems with blood pressure. Calcium from food falls in both older men and women, suggesting lower intakes of dairy or

---

BOX 13-2   Signs of Failure to Thrive

Children

Failure to grow normally
Failure to develop physically for self-care
Failure to develop social skills
Failure to develop cognitive skills

Older Adults

Weight loss
Loss in physical function for self-care
Social withdrawal
Loss of cognitive function
Decline leading to death

Modified from Egbert AM: The dwindles: failure to thrive in older patients, *Postgrad Med* 94(5):200, 1993.

BOX 13-3   Physical Characteristics of Frailty

Unintentional weight loss of 10 lb or more in the previous year
General weakness (can be measured using grip strength)
Problems with balance and gait
Slow motor function (can be measured by time required to walk 15 ft)
Low physical activity

Data from Fried LP et al: Untangling the concepts of disability, frailty, and comorbidity: implications for improved targeting and care, *J Gerontol A Biol Sci Med Sci* 59:M255, 2004.

PERSPECTIVES IN PRACTICE
Involuntary Weight Loss: Danger Sign in Older Adults

Unwanted and inappropriate weight loss is a nutritional risk factor for older adults. Although weight loss in younger persons can be a positive step toward well-being, this is not necessarily the case in older adults. For the older person who is overweight, achieving even a modest weight loss by increasing physical activity and eating a healthy diet can improve mobility, blood pressure and blood lipid levels, and glucose utilization. In contrast, involuntary weight loss brought about by inadequate energy intake and associated disease leads to functional disability, a lack of nutrient reserves, and a poor prognosis. In this situation not only fat but also important muscle tissue is lost. Failure to thrive and frailty are two conditions characterized by involuntary weight loss that offer opportunities for intervention.

Defining Weight Loss

Clinical care specialists have taken several approaches to describing serious weight loss. Long-term care facilities often use as the standard for intervention the loss of 10 lb or more over 6 months or the loss of 5% or more of total body weight over 1 year. The Nutrition Screening Initiative (NSI) for older adults living in the community recommends that individuals who lose 10 lb or more over 6 months receive nutrition counseling and intervention.[1] Caregivers should monitor body weight in chronically ill family members being cared for at home.

Failure to Thrive

Failure to thrive has long been recognized in neglected infants and children who lack both physical care and social interaction. In the developing child, failure to thrive is recognized by a failure to grow and develop in both physical and social skills (see Box 13-2). In older persons the opposite occurs; the individual fails to maintain and regresses in both physical and cognitive function. The signifying characteristic of failure to thrive in older adults is weight loss with a downhill progression of physical loss ending in death. These older people have been referred to as the "dwindles," and in most cases they live in the community.[2]

It is important to distinguish the physical changes observed in failure to thrive from those associated with terminal illness. In failure to thrive there is no biologic or physiologic explanation for the observed weight loss and downhill spiral. Rather, they are directly related to low energy intake brought about by a lack of financial resources, social isolation, limited ability to obtain groceries or prepare meals, chronic disease and disability, failing eyesight, or other circumstance that limits food intake. If detected early, intervention is both possible and effective.

Frailty

Frailty is another clinical condition associated with weight loss and physical disability that occurs in older adults. Frail older adults are at high risk for falls, loss of independence, need for long-term care, and death.[3] The characteristics of frailty (see Box 13-3) are sometimes associated with chronic disease, but this is not always true. Although underlying disease must be ruled out as the cause of these physical losses, frailty still confers special care needs over and above any medical treatment that may be required. Nutrition intervention to prevent further weight loss and resistance training to improve muscle size and muscle strength can prevent or reverse the signs of frailty.

Consequences of Involuntary Weight Loss

Older adults who experience rapid and substantial weight loss have poor health outcomes. They are more likely to fall and, if injured, are less likely to survive or return to their own homes. The loss of muscle mass that occurs with involuntary weight loss limits mobility and the capacity for self-care, and the downhill spiral of disability often leads to institutionalization. Older individuals who lose large amounts of weight are more likely to develop pressure ulcers or experience hip fractures.[4] Among homebound older adults receiving delivered meals, those losing weight were more likely to need help with activities of daily living such as self-feeding, getting dressed, or getting in and out of bed[5] (see the To Probe Further box, "Community-Based Long-Term Care: Access to Nutrition Services"). Older adults experiencing weight loss are more likely to die within 1 year after release from an acute care hospital.[6] Unwanted weight loss may begin with hospitalization if the diet provided does not meet energy needs. We must be vigilant to inappropriate weight loss among older persons in our care and implement intervention strategies to reverse the situation.

References

1. American Academy of Family Physicians, American Dietetic Association: *Nutrition Screening Initiative,* Washington, DC, 2005, Authors. Available at *www.aafp.org/nsi.xml.* Accessed November 13, 2005.
2. Egbert AM: The dwindles: failure to thrive in older patients, *Nutr Rev* 54(2):S26, 1996.
3. Fried LP et al: Untangling the concepts of disability, frailty, and comorbidity: implications for improved targeting and care, *J Gerontol A Biol Sci Med Sci* 59:M255, 2004.
4. Wilson M-M G, Morley JE: Invited review: aging and energy balance, *J Appl Physiol* 95:1728, 2003.
5. Sharkey JR: The interrelationship of nutritional risk factors, indicators of nutritional risk, and severity of disability among home-delivered meal participants, *Gerontologist* 42:373, 2002.
6. Liu LJ et al: Undernutrition and risk of mortality in elderly patients within 1 year of hospital discharge, *J Gerontol A Biol Sci Med Sci* 57:M741, 2002.

calcium-fortified foods;[9] however, nonfood calcium rises with over half of this age-group using either calcium supplements or calcium-containing antacids.[26] One fourth of older adults take a vitamin E supplement.

Chronic Disease. The burden of chronic disease continues to grow as the years go on, although individual risk factors are somewhat modified. Elevated blood cholesterol levels and overweight appear to diminish in importance as risk factors for cardiovascular disease in older versus middle adults, although elevated blood pressure continues to increase vulnerability to heart attack or stroke. A stroke (or cerebrovascular accident) caused by blockage or bursting of a blood vessel in the brain damages nearby brain cells and can seriously impact an individual's quality of life. Paralysis affecting speech, mobility, movement, or

FOCUS ON CULTURE

Acculturation and Food Intake

Acculturation refers to the changes in dietary habits and general patterns of behavior that occur when individuals move to a different location and take on the customs common to that area. Changes in food habits associated with relocation to the United States can be positive or negative, and this may depend on the extent to which individuals abandon their traditional food patterns in favor of the high-sugar, high-fat, and low-fiber diets followed by many Americans.

Among older Hispanic adults both the number of years they lived in the United States and their degree of acculturation influenced their food choices. Their degree of acculturation was evaluated on their use of Spanish versus English in speaking and writing. Older Hispanic persons who lived in the United State for 20 years or more and were more likely to use English rather than Spanish had diets more like the non-Hispanic older adults with similar incomes living in the same neighborhood.[1,2] The less-acculturated Hispanic men and women who were more likely to use Spanish rather than English had higher intakes of complex carbohydrates and lower intakes of sugar, saturated fat, and alcohol than their more acculturated Hispanic neighbors. They ate more rice and beans and milk and seldom had sweet desserts. In contrast, the non-Hispanic older adults in their neighborhood obtained 9% of their kcalories from cake, pastry, and quick breads. Although fiber intake was similar among all groups, the more traditional Hispanic adults obtained most of their fiber from beans and rice, whereas the non-Hispanic older adults and more acculturated older Hispanics obtained more of their fiber from bread, vegetables, or high-fiber cereals.

As individuals move away from their former diet patterns, it is important that we help them substitute items that represent healthy eating and supply the nutrients contributed by their traditional foods. Adopting new food habits that emphasize sugar and fat will compromise health and likely lead to unwanted weight gain.

References

1. Bermudez OI, Falcon LM, Tucker KL: Intake and food sources of macronutrients among older Hispanic adults: association with ethnicity, acculturation, and length of residence in the United States, *J Am Diet Assoc* 100:665, 2000.
2. Lin H, Bermudez OI, Tucker KL: Dietary patterns of Hispanic elders are associated with acculturation and obesity, *J Nutr* 133:3651, 2003.

loss of some degree of cognitive function often results from a stroke. Aggressive treatment of hypertension in older adults is now a practice standard. Deaths from cancer rise in older age-groups, pointing to the continuing need for fruits, vegetables, and whole grains supplying plant-based, cancer-fighting components. Intakes of healthy foods may change as older persons move away from their traditional food patterns and adopt foods higher in sugar and lower in fiber (see the *Focus on Culture* box, "Acculturation and Food Intake").

Obesity, especially severe obesity, in middle age is a major contributor to morbidity and complications of cardiovascular disease and diabetes in older age. Persons with a BMI over 30 in their middle years had annual medical costs more than $6500 higher in their later years than those whose BMI fell between 18.5 and 29.[48] Even small differences in BMI resulted in lower medical costs. Helping the severely obese lose even modest amounts of weight at any stage of adulthood can have positive dividends for long-term health.

Interest in Health Improvement.   Older adults are an important target audience for health education. Over a 10-year interval older adults were the most likely to make positive changes in health behavior as compared to young and middle age-groups.[12] Such changes included smoking cessation, increasing physical activity, and increasing intakes of fruits and vegetables. Older people have a strong interest in health and should be encouraged that it is never too late to reap positive benefits from making better food choices or increasing physical activity.

Oldest-Old: 85 Years and Older

Population Projections

As a nation we continue to grow older. To better characterize the changing nature of the older population the U.S. Census Bureau developed the following three categories for persons ages 65 and older:

1. *The young-old:* ages 65 through 74 years
2. *The old-old:* ages 75 through 84 years
3. *The oldest-old:* ages 85 years and older

More than 4 million people in the United States are now age 85 or older.[3] Approximately 52,000 persons have reached the age of 100.[4] Given the rapid pace of biomedical research, experts anticipate that life expectancy will continue to rise and the actual numbers of older adults will even surpass current projections.[4] The oldest age-group—those 85 and older—is the fastest growing age cohort, and its numbers are expected to double over the next 25 years. Because this increase is so recent, the physical characteristics and physical needs of the "oldest-old" are poorly understood.

Nutritional Needs

As older adults continue to age, they become less efficient in nutrient absorption and utilization, and this becomes most apparent in illness or stress. Nutrient stores undergo rapid loss in acute illness or long-term disease and can be difficult to replace. When developing the DRIs, nutrition scientists gave careful attention to the needs of persons ages 71 and older. Unfortunately, we know very little about the interactions between the aging process and chronic disease and how they might influence nutritional needs. Because more and more of the future practice of health professionals will be devoted to care of the aging, we will explore below some of the issues and theories about how and why we age.

THE AGING PROCESS

The Study of Gerontology

When studying aging the first step is to distinguish among terms. Researchers use the term *aging* to refer to all changes that occur in an individual over time—from the moment of conception until death. When studying health we usually think about aging as those changes that occur later in life and lead to increased vulnerability, frailty, or risk of death. The term gerontology refers to the study of aging and is different from the term geriatrics, which refers to the diseases and medical conditions common to older people.[1] The field of gerontology includes the biologic, physiologic, sociologic, and behavioral aspects of the aging process and how they play out in each individual. We are learning more about how people change as they age and the types of services that can help them remain independent. We also need to recognize how younger people can support their older neighbors as well as learn from them. Studies of nutrition and health are evaluating the genetic and environmental factors that influence physical aging and the length and quality of life.

Length of Life

Over the past century the life expectancy of Americans at birth has increased from 49 years to 77 years.[3] Advances in public health, bringing clean water and appropriate sewage and garbage systems, and the development of antibiotics that eliminated the scourges of various infectious diseases contributed to this change. Reducing the infant death rate and preventing the early deaths of young adults effectively increased life expectancy at birth. The harder work of increasing life expectancy at older ages still lies ahead as we try to understand normal aging and the impact of chronic disease. The new tools of molecular biology allow us to study aging as it occurs in the cell and the gene and separate out the many factors—genetic and environmental—that cause cells to change and grow old.

Our genetic inheritance controls to some extent our susceptibility or resistance to particular disease conditions and thus our length of life; however, environmental factors such as pollution or personal lifestyle, including diet, smoking habits, alcohol use, or activity level, also have a role in human aging. Oxidative damage to cells influences aging and affects both physiologic and cognitive functions. Our genes and the biologic limits to cell replication, not our age in years, control the changes in human cells and systems and the functional decline that occurs with age. In fact chronologic age is the least suitable measure of human aging. As we begin to separate the effects of chronic diseases from the effects of normal aging, we can lay the groundwork for an improved end of life in humans.

Quality of Life

An increasing life span and rapidly growing older population worldwide have focused attention on the quality of extended life. In the United States persons ages 65 and older make up only 13% of the population but incur more than one third of the nation's healthcare expenditures.[49] Average healthcare costs for adults ages 65 to 74 are $8297 per year; these costs increase to $18,353 for those ages 85 and older.[3] The healthcare needs of the oldest-old will become especially evident when the first of the baby boomer generation turns 85 in 2031.

Researchers are studying both the nature and rate of physiologic aging, looking for possible means of slowing or preventing these changes and related diseases. Nonfatal but highly disabling age-dependent conditions, including osteoarthritis, osteoporosis, blindness and other sensory impairments, and Alzheimer's disease, are the subjects of intensive study by workers at the National Institute on Aging and universities across the world.

Biologic Changes in Aging

The biologic process of growth, maturation, and gradual decline extends over the entire life span. The rate of biologic aging is conditioned by all previous life experiences and the imprint of these experiences on an individual's genetic heritage.

Nature of Biologic Changes

The gradual loss of cells and impaired function in remaining cells begins in middle age and brings about a

cognitive Pertaining to mental processes such as memory, judgment, and reasoning.

life expectancy The number of years a person of a given age, gender, race, or ethnic group can expect to live.

gerontology Study of the physiologic, biologic, psychologic, and sociologic aspects of the aging process, their effects on individuals, and potential preventive or intervention strategies.

geriatrics Branch of medicine specializing in medical problems of older adults.

chronologic age A person's age in years.

gradual reduction in the performance capacity of most organ systems. These changes may occur rapidly in one organ system but slowly in another, and the rate at which they occur varies widely among individuals. Losses in lean body mass happen slowly at first, but accelerate as the years go on. By the age of 70 the kidneys will have lost about 28% of their weight and the liver approximately 25% of its weight; skeletal muscle will have decreased by almost half, as compared to a young adult.[19,34,50] The gradual loss of cellular units across organ systems results in an overall reduction in the body's reserve capacity, making the older adult less able to respond to environmental changes, physical stress, infection, or disease.

Individuality of the Aging Process

The aging process moves forward in each of us, but at very different rates. Lifestyle choices, disease history, and exposure to environmental hazards or pollution act on each person's unique set of genes to determine the rate and severity of aging changes. For this reason older people of a certain age are less alike than younger people of a certain age, because each has experienced a different set of genetic and environmental influences over his or her lifetime. As a result some individuals are physically old at age 50, whereas others maintain an active pace into their 80s or 90s. Although we discuss aging and its nutritional implications in general terms, individual needs vary widely and must be independently assessed. The greatest influence of nutrition on the aging process may occur in the early growth years, even as early as fetal life, when tissues and metabolic systems are being built.[51] Nutrition in the growth and middle years prepares us to meet the cellular and metabolic changes of older age.

Normal Versus Successful Aging

Researchers who studied the aging process have defined two types of human aging: normal aging and successful aging. In normal aging both genetic and environmental influences interact to produce degenerative changes in body systems. In successful aging regressive changes are slowed or prevented by positive lifestyle choices and health interventions.[1] A healthy diet, regular physical activity, a positive mental outlook, appropriate healthcare, and avoidance of addictive behaviors such as smoking or alcohol abuse contribute to successful aging.

Health Promotion

Older Americans are not only living longer but also in many instances enjoying robust and active lives. More than 80% of even the oldest-old still live in the community, and less than 5% of all persons age 65 and older live in long-term care facilities.[4] Nutrition and health education should support positive lifestyle interventions relating to diet and physical activity—the keys to reducing chronic disease risk.

Dietary Pattern for Adult Health

Two basic tools issued by the U.S. Department of Agriculture (USDA) and the U.S. Department of Health and Human Services (USDHHS) provide a framework for planning healthy diets across the adult years. The *Dietary Guidelines for Americans*[52] and MyPyramid[53] emphasize moderation and variety and provide an outline for food selection (see Chapter 1 for a review of these materials). Food guides are especially helpful as energy needs decline and persons decrease the amount of food they eat from day to day. Eating a low variety of foods, even micronutrient-dense foods, in an effort to reduce kcalorie intake can lead to intakes below the recommended levels for energy, protein, vitamins, and minerals. Nutrition education messages emphasizing low-kcalorie foods, intended to prevent weight gain among younger individuals, may be having a negative influence on older persons, causing them to decrease kcalories below the amount needed and resulting in unwanted weight loss.[54]

Physical Activity for Optimal Function

There are two types of physical activity that promote fitness and well-being in both younger and older adults and each has its individual benefits, as follows:

1. *Endurance exercise:* The rhythmic use of the large muscles in walking, running, or jogging promotes cardiovascular fitness. For older individuals who have been sedentary, walking is a safe form of endurance exercise that supports cardiovascular health, weight management, and independent living. Endurance exercise increases the heart rate and over time strengthens heart and lung response to exercise and efficient use of oxygen.[1] Figure 13-8 illustrates endurance exercises for the upper and lower body.

2. *Resistance exercise:* Strength training, as it is sometimes called, is a form of exercise in which the individual pushes against or lifts a set weight. Gradually more weight is added. This stimulates the muscle cells bringing about an increase in both muscle cell size and cell number.[55] Resistance exercise has been successful in increasing the size of the thigh muscle in persons up to 100 years of age.[56] Any increase in the size or strength of a muscle improves functional capacity and the ability to remain independent.[57] Older residents in a long-term care facility who had required help to rise from a chair or walk across a room were able to perform these tasks independently

after completing a resistance exercise program.[56] Strengthening arm muscles could enable an older person to continue to carry groceries or lift cooking pots. Figure 13-9 illustrates an example of resistance training.

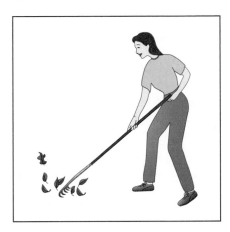

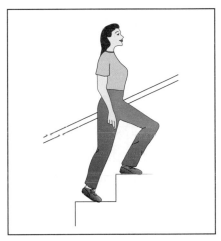

FIGURE 13-8 Everyday activities can provide endurance exercise. *(From U.S. National Institute on Aging, National Institutes of Health: Exercise: a guide from the National Institute on Aging, Publication No. NIH 98-4258, Washington, DC, 1998, U.S. Government Printing Office.)*

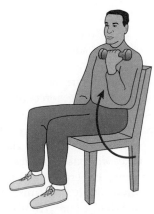

FIGURE 13-9 Use weights to perform resistance exercise in your own home. *(From U.S. National Institute on Aging, National Institutes of Health: Exercise: a guide from the National Institute on Aging, Publication No. NIH 98-4258, Washington, DC, 1998, U.S. Government Printing Office.)*

Both adequate protein and kcalories are needed to support an increase in muscle protein. A protein intake of 1.2 g/kg body weight and added kcalories sufficient to prevent unwanted weight loss are recommended for older people beginning strength training.[19]

NUTRITIONAL NEEDS OF OLDER ADULTS: AN INDIVIDUAL APPROACH

Energy

Maintaining Energy Intake

Individual needs vary with body size and physical activity, but for most reasonably healthy and moderately active older adults, daily energy needs range from 1600 to 2200 kcal for women and 2000 to 2800 kcal for men.[53] However, national surveys tell us that many older adults consume less than suggested amounts,[9] and black and Hispanic older adults have lower intakes than white older adults (Table 13-4).[7,58] Among the homebound, daily energy intake can fall below 1000 kcal.[40] In a follow-up study of older people continued for 7 years, mortality was highest for those reaching only 65% of their recommended energy intake.[59] Diets very low in kcalories are also limiting in protein and important vitamins and minerals. Chronic conditions common in older adults, including cancer, cardiac failure, and chronic obstructive pulmonary disease, increase energy needs.

Physical activity is a highly variable component of the energy requirement, and a nutrition assessment should include information about daily lifestyle and activity. It appears that older adults, even relatively inactive older adults, have higher energy requirements than predicted,[60] because they expend more energy in performing a given activity such as walking than younger adults with greater muscle coordination.[60,61]

Researchers are also reviewing body weight standards for later life. For persons above age 59 underweight

TABLE 13-4	Mean Energy Intakes of Persons Ages 60 and Older	
	Men	**Women**
White	1986 kcal	1446 kcal
Black	1686 kcal	1331 kcal
Hispanic	1748 kcal	1419 kcal

Data from Agricultural Research Service, U.S. Department of Agriculture: *Continuing survey of food intake by individuals, 1994-1996,* Washington, DC, 1994-1996, Authors. Retrieved December 19, 2005, from *www.ars. usda.gov/Services/docs.htm?docid=7716;* and Bermudez OI, Falcon LM, Tucker KL: Intake and food sources of macronutrients among older Hispanic adults: association with ethnicity, acculturation, and length of residence in the United States, *J Am Diet Assoc* 100:665, 2000.

carries great risk.[62] Men and women ages 60 to 69 with a BMI below 18.5 (indicative of underweight) had a mortality risk over twice that of their normal weight counterparts. Geriatric physicians recommend that older adults maintain a BMI of 22 or higher.[63] Preventing unintentional weight loss is key to continued physical and mental well-being in older adults in community settings or long-term care facilities.[42]

Planning an Adequate Diet

An appropriate diet for an older individual does not differ from one for a younger individual. Providing a variety of nutrient-dense foods in sufficient quantity to meet the following energy needs remains the goal:

- *Carbohydrates:* Persons of all ages should obtain 45% to 65% of their total energy from carbohydrates, with an emphasis on complex carbohydrates.[6] Diets rich in fiber support gastrointestinal function and reduce the need for laxatives and their potential for metabolic disruption. Complex carbohydrates found in legumes and whole grains help modulate postprandial blood glucose levels.[64,65] Carbohydrate kcalories should be sufficient to spare protein for body growth and repair.

- *Fats:* Fat intake is best contained within the range of 20% to 35% of total kcalories.[6] Fat supplies energy and essential fatty acids and is required for the absorption of fat-soluble vitamins. Fat adds to the palatability, pleasing mouth feel, and flavor of food and encourages food intake. A diet in which fat contributes 35% of total kcalories (with an emphasis on unsaturated fats) can assist in maintaining body weight in frail older adults. Fats are generally well digested and absorbed at older ages, although the rate of fat breakdown may be slowed; dividing fat intake among all meals and snacks enhances digestion and utilization.

- *Protein:* Adequate amounts of protein are needed to preserve muscle mass, support optimum immune function, and maintain body tissues. Preservation of muscle mass is important to sustain functional capacity for independent living and self-care. The current RDA of 0.8 g/kg body weight,[6] may not be sufficient for frail or chronically ill older adults. Protein turnover, the rate of protein breakdown and synthesis, is more rapid in debilitated older adults and over time contributes to a growing loss of muscle mass. Protein intakes of 1.25 g/kg not only reduce the net loss of body nitrogen, but also support the production of new proteins and addition of lean tissue.[66] When protein intake is inadequate, even healthy older adults are likely to have poorer immune response that improves with additional protein. Older individuals recovering from surgery or acute illness may require as much as 1.5 g/kg for optimal recovery.[67] A general protein standard of

1.0 g/kg has been suggested for persons over age 70 as metabolic systems become less efficient.[68] Overall, 10% to 35% of total kcalories should be supplied by good-quality protein.

Vitamins

At one time we believed that lower-than-normal blood and tissue vitamin levels in older adults were a normal consequence of aging. We now recognize that such levels in older people are the result of poor intakes, ineffective absorption, or elevated needs and require immediate attention. Vitamins of special importance to the aging adult include the following:

- *Folate:* Optimum folate intake prevents a rise in blood homocysteine levels that damage the blood vessels and accelerate atherosclerosis.[47]

- *Vitamin B_6:* As an active coenzyme in protein synthesis, vitamin B_6 is important to preserve or increase muscle mass.[47]

- *Vitamin B_{12}:* The age-related decrease in gastric acid hinders the release of vitamin B_{12} from animal protein foods. Vitamin B_{12}-fortified breads and cereals or vitamin B_{12} supplements can supply the amount needed.[47] Vitamin B_{12} deficiency leads to not only a megaloblastic anemia but also changes in cognitive function in older adults.

- *Vitamin D:* Vitamin D deficiency occurs in older persons who spend most of their time indoors and do not eat vitamin D–fortified foods.[11] Aging changes in the skin also reduce vitamin D synthesis regardless of sun exposure.

Minerals and Electrolytes

In planning diets for older adults, calcium and the electrolytes potassium and sodium require particular attention, as follows:

- *Calcium:* The AI for calcium is 1200 mg for those ages 51 and older.[8] Fluid milk, fortified soy milk, or fortified yogurt, good sources of calcium, also contain added vitamin D.

- *Potassium:* This electrolyte helps to regulate blood pressure. As an opposing force to sodium, which tends to raise blood pressure levels, potassium is especially important in the diets of older people. Elevated blood pressure increases the risk of both heart attack and stroke. Various diuretics commonly prescribed to manage hypertension or cardiac failure bring about a loss of body potassium, which must be replenished by diet. The AI for potassium is 4700 mg and can be obtained with the recommended servings of fruits and vegetables.[69] Potassium supplements can raise blood potassium to dangerous levels and should be avoided.

- *Sodium:* Sodium works in opposition to potassium and can raise blood pressure levels. Daily intakes should be limited to 2300 mg or less[69] to avoid unwanted fluid retention or increase in blood pressure. Lowering sodium intake can be difficult for the older adult who is dependent on heat-and-serve food items, which tend to be high in sodium-containing additives.

Water

Dehydration is a concern for both healthy and chronically ill older adults.[34,70] Physiologic changes, disease effects, and environmental circumstances can predispose older people to inadequate fluid intake (Box 13-4). Changes in the hypothalamus alter the thirst mechanism such that older persons do not always get thirsty and drink when or as much as they should. Age-related alterations in kidney function increase water loss, and body water serves as the medium for the dilution of medications. Dehydration exerts an effect on alertness and cognitive function.[71] The general fluid requirement of 1500 ml/day increases when either the outside or inside temperature rises. In patients with fever, daily fluid needs increase by 500 ml per degree Centigrade above normal temperature.[70] Older adults are also at risk of overhydration because regulatory mechanisms are less efficient in bringing about the excretion of excess water. Older people and their caregivers should monitor their fluid intake.

Nutrient Supplementation

Healthy older adults who consume a variety of foods, including fortified foods, and meet the DRIs for energy are unlikely to require nutrient supplements. However, older adults with low energy intakes can benefit from prudent, individually assessed supplementation. Individuals using multiple prescription and over-the-counter medications, those who eat a limited variety of foods, and isolated older people with little social support are at exceptional nutritional risk.[38-41] Nutrient supplements may be needed to replenish losses following critical or debilitating illness. But nutritional supplements should add to—not replace—food. Using food money to purchase supplements rather than nutritious food is not a solution.

Older adults should be guided in their use of supplements. Surveys indicate that older persons with better diets who are obtaining more nutrients from food are also the most likely to use vitamin or mineral supplements.[72] Three times as many older women as older men take calcium supplements, although both sexes have increased calcium needs after age 50. Despite the relatively low iron requirement of both men and women in their later years, some still use supplemental iron, presenting the risk of iron overload. On the other hand, vitamin D, low in the diets of most older persons, is seldom taken as a supplement. The use of nutrient supplements should be based on an individual assessment and advice of a healthcare professional. Supplements should supply those nutrients that (1) are not present in the diet in sufficient amounts and (2) are appropriate to meet the dietary requirements of that individual (see Chapter 7, *Perspectives in Practice* box, "Do I Need a Vitamin-Mineral Supplement?").

NUTRITION AND PREVENTIVE CARE

Influences on Food Intake

Many physical, social, and environmental factors relating to the individual and the community converge to support the health and quality of life of older people (Figure 13-10). Personal characteristics relating to health, relationships, and economic situation determine nutrient intake and physical well-being, but so do community resources such as available transportation to the grocery store or doctor, safe neighborhoods for walking, or meal programs, as will be discussed later in this chapter. Warning signs, such as the following, can alert us to developing problems, before nutritional and physical health is compromised[63]:

- *Physical changes:* Both chronic disease and physical changes related to normal aging can adversely affect food intake. Periodontal disease and decayed teeth, or tooth loss and poorly fitting dentures, or no dentures at all make chewing and eating both painful and difficult. Losses in taste, smell, or sight reduce the enjoyment of eating and lower appetite. In Chapter 8 we noted the changes in salivary secretions that lead to xerostomia (dry mouth) and make eating and swallowing painful and difficult. Radiation treatment or a stroke that damages the nerves in the head and neck, diabetes, or Parkinson's disease can interfere with the swallowing reflex and lead to fear of choking. Aging changes in the appetite control center of the hypothalamus can reduce food intake.
- *Multiple medications:* Treatment regimens involving multiple drugs, termed *polypharmacy,* can lower food

---

BOX 13-4	Risk Factors for Dehydration in Older Adults

Advanced age (85 and older)
Loss of thirst sensation
Problems with mobility hindering access to fluids
Confusion or cognitive changes
Problems in swallowing
Medications promoting fluid loss (diuretics, laxatives)
Incontinence leading to self-imposed fluid restriction

Modified from Ferry M: Strategies for ensuring good hydration in the elderly, *Nutr Rev* 63(suppl 6):S22, 2005. Copyright 2005 International Life Sciences Institute.

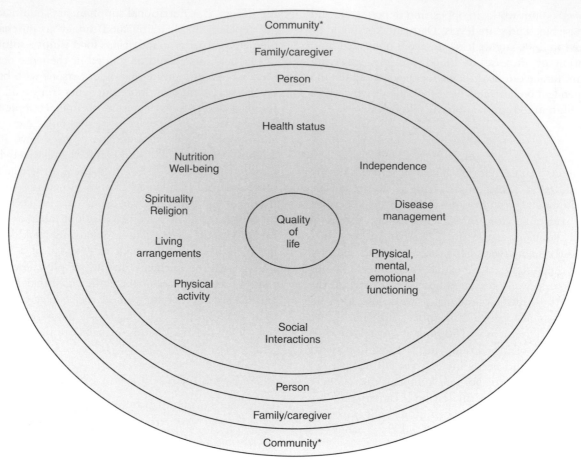

FIGURE 13-10   Many factors influence the quality of life of older adults. Personal characteristics, nearby neighbors or family caregivers, and support services available in the community help an older person remain independent. *The term *community* includes health and supportive services at local, state, and federal levels and health professionals and researchers. (*From American Dietetic Association: Position paper of the American Dietetic Association: nutrition across the spectrum of aging,* J Am Diet Assoc 105:616, 2005, with permission from the American Dietetic Association.)*

intake by producing anorexia, nausea, or an unpleasant taste. At the other extreme, certain drugs increase appetite, leading to intakes of greater amounts of food than needed. (We discuss more nutrient-medication effects in Chapter 17.)

- *Psychosocial distress:* Emotional loss arising from the death of a spouse or physical separation from family and friends causing depression can lead to disinterest in food. Older persons living alone, especially men who are unaccustomed to preparing food, may not go to the trouble of planning and cooking a meal for one person. Alcohol sometimes displaces food in the diet. A distorted body image with self-imposed food restriction (anorexia nervosa) is known to occur in older women and men.

- *Economic problems:* Older persons with incomes below the poverty level often lack the resources to purchase the quantity or quality of food they should have. Even those with higher incomes with costly medications or other out-of-pocket medical expenses may compromise on food. Inadequate housing with non-working appliances for food storage and preparation or homelessness put older individuals at risk.

- *Chronic illness and disability:* Food shopping and meal preparation can be difficult or impossible for individuals who must use a cane or walker, can no longer drive, or have visual losses. Those who are dependent on others for transportation and shop irregularly have limited fresh fruits, vegetables, or fluid milk available to them. An inappropriately restrictive therapeutic diet that forbids favorite ethnic or comfort foods often lowers food intake. (See the *Case Study* box, "An Older Adult Woman Living Alone," to review these problems.)

Development of Overt Malnutrition

Protein-energy malnutrition occurs in many older adults, including those living at home, those living in skilled nursing facilities, and those in the hospital (Table 13-5).[73-75] Medical problems accentuate the problems of undernutrition. Immune factors called cytokines, released

CASE STUDY

An Older Adult Woman Living Alone

Miss E is 81 years of age and lives in public housing. Her apartment kitchen has a two-unit cooking top and a small refrigerator but very little storage space. She prepares and eats all of her meals alone. She has always enjoyed mealtime but now has trouble with food sticking in her throat, so she cooks everything until it is very soft and seldom eats meat. She feels very tired much of the time, and on days when she is not well enough to fix meals, she just has cereal and milk. She likes fruit and vegetables but always buys canned because they are easier to swallow and cost less than fresh or frozen. Miss E does her own shopping at a supermarket about a half mile away. It has been her custom to walk to the market and take the bus home, but she is finding it increasingly difficult to walk and now generally rides both ways. She makes the trip twice a week, because it is difficult to carry more than a few items at a time. Because she has always liked to walk, she maintained a healthy body weight, but recently she has begun to lose weight and worries about her health. She wonders if she should be taking a vitamin supplement to increase her energy level.

Questions for Analysis

1. What are some physical changes that are influencing Miss E's food intake?
2. What are some socioeconomic or psychologic changes that may be affecting her food intake?
3. What nutrients are likely to be low in her diet? Why?
4. What might be causing her tiredness?
5. What are your general concerns about her physical condition? What are the implications of her recent weight loss?
6. Would you recommend that Miss E begin to take a vitamin or mineral supplement? If so, what might she take? Why would you recommend this?
7. What food assistance or other programs for older persons might help Miss E improve her nutrient intake or enable her to remain independent?

TABLE 13-5 | **Where Do We Find Undernourished Older Adults?**

Location	Estimated Proportion Undernourished (%)
Living independently in the community	5-12
Receiving hospital care	40-65
Living in long-term care facilities	30-61

Data from Thomas DR: Distinguishing starvation from cachexia, *Clin Geriatr Med* 18:883, 2002.

BOX 13-5 | **Nutrition Alerts for Older Adults in Long-Term Care**

Involuntary loss of 5% of body weight in 1 month or 10% in 6 months

Leaving uneaten 25% or more of served food over the past 7 days

BMI ≤ 21

Data from Thomas DR et al: Nutritional management in long-term care: development of a clinical guideline, *J Gerontol A Biol Sci Med Sci* 55A(12):M725, 2000.
   BMI, Body mass index.

in response to chronic disease or tissue injury, not only lower food intake but also interfere with the utilization of nutrients that are available, such that even aggressive efforts at nutrition intervention cannot always reverse the continuing weight loss. Congestive heart failure and cancer cause profound anorexia and weight loss, and these forms of malnutrition are referred to as cardiac and cancer cachexia.[73] Undernutrition in the aging adult results in lowered immune function, slowed production of red blood cells, and accelerated loss of body muscle. (See the *Perspectives in Practice* box, "Involuntary Weight Loss: Danger Sign in Older Adults," for further discussion of unintentional weight loss.)

Nutrition Screening

The Nutrition Screening Initiative (NSI) promotes routine nutrition screening of older persons in both community and institutional settings through a network of registered dietitians, public health nutritionists, physicians, nurses, and community workers.[76] This multidisciplinary project is a combined effort of the American Dietetic Association, the American Academy of Family Physicians, and 25 other organizations interested in older adults. It targets warning signs of malnutrition that increase the risk of chronic disease, physical disability, and loss of independence in community-living older adults

(Figure 13-11). The DETERMINE Your Nutritional Health checklist containing seven warning signs associated with poor nutritional health is a tool that can be used in senior centers, congregate meals sites, doctors' offices, or home-delivered meals programs to identify older adults at risk for low nutrient intake. The goal of the NSI is to identify vulnerable older persons and apply intervention strategies before they develop overt undernutrition. A set of warning signs for use with older people confined to skilled nursing facilities is found in Box 13-5.

Clinical Applications

Medical Nutrition Therapy

Physicians specializing in geriatrics and clinical dietitians working with older adults recommend that medically indicated diets for older adult patients be liberalized to the extent possible.[77,78] At older ages the benefits of dietary intervention for lowering blood lipid levels are less clear-cut than at younger ages. For the older adult malnutrition and serious weight loss can have more immediate consequences than elevated blood cholesterol levels[77]; therefore, severely restricting fat to the point of lowering food or energy intake can be counterproductive. Older patients with insulin-dependent diabetes are well managed on a less-restricted diet.[78] A

The Warning Signs of poor nutritional health are often overlooked. Use this checklist to find out if you or someone you know is at nutritional risk.

DETERMINE YOUR NUTRITIONAL HEALTH

Read the statements below. Circle the number in the "YES" column for those that apply to you or someone you know. For each yes answer, score the number in the box. Total your nutritional score.

	YES
I have an illness or condition that made me change the kind and/or amount of food I eat.	2
I eat fewer than 2 meals per day.	3
I eat few fruits or vegetables or milk products.	2
I have 3 or more drinks of beer, liquor, or wine almost every day.	2
I have tooth or mouth problems that make it hard for me to eat.	2
I don't always have enough money to buy the food I need.	4
I eat alone most of the time.	1
I take 3 or more different prescribed or over-the-counter drugs a day.	1
Without wanting to, I have lost or gained 10 pounds in the last 6 months.	2
I am not always physically able to shop, cook, and/or feed myself.	2
TOTAL	

Total Your Nutritional Score. If it's—

0-2   **Good!** Recheck your nutritional score in 6 months.

3-5   **You are at moderate nutritional risk.** See what can be done to improve your eating habits and lifestyle. Your office on aging, senior nutrition program, senior citizens center or health department can help. Recheck your nutritional score in 3 months.

6 or more   You are at high nutritional risk. Bring this checklist the next time you see your doctor, dietitian, or other qualified health or social service professional. Talk with them about any problems you may have. Ask for help to improve your nutritional health.

These materials developed and distributed by the Nutrition Screening Initiative, a project of:

 AMERICAN ACADEMY OF FAMILY PHYSICIANS

 THE AMERICAN DIETETIC ASSOCIATION

 NATIONAL COUNCIL ON THE AGING, INC.

Remember that warning signs suggest risk but do not represent diagnosis of any condition. Turn the page to learn more about the Warning Signs of poor nutritional health.

FIGURE 13-11   DETERMINE Your Nutritional Health checklist. *(From Nutrition Screening Initiative:* DETERMINE *your nutritional health checklist, Washington, DC, 2005, Author. The Nutrition Screening Initiative is a joint project of the American Academy of Family Physicians and the American Dietetic Association, funded in part by a grant from Ross Products Division, Abbott Laboratories Inc.)*

regular diet—well-balanced nutritionally—that offers a wide variety of foods with moderation in fats and sweets has the best outcomes. Frail or chronically ill older adults eating less than 2000 kcal/day will not be meeting the portions of fruits, vegetables, and milk recommended in the *Dietary Guidelines for Americans 2005.*[52] Special diet patterns emphasizing nutrient-dense foods or a carefully planned regimen of vitamin and mineral supplements may be needed for institutionalized or cognitively impaired older adults with low energy intakes.[79]

Support Programs for Self-Care

An individual's quality of life is magnified by the opportunity to live independently in safety and comfort or perform self-care to the extent possible in a supervised setting. Chronic diseases such as osteoporosis, osteoarthritis, Parkinson's disease, or congestive heart failure often require some adaptation of the living situation. Support programs for patients and their families expand their knowledge about a condition and its management, build emotional support, and promote creative decision making. Both individual and group sessions that focus on nutrition assessment and nutrition counseling, physical therapy, and medical information have a positive impact on both physical and psychologic well-being. This mutual intervention and support help both patients and caregivers cope with the chronic nature of the condition.

COMMUNITY RESOURCES FOR THE AGING

Food Assistance Programs for Older Americans

Government-supported food assistance programs including the Food Stamp Program and the surplus commodities distribution program serve older as well as younger Americans (see Chapter 10). Many older adults extend their food-buying power and obtain needed food using these resources. However, the program with the greatest impact on the nutritional status of older Americans is the national Elderly Nutrition Program.

Older Americans Act

The Elderly Nutrition Program funded under the Older Americans Act was first authorized in 1972. It was intended to meet both the nutritional and social needs of older adults who (1) could not afford adequate diets, (2) were unable to prepare adequate meals for themselves, (3) had limited mobility, or (4) were isolated and lacked incentive to prepare meals and eat alone. In 1978 specific funding was established for both congregate and home-delivered meals under Title III-C of the Older Americans Act.

Elderly Nutrition Program

The Elderly Nutrition Program operates in all 50 states and provides various nutrition services based on local needs and the funds available (Box 13-6). All persons ages 60 and over are eligible to participate regardless of income. Typically meals are served at congregate sites or home delivered at noon, Monday through Friday, although the increasing demand for home-delivered meals has led many programs to adopt more cost-effective delivery patterns. The meals provided through the Elderly Nutrition Program help older adults remain independent in the community. (Learn more about the Elderly Nutrition Program and community-based long-term care in the *To Probe Further* box, "Community-Based Long-Term Care: Access to Nutrition Services.")

Government Research and Education Services

Research Centers of the United States Department of Agriculture

The USDA has collaborated with several universities to establish human nutrition research centers on aging. These centers are authorized by Congress to study the role of nutrition in the aging process and help us learn more about nutritional requirements at older ages.

Extension Services of the United States Department of Agriculture

The USDA supports Cooperative Extension services at state universities and in county offices across all 50 states. Food and nutrition educators from these agencies provide nutrition education classes and practical nutrition materials for older adults and community workers.

State Public Health Departments

Public health nutritionists under the direction of local and state health departments provide nutrition education and oversee nutrition and health screening of older people in the community. State health department inspectors monitor food safety practices in adult day care centers, congregate meal sites, home-delivered meals kitchens, and long-term care facilities licensed by the state.

State Departments for the Aging

All states receive funds under the Older Americans Act to provide nutrition services to their older citizens. A Department on Aging within state government administers the program with responsibility for supervision, monitoring, and technical assistance. Area agencies on aging manage congregate and home-delivered meals programs on the local level under the guidelines of the state unit.

Professional Organizations and Resources

National Council on the Aging

The National Council on the Aging (NCOA) is a nonprofit organization that promotes research, training, technical assistance, advocacy and public policy, program standards, and publications relating to all aspects of aging. Members include professionals and volunteers from many different disciplines that work on many fronts to improve the quality of life for older Americans. This organization partnered with the American Dietetic Association and the American Academy of Family Physicians to establish the NSI discussed earlier in this chapter.

BOX 13-6	Services Provided by the Older Americans Act

Congregate meals
Home-delivered meals
Transportation services (to congregate meals or medical appointments)
Nutrition education
Nutrition and health screening

COMMUNITY-BASED LONG-TERM CARE: ACCESS TO NUTRITION SERVICES

As government and health leaders develop strategies for cost-effective services for the growing older population, community-based care has emerged as an alternative to institutional care for those who can remain independent given some level of help.[1] A dependable supply of nutritious food is the cornerstone to independent living and continuing physical health and quality of life. Providing for food and nutritional needs is especially critical in discharge planning before release from an acute care hospital.[2] Meal delivery, grocery delivery, or transportation to a congregate site where wholesome meals are served can help provide a day-to-day food supply. Other nutrition services, including nutrition screening, assistance with meal planning, and medical nutrition therapy, if warranted, support early intervention and help prevent the worsening of chronic health problems. As people continue to age, declining health, frailty, and physical disability may require assistance with personal care or household chores.

Evaluating the Need for Services

The first step in planning for community-based care is evaluating the individual's physical and cognitive abilities and limitations. An older individual's capacity to live independently is evaluated using the activities of daily living (ADLs) and the instrumental activities of daily living (IADLs). The ADLs, listed as follows, evaluate a person's ability to perform personal care either independently, with some amount of help, or not at all:

- Bathing
- Dressing
- Feeding
- Using the toilet
- Transferring between bed and chair

The IADLs, listed as follows, evaluate a person's ability to perform housekeeping tasks and other chores required for independent living:

- Preparing meals
- Performing housecleaning chores
- Handling money and balancing a checkbook
- Shopping without help
- Using the telephone
- Leaving home without help

Such an evaluation is carried out by a nurse, occupational therapist, or trained social worker.

Goals for Community-Based Long-Term Care

At one time *long-term care* referred only to medical, social, or personal services provided to individuals in skilled nursing facilities or settings giving personal care. Older people needing help with ADLs or IADLs were moved from their homes to such a facility depending on the level of care required. Today we place more emphasis on community-based long-term care and services that will enable older persons to remain in the community in their own homes or in the home of a family member. Many older people needing help with ADLs or IADLs are cared for by their families; however, increasing numbers of adult children live at some distance from their parents. Some older adults do not have children or other close family. To meet this need, community and in-home services are provided by home care agencies, area agencies on aging, and for-profit home care companies.

Food and Nutrition Services for Older Adults

Nutrition services are an important component of community-based long-term care. You will notice that several ADLs and IADLs relate to food and nutrition. For most older persons living in the community, self-feeding is not a problem; however, obtaining groceries and preparing adequate meals can be difficult or impossible for those with some degree of physical disability. When older people are able to leave their homes, congregate meals offering socialization and health-related services can improve their quality of life and prevent further deterioration in physical health.

The Older Americans Act (OAA) provides for a wide range of services to support independent living (see Box 13-6). The specific services offered depend on local needs and available funds, although most localities at a minimum provide both congregate and home-delivered meals. All persons ages 60 and older are eligible to participate regardless of income. Special funding is designated for Native Americans, Native Hawaiians, and Alaska Natives. The Administration on Aging of the U.S. Department of Health and Human Services is the agency with responsibility for setting guidelines and procedures for programs using OAA funds. Approximately 250 million meals are served each year to 2.6 million older adults.[3]

Congregate (Group) Meals

Congregate meal sites operate in senior centers, churches, municipal buildings, and high-rise apartment complexes—any location that is within easy access to older adults. Generally meals are served at noon, 5 days a week. Each meal is expected to supply at least one third of the Dietary Reference Intakes (DRIs) for the 60 and older age-group. Because the levels of energy, protein, and some micronutrients are higher for men, that is the standard used. When funding is available, meal sites provide transportation for those who may not have a car or no longer drive. For many congregate meal participants, particularly those living alone, the meal site is an important source of social support.

Home-Delivered Meals

To be eligible for home-delivered meals an individual must be physically unable to leave home or homebound as a result of caring for a disabled spouse. Traditionally a hot meal was delivered at noon, Monday through Friday. Volunteers donated their time and vehicles to deliver meals. However, with more women working outside the home and more older persons remaining in the work force beyond the usual retirement age, programs find it increasingly difficult to recruit volunteers. The cost of paying persons to deliver meals has forced many agencies to turn from daily delivery of a hot meal to weekly or biweekly delivery of frozen meals. Also, the rising numbers of homebound older adults and the earlier release of older patients from acute care facilities have fueled the growing demand for home-delivered meals. Based on client needs some programs deliver extra cold or frozen meals for use on weekends or as second meals on weekdays.

Evaluation of the Elderly Nutrition Program

Both congregate and home-delivered meals programs are mandated to target low-income and frail older adults. Most program participants have two to three chronic conditions, and those receiving meals are older than the general population of aging adults. The average age of the 60 and older group is 72 years; however, the average age of congregate meal participants is 76 years and that of home-delivered meal recipients is 78 years.[4]

Nutritional objectives are also being met. Meal recipients have better diets than other adults of similar age and socioeconomic status. For all major nutrients, with the exception of iron and vitamin B_{12}, program participants have higher intakes than nonparticipants. For most participants the program meal provides 30% to 50% of their total nutrient intake for the day.[4]

TO PROBE FURTHER—cont'd

COMMUNITY-BASED LONG-TERM CARE: ACCESS TO NUTRITION SERVICES

Current Issues

Despite the success of the Elderly Nutrition Program, program administrators still face difficult problems, as follows:

- *Funds for congregate versus home-delivered meals:* The growing demand for meals and the limited resources available pose a difficult dilemma for program administrators. Both congregate and home-delivered meals support independent living. Congregate meals have a role in preventive care, slowing the downhill spiral leading to increasing frailty and disability; home-delivered meals enable physically impaired older adults to remain in the community. The sharp rise in requests for home-delivered meals has diverted funds from congregate programs. Currently 54% of meals are home delivered, and 41% of home meal programs have waiting lists.[3] Funding is needed for both programs.
- *Number of meals provided per day:* When the Elderly Nutrition Program began, the goal was to supplement the food resources of older adults, not serve as their major food resource. However, for many participants, especially the homebound, program meals are their major source of food and these meals are divided across the day and/or the week.

- *Needs of diverse populations:* The increasing diversity of the older population will require meals appropriate for groups with a wide variety of food preferences. As the numbers of Hispanic and Asian older adults increase, meals reflecting their traditional food patterns must become available if their nutritional needs are to be met.

Health and social service professionals working with older adults should become familiar with the Elderly Nutrition Program and the services available in their communities.

References

1. American Dietetic Association: Position paper of the American Dietetic Association: nutrition across the spectrum of aging, *J Am Diet Assoc* 105:616, 2005.
2. Baker EB, Wellman NS: Nutrition concerns in discharge planning for older adults: a need for multidisciplinary collaboration, *J Am Diet Assoc* 105:603, 2005.
3. Wellman NS, Rosenzweig LY, Lloyd JL: Thirty years of the older Americans nutrition program, *J Am Diet Assoc* 102(3):348, 2002.
4. Millen BE et al: The Elderly Nutrition Program: an effective national framework for preventive nutrition interventions, *J Am Diet Assoc* 102(2):234, 2002.

American Geriatrics Society

The American Geriatrics Society is made up of physicians who provide medical care to older patients. They encourage research in geriatrics that will advance our knowledge about aging and the treatment of its diseases. This organization publishes the *Journal of the American Geriatrics Society.*

The Gerontological Society

Membership in the Gerontological Society includes a wide range of health and social service professionals. They have stimulated interest in gerontology and aging among other professional organizations and joined with community and government agencies to advocate for older adults. The group sponsors two publications, the *Journal of Gerontology* and *The Gerontologist.*

Volunteer Health Organizations

Volunteer health organizations such as the American Heart Association and the American Diabetes Association support health and nutrition programs of interest to older adults. These groups include both professional and public members and operate at national and community levels to fund research and provide education.

Community Groups

Local community groups representing health professions—medical societies, nursing organizations, and dietetic associations—sponsor classes and programs to help meet the needs of older adults in their communities. Professionals volunteer their time in community program support. Senior citizens centers and local service and religious organizations provide a broad range of services that may include nutrition education.

TO SUM UP

Throughout adult life, nutrient needs are influenced by the continuing maturation and eventual decline of body systems. In young adults nutrients support the physical body that has reached its full growth and sustain the reserves needed for active living. Lifestyle patterns formed by young adults will likely continue throughout the life span, and the unwanted gain in body weight and sedentary living that characterizes young adults is a matter for concern. Middle age begins the period of physical decline, although such changes occur slowly at the onset. The loss of muscle mass and bone mass can limit functional capacity and independent living in later years if allowed to continue unchecked. Attention to protein, calcium, and vitamin D, and participation in both endurance and resistance exercise can prevent or slow the aging process.

The nutritional needs of older adults are influenced by the biologic changes of aging that affect both body composition and organ function. The aging process is often complicated by chronic disease, associated with malnutrition and weight loss. Physical disability, poverty, chewing or swallowing problems, loneliness and isolation, and multiple medications can lower food intake and increase nutritional risk. The NSI offers a tool to identify older adults at risk and educate individuals and communities in preventive care.

QUESTIONS FOR REVIEW

1. Briefly describe the changes in age-groups now occurring in the United States population. Why are these changes occurring? What are the implications for healthcare and support services?

2. Discuss the economic status, ethnic and racial composition, and living arrangements of the aging population. How might these factors influence an older person's diet or health status?

3. Select one of the adult age-groups, and describe the group's physical growth, psychosocial development, socioeconomic status, and nutritional needs. What do you see as the most urgent topic for health promotion in this age-group? Why?

4. What is meant by the aging process? What are some physiologic changes that occur as we age? How do they influence food intake or nutritional status?

5. Interview an older member of your family or a neighbor or family friend who is over age 65. What are some changes in health, living arrangements, or employment that have influenced their lifestyle over the past 10 years? How might these changes have influenced their food habits?

6. You are helping a 75-year-old retired couple on a limited income with their diet. Both appear to be underweight, and you suspect that their food supplies have been limited. Using the MyPyramid, plan a 3-day menu for them that will supply each food group in the appropriate amounts. How might you increase their energy intake and still remain within the suggested ranges for the three macronutrients? What are some food assistance programs that might increase their food resources?

7. Distinguish between the terms *gerontology* and *geriatrics*. Go to your school library and find the *Journal of Gerontology* and the *Journal of the American Geriatrics Society*. Look for an article in each journal that discusses nutrition problems or nutrition-related diseases in older people. Compare the articles as to the type of information presented and the intended audience.

8. Identify a food-related program for older adults in your community, and interview the director to determine (a) the target audience, (b) the food provided, (c) any major problems associated with the program, and (d) the major successes of the program. If possible, administer the Determine Your Nutritional Health checklist to some of the participants. How would you characterize their nutritional risk?

9. You are working with a middle-age adult who is overweight, sedentary, and eats mostly meat, bread, potatoes, and desserts. Is this person an example of normal aging or successful aging? Why? What suggestions would you have for improvement?

10. Visit your local drug store, and review the liquid supplements being marketed to older adults. Make a table describing four different supplements listing the cost and amounts of kcalories, protein, calcium, vitamin D, vitamin B_6, vitamin B_{12}, and folate per 1-cup serving. Using the nutrient analysis program on the CD-ROM that accompanied your textbook, select a fortified cereal that would be eaten with 1 cup of milk. Compare the cost, kcalories, and nutrients listed above in a 1-cup serving of supplement with the usual serving size of the cereal with 1 cup of milk. Based on your findings, would you recommend the cereal serving or the liquid supplement as an evening snack? Explain.

REFERENCES

1. Timiras PS: *Physiological basis of aging and geriatrics,* ed 3, Boca Raton, Fla, 2003, CRC Press.
2. Butler RN: *Why survive? Being old in America,* Baltimore, 2002, Johns Hopkins University Press (originally published in 1975).
3. Federal Interagency Forum on Aging-Related Statistics: *Older Americans 2004: key indicators of well-being,* Washington, DC, 2004, U.S. Government Printing Office.
4. Administration on Aging, United States Department of Health and Human Services: *A profile of older Americans: living arrangements,* Washington, DC, 2004, Author. Retrieved December 15, 2005, from *www.aoa.gov/prof/Statistics/profile/2004/6.asp.*
5. Kobau R et al: Sad, blue, or depressed days, health behaviors and health-related quality of life, Behavioral Risk Factor Surveillance System, 1995-2000, *Health Qual Life Outcomes* 2(1):40, 2004.
6. Food and Nutrition Board, Institute of Medicine: *Dietary Reference Intakes for energy, carbohydrate, fiber, fat, fatty acids, cholesterol, protein, and amino acids (macronutrients),* Washington, DC, 2002, National Academies Press.
7. Beltsville Human Nutrition Research Center, Agricultural Research Service, United States Department of Agriculture: *Continuing survey of food intake by individuals, 1994-1996,* Table Set 16, Beltsville, Md, 1998, Author. Retrieved November 15, 2005, from *www.ars.usda.gov/Services/docs.htm?docid=7716/.*
8. Food and Nutrition Board, Institute of Medicine: *Dietary Reference Intakes for calcium, phosphorus, magnesium, vitamin D, and fluoride,* Washington, DC, 1997, National Academies Press.
9. Wright JD et al: *Dietary intake of ten key nutrients for public health, United States: 1999-2000,* Advance Data, Vital and Health Statistics, No. 334, Washington, DC, 2003 (April 17), U.S. Department of Health and Human Services.
10. Food and Nutrition Board, Institute of Medicine: *Dietary Reference Intakes for vitamin A, vitamin K, arsenic, boron, chromium, copper, iodine, iron, manganese, molybdenum, nickel, silicon, vanadium, and zinc,* Washington, DC, 2001, National Academies Press.
11. Park S, Johnson MA: Living in low-latitude regions in the United States does not prevent poor vitamin D status, *Nutr Rev* 63(6, pt 1):203, 2005.
12. Winkleby MA, Cubbin C: Changing patterns in health behaviors and risk factors related to chronic diseases, 1990-2000, *Am J Health Promot* 19(1):19, 2004.
13. Nielsen SJ, Siega-Riz AM, Popkin BM: Trends in energy intake in U.S. between 1977 and 1996: similar shifts seen across age groups, *Obes Res* 10(5):370, 2002.
14. Kant AK, Graubard BI: Eating out in America, 1987-2000: trends and nutritional correlates, *Prev Med* 38:243, 2004.

15. Gordon-Larsen P, Nelson MC, Popkin BM: Longitudinal physical activity and sedentary behavior trends: adolescence to adulthood, *Am J Prev Med* 27(4):277, 2004.

16. Burke V et al: Changes in health-related behaviours and cardiovascular risk factors in young adults: associations with living with a partner, *Prev Med* 39(4):722, 2004.

17. Kahn R et al: The metabolic syndrome: time for a critical appraisal, *Diabetes Care* 28(9):2289, 2005.

18. Yoo S et al: Comparison of dietary intakes associated with metabolic syndrome risk factors in young adults: the Bogalusa Heart Study, *Am J Clin Nutr* 80:841, 2004.

19. Roubenoff R, Hughes V: Sarcopenia: current concepts, *J Gerontol A Biol Sci Med Sci* 55:716, 2000.

20. Hughes VA et al: Longitudinal changes in body composition in older men and women: role of body weight change and physical activity, *Am J Clin Nutr* 76:473, 2002.

21. Kyle UG et al: Sedentarism affects body fat mass index and fat-free index in adults aged 18 to 98 years, *Nutrition* 20(3):255, 2004.

22. Newby PK et al: Dietary patterns and changes in body mass index and waist circumference in adults, *Am J Clin Nutr* 77:1417, 2003.

23. Nordin BEC et al: A longitudinal study of bone-related biochemical changes at the menopause, *Clin Endocrinol* 61:123, 2004,

24. Macdonald HM et al: Nutritional associations with bone loss during the menopausal transition: evidence for a beneficial effect of calcium, alcohol, and fruit and vegetable nutrients and of a detrimental effect of fatty acids, *Am J Clin Nutr* 79:155, 2004.

25. Centers for Disease Control and Prevention, United States Department of Health and Human Services: Trends in intake of energy and macronutrients—United States, 1971-2000, *MMWR Morb Mortal Wkly Rep* 53(4, Feb 6), 2004.

26. Radimer K et al: Dietary supplement use by US adults: data from the National Health and Nutrition Examination Survey, 1999-2000, *Am J Epidemiol* 160:339, 2004.

27. U.S. Department of Health and Human Services, Centers for Disease Control and Prevention: Racial/ethnic and socioeconomic disparities in multiple risk factors for heart disease and stroke—United States, 2003, *MMWR Morb Mortal Wkly Rep* 54(5, Feb 11), 2005.

28. Koopman RJ et al: Changes in age at diagnosis of type 2 diabetes mellitus in the United States, 1988 to 2000, *Ann Fam Med* 3:60, 2005.

29. Kant AK, Graubard BI, Schatzkin A: Dietary patterns predict mortality in a national cohort: the National Health Interview Surveys, 1987 and 1992, *J Nutr* 134:1793, 2004.

30. Suter PM: Alcohol: its role in health and nutrition. In Bowman BA, Russell RM, eds: *Present knowledge in nutrition,* ed 8, Washington, DC, 2001, International Life Sciences Institute.

31. Hughes VA et al: Anthropometric assessment of 10-y changes in body composition in the elderly, *Am J Clin Nutr* 80:475, 2004.

32. Pi-Sunyer FX: The epidemiology of central fat distribution in relation to disease, *Nutr Rev* 62(7, part 2):S120, 2004.

33. Fried LP et al: Untangling the concepts of disability, frailty, and comorbidity: implications for improved targeting and care, *J Gerontol A Biol Sci Med Sci* 59:M255, 2004.

34. Kane RL, Ouslander JG, Abrass IB: *Essentials of clinical geriatrics,* ed 5, New York, 2004, McGraw-Hill.

35. Morley J: Anorexia and weight loss in older persons, *J Gerontol A Biol Sci Med Sci* 58A:131, 2003 (editorial)

36. Egbert AM: The dwindles: failure to thrive in older patients, *Nutr Rev* 54(1, part 2):S25, 1996.

37. Center for Nutrition Policy and Promotion, U.S. Department of Agriculture: *Quality of diets of older Americans,* Nutrition Insight 29, Washington, DC, 2004 (June), Author.

38. Sharkey JR: Risk and presence of food insufficiency are associated with low nutrient intakes and multimorbidity among homebound older women who receive home-delivered meals, *J Nutr* 133:3485, 2003.

39. Gollub EA, Weddle DO: Improvements in nutritional intake and quality of life among frail homebound older adults receiving home-delivered breakfast and lunch, *J Am Diet Assoc* 104:1227, 2004.

40. Hughes G, Bennett KM, Hetherington MM: Old and alone: barriers to healthy eating in older men living on their own, *Appetite* 43:269, 2004.

41. American Dietetic Association: Position paper of the American Dietetic Association: nutrition across the spectrum of aging, *J Am Diet Assoc* 105:616, 2005.

42. Wilson M-M G, Morley JE: Invited review: aging and energy balance, *J Appl Physiol* 95:1728, 2003.

43. Blanc S et al: Energy requirements in the eighth decade of life, *Am J Clin Nutr* 79:303, 2004.

44. Campbell WW et al: Dietary protein adequacy and lower body versus whole body resistive training in older humans, *J Physiol* 542(2):631, 2002.

45. Borst SE: Interventions for sarcopenia and muscle weakness in older people, *Age Ageing* 33:548, 2004.

46. Fukagawa NK, Galbraith RA: Advancing age and other factors influencing the balance between amino acid requirements and toxicity, *J Nutr* 134:1569S, 2004.

47. Food and Nutrition Board, Institute of Medicine: *Dietary Reference Intakes for thiamin, riboflavin, niacin, vitamin B-6, folate, vitamin B 12, pantothenic acid, biotin, and choline,* Washington, DC, 1998, National Academies Press.

48. Daviglus ML et al: Relation of body mass index in young adulthood and middle age to Medicare expenditures in older age, *JAMA* 292:2743, 2004.

49. U.S. Department of Health and Human Services: *Health: United States, 1999 with chartbook on aging,* Rockville, Md, 1999, U.S. Government Printing Office.

50. Beers MH, Berkow R, eds: *The Merck manual of geriatrics,* ed 3, Whitehouse Station, NJ, 2000, Merck Research Laboratories.

51. Barker DJ et al: Fetal origins of adult disease, *Int J Epidemiol* 31:1235, 2002.

52. U.S. Department of Health and Human Services, U.S. Department of Agriculture: *Dietary Guidelines for Americans 2005,* ed 6, Washington, DC, 2005, U.S. Government Printing Office. Available at *www.healthierus.gov/dietaryguidelines.* Accessed July 18, 2005.

53. U.S. Department of Agriculture, Center for Nutrition Policy and Promotion: *MyPyramid food guidance system,* Washington, DC, 2005, Author. Available at *www.mypyramid.gov/.* Accessed July 17, 2005.

54. Roberts SB et al: Dietary variety predicts low body mass index and inadequate macronutrient and micronutrient intakes in community-dwelling older adults, *J Gerontol A Biol Sci Med Sci* 60A:613, 2005.

55. Seguin R, Nelson ME: The benefits of strength training for older adults, *Am J Prev Med* 25(3, suppl 2):141, 2003.

56. Kamel HK: Sarcopenia and aging, *Nutr Rev* 61(5):157, 2003.

57. Janssen I et al: Skeletal muscle cutpoints associated with elevated physical disability risk in older men and women, *Am J Epidemiol* 159(4):413, 2004.

58. Bermudez OI, Falcon, LM, Tucker KL: Intake and food sources of macronutrients among older Hispanic adults: association with ethnicity, acculturation, and length of residence in the United States, *J Am Diet Assoc* 100:665, 2000.

59. Leosdottir M et al: The association between total energy intake and early mortality: data from the Malmo Diet and Cancer Study, *J Intern Med* 256:499, 2004.

60. Roberts SB, Dallal GE: Effects of age on energy balance, *Am J Clin Nutr* 68(suppl):975S, 1998.

61. Roberts SB: Energy regulation and aging: recent findings and their implications, *Nutr Rev* 58:91, 2000.

62. Flegal KM et al: Excess deaths associated with underweight, overweight, and obesity, *JAMA* 293:1861, 2005.

63. Thomas DR et al: Nutritional management in long-term care: development of a clinical guideline, *J Gerontol A Biol Sci Med Sci* 55A(12):M725, 2000.

64. Schulze MB et al: Glycemic index, glycemic load, and dietary fiber intake and incidence of type 2 diabetes in younger and middle-aged women, *Am J Clin Nutr* 80:348, 2004.

65. McKeown NM: Whole grain intake and insulin sensitivity: evidence from observational studies, *Nutr Rev* 62(7):286, 2004.

66. Chevalier S et al: Frailty amplifies the effects of aging on protein metabolism: role of protein intake, *Am J Clin Nutr* 78:422, 2003.

67. Neumann M et al: Provision of high-protein supplement for patients recovering from hip fracture, *Nutrition* 20(5):415, 2004.

68. Chernoff R: Protein and older adults, *J Am Coll Nutr* 23(6, suppl):627S, 2004.

69. Food and Nutrition Board, Institute of Medicine: *Dietary Reference Intakes for water, potassium, sodium, chloride, and sulfate,* Washington, DC, 2004, National Academies Press.

70. Ferry M: Strategies for ensuring good hydration in the elderly, *Nutr Rev* 63(6, part 2):S22, 2005.

71. Wilson M-M, Morley JE: Impaired cognitive function and mental performance in mild dehydration, *Eur J Clin Nutr* 57(suppl 2):S24, 2003.

72. Foote JA et al: Factors associated with daily supplement use among healthy adults of five ethnicities, *Am J Epidemiol* 157:888, 2003.

73. Thomas DR: Distinguishing starvation from cachexia, *Clin Geriatr Med* 18:883, 2002.

74. Wilson M-M: Undernutrition in medical outpatients, *Clin Geriatr Med* 18:759, 2002.

75. Johnson KA, Bernard MA, Funderburg K: Vitamin nutrition in older adults, *Clin Geriatr Med* 18:773, 2002.

76. American Academy of Family Physicians, American Dietetic Association: *Nutrition Screening Initiative,* Washington, DC, 1989-2005, Authors. Materials available at *www.aafp.org/nsi.xml.* Accessed August 1, 2005.

77. American Dietetic Association: Position of the American Dietetic Association: liberalized diets for older adults in long-term care, *J Am Diet Assoc* 98:201, 1998. (Affirmed until 2005.)

78. Tariq SH: Dietary prescription in diabetes mellitus, *Clin Geriatr Med* 18:827, 2002.

79. Wendland BE et al: Malnutrition in institutionalized seniors: the iatrogenic component, *J Am Geriatr Soc* 51:85, 2003.

FURTHER READINGS AND RESOURCES

Readings

Bermudez OI, Falcon LM, Tucker KL: Intake and food sources of macronutrients among older Hispanic adults: association with ethnicity, acculturation and length of residence in the United States, *J Am Diet Assoc* 100:665, 2000.

Sharkey JR, Schoenberg NE: Prospective study of black-white differences in food insufficiency among homebound elders, *J Aging Health* 17(4):507, 2005.

Bailey RL et al: Persistent oral health problems associated with co-morbidity and impaired diet quality in older adults, *J Am Diet Assoc* 104:1273, 2004.

Keller HH et al: Prevention of weight loss in dementia with comprehensive nutritional treatment, *J Am Geriatr Soc* 51:945, 2003.

Mattes RD: The chemical senses and nutrition in aging: challenging old assumptions, *J Am Diet Assoc* 102(2):192, 2002.

Egbert AM: The dwindles: failure to thrive in older patients, *Nutr Rev* 54(1, part 2):S25, 1996.

These articles discuss some of the physical, financial, social, cognitive, ethnic, and racial influences on food habits of older persons and help us understand how we can assist older adults in selecting and obtaining nutrient-dense foods.

Morley JE: The top 10 hot topics in aging, *J Gerontol A Biol Sci Med Sci* 59A:24, 2004.

Dr. Morley is an internationally recognized expert in the nutritional and medical problems of older persons. His 10 hot topics include several nutrition issues, and he describes the research that is needed to solve these problems.

Minkler M, Schauffler H, Clements-Nolle K: Health promotion for older Americans in the 21st century, *Am J Health Promot* 14:371, 2000.

This article by Minkler and her colleagues gives us some good ideas for developing health promotion programs for older adults.

Wellman NS, Rosenzweig LY, Lloyd JL: Thirty years of the older Americans nutrition program, *J Am Diet Assoc* 102(3):348, 2002.

Baker EB, Wellman NS: Nutrition concerns in discharge planning for older adults: a need for multidisciplinary collaboration, *J Am Diet Assoc* 105:603, 2005.

Dr. Wellman and her co-workers help us understand the breadth and importance of the Elderly Nutrition Program for older Americans living in the community.

Websites of Interest

- Administration on Aging (AoA); this website describes many activities and health-related materials that are available to assist older adults: *www.aoa.dhhs.gov.*

- Florida International University, National Resource Center on Nutrition, Physical Activity, and Aging; this website provides many resource materials for nutrition and activity programs for older adults, as well as AoA policy guidelines and evaluation reports for the Elderly Nutrition Program: *http://nutritionandaging.fiu.edu.*

- National Institutes of Health, Health Information; this website is intended to assist consumers seeking information about healthy lifestyles and specific diseases; click on the quick link to *Seniors' Health* to find a wealth of materials pertaining to aging and health issues of older adults: *http://health.nih.gov.*

- Nutrition Screening Initiative: *www.aafp.org/x16081.xml.*

CHAPTER 14

Nutrition and Physical Fitness

Staci Nix

This chapter relates two basic factors—(1) nutrition and (2) physical fitness—to health maintenance throughout the life cycle. In an increasingly fast-paced and technology-dependent society, building regular physical activity into our busy lives requires commitment and effort. However, physical fitness is a vital cornerstone in the preventive approach to controlling the chronic diseases of modern civilization.

We examine first how nutrition works to provide energy fuels for muscle action. Then we apply these principles to enhancing athletic performance and to building a reasonable and appropriate personal exercise program.

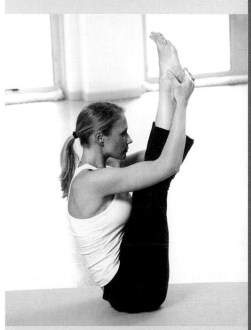

MODERN CIVILIZATION, CHRONIC DISEASE, AND PHYSICAL ACTIVITY

Modern Developed Nations and Diseases of Civilization

Over thousands of years the human body has evolved from earlier ages when survival in agriculture-based societies required constant physical exertion and energy expenditure. Now, over only a few generations, the developed nations of the world have come to live in very different circumstances. Our knowledge-based societies demand little, if any, physical activity in our daily work or lifestyles. As a result, although life expectancy continues to rise, overall quality of life and health are paying a price. Our inactivity contributes to a host of modern illnesses, the so-called diseases of civilization, including coronary heart disease, diabetes, hypertension, osteoporosis, and obesity.[1]

The Physical Fitness Movement and Health

Physical inactivity is a global problem and is estimated by the World Health Organization to cause 2 million deaths annually.[2] Physical fitness is no longer just a fad or a trend; increased participation in regular physical activity as a part of everyday life remains a national health goal, especially with healthy weight being of national concern. The U.S. Department of Health and Human Services, in its report *Healthy People 2010: Understanding and Improving Health,* has set health-related goals for Americans in nutrition and physical fitness. The 2010 target is for 30% of adults and 85% of adolescents to participate in regular moderate-to-vigorous physical activity.[3] Walking, swimming, biking, and jogging are some of the most popular outdoor activities. Athletics, both amateur and professional, have become big business, and the health specialty of sports medicine has grown dramatically.

The health benefits of physical activity are not reserved just for athletes. In everyday life the need for exercise is serious. The modern healthcare approach of preventive medicine, as well as the necessity of dealing with chronic disease, demands attention to the related roles of nutrition and physical fitness in healthcare. The U.S. Department of Agriculture has published national dietary guidelines every 5 years since 1980. Starting with the *Dietary Guidelines for Americans 2000,*[4] a new "Aim for Fitness" category was added to the well-established guidelines for what we eat. These guidelines encourage all people, in addition to practicing healthy eating choices, to be physically active each day and to aim for a healthy weight. Fitness has definite health benefits. Aerobic exercise, combined with weight training, increases fitness for all aspects of life.

The 2005 *Dietary Guidelines for Americans* recommends 30 to 60 minutes of moderate physical activity per day to prevent weight gain, and 60 to 90 minutes per day to sustain weight loss.[5] Exercise also has emerged as an effective therapy, along with nutrition care and weight management, in the control of hypertension, diabetes, cancer risk, and elevated blood lipids.[6] Moderate exercise helps control the health problems of many older adults. Regardless of the level of exercise or active pursuits that a person can achieve, even a limited beginning builds into consistent habits. The longer people follow some form of regular exercise, the more committed they become. For many, it is a matter of life and health.

BODY IN MOTION

The Nature of Energy

The term *energy* refers to the body's ability, or power, to do work. The energy required to do body work takes several different forms: mechanical, chemical, electrical, radiant, and heat. Energy, like matter, can neither be created nor destroyed. It can only be changed into another form; therefore energy is constantly cycled in the body and environment. We also speak of energy as being potential or kinetic. Potential energy is stored energy, ready to be used. Kinetic energy is active energy, being used to do work. Energy balance in physical activity requires a base of sound nutrition to supply the substrate fuels, which along with oxygen and water meet widely varying levels of energy demands for body action.

Muscle Physiology

Muscle Structure

The synchronized action of millions of specialized cells and structures that make up our skeletal muscle mass makes possible all forms of physical activity. A finely coordinated series of small bundles within the muscle fibers (Figure 14-1) triggered by nerve endings produces a smooth symphony of action through simultaneous and alternating contraction and relaxation. These successively smaller muscle structures include the following:

- *Skeletal muscle:* The largest bundle in the series is the complete muscle. Each particular muscle is composed of muscle fibers called fasciculi.
- *Muscle fiber:* Each muscle fiber is composed of bundles of still smaller strands called myofibrils.
- *Myofibril:* Each single myofibril strand of the muscle fiber is made up of the smallest of all the fiber bundles, called myofilaments. Muscular contraction occurs here.
- *Myosin and actin:* Within each myofilament are the contractile proteins, myosin and actin, which are the smallest moving parts of every muscle.

Muscle Action

Inside the cell membrane, these contractile proteins, myosin and actin, are arranged in long parallel rows.

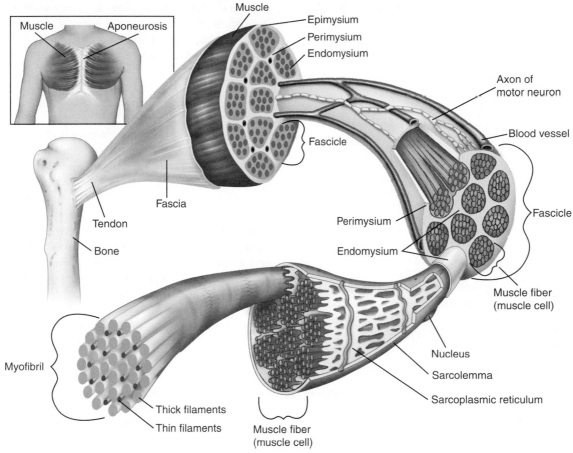

FIGURE 14-1 Skeletal muscle, showing the progressively smaller bundles within bundles. *(From Thibodeau GA, Patton KT:* Anatomy & physiology, *ed 5, St. Louis, 2003, Mosby/Elsevier.)*

These parallel rows slide together and mesh tightly when the muscle contracts and then pull apart when the muscle relaxes, allowing the muscle to shorten or lengthen as needed. When a specific motor nerve impulse excites these molecules of myosin and actin in a myofilament, they mesh together and thereby shorten the muscle. This contraction of the muscle bundles occurs instantly and simultaneously. Periods of relaxation occur between contractions. This alternating process of muscle contraction/relaxation can continue until muscle glycogen is depleted and muscle fatigue sets in.

Fuel Sources

Fuel sources are the basic energy nutrients in the diet, primarily carbohydrate and some fat. Their metabolic products—glucose, glycogen, and fatty acids—provide ready fuel sources for the chemical energy reactions within cells. Phosphate bonds form high-energy chemical compounds in body metabolism (see Chapter 5). The main high-energy compound of the body cells is *adenosine triphosphate (ATP)*. It has rightly been called the "energy currency" of the cell. Various forms of en-

potential Energy existing in stored fuels and ready for action but not yet released and active.

kinetic Energy released from body fuels by cell metabolism and now active in moving muscles and energizing all body activities.

substrate The specific organic substance on which a particular enzyme acts to produce new metabolic products.

fasciculi A general term for a small bundle or cluster of muscle, tendon, or nerve fibers.

myofibril Slender thread of muscle; runs parallel to the long axis of the muscle fiber.

myofilaments Threadlike filaments of actin or myosin, which are components of myofibrils.

myosin Myofibril protein whose synchronized meshing action in conjunction with actin causes muscles to contract and relax.

actin Myofibril protein whose synchronized meshing action in conjunction with myosin causes muscles to contract and relax.

ergy are called on for successive energy needs, as follows:

- *Immediate energy:* High-power or immediate energy demands over a short time depend on ATP being readily available within the muscle tissue. This amount is used up rapidly, and a backup compound, *creatine phosphate (CP),* is made available. These high-energy phosphate compounds, however, will sustain exercise for only approximately 5 to 8 seconds.
- *Short-term energy:* If an activity lasts longer, between 30 seconds and 2 minutes, *muscle glycogen* provides the needed energy source through the lactate pathway. Although the amount of available glycogen is small, it is an important rapid source of energy for brief muscular effort.
- *Long-term energy:* Exercise continuing more than 2 minutes requires an oxygen-dependent, or *aerobic,* energy system. A constant supply of oxygen in the blood is necessary for continued exercise. Special cell organelles, the *mitochondria,* located within each cell, produce large amounts of ATP. The ATP is produced mainly from glucose and fatty acids and supplies the continued energy needs of the body (Figure 14-2).

Exercise intensity will also affect the preferred source of fuel for the active muscles. More sustained, low-intensity exercises rely primarily on muscle fat stores for energy through the aerobic pathway. As intensity increases, measured through VO₂max (discussed below), the source of energy gradually shifts to carbohydrates and utilizes the lactate system more (Table 14-1).

Nutrients become depleted during continued exercise as the body draws on its stored energy. As demands for cell ATP increase, the body metabolizes blood glucose

and muscle glycogen to provide energy via anaerobic glycolysis. With prolonged exercise of greater intensity, however, the levels of these nutrients fall too low to sustain the body's demands. Fatigue follows, and exercise cannot continue.

Oxygen Use and Physical Capacity

The most profound limit to exercise is the person's ability to deliver oxygen to the tissues and use it for the production of energy. This vital ability depends on the fitness of the pulmonary and cardiovascular systems. Because the heart is a muscle, exercise strengthens it, enabling it to pump more blood per beat, a capacity called stroke volume. The cardiac output—how much the heart pumps out in a given period—depends on the amount of blood per contraction and on the cardiac rate—the number of contractions in a given time. Fitness levels depend on the following factors:

- *Body fitness:* Physical fitness is defined in terms of aerobic capacity, which depends on the body's ability to deliver and use oxygen in sufficient quantities to meet the demands of increasing levels of exercise. Oxygen uptake increases with exercise intensity until either the demand is met or the ability to supply it is exceeded. The maximum rate the body can take in oxygen (O₂), or aerobic capacity, is called the VO₂max—the maximum uptake volume of oxygen. This capacity determines the intensity and duration of exercise that a person can perform. From the resting level, there is a steep rise in oxygen consumption during the first 3 minutes of exercise. After approximately 6 minutes the rate levels off into a steady state, indicating equilibrium between the energy required by the exercising muscles and the aerobic energy-producing system. The aerobic capacity of an individual is measured in terms of milliliters of oxygen consumed per kilogram of body weight per minute. Thus persons of differing sizes can be compared equally.
- *Body composition:* Gender differences in aerobic capacity reflect differences in body composition. In general, men have a higher aerobic capacity because of their larger lean body mass, the active metabolic body tissue. These highly metabolic tissues of the body thus

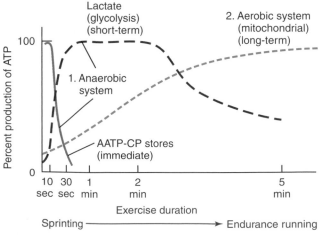

FIGURE 14-2 Contribution of the two energy systems during exercise of increasing duration. The anaerobic energy system provides ATP to the working myofilaments from ATP-CP stores and the lactate or glycolysis path. The aerobic system supplies ATP from mitochondria, which require oxygen to burn carbohydrates and fats. *(Redrawn from Nieman DC: Exercise testing and prescription, ed 5, Boston, 2003, McGraw-Hill.)*

TABLE 14-1	Effect of Intensity on Fuel Type
Exercise Intensity	**Fuel Used by Muscle**
<30% VO₂max (easy walking)	Mainly muscle fat stores
40%-60% VO₂max (jogging, brisk walking)	Fat and carbohydrate used evenly
75% VO₂max (running)	Mainly carbohydrate
≥80% VO₂max (hard running)	Nearly 100% carbohydrate

use more oxygen than other tissues such as fat. When oxygen consumption is expressed only in terms of lean body mass instead of body weight, however, men and women have a similar aerobic capacity. In general, women carry more body fat, a gender difference in body composition that serves critical biologic functions. Apart from stored adipose tissue fuel, essential structural and functional body fat in women is about 12% of their body weight; in men it is only 5%.[7] And because women must, of course, carry their entire body weight as part of their total workload, their performance will be affected accordingly.

- *Genetic influence:* A person's aerobic capacity is mainly genetically determined. But the genetic heritage is influenced, as indicated, by body composition, which is associated with sex, and by aerobic training and age. Before puberty, lean body mass is about equal in boys and girls of comparable body size, but it increases rapidly in boys at puberty under the anabolic effect of testosterone. Maximal aerobic capacity then peaks at 18 to 20 years of age and declines gradually thereafter, largely as a result of age-related losses in lean body mass.

NUTRITIONAL NEEDS DURING PHYSICAL ACTIVITY

Carbohydrates

Carbohydrates as Fuel Substrate

Although fat and protein have their special roles to play in maintaining general health, the major nutrient for energy support in exercise is carbohydrate. Carbohydrate fuels come from two sources: (1) the circulating blood glucose and (2) glycogen stored in muscle and the liver.

Carbohydrates in the Diet

Carbohydrates are the preferred energy nutrient. For active persons, carbohydrate energy should contribute about 45% to 65% of the kilocalories (kcalories or kcal) in the daily diet. Athletes competing in prolonged endurance events should increase their energy from carbohydrates to 60% to 70% of their daily total (6 to 10 g/kg body weight).[7] Complex carbohydrates (starches) are preferable to simple carbohydrates (sugars). Starches break down more slowly and help maintain blood glucose levels more evenly, avoiding low blood sugar drops, as well as maintain glycogen storage as a constant primary fuel. Simple sugars, however, can supply important energy, especially for athletes in endurance events who may require as much as 5000 kcal/day. Simple sugars may also trigger a sharper insulin response, which in some persons may contribute to the dangers of follow-up hypoglycemia.

Many studies have shown that low-carbohydrate diets hinder exercise performance. In repeated bouts of intense exercise, diets low in carbohydrate have proved to be less efficient at restoring tissue glycogen levels.[7,8] A low-carbohydrate diet decreases the body's capacity for work, which intensifies over time. Conversely, a high-carbohydrate diet restores glycogen concentrations to their regular levels. Athletes on a low-carbohydrate diet are susceptible to fatigue, ketoacidosis, dehydration, and hypoglycemia. However, athletes given carbohydrate feedings before and during exercise maintain glucose concentrations and rates of glucose oxidation necessary to exercise strenuously and thus are able to delay fatigue.[9]

Glycogen loading is a popular practice among endurance athletes. The idea is to allow the muscle to deposit more glycogen than normal immediately before an endurance event for extra stored energy. The initial method of glycogen loading was a two-step procedure. First, athletes consumed a diet higher than usual in fat and protein and lower in carbohydrates, while simultaneously exercising at high intensity, thus muscle glycogen stores were rapidly depleted. The next step is to do just the opposite: gradually decrease exercise intensity while consuming a diet high in carbohydrates (approximately 70% to 75% of total caloric intake). Table 14-2 illustrates the second phase of this procedure. There is evidence that glycogen storage capacity and rates are higher following glycogen depletion; however, there is also evidence that a substantial increase in glycogen storage will still occur without the stringent first step of this plan.[10] Because every gram of glycogen stored requires 2.7 ml of water, potential side effects may occur. Extra water weight in muscles may result in tight or sore muscles that could ultimately hinder performance.

Fat

Fat as Fuel Substrate

Fatty acids serve as a fuel source from stored fat tissue. In the presence of oxygen, fatty acids are oxidized to provide energy. The rate at which this can occur is determined in part by the rate of mobilization of fatty acids from storage, but not all stored fat is alike. Actually, the body stores fat in two ways: (1) *depot* fat in adipose tissue, which is destined for transport back and forth to other tissues as needed for energy, and (2) *essential* fat in metabolically active tissue,

---

VO$_2$max Maximal uptake volume of oxygen during exercise; used to measure the intensity and duration of exercise a person can perform.

stroke volume The amount of blood pumped from a ventricle (chamber of the heart releasing blood to body circulations) with each beat of the heart.

cardiac output Total volume of blood pumped by the heart in 1 minute.

aerobic capacity Milliliters of oxygen consumed per kilogram of body weight per minute; influenced by body composition and fitness level.

TABLE 14-2	Modified Depletion-Taper Precompetition Program for Glycogen Loading

Day	Exercise	Diet
1	90-minute period at 70%-75% VO₂max	Mixed diet; 50% carbohydrate (350 g)
2-3	Gradual tapering of time and intensity	Day 1 diet continued
4-5	Tapering of exercise time and intensity continues	Mixed diet, 70% carbohydrate (550 g)
6	Complete rest	Days 4 and 5 diet continued
7	Day of competition	High-carbohydrate pre-event diet

From Wright ED: Carbohydrate nutrition and exercise, *Clin Nutr* 7(1):18, 1988, with permission from Elsevier.

such as bone marrow, heart, lungs, liver, spleen, kidneys, intestines, muscles, and nervous system, which is reserved in these places for necessary structural and functional use only. Although storage depot fat in men and women is roughly comparable, essential fat reserves make the big difference; they are about three times greater in women.

Free fatty acids, the fat fuel, are stored with glycerol as triglycerides in the body's adipose tissue. The enzyme *lipoprotein lipase* allows for the mobilization of these stored fatty acids throughout the body. This lipase is stimulated by exercise. Its activity is affected by levels of hormones also involved in exercise, especially growth hormone and epinephrine.

Fat in the Diet

It is important to recognize that fat as a fuel substrate is not drawn from the diet directly but rather from the body's stored adipose fat. It is not necessary to consume fat directly in food to maintain the body's adipose tissue depot fat stores because excess kcalories in the diet will be converted to fat and stored on the body regardless of the dietary source. We do not need to eat in excess of our dietary needs to burn fat, and there is no danger of depleting our fat stores before exercise has proceeded to exhaustion. Thus there is no basis for increased levels of fat in the diet. On the other hand, a moderate level of fat in the diet is needed for essential fat purposes, especially as a source of the essential fatty acids, alpha-linolenic and linoleic acid. An extremely low fat intake can be medically dangerous by creating a dangerous linoleic acid deficiency. Because the heart muscle prefers fatty acids as an energy source, there have been reports of deaths from cardiac arrest in some cases of essential fatty acid deficiency. The standard recommendation that dietary fat should not exceed 20% to 35% of the total daily kcaloric intake, per the Acceptable Macronutrient Distribution Range (AMDR), is ample for most healthy individuals.

Protein

Protein as Fuel Substrate

Dietary protein has only a small role as a fuel substrate in energy production during exercise. Although some amino acids can feed into the basic energy cycle, the extent of this input during exercise is minimal. There is evidence that some amino acid breakdown occurs during exercise, and there is some nitrogen loss in sweat. But authorities agree that under normal circumstances protein makes a relatively insignificant contribution to energy during exercise. In endurance events, however, somewhat more protein may be used, especially when carbohydrate resources are exhausted.

Protein in the Diet

A daily intake of 0.8 to 1 g of protein/kg of body weight is sufficient to meet the general needs of the physically active person. This amounts to the recommended daily dietary intake standard for adults, with about 10% to 35% of the kcalories in the diet coming from protein. Ill-informed athletes who purchase and use excess protein supplements in various forms are subjecting their bodies to an even greater taxing load and the dangers of abnormal metabolic stress. Nitrogen consumed in excess of need must be excreted. This puts a burden on the kidneys to excrete the increased urea coming from the liver, which contributes to dehydration, a serious factor during strenuous exercise. Chronic high-protein diets and supplements can also lead to increased excretion of calcium in the urine, particularly in women, and can have long-term detrimental effects on bone structure.[11-13] Protein from animal sources, versus plant-based proteins, elicit a more acidic by-product. This metabolic acid load from animal protein metabolism is thought to be the cause of excess calcium excretion and bone resorption.[13]

Micronutrients

Vitamins and Minerals as Catalytic Cofactors

Vitamins and minerals cannot be used as fuel substrates. They are not oxidized or used up in the process of energy production. Vitamins and minerals are, however, essential as catalytic cofactors in enzyme reactions.

Vitamins and Minerals in the Diet

Increased physical exertion during exercise or athletic training does not require a greater intake of vitamins and minerals beyond currently recommended intakes. A well-balanced diet will supply adequate amounts of vitamins and minerals, and exercise may well improve the body's efficient use of them. Because athletes, for example, have an increased dietary need for energy, their larger kcaloric intake from good food sources would automatically boost their general intake of vitamins and minerals. Multivitamin and mineral supplementation does not improve physical performance in healthy athletes eating a well-balanced

CASE STUDY

Fluid and Energy Needs for Endurance Athletes

Jamie is a 25-year-old man training for an ultramarathon race of 50 miles. He is 5 ft 10 in tall and currently weighs 170 lb. On his long runs of 3 hours and more, he has been drinking nothing but water, approximately 30 oz, and consuming one Gu (100 kcal, all from simple carbohydrates) at once at the 2-hour mark. He is coming to you for advice because he is becoming increasingly weak and nauseous toward the end of his runs. He reports feeling light-headed and irritable on his long training days. Jamie states that he is eating an egg salad sandwich with two hard boiled eggs mixed with 3 tbsp of mayonnaise on whole wheat bread about 20 minutes before his run.

Questions for Analysis

1. What sources of fuel is Jamie predominately using in this type of exercise?
2. How much fluid should Jamie be consuming during a 3-hour run?
3. Based on his weight, how many calories and grams of carbohydrate should he consume during his run?
4. On what time schedule would you recommend he consume his fluid and carbohydrate?
5. What would you recommend regarding his preexercise meal?

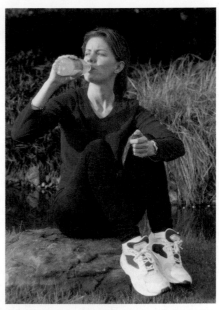

FIGURE 14-3   Frequent small drinks of cold water during extended exercise prevent dehydration. *(Credit: PhotoDisc.)*

diet; and the potential side effects from megavitamin supplements are well known (see Chapters 6 and 7). However, *therapeutic* iron supplements may be necessary for some athletes who experience iron deficiency anemia. Also, special assessment of nutrient-energy status is needed for young adolescent amenorrheic female athletes such as gymnasts, ballet dancers, and runners, who may be experiencing eating disorders such as anorexia nervosa. Such disordered eating patterns may involve low calcium intake, which can have serious consequences for bone development (see the *Perspectives in Practice* box, "The Female Athlete Triad: How Performance and Social Pressure Can Lead to Low Bone Mass").[13]

Hydration: Water and Electrolytes

Water and Dehydration

Dehydration can be a serious problem for athletes and may greatly limit exercise capacity.[14,15] Its extent depends on the intensity and duration of the exercise, the surrounding temperature, the level of fitness, and the preexercise or pregame state of hydration. It is especially severe in endurance events (see the *Case Study* box, "Fluid and Energy Needs for Endurance Athletes"). Athletes may experience problems such as cramps, delirium, vomiting, hypothermia, or hyperthermia—all caused by dehydration. With careful planning ahead of athletic events and providing fluid replacement throughout, many of these problems can be prevented. Regular fluid intake should be planned for all types of athletes, not just runners. Some strategies to increase fluid intake by athletes are given in Box 14-1. A useful tool that many coaches use is mandatory weighing before and after the athletic event; then each pound (2.2 kg) of weight lost by a player during the event should be replaced by 16 oz (480 to 500 ml) of fluid.

BOX 14-1	Strategies for Sports Team Members to Increase Fluid Intake

- Establish a regular schedule; drink during warm-up exercises and between periods of play.
- Give each player a sports squeeze bottle.
- Supply players with a sports drink that tastes good while exercising.
- Make available a choice of fluids to drink.
- Offer cool fluids, which are preferred over warm fluids.
- Avoid carbonated beverages because athletes tend to drink less when the beverage is carbonated.

From Palumbo CM: Nutrition concerns related to the performance of a baseball team, *J Am Diet Assoc* 100(6):704, 2000, Copyright with permission from the American Dietetic Association.

Cause of Dehydration.   Approximately 60% of the energy from the breakdown of glucose is released as heat. In minimal physical exercise this heat production maintains desirable body temperature. During heavier exercise it exceeds the body's needs and sometimes even exceeds the body's heat tolerance capacity. Sweating is our main mechanism for dissipating body heat. The major source of fluid loss in sweat is plasma fluid. Endurance events can cause the loss of several liters of water as sweat, which is pulled from the plasma fluid to control body heat. Unless this amount is replaced, serious consequences can follow.

Prevention of Dehydration.   The thirst mechanism fails to keep pace with the body's increased need for fluid during exercise. To prevent dehydration, athletes are advised to drink more water than they think is needed, in frequent small amounts (4 oz every 15 minutes), without dependence on the normal thirst mechanism (Figure 14-3). Cold water, 15° to 21° C, will stimulate intake and is generally

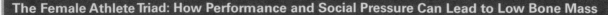

PERSPECTIVES IN PRACTICE
The Female Athlete Triad: How Performance and Social Pressure Can Lead to Low Bone Mass

Meredith Catherine Williams

The female athlete triad consists of three health afflictions faced by women who are extremely physically active: disordered eating, menstrual disturbances and irregularity, and osteopenia (low bone mass) or even osteoporosis. Low bone mineral density (BMD) is often the final result of the triad that affects women, and it is the leading cause of stress fractures and injuries throughout the body, some of which may be irreversible. Many women who are in top physical form are ironically the most likely to develop these three linked complications and health problems because social and performance pressure may steer women to extreme eating habits and exercise regimens. The dilemma facing women athletes today is how to maintain optimal physical performance while not tampering with health risks.

Women who participate in competitive sports that require endurance, such as rowing or long distance running, or who are judged partially on physical appearance, such as in ice skating, diving, or dancing, are more likely to be preoccupied with their weight and to have self-image issues. Social and competitive pressure for a woman to be thin can contribute to her sense of imperfection. These demands and pressures can lead some women to develop disordered eating patterns, which in combination with strenuous exercise will result in low energy levels. This drop in energy will be followed by a drop in performance as the athlete loses focus and concentration and is fatigued. Some women develop extreme dietary conditions, such as bulimia nervosa, which is characterized by binge eating followed by forced vomiting, purging, or excessive laxative intakes, or anorexia nervosa, which is characterized by the refusal or inability to consume sufficient calories for daily requirements. These more serious disorders can progress to psychologic problems (depression or low self-esteem), seizures, cardiac arrhythmia, myocardial infarction, or other health complications. The seriousness of the eating disorder is linked to the amount of stress and concern the woman feels over her body image combined with the amount of emphasis put on weight by trainers, coaches, and instructors. Athletes often believe that leanness enhances performance, and some are willing to take health risks to satisfy perfectionist needs and habits.

Poor caloric intake and disordered eating can cause menstrual irregularity. Amenorrhea is the suppression of menstrual cycles to a level of zero to three menses a year, and primary amenorrhea is the repression of all menstrual cycles until the age of 16 years. This condition is often found in young female gymnasts who, in the most competitive circles, may actually strive to delay the onset of puberty to maintain small, childlike physiques. Some women may experience oligomenorrhea instead, which are sporadic cycles that occur 3 to 9 times a year. The levels of estrogen and progesterone that regulate menses can be affected by metabolism, intensive exercise, dieting, or stress.

There are several treatments available for female athletes: sex steroid replacement, increased caloric intake, decreased exercise, weight gain, and calcium supplements. Evidence suggests that raising estrogen and progesterone levels and increasing caloric intake are the most effective measures, yet there is a wide range of treatment prescribed. Education and further research are needed to find the optimal course.

Menstrual irregularities are related to low bone density. Before the age of 30, bone density reaches its peak, and it is vital for young women to strive for dense bones in early adulthood so as to have healthy bone density later in life. If the density of bones is diminished early on, osteopenia occurs, and if severe enough, it can be a signal of future osteoporosis. Although women who were once athletes seem to recover some of their bone density loss, vertebral bone normalization is uncommon. In active young females with tightly regulated diets and menstrual inconsistency, there can be bone density as low as that of a 70-year-old woman. These thin bones increase the likelihood of stress fractures and injuries, and women are far more likely to incur such injuries than men.

Some studies, however, indicate that weight-bearing activities, such as gymnastics, seem to actually improve bone density, even perhaps in vertebrae, and may help prevent density decreases later in life. Yet the problem facing women athletes who are eating improperly is that the rate of decrease in BMD increases as menstrual cycles continue to be erratic. The longer the menstrual cycles are inconsistent; the sooner bone density is lost. Weight-bearing sports will not overcome the tendency toward low BMD if diet and exercise levels are not carefully monitored.

The best course of action is to have women athletes monitor their diet to include substantial caloric intake and sufficient micronutrient consumption. The prevention of osteoporosis later in life lies in the habits of the individual and the modification of factors that can lead to the triad of eating disturbances, menstrual irregularity, and low bone density. Body weight is individual, depending on height and skeletal structure, and there should not be one specific weight goal for all female athletes.

However, the societal and competitive pressures that cause the initial step in this three step process must also be addressed. Asking female athletes to sacrifice their health for an unrealistic image projected on them and the need for vicarious victory must not dominate the standards of what are acceptable eating habits. In today's weight conscious society, the emphasis must not be on a perfect image, size, or body but rather on the perfect balance of health and training. The female athlete's skeletal integrity suffers as she resorts to drastic measures in her aspiration for a perfect lean physical image, but her male athlete counterpart has no such risk because his bone density is not dependent on menstrual regularity.

The need now is to educate trainers, athletes, and health professionals about the consequences of neglected nutrition. There should be no one image of the perfect female body, and young female athletes must understand that deprivation of life's essential nutrients ultimately only does more harm than good.

References

Iacopino L et al: Body composition differences in adolescent female athletes and anorexic patients, *Acta Diabetol* 40(1 suppl):S180, 2003.

Kerstetter JE et al: Dietary protein, calcium metabolism, and skeletal homeostasis revisited, *Am J Clin Nutr* 78(3 suppl):584S, 2003.

Lloyd T et al: Lifestyle factors and the development of bone mass and bone strength in young women, *J Pediatr* 144(6):776, 2004.

Miller KK: Mechanisms by which nutritional disorders cause reduced bone mass in adults, *J Womens Health* 12(2):145, 2003.

Thrash LE, Anderson JJB: The female athlete triad: nutrition, menstrual disturbances, and low bone mass, *Nutr Today* 35(5):168, 2000.

Zeni AI et al: Stress injury to the bone among women athletes, *Phys Med Rehabil Clin North Am* 11(4):929, 2000.

TO PROBE FURTHER

SORTING OUT THE SPORTS DRINKS SAGA

The first of the so-called sports drinks hit the market about 25 years ago, and now, with all its followers, these beverages have spawned a multimillion-dollar industry. Their claims abound, and sorting them out is not always easy for athletes and their coaches, who forever seek that prize of the competitive edge.

The current saga of the sports drinks began with a solution called Gatorade, a beverage its developers named for their university's football team. They reasoned that if they analyzed the sweat of their players, they could replace the lost minerals and water in a drink containing some flavoring, coloring, and sugars to make it acceptable, and it would taste better and do a better job than plain water. Although it is beneficial for some athletes, most do not need it during general exercise. Physically fit athletes engaged in regular nonendurance exercise generally do as well on plain water as on a solution such as this product and obtain their minerals from their regular diets.

However, what long-term endurance athletes do need, especially in hot weather, is water and fuel, that is, carbohydrates. For example, so much water is lost by a runner in a long-distance marathon—when the body sweats 2% to 6% of its weight—that it cannot keep cool enough and the overall system overheats, leading to heat stroke and collapse. Also, without adequate carbohydrate replacement, the muscles soon run out of glycogen stores and slow down. For athletes losing substantial amounts of water and sodium through sweat, electrolyte replacement is also an important consideration. Hyponatremia (plasma sodium concentration less than 135 mEq/L), although rare, can be fatal. The most common cause of hyponatremia in endurance athletes is caused from excess sodium loss through sweat combined with fluid replacement of plain water. Water dilutes the plasma volume of sodium even more, thus exacerbating the condition. Thus sports drinks with simple carbohydrates and electrolytes are necessary for endurance athletes.

Simply adding sugar to water holds it in the stomach longer, where it does the body tissues no good for immediate needs. To meet the body's dual need during such marathon events, a second category of sports drinks has now been developed, using glucose polymers instead of sugar and adding less sodium. These short chains of about five glucose molecules—maltodextrins—are produced in the breakdown of starch. These drinks are less concentrated and are only slightly sweetened and flavored, and they leave the stomach rapidly, thus making them ideal as a continuing fuel source for the endurance athlete.

Other sports drinks to enter the market have been Gatorade clones such as the product Recharge, which claims to add no sugar yet supplies an ample amount of it as fructose and glucose in its fruit juice base. And still another category has emerged in products such as Gear Up, which adds to its base of 10 fruit juices 10 vitamins in amounts yielding 137% of the RDAs in a single 10-ounce bottle but contains no minerals. All of these extra vitamins do not help an athlete's performance, and on a hot day a perspiring athlete could easily down a megadose in four or five bottles. However, recent studies indicate that controlled use in intermittent moderate-to high-intensity exercise improves the athlete's performance.

So sort out the costs and claims of sports drinks. They are not for everyone. For the long run, special ones may meet the needs of the athlete in endurance events. But for nonendurance activities most persons do not need them. After all, water is the best solution for regular needs—and it costs far less.

References

American College of Sports Medicine, American Dietetic Association, Dietitians of Canada: Joint position statement: nutrition and athletic performance. *Med Sci Sports Exerc* 32(12):2130, 2000.

Rehrer NJ: Fluid and electrolyte balance in ultra-endurance sport, *Sports Med* 31(10):701, 2001.

Von Duvillard SP et al: Fluids and hydration in prolonged endurance performance, *Nutrition* 20(7-8):651, 2004.

more palatable for individuals exercising. It is important to speed rehydration and to minimize the discomfort that a full stomach gives the athlete. During longer events, lasting several hours, small cups of cold water, or sports drinks with mild solutions of saline and glucose (600 to 1200 ml/hr containing 4% to 8% carbohydrates), should be taken frequently. Until quite recently it was thought that drinking water immediately before or during an athletic event would cause cramps; there is no basis for this claim.

Electrolytes

A number of special sports drinks are now being marketed with the indication that the electrolytes lost in sweat must be replaced (see the *To Probe Further* box, "Sorting Out the Sports Drinks Saga"). This is true, but how? Sweat is more dilute than our internal fluids, and thus we lose proportionately, not just absolutely, much more water than anything else. In most instances, water is the rehydration fluid of choice; electrolytes are replaced with the athlete's next meal. However, during longer and more demanding endurance events (1 to 2 hours), especially in a warm environment, a mild saline and glucose (0.5 to 0.7g NaCl/L and 4% to 8% glucose solution) sports drink that has rapid gastric emptying and intestinal absorption times may be used. For ultraendurance events lasting between 3 and 24 hours, a higher concentration of sodium (1.7 to 2.9 g NaCl/L) is recommended to adequately replace sodium losses and to avoid the risk of hyponatremia.[16]

---

hyponatremia Serum sodium less than 135 mEq/L; a relative excess of body water compared with sodium.

TABLE 14-3	Approximate Energy Expenditure per Hour During Various Activities

Activity	Kcalories per Hour*
Sleeping	63
Lying/sitting, awake	70
Standing, relaxed	84
Rapid typing, sitting	105
Dressing and undressing	140
Walking slowly (24 min/mile)	210
Water aerobics	280
High-impact aerobics	490
Football, flag/tough	560
Walking very fast (12 min/mile)	560
Stair, treadmill	630
Swimming, vigorous effort	700
Running (8 min/mile)	875

From Nix S: *Williams' basic nutrition & diet therapy*, ed 12, St. Louis, 2005, Mosby/Elsevier.

*For an adult weighing 70 kg (154 lb).

NUTRITION AND ATHLETIC PERFORMANCE

Exercise and Energy

Exercise raises the body's kcalorie need and has the additional benefit of helping to regulate appetite to meet these needs. Table 14-3 gives some examples of the amount of kcalories expended in various activities. The building of glycogen reserves in particular is important for athletes such as long-distance runners who compete in endurance events. Persons at moderate exercise levels have actually been shown to eat less than inactive persons. This may relate to an internal "set point" regulating the amount of body fat the person will carry. According to this theory, the set point is raised—that is, more body fat is stored—when the individual becomes inactive. In any case, when exercise levels rise from mild or moderate amounts up to strenuous levels, kcaloric needs also rise to supply needed fuel.

Active persons, even athletes, require no more fat than inactive persons. Carbohydrate is the preferred fuel and is the critical food for the active person—not only before an exercise period but also during the recovery period. The complex carbohydrate forms (i.e., starches) not only sustain energy needs but also supply added fiber, vitamins, and minerals. Thus the recommended composition of energy nutrients to support physical activity in highly active persons is approximately the following[7]:

- *Carbohydrate:* 6 to 10 g/kg body weight per day
- *Protein:* 1.2 to 1.4 g/kg of body weight per day for endurance athletes and 1.6 to 1.7 g/kg body weight per day for resistance and strength-trained athletes
- *Fat:* 15% to 25% of total kcalories

BOX 14-2	Sample Pregame Meal

This following sample pregame meal includes approximately 320 kcal; high complex carbohydrate; and low protein, fat, and fiber:
- ¾ cup spaghetti (150 kcal, 30 g CHO)
- ¼ cup tomato sauce (23 kcal, 4.5 g CHO)
- 1 slice French bread, small (88 kcal, 17 g CHO)
- ½ cup apple juice (58 kcal, 15 g CHO)

CHO, Carbohydrate.

Pregame and Training Meals

Protein and fat delay the emptying of the stomach, and neither contributes to the glycogen stores needed during exercise. Therefore the ideal pregame meal is now known to be a light one of approximately 200 to 300 kcal that is eaten about 3 to 4 hours before the event, such as the meal illustrated in Box 14-2.[7] This meal should be high in complex carbohydrates, moderate in protein, and with little fat or fiber. This meal schedule gives the body time to digest, absorb, and transform it into stored glycogen. Good food choices include pasta, bread, bagels, muffins, and cereal with nonfat milk. Throughout the period of vigorous training, a high-carbohydrate diet with 500 to 600 g/day is recommended, such as that illustrated in Table 14-4. In addition, nutrient information may be used to calculate such diets. Small amounts of carbohydrate-containing foods or drinks may be consumed briefly before the event without affecting the performance. A total carbohydrate intake of 1 to 5 g/kg body weight taken from 5 minutes to 4 hours before the exercise is sufficient to enhance performance.[17]

Energy During Exercise

For activities lasting less than 1 hour, most athletes do not need exogenous sources of energy during the exercise period. However, it is well known that performance is enhanced during longer endurance events with the interval consumption of carbohydrates. The American College of Sports Medicine, the American Dietetic Association, and the Dietitians of Canada recommend eating or drinking 0.7 g of carbohydrate per kilogram of body weight per hour (approximately 30 to 60 g/hr) during long events.[7] It is most effective to consume equal amounts of the preferred food every 15 to 20 minutes throughout the event rather than consuming the entire 30 to 60 g at once. Athletes should experiment with various forms of glucose before competition to determine what is best tolerated. There are a large variety of sports drinks, gels, and other forms of carbohydrates that the athlete may choose from. The food of choice should provide carbohydrates primarily from glucose, with little or no fat, protein, or fiber.

Energy After Exercise: Recovery

Proper nutrition not only is important to the athlete before and during exercise, but also plays a major role in

TABLE 14-4 | 600-g Carbohydrate Diet

Menu	Carbohydrates (g)
Breakfast	
1 orange, 2⅝-in diameter	16
2 cups plain oatmeal, cooked	45
1 cup skim milk	12
1 oat bran muffin, medium	55
1 tbsp jam	14
Snack	
½ cup seedless raisins	57
Lunch	
Lettuce salad	
1 cup romaine lettuce	2
½ cup garbanzo beans	27
½ cup tomatoes chopped	4
2 tbsp French dressing	5
2 cups macaroni and cheese	94
1½ cups apple juice	43
Snack	
2 slices whole wheat bread	24
1 tbsp peanut butter	3
Dinner	
2 oz turkey breast (no skin)	—
2 cups mashed potatoes with whole milk	74
1 cup peas and onions	16
¾ cup fruit salad (banana, pineapple, papaya, guava)	43
1 cup skim milk	12
Snack	
1 cup cranberry juice, unsweetened	33
1 oz pretzels	22
TOTAL	601

Data from U.S. Department of Agriculture, Agricultural Research Service: *National nutrient database for standard reference,* Release 18, Washington, DC, 2005, Author. Accessible at *www.nal.usda.gov/fnic/foodcomp/search/index.html.*

recovery after the event. It is well accepted that fluid and carbohydrate replacement beverages consumed immediately after a glycogen-depleting endurance event will result in higher glycogen synthesis and muscle recovery than if replacement beverages are delayed for 2 hours or more.[7] Beverages of 6% glucose concentration are adequate during this period, but higher concentrations may be consumed depending on the tolerance of the athlete. For athletes taking only a short break in between events (e.g., triathletes), foods and beverages ingested should be limited to primarily carbohydrate-containing substances. For athletes recovering for longer periods of time, a replacement beverage containing at least 0.8 g of carbohydrate per kilogram body weight results in a greater rate of muscle glycogen recovery.[18]

Myths and Misinformation

Athletes and their coaches are particularly susceptible to myths and claims about foods and dietary supplements. They search relentlessly for the competitive edge (see the *Focus on Culture* box, "The Winning Edge—or Over the Edge?"). Knowing this, marketers unremittingly exploit this search. Manufacturers sometimes make distorted and false claims for products. For example, pangamic acid, marketed as "vitamin B_{15}" although it is not a vitamin at all, carried claims about its ability to enhance oxygen transport during exercise. Naturally, if there were such a compound, it would be of interest to athletes and their trainers. However, scientific research has exposed these claims as unfounded.

In addition to specific fraud, the world of athletics is beset with superstitions and misconceptions such as the following:

- Athletes need protein for energy.
- Protein supplements are needed to build bigger and stronger muscles.
- Vitamin supplements are needed to enable athletes to use more energy.
- Vitamins and minerals are burned up in workouts and training sessions.
- Electrolyte solutions are always needed during exercise to replace sweat losses.
- A pregame meal of steak and eggs ensures maximal performance.
- Drinking water during exercise will cause cramps.

Training and Precompetition Abuses Among Athletes

Weight Control Measures

The sport of wrestling has a long history of widely fluctuating weight patterns among its athletes. Wrestlers often restrict food and fluid intake to qualify for a weight classification that is below their off-season weight, seeking to gain advantages in strength, speed, and leverage over a smaller opponent. This practice of "making weight" still seems to be an ingrained tradition that produces large, frequent, and rapid weight loss/regain cycles, with methods such as dehydration, severe food restriction, and loss of food and fluid through induced vomiting and use of laxatives and diuretic drugs. Such disordered eating affects normal growth, and progressive dehydration impairs regulation of body temperature and cardiovascular function. Other sports such as bodybuilding and gymnastics often follow similar routines, especially before competition. In gymnastics, for example, young preadolescent girls who must maintain a small body size in the face of advancing age increasingly reduce food intake and body fat, sometimes developing eating disorders. As a result, a cascade of events may follow—impaired growth,

FOCUS ON CULTURE

The Winning Edge—or Over the Edge?

Athletes, their coaches, and our entire culture have become increasingly aware that the percentage of body fat versus the percentage of lean body mass is a major influence on athletic performance. Each extra pound of body fat an athlete carries into competition is nonproductive weight. It is the muscles, the lean body mass, that provide the strength, agility, and endurance required to win.

Because of this, athletes strive to achieve as low a percentage of body fat as possible while still maintaining good health. In reaching for such a goal, however, many young athletes develop an abhorrence of body fat, resulting in food aversion and the undertaking of excessive weight loss regimens. These self-generated excesses are commonly reinforced by those surrounding the young athletes: coaches, teammates, and, perhaps the most demanding of all, parents. Such an all-consuming focus results in compulsive behaviors, leading the young person to set unrealistic goals and resulting in abusive weight losses.

Fortunately, such excessive voluntary weight losses in young athletes are not usually caused by chronic emotional problems. The reasons typically are more superficial, resulting from an accumulation of immediate and short-term goals and concerns. These athletes usually respond well to counseling and can reverse the excessive behavior with the support of concerned friends and teammates.

Yet for a few individuals, excessive, compulsive fixation on lean body mass and the loss of body fat becomes obsessive and enduring. For example, a compulsive runner's ideal of 5% body fat is regularly found only in ballet dancers, gymnasts, fashion models, and victims of anorexia nervosa. Our mass media culture unfortunately reinforces the view that the most desirable attributes of beauty are slimness in women and physical prowess in men. When a susceptible individual enters a time of stress in search of a firm identity, he or she may turn toward cultural and media stereotypes to provide a positive self-concept. For women this stress is usually encountered during adolescence, when being physically attractive is thought by some women to be the key to social acceptance. For men the sense of self is more closely tied to their vocational and sexual effectiveness, both of which some men relate to their physical abilities. Thus the test of a man's abilities tends to occur more often in adulthood, which may result in his preoccupation with physical fitness as a way to deny any decline in strength or ability. This may be why the majority of compulsive runners, those who feel they must run despite everything, including injury or ill health, are men. Such compulsive fixation on body image in susceptible individuals often results in disordered eating that may require extensive counseling.

Our culture views compulsive dieting, as in anorexia nervosa, as a serious emotional disorder; compulsive training, on the other hand, is seen as a positive personality trait showing dedication. In reality, both may be symptomatic of unstable self-concepts and attempts to establish a firm sense of identity. They are perceptual disorders: the anorexia nervosa victim always sees herself as fat; the compulsive runner always sees himself as out of shape. Such risk factors are not necessarily true for all competitive athletes. White female athletes reported the highest prevalence of disordered eating and the lowest level of self-esteem in a 2004 study examining the cultural and ethnic differences in collegiate athletes. For these individuals, no goal, once attained, is sufficiently satisfying. If 5% body fat is achieved, the person strives for 4%. Such striving, often despite physical indications against it, has resulted in permanent disabilities and even death, sometimes from cardiac arrest caused by a linoleic acid deficiency.

The danger of athletic compulsion leading to eating disorders was highlighted by the 1994 death from anorexia nervosa of 22-year-old Christy Henrich, a world-class American gymnast. At 4 ft 10 in (147 cm) and 95 lb (43 kg), Christy won a silver medal at the 1989 U.S. national championships. She was known as a perfectionist who pushed herself hard, a characteristic that, when extreme, is often associated with eating disorders in athletes. She felt compelled to lose more weight and at times limited herself to only an apple a day even while continuing to train. Because of her eating disorder, she eventually lost the strength to perform her routines and was forced to retire from competition. She weighed only 60 pounds (27 kg) when she died. Although her death marked the first time an American gymnast had died from an eating disorder, such problems are widely known in competitive women's gymnastics, especially at the national and international levels.

Although physical fitness and athletic accomplishments may be admirable goals, the thrill of victory for a small percentage of participants may be a hollow one if the victory is at the expense of their health and peace of mind. These driven individuals have a strict sense of self-denial and are unable to enjoy life's more receptive pleasures. The ability to slow down, stop, and enjoy smelling the roses may mean more in the long run to the quality and quantity of a person's life span than the color of a coveted ribbon or medal that may be won.

References

Johnson C et al: Gender, ethnicity, self-esteem and disordered eating among college athletes, *Eat Behav* 5(2):147, 2004.
Obituary: Christy Henrich 1972-1994, *Int Gymnast* 36(10):1, 1994.

delayed puberty, induced amenorrhea from low estrogen levels, disruption or delay in bone density development, and even later osteoporosis. A similar pattern has been observed among young runners.

Drug Abuse

From ancient Greek runners and discus throwers in the first Olympian contests to top competitors from around the world in current Olympic events, athletes have experimented with various ergogenic aids in their eternal search for the competitive edge or the perfect body. Modern athletes—from professional football players to their aspiring high school counterparts—are doing the same thing, trying to find the magic potion in everything from bee pollen and seaweed to freeze-dried liver flakes, gelatin, amino acid supplements, and ginseng. Such efforts have been worthless in most cases but fortunately not particularly harmful. However, in the case of the group of drugs called *anabolic-androgenic steroids,* which are now epidemic in the sporting world, great danger and even death may lie ahead for the user. These dangers have included adverse effects to the liver, heart, and reproductive system, with additional disturbances in psychology and dermatology.[19]

The use of legal pharmacologic agents in an illegal manner has created a black market network, which adds criminal jeopardy and street preparation impurities to the drug's inherent dangers. Abuse of ergogenic aids in the United States has moved from its early use among bodybuilders to invade almost all areas of athletics, becoming epidemic among football players, significantly young junior and senior high school boys.[20,21] In addition, other abuses amplify the dangers of steroids. For example, a large dose of a diuretic such as furosemide (Lasix, 80 to 120 mg) is taken on the day of drug testing to dilute the urine and decrease the risk of detection. Also, large megadoses of vitamins and minerals become abused drugs and as such are used as ergogenic aids in all areas and levels of sports. Such megadoses of nutrients alter normal metabolic processes and may cause severe disturbances.

Risks for Female Athletes

Some women athletes who enter highly competitive and demanding sports beginning in their preadolescent and young adolescent years could face significant health risks related to anemia and low bone mineral density if their dietary habits are not sufficient to meet increased calorie needs. These risks are especially prevalent for women athletes in sports with intensive training and with endurance events, such as gymnastics and running. Highly skilled dancers in the performing arts world often face similar risks.

Sports Anemia and Iron Deficiency Anemia

Normal hemoglobin (Hb) values are 12 to 15 g/dl for women and 13.8 to 17.2 g/dl for men. Anemia is defined as Hb levels below these ranges. Although absolute anemia is rare among competitive athletes, low normal values are typical. As baseline plasma volume increases with aerobic training, the concentration of Hb (found within red blood cells) is reduced as a percentage of total blood. Such a situation is more appropriately referred to as sports anemia rather than iron deficiency anemia because the total volume of red blood cells is normal. Additional iron intake, whether through food or supplementation, is not needed in sports anemia. However, care must be taken to appropriately distinguish sports anemia from other forms of true anemias.

True iron deficiency anemia is typically a result of inadequate iron in the diet, decreased iron absorption, or increased iron losses. Reduced hemoglobin in an athlete's blood means reduced oxygen-carrying capacity; with obvious implications for aerobic capacity and the ability to sustain an exercise workload.[22] One of the first implications for iron deficiency anemia is exertional fatigue. Women athletes have cyclic menstrual loss of iron unless they experience amenorrhea. Some iron is lost in profuse sweating and occasionally because of *intravascular hemolysis,* which is the rupture of red blood cells caused by the stresses of heavy exercise. Neither sweat nor intravascular hemolysis is believed to be a major contributor to iron loss. Thus iron intake should be evaluated and addressed regularly.

Low Bone Mineral Density

Many young women athletes, as they strive for the perfect body shape and the perfect performance, do not realize the great danger they face of creating long-term irreversible damage to their bones. An inadequate diet, because of weight control efforts or disordered eating, combined with an interrupted menstrual and estrogen cycle can lead to lower-than-normal bone mineral density (osteopenia) and even in some cases to a state of osteoporosis at an abnormally young age (Figure 14-4). Because this pattern affects primarily athletes, it has been called the "female athlete triad" (see the *Perspectives in Practice* box, "The Female Athlete Triad: How Performance and Social Pressure Can Lead to Low Bone Mass").[23]

An estimated 40% to 60% of a woman's normal bone mineral density for her lifetime is created during adolescence, when her sex hormone estrogen becomes active. The diet and hormones must work together. There must be an adequate amount of calcium in the diet, as well as normal functioning of the female estrogen cycle that stimulates osteoblastic activity (bone growth). Unfortunately, many young female athletes and dancers restrict their diets in an effort to control their weight, growth, and optimal body fat, with resulting inadequate dietary energy and calcium.[24] Some may have more profound eating disorders, such as anorexia nervosa. At the same time, intense athletic training in young women can lead to amenorrhea, which is defined as the absence of menses

---

amenorrhea The absence of menses (menstrual cycle) entirely or no more than three periods in a year; associated with lower-than-normal estrogen levels in women.

ergogenic Tendency to increase work output; various substances that increase work or exercise capacity and output.

osteopenia Below-normal level of bone mineral density, which increases the risk of stress fractures; the bone thinning is not as severe as that found in osteoporosis.

osteoporosis Abnormal thinning of bone, producing a porous, fragile, latticelike bone tissue of enlarged spaces that is prone to fracture or deformity.

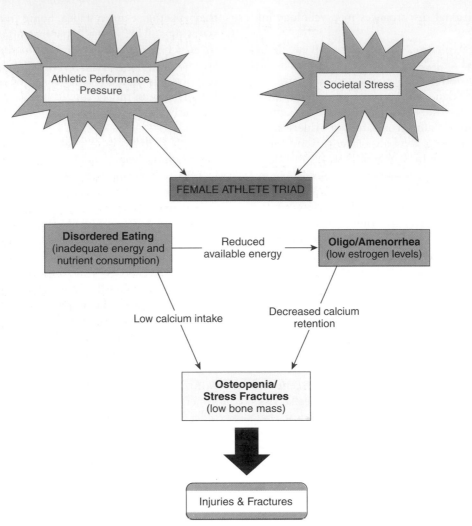

FIGURE 14-4 The female athlete triad. *(From Thrash LE, Anderson JJB: The female athlete triad: nutrition, menstrual disturbances, and low bone mass,* Nutr Today 35{5}:168, 2000, with permission from Lippincott Williams & Wilkins.)

entirely or no more than three periods in a year. Amenorrhea or missed periods are much more common in athletes than in nonathletes and are especially prevalent among endurance athletes such as runners. When athletic training begins at an early age before normal menarche, that onset of puberty with its normal growth and development pattern is delayed, along with the secondary sex characteristics shaping the female figure, as evidenced in the petite bodies of young gymnasts. Older amenorrheic adolescent runners have usually entered training after menarche and then stopped menstruating after beginning their running program. When the menstrual cycle is delayed or interrupted, normal estrogen levels are depressed. As a result, these young women athletes are at a high risk for low bone mineral density and for stress fractures.[25,26] Injuries and fractures can interrupt or permanently end an athletic career, and bone mineral loss may be irreversible and become a lifelong risk.

Health Promotion

Building a Personal Exercise Program

Exercise is a critical component in health promotion and disease prevention. The current *Dietary Guidelines for Americans* (see Chapter 1) state the following[5]:

- Moderate physical activity for 30 minutes most days provides important health benefits; more than 30 minutes provides additional benefits.
- Adults need 60 minutes of moderate to vigorous physical activity most days to prevent unhealthy weight gain.
- Children and adolescents should aim for 60 minutes of moderate to vigorous physical activity most days to maintain good health and fitness and for healthy weight during growth.

- Resistance exercise training is recommended to increase muscular strength and endurance and to maintain or increase lean body weight.

Coronary Heart Disease

Exercise reduces risks for heart disease in several ways related to heart function, blood cholesterol levels, and oxygen transport, as follows:

- *Heart muscle function:* The heart is a four-chambered organ of muscle that is about the size of an adult fist. Exercise, especially aerobic conditioning, strengthens the heart, thereby enabling the heart to pump more blood per beat (stroke volume). A heart strengthened by exercise has an increased aerobic capacity; that is, the heart can pump more blood per minute without an undue increase in the heart rate. Therefore exercises relying primarily on the aerobic oxygen system for energy such as walking, jogging, and light cardio machines would improve heart function.
- *Blood cholesterol levels:* Exercise raises blood levels of high-density lipoprotein (HDL), referred to as "good cholesterol" because it carries surplus cholesterol from the tissues to the liver for breakdown and removal from the body. Exercise also lowers blood levels of low-density lipoprotein (LDL). LDL cholesterol is referred to as "bad cholesterol" because it carries at least two thirds of the total blood cholesterol to body tissues, raising the potential of cholesterol deposits in major arteries of the heart. Both of these exercise effects lower the risks for diseased arteries.
- *Oxygen-carrying capacity:* Exercise also enhances the circulatory system by increasing the oxygen-carrying capacity of the blood. As training continues, a person's VO_2max will improve, thus increasing the efficiency of oxygen use and uptake.

Hypertension

The risk for cardiovascular complications increases continuously with increasing levels of blood pressure. When blood pressure is measured, persons with stage 1 hypertension show a systolic blood pressure (the upper notation) of 140 to 159 mm Hg or a diastolic blood pressure (the lower notation) of 90 to 99 mm Hg, or both. Persons with stage 1 hypertension represent the overwhelming majority of hypertensive individuals in the general population, and exercise has become one of the most effective nondrug treatments. Even for persons with higher levels of blood pressure, exercise has proved to be an important adjunct to drug therapy, offsetting adverse drug effects and lowering drug needs. There are normal rises in blood pressure during both dynamic (walking, cycling) and resistance (strength training) type of exercises. Both forms of exercise are beneficial for individuals with hypertension. However, exercisers with diagnosed hypertension should avoid excess exertion, as with heavy weight lifting, and holding their breath during the exertion phase of the exercise to prevent severe stress on the cardiovascular system.

Diabetes

Regular, moderate-intensity exercise programs help individuals with type 2 diabetes control blood glucose levels and reduce the risk of chronic complications associated with diabetes. Exercise improves the action of a person's naturally produced insulin by increasing the number of insulin receptor sites (i.e., areas where insulin may be carried into cells). In managing type 1 diabetes mellitus, the type of exercise and when it is done must be balanced with food and insulin to prevent reactions caused by drops in blood glucose. (See Chapter 21 for a more detailed discussion of diabetes.)

Weight Management

Exercise is extremely beneficial in weight management because it (1) helps to regulate appetite, (2) increases the basal metabolic rate, and (3) reduces the genetic fat deposit set-point level. Together with a well-planned diet, physical exercise corrects the energy balance in favor of increased energy output and decreased energy intake (see Chapter 5). Fat is used efficiently as the fuel source for muscles during lower intensity (30% to 60% VO_2max) aerobic exercise such as walking, jogging, swimming, and light cycling.

Stress Management

Exercise helps reduce stress-related eating. It also provides a physical outlet for working off the hormonal physiologic effects of catecholamines and corticoid hormones produced in the body by stress, thus helping to reduce a major risk factor in the development of chronic disease.

Bone Disease

Weight-bearing exercises improve bone mineralization, thus reducing the risk of bone weakness and of potential osteoporosis.[27]

Mental Health

Exercise stimulates the production of brain opiates, which are substances called *endorphins.* These natural substances decrease pain (this is how aspirin works, by stimulating production of endorphins) and improve the mood, including an exhilarating kind of "high."

Assessment of Personal Health and Exercise Needs

There are many kinds of exercise. Choosing the best form depends on individual health, personal needs, the aerobic benefits involved, and personal enjoyment.

Health and Personal Needs

In planning an exercise program, it is important to assess individual health status, personal needs, present level of fitness, and resources required. Discussing an exercise program with a medical practitioner is always recommended, and getting a medical clearance before beginning an exercise program is especially important for older persons or those with chronic disease. It is wise to start slowly and build gradually rather than risk injury and discouragement. Moderation and consistency are the key guides.

Beginning a Program

There are many options to choose from regarding where, what, when, and how one exercises. It is important to evaluate these options before committing to any one routine. As a healthcare professional, you may have the responsibility of helping design exercise programs for your clients or patients. One golden rule for success is that if your clients enjoy the activity they are doing, they are much more likely to make it part of their everyday schedule. Some individuals benefit from joining a fitness facility where they feel encouraged by others. Others, however, may shy away from fitness facilities for fear of discomfort. It is not necessary to join a fitness facility or hire a personal trainer to start an exercise program. Keeping the following questions in mind while designing an exercise program can be helpful:

1. Which is better—a fitness facility or home program?
    *   Is external encouragement needed to exercise? Is company and interaction with others desirable during exercise? Or is exercising alone preferable?
    *   Is sticking to a schedule ideal and easy? Or is it more realistic to need to work around other obligations and exercise when and where possible?
    *   Is there a fitness facility located near home or work? How much does it cost?
    *   Is the office or home in an area that can provide uninterrupted bouts of exercise?
2. What kind of exercise best fits the needs of your client?
    *   It is important for everyone to determine independently what it is he or she *likes* to do. If the exercise chosen is not fun, the patient or client will soon stop doing it, and it will be of no benefit. Encourage someone who has little exposure to various forms of physical activity to experiment with a variety of activities before committing to any one.
    *   While exercising at a fitness facility, the question for your client or patient to consider is, Would you enjoy aerobic workouts on a bike or treadmill or in a group class?
    *   While exercising at home, questions for your client or patient to consider are, Do you live in an area that you can run, walk, or bike in? If not, do you have access to a stationary bike, treadmill, or other aerobic machine? Try to choose an activity that you can stick with year round, or choose a variety of activities that you can alternate throughout the year. For instance, perhaps swimming or biking in the summer and then running or participating in aerobic classes in the winter would work.
    *   For strength training, fitness facilities usually provide an assortment of free weights and resistance machines. Always encourage your client or patient to ask for help if he or she is not sure how to correctly perform any exercise. Resistance training can be done effectively at home as well with a combination of resistance bands, small hand weights, or even cans of beans!

Aerobic Benefits

To build aerobic capacity, the level of exercise must raise the pulse rate to within 70% of maximal heart rate (Table 14-5). Unless an exercise tolerance or stress test has been performed and the precise maximal exercising heart rate is known, an acceptable calculation to estimate maximum heart rate is 220 minus age. For aerobic benefits, 70% of maximal heart rate should then be maintained for approximately 20 minutes about 3 times per week. Check resting pulse before starting the exercise period, then again during and immediately afterward, to monitor progress in developing target exercising heart rate and aerobic capacity. Heart rate monitors are a convenient way to monitor and keep track of heart rate.

Types of Exercise

There are many exercises to choose from. Many of them are enjoyable and healthful but do not reach aerobic levels. For example, golf is a passion for many and gets them outdoors, but it is far too slow and sporadic to be aerobic. It is best to have a variety of exercises in any exercise plan (Figure 14-5). Even though many sports do not reach aerobic levels, if they are enjoyable they should be included.

Aerobic Exercise

Forms of exercise that can be sustained at a necessary level of intensity to provide aerobic benefits include such activities as swimming, running, jogging, bicycling, and aerobic dancing routines and workouts (Table 14-6). Perhaps the simplest and most popular form of stimulating exercise is *walking*. Figure 14-6 illustrates that aerobic walking can fit into almost anyone's lifestyle. If the pace is fast enough to elevate your pulse and it is maintained for at least the required 20 minutes, walking can be an excellent form of aerobic exercise. It is convenient and requires no equipment other than good walking shoes. It is appropriate for and available to many persons.

Resistance Exercise

Resistance type of exercises are designed to increase muscle strength and endurance. An ideal program would consist of 8 to 10 separate exercises (with 8 to 12 repetitions of each) focusing on the major muscles of the body,

TABLE 14-5	Target Zone Heart Rate According to Age to Achieve Aerobic Physical Effect of Exercise		

Age (yr)	Maximal Attainable Heart Rate (Pulse: 220 Minus Age)	Target Zone	
		70% Maximal Rate	85% Maximal Rate
20	200	140	170
25	195	136	166
30	190	133	161
35	185	129	157
40	180	126	153
45	175	122	149
50	170	119	144
55	165	115	140
60	160	112	136
65	155	108	132
70	150	105	127
75	145	101	124

TABLE 14-6	Aerobic Exercises for Physical Fitness*

Type of Exercise	Aerobic Forms
Ball playing	Handball
	Racquetball
	Squash
Bicycling	Stationary
	Touring
Dancing	Aerobic routines
	Ballet
	Disco
Jumping rope	Brisk pace
Running or jogging	Brisk pace
Skating	Ice-skating
	Roller-skating
Skiing	Cross-country
Swimming	Steady pace
Walking	Brisk pace

*Maintained at aerobic level for at least 20 minutes.

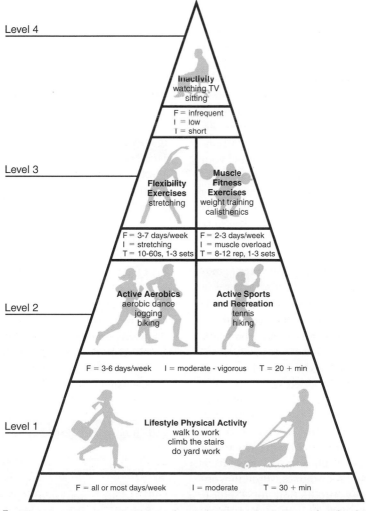

FIGURE 14-5   Physical activity pyramid. (*Redrawn from Corbin RB, Lindsey R: Fitness for life, ed 5, p. 64, Champaign, Ill, 2005, Human Kinetics.*)

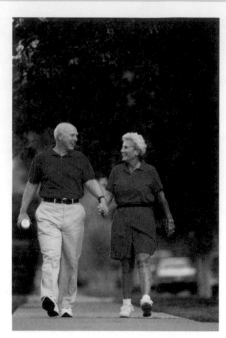

FIGURE 14-6   Aerobic walking is an enjoyable exercise that can fit into almost anyone's lifestyle. *(Credit: PhotoDisc.)*

performed 2 to 3 days per week. For an individual whose primary goal is to gain strength and power, the repetitions should be of high intensity with less than 6 repetitions to muscle fatigue. For improved endurance, a lower weight should be used that will allow at least 15 repetitions before muscle fatigue.

Weight-Bearing Exercise

Weight-bearing exercises, such as walking, jogging, aerobic dancing, or jumping rope, are important for bone structure and strength. In each of these exercises, your muscles are working against gravity. Bones will adapt to their environment and the load put on them during weight-bearing exercises to build more bone cells. Resistance exercises are also beneficial to bone health because the muscle pulls on the bone to increase bone density.

TO SUM UP

The energy molecule of the body is ATP, and the powerhouse of the cell is the mitochondrion. The cell's storehouse of energy is CP. These two high-energy phosphate compounds are in limited supply. They can produce energy for only a brief initial period and need to be replenished for exercise to continue. This added supply is made available by anaerobic glycolysis, with added energy made available for continued exercise by the body's aerobic system of energy production. The process of glycolysis metabolizes only carbohydrate substrate, furnished by either blood glucose or stored glycogen. Dietary carbohydrate is necessary to replenish these fuel sources. Protein contributes little to total energy production for exercise, whereas the body's ability to burn fat as fuel depends on

the level of fitness. The higher the body's efficiency in using oxygen, the more fatty acids will contribute to the energy supply. Even in the best-trained athletes, fatty acid oxidation must be accompanied by glucose metabolism.

Contrary to popular belief, exercise does not require an increased intake of protein, vitamins, or minerals. The body's increased needs are well supplied by a normal healthy diet. Exercise increases the body's need for kcalories and water. Cold water taken in small, frequent amounts is the best way to prevent dehydration in most athletic events and exercise. In most cases, electrolytes lost in sweat are replaced by a continuing diet of adequate quality and quantity. Depending on the amount added, electrolytes or sugar in water may delay its emptying from the stomach and thus delay rehydration. A mild saline and glucose solution (4% to 8%) may supply fluid and fuel to sustain energy during longer endurance events. Some highly competitive athletes use harmful practices such as food and fluid deprivation for controlling weight and such ergogenic aids as illegal steroid drugs for bulking muscles.

The optimal diet for the athlete is moderate in protein and fat, with to 6 to10 g/kg body weight per day coming from carbohydrates. The pregame meal should be small, having little or no protein or fat and relying mainly on complex carbohydrates (starches).

The health benefits of general and aerobic exercise are many and increase with practice up to the point of overdoing. Excellent aerobic exercises include sustained fast walking, swimming, jogging, running, and aerobic dancing or workouts. Approach any exercise sensibly, and choose those activities that are enjoyable.

QUESTIONS FOR REVIEW

1. What are the component muscle structures, and how do they produce muscle action?
2. What type of substrate fuel does the body use for immediate energy needs? For short-term needs? For long-term needs?
3. How does oxygen relate to physical activity capacity and aerobic effect?
4. Outline the nutrition and physical fitness principles you would discuss with a client who is an athlete. Plan a diet for this client that would meet nutrient and energy needs.
5. Why is fluid balance vital during exercise periods? How is water and electrolyte balance achieved?
6. Describe the dangers of anabolic steroids used by some athletes for bulking muscles and gaining an edge in strength over an opponent.

REFERENCES

1. Centers for Disease Control and Prevention, Council of State and Territorial Epidemiologists, Association of State and Territorial Chronic Disease Program Directors: Indicators for chronic disease surveillance, *MMWR Recomm Rep* 53(RR-11):1, 2004.

2. World Health Organization: *Global strategy on diet, physical activity and health,* Geneva, Switzerland, 2003, Author. Retrieved January 6, 2005, from *www.who.int/dietphysicalactivity/media/en/gsfs_pa.pdf.*

3. U.S. Department of Health and Human Services: *Healthy people 2010: understanding and improving health,* Washington, DC, 2000, U.S. Government Printing Office.

4. U.S. Department of Agriculture: *Dietary Guidelines for Americans 2000,* ed 5, Washington, DC, 2000, U.S. Government Printing Office.

5. U.S. Department of Agriculture: *Nutrition and your health: Dietary Guidelines for Americans 2005,* Washington, DC, 2005, Author. Accessible at *www.health.gov/dietaryguidelines/dga2005/backgrounder.htm.*

6. Bauman AE: Updating the evidence that physical activity is good for health: an epidemiological review 2000-2003, *J Sci Med Sport* 7(1 suppl):6, 2004.

7. American College of Sports Medicine, American Dietetic Association, Dietitians of Canada: Joint position statement: nutrition and athletic performance, *Med Sci Sports Exerc* 32(12):2130, 2000.

8. Walker JL et al: Dietary carbohydrate, muscle glycogen content, and endurance performance in well-trained women, *J Appl Physiol* 88(6):2151, 2000.

9. Utter AC et al: Carbohydrate supplementation and perceived exertion during prolonged running, *Med Sci Sports Exerc* 36(6):1036, 2004.

10. Price TB et al: Glycogen loading alters muscle glycogen resynthesis after exercise, *J Appl Physiol* 88:698, 2000.

11. Ince BA et al: Lowering dietary protein to U.S. Recommended Dietary Allowance levels reduces urinary calcium excretion and bone resorption in young women, *J Clin Endocrinol Metab* 89(8):3801, 2004.

12. Barzel US, Massey LK: Excess dietary protein can adversely affect bone, *J Nutr* 128(6):1051, 1998.

13. Kerstetter JE et al: Dietary protein, calcium metabolism, and skeletal homeostasis revisited, *Am J Clin Nutr* 78(3 suppl):584S, 2003.

14. Von Duvillard SP et al: Fluids and hydration in prolonged endurance performance, *Nutrition* 20(7-8):651, 2004.

15. Shirreffs SM, Armstrong LE, Cheuvront SN: Fluid and electrolyte needs for preparation and recovery from training and competition, *J Sports Sci* 22(1):57, 2004.

16. Rehrer NJ: Fluid and electrolyte balance in ultra-endurance sport, *Sports Med* 31(10):701, 2001.

17. American Dietetic Association Sports Cardiovascular and Wellness Nutritionists Dietetic Practice Group: *Sports nutrition: a guide for the professional working with active people,* ed 3, Chicago, 2000, American Dietetic Association.

18. Williams MB et al: Effects of recovery beverages on glycogen restoration and endurance exercise performance, *J Strength Cond Res* 17(1):12, 2003.

19. Kutscher EC et al: Anabolic steroids: a review for the clinician, *Sports Med* 32(5):285, 2002.

20. Gomez JE: Performance-enhancing substances in adolescent athletes, *Tex Med* 98(2):41, 2002.

21. Ray TR et al: Use of oral creatine as an ergogenic aid for increased sports performance: perceptions of adolescent athletes, *South Med J* 94(6):608, 2001.

22. Beard J, Tobin B: Iron status and exercise, *Am J Clin Nutr* 72(2 suppl):594S, 2000.

23. Thrash LE, Anderson JJB: The female athlete triad: nutrition, menstrual disturbances, and low bone mass, *Nutr Today* 35(5):168, 2000.

24. Miller KK: Mechanisms by which nutritional disorders cause reduced bone mass in adults, *J Womens Health* 12(2):145, 2003.

25. Zeni AI et al: Stress injury to the bone among women athletes, *Phys Med Rehabil Clin N Am* 11(4):929, 2000.

26. Iacopino L et al: Body composition differences in adolescent female athletes and anorexic patients, *Acta Diabetol* 40(1 suppl):S180, 2003.

27. Lloyd T et al: Lifestyle factors and the development of bone mass and bone strength in young women, *J Pediatr* 144(6):776, 2004.

FURTHER READINGS AND RESOURCES

Readings

Kutscher EC et al: Anabolic steroids: a review for the clinician, *Sports Med* 32(5):285, 2002.

Anabolic steroid use continues to be a problem in the world of competitive sports. This review explores the many misconceptions regarding self-administered ergogenic aids by addressing the epidemiology, physiology, efficacy, and the adverse effects of such products.

Schwenk TL, Costley CD: When food becomes a drug: nonanabolic nutritional supplement use in athletes, *Am J Sports Med* 30(6):907, 2002.

A discussion and review of some of the most commonly used nutritional supplements in the athletic world. Misconceptions, validity, and proper use are addressed.

American College of Sports Medicine, American Dietetic Association, Dietitians of Canada: Joint position statement: nutrition and athletic performance, *Med Sci Sports Exerc* 32(12):2130, 2000.

This joint position statement emphasizes the importance of nutrition in physical activity, athletic performance, and recovery from exercise. The experts specifically address nutrient and fluid needs, body composition, supplements and ergogenic aids, and the roles and responsibilities of healthcare professionals.

Keim NL et al: America's obesity epidemic: measuring physical activity to promote an active lifestyle, *J Am Diet Assoc* 104:1398, 2004.

The authors discuss the health benefits of physical activity, the recommendations to the public for health promotion and disease prevention, and methods of balancing the equation of energy intake versus energy output. Both the prevalence of overweight and inactivity are reviewed.

Websites of Interest

- Centers for Disease Control and Prevention, National Center for Chronic Disease Prevention and Health Promotion: *Physical activity and health: a report of the surgeon general: www.cdc.gov/nccdphp/sgr/sgr.htm.*
- American College of Sports Medicine: *www.acsm.org.*
- Washington Coalition for Promoting Physical Activity: *www.be-active.org.*

CHAPTER 15

The Complexity of Obesity: Beyond Energy Balance

George A. Bray and Catherine M. Champagne

In this chapter, we look at the complex issue of obesity. In recent years the prevalence of obesity has grown to epidemic proportions. Linked as a risk factor for many chronic disorders in the United States, the magnitude of this healthcare problem and its impact on the healthcare system is immense.

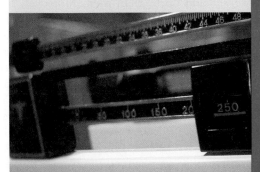

Chapter authors are affiliated with the Pennington Biomedical Research Center, Baton Rouge, La, supported in part by U.S. Department of Agriculture grant #DK 32089.

We are living in a time when the number of overweight individuals is increasing more rapidly than in earlier decades. This chapter is intended to help you understand this problem. Using an epidemiologic model of the interactions between environmental agents and the human host to explain obesity, we explore food, medications, physical inactivity, toxins, and viruses as environmental agents that interact with the genetically programmed host to disturb energy balance as causal factors in obesity. Large portion size, high fat intake, easy access to calorically sweetened beverages, and lack of any need to be physically active all play a role in the toxic environment that leads to obesity. The genetic and physiologic responses of the host determine whether or not this "toxic environment" will produce obesity. Reversing the current trends of obesity requires a new look at the limits of the energy balance concept and a better understanding of how environmental factors acutely and chronically change the responses of the susceptible host so that obesity becomes a chronic, relapsing disease.

REALITIES OF OBESITY

During the early part of the twentieth century the prevalence of obesity rose slowly, but around 1980 it began to rise more rapidly.[1-4] As illustrated in Figure 15-1, the rise has continued to the present time. In the period between 1999 and 2002 the prevalence of overweight was 65.1% and the prevalence of obesity was 31.7%. This means that within current definitions nearly two thirds of American adults are defined as overweight. Prevalence of obesity and overweight increases with age. Peak age in women is between ages 60 and 70 and in men between ages 50 and 60. A higher percentage of women are overweight and obese than men. Moreover, black and Hispanic women have a higher prevalence of obesity than white women. This racial disparity is larger in women than in men. Overweight is also higher among people who make less money and have less education than it is among those who have a higher education and income.

Children are also affected by obesity. The prevalence was about 5% in 1960 and has risen to more than 15% in 2000.[5] For children as well as adults a social stigma is associated with this weight problem. Overweight children are less liked as playmates and tend to view themselves less favorably than normal-weight children. Being called "fatty" jeopardizes feelings of self-confidence. Many overweight children and adults are traumatized by the stigma of obesity. Children are often teased at school by being labeled "fatty" and other derogatory terms. Adults experience prejudice in social and economic situations. Measures of quality of life show that the obese score lower on many scales and that weight loss improves their quality of life (see the *Focus on Culture* box, "Antifat Bias: The Last Acceptable Form of Cultural Discrimination").

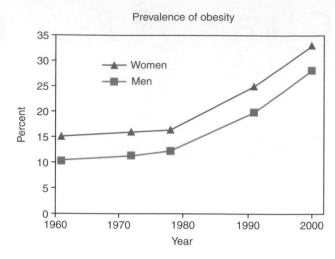

Prevalence of obesity

| NHES I | NHANES | NHANES II | NHANES III | NHANES III |
| 1960-1962 | 1970-1974 | 1976-1980 | 1988-1994 | 1999-2000 |

FIGURE 15-1   Graph illustrating the prevalence of obesity. The upper line shows the prevalence of obesity for women and the lower line for men using data from several surveys of obesity done by the U.S. government beginning in the years 1960 to 1962. Obesity rose slowly from 1960 until approximately 1980, when the rate for both men and women began to increase. *(Data from National Center for Health Statistics:* National Health and Examination Survey I, *1962-1962 and* National Health and Nutrition Examination Surveys *1970-1974, 1976-1980, 1988-1994, and 1999-2000, Hyattsville, Md, 1960-2000, Centers for Disease Control and Prevention.)*

Overweight increases the risk of developing many chronic diseases. Prominent among these is type 2 diabetes mellitus in children and adolescents.[6] This disease most often occurs in overweight or obese adolescents and adults and presages a dire future, particularly for these children as the complications of blindness, heart disease, renal failure, and amputation disable them in the next 20 years or so. Overweight also increases the risk of gallbladder disease, heart disease, high blood pressure, and some forms of cancer. Through the development of these diseases, being overweight reduces life expectancy and shortens life span by 3 to 7 years for an individual age 40 with a body mass index (BMI) of 30 or more.

Obesity increases the cost of healthcare.[7] Frequency of hospital and medical office visits is increased with increasing body weight. Use of drugs to treat the complications associated with obesity also increases. The extra burden to Medicare after age 65 rises with each increase in the class of obesity.

Risks associated with obesity are generally reversed by modest weight loss. A weight loss of 5% to 10% of initial body weight is sufficient to reduce the development of diabetes in people with prediabetes by up to 58%.[8] Weight loss that is maintained is an effective treatment for hypertension. Risks from abnormal blood lipids (dyslipidemia) are also reduced with weight loss.

To tackle the hazards of obesity for children, adolescents, and adults, we need to adopt effective strategies for prevention and, where prevention fails, for treatment of obesity.

FOCUS ON CULTURE

Antifat Bias: The Last Acceptable Form of Cultural Discrimination

Our culture idealizes slimness and denigrates obesity. Discrimination based on weight bias has been recognized in many different areas of our society, including representation of obese persons in our culture. Common stereotypes of obese persons include the following:
- Warm
- Dependable
- Gluttonous
- Lazy
- Stupid
- Worthless

Popular messages in the media promote fat jokes and idealization of thin women and muscular men. It appears that it is a socially acceptable cultural value in the United States that obese people are responsible for their condition. But surely healthcare professionals, who understand that obesity is caused by hereditary and environmental factors and is not merely a function of personal behavior (overeating and/or lack of exercise), do not express these biases. Or do they?

Regrettably, research shows that health professionals are not immune to overt as well as inherent antifat bias. The very people who are responsible for caring for individuals who are obese demonstrated the following attitudes toward obese patients[1-8]:
- Family practice physicians described obese patients with negative terms such as "lacking self-control."
- Physicians reported that they would feel more negatively toward overweight patients and spend less time with them but would order more tests.
- Nurses reported the following:
  - Feeling uncomfortable caring for obese patients
  - Being "repulsed" by obese persons
  - Having a preference not to care for obese patients
- Medical students described obese patients as follows:
  - Less attractive
  - More depressed
  - Less compliant

- Registered dietitians and dietetic students reported negative attitudes toward obese individuals.
- Overweight and obese women are less likely to be screened for cervical and breast cancer.

Thus it appears the physical and psychologic consequences of obesity may stem from not only the Western culture's weight-related bias and stigma, but also from the biases of health professionals. It is obvious Schwartz and colleagues[6] are right: "Much more work is needed to understand and ameliorate this bias." How about you? Are you part of the solution or part of the problem?

References

1. Bagley CR et al: Attitudes of nurses toward obesity and obese patients, *Percept Mot Skills* 68:954, 1989.
2. Hebl MR, Xu J: Weighing the care: physicians' reaction to the size of a patient, *Int J Obes Relat Metab Disord* 25:1246, 2001.
3. Loomis GA et al: Attitudes and practices of military family physicians regarding obesity, *Mil Med* 166:121, 2001.
4. Maroney D, Golub S: Nurses' attitudes toward obese persons and certain ethnic groups, *Percept Mot Skills* 75:387, 1992.
5. Oberrieder H et al: Attitude of dietetics students and registered dietitians toward obesity, *J Am Diet Assoc* 95:914, 1995.
6. Schwartz M et al: Weight bias among health professionals specializing in obesity, *Obes Res* 11:1033, 2003.
7. Techman BA et al: Demonstrations of implicit anti-fat bias: the impact of providing causal information and evoking empathy, *Health Psychol* 22:68, 2003.
8. Wigton RS, McGaghie WC: The effects of obesity on medical students' approach to patients with abdominal pain, *J Gen Intern Med* 16:262, 2001.

---

overweight A weight above the upper limit of some arbitrarily set standard (see also *obesity*).

obesity An excess amount of body fat. Operationally it is usually defined by a body mass index (BMI) of 30 kg/m^2 or greater, which uses height and weight. Three subclasses of obesity are defined as follows:
- Class 1 = BMI 30-34.9 kg/m^2
- Class 2 = BMI 35-39.9 kg/m^2
- Class 3 = BMI ≥40 kg/m^2

prevalence This term relates the number of individuals with a particular condition at a particular time to the total number of people. If 10 people were overweight in a population of 1000, this would indicate a prevalence of 1%.

stigma A mark or identification marking. In this context it is an increased body fat that is obvious to the viewer and that elicits emotional feelings, which are usually negative.

diabetes mellitus A disease defined by a high level of glucose in the blood, which often appears in the urine if it is high enough. There are two general types of diabetes mellitus—(1) type 1, which refers to the disease normally diagnosed in younger individuals (less than 30 years of age) in which the pancreas cannot produce enough insulin and there is thus not enough circulating insulin, and (2) type 2, which refers to the disease normally diagnosed in older people who are often overweight or obese and in which there is more than enough circulating insulin but relatively poor response to this insulin.

body mass index (BMI) Body weight in kilograms divided by the height in square meters (kg/m^2). It can be calculated from pounds and inches as 703 times body weight in pounds divided by the height in inches squared. This is the usual measurement to define overweight and obesity.

prediabetes A condition also known as *impaired glucose tolerance* and defined as a fasting glucose between 100 and 126 mg/dl and a blood glucose between 140 and 1999 mg/dl 2 hours after ingestion of 75 g of glucose.

ENERGY INTAKE, ENERGY EXPENDITURE, AND DEVELOPMENT OF OBESITY

One easy way to view the problem of obesity is with the aid of a teeter-totter—the childhood toy. On one side is the amount of food we eat expressed in calories (joules). On the other side is the energy we expend during the day for our various activities. This includes the energy needed to heat our bodies and keep the body temperature at 37° C (98.6° F), the energy needed to keep our hearts beating, our brains working, our kidneys excreting urine, and our intestines digesting food whether we are awake or not. Energy is also used for physical activity when we sit, stand, walk, run, or do other daily activities. When the two sides of the teeter-totter are in balance, that is, when the energy on one side is equal to the energy on the other side, we are in "energy balance." As long as we are in energy balance we will not gain or lose weight. Overweight develops when the energy on the intake side is more than on the expenditure side. This can occur because energy intake rises or because energy expenditure falls, or both. The conservation of energy implied by the energy balance equation is often referred to as the First Law of Thermodynamics applied to human energy consumption and expenditure. It was first demonstrated for human beings more than 100 years ago, and there is no reason to doubt that it provides the overall framework for understanding the way in which obesity develops. However, as we will show, it is in the details of the relation of energy intake and energy expenditure that the problem of obesity lies.

OBESITY AS A DISEASE

Obesity can be viewed as a disease. What do we mean by this? A disease has several components. It has a cause. As noted previously, this is the result of an imbalance between energy intake and energy expenditure. It has clinical signs and symptoms such as increased amount of fatness that is usually visible to the eye. No one would have difficulty distinguishing between an overweight and normal-weight individual walking down the street. Obesity also has a "pathology," by which we mean the presence of some unique features that allow one to diagnose it under a microscope, at an autopsy examination, or by defined blood tests. For obesity this is the large fat cell.

All forms of obesity have as one characteristic an enlargement of the individual fat cells all over the body. The adult human has close to 60 billion fat cells. As people gain weight, the first change in these cells is to enlarge to accommodate the extra fat. As the cells reach their maximal size, additional cells may be recruited to store the extra fat. Fat cells are remarkable cells. They are part of the larger endocrine cellular system that secretes products into the bloodstream that have effects elsewhere. In the case of fat cells, there are many secreted products that can affect blood clotting (plasminogen activator inhibitor-1), the removal of fats from the blood (lipoprotein lipase), inflammation (interleukin-1, interleukin-6, tumor necrosis factor-alpha), blood pressure (angiotensinogen), and the body's recognition of the amount of its body fat (leptin). This latter hormone, leptin, is an important signal from the fat cells to the brain about the amount of body fat. Circulating levels of leptin are directly related to amount of body fat. Until the amount of body fat reaches a "critical" level in women, menstruation does not occur, and in many women who are ballet dancers or gymnasts with small amounts of body fat, menstrual periods cease because leptin is too low. The many hormones produced and secreted from the fat cells in the body produce the pathophysiologic responses that lead to the associated diseases that we described above. Thus obesity can be described as a chronic, relapsing, neurochemical disease.

BEYOND ENERGY BALANCE

There is no doubt that obesity results from energy imbalance and that we can predict the magnitude of the weight change over time if we know the net energy balance. However, it is what the energy balance concept *does not tell us* that is most important in dealing with obesity. The First Law of Thermodynamics does not tell us anything about the regulation of food intake or the way in which genes are involved in this process. It does not help us to understand why men and women distribute fat in different places on their bodies or to understand how fat distribution changes with age. The First Law of Thermodynamics also does not help us to understand why some drugs produce weight gain and others weight loss or why weight loss stops after a period of treatment with diet or medication. It is the understanding of these mechanisms that will allow us to tackle the epidemic of obesity.

One problem with the concept of energy balance is that we are never in energy balance. To study energy balance, we housed healthy men in small rooms (respiration calorimeters) in which we manipulated food intake and exercise to get as close as possible to zero energy balance—that is, when energy intake equals energy expenditure.[9] In fact, we rarely got closer than 50 kcal/day, or about 2.5% out of an intake of 2000 kcal/day. The values of energy imbalance for these healthy men ranged from 50 to 150 kcal/day. Had these differences been maintained for 1 year, these men would be expected to gain about 2.5 kg (5.5 lb) at the smaller error and 7.5 kg (16.5 lb) at the larger error.

To keep from gaining weight, we must make "corrective" responses in energy intake or energy expenditure to counterbalance the error that occurred on previous days.

These corrective responses around a weight of relative stability make it look as though there is "weight regulation." For some people the oscillations around this balance point can keep weight stable for many years. For others there is a slow upward drift in this regulatory point, and weight is gradually gained. If you are fortunate enough to have robust corrective responses, you can maintain a stable weight over many years. If it is not stable, the following two strategies are available:

1. *Conscious control:* This method is exhibited in some people who have a pattern of eating called *restrained eating.*
2. *Regular weighing:* This second and perhaps best way to maintain weight over a long period is not to count calories but to weigh oneself regularly at the same time of day on an accurate scale and address weight increases in a timely fashion.

Consequences of energy imbalance are graphically illustrated in the movie by Morgan Spurlock entitled *Supersize Me,* in which the protagonist gained 25 lb in one month by eating all of his meals at McDonald's restaurants. Because we are never in energy balance, we need to view energy balance as an ideal—not a realistic goal to be obtained by counting calories.

From the perspective of energy balance, the solution to obesity should be simple: eat less and exercise more. The truth of this advice was shown by Kinsell et al for overweight individuals housed in a metabolic ward and provided with all of their food.[10] During the course of several months these patients ate diets with 1200 kcal/day. After the initial rapid weight loss due to rebalancing body fluids, subsequent weight loss was linear and was not affected by wide variations in macronutrient content of the diet. More recent studies using foods that were tagged with a nonradioactive isotopic carbon-13 showed that the better the adherence to a diet, the greater the weight loss.[11] Thus it is adherence to diets, not diets themselves, that make the difference.

Another limitation to the concept of energy balance as the cause of obesity is the implication that if you are getting fatter, it is your fault. You only need to control your calorie intake (food) and calorie expenditure to control the problem. This implies that we should blame our children for their obesity. This seems grossly inappropriate. If obesity were easily controlled by moderating calorie intake, the U.S. military would not discharge up to 5000 men and women yearly for failing to meet its weight standards. If loss of livelihood is not sufficient motivation to lose weight, the problem must be more complex.

The cure of obesity in leptin-deficient human beings treated with leptin shows a genetic basis for some obesity, more than simply lack of "willpower."[12] Although simple in theory, applying the ideas of energy balance and calorie counting to body weight control has proven unsuccessful. More than 95% of people using dietary, behavior, and lifestyle approaches to lose weight regained it within less than 5 years.[13]

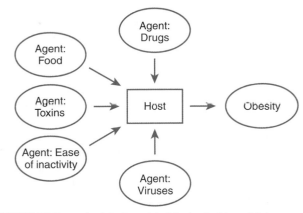

FIGURE 15-2   Epidemiologic model of obesity. In this model the agent that produces obesity is "food" or food-related products. If food is in limited supply, obesity does not develop. The food that is ingested interacts with the host. In a susceptible host the toxic effects of food produce obesity, the disease.

AN EPIDEMIOLOGIC MODEL

The current epidemic can be viewed from the perspective of an epidemiologic model, shown in Figure 15-2. Food, drugs, viruses and toxins, and low physical activity are the environmental agents that facilitate the development of obesity. One or more these factors acting on a susceptible host can produce obesity. As the spokesperson for the Grocery Manufacturers of America said in the movie *Supersize Me,* "The food industry is part of the problem." Using this model, we can approach the problem by manipulating either the environment or the host.

---

calorie   The amount of heat energy needed to raise the temperature of water from 14° C to 15° C. Because this is a small unit, we usually use *kilocalories,* which are 1000 of these small calories (see also *joule*).

joule   A unit of energy. The International System of Units uses joules in place of calories to refer to food energy, and most nutrition journals require its use instead of calories (1 kcal = 4.184 kilojoules [kJ], often rounded to 4.2 kJ for ease in calculation.) A 1000-kcal diet would be equivalent to a 4200 kJ or 4.2 megajoule (MJ) diet.

pathology   The science of disease. Changes that reflect disease can be in organs (liver disease), tissues (skin disease), cells, or parts of cells.

leptin   A peptide of 167 amino acids that is produced primarily in fat cells and released into the blood to circulate as a hormone to the brain to tell the body about long-term regulation of body fat.

pathophysiologic   Term referring to the processes by which the disease develops.

ENVIRONMENTAL AGENTS

Food and Its Costs as a Major Environmental Agent

Several components of our food supply may be important in determining whether or not obesity develops. The first of these is the portion size of packages and servings. There is convincing evidence that when larger portion sizes are provided, more food is eaten. Portion sizes have dramatically increased in the past 40 years[14] and now need reduction. Calorically sweetened beverages that contain 10% high fructose corn syrup (HFCS) and are available in containers with 12, 20, or 32 oz provide 150, 250, or 400 kcal if all is consumed. Many foods list the calories per serving, but the package often contains more than one serving.

Patterns of food consumption have changed during the past 30 years.[15] The most striking change from 1970 to 2000 was in the rising consumption of HFCS.[16] HFCS is now used as the caloric sweetener in almost all soft drinks, as well as in reconstituted juice drinks and many solid foods. The rise in HFCS consumption occurred over the same time interval as the rapid rise in the prevalence of obesity.[16] On the one hand, this relationship may be strictly coincidental. However, on the other hand, it may not be (Figure 15-3). Fructose is sweeter than either glucose or sucrose, a molecule that is a combination of fructose and glucose. In addition, HFCS is a solution of both fructose and glucose as separate molecules, and thus it differs in osmotic properties from a solution with the same concentration of sucrose.

The intake of calorically sweetened beverages has been related to the epidemic of obesity.[16-18] Ludwig, Peterson, and Gortmaker[17] reported that the intake of soft drinks was a predictor of initial BMI in children in the Planet Health Study. They also showed that higher soft drink consumption also predicted an increase in BMI; during

nearly 2 years of follow-up, those with the highest soft drink consumption at baseline had the highest increase in BMI. A Danish study[18] showed that individuals consuming calorically sweetened beverages during 10 weeks gained weight, whereas subjects drinking the same amount of artificially sweetened beverages lost weight. In one study, children who were focusing on reducing intake of "fizzy" drinks and replacing them with water showed slower weight gain than those not advised to reduce the intake of fizzy drinks.[19]

These studies strongly suggest that calorie-containing soft drinks could play a role in the epidemic of obesity. If so, then their consumption should be curtailed, particularly for very young children, in whom neuronal changes may reflect the response of insulin to these beverages, and for schoolchildren, for whom beverages are a ready source of energy with few other nutrients.

Dietary fat is another component that may be related to the epidemic of obesity.[20] Foods combining fat and sugar may be a particular problem because they are often very palatable and usually inexpensive.[21] The Leeds Fat Study shows that people who were high-fat consumers have an increased incidence of obesity.[22] Providing palatable low-fat foods is important.

There are now several studies showing that when breast feeding is the sole source of nutrition for more than 3 months, the risk of obesity is significantly reduced at the time of entry into school and in adolescence when compared to infants who are not breast-fed at all or for less than 3 months.[23] This may be an example of "infant imprinting." The composition of the breast milk may also be important. Over the past 50 years the proportion of n-6 fatty acids in human breast milk has increased, reflecting changes in dietary fat composition. The amount of n-3 fatty acids in breast milk has remained constant. A higher amount of n-6 fatty acids provides prostaglandin derivatives that stimulate fat cell proliferation in infants.[24] This is a concept that needs further evaluation. The rate of weight gain between ages 2 and 12 years also predicts future obesity; those children who gain the most weight have the highest risk of becoming obese.[25] Monitoring weight change early can be predictive of future obesity.

Calcium intake is another dietary factor that may be related to the development of obesity in children and adults. The level of calcium intake in population studies is inversely correlated with the risk of being overweight. In other epidemiologic studies and in feeding trials, higher dietary calcium is associated with reduced BMI or reduced incidence of insulin resistance.[26]

The cost of food is another factor in the cause of obesity. The price of items we buy influences our choices and the amount we buy. During the period from 1960 to 1980 the price of food rose more slowly than the other components in the consumer price index. Real wages also rose, providing additional money for consumption, some of which could buy a wider variety of healthy foods such

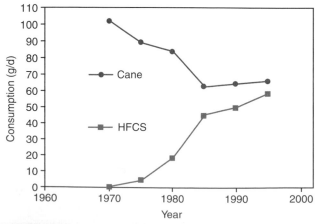

FIGURE 15-3   The consumption of high-fructose corn syrup (HFCS) and sugar (sucrose) over the years when the obesity epidemic developed. *(Copyright 2005, George A. Bray, Baton Rouge, La.)*

as fresh fruits and vegetables, fish, and dairy products. This was a time when the rise in the prevalence of obesity was slow. However, between 1985 and 2000 the relative cost increase in these food items was much faster than the foods with higher energy density, which contain more fat and sugar. In this period the price of fresh fruits and vegetables rose 117%, fish by 77%, and dairy products by 56%. Contrast this with sugar and sweets, which increased 47%; fats and oils, 37%; and carbonated beverages, 20%.[7] This means that your food dollar will buy relatively more food energy if the foods contain more sugar and fat or are carbonated beverages.

Low Levels of Physical Activity

Epidemiologic data show that low levels of physical activity and watching more television predict higher body weight.[27] Recent studies suggest that individuals in American cities where they had to walk more than people in other cities tended to weigh less. Low levels of physical activity also increase the risk of early mortality. Using normal weight, physically active women as the comparison group, Hu et al[28] found that the relative risk of mortality increased to 1.55 in inactive lean women, to 1.92 in active obese women, and to 2.42 in women who are obese but physically inactive. It is thus better to be thin than fat and to be physically active rather than inactive.

Drugs and Chemicals That Produce Weight Gain

Several drugs can cause weight gain, including a variety of hormones and psychoactive agents.[29] The degree of weight gain is generally not sufficient to cause substantial obesity, except occasionally in patients treated with high-dose corticosteroids, some psychoactive drugs, or valproate. These drugs can also increase the risk of future type 2 diabetes mellitus. Cessation of smoking is another environmental agent that will affect body fat stores. Partially mediated by nicotine withdrawal, a weight gain of 1 to 2 kg (2.2 to 4.4 lbs) is seen in the first few weeks and is often followed by an additional 2- to 3-kg weight gain over the next 4 to 6 months, resulting in an average weight gain of 4 to 5 kg or more.[30] This concept that increasing energy expenditure through drugs that act like physical activity to increase energy expenditure is being tested in several ways, but as yet no effective agents have been identified.

Viruses as Environmental Causes of Obesity

The injection of several viruses into the central nervous system produces obesity in mice. Recent findings of antibodies to one of the adenoviruses (AD-36) in larger amounts in obese humans raises the possibility that viruses are involved in some cases.[31] The adenoviral syndrome can be replicated in nonhuman primates and is characterized by modest obesity and a low circulating cholesterol concentration. Further studies are needed to establish that a syndrome of obesity associated with low concentrations of cholesterol clearly exists in human beings. If so, this would enhance the value of the epidemiologic model.

Toxins

In experimental animals, exposure in the neonatal period to monosodium glutamate, a common flavoring ingredient in food, will produce obesity. A similar effect of reduction in glucose can also produce obesity, suggesting that the brain of the growing animal, and possibly that of human beings, may respond with damage to the "metabolic sensors" that regulate food needs. In human beings, we know that body fat stores many "toxic" chemicals and that they are mobilized with weight loss. The metabolic rate can be reduced by organochlorine molecules,[32] and conceivably prolonged exposure to many chlorinated chemicals in our environment has affected metabolic pathways and energy metabolism. Food additives are another class of chemicals that are widely distributed and may be involved in the current epidemic of obesity.

The Host

Genetic Factors

Several kinds of research indicate that genetic factors are important in regulating body weight and in whether we develop obesity. The first is family studies. For more than 75 years we have known that individuals from families with overweight parents are likely to be overweight. In contrast, individuals from families where the parents are lean are likely to be lean. Adoption studies where children adopted by one family can be traced show that they are more like their biologic parents than the parents that adopt them. Finally, studies in identical and nonidentical twins provide the icing on the cake, so to speak. When identical twins that have been reared in separate families from birth are identified, they are found to be more like

---

insulin Hormone produced by the pancreas that lowers blood glucose by enhancing its entry into cells.

incidence The number of new cases of a particular condition that develop over time. If among 1000 people, 10 people who were not overweight initially become overweight in 1 year, the incidence rate would be 10 cases per 1000 person-years.

energy density The amount of energy or calories in a good compared to the weight of the food.

each other than are nonidentical twins similarly reared apart. From these data we can place the role of genetic factors between 35% and 70% of the inheritance of obesity. This means that if one individual in a given environment becomes overweight, it is highly likely that his or her identical twin would also become overweight. If one twin resists obesity, the other identical twin would be very likely to resist obesity as well.

Further insight into the genetic causes of obesity has come from the cloning of several genes that produce obesity in human beings. Leptin, identified in 1994, was the first of these important gene products to be identified. As noted previously, it is produced in adipose tissue and secreted into the blood in relation to the amount of body fat.[33] Leptin-deficient individuals are massively obese. When they are treated with leptin, food intake falls and body fat is mobilized until body weight is nearly normalized, indicating that this is an important metabolic pathway for which the gene has been identified. The most common single gene defect in obese children and adults is in the melanocortin-4 receptor, a key regulator of food intake.[34] When this receptor is inactive, food intake is nearly as high as when leptin is deficient. When this receptor is only partially inactivated, the food intake is only modestly above control levels.[35] Several other rare genetic defects have been identified in the regulatory process for controlling food intake that when abnormal lead to obesity. These basic biologic insights tell us that body fat has important regulation that is largely, if not completely, independent of willpower.

Intrauterine Imprinting

Several intrauterine events may lead to obesity later in life, probably due to fetal imprinting as a result of early exposure that affects brain plasticity. The Dutch winter famine of 1945 showed that starvation of infants in utero could affect long-term postnatal weight status. Another example is the infants of mothers who smoked during pregnancy, who have an increased risk of becoming overweight during their first three decades of life when compared to infants of mothers who did not smoke during pregnancy.[36] Similarly, infants of mothers who have diabetes are at higher risk of developing obesity than infants born to mothers who did not have diabetes during pregnancy.[37] Infants who are small for their birth date are at higher risk of developing central adiposity and diabetes than normal-weight infants.[25] Finally, experimental studies teach us that exposure to high levels of insulin during the period of brain plasticity can lead to obesity later in life.

Physiologic Control

To maintain a stable body weight over time, the body must correct daily errors in energy balance. A number of physiologic factors are known to disturb this correction. A high rate of carbohydrate oxidation, as measured by a high respiratory quotient (RQ) predicts future weight gain.[38] One explanation is that when carbohydrate oxidation is higher than carbohydrate intake, carbohydrate stores are depleted and we must eat to replace them. Obese individuals who have lost weight are less effective in increasing fat oxidation in the presence of a high-fat meal than normal-weight individuals, and this may be one reason why they are so susceptible to weight regain. Low metabolic rate may also predict future weight gain.[39]

Physical activity gradually declines with age, accounting for some increase in body fat. Recent studies suggest moderate exercise is beneficial in reducing risk of cardiovascular disease[40] and type 2 diabetes and in facilitating the oxidation of fat in the diet.[9]

Fat cells in our body serve two major functions. They store and release fatty acids ingested from food or from liver or fat cells, and they secrete many important hormones and chemicals. The discovery of leptin catapulted the fat cell into the arena of endocrine cells.[41] In addition to leptin, the fat cell secretes a variety of other peptides (lipoprotein lipase, adipsin [complement D], complement C, adiponectin, tumor necrosis factor-α [TNF-α], interleukin-6 [IL-6], plasminogen activator inhibitor-1 [PAI-1], angiotensinogen, bradykinin, and resistin). The fat cell also releases other metabolites such as lactate, fatty acids, glycerol, and prostacyclin formed from arachidonic acid. Our understanding of fat cells as important endocrine cells continues to expand.

Production of cortisol from inactive cortisone in fat cells by the enzyme 11-β-hydroxysteroid dehydrogenase type 1 may be important in determining the quantity of visceral adipose tissue.[42] Changes in this enzyme may contribute to the risk for menopausal women to develop more visceral fat. High levels of this enzyme keep the quantity of cortisol in visceral fat high, providing a fertile environment for developing new fat cells.

Information about hunger and satiety comes from the gastrointestinal (GI) tract, where several peptides signal the body to stop or start eating. Ghrelin has received recent attention because, in contrast to other GI hormones, it stimulates food intake.[43] Levels of ghrelin are low in obesity, except for the Prader-Willi syndrome, suggesting that it may play a role.

The brain is a receiver, transducer, and transmitter of information about hunger and satiety. Several neurotransmitter systems are involved in regulation of food intake.[44] Receptors for serotonin modulate both the quantity of food eaten and macronutrient selection, and their loss through genetic targeting produces obesity. Peptide neurotransmitters also play a very important role in the regulation of feeding. Sleep deprivation is one way to enhance the release of peptides that produce hunger.[45] In young men allowed to sleep only 4 hours per night for 2 days, the leptin decreased and ghrelin increased relative to the pattern seen with 10 hours of sleep on each of 2 nights.

AN OVERVIEW OF TREATING THE DISEASE OF OBESITY

Prevention of the Current Epidemic

The epidemic of obesity occurs on a genetic background that has not changed significantly in the last 100 years and certainly not since the epidemic began 20 years ago. Nonetheless, it is clear that genetic factors play a critical role in the susceptibility of becoming obese in a "toxic environment."[46] One analogy is that "genes load the gun and a permissive or toxic environment pulls the trigger." Modification of environmental factors acting on our ancient genes must be the strategy to prevent the disease. The belief that this can be done by the individual alone is to miss the argument of how environmental factors have acted on these genes to produce the current epidemic, with major emphasis on the imprinting of the plastic brain of the growing child and adolescent.

We argue that the First Law of Thermodynamics has lulled us into the uncomfortable place of believing that individuals through "willpower," increased food choices, or more places to exercise can overcome the current epidemic of obesity. "Cognitive" approaches relying on individual commitment and resolve have been unsuccessful in stemming the epidemic, and nothing suggests that they will be more successful in the future.

We also argue that it is what the First Law of Thermodynamics does not tell us that is important. In this context it is the unconscious host systems on which environmental factors operate that produces the disease. If the vending machines that now provide kickbacks to schools contained beverages with no added sugar or HFCS, available calories would be reduced. We have argued that the exposure of young children to HFCS may produce detrimental imprinting of the brain, making obesity more likely and more difficult to control.

At least three preventive strategies are available to deal with the epidemic: education, regulation, and modification of the food supply. Education in the school curriculum about good nutrition and healthy weight would be beneficial in helping all children learn how to select appropriate foods. School breakfast and lunch programs would match the educational messages.

However, it is unwise to rely on educational strategies alone, because they have not prevented the epidemic of obesity. Regulation is a second strategy. Regulating an improved food label would be one good idea. Regulations on appropriate serving sizes might be part of the information provided by restaurants when requested.

Modification in some components of the food system is a third and most important strategy. Because the energy we eat comes from food, we need to modify this system to provide smaller portions and less energy density if we are to succeed in combating the epidemic of obesity.

Treatment of Overweight People When Prevention Fails

A detailed discussion of treatment for obesity is beyond the scope of this chapter, but a few general comments about the major approaches are essential because they involve food intake and exercise. Although prevention is unlikely to be successful by relying solely on individual initiative, treatment requires individual initiative. For any change to occur, the individual must be ready for change. This idea of "stages of change" is a key component of any individual approach. The overweight individual must be aware that he or she has a problem and must have moved beyond the stage of precontemplation, that is, the stage of denial before the person is willing to do anything about it, into a stage of contemplation and then to action. When overweight individuals are in this state, they are ready to move forward. Their options are diet, exercise, behavioral therapy, medication, and surgery. These are the principal approaches available to individuals who have a weight problem that they want to address. The use of diet, exercise, and behavioral therapy are appropriate for all levels of overweight.

Dietetic professionals can play an important role in all of these approaches. First, the educated dietetic professional needs to be keenly aware of the complexity of the obesity problem. The dietitian obviously cannot alter the genetic makeup of an individual but is able to address the environmental aspects that serve to exacerbate the situation. Simply handing out diet sheets should be discouraged. Helping the obese patient requires attention to his or her overall diet history, current eating and activity patterns, and behavioral obstacles that either cause problems or prevent change. Although quick weight loss may be the patient's immediate desire, the need for permanent lifestyle changes should be the primary objective. Tips for addressing this have been outlined by Bray and Champagne previously (Box 15-1).[47] Finally, the dietitian can be an instrument of change by appealing to policymakers to modify environmental conditions such as the school vending machine situation cited above. We can think of no better professional to craft this effective message to both lawmakers and school officials alike.

Diet

Popular diets have been published for more than 150 years, and obviously if any diet were significantly better than the others it would have "won the battle" and the others would have disappeared. The popular diets can be grouped into several categories: low-energy (calorie) diets, low-fat diets, low-carbohydrate diets, and high-

BOX 15-1 | Practice Points for the Clinical Dietitian

- *Focus on personal history:* More than ever, the personal history of the patient is a critical focus area for the dietitian in clinical practice who deals with patients diagnosed with the metabolic syndrome. In particular, assessment of past dietary habits using a valid food frequency questionnaire is warranted. The current dietary practices of the patient can help to highlight target areas; collecting a food record for as many days as the patient is willing to keep it will be instrumental in future counseling efforts.
- *Obtain thorough information:* Encouraging the patient to provide as much dietary information as possible will make a measurable difference in the accuracy of the dietary data for evaluation purposes. Remember to focus on the fact that no judgments will be formed, only areas of diet for targeting change.
- *Assess exercise habits:* Physical activity patterns are useful for designing the total lifestyle program. The dietitian may choose to collect a physical activity questionnaire from the patient and, in addition, provide the patient with an activity monitor to assess actual physical activity steps for a more accurate appraisal of daily activity levels.
- *Customize:* For greater success, the dietary treatment needs to be highly individualized. It may be helpful to include a variety of weight loss strategies, such as meal replacements (for quicker initial weight loss), slightly higher protein diets, low-fat diets, and perhaps even a Mediterranean diet approach. It is key to remember that what works for one patient may not necessarily be ideal for another.
- *Consult the physician:* Working with the patient's physician to provide the ideal combination of diet, physical activity suggestions, behavior changes, and drug (if prescribed by the physician) is key to the patient's success.
- *Follow up:* Regular evaluations to monitor progress are key to weight management, both on the part of the physician and the dietitian in clinical practice.

protein diets. A summary of data abstracted by the U.S. Department of Agriculture is shown in Table 15-1.

Several popular diets, including the Atkins Diet (low carbohydrate), the Ornish (low fat), the American Heart Association diet (balanced low calorie), and the Zone diet (high protein), were recently compared and found to produce comparable weight loss, suggesting that none of these diets has any greater effect than the others.[48] In a large and extensive analysis of 26 studies of diets in which treatment lasted at least 12 months, the results showed that the low-fat diets were superior to the control diet and that very-low-calorie diets produced the most weight loss at 1 year.[49]

Exercise

Increased movement, both modest and vigorous, is a way to increase energy expenditure that will burn fat deposits. Human beings expend approximately two thirds of their energy with basal activities, including maintaining body temperature, and only approximately one third in various activities. Thus to expend a significant number of calories

through exercise takes time. As a rule of thumb approximately 100 kcal are expended for each mile walked. If it takes 15 minutes to walk a mile, you could expend up to 400 kcal in an hour of brisk walking. From a practical point of view it is often easier to eat 400 kcal less than to exercise for the extra 400 kcal. Over and above any effect on body weight, regular activity can have beneficial effects on improving cardiovascular health.

Behavioral Therapy

Since their introduction in 1967, behavioral approaches to helping overweight individuals focus on the issues that revolve around eating have been a cornerstone in the treatment of obesity. These techniques are adapted from psychologic learning theory, where rewarding appropriate behavior tends to reinforce that behavior. The process involves familiarity with the activities associated with learning and providing consequences of eating and rewards that reinforce appropriate behaviors. Among the successful techniques in this area are self-monitoring, increased physical activity, and eating a lower-fat diet. People who are successful at maintaining a lowered body weight over time utilize these techniques as well as others.

Medication

There are currently only four medications approved by the U.S. Food and Drug Administration for the treatment of obesity. These include four drugs that have only been approved for short-term use (benzphetamine [Didrex], diethylpropion [Tenuate], phendimetrazine [*Adipost, Anorex-SR, Appecon, Bontril PDM, Bontril Slow-Release, Melfiat, Obezine, Phendiet, Plegine, Prelu-2, Statobex*], and phentermine [*Adipex-P, Fastin, Ionamin, Obenix, Obephen, Oby-Cap, Oby-Trim, Panshape M, Phentercot, Phentride, Pro-Fast HS, Pro-Fast SA, Pro-Fast SR, Teramine, Zantryl*]) and two drugs that have been approved for longer-term use—orlistat (Xenical) and sibutramine (Meridia). The four short-term drugs and sibutramine are thought to work by modifying the neurotransmitters in the central nervous system. Each of these drugs works in part by binding to molecules on the surface of brain cells (neurons) that transport neurotransmitters back into these neurons after they have been secreted. Because they are related to the addictive drugs amphetamine, albeit quite indirectly, the U.S. government regulated their use through the Drug Enforcement Agency (DEA). In clinical studies with these drugs the weight loss is approximately 4 to 5 kg (8.8 to 11 lb) more than with placebo controls after 6 to 12 months of treatment. To be eligible for use of medications, an individual needs to have a BMI above 30 kg/m^2, unless there are associated problems such as diabetes, heart disease, high blood pressure, or other problems that would benefit from weight loss; then the lower limit for use of medications may be 27 kg/m^2 (see the *Diet-Medications Interactions* box, "Drugs Used to Treat Obesity").

TABLE 15-1	Features of the Major Diets Used by Americans			
Type of Diet	**Calories**	**Fat, g (%)**	**Carbohydrate, g (%)**	**Protein, g (%)**
Typical American	2200	85 (35)	274 (50)	82 (15)
High-fat, low- carbohydrate	1400	94 (60)	35 (10)	105 (30)
Moderate-fat	1450	40 (25)	218 (60)	54 (15)
Low-fat and very-low-fat	1450	16-24 (10-15)	235-271 (65-75)	54-72 (15-20)

Modified from Freedman MR, King J, Kennedy E: Popular diets: a scientific review, *Obes Res* 9(suppl):1S, 2001, with permission from NAASO, The Obesity Society.

Orlistat contrasts with these centrally acting drugs. It works in the intestine to block an enzyme called lipase, which is produced and secreted from the pancreas. At clinically used doses, it blocks digestion of approximately one third of the dietary fat. This dietary fat then passes through the intestinal tract and exits the body in the feces. When used improperly, this drug can produce significant GI tract symptoms. In clinical studies this drugs produces 2 to 4 kg (4.4 to 8.8 lb) more weight loss than placebo-treated groups and appears to be slightly less effective.[50]

A new class of drugs called the *cannabinoid receptors antagonists* (rimonabant [Acomplia]) are on their way to approval by the Food and Drug Administration. They work by blocking the receptor that binds endocannabinoids (anandamide and 2-arachidonoyl glycerol). The clinical studies with this drug show that it produces weight loss that is about 5 kg (11 lb) more than placebo, which is similar to the other drugs that are available. Other new drugs are under trial and may become available in the not-too-distant future.

In addition to prescription medication, a variety of herbs and supplements are used to help individuals lose weight (see the Complementary and Alternative Medicine [CAM] box, "Common Herbs and Supplements Used for Weight Loss").

Surgery

Use of surgery for treatment of obesity has expanded greatly in the last decade of the twentieth century.[51] Several different types of operations are currently in use for treatment of obesity. To be eligible for surgical intervention, an overweight individual needs to have a BMI above 40 kg/m^2, unless the person has associated diseases such as diabetes, heart disease, sleep apnea, or osteoarthritis, in which case the BMI for considering therapy can be lowered to 35 kg/m^2.

Health Promotion

Our lives are constrained by the laws of nature—gravity, momentum, and thermodynamics—with which we have been dealing in this chapter. The strategies we take to deal with the impact of these laws on our lives include

benzphetamine One of the appetite-suppressant drugs that has been approved for more than 30 years for short-term use but that is regulated by the Drug Enforcement Agency because of potential for addictive abuse; trade name Didrex.

diethylpropion One of the appetite-suppressant drugs that has been approved for more than 30 years for short-term use but that is regulated by the Drug Enforcement Agency because of potential for addictive abuse; trade name Tenuate.

phendimetrazine One of the appetite-suppressant drugs that has been approved for more than 30 years for short-term use but that is regulated by the Drug Enforcement Agency because of potential for addictive abuse; trade names Adipost, Anorex-SR, Appecon, Bontril PDM, Bontril Slow-Release, Melfiat, Obezine, Phendiet, Plegine, Prelu-2, and Statobex.

phentermine One of the appetite-suppressant drugs that has been approved for more than 30 years for short-term use but that is regulated by the Drug Enforcement Agency because of potential for addictive abuse; trade names Adipex-P, Fastin, Ionamin, Obenix, Obephen, Oby-Cap, Oby-Trim, Panshape M, Phentercot, Phentride, Pro-Fast HS, Pro-Fast SA, Pro-Fast SR, Teramine, and Zantryl.

orlistat Drug (trade name Xenical) that partially blocks pancreatic lipase, thus decreasing digestion of dietary fat. It is available by prescription and over the counter.

sibutramine A newer appetite-suppressant drug that has been approved for long-term use but that is still regulated by the Drug Enforcement Agency because of potential for addictive abuse; trade name Meridia.

pancreas Gland located near the duodenum and small intestine that has two sets of cells: (1) acinar cells, which secrete digestive enzymes into the intestine, and (2) beta cells, which produce and secrete insulin into the blood.

⬤ DIET-MEDICATIONS INTERACTIONS

Drugs Used to Treat Obesity

Generic Name	Trade Name	Mechanism of Action	Food-Drug Interactions
Benzphetamine	Didrex	Appetite suppressant, stimulates CNS and decreases appetite (similar to amphetamine); short-term use only	Alcohol may increase the dizziness effects of this medicine.
Diethylpropion	Tenuate, Tenuate Dospan		A reduced-calorie diet must be followed while using an appetite suppressant in order to lose weight. Also, in order to keep the lost weight from returning, changes in diet and exercise must be continued after the weight has been lost.
Phendimetrazine	Adipost, Anorex-SR, Appecon, Bontril PDM, Bontril Slow-Release, Melfiat, Obezine, Phendiet, Plegine, Preu-2, Statobex		
Phentermine	Adipex-P, Fastin, Ionamin, Obenix, Obephen, Oby-Cap, Oby-Trim, Panshape M, Phentercot, Phentride, Pro-Fast HS, Pro-Fast SA, Pro-Fast SR, Teramine, Zantryl		
Orlistat	Xenical	Blocks fat from being absorbed in intestine	Prevents absorption of some dietary fat; should be taken during the meal or within 1 hr of eating; may decrease absorption of fat-soluble vitamins from food; multivitamin supplement should be taken once a day at least 2 hr before or after taking orlistat. Diet should contain no more than 30% of calories as fat. More fat in the diet will increase side effects. Patients who have DM may need to have their insulin or oral hypoglycemic agents adjusted. May experience gas with leaky bowel movements; inability to hold bowel movement; increases in bowel movements; oily bowel movements; oily spotting of underclothes.
Sibutramine	Meridia	Boosts levels of serotonin, dopamine, and norepinephrine in the body	Reduced-calorie diet must be followed in conjunction with medication to lose weight and keep it off. Do not drink alcohol.

CNS, Central nervous system; *DM,* diabetes mellitus.

education, regulation, and product design. Deaths from the effects of the laws of momentum produced by automobile accidents provide a glimpse into the strategies we could use to minimize this effect. They also provide insights into the strategies that may be needed to deal with the epidemic of obesity. Although the laws of momentum or the laws of thermodynamics cannot be changed, their impact on producing automobile accidents and obesity can be mitigated. This can be done through better education about driving and about nutritional needs to

prevent obesity. Education can be complemented in the case of cars by regulations that require seat belts, airbags, and other safety devices. In the case of obesity it can be complemented by limiting access to large portion sizes and to high-energy-density foods and having an environment where physical activity is more prevalent. Finally, product design to make cars safer partly addresses the driving problem, and modifying the types of foods that are available provides strategies to combat the obesity epidemic by redesigning the food environment.

COMPLEMENTARY AND ALTERNATIVE MEDICINE (CAM)
Common Herbs and Supplements Used for Weight Loss

Herb/Supplement	Common Uses	Drug/Herb Interactions	Interaction	Safety	Efficacy
Chromium	Thought to improve insulin sensitivity, causing insulin levels to fall, thereby initiating lipolysis	Hypoglycemic agents	Possible potentiation of drug, increasing risk of hypoglycemia.	Safe.	Strong evidence.
		Calcium carbonate and antacids	Reduce chromium absorption.		
Pyruvate	Enhance fat metabolism	No known drug interactions		Formal toxicologic studies have not been reported.	Some evidence of weight loss when used in conjunction with low-calorie diet.
5-HTP (5-hydroxy-tryptophan)	Serotonin precursor	Levodopa-carbidopa	Possible increased risk of scleroderma-like syndrome.	No significant adverse effects reported in clinical trials.	Some evidence that it is helpful in weight loss.
		SSRIs, other serotonergic drugs	Possible risk of serotonin syndrome.		
Hydroxycitric acid (HCA)		No known drug interactions.		No serious side effects have been reported, but formal safety studies have not been performed.	Weak evidence it may be useful for weight loss.
Caffeine-ephedrine	Stimulant	CNS stimulants	Potentiation of stimulant side effects. Death.	Use of herb ephedra instead of ephedrine may present unpredictable risks.	Strong evidence it promotes short- and long-term weight loss.
Conjugated linolenic acid (CLA)	Reduce body weight while retaining muscle mass	None known.		Appears to be a safe nutritional substance.	Contradictory evidence that CLAs might help reduce fat mass.
Calcium	Weight and fat loss	Calcium channel blockers	Action may be affected by combination calcium supplements and high-dose vitamin D.	Calcium supplements may increase kidney stone risk, whereas dietary calcium reduces risk of kidney stones.	Dietary calcium facilitates greater weight loss than calcium supplements (calcium carbonate).
		Beta-blockers	May decrease blood levels.		
		Tetracycline and fluoroquinolone antibiotics	May interfere with absorption; take calcium supplements at least 2 hr before antibiotic dosing.		

Data from Bratman S, Girman AM, for HealthGate Data Corp: *Mosby's handbook of herbs and supplements and their therapeutic uses,* St. Louis, 2003, Mosby; Contributors and consultants: *Professional guide to complementary and alternative therapies,* Springhouse, Pa, 2001, Springhouse; Kuhn MA, Winston D: *Herbal therapy and supplements: a scientific and traditional approach,* Philadelphia, 2001, Lippincott; and Zemel MB et al: Calcium and dairy acceleration of weight and fat loss during energy restriction in obese adults, *Obesity Res* 12(4):582, 2004.

SSRI, Selective serotonin reuptake inhibitor; *CNS,* central nervous system; *MAOI,* monamine oxidase inhibitor.

Continued

COMPLEMENTARY AND ALTERNATIVE MEDICINE (CAM)—cont'd
Common Herbs and Supplements Used for Weight Loss

Herb/Supplement	Common Uses	Drug/Herb Interactions	Interaction	Safety	Efficacy
Calcium—cont'd		Thiazide diuretics	Long-term use of thiazide diuretics tends to increase serum calcium levels by decreasing calcium excretion.		
		Corticosteroids and anticon-vulsants	Interfere with absorption of calcium.		
Gymnema (*Gymnema sylvestre*)	Diminish ability to taste sweet substances and decrease appetite for up to 90 minutes	Hyperglycemic drugs or insulin	Blood glucose levels should be monitored closely.	Not known.	May be useful in reducing cravings for sweets.
Yohimbe (*Pausinystalia yohimbe*)	CNS stimulant	Phenothiazines (chlorpromazine)	Increases yohimbe toxicity.	Inappropriate for long-term use. Side effects: priapism, hypertension or hypotension depending on dosage, irritability, migraines, dizziness, tremors, bronchospasm, insomnia, tachycardia, nausea and vomiting.	Inhibits hunger.
		MAOIs, tricyclic antidepressants	Hypertensive crisis.		
		Antihypertensive medications (e.g., clonidine)	Antagonizes effects of drugs		

REFERENCES

1. World Health Organization: *Diet, nutrition and the prevention of chronic diseases: WHO technical report series, Report No. 916,* Geneva, Switzerland, 2003, Author.
2. Bray GA: Obesity is a chronic, relapsing neurochemical disease, *Int J Obes Relat Metab Disord* 28(1):34, 2004.
3. Hedley AA et al: Prevalence of overweight and obesity among U.S. children, adolescents, and adults, 1999-2002, *JAMA* 291(23):2847, 2004.
4. Flegal KM et al: Excess deaths associated with underweight, overweight, and obesity, *JAMA* 293(15):1861, 2005.
5. Ogden CL et al: Prevalence and trends in overweight among U.S. children and adolescents, 1999-2000, *JAMA* 288(14):1728, 2002.
6. Klein S et al: Clinical implications of obesity with specific focus on cardiovascular disease: a statement for professionals from the American Heart Association Council on Nutrition, Physical Activity, and Metabolism: endorsed by the American College of Cardiology Foundation, *Circulation* 110(18):2952, 2004.
7. Finkelstein EA, Ruhm CJ, Kosa KM: Economic causes and consequences of obesity, *Annu Rev Public Health* 26:239, 2005.
8. Knowler WC et al. Reduction in the incidence of type 2 diabetes with lifestyle intervention or metformin, *N Engl J Med* 346(6):393, 2002.
9. Smith SR et al: Concurrent physical activity increases fat oxidation during the shift to a high-fat diet, *Am J Clin Nutr* 72(1):131, 2000.
10. Kinsell LW et al: Calories do count, *Metabolism* 13:195, 1964.
11. Lyon XH et al: Compliance to dietary advice directed towards increasing the carbohydrate to fat ratio of the everyday diet, *Int J Obes Relat Metab Disord* 19(4):260, 1995.
12. Licinio J et al: Phenotypic effects of leptin replacement on morbid obesity, diabetes mellitus, hypogonadism, and behavior in

leptin-deficient adults, *Proc Natl Acad Sci U S A* 101(13):4531, 2004.

13. Institute of Medicine: *Weighing the options: criteria for evaluating weight-management programs,* Washington, DC, 1995, National Academies Press.

14. Nielsen SJ, Popkin BM: Patterns and trends in food portion sizes, 1977-1998, *JAMA* 289(4):450, 2003.

15. Putnam J, Allshouse JE: *Food consumption, prices and expenditures, 1970-1997: statistical bulletin, Report No. 965,* Washington, DC, 1999 (April), Economic Research Service, U.S. Department of Agriculture.

16. Bray GA, Nielsen SJ, Popkin BM: Consumption of high-fructose corn syrup in beverages may play a role in the epidemic of obesity, *Am J Clin Nutr* 79(4):537, 2004.

17. Ludwig DS, Peterson KE, Gortmaker SL: Relation between consumption of sugar-sweetened drinks and childhood obesity: a prospective, observational analysis, *Lancet* 357(9255):505, 2001.

18. Raben A et al: Meals with similar energy densities but rich in protein, fat, carbohydrate, or alcohol have different effects on energy expenditure and substrate metabolism but not on appetite and energy intake, *Am J Clin Nutr* 77(1):91, 2003.

19. James J et al: Preventing childhood obesity by reducing consumption of carbonated drinks: cluster randomised controlled trial, *BMJ* 328(7450):1237, 2004.

20. Bray GA, Popkin BM: Dietary fat intake does affect obesity! *Am J Clin Nutr* 68(6):1157, 1998.

21. Drewnowski A, Specter SE: Poverty and obesity: the role of energy density and energy costs, *Am J Clin Nutr* 79(1):6, 2004.

22. Blundell JE, MacDiarmid JI: Fat as a risk factor for overconsumption: satiation, satiety, and patterns of eating, *J Am Diet Assoc* 97(7 suppl):S63, 1997.

23. von Kries R et al: Breast feeding and obesity: cross sectional study, *BMJ* 319(7203):147, 1999.

24. Ailhaud G, Guesnet P: Fatty acid composition of fats is an early determinant of childhood obesity: a short review and an opinion, *Obes Rev* 5(1):21, 2004.

25. Bhargava SK et al: Relation of serial changes in childhood body-mass index to impaired glucose tolerance in young adulthood, *N Engl J Med* 350(9):865, 2004.

26. Pereira MA et al: Dairy consumption, obesity, and the insulin resistance syndrome in young adults: the CARDIA Study, *JAMA* 287(16):2081, 2002.

27. Hancox RJ, Milne BJ, Poulton R: Association between child and adolescent television viewing and adult health: a longitudinal birth cohort study, *Lancet* 364(9430):257, 2004.

28. Hu FB et al: Adiposity as compared with physical activity in predicting mortality among women, *N Engl J Med* 351(26):2694, 2004.

29. Allison DB et al: Antipsychotic-induced weight gain: a comprehensive research synthesis, *Am J Psychiatry* 156(11):1686, 1999.

30. O'Hara P et al: Early and late weight gain following smoking cessation in the Lung Health Study, *Am J Epidemiol* 148(9):821, 1998.

31. Dhurandhar NV et al: Increased adiposity in animals due to a human virus, *Int J Obes Relat Metab Disord* 24(8):989, 2000.

32. Tremblay A et al: Thermogenesis and weight loss in obese individuals: a primary association with organochlorine pollution, *Int J Obes Relat Metab Disord* 28(7):936, 2004.

33. Zhang Y et al: Positional cloning of the mouse obese gene and its human homologue, *Nature* 372(6505):425, 1994.

34. Farooqi IS et al: Clinical spectrum of obesity and mutations in the melanocortin 4 receptor gene, *N Engl J Med* 348(12):1085, 2003.

35. Farooqi IS, Yeo GS, O'Rahilly S: Binge eating as a phenotype of melanocortin 4 receptor gene mutations, *N Engl J Med* 349(6):606, 2003.

36. Toschke AM et al: Maternal smoking during pregnancy and appetite control in offspring, *J Perinat Med* 31(3):251, 2003.

37. Dabelea D et al: Birth weight, type 2 diabetes, and insulin resistance in Pima Indian children and young adults, *Diabetes Care* 22(6):944, 1999.

38. Zurlo F et al: Low ratio of fat to carbohydrate oxidation as predictor of weight gain: study of 24-h RQ, *Am J Physiol* 259(5, part 1):E650, 1990.

39. Astrup A et al: Meta-analysis of resting metabolic rate in formerly obese subjects, *Am J Clin Nutr* 69(6):1117, 1999.

40. Blair SN, LaMonte MJ, Nichaman MZ: The evolution of physical activity recommendations: how much is enough? *Am J Clin Nutr* 79(5 suppl):913S, 2004.

41. Spiegelman BM, Flier JS: Obesity and the regulation of energy balance, *Cell* 104(4):531, 2001.

42. Hochberg Z et al: Hypothalamic regulation of adiposity: the role of 11-beta-hydroxysteroid dehydrogenase type 1, *Horm Metab Res* 36(6):365, 2004.

43. Cummings DE, Shannon MH: Roles for ghrelin in the regulation of appetite and body weight, *Arch Surg* 138(4):389, 2003.

44. Cowley MA et al: Electrophysiological actions of peripheral hormones on melanocortin neurons, *Ann N Y Acad Sci* 994:175, 2003.

45. Spiegel K et al: Brief communication: sleep curtailment in healthy young men is associated with decreased leptin levels, elevated ghrelin levels, and increased hunger and appetite, *Ann Intern Med* 141(11):846, 2004.

46. Perusse L et al: The human obesity gene map: the 2004 update, *Obes Res* 13(3):381, 2005.

47. Bray GA, Champagne CM: Obesity and the metabolic syndrome: implications for dietetics practitioners, *J Am Diet Assoc* 104(1):86, 2004.

48. Freedman MR, King J, Kennedy E: Popular diets: a scientific review, *Obes Res* 9(1 suppl):1S, 2001.

49. Avenell A et al: What are the long-term benefits of weight reducing diets in adults? A systematic review of randomized controlled trials, *J Hum Nutr Diet* 17(4):317, 2004.

50. Padwal R, Li SK, Lau DC: Long-term pharmacotherapy for overweight and obesity: a systematic review and meta-analysis of randomized controlled trials, *Int J Obes Relat Metab Disord* 27(12):1437, 2003.

51. Buchwald H et al: Bariatric surgery: a systematic review and meta-analysis, *JAMA* 292(14):1724, 2004.

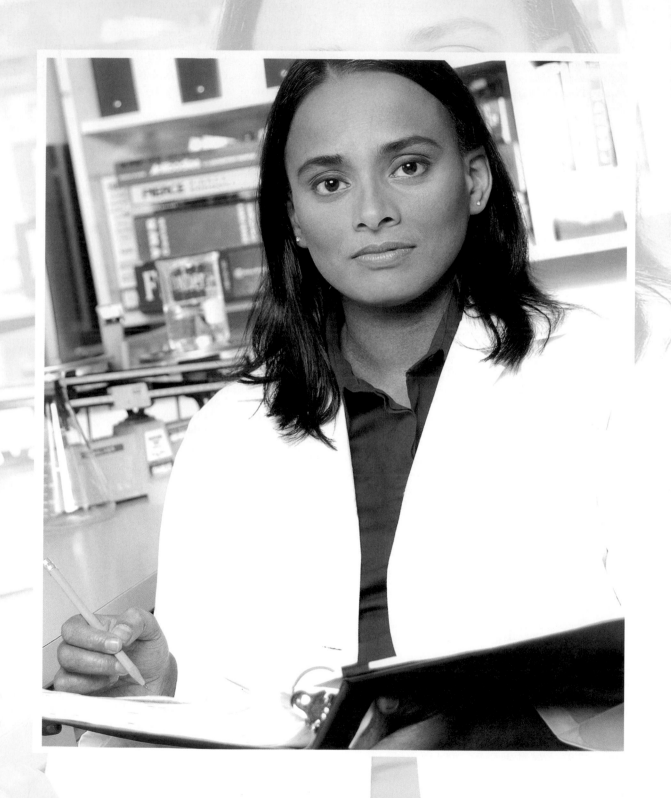

PART 3

Introduction to Clinical Nutrition

CHAPTER 16

Nutrition Assessment and Nutrition Therapy in Patient Care

Sara Long

In this chapter, we focus on the foundation for nutrition therapy—nutrition assessment. Information gathered during nutrition assessment is used to establish goals for nutrition intervention. Once interventions are initiated, nutrition assessment data functions as the point of reference from which to determine efficacy of treatment.[1]

Nutrition assessment is defined as "an evaluation of the nutritional status of individuals or populations through measurements of food and nutrient intake and evaluation of nutrition-related health indicators."[2] Because there is no single test that measures nutritional status, nutrition assessment draws from numerous indexes to provide a complete picture of nutritional health.[1]

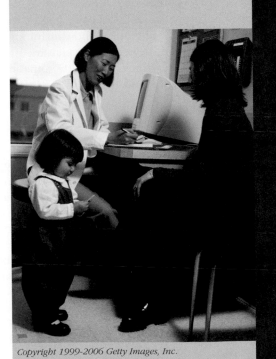

ROLE OF NUTRITION IN CLINICAL CARE

Nutrition therapy plays an essential role in disease management, healthcare, and preventive healthcare and should be provided by a qualified nutrition professional.[1,3,4] Comprehensive nutrition assessment provides the necessary basis for appropriate nutrition therapy based on identified needs. Nutrition assessment and medical nutrition therapy promote multiple goals: assisting patients in recovery from illness or injury, helping persons maintain follow-up care to promote health, and helping to control healthcare costs.[3] Clinical nutritionists, all registered dietitians (RDs), and many with advanced degrees in nutrition science, use their expertise and skills to make sound clinical judgments and to work effectively with the clinical care team. These professionals provide an essential component for the successful management of the patient's plan of care.

Stress of the Therapeutic Encounter

In the modern hospital setting the patient experiences a great deal of stress because he or she is sick, upset, or scared. Even the most ideal hospital stay is a very emotional experience.[5] Encounters between healthcare providers and their patients occur, unavoidably, under stressful conditions. Several factors can contribute to added nutritional toll. (See the *Diet-Medications Interactions* box, "Assess Your Knowledge of Food-Drug Interactions.")

Bed Rest

Even though the reason for the hospitalization may indicate need for bed rest, at the same time it has long been known that bed rest itself can result in detrimental effects on the human body.[6] For example, after just 3 days of lying supine in bed the body begins to lose its resistance to the pull of gravity, and continuing inactivity diminishes muscle tone, bone calcium, plasma volume, and gastric secretions, bringing some impairment in glucose tolerance and shifts in body fluids and electrolytes.

Hospital Malnutrition

Hospital, or iatrogenic, malnutrition has been widely documented. Hospitalized patients with hypermetabolic and physiologic stress of illness or injury can be at risk for malnutrition from increased nutritional needs. Hospital operating guidelines that provide for nutrition screening on admission combined with follow-up monitoring will identify patients at malnutrition risk and provide essential medical nutrition therapy.[7] However, potential problems arising from hospital routines may contribute to a lack of adequate nourishment in some cases, including the following:

- Highly restricted diets remaining on order and unsupplemented too long

- Unserved meals due to interference of medical procedures and clinical tests
- Unmonitored patient appetite

Hospital Setting and System

Each injured or ill patient is a unique person and requires special treatment and care. A formidable array of staff persons seek to determine needs and implement what each patient needs as appropriate care. When individual human needs are met with personal care, within the context of carefully developed care protocols, patients will not feel intimidated and powerless.

Constant open and validating communication is essential, both among the healthcare team members and between the healthcare provider and the patient and family. It is at such times we need to remind ourselves of the time-tested fundamental ethical principles guiding all our patient care,[8,9] principles that ensure that all we do performs the following functions:

- *Benefit* the patient.
- Do no *harm*.
- Preserve the patient's *autonomy*.
- *Disclose* full and truthful information for patient decisions concerning personal care.
- Provide *social justice*.

Such ethical behavior is based on the overriding fundamental principles of right action found within Anglo-American common law, which emphasizes the basic rights of privacy and free choice.[9] Continuing open communication provides the basis for such ethical practices among the healthcare team members and between healthcare providers and patient and family. This is especially important for many stressed older adult patients who fail to thrive. In this team effort for quality nutrition care the RD, along with physician, carries primary responsibility. Nurses and other primary care practitioners provide essential support.

Focus of Care: The Patient

Patient-Centered Care

The primary principle of nutrition practice, too often overlooked in the many routine procedures of the hospital setting, is evident: to be valid, nutrition care must be person centered. In this renewed partnership paradigm for patient-centered healthcare, the patient must always be a senior partner. Care must be based on initial identified

---

iatrogenic Describes a medical disorder caused by physician diagnosis, manner, or treatment.
paradigm A pattern or model serving as an example; a standard or ideal for practice or behavior based on a fundamental value or theme.

● DIET-MEDICATIONS INTERACTIONS

Assess Your Knowledge of Food-Drug Interactions

Medications can treat and cure many health problems, but they must be taken properly to be effective. Many medications interact with foods, beverages, alcohol, and caffeine to make them less effective or cause dangerous side effects. Assess your knowledge of food drug interactions by answering the questions below.

1. There is no risk of food drug interactions when taking over-the-counter medications.
   a. True
   b. False
2. Your neighbor, Greta, has serious allergies. Her physician prescribed an antihistamine to control her symptoms. Which of the following labels may appear on her prescription bottle?
   a. Take on an empty stomach.
   b. Take with food.
   c. Take only at bedtime.
   d. Take with coffee.
3. The above label is on Greta's prescription antihistamine because:
   a. Effectiveness is increased when taken on an empty stomach
   b. Effectiveness is increased when taken with food
   c. The drug is metabolized more efficiently when taken at bedtime
   d. Caffeine enhances absorption of the medication
4. Your other neighbor, Abdul, has a horrible headache from studying too hard last night. He asks you if he should take his over-the-counter nonsteroidal antiinflammatory drug (NSAID) on an empty stomach or with a meal. He should take the NSAID with food because:
   a. These medications can irritate the stomach
   b. Food will increase effectiveness
   c. It is easier to remember to take them with a meal
5. Combining NSAIDs or acetaminophen with alcohol will:
   a. Decrease stomach irritation
   b. Increase risk of liver damage
   c. Protect the liver from the effects of alcohol
   d. Have no effect whatsoever.
6. Your cousin Vinny is dining on a super-sized meal at the local fast-food restaurant. Which of the following prescription medications should he avoid taking with the meal because high-fat meals may increase levels in the body?
   a. Hydrochlorothiazide (diuretic)
   b. Tetracyclines (antibiotic)
   c. NSAIDs
   d. Some forms of theophylline (bronchodilator)
7. Grandma Minnie takes a diuretic to control hypertension. Her physician told her this drug could cause hypokalemia. Which of the following foods should she eat on a regular basis to avoid hypokalemia?
   a. Hamburgers and hot dogs
   b. Twinkies and Ding Dongs
   c. Low-fat dairy products
   d. Bananas, oranges, and potatoes
8. Uncle Joe is taking captopril (an angiotensin-converting enzyme [ACE] inhibitor) for his high blood pressure. He cannot remember if his physician told him to take the captopril with a meal or on an empty stomach. What can you tell him?
   a. Take it with meals to increase absorption.
   b. Take it 1 hour before or 2 hours after meals so as to not affect absorption.
   c. Take it with breakfast, but not with dinner.

9. Your roommate's cousin's uncle is taking a "statin" medication to lower serum cholesterol. Which of the following statements is true about statin medications?
   a. Avoid drinking large amounts of alcohol because it may increase risk of liver damage.
   b. Take with breakfast to enhance absorption.
   c. Take with the evening meal to decrease absorption.
10. High doses of vitamin E may prolong clotting time and increase risk of bleeding. Large doses of vitamin E should be avoided when taking which of the following drugs?
    a. Warfarin (anticoagulant)
    b. Lovastatin (HMG-CoA reductase inhibitor)
    c. Furosemide (diuretic)
    d. NSAIDs
11. Your cousin Bunny is taking oral contraceptives. Which of the following drugs may decrease effectiveness of "the pill," thereby increasing her chance of pregnancy?
    a. Anticoagulants
    b. NSAIDs
    c. Antibiotics
    d. Antidepressants
12. Bunny's pet turtle, Speedy, died. She wants to take St. John's wort because her roommate told her it would help with her depression. Are there any problems with her taking St. John's wort while she is taking oral contraceptives?
    a. No. St. John's wort is an herb and sold at the Universal Nutrition Center at the mall. Herbal and dietary supplements cannot be sold if they are not safe.
    b. Yes. St. John's wort will decrease effectiveness of the oral contraceptives.
13. Mr. Wilson is very excitable and nervous. Which of the following might be an explanation for this?
    a. He took Cipro (quinolone) with his morning coffee.
    b. He took penicillin at breakfast, which included yogurt.
    c. He took aspirin on an empty stomach.
    d. He just received a call from the IRS to schedule an audit of last year's tax return.
14. Curt is taking tetracycline to control acne. Which of the following should he avoid?
    a. Dairy products
    b. Antacids
    c. Vitamins containing iron
    d. All of the above
15. Your favorite aunt, Constance, takes a monoamine oxidase inhibitor (MAOI). Her pharmacist cautioned her about eating foods high in tyramine (an amino acid). Why?
    a. MAOIs combined with tyramine cause hiccups.
    b. A rapid, potentially fatal decrease in blood pressure can occur.
    c. A rapid, potentially fatal increase in blood pressure can occur.
    d. None of the above will happen. Her pharmacist is mistaken.
16. Your nervous neighbor, Biff, takes alprazolam (Xanax), an antianxiety drug. He was told he should not take the Xanax with Mountain Dew. Why?
    a. Carbonation in the soft drink will enhance effects of the Xanax.
    b. Carbonation in the soft drink will decrease effects of the Xanax.
    c. Caffeine in Mountain Dew may lessen the antianxiety effect of Xanax.
    d. Caffeine in the Mountain Dew may enhance the antianxiety effect of Xanax.

Continued

needs, updated constantly with the patient, with results monitored continuously in relation to therapy goals. This is necessary, of course, to providing essential physical care. But it is also necessary to supporting the patient's personal need to maintain self-esteem and control as much as possible. In addition, a second fundamental fact needs emphasis: despite all methods, tools, and technologies described here or elsewhere, the most therapeutic instrument of such person-centered care is yourself. It is to this seemingly simple yet profoundly personal healing encounter that you bring your skills and your dedication.

Communication with the patient at its best is an interactive, two-way process. This ideal is not always easy to achieve, however, and means much more than simply having the patient answer a few questions. All medical communication, including clinical nutrition therapies, is a form of teaching. The patient in almost all cases needs to learn new information and make the attitudinal and lifestyle changes necessary to put new knowledge to effective therapeutic use. Such teaching can take different forms, from a simple prescription concerning diet, to a persuasive appeal to emotions and attitudes, to a two-sided personal interaction (see the *Focus on Culture* box, "Cultural Stereotyping: Melting Pot or Salad Bowl?"). Patients today are more interested in nutrition than ever before and have more sources of information, from the media to the Internet. The websites on the Internet sponsored by Tufts University and by the Hardin Library of the University of Iowa[10] are excellent sources of medically accurate nutrition information. For finding broader medical information, trustworthy advice on safe Internet searching exists for interested patients, such as the guide from Yale-New Haven Hospital.[11] The patient's personal knowledge may be accurate or erroneous, but either way it will in-

fluence the patient's behavior and receptivity. Clinical practitioners often have severe time constraints in the contemporary medical environment. They nonetheless need to strive to interact with patients as sensitively and respectfully as possible.[12]

Healthcare Team

In the setting of the individual medical center and within the essential team care provided in a managed care system, the clinical dietitian must care for the patient's fundamental nutritional needs in close relationship with the medical and nursing care.[13] Sensitive communication skills are essential for all ages and degrees of health problems. Determining the patient's initial nutritional status and ongoing medical nutrition therapy needs is a primary responsibility for supporting healing and avoiding malnutrition.[7]

THE NUTRITION CARE PROCESS

Patients entering the healthcare system are prone to having nutrition problems. As a result, those patients at nutritional risk need to be identified so that high-quality nutrition care can be provided.[14]

Nutrition Screening

Although nutrition screening and referral are not part of the American Dietetic Association's (ADA's) Nutrition Care Process (NCP), they are essential antecedent steps in the overall NCP.[14] It is not possible or necessary to complete a full nutrition assessment on every patient. It is necessary, however, to have a system in place to quickly identify patients at risk for nutrition problems, such as

✦ FOCUS ON CULTURE

Cultural Stereotyping: Melting Pot or Salad Bowl?

Do all Southerners eat grits? Do all those who practice the Jewish religion follow orthodox food laws? Do all people of Hispanic origin eat tortillas and beans? Should you address your patient informally (by his or her first name) or more formally (Mrs. Garcia or Mr. Sato)? If your patient does not look you in the eye while talking, is he or she being deceitful or showing respect? Why do you need to know the answer to these questions and others?

The population of the United States is growing more and more culturally diverse. Almost 25% of the population is non–Anglo-American. By 2050, Latinos will be the largest minority group. By 2065, non-Hispanic whites will most likely be a minority group. So what does this mean to you?

In terms of nutrition assessment and nutrition counseling, cultural diversity is a fact. Cultural competency is a necessity.

Cultural competency is more than recognizing and accepting cultural diversity. It is a skill critical to all dietitians and healthcare professionals. What good does it do to conduct a nutrition assessment or provide nutrition education if the patient's cultural background is not considered? Culture includes language, lifestyle, values, beliefs, and attitudes. These and other elements of culture influence how patients might experience illness, how they might access healthcare, and how they get well.

To deliver culturally competent care, dietitians and healthcare providers must understand beliefs, values, traditions, cultural practices. Consider the following differences in the dominant American cultural paradigm, the Anglo-American culture, and more traditional cultural populations:

Anglo-American	More Traditional Cultures	What This May Mean to You
Personal control over environment	Fate	Many traditional cultures believe fate, God, or other supernatural factors determine a person's destiny and directly influence health. The way they eat and exercise cannot have any influence of whether or not they develop complications of diabetes, for example.
Change	Tradition	Tradition and continuity are valued over change. A reverence for the past takes precedence over efficiency of striving.
Time dominates	Human interaction dominates	Personal relationships determine self-worth and take priority over time schedules—promptness is not always a priority.
Human equality	Hierarchy/rank/status	In some cultures, healthcare professionals are more highly respected than other professionals. This may result in patients being less forthcoming if they disagree with a healthcare professional.
Individualism/privacy	Group or family welfare	Decision making about health issues may be a family affair.
Self-help	Birthright inheritance	Individuals may not believe they can help themselves in terms of their health.
Competition	Cooperation	Cooperation is preferred to competition
Future orientation	Past orientation	Preventative care may not be a priority.
Action/goal/work orientation/informality	"Being" orientation	Informality (calling people by their first name, for example) is associated with rudeness in many traditional cultures. Clarify the patient's reference early.
Directness/openness/honesty	Formality	Individuals may not "volunteer" information.
Practicality/efficiency	Idealism/spiritualism	Idealism is stressed over practicality or expedience.

There was a time when minorities in the United States tended to imitate the dominant middle-class culture, but this is no longer the case. Individual and cultural expression is becoming desirable. It is an expression of respect to learn about different cultures, to develop flexibility in how to approach clients and patients, and to develop cultural competency.

How Culturally Competent Are You?*

1. When the patient and dietitian come from different cultural backgrounds, the nutrition history obtained may not be accurate.
   a. True
   b. False
2. Which of the following are the correct ways to communicate with a patient through an interpreter?
   a. Making eye contact with the interpreter when you are speaking, then looking at the patient while the interpreter is telling the patient what you said
   b. Speaking slowly, pausing between words
   c. Asking the interpreter to further explain the patient's statement in order to get a more complete picture of the patient's condition
   d. None of the above

3. Which of the following statements is *not* true?
   a. Friendly (nonsexual) physical contact is an important part of communication for many Latin American people.
   b. Many Asian people think it is disrespectful to ask questions of a healthcare professional.
   c. Most African people are either Christian or follow a traditional religion.
   d. Eastern Europeans are highly diverse in terms of customs, language, and religion.
4. Which of the following is good advice for a healthcare professional attempting to use and interpret nonverbal communication?
   a. The provider should recognize that a smile may express unhappiness or dissatisfaction in some cultures.
   b. To express sympathy, a healthcare professional can lightly touch a patient's arm or pat the patient on the back.
   c. If a patient will not make eye contact with a healthcare professional, it is likely the patient is hiding the truth.
   d. When there is a language barrier, the provider can use hand gestures to bridge the gap.

Continued

FOCUS ON CULTURE—cont'd

Cultural Stereotyping: Melting Pot or Salad Bowl?

5. Some symbols—a positive nod of the head, a pointing finger, a "thumbs-up" sign—are universal and can help bridge the language gap.
   a. True
   b. False

6. A female Muslim patient may avoid eye contact and/or physical contact because:
   a. She does not want to spread germs
   b. Muslim women are taught to be submissive
   c. Modesty is very important in Islamic tradition
   d. She does not like the healthcare professional

7. When a patient is not compliant with prescribed nutrition therapy after several visits, which of the following approaches is *not* likely to lead to compliance?
   a. Involving family members
   b. Repeating the instructions very loudly and several times to emphasize the importance of the nutrition therapy
   c. Agreeing to a compromise in the recommended nutrition therapy
   d. Spending time listening to discussions of folk and alternative remedies

8. If a family member speaks English as well as the patient's native language and is willing to act as interpreter, this is the best possible solution to the problem of interpreting.
   a. True
   b. False

9. Which of the following is *true?*
   a. People who speak the same language have the same culture.
   b. The people living in the African continent share the main features of African culture.
   c. Cultural background, diet, religious, and health practices, as well as language, can differ widely within a given country or part of the country.

   d. An alert healthcare professional can usually predict a patient's health behaviors by knowing what country he or she comes from.

10. Out of respect for a patient's privacy, the healthcare professional should always begin a relationship by seeing an adult patient alone and drawing the family in as needed.
    a. True
    b. False

Answers: 1.a., 2.d., 3.c., 4.a., 5.b., 6.c., 7.b., 8.b., 9.c., 10.b.
    *Quiz modified from Management Sciences for Health and the U.S. Department of Health and Human Services, Health Resources and Administration, Bureau of Primary Healthcare: *The provider's guide to quality & culture,* Boston, 2005, Management Sciences for Health. Retrieved December 1, 2005, from *http://erc.msh.org/mainpage.cfm?file= 3.0.htm&module=provider&language=English.*

References

Betterley C: Increasing *cultural competency of nutrition educators through travel study programs,* Unpublished paper, July 6, 2001.

Brannon C: Cultural competency—values, traditions, and effective practice, *Today's Dietitian* 6(11):14, 2004. Retrieved December 1, 2005, from *www.todaysdietitian.com/archives/td_1104p14.shtml.*

Curry KR: Multicultural competence in dietetics and nutrition, *J Am Diet Assoc* 100:1142, 2000.

U.S. Census Bureau: *Census 2000 data for the United States,* Washington, DC, 2000, Author. Available at *www.census.gov.*

Hall GG: *Culturally competent patient care: a guide for providers and their staff,* Modesto, CA, 2001, Institute for Health Professions Education. Retrieved December 1, 2005, from *http://www.ecu.edu/ascc/ CultCompCare.pdf.*

National Center for Cultural Competence: *Health disparities among ethnic and racial groups* [policy brief], Washington, DC, 1999, Georgetown University. Retrieved July 18, 2005, from *http://gucchd. georgetown.edu//nccc/cultural6.html*

---

malnutrition or nutritional risk.[1] "Nutrition screening is the process of identifying characteristics known to be associated with nutrition problems."[15] The Joint Commission on Accreditation of Healthcare Organizations requires all patients admitted to a hospital to be screened within 48 hours of admission.[16]

Nutrition screening can be executed by RDs, dietetic technicians, dietary managers, nurses, physicians, or other trained personnel.[1,14,15] Whether or not RDs are engaged in performing nutrition screening, they are responsible for providing input into development of suitable screening parameters to make certain the screening process addresses the correct parameters.[14] The nutrition screening process has the following characteristics[15]:

- May be completed in any setting
- Facilitates completion of early intervention goals
- Includes collection of relevant data on risk factors and interpretation of data for intervention/treatment
- Determines need for a nutrition assessment
- Is cost-effective

A referral process may be necessary to ensure a patient is referred to an RD, who will conduct the nutrition assessment, make nutrition diagnoses, and provide nutrition care.

Definition of the American Dietetic Association's Nutrition Care Process

Providing nutrition care employing the ADA's NCP starts when a patient is recognized as being at nutritional risk and requiring additional support to attain or maintain positive nutritional status. The ADA's NCP is defined "as a systematic problem-solving method that dietetics professionals use to critically think and make decisions to address nutrition-related problems and provide safe and effective quality nutrition care." It is composed of the following four separate but interrelated and associated steps[14]:

1. Nutrition assessment
2. Nutrition diagnosis
3. Nutrition intervention
4. Nutrition monitoring and evaluation

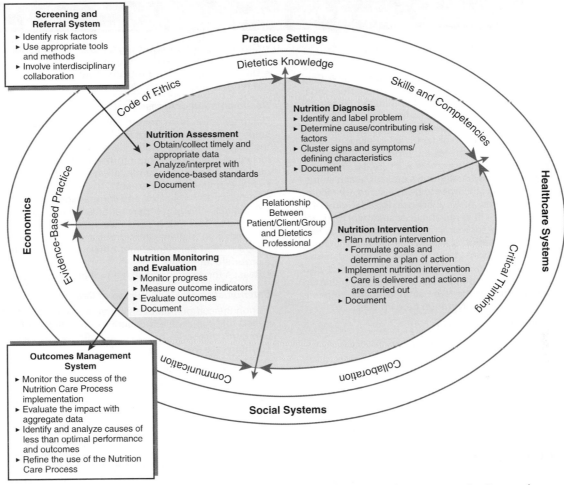

Screening and Referral System
- ▶ Identify risk factors
- ▶ Use appropriate tools and methods
- ▶ Involve interdisciplinary collaboration

Nutrition Assessment
- ▶ Obtain/collect timely and appropriate data
- ▶ Analyze/interpret with evidence-based standards
- ▶ Document

Nutrition Diagnosis
- ▶ Identify and label problem
- ▶ Determine cause/contributing risk factors
- ▶ Cluster signs and symptoms/ defining characteristics
- ▶ Document

Nutrition Intervention
- ▶ Plan nutrition intervention
  - • Formulate goals and determine a plan of action
- ▶ Implement nutrition intervention
  - • Care is delivered and actions are carried out
- ▶ Document

Nutrition Monitoring and Evaluation
- ▶ Monitor progress
- ▶ Measure outcome indicators
- ▶ Evaluate outcomes
- ▶ Document

Outcomes Management System
- ▶ Monitor the success of the Nutrition Care Process implementation
- ▶ Evaluate the impact with aggregate data
- ▶ Identify and analyze causes of less than optimal performance and outcomes
- ▶ Refine the use of the Nutrition Care Process

Relationship Between Patient/Client/Group and Dietetics Professional

Practice Settings
Dietetics Knowledge
Code of Ethics
Skills and Competencies
Economics
Evidence-Based Practice
Healthcare Systems
Critical Thinking
Communication
Collaboration
Social Systems

FIGURE 16-1 The Nutrition Care Process model. (*Redrawn from Lacey K, Pritchitt E: Nutrition Care Process and model: ADA adopts road map to quality care and outcomes management,* J Am Diet Assoc 103{8}:1061, 2003, with permission from the American Dietetic Association.)

Each stage builds upon the preceding one, but the process is not necessarily linear.[14] Box 16-1 describes each step of this process, and Figure 16-1 provides a visual illustration of the model.

Nutrition Assessment

The fundamental purpose of nutrition assessment in general clinical practice is to determine the following three factors:

1. Overall nutritional status of the patient
2. Current healthcare needs—physical, psychosocial, and personal
3. Related factors influencing these needs in the person's current life situation

The first step in nutrition assessment, as with assessing any situation to determine needs and actions, is to collect pertinent information—a database—for use in identifying needs. The clinical dietitian, assisted by other healthcare team members as needed, uses several basic types of activities for nutrition assessment of patients' needs, as follows:

- Anthropometric data
- Biochemical tests
- Clinical observations
- Diet evaluation and personal histories (medical, social, medications) (See the *To Probe Further* box, "Selecting Computer Nutrient-Calculation Software" on p. 400.)

Each part of this approach is important because no single parameter alone directly measures individual nutritional status or determines problems or needs. Further, the overall resulting picture must be interpreted within the context of personal social and health factors that may alter nutritional requirements. Procedures outlined here provide a good base in general practice.

Anthropometric Indexes

Skill gained through careful practice is necessary to minimize the margin of error in making body measurements.
Text continued on p. 398.

BOX 16-1 | American Dietetic Association's Nutrition Care Process

Step 1. Nutrition Assessment
Basic Definition and Purpose

"Nutrition Assessment" is the first step of the Nutrition Care Process. Its purpose is to obtain adequate information in order to identify nutrition-related problems. It is initiated by referral and/or screening of individuals or groups for nutritional risk factors. Nutrition assessment is a systematic process of obtaining, verifying, and interpreting data in order to make decisions about the nature and cause of nutrition-related problems. The specific types of data gathered in the assessment will vary depending on (a) practice settings, (b) individual/group's present health status, (c) how data are related to outcomes to be measured, (d) recommended practices such as ADA's Evidence Based Guides for Practice, and (e) whether it is an initial assessment or a reassessment. Nutrition assessment requires making comparisons between the information obtained and reliable standards (ideal goals). Nutrition assessment is an ongoing, dynamic process that involves not only initial data collection, but also continual reassessment and analysis of patient/client/group needs. Assessment provides the foundation for the nutrition diagnosis at the next step of the Nutrition Care Process.

Data Sources/Tools for Assessment

- Referral information and/or interdisciplinary records
- Patient/client interview (across the lifespan)
- Community-based surveys and focus groups
- Statistical reports; administrative data
- Epidemiological studies

Types of Data Collected

- Nutritional Adequacy (dietary history/detailed nutrient intake)
- Health Status (anthropometric and biochemical measurements, physical and clinical conditions, physiological and disease status)
- Functional and Behavioral Status (social and cognitive function, psychological and emotional factors, quality-of-life measures, change readiness)

Nutrition Assessment Components

- Review dietary intake for factors that affect health conditions and nutritional risk
- Evaluate health and disease condition for nutrition-related consequences
- Evaluate psychosocial, functional, and behavioral factors related to food access, selection, preparation, physical activity, and understanding of health condition
- Evaluate patient/client/group's knowledge, readiness to learn, and potential for changing behaviors
- Identify standards by which data will be compared
- Identify possible problem areas for making nutrition diagnoses

Critical Thinking

The following types of critical thinking skills are especially needed in the assessment step:
- Observing for nonverbal and verbal cues that can guide and prompt effective interviewing methods
- Determining appropriate data to collect
- Selecting assessment tools and procedures (matching the assessment method to the situation)
- Applying assessment tools in valid and reliable ways
- Distinguishing relevant from irrelevant data
- Distinguishing important from unimportant data
- Validating the data

- Organizing and categorizing the data in a meaningful framework that relates to nutrition problems
- Determining when a problem requires consultation with or referral to another provider

Documentation of Assessment

Documentation is an ongoing process that supports all of the steps in the Nutrition Care Process. Quality documentation of the assessment step should be relevant, accurate, and timely. Inclusion of the following information would further describe quality assessment documentation:
- Date and time of assessment
- Pertinent data collected and comparison with standards
- Patient/client/group's perceptions, values, and motivation related to presenting problems
- Changes in patient/client/group's level of understanding, food-related behaviors, and other clinical outcomes for appropriate follow-up
- Reason for discharge/discontinuation if appropriate

Determination for Continuation of Care

If upon the completion of an initial or reassessment it is determined that the problem cannot be modified by further nutrition care, discharge or discontinuation from this episode of nutrition care may be appropriate.

Step 2. Nutrition Diagnosis
Basic Definition and Purpose

"Nutrition Diagnosis" is the second step of the Nutrition Care Process, and is the identification and labeling that describes an actual occurrence, risk of, or potential for developing a nutrition problem that dietetics professionals are responsible for treating independently. At the end of the assessment step, data are clustered, analyzed, and synthesized. This will reveal a nutrition diagnostic category from which to formulate a specific nutrition diagnostic statement. Nutrition diagnosis should not be confused with medical diagnosis, which can be defined as a disease or pathology of specific organs or body systems that can be treated or prevented. A nutrition diagnosis changes as the patient/client/group's response changes. A medical diagnosis does not change as long as the disease or condition exists. A patient/client/group may have the medical diagnosis of "Type 2 diabetes mellitus"; however, after performing a nutrition assessment, dietetics professionals may diagnose, for example, "undesirable overweight status" or "excessive carbohydrate intake." Analyzing assessment data and naming the nutrition diagnosis(es) provide a link to setting realistic and measurable expected outcomes, selecting appropriate interventions, and tracking progress in attaining those expected outcomes.

Data Sources/Tools for Diagnosis

- Organized and clustered assessment data
- List(s) of nutrition diagnostic categories and nutrition diagnostic labels
- Currently the profession does not have a standardized list of nutrition diagnoses. However ADA has appointed a Standardized Language Work Group to begin development of standardized language for nutrition diagnoses and intervention. (June 2003)

Nutrition Diagnosis Components (3 distinct parts)

1. Problem (Diagnostic Label)

The nutrition diagnostic statement describes alterations in the patient/client/group's nutritional status. A diagnostic label

From Lacey K, Pritchitt E: Nutrition Care Process and model: ADA adopts road map to quality care and outcomes management, *J Am Diet Assoc* 103(8):1061, 2003, with permission from the American Dietetic Association.
ADA, American Dietetic Association; *MNT*, Medical nutrition therapy.

BOX 16-1 | American Dietetic Association's Nutrition Care Process—cont'd

(qualifier) is an adjective that describes/qualifies the human response such as:

- Altered, impaired, ineffective, increased/decreased, risk of, acute or chronic.

2. Etiology (Cause/Contributing Risk Factors)

The related factors (etiologies) are those factors contributing to the existence of, or maintenance of pathophysiological, psychosocial, situational, developmental, cultural, and/or environmental problems.

- Linked to the problem diagnostic label by words "related to" (RT)
- It is important not only to state the problem, but to also identify the cause of the problem.
  - This helps determine whether or not nutrition intervention will improve the condition or correct the problem.
  - It will also identify who is responsible for addressing the problem. Nutrition problems are either caused directly by inadequate intake (primary) or as a result of other medical, genetic, or environmental factors (secondary).
  - It is also possible that a nutrition problem can be the cause of another problem. For example, excessive caloric intake may result in unintended weight gain. Understanding the cascade of events helps to determine how to prioritize the interventions.
  - It is desirable to target interventions at correcting the cause of the problem whenever possible; however, in some cases treating the signs and symptoms (consequences) of the problem may also be justified.
- The ranking of nutrition diagnoses permits dietetics professionals to arrange the problems in order of their importance and urgency for the patient/client/group.

3. Signs/Symptoms (Defining Characteristics)

The defining characteristics are a cluster of subjective and objective signs and symptoms established for each nutrition diagnostic category. The defining characteristics, gathered during the assessment phase, provide evidence that a nutrition-related problem exists and that the problem identified belongs in the selected diagnostic category. They also quantify the problem and describe its severity:

- Linked to etiology by words "as evidenced by" (AEB);
- The symptoms (subjective data) are changes that the patient/client/group feels and expresses verbally to dietetics professionals; and
- The signs (objective data) are observable changes in the patient/client/group's health status.

Nutrition Diagnostic Statement (PES)

Whenever possible, a nutrition diagnostic statement is written in a PES format that states the Problem (P), the Etiology (E), and the Signs & Symptoms (S). However, if the problem is either a risk (potential) or wellness problem, the nutrition diagnostic statement may have only two elements, Problem (P), and the Etiology (E), since Signs & Symptoms (S) will not yet be exhibited in the patient. A well-written Nutrition Diagnostic Statement should be:

1. Clear and concise
2. Specific: patient/client/group-centered
3. Related to one client problem
4. Accurate: relate to one etiology
5. Based on reliable and accurate assessment data

Examples of Nutrition Diagnosis Statements (PES or PE)

- Excessive caloric intake (problem) "related to" frequent consumption of large portions of high fat meals (etiology) "as evidenced by" average daily intake of calories exceeding recommended amount by 500 kcal and 12-pound weight gain during the past 18 months (signs)
- Inappropriate infant feeding practice RT lack of knowledge AEB infant receiving bedtime juice in a bottle
- Unintended weight loss RT inadequate provision of energy by enteral products AEB 6-pound weight loss over past month
- Risk of weight gain RT a recent decrease in daily physical activity following sports injury

Critical Thinking

The following types of critical thinking skills are especially needed in the diagnosis step:

- Finding patterns and relationships among the data and possible causes
- Making inferences ("if this continues to occur, then this is likely to happen")
- Stating the problem clearly and singularly
- Suspending judgment (be objective and factual)
- Making interdisciplinary connections
- Ruling in/ruling out specific diagnoses
- Prioritizing the relative importance of problems for patient/client/group safety

Documentation of Diagnosis

Documentation is an ongoing process that supports all of the steps in the Nutrition Care Process. Quality documentation of the diagnosis step should be relevant, accurate, and timely. A nutrition diagnosis is the impression of dietetics professionals at a given point in time. Therefore, as more assessment data become available, the documentation of the diagnosis may need to be revised and updated.

Inclusion of the following information would further describe quality documentation of this step:

- Date and time
- Written statement of nutrition diagnosis.

Determination for Continuation of Care

Since the diagnosis step primarily involves naming and describing the problem, the determination for continuation of care seldom occurs at this step. Determination of the continuation of care is more appropriately made at an earlier or later point in the Nutrition Care Process.

Step 3. Nutrition Intervention

Basic Definition and Purpose

"Nutrition Intervention" is the third step of the Nutrition Care Process. An intervention is a specific set of activities and associated materials used to address the problem. Nutrition interventions are purposefully planned actions designed with the intent of changing a nutrition-related behavior, risk factor, environmental condition, or aspect of health status for an individual, target group, or the community at large. This step involves (a) selecting, (b) planning, and (c) implementing appropriate actions to meet patient/client/group's nutritional needs. The selection of nutrition interventions is driven by the nutrition diagnosis and provides the basis upon which outcomes are measured and evaluated. Dietetics professionals may actually do the interventions, or may include delegating or coordinating the nutrition care that others provide. All interventions must be based on scientific principles and rationale and, when available, grounded in a high level of quality research (evidence-based interventions).

Dietetics professionals work collaboratively with the patient/client/group, family, or caregiver to create a realistic plan

Continued

BOX 16-1 | American Dietetic Association's Nutrition Care Process—cont'd

that has a good probability of positively influencing the diagnosis/problem. This client-driven process is a key element in the success of this step, distinguishing it from previous planning steps that may or may not have involved the patient/client/group to this degree of participation.

Data Sources/Tools for Interventions

- Evidence-based nutrition guides for practice and protocols
- Current research literature
- Current consensus guidelines and recommendations from other professional organizations
- Results of outcome management studies or Continuous Quality Index projects
- Current patient education materials at appropriate reading level and language
- Behavior change theories (self-management training, motivational interviewing, behavior modification, modeling)

Nutrition Intervention Components

This step includes two distinct interrelated processes.

1. **Plan the nutrition intervention:** Formulate and determine a plan of action.
   - Prioritize the nutrition diagnoses based on severity of problem; safety; patient/client/group's need; likelihood that nutrition intervention will impact problem and patient/client/group's perception of importance.
   - Consult ADA's *MNT Evidence-Based Guides for Practice* and other practice guides. These resources can assist dietetics professionals in identifying science-based ideal goals and selecting appropriate interventions for MNT. They list appropriate value(s) for control or improvement of the disease or conditions as defined and supported in the literature.
   - Determine patient-focused expected outcomes for each nutrition diagnosis. The expected outcomes are the desired change(s) to be achieved over time as a result of nutrition intervention. They are based on nutrition diagnosis; for example, increasing or decreasing laboratory values, decreasing blood pressure, decreasing weight, increasing use of stanols/sterols, or increasing fiber. Expected outcomes should be written in observable and measurable terms that are clear and concise. They should be patient/client/group-centered and need to be tailored to what is reasonable to the patient's circumstances and appropriate expectations for treatments and outcomes.
   - Confer with patient/client/group, other caregivers or policies and program standards throughout planning step.
   - Define intervention plan (for example write a nutrition prescription, provide an education plan or community program, create policies that influence nutrition programs and standards).
   - Select specific intervention strategies that are focused on the etiology of the problem and that are known to be effective based on best current knowledge and evidence.
   - Define time and frequency of care including intensity, duration, and follow-up.
   - Identify resources and/or referrals needed.
2. **Implement the nutrition intervention:** Care is delivered and actions are carried out.
   - Implementation is the action phase of the nutrition care process. During implementation, dietetics professionals:
     - Communicate the plan of nutrition care
     - Carry out the plan of nutrition care
     - Continue data collection and modify the plan of care as needed

- Other characteristics that define quality implementation include:
  - Individualize the interventions to the setting and client
  - Collaborate with other colleagues and healthcare professionals
  - Follow up and verify that implementation is occurring and needs are being met
  - Revise strategies as changes in condition/response occurs.

Critical Thinking

Critical thinking is required to determine which intervention strategies are implemented based on analysis of the assessment data and nutrition diagnosis. The following types of critical thinking skills are especially needed in the intervention step:
- Setting goals and prioritizing
- Transferring knowledge from one situation to another
- Defining the nutrition prescription or basic plan
- Making interdisciplinary connections
- Initiating behavioral and other interventions
- Matching intervention strategies with client needs, diagnoses, and values
- Choosing from among alternatives to determine a course of action
- Specifying the time and frequency of care.

Documentation of Nutrition Interventions

Documentation is an ongoing process that supports all of the steps in the Nutrition Care Process. Quality documentation of nutrition interventions should be relevant, accurate, and timely. It should also support further intervention or discharge from care. Changes in patient/client/group's level of understanding and food-related behaviors must be documented along with changes in clinical or functional outcomes to assure appropriate care/case management in the future. Inclusion of the following information would further describe quality documentation of this step:
- Date and time
- Specific treatment goals and expected outcomes
- Recommended interventions, individualized for patient
- Any adjustments of plan and justifications
- Patient receptivity
- Referrals made and resources used
- Any other information relevant to providing care and monitoring progress over time
- Plans for follow-up and frequency of care
- Rationale for discharge if appropriate.

Determination for Continuation of Care

If the patient/client/group has met intervention goals or is not at this time able/ready to make needed changes, the dietetics professional may include discharging the client from this episode of care as part of the planned intervention.

Step 4. Nutrition Monitoring and Evaluation

Basic Definition and Purpose

"Nutrition Monitoring and Evaluation" is the fourth step of the Nutrition Care Process. *Monitoring* specifically refers to the review and measurement of the patient/client/group's status at a scheduled (preplanned) follow-up point with regard to the nutrition diagnosis, intervention plans/goals, and outcomes, whereas *Evaluation* is the systematic comparison of current findings with previous status, intervention goals, or a reference standard. Monitoring and evaluation use selected outcome indicators (markers) that are relevant to the patient/client/group's defined needs, nutrition diagnosis, nutrition goals, and disease state. Recommended times for follow-up, along with relevant outcomes to be monitored, can be found in ADA's Evidence Based Guides for Practice and other evidence-based sources.

The purpose of monitoring and evaluation is to determine the degree to which progress is being made and goals or desired outcomes of nutrition care are being met. It is more than just "watching" what is happening, it requires an active commitment to measuring and recording the appropriate outcome indicators (markers) relevant to the nutrition diagnosis and intervention strategies. Data from this step are used to create an outcomes management system. Refer to Outcomes Management System in text.

Progress should be monitored, measured, and evaluated on a planned schedule until discharge. Short inpatient stays and lack of return for ambulatory visits do not preclude monitoring, measuring, and evaluation. Innovative methods can be used to contact patients/clients to monitor progress and outcomes. Patient confidential self-report via mailings and telephone follow-up are some possibilities. Patients being followed in disease management programs can also be monitored for changes in nutritional status. Alterations in outcome indicators such as hemoglobin A_{1c} or weight are examples that trigger reactivation of the nutrition care process.

Data Sources/Tools for Monitoring and Evaluation

- Patient/client/group records
- Anthropometric measurements, laboratory tests, questionnaires, surveys
- Patient/client/group (or guardian) interviews/surveys, pretests, and posttests
- Mail or telephone follow-up
- ADA's *Evidence Based Guides for Practice* and other evidence-based sources
- Data collection forms, spreadsheets, and computer programs

Types of Outcomes Collected

The outcome(s) to be measured should be directly related to the nutrition diagnosis and the goals established in the intervention plan. Examples include, but are not limited to:

- Direct nutrition outcomes (knowledge gained, behavior change, food or nutrient intake changes, improved nutritional status)
- Clinical and health status outcomes (laboratory values, weight, blood pressure, risk factor profile changes, signs and symptoms, clinical status, infections, complications)
- Patient/client-centered outcomes (quality of life, satisfaction, self-efficacy, self-management, functional ability)
- Health care utilization and cost outcomes (medication changes, special procedures, planned/unplanned clinic visits, preventable hospitalizations, length of hospitalization, prevent or delay nursing home admission)

Nutrition Monitoring and Evaluation Components

This step includes three distinct and interrelated processes:

1. Monitor Progress

- Check patient/client/group understanding and compliance with plan
- Determine if the intervention is being implemented as prescribed
- Provide evidence that the plan/intervention strategy is or is not changing patient/client/group behavior or status

- Identify other positive or negative outcomes
- Gather information indicating reasons for lack of progress
- Support conclusions with evidence

2. Measure Outcomes

- Select outcome indicators that are relevant to the nutrition diagnosis or signs or symptoms, nutrition goals, medical diagnosis, and outcomes and quality management goals.
- Use standardized indicators to:
  - Increase the validity and reliability of measurements of change
  - Facilitate electronic charting, coding, and outcomes measurement.

3. Evaluate Outcomes

- Compare current findings with previous status, intervention goals, and/or reference standards.

Critical Thinking

The following types of critical thinking skills are especially needed in the monitoring and evaluation step:

- Selecting appropriate indicators/measures
- Using appropriate reference standard for comparison
- Defining where patient/client/group is now in terms of expected outcomes
- Explaining variance from expected outcomes
- Determining factors that help or hinder progress
- Deciding between discharge or continuation of nutrition care

Documentation of Monitoring and Evaluation

Documentation is an on-going process that supports all of the steps in the Nutrition Care Process and is an integral part of monitoring and evaluation activities. Quality documentation of the monitoring and evaluation step should be relevant, accurate, and timely. It includes a statement of where the patient is now in terms of expected outcomes. Standardized documentation enables pooling of data for outcomes measurement and quality improvement purposes. Quality documentation should also include:

- Date and time
- Specific indicators measured and results
- Progress toward goals (incremental small change can be significant therefore use of a Likert type scale may be more descriptive than a "met" or "not met" goal evaluation tool)
- Factors facilitating or hampering progress
- Other positive or negative outcomes
- Future plans for nutrition care, monitoring, and follow up or discharge

Determination for Continuation of Care

Based on the findings, the dietetics professional makes a decision to actively continue care or discharge the patient/client/group from nutrition care (when necessary and appropriate nutrition care is completed or no further change is expected at this time). If nutrition care is to be continued, the nutrition care process cycles back as necessary to assessment, diagnosis, and/or intervention for additional assessment, refinement of the diagnosis and adjustment and/or reinforcement of the plan. If care does not continue, the patient may still be monitored for a change in status and reentry to nutrition care at a later date.

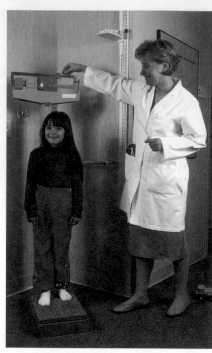

FIGURE 16-2   Balance beam scale. *(From Jarvis C:* Physical examination and health assessment, *ed 3, Philadelphia, 2000, WB Saunders.)*

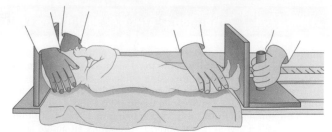

FIGURE 16-3   Measuring a baby's stature. *(From Mahan LK, Escott-Stump S:* Krause's food, nutrition, & diet therapy, *ed 11, Philadelphia, 2004, Saunders/Elsevier.)*

Selection and maintenance of proper procedures and equipment, as well as attention to careful technique, are essential in securing accurate data.

Weight.   Hospitalized patients should be weighed at consistent times—for example, before breakfast after the bladder has been emptied. Clinic patients should be weighed without shoes in light, indoor clothing or an examining gown. For accuracy, use regular clinic beam scales with nondetachable weights (Figure 16-2). An additional weight attachment is available for use with very obese persons. Metric scales with readings to the nearest 20 g provide specific data; however, the standard clinic scale is satisfactory. Check all scales frequently, and have them calibrated every 3 or 4 months for continued accuracy.

After careful reading and recording of the patient's weight, ask about usual body weight and compare it with standard height-weight tables, remembering that these tables are general guidelines. Interpret present weight in terms of percentage of usual and standard body weight for height. Check for any recent weight loss: 1% to 2% in the past week, 5% over the past month, 7.5% during the previous 3 months, or 10% in the past 6 months is significant. Unintentional weight loss greater than this rate can be severe. Unexplained weight loss is a problem with persons of any age. It is particularly important in older adults because it may be a clue to depression or a wasting disease such as cancer and needs to be on record and followed up. Values charted in the patient's record should indicate percentage of weight change.

Height.   If possible, use a fixed measuring stick or tape on a true vertical flat surface. Have the patient stand as straight as possible, without shoes or cap, heels together, and looking straight ahead. The heels, buttocks, shoulders, and head should be touching the wall or vertical surface of the measuring rod. Read the measure carefully, and compare it with previous recordings. Children under the age of 2 years should be measured using a stationary headboard and movable footboard (Figure 16-3). Note growth of children or the diminishing height of adults. Metric measures of height in centimeters provide a smaller unit of measure than inches.

Body Mass Index.   Weight and height measures are used to calculate the patient's body mass index (BMI): weight (kilograms) divided by the square of the height (meters). This ratio is commonly used in evaluating obesity states in relation to risk factors.

Body Frame.   The Metropolitan Life Insurance Company's widely used tables for height and weight of men and women use very general arbitrary categories of body frame size. Data on which these height-weight tables are based are not representative of the entire population, making it difficult to extrapolate recommendations. Quality of the data is variable because there was no consistency in determining frame size, and standardized procedures were not used when collecting height and weight data.[2]

Two more precise methods of establishing body frame size have been developed, as follows, based on specific body joint measurements[2]:

1. *Elbow breadth:* Standards of weight and body composition by frame size and height have been developed with frame size based on measurement of elbow breadth. With the patient's arm extended and forearm bent upward to form a 90-degree angle, elbow breadth is measured with a specially developed instrument such as the Frameter, which measures the distance in centimeters between the two outer bony landmarks (medial and lateral epicondyles of the humerus) (Figure 16-4).

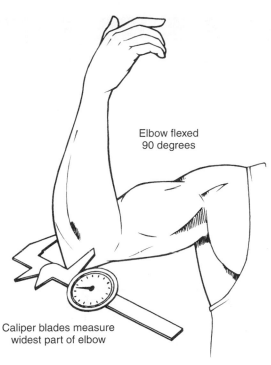

FIGURE 16-4   Elbow breadth. *(From Lee RD, Nieman DC: Nutritional assessment, ed 3, New York, 2003, McGraw-Hill.)*

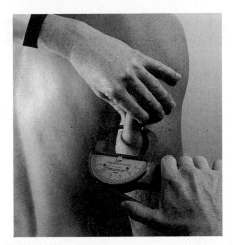

FIGURE 16-5   Assessment tools include skinfold calipers, shown here, which measure the relative amount of subcutaneous fat tissues at various body sites. *(From Mahan LK, Escott-Stump S: Krause's food, nutrition, & diet therapy, ed 11, Philadelphia, 2004, Saunders/Elsevier.)*

2. *Wrist circumference:* This is a measure of height (in centimeters) divided by wrist circumference (in centimeters). To measure the right wrist, the arm should be flexed at the elbow with the palm facing upward and hand muscles relaxed. Using a nonstretchable metric tape (no wider than 0.7 cm), measure the wrist circumference at the joint just distal (toward the fingers) to the bony wrist bone protrusion (the styloid process).[2] The tape should touch the skin but not compress soft tissues. Interpret results by the following standard:

Frame Size	Male Ratio Values	Female Ratio Values
Small	>10.4	>10.9
Medium	10.4-9.6	10.9-9.9
Large	<9.6	<9.9

Body Measures. In general clinical practice the clinician rarely uses body measurements to assess nutritional status because they are not practical measures due to shortened hospital stays. But in practice settings (such as long-term care) where serial measures can be useful in assessing nutritional status, two basic body measurements can be used—the midarm circumference and the triceps skinfold thickness—and from these a third measure, the mid-upper-arm muscle circumference, can be calculated. First, using a nonstretchable centimeter tape, locate the

midpoint of the upper arm on the nondominant arm, unless it is affected by edema. The midarm circumference (MAC) is measured at this midpoint and read accurately to the nearest tenth of a centimeter and recorded. The resulting measure is compared with previous measurements to note possible changes. Second, using a standard millimeter skinfold caliper, take a measure of the triceps skinfold thickness (TSF) at this same midpoint of the upper arm (Figure 16-5). This measure provides an estimate of the subcutaneous fat reserves. Then, together with the midpoint circumference value at this same point, midarm muscle circumference (MAMC) is calculated by the following formula:

$$\text{MAMC (cm)} = \text{MAC (cm)} - [3.14 \times \text{TSF (cm)}]$$

In this equation, the calculation constant 3.14 represents the value of pi (π). Because calipers measure in millimeters, for ease of using the equation TSF may be left in mm, with the other units remaining in cm; the calculation constant in this case is changed to 0.314.

This final derived value gives an indirect measure of the body's skeletal muscle mass, a good indicator of body composition. Finally, to interpret the patient's measurements for monitoring nutritional status, these values are compared as percentages of standards in reference tables (see Appendix E).

Alternative Measures for Nonambulatory Patients. Several alternative measures can provide values for estimating height and weight of persons confined to bed, as follows:

- *Total arm length:* Have the patient hold the arm straight down by the side of the body, and, using a nonstretchable metric tape, measure arm length

TO PROBE FURTHER

SELECTING COMPUTER NUTRIENT-CALCULATION SOFTWARE

In our modern age of electronics the computer has become a standard tool for rapid calculation procedures. In clinical and community nutrition practices, as well as in population studies, it saves valuable time and provides a precise nutrient analysis of an individual's reported food intake.

Certainly computerized nutrient analyses are time-savers compared with the previous tedious manual calculations using published food value tables. But just how precise are the results? This depends on the heart of any nutrient-analysis software program—its nutrient database.

During the past few years of computer use by clinicians, researchers, and educators, it has become increasingly evident that the quality of the nutrient database on which all calculations are based determines the quality of the resulting output. Important questions that should be asked when evaluating the nutrient database in any software package being considered for purchase include the following from the University of Minnesota School of Public Health.

Does the Database Contain All Foods and Nutrients of Interest?

Most databases contain the most common foods, but you may require particular foods such as ethnic, vegetarian, or fast-food items; brand-name products; and infant or nontraditional foods. The number of food items in a database does not necessarily indicate how comprehensive the system is, and adding your own foods to the database requires considerable effort.

Is the Database Complete for Nutrients of Interest?

Missing or not available values exist in available software packages and often are not flagged; therefore you may be unaware of this source of error. Inappropriate patient counseling may result. Such missing value errors in small items such as spices or other condiments may not matter, but value that is missing for total saturated fatty acids in a fast-food hamburger because the food manufacturers have not supplied it is not acceptable.

Do Foods Included in the Database Provide Sufficient Specific Data to Accurately Assess Nutrients of Interest?

For example, if total fat and fatty acids are of concern, separate database entries must be included for such items as regular, low-fat, and nonfat dairy products and brand-name high-fat items such as margarines and salad dressings. In other cases, inclusion of food items according to preparation method, or of any dietary supplements for vitamin-mineral calculations, may be required.

Is the Nutrient Database Current With the Changing Marketplace and Availability of New Nutrient Data?

The U.S. Department of Agriculture (USDA) routinely releases updates of the USDA Nutrient Data Base, the common source of data for nutrient-calculation systems, as new information becomes available. Information from food manufacturers is also available. A well-maintained software product's database should include all such data updates, and the vendor should supply information about frequency of updating and sources of data.

Are Manufacturers Contacted Routinely for New Information or Reformulations of Existing Products?

This question extends the previous question to emphasize the still-too-frequent neglect of brand-name product–updating practices of software developers. Routine contact with food manufacturers is essential to maintaining an acceptable quality standard.

What Quality-Control Procedures Are Used to Ensure Database Accuracy?

Because there are thousands of values for nutrients and non-nutrient information, such as food-specific serving sizes, the margin for error is great and built-in maintenance procedures for checking such errors should be present.

Vendors of nutrient-calculation software packages should be able to give answers to these important questions. Ask before you buy!

References

Buzzard IM et al: Considerations for selecting nutrient-calculation software: evaluation of the nutrient database, *Am J Clin Nutr* 54:7, 1991.

Byrd-Bredbenner C, Juni RP: How should nutrient databases be evaluated? *J Am Diet Assoc* 96(2):120, 1996.

Haytowitz DB: Information from USDA's Nutrient Data Bank, *J Nutr* 125(7):1952, 1995.

Lee RD et al: Comparison of eight microcomputer dietary analysis programs with the USDA Nutrient Data Base for Standard Reference, *J Am Diet Assoc* 95(8):858, 1995.

from attachment at the shoulder to the end of the arm at the wrist. Reference standards indicate relation of this measure to height equivalents.[17] This is also a useful alternative to standing body height when body conditions distort usual standing height of ambulatory patients. For example, this measure is helpful with older persons, in whom a general thinning of weight-bearing cartilage, the bent-knee gait, and a possible kyphosis of the spine may make standing height measurement inaccurate.

- *Arm span:* Full arm span measure is an alternate to height in adults; it is especially practical for older adults. Tests indicate it may give a more accurate result than height in calculating BMI in older adult patients. Using a flexible metric tape, measure full arm span from fingertip to fingertip in centimeters, passing the tape in front of the clavicles. A recumbent half-span measure from fingertip to body midline at the sternal notch may be used for patients with limited movement in one arm and then doubled to achieve the same result.

- *Knee height:* With the patient lying in the supine position and the left knee and ankle each bent at a 90-degree angle, the knee height is measured with a special caliper (Figure 16-6). A simple comparative measure of knee-to-floor height in the sitting position, from the outside bony point just under the kneecap, indicating the head of the tibia, down to

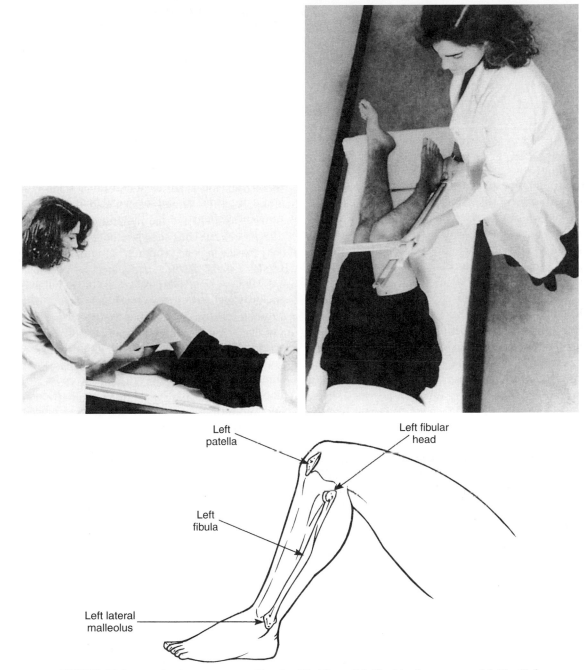

FIGURE 16-6 Knee height measurement. *(From Lee RD, Nieman DC:* Nutritional assessment, *ed 3, New York, 2003, McGraw-Hill.)*

the floor surface, may also be used. The knee height (KH) measurement is then used to calculate the value for deriving body height equivalent, as follows:

Height (women) =
$$[(1.833 \times KH) - (0.24 \times Age)] + 84.88$$
Height (men) =
$$[(2.02 \times KH) - (0.04 \times Age)] + 64.19$$

- *Calf circumference:* With the patient in the same supine position and the left knee bent at a 90-degree angle, and using nonstretchable metric tape, measure the calf circumference (CC) at the largest point. This

measurement is then used with three other values—KH, MAC, and subscapular skinfold (SSF)—to derive body weight value, as follows:

Weight (women) = $(1.27 \times CC) + (0.87 \times KH) +$
$$(0.98 \times MAC) + (0.4 \times SSF) - 62.35$$
Weight (men) = $(0.98 \times CC) + (1.16 \times KH) +$
$$(1.73 \times MAC) + (0.37 \times SSF) - 81.69$$

---

kyphosis Increased, abnormal convexity of the upper part of the spine; hunchback.

Biochemical Tests

A number of laboratory tests are available for studying nutritional status. The most commonly used ones for assessing and monitoring nutritional status and planning nutrition care in clinical practice are listed here. General ranges for normal values are given in standard texts.

Measures of Plasma Protein.
Basic measures include serum albumin, prealbumin, hemoglobin, and hematocrit. Additional ones may include prealbumin (PAB), a thyroxin-binding protein, serum transferrin, or total iron-binding capacity (TIBC) and ferritin.

Measures of Protein Metabolism.
Basic 24-hour urine tests are used to measure urinary creatinine and urea nitrogen levels; these materials are products of protein metabolism. The patient's 24-hour excretion of creatinine is interpreted in terms of ideal creatinine excretion for height—the creatinine-height index (CHI). Comparison is made with standard values for this index. The patient's 24-hour urea nitrogen excretion is used with the calculated dietary nitrogen intake over the same 24-hour period to calculate nitrogen balance, as follows:

$$\text{N balance} = (\text{Protein intake} \times 6.25) -$$
$$(\text{Urinary urea nitrogen} + 4)$$

The formula factor of 4 represents additional nitrogen loss through feces and skin. Urinary urea nitrogen excretion reflects metabolism of dietary nitrogen, as the nitrogen balance formula indicates, and is a measure of the adequacy of protein nutrition.

Measures of Immune System Integrity: Anergy.
Basic measures are made of the lymphocyte count. Additional measures may be made by skin testing, observing delayed sensitivity to common recall antigens such as mumps or purified protein derivative of tuberculin (PPD). Skin tests are read at 24 and 48 hours, with greater than 5 mm considered positive and the presence of one positive test indicating intact immunity. For hospitalized patients, this test is used with caution because there are often confounding factors that may offset the results.

Clinical Observations and Nutrition Physical Assessment

For hospitalized patients, clinical practitioners make use of detailed observations, looking for signs of possible malnutrition. These observations are combined with indications gained from measured vital signs and medical and nursing physical examinations. Furthermore, RDs carry out nutrition physical assessments to assess the patient for signs and symptoms consistent with specific nutrient deficiency or malnutrition.[18]

Clinical Signs of Malnutrition.
Careful attention to physical signs of possible malnutrition provides an added dimension to the overall assessment of general nutritional status. A guide for a general examination of such signs is given in Table 16-1. A careful description of any such observations is documented in the patient's medical record.

Nutritional Physical Examination.
Certain information used to assess nutritional status is taken from physical examinations performed by physicians and nurses. Furthermore, Registered Dietitians (RDs) perform nutritional physical examinations to assess patients for signs and symptoms consistent with malnutrition or specific nutrient deficiency.[1,13] Techniques used in nutritional physical examinations are summarized in Table 16-2.

Dietary Assessment.

Collecting Information.
A careful nutrition history, including nutrition information related to living situation and other personal, psychosocial, and economic problems, is a fundamental part of nutrition assessment. Obtaining accurate information about basic food patterns and actual dietary intake is not a simple matter because some individuals misreport or underreport what they eat. Each method of diet evaluation has particular strengths and limitations.[2] However, a sensitive practitioner may obtain useful information by using one or more of the basic tools described in Table 16-3.

Problems With Underreporting.
Eating is one of life's most fundamental and universal pleasures. Is it any wonder then that many people are reluctant to divulge to others true intimate details of what and how much they consume? Nutrition research scientists and clinical practitioners alike have long had to grapple with the psychology of eating and the emotions aroused by food.[19] Underreporting of what is actually eaten is a recurring problem in nutrition assessment.[20-23] Degree and type of underreporting vary. Influences on eating habits and reporting of dietary intakes include educational level, sex, race, age, and weight.[24-26] Obese individuals (those with a high body mass index) are much more likely to underreport their food intake than are persons of normal weight.[22] In addition, women are more likely to underreport than are men.[19]

Type of underreporting typically varies with assessment instrument used. Recall techniques are most likely to have simply underrecording, which in many cases can be as high as 25% of total dietary intake. Food diary methods, by contrast, can have the dual problems of both underrecording what is eaten and undereating during the period of recording in the food diary. One study found that during a period of using food diaries, obese men reduced their usual food intake by 26% (undereating) and did not record 12% of what they actually ate (underrecording).[27] A similar pattern was observed in a study of

| TABLE 16-1 | **Clinical Signs of Nutritional Status** |

Body Area	Signs of Good Nutrition	Signs of Poor Nutrition
General appearance	Alert, responsive	Listless, apathetic, cachectic
Weight	Normal for height, age, body build	Overweight or underweight (special concern for underweight)
Posture	Erect, arms and legs straight	Sagging shoulders, sunken chest, humped back
Muscles	Well-developed, firm, good tone, some fat under skin	Flaccid, poor tone, undeveloped, tender, "wasted" appearance, cannot walk properly
Nervous control	Good attention span, not irritable or restless, normal reflexes, psychologic stability	Inattentive, irritable, confused, burning and tingling of hands and feet (paresthesia), loss of position and vibratory sense, weakness and tenderness of muscles (may result in inability to walk), decrease or loss of ankle and knee reflexes
Gastrointestinal function	Good appetite and digestion, normal regular elimination, no palpable (perceptible to touch) organs or masses	Anorexia, indigestion, constipation or diarrhea, liver or spleen enlargement
Cardiovascular function	Normal heart rate and rhythm, no murmurs, normal blood pressure for age	Rapid heart rate (above 100 beats/min tachycardia), enlarged heart, abnormal rhythm, elevated blood pressure
General vitality	Endurance, energetic, sleeps well, vigorous	Easily fatigued, no energy, falls asleep easily, looks tired, apathetic
Hair	Shiny, lustrous, firm, not easily plucked, healthy scalp	Stringy, dull, brittle, dry, thin and sparse, depigmented, easily plucked
Skin (general)	Smooth, slightly moist, good color	Rough, dry, scaly, pale, pigmented, irritated, bruises, petechiae
Face and neck	Skin color uniform, smooth, healthy appearance, not swollen	Greasy, discolored, scaly, swollen, skin dark over cheeks and under eyes, lumpiness or flakiness of skin around nose and mouth
Lips	Smooth, good color, moist, not chapped or swollen	Dry, scaly, swollen, redness and swelling (cheilosis), or angular lesions at corners of the mouth or fissures or scars (stomatitis)
Mouth, oral membranes	Reddish pink mucous membranes in oral cavity	Swollen, boggy oral mucous membranes
Gums	Good pink color, healthy, red, no swelling or bleeding	Spongy, bleed easily, marginal redness, inflamed, gums receding
Tongue	Good pink color or deep reddish in appearance, not swollen or smooth, surface papillae present, no lesions	Swelling, scarlet and raw, magenta color, beefy (glossitis), hyperemic and hypertrophic papillae, atrophic papillae
Teeth	No cavities, no pain, bright, straight, no crowding, well-shaped jaw, clean, no discoloration	Unfilled caries, absent teeth, worn surfaces, mottled (fluorosis), malpositioned
Eyes	Bright, clear, shiny, no sores at corner of eyelids, membranes moist and healthy pink color, no prominent blood vessels or mound of tissue or sclera, no fatigue circles beneath	Eye membranes pale (pale conjunctivae), redness of membrane (conjunctivae), redness of membrane (conjunctival infection), dryness, signs of infection, Bitot's spots, redness and fissuring of eyelid corners (angular palpebritis), dryness of eye membrane (conjunctival xerosis), dull appearance of cornea (corneal xerosis), soft cornea (keratomalacia)
Neck (glands)	No enlargement	Thyroid enlarged
Nails	Firm, pink	Spoon-shaped (koilonychia), brittle, ridged
Legs, feet	No tenderness, weakness, or swelling; good color	Edema, tender calf, tingling, weakness
Skeleton	No malformations	Bowlegs, knock-knees, chest deformity at diaphragm, beaded ribs, prominent scapulas

Modified from Williams SR: Nutrition assessment and guidance in prenatal care. In Worthington-Roberts BS, Williams SR: *Nutrition in pregnancy and lactation,* ed 5, New York, 1993, McGraw-Hill.

TABLE 16-2	Nutritional Physical Examination	
Technique	**Skill**	**Used to Measure**
Inspection	Systematic visual inspection	Changes from normal features
Palpation	Examination of the body using touch	Conditions that have nutritional implications such as abdominal tenderness, ascites, distention, peripheral edema, nail integrity, and skin turgor
Percussion	Use of sound to distinguish deviations from standard sounds created by presence of body organs and cavities	Identify gastric air bubble or intestinal air or identify fluid present in lungs
Auscultation	Using a stethoscope and naked ear to identify deviations from standard sounds	Evaluate sounds produced by heart, lungs, and gastrointestinal tract such as bowel sounds

Data from Nelms MN, Sucher K, Long S: *Understanding nutrition therapy and pathophysiology,* Belmont, Calif, 2007, Wadsworth; and Dietitians in Nutrition Support: *Study guide: nutrition focused physical assessment skills for dietitians,* Chicago, 1998, The American Dietetic Association.

TABLE 16-3	Strengths and Limitations of Techniques Used to Measure Dietary Intake		
Technique	**Brief Description**	**Strengths**	**Limitations**
24-Hour food record	Trained interviewer asks respondent to recall, in detail, all food and drink consumed during a period of time in the recent past.	• Requires <20 min to administer • Inexpensive • Easy to administer • Can provide detailed information on types of foods consumed • Low respondent burden • More objective than dietary history • Does not alter usual diet • Useful in clinical settings	• One recall rarely illustrative of typical intake • Under/over-reporting occurs • Dependent on memory • Omissions of sauces, dressings, and beverages can lead to low estimates of energy intake • Data entry can be labor intensive
Food record or diary	Respondent records, at time of consumption, identity and amounts of all foods and beverages consumed for a period of time, usually ranging from 1-7 days.	• Does not rely on memory • Can provide detailed intake data • Can provide information about eating habits • Multiple-day data more representative of usual intake • Reasonably valid up to 5 days	• Requires high degree of cooperation • Subject must be literate • Takes more time to obtain data • Act of recording may alter usual intake
Food frequency questionnaires	Respondents indicate how many times a day, week, month or year they usually consume foods using a questionnaire consisting of a list of approximately ≤150 foods or food groups that are important contributors to the population's intake of energy and nutrients.	• Can be self-administered • Machine readable • Modest demand on respondents • Relatively inexpensive • May be more representative of usual intake than a few days of diet records	• May not represent usual food or portion sizes chosen by respondent • Intake data can be compromised when multiple foods are grouped within single listings • Depends on ability of respondent to describe diet
Diet history	Respondents are interviewed by a trained interviewer about number of meals eaten per day; appetite; food dislikes; presence/absence of nausea and/or vomiting; use of nutritional supplements and/or herbal products; cigarette smoking; habits related to sleep, rest, work, and exercise.	• Assess usual nutrient intake • Can detect seasonal changes • Data on all nutrients can be obtained • Can correlate well with biochemical measures	• Lengthy interview process • Requires highly trained interviewers • May overestimate nutrient intake • Requires cooperation of respondent with ability to recall usual diet

Modified from Lee RD, Neiman DC: *Nutrition assessment,* ed 3, New York, 2003, McGraw-Hill.

postmenopausal women; all of the women tended to undereat during the record-keeping period, whereas underrecording was most common among those who reported they were controlling their food intake to lose or maintain weight.[28]

Because underreporting of food intake is a common problem and one intimately connected with human psychology, what measures can a dietitian or other health practitioner take to compensate? Being a careful observer is important, from initial contact with a patient on. It is often possible in reality to identify individuals who are likely to underreport. When follow-up interviews are done, these individuals will usually admit their underreporting voluntarily to the practitioner and frequently will even provide information about both undereating and underrecording and what foods are involved.[19] The dietitian can then make reasonably informed adjustments to food records on a case-by-case basis.

Evaluation of Dietary Intake.   Valid patient care planning requires analysis of all nutrition data collected. On this basis, problems requiring solutions can be identified. A detailed analysis of all available nutrition information helps determine nutrition diagnosis, any primary or secondary nutritional disease, and any underlying nutrition-related conditions.

Medical tests used for nutrition assessment are generally reliable in persons of any age, but conditions in older adult patients may interfere and need to be considered in evaluating test results. For example, laboratory values are affected by hydration status, presence of chronic diseases, changes in organ function, and drugs. Nutrition assessment is an important part of the general healthcare of everyone, especially of older adults. Health outreach programs for older persons, such as in rural areas, can use brief, easily administered tools for screening and assessing nutritional status and risk of malnutrition as part of geriatric care.

NUTRITION DIAGNOSIS

Nutrition diagnosis is not to be confused with medical diagnosis. Medical diagnosis is a disease or pathologic condition that can be treated or prevented, and the diagnosis does not change as long as the condition exists.[14] Nutrition diagnosis is "identification and labeling an actual occurrence, risk of, or potential for developing a nutrition problem that dietetics professionals are responsible for treating independently."[14] Nutrition diagnoses change as patients' nutritional needs change.[14] Nutrition diagnoses provide a mechanism for dietetics practitioners to document the link between nutrition assessment and nutrition intervention and to set realistic and measurable expected outcomes for patients. Identifying diagnoses also assists dietetics practitioners in

establishing priorities when planning nutrition care.[29] Nutrition diagnoses are dependent upon evidence-based practice and standardized language.[1,14] (More information on evidence-based practice is available at *http://adaevidencelibrary.com/default.cfm* for ADA members.)

Sixty-two nutrition diagnoses have been developed through use of standardized language. Standardized language provides a means for dietetics professionals to communicate with each other and other healthcare professionals. It is a fundamental part of the NCP and assists dietetics professionals to better document their nutrition care.[29] See Box 16-1 for more in-depth information and to determine how a nutrition diagnosis is written.

NUTRITION INTERVENTION: FOOD PLAN AND MANAGEMENT

Basic Concepts of Nutrition Therapy

Nutrition therapy is always based on normal nutritional requirements and personal needs for each particular patient. It is modified only as the specific disease in the specific individual necessitates. In planning and counseling for nutrition care this is an important initial fact to grasp and impart to patients and clients. For example, it is a great source of encouragement to the parents of a child newly diagnosed with diabetes to know the food plan will be based on individual growth and development needs and will make use of regular foods.

Disease Application

Principles of a nutrition therapy will be based on modifications of nutritional components of the normal diet as a particular disease condition may require. These changes may include the following types of modifications:

- *Nutrients:* modification of one or more of the basic nutrients—protein, carbohydrate, fat, minerals, and vitamins
- *Energy:* modification in energy value as expressed in kilocalories (kcalories or kcal)
- *Texture:* modification in texture or seasoning, such as liquid or low residue

Individual Adaptation

Nutrition therapy may be theoretically correct and have well-balanced food plans, but if these plans are unacceptable to the patient, they will not be followed. A workable plan for a specific person must be based on individual food habits within the specific personal life situation. This can be achieved only through careful planning with the patient, or with the parents of a child requiring a special diet, based on an initial interview to obtain a diet history, knowledge of personal food habits,

TABLE 16-4	Routine Hospital Diets			
Food	**Clear Liquid**	**Full Liquid**	**Soft**	**Regular**
Soup	Clear fat-free broth, bouillon	Same, plus strained or blended cream soups	Same, plus all cream soups	All
Cereal		Cooked refined cereal	Cooked cereal, cornflakes, rice, noodles, macaroni, spaghetti	
Bread			White bread, crackers, melba toast, zwieback	All
Protein foods		Milk, cream, milk drinks, yogurt	Same, plus eggs (not fried), mild cheese, cottage and cream cheese, fowl, fish, sweetbreads, tender beef, veal, lamb, liver, bacon, gravy	All
Vegetables			Potatoes: baked, mashed, creamed, steamed, scalloped; tender cooked whole bland vegetables; fresh lettuce, tomatoes	All
Fruit and fruit juices	Fruit juices (as tolerated), flavored fruit drinks	All	Same, plus cooked fruit: peaches, pears, applesauce, peeled apricots, white cherries; ripe peaches, pears, banana, orange and grapefruit sections without membrane	
Desserts and gelatin	Fruit-flavored gelatin, fruit ices, and Popsicles	Same, plus sherbet, ice cream, puddings, custard, frozen yogurt	Same, plus plain sponge cakes, plain cookies, plain cake, puddings, pie made with allowed foods	All
Miscellaneous	Soft drinks (as tolerated), coffee and tea, decaffeinated coffee and tea, cereal beverages such as Postum, sugar, honey, salt, hard candy, Poly cose (Ross), residue-free supplements	Same, plus margarine, pepper, all supplements	Same, plus mild salad dressings	

living conditions, and food security. In this way, diet principles can be understood and motivation secured to follow through. Regardless of the problems, nutrition therapy is valid only to the extent it involves this kind of knowledge, skills, and insights. Individual adaptations of the diet to meet individual needs are imperative for successful therapy.

Routine House Diets

A schedule of routine "house" diets, based on some type of cycle menu plan, is usually followed in hospitals for patients who do not require a special diet modification. According to general patient need and tolerance, the diet order may be liquid (clear liquid or full liquid), soft (in texture), and regular (a full, normal-for-age diet) (Table 16-4).

Managing the Mode of Feeding

Depending on the patient's condition, the clinical dietitian may manage nutrition therapy by using any one of the following four feeding modes.

Oral Diet

As long as possible, of course, regular oral feeding is preferred. Supplements are added if needed. According to the patient's condition, there may also be a need for assistance in eating.

Tube Feeding

If a patient is unable to eat but the gastrointestinal tract can be used, enteral delivery, or tube feeding, may provide needed nutrition support. A number of commercial formulas are available.

Peripheral Vein Feeding

If the patient cannot take in food or formula via the gastrointestinal tract, intravenous feeding is used. Solutions of dextrose, amino acids, vitamins, and minerals, with lipids as appropriate, can be fed through peripheral veins when the need is not extensive or long term.

Total Parenteral Nutrition

If the patient's nutritional need is great and support therapy may be required for a longer time, parenteral feeding

CASE STUDY

Nutrition Assessment and Therapy for a Patient With Cancer

Esther is a 160-cm (5 ft 4 in)–tall, medium-frame, 43-year-old patient recovering from a *gastrectomy* performed 8 days ago to treat gastric cancer. Her weight has dropped gradually for the past 4 months from an average of 59 kg (130 lb) before her illness began. She continues to follow a full-liquid diet, consuming 60 to 120 ml (2 to 4 oz) of milk every few hours, plus one or two soft-boiled eggs each day. Today she informed the nutritionist that she consumed a total of 721 ml (24 oz) of milk and two eggs.

In reviewing Esther's records, the clinical dietitian found the following nutrition assessment data: weight, 46.8 kg (103 lb); triceps skinfold, 10 mm; and midarm circumference, 17 cm. Laboratory values include serum albumin, 3 g/dl; total iron-binding capacity (TIBC), 230 μg/dl; lymphocytes, 1200 cells/m³ (23%); hematocrit, 35%; and hemoglobin, 10.5 g/dl. Urinalysis (24 hours) included urea nitrogen, 16 g; and creatinine, 1.75 g.

After reviewing the data, the clinical dietitian calculated nitrogen balance, transferrin, and creatinine-height index, which were recorded on the patient chart. Basal energy expenditure needs and kcalories and protein needed to overcome catabolism were also calculated along with estimates for additional vitamin and mineral requirements.

The clinical dietitian noted the physician had ordered chemotherapy for the patient, continuing after discharge, and recommended use of TPN, also to be continued after discharge, as a means of meeting Esther's nutritional needs. In addition, the clinical dietitian planned ways of meeting any feeding problems that often accompany chemotherapy, such as sore mouth, nausea, and food intolerances. Following a carefully prepared protocol developed by the hospital nutrition support team, both Esther and her husband were instructed in procuring and using the home TPN treatment. The clinical dietitian also provided follow-up counseling for Esther and her husband at the office and in the group sessions for cancer patients and their families.

Questions for Analysis

1. Use a nutrition assessment data summary sheet from your hospital (or design your own) to record pertinent data given in this case study. What additional data would you collect? How would it be obtained?
2. For each test listed on your data sheet, explain what it measures and how that information contributes to an understanding of Esther's status.
3. What specific nutritional needs can you identify in this case? List them in order of priority.
4. Calculate Esther's nitrogen balance and transferrin for day 8. Why are these indexes important to assessing her nutritional status?
5. What is Esther's creatinine-height index? How does it reflect her nutritional status?
6. Interpret Esther's anthropometric data, including your calculations of her midarm muscle circumference.
7. What skin tests were probably ordered? How would the results contribute to the assessment of her nutritional status?
8. What nutrition problems do you expect Esther to encounter after discharge? How could they be resolved? What community agencies might contribute to her sense of well-being after discharge?

---

through a large central vein is needed. Placement of this catheter is a special surgical procedure. More concentrated special solutions can be used and monitored by a nutrition support team. Formulas are determined by the dietitian and physician and prepared by trained pharmacists. This specialized nutrition support method was originally used only in hospitals, but advances in total parenteral nutrition (TPN) administration now allow its use in many healthcare settings and even at home with some patients.

EVALUATION: QUALITY PATIENT CARE

General Considerations

When the nutrition care process is carried out, patient care activities need to be considered in terms of nutrition diagnosis and treatment objectives and the extent to which each of the care activities helps to meet the particular goals of the patient and the family. This evaluation is both continuous and thorough and requires careful, objective documentation (see the *Case Study* box, "Nutrition Assessment and Therapy for a Patient With Cancer"). It seeks to validate care while it is being given, as well as to determine the effectiveness of a particular course of care. Various areas need to be investigated, as follows:

- *Estimate the achievement of nutrition therapy goals:* What is the effect of diet or mode of feeding on the illness or patient's situation? Is there a need for any change in nutrient ratios of diet or formula as originally calculated, in meal-distribution pattern, or in feeding mode?
- *Judge the accuracy of intervention actions:* Is there a need to change any of the NCP components? For example, is there a need for a change in the type of food or feeding equipment, environment for meals, procedures for counseling, or types of learning activities for nutrition education and self-care procedures?
- *Determine the patient's ability to follow the prescribed nutrition therapy:* Are there any hindrances or disabilities that prevent the patient from following the treatment plan? What is the impact of nutrition therapy on the patient, family, or staff? Were the necessary nutrition assessment procedures for collecting nutrition data carried out correctly? Do patient and family understand the information given for self-care? Have community resources required by the patient and family been available and convenient for use? Has any needed food assistance program been sufficient to meet needs for the patient's ongoing care?

---

enteral A mode of feeding that uses the gastrointestinal tract; oral or tube feeding.
parenteral A mode of feeding that does not use the gastrointestinal tract, but instead provides nutrition by intravenous delivery of nutrient solutions.

Health Promotion

Collaborative Roles of the Dietitian and Nurse

The clinical dietitian works closely with the nurse in managing nutrition care of patients. At varying times, depending on need, the nurse may provide valuable nutrition assistance as coordinator, interpreter, or teacher. Skills in consultation and referral are therefore essential.

Coordinator

Nurses coordinate special services or treatment required because of their close relationship with patients and their constant attendance. The nurse may help schedule activities to prevent conflicts or secure needed consultation for the patient with the dietitian, social worker, or other healthcare team member. Sometimes in-hospital malnutrition can develop simply because meals are constantly being interrupted by various procedures, staff interviews, or medical rounds.

Interpreter

Because of a close relationship with the patient, the nurse may often reduce tension by helping the patient understand explanations concerning various treatments and plans of care. This will include basic interpretation of the therapeutic diet from the RD and of the resulting food selections on the tray. The nurse may sometimes assist the patient in making appropriate selections from the menus provided.

Teacher or Counselor

One of the nurse's most significant roles is that of healthcare educator and counselor. There will be innumerable informal opportunities during daily nursing care for planned conversation about sound nutrition principles, reinforcing counseling of the clinical dietitian. In addition, according to patient situations, the nurse may work with the clinical dietitian during periods of instruction about principles of the patient's nutrition therapy in relation to the disease process. The nurse will work in close cooperation with the clinical dietitian and the physician to coordinate nutritional and medical management of the patient's illness with overall nursing care. At all times the nurse will work closely with the hospital's clinical nutrition staff to support and reinforce primary nutrition education, as well as discharge planning for follow-up care. These clinical staff nutrition experts will always be excellent resources for needed nutrition consultation and referral.

Clearly, learning about the hospitalized patient's nutritional needs is a continuing activity beginning with admission. It should follow through and include plans for continuing application in the home environment. Follow-up care may be provided by the hospital's clinical dietitian, by consultation with clinical dietitians in community private practice, by public health dietitians and nurses, or by referrals to community agencies and resources.

TO SUM UP

The basis for an accurate assessment of the patient's nutritional needs begins with the individual patient and family. Physical as well as psychologic, social, economic, and cultural factors in and out of the clinical setting all play a role in evaluating the patient's health status and any possible problems with the nutrition care plan.

Nutrition assessment is based on a broad foundation of pertinent data, including food and drug uses and values. Effectiveness of an assessment based on analysis of these data depends in turn on effective communication with the patient, family members, and significant others in the development of an appropriate care plan, as well as with other members of the healthcare team. The patient's medical record is a basic means of communication among healthcare team members.

Nutrition therapy, based on a combination of personal and physiologic needs of the patient, requires a close working relationship among nutrition, medical, and nursing staff in the healthcare facility. The nurse's schedule offers many opportunities to reinforce nutrition principles of the diet. Nutrition therapy does not end with the patient's discharge. Outpatient nutrition services, appropriate social services, and food resources in the community help meet continuing needs of patients and their families.

QUESTIONS FOR REVIEW

1. Identify and discuss possible effects of various psychologic factors on the outcome of nutrition therapy.
2. Outline a general procedure for assessing nutritional needs for a 65-year-old widower hospitalized with coronary heart disease. Include appropriate community agencies to refer the patient for follow-up care, services, and information.
3. Describe commonly used anthropometric procedures, blood tests, and urine tests for nutritional status information in terms of significance of the measure or test—what is being measured and what the results tell you.
4. Select several clinical signs used to assess nutritional status, and describe what each sign shows in a malnourished person and why.
5. Describe the nature and purpose of quality assurance plans for standards of nutrition care.

REFERENCES

1. Nelms MN, Sucher K, Long S: *Understanding nutrition therapy and pathophysiology,* Belmont, Calif, 2007, Wadsworth.
2. Lee RD, Neiman DC: *Nutrition assessment,* ed 3, New York, 2003, McGraw-Hill.

3. Chima CS, Pollack HA: Position of the American Dietetic Association: nutrition services in managed care, *J Am Diet Assoc* 102(10):1471, 2002.

4. Larson E: Disease management, registered dietitians and medical nutrition therapy, *J Am Diet Assoc* 102(2):190, 2002.

5. Belanger MC, Dube L: The emotional experience of hospitalization: its moderators and its role in patient satisfaction with food services, *J Am Diet Assoc* 96(4):354, 1996.

6. Rubin M: The physiology of bed rest: how bed rest changes perception, *Am J Nurs* 88(1):50, 1988.

7. Gallagher-Allred CR et al: Malnutrition and clinical outcomes: the case for medical nutrition therapy, *J Am Diet Assoc* 96(4):361, 1996.

8. Bone RC: Ethical principles in critical care, *JAMA* 263(5):696, 1990.

9. Monsen ER et al: Ethics: responsible scientific conduct, *Am J Clin Nutr* 54:1, 1991.

10. The University of Iowa, Hardin Library for the Health Sciences: *Hardin MD: nutrition,* Iowa City, Iowa, 2005, Author. Available at *www.lib.uiowa.edu/hardin/md/nutr.html.* Accessed June 26, 2006.

11. Yale-New Haven Hospital: *Making the right choice on the web: safe surfing for health care information,* New Haven, Conn, 2001, Author. Available at *www.ynhh.org.*

12. Truswell AS: Family physicians and patients: is effective nutrition interaction possible? *Am J Clin Nutr* 71:6, 2000.

13. Laramee SH: Position of the American Dietetic Association: nutrition services in managed care, *J Am Diet Assoc* 96(4):391, 1996.

14. Lacey K, Pritchitt E: Nutrition Care Process and model: ADA adopts road map to quality care and outcomes management, *J Am Diet Assoc* 103(8):1061, 2003.

15. Identifying patients at risk: ADA's definitions for nutrition screening and nutrition assessment, *J Am Diet Assoc* 94(8):838, 1994.

16. Joint Commission on Accreditation of Healthcare Organizations: *2004 Comprehensive accreditation manual for hospitals: the official handbook (CAMH),* Oakbrook Terrace, Ill, 2004, Author.

17. Mitchell CO, Lipschitz DA: Arm length measurement as an alternative to height in the nutritional assessment of the elderly, *J Am Geriatr Soc* 39:492, 1991.

18. Mackle TJ, Touger-Decker R, Maillet JO: Registered dietitians' use of physical assessment parameters in professional practice, *J Am Diet Assoc* 103(12):1632, 2003.

19. Blundell JE: What foods do people eat? A dilemma for nutrition, an enigma for psychology, *Am J Clin Nutr* 71:3, 2000.

20. Schaefer EJ et al: Lack of efficacy of a food-frequency questionnaire in assessing dietary macronutrient intakes in subjects consuming diets of known composition, *Am J Clin Nutr* 71:746, 2000.

21. Mela DJ, Aaron JI: Honest but invalid: what subjects say about recording their food habits, *J Am Diet Assoc* 97:791, 1997.

22. Klesges RC et al: Who underreports dietary intake in a dietary recall? Evidence from the second National Health and Nutrition Survey, *J Consult Clin Psychol* 63:438, 1995.

23. Macdiarmid JI, Blundell JE: Assessing dietary intake: who, what, and why of underreporting, *Nutr Res Rev* 1:231, 1998.

24. Kristal AR et al: Associations for race/ethnicity, education, and dietary intervention with the validity and reliability of a food frequency questionnaire, *Am J Epidemiol* 146:856, 1997.

25. Sawaya AL et al: Evaluation of four methods for determining energy intake in young and older women: comparison with doubly labeled water measurements of total energy expenditure, *Am J Clin Nutr* 63:491, 1996.

26. Weber JL et al: Validity of self-reported energy intake in lean and obese young women, using two nutrient databases, compared with total energy expenditure assessed by doubly labeled water, *Eur J Clin Nutr* 55(11):940, 2001.

27. Goris AHC et al: Undereating and underrecording of habitual food intake in obese men: selective underreporting of fat intake, *Am J Clin Nutr* 71:130, 2000.

28. Bathalon GP et al: Psychological measures of eating behavior and the accuracy of 3 common dietary assessment methods in healthy postmenopausal women, *Am J Clin Nutr* 71:739, 2000.

29. American Dietetic Association: *Nutrition diagnosis: a critical step in the nutrition care process,* Chicago, 2006, Author. Retrieved July 14, 2005, from *www.eatright.org/Member/index_22405.cfm* (requires membership for access).

FURTHER READINGS AND RESOURCES

Readings

American Dietetic Association: Practice report of the American Dietetic Association: home care—an emerging practice area for dietetics, *J Am Diet Assoc* 99(11):1453, 1999.

> *Home care, especially for the growing numbers of older persons in our population, is increasing, and the accompanying need for nutrition and nursing care reflects this pressing situation. This excellent report identifies these needs and discusses possible ways of meeting them.*

Porter C et al: Dynamics of nutrition care among nursing home residents who are eating poorly, *J Am Diet Assoc* 99(11):1444, 1999.

> *This article provides insight into the common problem of malnutrition among nursing home residents and the apparently haphazard ways some staff members may respond, such as using liquid supplements for vitamins but not for minerals, replacing regular meals with liquid supplement drinks, or resorting to unpleasant and unethical measures such as force feeding.*

Websites of Interest

- U.S. Department of Agriculture, Food and Nutrition Information Center, Dietary Analysis and Intake Calculators; this website, hosted by the Food and Nutrition Information Center (FNIC) at the National Agricultural Library (NAL), provides links to numerous diet-analysis tools; *www.nal.usda.gov/fnic/etext/000108.html.*

- National Policy and Resource Center on Nutrition and Aging, Nutrition Screening and Assessment: Nutrition Screening Initiative and Mini Nutritional Assessment; this website provides a listing of research references and reports, many with additional links: *www.fiu.edu/~nutreldr/SubjectList/N/Nutrition_Screening_Assessment.htm.*

- Stanford University, HighWire Press, Nutrition Assessment; this interesting website provides links to peer-reviewed journals that publish articles on the topic of nutrition assessment: *http://highwire.stanford.edu/lists/topic_dir/608683/608684/617569/618062/alpha.dtl.*

CHAPTER 17

Drug-Nutrient Interactions

Sara Long

In this chapter, continuing our clinical nutrition sequence, we look briefly at some main effects of combining food and nutrients with drugs. We will see how these interactions affect nutrition therapy.

Today consumers are generally better informed about drug misuse. However, many are dangerously uninformed or misinformed about the specific drugs they may be taking, especially in relation to the food they eat.

All members of the healthcare team must have knowledge of drug actions and nutrition to make the wisest and most effective use of drugs and nutrition therapy. Here we examine some of these drug-nutrient effects and how these interactions affect nutrition therapy and education.

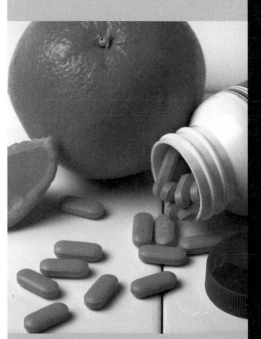

DRUG-NUTRIENT PROBLEMS IN MODERN MEDICINE

Problem Significance: Causes, Extent, and Effects

During this century, unprecedented medical progress has resulted in decreased childhood mortality rates and increased life expectancy. As we live longer, incidence of chronic diseases such as cardiovascular disease, type 2 diabetes mellitus, hypertension, and arthritis will continue to increase, often in comorbid manner. Furthermore, treatment of these and other chronic diseases often involves long-term use of medications, often resulting in polypharmacy.

Every year 25 to 30 new medications are introduced.[1-3] American physicians prescribe and pharmacists dispense a total amount of drugs sufficient to provide seven individual medications for each woman, man, and child in the United States (see the *Focus on Culture* box, "Are We Speaking the Same Language?"). To this amount, we can then add the large volume of nonprescription drugs Americans purchase over the counter (Figure 17-1).

Some concerned persons have come to view the proliferation of pills in our society with alarm. For example, epidemiologic studies in America and Europe indicate that cycles of repeated antibiotic prescriptions may increase the patient's risk of contracting an antibiotic-resistant disease organism.[4] Knowledgeable and concerned pharmacologists indicate that outside of extremely serious illness, most general medical problems can be treated with fewer than 25 drugs. The World Health Organization (WHO) has estimated that only some 150 to 200 drugs are actually needed to take care of almost all ordinary illnesses around the world. Yet on our American market there are about 54,000 drugs, many of them only slight variations of other drugs.

Drug Use and Nutritional Status

Older Adults at Risk

All of us, at any age, risk harmful drug-drug or drug-nutrient interactions. However, older adults are particularly vulnerable,[5] and this will only become more serious.

Today, adults over 65 represent approximately 12% of the U.S. population. It is projected this number will increase to 20% to 22% by 2050.[5,6] Older adults take a much larger percentage of prescription and nonprescription medications than their younger counterparts (Figure 17-2). Approximately 23% of women and 19% of older men over 65 years of age take five or more prescription medications a week.[7]

Several factors contribute to an increased risk among older adults, including the following:

- They are likely to be taking more drugs for longer periods to control chronic diseases.
- Their drugs are likely to be more toxic.
- They respond to drugs with greater variability.
- They have less capability of handling drugs efficiently.
- Their nutritional status is more likely to be deficient.
- They are more likely to make increased errors in self-care because of illness, mental confusion, or lack of drug information.

As a result of these problems, concerned physicians, nutritionists, pharmacists, and nurses are increasingly working together as a team to provide drug and nutrition education and therapy on a more sound basis. A number of drug-nutrient interactions demand this type of teamwork in patient care.

Nutritional Status

Well-nourished individuals are less likely to acquire diseases necessitating treatment with medication, and when they encounter specific diseases, the illness is usually less severe and responds to medication more favorably.[8] Thus poor nutritional status can have a major impact on risk for complications of drug-nutrient reactions. Nutrient-drug mechanisms that influence nutritional status include those affecting the following:

- Stimulated or suppressed appetite
- Decreased intestinal absorption

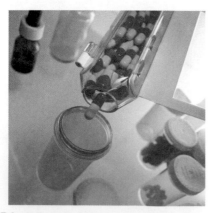

FIGURE 17-1   Prescription and nonprescription drugs have become part of American life. *(Copyright 2006 JupiterImages Corporation.)*

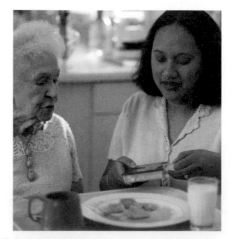

FIGURE 17-2   Older adults make up a large percentage of those taking both prescription and nonprescription medications in the United States.

- Increased renal excretion
- Competition or displacement of nutrients for carrier protein sites
- Interference with synthesis of necessary enzyme, coenzyme, or carrier
- Hormonal effects on genetic systems
- The drug delivery system
- Components in drug formulation

In general, drugs are grouped according to primary action. Here we review briefly various effects of drugs on food and nutrients and effects of food and nutrients on drugs. In each case, we give some examples for your reference in patient care.

DRUG EFFECTS ON FOOD AND NUTRIENTS

Drug Effects on Food Intake

Appetite Changes

The following drugs may stimulate appetite and/or weight gain[9]:

- *Antihistamines:* These drugs can lead to marked increase in appetite and subsequent weight gain. One of these agents, both an antihistamine and a serotonin antagonist, is cyproheptadine hydrochloride (Periactin).
- *Antianxiety drugs:* Some drugs in this classification may lead to hyperphagia, or excessive eating. Some of these drugs include chlordiazepoxide hydrochloride (Librium), diazepam (Valium), and alprazolam (Xanax).
- *Tricyclic antidepressants:* Tricyclic antidepressants and most antipsychotic drugs such as amitriptyline hydrochloride (Elavil), olanzapine (Zyprexa), chlorpromazine hydrochloride (Thorazine), and clozapine (Clozaril) may promote appetite and lead to significant weight gain.
- *Insulin:* Hypoglycemia can occur in persons with type 1 diabetes if food is not taken immediately after their insulin injection (see Chapter 21). If some food is not readily available to counteract the rapid progression of the unrelieved severe hypoglycemia, coma and death occur. If excess food is consumed to avoid or treat hypoglycemia, weight gain may occur.
- *Steroids:* Anabolic steroids, including testosterone, promote nitrogen retention, increased lean body mass, and subsequent weight gain.

The following drugs may depress appetite[9]:

- *Selective serotonin reuptake inhibitor (SSRI):* This class of antidepressants may cause anorexia and weight loss; an example is fluoxetine (Prozac). (See the *Case Study* box, "Drug-Herb Interaction," for an application of the use of SSRIs.)
- *Amphetamines:* These drugs act as stimulants to the central nervous system and have the effect of depressing desire for food, thus leading to marked loss of

weight. For this reason, they have been used in the past as appetite-depressant drugs in the treatment of obesity. However, long-term use of these drugs for such treatment has caused problems, such as addiction. For this reason, amphetamines are rarely used now for this purpose. Children taking amphetamines show dose-dependent growth retardation.

- *Alcohol:* Abuse of alcohol can lead to loss of appetite, reduced food intake, and malnutrition. The anorexia, or loss of appetite, can stem from various effects of alcoholism such as gastritis, hepatitis, cirrhosis, ketosis, pancreatitis, alcoholic brain syndrome, drunkenness, and withdrawal symptoms. The resulting reduced food intake can then lead to malnutrition, which further complicates the anorexia.

Taste and Smell Changes

Drugs such as the tricyclic antidepressant amitriptyline (Elavil) may impair salivary flow, causing dry mouth along with a sour or metallic taste.[9] The antibiotic clarithromycin (Biaxin) is secreted into saliva, causing a bitter taste.[9] Antibiotics such as tetracycline may suppress natural oral bacteria, resulting in oral yeast overgrowth or

---

CASE STUDY

Drug-Herb Interaction

Ivanna is a 20-year-old exchange student from Germany. She lives with three roommates and is in her junior year at the local university. Ivanna is seeking medical attention at the urging of her roommates, who report her mood has become increasingly depressed over the past two semesters. She has become withdrawn and moody; but is otherwise a healthy young woman. She is 5 ft, 11 in tall and weighs 160 lb on admission.

Ivanna reports a 5-lb weight loss in the past 3 months. She takes oral contraceptives, smokes ½ pack of cigarettes per day, and drinks four to five beers on the weekends. Her mother has been treated for depression with St. John's wort by the family physician in Germany for the past 10 years. Her admitting diagnosis is depression. Physician's orders are as follows: Zoloft, 50 mg every day, referral to house psychologist for counseling, and nutrition consult for her poor eating habits.

Questions for Analysis

1. Her physician ordered Zoloft to treat Ivanna's depression. Zoloft is a selective serotonin reuptake inhibitor (SSRI). Are there any pertinent nutritional considerations when using this medicine?
2. How do SSRIs work?
3. During the diet history, you ask Ivanna if she uses any over-the-counter (OTC) vitamins, minerals, or herbal supplements. She tells you her mother suggested she try *Hypericum perforatum* (St. John's wort) because in Germany it is prescribed to treat depression. Ivanna did as her mother suggested, because it is available without prescription in the United States. What is St. John's wort?
4. How is St. John's wort used in the United States?
5. How does St. John's wort work as an antidepressant?
6. Does St. John's wort have any side effects?
7. How is St. John's wort regulated in the United States? How is it used in Europe?
8. What is your immediate concern regarding Ivanna's use of St. John's wort?

Modified from Nelms MN, Long S: *Medical nutrition therapy: a case study approach,* ed 2, Belmont, Calif, 2004, Brooks/Cole, a division of Thomson Learning.

FOCUS ON CULTURE

Are We Speaking the Same Language?

Consider the following prescription label directions written half in English and half in Spanish:

Aplicarse once cada dia til rash is clear.

What does it mean to you? If you do not read Spanish, it probably does not mean much, although you can pick out the words *once* and *til rash is clear.* And if you study this phrase hard enough, you might figure out it says something about using the medication once a day until the rash is gone.

If you read Spanish, the meaning may be entirely different. "Once" means "eleven" in Spanish. If this is a topical medication, then no permanent harm may result in using it 11 times a day. If this is an oral medication, the results could be fatal.

Many people using prescription or over-the-counter (OTC) medications, herbal products, or vitamin/mineral supplements use a language other than English as their primary language. Foreign-born individuals make up 11% of the U.S. population. The majority of immigrants are of Hispanic origin. Although members of these groups have good reading and writing skills in their native language, they do not possess these skills in English. How then, are they supposed to read and understand directions on how to take medications or supplements? How can they adhere to prescribed medical regimens? They may be more susceptible to food-drug interactions because of this.

Another barrier to health is literacy. More than 40% of patients with chronic illnesses are functionally illiterate. Almost 25% of all adult Americans read at or below a fifth-grade level, whereas medical information is typically written at a tenth-grade level or above. The National Adult Literacy Survey (NALS) found almost 25% of patients with inadequate functional health literacy did not know how to take medications.

Limited health literacy and language barriers have many consequences. Patients who do not understand prescription directions and instructions for preventative care and self-care may make the following mistakes:

- Incorrect dosages (e.g., improper infant formula preparation and feeding)
- Incorrect schedules of administration (e.g., 4 times a day versus 4 pills at one time)
- Incorrect routes of administration (e.g., teens who have misunderstood directions for contraceptive jelly and have eaten it on toast every morning to prevent pregnancy)

Low health literacy risk groups include pediatric patients, older adult patients, and patients with language barriers. Pediatric patients are at increased risk of incorrect dosages. Older adult patients take multiple medications, which increases risk for errors. In addition, patients over the age of 60 years may have hearing loss, memory loss, short attention span, and low energy levels, thus exacerbating the problems. Patients who speak English as their second language are vulnerable to misinterpretation of information.

What are some solutions?

- Provide written materials in several languages and at a fifth-grade reading level or lower.
- Offer small amounts of information at a time.
- Avoid using "medical speak" (medical terms that are used every day in the clinical setting, but are unfamiliar to patients).
- Employ a multilingual staff.
- Have patients repeat instruction to ensure the message was received and understood.
- Use identifiers such as time-of-day references (e.g., "Take one tablet in the morning when you wake up and the second tablet at bedtime.").
- Use visual images when possible.

References

Hardin LR: Frontline pharmacist: counseling patients with low health literacy, *Am J Health Syst Pharm* 62:364, 2005.

Institute for Safe Medication Practices: Hospitals need to take action now to reduce threat of medication errors with magnesium sulfate, *ISMP Medication Safety Alert!* March 12, 1997. Retrieved November 27, 2005, from *www.ismp.org/MSAarticles/calendar/Mar97.html.*

Institute for Safe Medication Practices: To promote understanding, assume every patient has a health literacy problem, *ISMP Medication Safety Alert!* October 31, 2001. Retrieved November 27, 2005, from *http://www.ismp.org/MSAarticles/calendar/Oct01.html#Oct31,2001.*

Literacy Partners of Manitoba: *Literacy and health resources,* Manitoba, Canada, 2005, Author. Retrieved November 27, 2005, from *www.health.mb.literacy.ca/health.htm.*

National Institute for Literacy: *Literacy fact sheets: scope of the literacy need,* Washington, DC, 2001, Author. Available at *www.nifl.gov.*

New York State Department of Health AIDS Institute: Promoting adherence to HIV antiretroviral therapy, New York, NY, 2001, Author. Retrieved November 27, 2005, from *www.hivguidelines.org/public_html/center/best-practices/best-practices.shtml.*

U.S. Census Bureau: Profile of selected social characteristics: 2000, *Census 2000 supplementary survey summary tables,* Washington, DC, 2001, Author.

Wallendorf M: Literally literacy, *J Consum Res* 27:505, 2001.

candidiasis. Metronidazole (Flagyl), an antibiotic, may cause *dysgeusia* (abnormal or impaired sense of taste) by causing a metallic taste in the mouth.[9] Antineoplastic medications (cisplatin or methotrexate) may damage rapidly growing cells, causing stomatitis, glossitis, and/or esophagitis[9] (see the *Perspectives in Practice* box, "The Proof of the Pudding").

Gastrointestinal Effects

Many drugs can affect the stomach and cause nausea, vomiting, bleeding, or ulceration; intestinal peristalsis; or changes in intestinal flora. Nonsteroidal antiinflammatory drugs (NSAIDs) such as acetylsalicylic acid (aspirin), ibuprofen (Advil, Motrin), and naproxen (Aleve, Anaprox) cause stomach irritation.[9] Sometimes the irritation is so severe as to cause sudden and serious gastric bleeding.[9] Anticholinergic medications (antipsychotics, antidepressants, antihistamines) slow peristalsis, resulting in constipation. Ciprofloxacin (Cipro) is an antibiotic that can allow for the overgrowth of *Clostridium difficile,* resulting in pseudomembranous colitis.[9]

Drug Effects on Nutrient Absorption and Metabolism

Nutrient Absorption

A number of drugs can increase nutrient absorption and thus benefit nutritional status. For example, cimetidine

PERSPECTIVES IN PRACTICE
The Proof of the Pudding

The senses of taste and smell greatly affect our responses to various foods. Loss of these senses may drive persons to constantly seek elusive satisfaction by overeating, or it may stop them from eating entirely. In either case, the pleasure of eating is gone, and nutritional status suffers. The following are examples of drugs that affect taste and smell:

Anesthetics, local—benzocaine, cocaine, procaine
Antibiotics—amphotericin B, ampicillin, griseofulvin, lincomycin, streptomycin, tetracyclines
Anticoagulant—phenindione
Antihistamine—chlorpheniramine maleate
Antihypertensive agents—captopril, diazoxide, ethacrynic acid
Antiinfective agent—metronidazole
Cholesterol-lowering agent—clofibrate
Hypoglycemic agent—glipizide
Psychoactive agents—carbamazepine, lithium carbonate, phenytoin, amphetamines
Toothpaste ingredient—sodium lauryl sulfate

The proof of the pudding—our food—is in the tasting, which is easily affected by a variety of drugs, resulting in diminished appetite and necessary food intake. Patients taking these drugs that affect taste and smell may benefit from counseling about these taste effects, along with other effects, and ways of counteracting them in food selection, seasoning, and serving.

References

Powers D, Moore A: *Food medication interactions,* ed 6, Phoenix, Ariz, 1988, Food Medication Interactions.
Roe DA: *Diet and drug interactions,* ed 2, New York, 1989, AVI Books.
Thomas JA: Drug-nutrient interactions, *Nutr Rev* 53(10):271, 1995.
Trovato A et al: Drug-nutrient interactions, *Am Fam Physician* 44(5):1651, 1991.

(Tagamet), a gastric antisecretory agent, helps patients with bowel resection in several ways.[9] The drug reduces gastric acid and volume output; it also lowers duodenal acid load and volume and reduces jejunal flow.[9] It maintains pH of secretions and decreases fecal fat, nitrogen, and volume, thus improving absorption of macronutrients.[9] This drug is therefore helpful in the treatment of various gastrointestinal disorders, including peptic ulcer disease (see Chapter 19).[9] On the other hand, prolonged use of cimetidine may cause decreased absorption of vitamin B_{12}, thiamin, and iron.[9]

A number of drugs can contribute to primary malabsorption. Questran (antihyperlipidemic, bile acid sequestrant [cholestyramine]) binds vitamins A, D, E, and K in the gastrointestinal tract, preventing absorption of these nutrients.[9] Colchicine, a drug used in the treatment of gout, leads to vitamin B_{12} deficiency, causing megaloblastic anemia.[9] Alcohol abuse can provoke malabsorption of thiamin and folic acid, causing peripheral neuritis and anemia.[9] Laxatives can produce severe malabsorption, leading to conditions such as osteomalacia.[9]

Secondary malabsorption may also be drug induced. For example, the antibiotic neomycin causes tissue changes in the intestinal villi, precipitates bile salts, prevents fat breakdown by inhibiting pancreatic lipase, and decreases bile acid absorption.[9] These effects can lead to steatorrhea and failure to absorb the fat-soluble vitamins A, D, E, and K.[9] Malabsorption of vitamin D in turn leads to a calcium deficiency. Other drugs cause malabsorption of folic acid or impair its utilization. Methotrexate, for example, used in cancer chemotherapy, is a folic acid antagonist that impairs the intestinal absorption of calcium.[9]

Summaries of medications affecting food and/or nutrients can be found in Table 17-1.

Mineral Depletion

Certain drugs can lead to mineral depletion through induced gastrointestinal losses or renal excretion, as follows[10]:

- *Diuretics:* Diuretic drugs are intentionally used to reduce levels of excess tissue water and sodium, but they may also result in loss of other minerals, such as potassium, magnesium, and zinc. Potassium deficiency brings weakness, anorexia, nausea, vomiting, listlessness, apprehension, and sometimes diffuse pain, drowsiness, stupor, and irrational behavior. On the contrary, potassium-retaining diuretics such as spironolactone, as well as overuse of potassium supplementation, may cause the opposite effect of hyperkalemia.
- *Chelating agents:* Penicillamine attaches to metals and can lead to the deficiency of such key trace elements as zinc and copper.
- *Alcohol:* Abuse of alcohol can lead to diminished levels of potassium, magnesium, and zinc.
- *Antacids:* These commonly used over-the-counter medications are of concern because they can produce phosphate deficiency, with symptoms of anorexia, malaise, paresthesia, profound muscle weakness, and convulsions, as well as calcification of soft tissues from the prolonged hypercalcemia.

---

paresthesia Abnormal sensations such as prickling, burning, and crawling of skin.

TABLE 17-1	Medications Affecting Food and/or Nutrients			
Drug Class	**Examples**	**Use**	**Action**	**Nutrients Affected**	**How to Avoid**
Alcohol, particularly excessive use	Beer, wine, spirits	Lower inhibitions, CNS depressant	Increases turnover of some vitamins; substitution of alcohol for food	Vitamin B$_{12}$, folate, and magnesium	Limit alcohol consumption to ≤2 drinks per day for men, ≤1 drink per day for women
Analgesics, NSAIDs, and antiinflammatory agents	Salicylates (aspirin), ibuprofen (Motrin, Advil), naproxen (Anaprox, Aleve, Naprosyn), acetaminophen (Tylenol)	Pain and fever	Increases loss of vitamin C and competes with folate and vitamin K	Vitamin C, folate, vitamin K	Increase intake of foods high in vitamin C, folate, and vitamin K; take with 8 oz water
Antacids	Aluminum antacids, H$_2$ blockers	Stomach upset	Inactivates thiamin; decreased absorption of some nutrients	Thiamin B$_1$	Foods containing thiamin (B$_1$) should be consumed at a different time; depending on antacid, possibly magnesium, phosphorus, iron, vitamin A, and folate

Take antacid after meals; take iron, magnesium, or folate supplements separately by 2 hours; take separately from citrus fruit or juices or calcium citrate by 3 hours |
Antiulcer agents (histamine blockers)	Ranitidine (Zantac), Cimetidine (Tagamet), famotidine (Pepcid)	Ulcers	Decreases vitamin absorption	Vitamin B$_{12}$	Consult physician or registered dietitian regarding vitamin B$_{12}$ supplementation
Antibiotics	Tetracycline, Ciprofloxacin (Cipro)	Infection	Chelation of minerals; ingestion with caffeine may increase excitability and nervousness	Calcium, magnesium, iron, and zinc; caffeine	Take tetracycline at least 1 hr before or 2 hr after a meal; do not take with caffeine-containing products
Antineoplastic drugs	Methotrexate	Cancer	Causes mucosal damage, which may cause decreased nutrient absorption	Folate and vitamin B$_{12}$, also see *Antibiotics*	Consult physician or registered dietitian regarding supplementation
Anticholinergics	Amitriptyline (Elavil), chlorpromazine (Thorazine)		Saliva thickens and loses ability to prevent tooth decay	Fluids	Increase intake of fluids
Anticonvulsants	Phenobarbital, Phenytoin (Dilantin)	Seizures, epilepsy	Increases metabolism of folate (possibly leading to megaloblastic anemia), vitamin D (especially in children), and vitamin K	Folate, vitamin D, and vitamin K	Increase folate, vitamins D and K intake
Antidepressants	Lithium carbonate, Lithane, Lithobid, Lithonate, Lithotabs, Eskalith	Depression, anxiety	May cause metallic taste, nausea, vomiting, dry mouth, anorexia, weight gain, and increased thirst	Fluids	Drink 2-3 L of water per day and take with food, consistent sodium intake

Category	Drug	Use/Condition	Effect	Nutrient(s)	Recommendation
Antihyperlipidemics	Cholestyramine (Questran), colestipol (Colestid)	High serum cholesterol	Binds bile salts and nutrients	Fat-soluble vitamins (A, D, E, K), folate, vitamin B$_{12}$, and iron	Include rich sources of these vitamins and minerals in diet
Antituberculosis	Isoniazid (INH)	Tuberculosis	Inhibits conversion of vitamin B$_6$ to active form	Vitamin B$_6$	Vitamin B$_6$ supplementation is necessary to prevent deficiency and peripheral neuropathy
Corticosteroids	Prednisone, Solu-Medrol, hydrocortisone	Antiinflammatory, immunosuppression	Increases excretion	Protein, potassium, calcium, magnesium, zinc, vitamin C, and vitamin B$_6$	Increase intake of foods high in protein, potassium, calcium, magnesium, zinc, vitamin C, and vitamin B$_6$
Loop diuretics	Furosemide (Lasix)	Water retention, hypertension	Increases mineral excretion in urine	Potassium, calcium, magnesium, zinc, sodium, and chloride	Include fresh fruits and vegetables in diet
Thiazide diuretics	Hydrochlorothiazide (HCTZ)	Water retention, hypertension	Increases excretion of most electrolytes, but enhances reabsorption of calcium	Potassium, calcium, magnesium, zinc, sodium, chloride, and calcium	Increase intake of foods high in potassium, calcium, magnesium, zinc, sodium, chloride, and calcium
Potassium-sparing diuretics	Triamterene (Dyrenium)	Water retention, hypertension	Hyperkalemia	Potassium	Avoid potassium-based salt substitutes
Laxatives	Fibercon, Mitrolan	Constipation	Decreases nutrient absorption	Vitamins and minerals	Consult physician or registered dietitian regarding supplementation
Sedatives	Barbiturates	Sedation	Increases metabolism of vitamins	Folate, vitamin D, vitamin B$_{12}$, thiamin, and vitamin C	Increase intake of foods high in folate, vitamin D, vitamin B$_{12}$, thiamin, and vitamin C
Mineral oil	Agoral Plain	Lubricant laxative	Decreases absorption	Fat-soluble vitamins (A, D, E, K), betacarotene, calcium, phosphorus, and potassium	Take 2 hr apart from food and fat-soluble vitamins
Oral contraceptives	Estrogen/progestin	Birth control	May cause selective malabsorption or increased metabolism and turnover	Vitamin B$_6$ and folate	Increase foods high in B$_6$ and folate

Data from Anderson J, Hart H: *Nutrient-drug interactions and food*, Fort Collins, 2004, Colorado State University Cooperative Extension. Retrieved November 27, 2005, from *www.ext.colostate.edu/pubs/foodnut/09361.html*; Bland SE: Drug-food interactions, *J Pharm Scc W'sc*, p 28, Nov/Dec1998; Bobroff LB, Lentz A, Turner RE: *Food/drug and drug/nutrient interactions: what you should know about your medications*, Gainesville, 1994, University of Florida Cooperative Extension Service, Institute of Food and Agricultural Science. Available at *http://edis.ifas.ufl.edu*; Brown CH: Overview of drug interactions, *US Pharm* 25(5), 2000. Retrieved November 27, 2005, from *www.uspharmacist.com/index.asp?show=archive&issue=5_2000*; Kuhn MA: Drug interactions with medications and food [online course], Hoffman Estates, Ill, 2005, Nursing Spectrum Online. Available at *http://nsweb.nursingspectrum.com/ce/ce174.htm*; and Food and Drug Administration/National Consumers League: *Food & drug interactions* [brochure], Washington, DC, Authors. Retrieved November 27, 2005, from *www.nclnet.org;Food%20&%20Drug.pdf*.

CNS, Central nervous system; *NSAID,* nonsteroidal antiinflammatory drug.

- *Aspirin:* Salicylates such as aspirin (acetylsalicylic acid [ASA]) can induce iron deficiency by causing low-level blood loss from erosions in the stomach or intestinal tissue when taken incorrectly (see the discussion under the heading "Health Promotion").

Vitamin Depletion

Certain drugs act as metabolic antagonists and can cause deficiencies of the vitamins involved, as follows:

- *Vitamin antagonists:* Various drugs have been used successfully to treat disease because they are antagonists of certain vitamins and thus can control key metabolic reactions in which that vitamin is involved. For example, warfarin (Coumadin) anticoagulants inhibit regeneration of vitamin K, which is necessary for blood clotting. Also, some cancer chemotherapy drugs such as methotrexate have multiple antagonist effects on folate metabolism, thus inhibiting the synthesis of cell reproduction substances—deoxyribonucleic acid (DNA) and ribonucleic acid (RNA)—and protein. In a similar manner, the antimalaria drug pyrimethamine inhibits the action of folate in protein synthesis.
- *Hypovitaminosis from use of oral contraceptives:* Some women using oral contraceptive agents (OCAs) have developed subclinical deficiencies of the vitamins folate, riboflavin, pyridoxine (B_6), cobalamin (B_{12}), and ascorbic acid (C). Apparently OCAs induce a greater demand for these vitamins.[11] However, a Canadian/U.S. study has shown that this effect does not hold true with folate.[12]

Special Adverse Reactions

Several reactions are related to specific drug interactions with particular nutrients, as follows:

- *Monoamine oxidase inhibitors (MAOIs):* These antidepressant drugs can increase the vascular effect of simple vasoactive amines, such as tyramine and dopamine, from food.[13] The resulting tyramine syndrome is marked by headache, pallor, nausea, and restlessness. With increased absorption, symptoms may escalate to apprehension, sweating, palpitations, chest pain, fever, and increased blood pressure, at times, although rarely, to the extent of hypertensive crisis and stroke. A low-tyramine food list (see Table 17-3) is provided for use by any patient taking one of these antidepressant drugs.
- *Flushing reaction:* A number of drugs react with alcohol to produce a flushing reaction along with dyspnea and headache (Table 17-2). Central nervous system depressants, including hypnotic sedatives, antihistamines, phenothiazines, and narcotic analgesics, may cause a loss of consciousness if taken in combination with alcohol. Extreme caution must be exercised with these medications, and patients should be alerted to the dangers of mixing them with alcohol.
- *Hypoglycemia:* Drugs such as chlorpropamide (Diabinese) and similar oral medications used to control type 2 diabetes mellitus are hypoglycemic agents. They precipitate a rapid release of insulin, which may provoke a hypoglycemic reaction. This response of a rapidly reduced blood glucose level is especially strong when the drugs are used with alcohol. Symptoms of hypoglycemia include weakness, mental confusion, and irrational behavior. If not treated, loss of consciousness can follow.
- *Disulfiram reaction:* The drug disulfiram, commonly called Antabuse, is used in the treatment of alcoholism. It combats alcohol consumption by producing extremely unpleasant side effects when taken with alcohol. Within 15 minutes, flushing ensues, followed by headache, nausea, vomiting, and chest or abdominal pain. Other drugs, including aldehyde dehydrogenase inhibitors, may have this similar disulfiram effect.

TABLE 17-2	Adverse Drug Reactions Caused by Alcohol and Specific Foods		
Type of Reaction	**Drugs**	**Alcohol/Foods**	**Effects**
Flushing	Chlorpropamide (diabetes), griseofulvin, tetrachloroethylene	Alcohol	Dyspnea, headache, flushing
Disulfiram reaction	Aldehyde dehydrogenase inhibitors: disulfiram (Antabuse), calcium carbamide, metronidazole, nitrofurantoin, sulfonylureas	Alcohol, foods containing alcohol	Abdominal and chest pain, flushing, headache, nausea and vomiting
Hypoglycemia	Insulin-releasing agents: oral hypoglycemic drugs	Alcohol, sugar, sweets	Mental confusion, weakness, irrational behavior, unconsciousness
Tyramine reaction	Monoamine oxidase inhibitors (MAOIs): antidepressants such as phenelzine, procarbazine, isoniazid (isonicotinic acid hydrazide)	Foods containing large amounts of tyramine: cheese, red wines, chicken liver, broad beans, yeast	Cerebrovascular accident, flushing, hypertension

Modified from Roe DA: Interactions between drugs and nutrients, *Med Clin North Am* 63:985, 1979; and Roe DA: *Diet and drug interactions,* ed 2, New York, 1979, AVI Books.

FOOD AND NUTRIENT EFFECTS ON DRUGS

Physiologic Factors in Drug Absorption

Absorption of drugs is a complex matter. Physiologic events are important in a number of ways.

Solution

Before an orally administered tablet or capsule can dissolve, it must first disintegrate. The absorption of the drug, either from solution in acid gastric secretions or in the more alkaline medium of the intestine, may be more or less complete depending on its degree of solubility (see the *To Probe Further* box, "Grapefruit 'Juices' Certain Medications"). Food may affect eventual drug absorption at any of these points. Table 17-3 provides some examples of drugs that are better utilized when taken without food and those that should be taken with food. The drug then passes through the intestinal mucosa and liver circulation before entering systemic circulation. In the systemic blood circulation system, it may be subject to metabolism, deactivation, and elimination through the so-called first-pass mechanism.

Stomach-Emptying Rate

Composition of the diet affects the rate at which food enters the small intestine from the stomach. Slow emptying of food from the stomach has the effect of doling out small portions of a drug, creating more optimal saturation rates on the absorptive sites in the small intestine. Fats, high temperatures, and solid meals prolong the time the food stays in the stomach. Food usually increases secretion of bile, acid, and gut enzymes. It also enhances intestinal motility and splanchnic blood flow. Drugs may adsorb to certain food particles.

Clinical Significance

Whether these physiologic events have clinical significance depends on the extent of the effect and nature of the drug. A small change in absorption is critical for a drug with a steep dose-response curve but perhaps unnoticeable for a drug with a wide range of effective concentrations. In general, the amount of absorption is clinically more important than the rate because it has greater impact on the steady-state plasma concentration of the drug after multiple doses.

Effects of Food on Drug Absorption

Increased Drug Absorption

In summary, the following five basic circumstances contribute to increased absorption of a drug:

1. *Dissolving characteristics:* When a drug does not dissolve rapidly after it has been taken, the time it remains in the stomach with food is prolonged. This increased time in the stomach may increase its effective dissolution and consequent absorption. In some instances, the drug may not dissolve properly because of either the drug or gastric pH and is excreted, thus decreasing absorption of the drug.

2. *Gastric-emptying time:* Delayed emptying of food from the stomach can have the effect of doling out small portions of a drug, creating more optimal saturation rates on the absorption sites in the small intestine.

3. *Nutrients:* Some nutrients can promote absorption of certain drugs. For example, high-fat diets increase absorption of the antifungal drug griseofulvin. This drug is fat soluble, and high-fat diets stimulate the secretion of bile acids, which aid in absorption of the drug. Vitamin C, as well as gastric acid, enhances iron absorption. Recent studies indicate that citrus fruit reduced lipoprotein oxidation in persons consuming a high-saturated fat diet.[14] Anticoagulant drugs interact with dietary factors, and a consistent dietary intake of vitamin K is important.[15,16] Folic acid supplementation is needed when phenytoin is used for seizure control in epileptic patients.[17]

4. *Blood flow:* Food intake increases splanchnic blood flow carrying any ingested drugs. This direct circulation to abdominal visceral organs stimulates absorption and results in an increased availability of the accompanying drugs.

5. *Nutritional status:* In addition to the presence of specific nutrients, nutritional status may also affect the bioavailability of certain drugs in different ways. For example, the antibiotic chloramphenicol is absorbed more slowly in children with protein-energy malnutrition, but elimination of the drug is slower in well-nourished children. In both cases the effect is a net increased bioavailability of the drug.

vasoactive Having an effect on the diameter of blood vessels.

flushing reaction Short-term reaction resulting in redness of neck and face.

dyspnea Labored, difficult breathing.

disulfiram White to off-white crystalline antioxidant; inhibits oxidation of the acetaldehyde metabolized from alcohol. It is used in the treatment of alcoholism, producing extremely uncomfortable symptoms when alcohol is ingested after oral administration of the drug.

TO PROBE FURTHER

GRAPEFRUIT "JUICES" CERTAIN MEDICATIONS

Almost all oral drugs are subject to first-pass metabolism. That is, any substance the body views as a toxin (e.g., drugs, alcohol) goes through the liver via hepatic portal circulation, thus removing some of the active substance from blood before it enters general circulation. This means a fraction of the original dose of the drug will not be "available" to systemic circulation because it has undergone biotransformation. In other words, bioavailability of the drug has been altered, or lowered. One mechanism responsible for this is an enzyme system found in the intestinal wall and liver. The cytochrome P450 3A4 system (specifically CYP3A4-mediated drug metabolism) is responsible for first-pass metabolism of many medications. Most medications are lipid soluble and readily absorbed. To eliminate toxins (i.e., drugs) from the body, however, the cytochrome P450 system either breaks them down in the gut or changes the drug into a more water-soluble version in the liver, allowing it to be eliminated via urine.

Where does grapefruit juice come into play? Grapefruit juice blocks CYP3A4 enzyme in the wall of the small intestine, thus increasing bioavailability of the drug. This means a higher serum drug level, which may cause unpleasant consequences, including side effects and/or toxicity.

What is it in grapefruit juice that does this? The precise chemical nature of the substance responsible for inhibiting gut wall CYP3A4 enzyme is unknown, but it is believed that more than one component present in grapefruit juice may contribute to the inhibitory effect on CYP3A4.

A single glass (8 oz) of grapefruit juice has the potential to increase bioavailability and enhance beneficial or adverse effects of a broad range of medications. These effects can persist up to 72 hours after grapefruit consumption, until more CYP3A4 has been metabolized. Interactions have been found between grapefruit juice and drugs, as outlined in the following table:

Interactions Between Grapefruit Juice and Medications

Category	Generic Name	Brand Name	Effect
Antihypertensive (calcium channel blockers)	Felodipine	Plendil	Flushing, headache, tachycardia, decreased blood pressure
	Nifedipine	Procardia, Adalat	
	Nimodipine	Nimotop	
	Nisoldipine	Sular	
	Nicardipine	Cardene	
	Isradipine	DynaCirc	
	Verapamil	Calan, Isoptin	Same as above plus bradycardia and atrioventricular (AV) block
Nonsedating antihistamines	Astemizole	Hismanal	No studies, but recommended to avoid taking grapefruit juice with astemizole
Immunosuppressant	Cyclosporine	Neoral, Sandimmune, SangCya	Kidney toxicity, increased susceptibility to infections
	Tacrolimus	Prograf	
Statin (HMG-CoA reductase inhibitors)	Atorvastatin	Lipitor	Headache, gastrointestinal complaints, muscle pain, increased risk of myopathy
	Lovastatin	Mevacor	
Caffeine	Simvastatin	Zocor	Nervousness, overstimulation
Antianxiety, insomnia, or depression	Buspirone	BuSpar	Increased sedation
	Diazepam	Valium	
	Alprazolam	Xanax	
	Midazolam	Versed	
	Triazolam	Halcion	
	Zaleplon	Sonata	
	Carbamazepine	Tegretol	
	Clomipramine	Anafranil	
	Trazodone	Desyrel	

TO PROBE FURTHER—cont'd

Interactions Between Grapefruit Juice and Medications—cont'd

Category	Generic Name	Brand Name	Effect
Protease inhibitors	Saquinavir	Fortovase, Invirase	Doubles bioavailability, resulting in increased efficacy or toxicity depending on dose and patient variability
Sexual dysfunction	Sildenafil	Viagra	Delayed absorption (takes longer to become effective)

Medications Considered Safe for Use With Grapefruit

	Cetirizine	Zyrtec, Reactine	
	Fexofenadine	Allegra	
	Fluvastatin	Lescol	
	Loratadine	Claritin	
	Pravastatin	Pravachol	

References

Bailey DG et al: Grapefruit juice-drug interactions, *Br J Clin Pharmacol* 46(2):101, 1998.

Guo L et al: Role of furanocoumarin derivatives on grapefruit juice–mediated inhibition of human CYP3A activity, *Drug Metab Dispos* 28:766, 2000.

Ho P et al: Inhibition of human CYP3A4 activity by grapefruit flavonoids, furanocoumarins and related compounds, *J Pharm Pharm Sci* 4(3):217, 2001.

Hyland R et al: Identification of the cytochrome P450 enzymes involved in the N-demethylation of sildenafil, *Clin Pharmacol* 51:239, 2000.

Jetter A et al: Effects of grapefruit juice on the pharmacokinetics of sildenafil, *Clin Pharmacol Ther* 71(1):21, 2002.

Kane GC, Lipsky JJ: Drug–grapefruit juice interactions, *Mayo Clin Proc* 75:933, 2000.

Muirhead GJ et al: Pharmacokinetic interactions between sildenafil and saquinavir/ritonavir, *Br J Clin Pharmacol* 50:99, 2000.

Pronsky ZM: *Food medication interactions*, ed 13, Birchrunville, Pa, 2004, Food Medication Interactions.

Schmiedlin-Ren P et al: Mechanisms of enhanced oral availability of CYP3A4 substrates by grapefruit constituents, *Drug Metab Dispos* 25(1):1228, 1997.

University of Illinois Chicago College of Pharmacy Drug Information Center: *Grapefruit juice interactions,* Chicago, 2005, Author. Retrieved November 27, 2005, from *www.uic.edu/pharmacy/services/di/grapefru.htm.*

University of Michigan Health System Drug Information Service: *Selected drugs interacting with grapefruit juice,* Ann Arbor, Mich, 1999, The Regents of the University of Michigan. Retrieved November 27, 2005, from *http://www-personal.umich.edu/~mshlafer/Lectures/grapefruit.pdf.*

Decreased Drug Absorption

Absorption of some drugs, as follows, is delayed or reduced by the presence of food:

- *Aspirin:* Absorption of aspirin is reduced or delayed by food. It should be taken on an empty stomach with ample water, preferably cold (see the discussion under the heading "Health Promotion").

- *Tetracycline:* Nutritional status may also have an impact on drug absorption. For example, tetracycline absorption is impaired in malnourished individuals. Absorption of this commonly used antibiotic is also hindered when it is taken with milk, as well as with antacids or iron supplements. The drug combines with these materials to form new insoluble compounds that the body cannot absorb, causing loss of the minerals involved, that is, calcium or iron.[14]

- *Phenytoin:* The presence of protein inhibits absorption of phenytoin. Carbohydrate increases its absorption, but fat has no impact.

Food Effects on Drug Distribution and Metabolism

Carbohydrate and Fat

Dietary carbohydrate and fat, especially their relative quantities, influence liver enzymes that metabolize drugs. For example, presence of fat increases the activity of diazepam (Valium). Fat increases the concentration of the unbound active drug by displacing it from binding sites in plasma and tissue protein.

Licorice

Licorice, a sweet-tasting plant extract used in making chewing tobacco, candy, and certain drugs, causes sodium retention and increased hypertension.[18] A person being treated for hypertension needs to avoid any natural licorice-containing product. The active ingredient in licorice is glycyrrhizic acid, which is named for its natural plant source, *Glycyrrhiza glabra,* meaning "sweet root," a member of the legume family. An analogue of this active part of licorice is marketed under the trade names Biogastrone and Duogastrone, which are widely used, especially in Europe, for healing gastric ulcers, but hypertension is a side effect.

TABLE 17-3 | **Foods and/or Nutrients Affecting Medications**

Drug Class	Examples	Use	Action	Food/Nutrients	How to Avoid
Alcohol, particularly excessive use	Beer, wine, spirits	Lower inhibitions, CNS depressant	Slows absorption	Food	Consume alcohol with food or meals
Analgesics and NSAIDs	Salicylates (aspirin), Ibuprofen (Motrin, Advil), naproxen (Anaprox, Aleve, Naprosyn), Acetaminophen (Tylenol)	Pain and fever	Alcohol ingestion increases hepatotoxicity, liver damage, or stomach bleeding	Alcohol	Limit alcohol intake to ≤2 drinks per day for men, <1 drink per day for women
Antiulcer agents (histamine blockers)	Cimetidine (Tagamet)	Ulcers	Increased blood alcohol levels; reduced caffeine clearance	Alcohol; caffeine-containing foods and beverages	Limit caffeine intake; limit alcohol intake to ≤2 drinks per day for men, <1 drink per day for women
Antibiotics	Ciprofloxacin (Cipro)	Infection	Decreases absorption	Dairy products	Avoid dairy products
Anticoagulant	Warfarin (Coumadin)	Blood clots	Reduced efficacy; increased anticoagulation	Vitamins K and E (supplements) may reduce efficacy; alcohol and garlic may increase anticoagulation	Limit foods high in vitamin K: broccoli, spinach, kale, turnip greens, cauliflower, brussels sprouts; avoid high dose of vitamin E (400 IU or more)
Antineoplastic drugs	Methotrexate	Cancer	Increased hepatotoxicity with chronic alcohol use	Alcohol	Avoid alcohol
Antiemetic	Amitriptyline HCl (Elavil), chlorpromazine HCl (Thorazine)	Antidepressant; antipsychotic/antiemetic	Increased sedation	Alcohol	Avoid alcohol
Anticonvulsants	Phenobarbital	Seizures, epilepsy	Increased sedation	Alcohol	Avoid alcohol
Antidepressants: monoamine oxidase inhibitors (MAOIs)	Phenelzine (Nardil), tranylcypromine (Parnate)	Depression, anxiety	Rapid, potentially fatal increase in blood pressure	Foods or alcoholic beverages containing tyramine	Avoid beer; red wine; American processed, cheddar, bleu, Brie, mozzarella, and Parmesan cheeses; yogurt; sour cream; beef or chicken liver; cured meats such as sausage and salami; game meats; caviar; dried fish; avocados; bananas; yeast extracts; raisins; sauerkraut; soy sauce; miso soup; broad (fava) beans; ginseng; caffeine-containing products (colas, chocolate, coffee, tea)

Antihistamine	Fexofenadine (Allegra), loratadine (Claritin), cetirizine (Zyrtec), astemizole (Hismanal)	Allergies	Increases drowsiness and slows mental and motor performance	Alcohol	Use caution when operating machinery or driving
Antihypertensives	ACE-inhibitors, angiotensin II receptor antagonists, beta blockers, verapamil HCl	Hypertension	Reduced effectiveness	Natural licorice (*glycyrrhiza glabra*) and tyramine-rich foods	Avoid these foods
Antihyperlipidemics (HMG-CoA reductase inhibitors) or statins	Atorvastatin (Lipitor), lovastatin (Mevacor), pravastatin (Pravachol), simvastatin (Zocor)	High serum LDL cholesterol	Enhances absorption; increases risk of liver damage	Food/meals; alcohol	Lovastatin should be taken with evening meal to enhance absorption; avoid large amounts of alcohol
Antiparkinson	Levodopa (Dopar, Larodopa)	Parkinson's disease	Decreased absorption	High-protein foods (eggs, meat, protein supplements); B_6	Spread protein intake equally in 3-6 meals per day to minimize reaction; avoid B_6 supplements or multivitamin supplement in doses >10 mg
Antituberculosis	Isoniazid (INH)	Tuberculosis	Reduced absorption with foods; increased hepatotoxicity and reduced INH levels with alcohol	Alcohol	Take on empty stomach; avoid alcohol
Bronchodilators	Theophylline (Slo-bid, Theo-Dur)	Asthma, chronic bronchitis, and emphysema	Increased stimulation of CNS; alcohol can increase nausea, vomiting, headache, and irritability	Caffeine, alcohol	Avoid caffeine-containing foods/beverages (chocolate, colas, teas, coffee); avoid alcohol if taking theophylline medications
Corticosteroids	Prednisolone (Pediapred, Prelone), methyl prednisolone (Solu-Medrol); hydrocortisone	Inflammation and itching	Stomach irritation	Food	Take with food or milk to decrease stomach upset
Hypoglycemic agents	Chlorpropamide (Diabinese), metformin (Glucophage)	Diabetes	Severe nausea and vomiting	Alcohol	Avoid alcohol

Data from Anderson J, Hart H: *Nutrient-drug interactions and food*, Fort Collins, 2004, Colorado State University Cooperative Extension. Retrieved November 27, 2005, from *www.ext.colostate.edu/pubs/foodnut/09361.html*; Bland SE: Drug-food interactions, *J Pharm Soc Wisc* p 28, Nov/Dec 1998; Bobroff LB, Lentz A, Turner RE: *Food/drug and drug/nutrient interactions: what you should know about your medications*, Gainesville, 1994, University of Florida Cooperative Extension Service, Institute of Food and Agricultural Science. Available at *http://edis.ifas.ufl.edu*; Brown CH: Overview of drug interactions, *US Pharm* 25(5), 2000. Retrieved November 27, 2005, from *www.uspharmacist.com/index.asp?show=archive&issue=5_2000*; Kuhn MA: Drug interactions with medications and food [online course], Hoffman Estates, Ill, 2005, Nursing Spectrum Online. Available at *http://nsweb.nursingspectrum.com/ce/ce174.htm*; and Food and Drug Administration/National Consumers League: *Food & drug interactions* [brochure], Washington, DC, Authors. Retrieved November 27, 2005, from *www.nclnet.org/Food/Food%20%20%20Drug.pdf*.

CNS, Central nervous system; *NSAID*, nonsteroidal antiinflammatory drug; *ACE*, angiotensin-converting enzyme; *LDL*, low-density lipoprotein.

Indoles

Indoles in cruciferous vegetables (e.g., cabbage, brussels sprouts, broccoli, cauliflower; Figure 17-3) can speed up rate of drug metabolism. They apparently induce mixed-function oxidase enzyme systems in the liver.

Cooking Methods

The method of cooking foods may alter rate of drug metabolism. Charcoal broiling, for example, increases hepatic drug metabolism through enzyme induction.

Vitamin Effects on Drug Action

Vitamin Effects on Drug Effectiveness

Pharmacologic doses or large megadoses beyond nutritional need of vitamins decrease blood levels of drugs when vitamins interact with the drugs. For example, large doses of folate or pyridoxine can reduce the blood level and effectiveness of anticonvulsive drugs such as phenytoin (Dilantin) or phenobarbital that are used for seizure control. Unwise self-medication with large drug-level doses of vitamins can cause severe toxic complications (see the *Complementary and Alternative Medicine (CAM)* box, "At Least It's Natural!"). On the other hand, vitamins themselves may become important medications when used as part of the medical treatment for a secondary deficiency induced by a childhood genetic or metabolic disease. Such is the case with biotin in treating certain organic acidemias or with riboflavin in treating certain defects in fatty acid metabolism.

Control of Drug Intoxication

Riboflavin is useful in treating boric acid poisoning. Boric acid combines with the ribitol side chain of riboflavin and is excreted in the urine. Also, vitamin E combats pulmonary oxygen toxicity. Premature human infants at risk for development of bronchopulmonary dysplasia by oxygen treatment have been protected by vitamin E administration during the acute phase of respiratory distress requiring oxygen treatment.

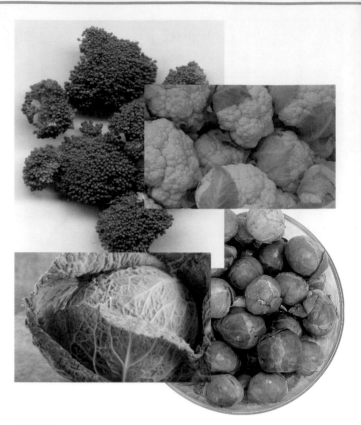

FIGURE 17-3   Examples of cruciferous vegetables. *(Copyright 2006 Jupiter-Images Corporation.)*

indole A compound produced in the intestines by the decomposition of tryptophan; also found in the oil of jasmine and clove.

cruciferous Bearing a cross; botanical term for plants belonging to the botanical family *Cruciferae* or *Brassicaceae*, the mustard family, so-called because of crosslike four-petaled flowers; name given to certain vegetables of this family, such as broccoli, cabbage, brussels sprouts, and cauliflower.

NUTRITION-PHARMACY TEAM

A decade or so ago hospitalized patients as a whole were less severely ill than they are today. Now, however, as a reflection of our more complex medical system and economic reform efforts, patients who are hospitalized are more acutely ill. They are more at risk for nutritional deficits and more likely to develop malnutrition, which leads to increased lengths of stay and higher costs. The task of monitoring food and drug interactions is complex and requires team responsibilities. Coordinating the pharmacy, food service, and clinical nutrition minimizes adverse drug-nutrient interactions.

Hospitals and other healthcare facilities concentrate on key processes and functions, such as drug-nutrient interactions in this case, rather than traditional strictly compartmentalized tasks of departments. Current standards focus still on departmental or service roles, but this is changing because of economic necessity as well as philosophy of care. This changing focus is being shaped, for example, in the work of the Joint Commission on Accreditation of Healthcare Organizations (JCAHO).[19]

COMPLEMENTARY AND ALTERNATIVE MEDICINE (CAM)
At Least It's Natural!

Herbal remedies and dietary supplements are not regulated by the Food and Drug Administration (FDA), so the purity, potency, and safety of these products can and do vary. Manufacturers' claims of efficacy and safety are not subject to the same rigorous testing mandatory for medications. It is likely for herbs and dietary supplements to be contaminated with other herbs, pesticides, herbicides, and other products during growth, harvesting, preparation, and storage. Moreover, active chemical components in the herb may not be standardized. This leads to dissimilar potencies from lot to lot or even from capsule to capsule within the same lot. Safety, toxicity, and the likelihood of adverse interactions with other medications or treatments frequently have not been tested, particularly in children. Patients contemplating use of herbs and dietary supplements should proceed with caution and seek out products only from reliable manufacturers.

The reason many people give for using herbal remedies and food supplements is based in tradition—the Chinese have been using this for thousands of years!—and extensive and aggressive marketing as "miracle cures" for what might ail a person rather than scientific data. Many turn to herbal remedies because they are "natural" and therefore seen as harmless. Well, hemlock, nightshade, mistletoe berries, belladonna, and poison ivy are all "natural" plants. What many do not realize is that "natural" is not synonymous with "safe"—especially when they combine herbs with medications.

Herb	Traditional Use*	Drug(s) That Interact With the Herb	Adverse Effects/Drug Interactions
Chamomile (English) (*Chamaemelum nobile, Matricaria recutita*)	Indigestion, reduce tension and induce sleep, eczema, irritation of mucous membranes following chemotherapy or radiation (for cancer)	Anticoagulants: heparin, warfarin (Coumadin)	May increase bleeding time
		Benzodiazepines: alprazolam (Xanax), chlordiazepoxide (Librium), diazepam (Valium), flurazepam (Dalmane), lorazepam (Ativan), temazepam (Restoril), triazolam (Halcion)	Binds to benzodiazepine receptors, which may alter effect of drug
		CNS depressants: alcohol, anticonvulsants, antiemetics, antihistamines, antipsychotics, antivertigo drugs, barbiturates, hypnotics, opioids, tricyclic antidepressants, paraldehyde (Paral)	May add to sedative effect
Chasteberry (*Vitex agnus-castus*)	Premenstrual syndrome (PMS), menopausal symptoms, amenorrhea, and other menstrual irregularities, fibrocystic breasts	Hormone replacement therapy, oral contraceptives	Herb binds to estrogen receptor, may counteract oral contraceptives
Dong quai (*Angelica sinensis*)	Menstrual irregularities and menopausal complaints	Anticoagulants	May increase bleeding time; if using concurrently, obtain prothrombin time and International Normalized Ratio (INR) to rule out interactions
Echinacea (*Echinacea angustifolia, E. pallida, E. purpurea*)	Decrease duration of colds	Immunosuppressants: azathioprine, basiliximab, cyclosporine, daclizumab, interferon, muromaonab-CD3, mycophenolate, sirolimus, tacrolimus, corticosteroids	May decrease immunosuppressant effect

Data from Herr SM: *Herb-drug interaction handbook,* ed 2, Nassau, NY, 2002, Church Street Books; Kuhn MA, Winston D: *Herbal therapy and supplements. a scientific and traditional approach,* Philadelphia, 2001, Lippincott; Brown CH: Overview of drug interactions, *US Pharm* 25(5), 2000. Retrieved November 27, 2005, from *www.uspharmacist.com/index.asp?show=archive&issue=5_2000*; Kemper K, Gardiner P, Chan E: "At least it's natural . . ." Herbs and dietary supplements in ADHD, *Contemp Ped* 9:116, 2000. Retrieved June 21, 2005, from *www.contemporarypediatrics.com*; Kemper K, Gardiner P, Conboy LA: Herbs and adolescent girls: avoiding the hazards of self-treatment, *Contemp Ped* 3:133, 2000. Retrieved June 21, 2005, from *www.contemporarypediatrics.com*.

*Not an exhaustive listing.

Continued

COMPLEMENTARY AND ALTERNATIVE MEDICINE (CAM)—cont'd
At Least It's Natural!

Herb	Traditional Use*	Drug(s) That Interact With the Herb	Adverse Effects/Drug Interactions
Ma Huang, Ephedra (*Ephedra sinica, E. equisetina, E. intermedia*)	Bronchodilator, decongestant, central nervous system (CNS) stimulant, diuretic	Amitriptyline (Elavil)	Drug may decrease hypertensive effect of ephedrine
		Anticonvulsants	Sympathomimetic effects, which may interfere with drug
		General anesthetics	Concurrent use may result in arrhythmias
		Caffeine and other xanthine alkaloids	Increased effects and potential toxicity
		Monoamine oxidase inhibitors (MAOIs)	Increased sympathomimetic effects
		Antihypertensives: angiotensin-converting enzyme (ACE) inhibitors, alpha blockers, angiotensin II receptor blockers, beta blockers, calcium channel blockers, diuretics	May decrease effectiveness of drug due to stimulant effect
		Insulin/oral hypoglycemic agents	Possible hyperglycemia with concurrent use
		Methylphenidate (Ritalin)	May displace drug from adrenergic neurons, which may decrease effectiveness of drug
		Morphine	Increases analgesic effect
		Oxytocin (Pitocin)	Possible hypertension
Evening primrose oil (*Oenothera biennis L*)	PMS, eczema, diabetic neuropathy, fibrocystic breasts, rheumatoid arthritis	Phenothiazines: chlorpromazine (Thorazine), fluphenazine (Prolixin), prochlorperazine (Compazine), promethazine hydrochloride (Phenergan)	May increase risk of seizures
		Anticoagulants	May increase risk of bleeding
Ginkgo (*Ginkgo biloba*)	Improved blood flow, protection against free-radical damage, attention-deficit/hyperactivity disorder (ADHD), dementia, macular degeneration, mental performance	Aspirin or Coumadin	May increase risk of bleeding
Ginseng American (*Panax quinquefolius*) Panax or Asian (*Panax ginseng*)	ADHD, stress reduction, chronic fatigue syndrome, fibromyalgia, age-related memory loss, menopausal cloudy thinking	Insulin/oral hypoglycemic agents	May enhance hypoglycemic effect
		Oral contraceptives/hormone replacement therapy	May alter effectiveness of exogenous hormones
		General anesthetics	Should be discontinued 7 days before surgery, herb increases risk of hypoglycemia and bleeding
		Caffeine and other stimulants	Red ginseng (steamed) may be additive to stimulant effect
		Immunosuppressants	Ginseng has immunostimulant activity and should not be used concurrently
		MAOIs	Potentiates phenelzine, causing manic symptoms

COMPLEMENTARY AND ALTERNATIVE MEDICINE (CAM)—cont'd
At Least It's Natural!

Herb	Traditional Use*	Drug(s) That Interact With the Herb	Adverse Effects/Drug Interactions
Kava (or kava kava) (*Piper methysticum*)	Sleep disorders, antianxiety, tension headaches, menopausal anxiety, fibromyalgia	Alprazolam (Xanax)	Synergistic CNS activity of alprazolam
		Alcohol, tranquilizers (barbiturates), and antidepressants	May potentiate action
		Antiparkinsonian drugs	May increase tremors and make medications less effective
Senna (*Cassia senna*)	Laxative, weight loss,	Any drug	May reduce intestinal absorption
		Antiarrhythmics	May potentiate drug
		Corticosteroids	May cause hypokalemia
		Digoxin/cardiac glycosides	May increase effects
		Diuretics	May interfere with potassium-sparing effect
St. John's wort	Depression, seasonal affective disorder	Theophylline and beta-2 agonists	Possibility of increased anxiety
		Selective serotonin reuptake inhibitors (SSRIs)	Serotonin syndrome (sweating, agitation, tremor)
Valerian (*Valeriana officinalis*)	Sleep disorders. ADHD, menstrual cramps	Sedatives, barbiturates, CNS depressants, general anesthetics, thiopental	May intensify effects

The JCAHO's accreditation manual reflects the philosophy that key functions often involve different disciplines coming together, partners with clearly defined responsibilities. The team of clinical nutritionist and clinical pharmacologist is clearly one of these partnerships. Current JCAHO guidelines mandate monitoring of drug therapy and counseling with patients about adverse drug-nutrient interactions.[20]

Health Promotion

"The Pain Reliever Doctors Recommend Most"

Aspirin (Figure 17-4) has a venerable history. Being a buffered form of salicylic acid, it is a modified version of an ancient folk remedy of willow bark that had been used for many hundreds of years for fever, aches, and pain. The acetyl group in acetylsalicylic acid makes aspirin easier on the stomach than willow bark.

Aspirin is an analgesic agent, an effect enhanced in combination with caffeine[21] that is used for the relief of minor aches and pains. Its mechanism of action is through inhibition of certain prostaglandins (see Chapter 4), which have a profound influence on a spectrum of physiologic functions, including blood clotting, blood pressure, inflammatory process, contraction of voluntary muscles, and transmission of nerve impulses (Table 17-4).

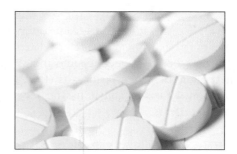

FIGURE 17-4   Aspirin remains one of the most popular pain relievers in the United States. (*Copyright 2006 JupiterImages Corporation.*)

Studies implicate aspirin in alleviating many disorders, dangers, and discomforts, including the following:

- Risk of repeated transient ischemic attacks (TIAs), or little strokes, is reduced by 50% in men (but not in women) who have already had one.
- Many studies indicate aspirin is effective in reducing risk for myocardial infarction.
- Aspirin is one of the most effective antiinflammatory drugs and is effective in long-term treatment of arthritis.
- Aspirin may play a role in inhibiting spread of some cancers through its action of inhibiting production of prostaglandin E_2.

TABLE 17-4	Is There a Difference in Pain Relievers?

Analgesic	Effects		Other Effects	Trade Names
	Pain Relief	**Fever Reduction**		
Aspirin (acetylsalicylic acid)	√	√	Antiinflammatory Reduces blood clotting Gastric irritation May cause Reye's syndrome in children with viral infection Allergic reaction	Ascriptin, Bayer, Bufferin, Ecotrin
Acetaminophen	√	√	Large doses can injure the liver or kidneys Use by persons who have 3 or more alcoholic drinks per day may cause liver damage	Tylenol
Ibuprofen	√	√	Antiinflammatory Gastric irritation Reduces blood clotting Worsens existing kidney problems	Advil, Motrin IB
Naproxen sodium	√	√	Antiinflammatory Reduces blood clotting Worsens existing kidney problems	Aleve
Ketoprofen	√	√	Antiinflammatory Gastric irritation Use by persons who have 3 or more alcoholic drinks per day may cause gastric bleeding	Orudis, Orudis KT

Data from Mayo Clinic Staff: *Over-the-counter pain reliever guide: compare before choosing,* Rochester, Minn, 2005 (April 11), MayoClinic.com *(www. mayoclinic.com).*

- Aspirin's effect as an anticoagulant is important in treatment of phlebitis and other clot-related disorders.
- Aspirin may be effective in promoting sleep. Many scientists now believe aspirin is as effective as most prescription sedatives, and it has far fewer and less serious side effects.

It is important to remember aspirin is a drug. Many of the benefits of aspirin stem from its systemic, wide-reaching effects on metabolism, which may have unforeseen short- and long-term detrimental results. We do know aspirin is to be strictly avoided by persons with hemophilia. Also, allergic reactions to aspirin can be severe. Aspirin seems to be implicated in asthma. Children are especially vulnerable to side effects and should not be given aspirin without a physician's instructions.

Aspirin is an irritant to the stomach and intestine. Its continuous use is associated with low-level chronic loss of iron caused by mucosal erosion. This can lead to iron deficiency anemia. Aspirin has been linked to birth defects, especially when it is taken later in the course of pregnancy. It increases risk of infant and neonatal mortality, low birth weight, and intracranial hemorrhage.

The best way to take aspirin is on an empty stomach with a full glass of water. This is important: absorption of aspirin is facilitated by a large volume of liquid and inhibited by the presence of food. In addition, taking aspirin—especially on an empty stomach—without a large fluid intake invites erosion of the stomach lining.[22] But aspirin should never be taken when using alcohol because it increases the bioavailability of alcohol, raising the blood concentration and thus the effect of alcohol on brain centers.[23]

TO SUM UP

Drugs can have multiple effects on the body's absorption, metabolism, retention, and nutrient status. They can provoke adverse reactions in combination with certain foods and can influence appetite, either repressing it or artificially stimulating it. Drugs can either increase an individual's absorption of nutrients or, more commonly, decrease absorption, sometimes leading to clinical deficiencies. Drugs can also induce mineral and vitamin deficiencies by their mode of action.

Just as drugs affect our use of food, food affects our use of drugs. Food can affect the absorption of drugs in a variety of ways. Foods also have an effect on subsequent distribution and metabolism of drugs. Vitamins may interfere with drug effectiveness, especially if they are taken in large doses. On the other hand, large doses of specific vitamins can be effective in countering certain toxicity conditions or a specific secondary deficiency induced by a genetic disease.

QUESTIONS FOR REVIEW

1. Name four ways food may affect drug use, and give examples of each.
2. If your patient were using a prescribed MAOI such as tranylcypromine sulfate (Parnate), what foods would you instruct the patient to avoid?
3. What is the most effective way to take aspirin? With what type of liquid? With or without food? Why?
4. What foods would you suggest to a hypertensive patient on the diuretic drug hydrochlorothiazide (HCTZ) as good sources of potassium replacement?
5. Outline suggestions you would discuss with a patient experiencing a drug-induced taste loss. How would you explain the cause of the taste loss?

REFERENCES

1. Ament PW, Bertolino JG, Liszewski JL: Clinically significant drug interactions, *Am Fam Physician* 61(6):1745, 2000.
2. Brown CH: Overview of drug interactions, *US Pharm* 25(5), 2000. Retrieved November 27, 2005, from *www.uspharmacist.com/index.asp?show=archive&issue=5_2000*.
3. Gnerali J: Avoiding drug interactions, *Am Fam Physician* 61(6):1628, 2000.
4. Smaglik P: Proliferation of pills, *Sci News* 151(20):310, 1997.
5. Woodard KW, Franklin RM: Treating elderly patients, *US Pharm* 24(8), 1999. Retrieved November 27, 2005, from *www.uspharmacist.com/index.asp?show=archive&issue=8_1999*.
6. U.S. Census Bureau: *Profiles of general demographic characteristics 2000*, Washington, DC, 2001, U.S. Department of Commerce.
7. Kaufman DW et al: Recent patterns of medication use in the ambulatory adult population of the United States: the Slone survey, *JAMA* 287(3):337, 2002.
8. Albion Research: Drug-nutrient interactions: this clinical consideration will continue to grow, *Albion Res Notes* 5(4):1, 1996.
9. Pronsky ZM: *Food medication interactions,* ed 13, Birchrunville, Pa, 2004, Food Medication Interactions.
10. Murray JJ, Healy MD: Drug-mineral interactions: a new responsibility for the hospital dietitian, *J Am Diet Assoc* 91(1):66, 1991.
11. Masse PG: Nutrient intakes of women who use oral contraceptives, *J Am Diet Assoc* 91(9):1118, 1991.
12. Green TJ et al: Oral contraceptives did not affect biochemical folate indexes and homocysteine concentrations in adolescent females, *J Am Diet Assoc* 98(1):50, 1998.
13. Merriman SH: Monoamine oxidase drugs and diet, *Hum Nutr Diet* 12:21, 1999.
14. Harats D et al: Citrus fruit supplementation reduces lipoprotein oxidation in young men ingesting a diet high in saturated fat: vitamin E presumptive evidence for an interaction between vitamins C and E in vivo, *Am J Clin Nutr* 67(2):240, 1998.
15. Harris JE: Interaction of dietary factors with oral anticoagulants: review and applications, *J Am Diet Assoc* 95(5):580, 1995.
16. Booth SL et al: Dietary vitamin K and stability of oral anticoagulation: proposal of a diet with constant vitamin K content, *Thromb Haemost* 77(3):408, 1997.
17. Lewis DP et al: Phenytoin-folic acid interaction, *Ann Pharmacother* 29(7/8):726, 1995.
18. Morris DJ et al: Licorice, chewing tobacco, and hypertension, *N Engl J Med* 151:733, 1991.
19. Kessler DA: Communicating with patients about their medications, *N Engl J Med* 325(23):1650, 1991.
20. Joint Commission on Accreditation of Healthcare Organizations: *Comprehensive accreditation manual for hospitals: the official handbook* (CAMH), Oakbrook Terrace, Ill, 2002, Author.
21. Schachtel BP et al: Caffeine as an analgesic adjuvant, *Arch Intern Med* 151:733, 1991.
22. Koch PA et al: Influence of food and fluid ingestion on aspirin bioavailability, *J Pharm Sci* 67(11):1533, 1978.
23. Roine R et al: Aspirin increases blood alcohol concentration in humans after ingestion of ethanol, *JAMA* 264(18):2406, 1990.

FURTHER READINGS AND RESOURCES

Readings

Ahmed FE: Effects of nutrition on the health of the elderly, *J Am Diet Assoc* 92(9):1102, 1992

Kerstetter JE et al: Malnutrition in the institutionalized adult, *J Am Diet Assoc* 92(9):1109, 1992.
These excellent companion articles speak to the twin problems of malnutrition and polypharmacy—multiple drug use—among older adults.

Clayman CB, ed: *Know your drugs and medications: the American Medical Association home medical library series,* Pleasantville, NY, 1991, Dorling Kindersly and Reader's Digest.

Herr SM: *Herb-drug interaction handbook,* ed 2, Nassau, NY, 2002, Church Street Books.

Kuhn MA, Winston D: *Herbal therapy and supplements: a scientific and traditional approach,* Philadelphia, 2001, Lippincott.
These resources, prepared for public education and patient-professional reference, provide useful information about effects and interactions of drugs in common use.

Thomas JA: Drug-nutrient interactions, *Nutr Rev* 53(10):271, 1995.
This is an excellent review with numerous tables. It is a "must read" for all persons taking care of patients and clients.

Websites of Interest

- U.S. Pharmacist; *U.S. Pharmacist* is a monthly journal dedicated to providing up-to-date, authoritative, peer-reviewed clinical articles relevant to contemporary pharmacy practice in a variety of settings: *www.uspharmacist.com/*.
- Grapefruit-Drug Interactions; created for pharmacists and other allied health professionals, this page is designed to provide up-to-date information in the large body of research on grapefruit-drug interactions: *www.powernetdesign.com/grapefruit/*.
- Center for Food-Drug Interaction Research and Education; this site, co-sponsored by the University of Florida and Tufts University, provides education about risk and potential significance of food-drug interactions based on scientifically-founded evidence: *www.druginteractioncenter.org/about.php.*
- Harvard University Health Services, Drug/Food Cautions; this website lists some common medications and specific interactions: *http://huhs.harvard.edu/HealthInformation/CWHCWellnessInformationFoodDrugInteractions.htm.*

- Food and Drug Administration, Center for Drug Evaluation and Research; in addition to offering a subscription service, this informative web page provides information on drug safety, quick information links, along with news from the Center for Drug Evaluation and Research: *www.fda.gov/cder/consumerinfo/druginteractions.htm.*
- American Academy of Family Physicians, familydoctor.org; this consumer-focused website provides links to the Family Doctor website: *http://familydoctor.org/121.xml.*

- Medline Plus; this website has gathered facts from the National Library of Medicine, National Institutes of Health, and other government agencies and health-related organizations to provide information on thousands of prescription and over-the-counter medicines: *www.nlm.nih.gov/medlineplus/druginformation.html.*
- Rx List: The Internet Drug List; sponsored by WebMD, this website provides food drug interaction information for consumers and health professionals: *www.rxlist.com/.*

CHAPTER 18

Nutrition Support: Enteral and Parenteral Nutrition

M. Patricia Fuhrman

In this chapter we look at alternate modes of feeding to provide nutrition support for patients with special needs. We examine ways of feeding when the gastrointestinal tract can be used—enteral nutrition given orally or through a feeding tube. Then we review nutrient feeding directly into a vein when the gastrointestinal tract cannot be used—parenteral nutrition (PN).

Malnutrition, preexisting and hospital-induced, is a serious concern in hospitalized patients, especially those with critical illness or injury. Nutrition care provided by a skilled nutrition support team or clinician can have a positive effect on patient survival and recovery. This chapter will examine enteral and PN support formulas, solutions, and delivery systems for use in hospital and home.

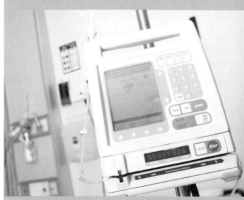

Copyright 2006 JupiterImages Corporation.

NUTRITION ASSESSMENT

Nutrition Support and Degree of Malnutrition

It is an easier task to maintain nutrition than to replenish body stores from malnutrition. The effect of starvation on the body, even during relatively brief periods, is well documented.[1] The small amount of glycogen stored in the liver is a crucial immediate energy source. Glycogen breakdown for fuel begins 2 to 3 hours after a meal, and glycogen stores are depleted after 30 hours of fasting in the absence of metabolic stress. Release of amino acids from body tissue proteins begins after 4 to 6 hours of fasting to provide a source of blood glucose. Also, fatty acids are mobilized from the body's adipose tissues to provide keto acids as a principal fuel for heart, brain, and other vital organs. As adaptation to starvation occurs, the body relies less on amino acids from protein for fuel and uses more ketones from fat to meet metabolic needs. This reduces nitrogen losses and preserves lean body mass. During critical illness this adaptation to insufficient energy to meet needs does not occur. Severely ill patients rely heavily on large amounts of glucose and protein for fuel. They often have elevated insulin levels, which inhibit the mobilization of fat for energy production and thus increase reliance on amino acids from protein with a urinary nitrogen loss of 10 to 15 g/day or greater that continues unchecked. Critical illness can lead to severe depletion of lean body mass. Nutrition provided during critical illness reduces but does not reverse the process.

For example, two healthy people are hiking in the mountains and get lost. They have a limited supply of food but adequate water available from mountain streams. Hiker #1 is severely injured in a fall while the two are searching for the way back to civilization. Both have inadequate food supply to meet their energy needs. Hiker #2 will initially use glycogen stores followed by breakdown of lean body mass and fat for energy needs. However, after several days the body will decrease its use of protein for energy and start relying on fat so lean body mass is preserved as long as possible. This is the adaptation to starvation. Hiker #1 will not adapt to starvation. He will continue to use protein for energy and rely much less on fat for fuel and thus will lose more lean body mass during the period of inadequate energy supply than Hiker #2.

Any medical treatment has less chance of success if the patient is malnourished. The patient who becomes malnourished during hospitalization (iatrogenic malnutrition) has been referred to as "the skeleton in the hospital closet" with several reports of general malnutrition among hospitalized patients.[2-6] Lack of adequate nutrition to meet metabolic demands is increasingly recognized as a serious concern in medical and surgical patients. Adult malnutrition can be defined as inadequate nutrient intake, digestion, absorption, or metabolism that results in a significant weight change from usual body or ideal body weight over a defined period.[7] Braunschweig and colleagues[6] reported that as many as 54% of patients admitted to the hospital were malnourished, and 31% of these patients declined nutritionally during hospitalization.

In addition, the disease process itself imposes a nutritional risk and affects nutrient requirements. Deterioration of a patient's nutritional status during hospitalization contributes to increased length of hospital stay, development of comorbidities, and increased cost.[6] Persons with underlying chronic disease, traumatic injury, and older adults are particularly at risk. Thus assessment, monitoring, and reassessment of nutritional status become an important part of overall care, especially for hospitalized patients (see Chapter 16). For the severely malnourished patient, especially those facing problems such as organ failure or extensive surgery, adequate and consistent provision of nutrition support is indicated. The guiding principle for provision of nutrition support is "If the gut works, use it." Studies have shown patients experience fewer infectious complications and shorter length of stay and recover more rapidly when fed enterally rather than parenterally.[8,9]

A general screening and assessment program at hospital admission should be a routine procedure to identify those already in states of malnutrition, as well as those at risk of potential malnutrition because of their underlying disease or injury.[6] In the hospital the attending nurse or another healthcare professional may discover eating problems or disorders in a patient and confer with the registered dietitian (RD), who can evaluate any malnutrition risks associated with the current hospitalization and perform a full nutrition assessment.

The RD conducts the initial nutrition assessment and performs ongoing monitoring of nutritional status. Initial assessment data supply the necessary basis for (1) identifying patients requiring nutrition intervention, (2) determining appropriate nutrition support route: enteral or parenteral, (3) calculating the patient's nutrient requirements, (4) determining specific formulations to meet requirements, and (5) identifying measurable nutrition-related outcomes for determining if the nutrition care plan is appropriate and effective. Once therapy begins, careful monitoring maintains optimal therapy and avoids metabolic, septic, and gastrointestinal complications.

Guidelines for Nutrition Assessment

Nutrition assessment is done through a standard approach and includes several key parameters: (1) evaluation of nutrient intake and adequacy, (2) nutrition-focused physical assessment, (3) biochemical laboratory data, (4) anthropometrics, (5) comprehensive review of medical and surgical histories, and (6) nutrition diagnosis.[10,11] Nutrition assessment techniques and parameters are described in detail in Chapter 16. However, standard nutrition assessment parameters are adversely affected by critical illness and inflammatory response. Weight is often affected by fluid status and may no longer reflect usual or current body weight. Laboratory values are often not reflective of nutrition, particularly if the patient has inadequate liver or renal function, acid-base imbalance, or abnormal hydration status. Constitutive hepatic proteins such as serum albumin, transferrin, and prealbumin are decreased as a result of inflammation and do not reflect nutritional status; therefore the clinician must rely primarily on subjective global assessment (Box 18-1) and astute clinical judgment to perform and interpret assessment of nutritional status.[5,12] Subjective global assessment focuses on two features: history and physical examination.[5] This technique eliminates the ambiguity and nonspecific, nonsensitive nature of laboratory values during critical illness and inflammation.

History

History includes all aspects of the patient's health: weight change, nutrient intake, gastrointestinal function and symptoms, functional capacity, and diagnosis, and its nutritional impact. The clinician should identify whether the patient has experienced an intentional or nonintentional weight change from normal or usual weight and time frame during which the weight change occurred. Quantifying weight loss is not always easy, particularly if the patient has lost lean body mass but weight is unchanged because the patient is retaining fluid as occurs with end-stage liver, heart, and kidney diseases. Current or actual body weight (ABW) and height are interpreted according to changes from usual body weight (UBW) and the percent of recent weight change:

$$\text{Percent usual body weight} = \text{ABW} \div \text{UBW} \times 100$$

$$\text{Percent weight change} = [(\text{UBW} - \text{ABW}) \div \text{UBW}] \times 100$$

BOX 18-1	Subjective Global Assessment Components

History

Change in weight
Change in dietary intake
Gastrointestinal symptoms
Functional capacity
Nutritional requirements of disease

Physical Assessment

Loss of subcutaneous fat
Muscle loss
Fluid retention
- Ankle and sacral edema
- Ascites

From Detsky AS et al: What is subjective global assessment of nutritional status? *JPEN J Parenter Enteral Nutr* 11(1):8, 1987, with permission from the American Society for Enteral and Parenteral Nutrition (A.S.P.E.N.). A.S.P.E.N. does not endorse the use of this material in any form other than its entirety.

The amount of recent weight change is compared with values associated with malnutrition (Table 18-1).

Changes in appetite and dietary intake must be assessed to identify overall nutrient adequacy of the diet and potential contributing factors for reported weight loss. It is important to identify diet modifications followed and nutritional supplements consumed by the patient. The clinician must verify whether nutritional supplements are being taken in addition to meals or used as a meal replacement. Gastrointestinal function determines the ability to assimilate nutrients. Presence of nausea, vomiting, diarrhea, and anorexia inhibits nutrient intake and availability. Assessment of functional capacity of the patient determines whether the patient can perform activities of daily living completely or in part or if the patient is bedridden and totally dependent on others for care. Medical and surgical history entails examination of the past and current medical problems and enables the clinician to identify potential risks for nutrient inadequacies, deficiencies, excesses, and toxicities.

Physical Examination

During the physical assessment the clinician looks for signs of muscle and fat wasting. Inspection of the upper body can identify temporal, clavicular, and torso wasting of skeletal muscle mass and subcutaneous fat. Signs of edema and ascites indicate inability to keep fluid in the vascular space with subsequent interstitial fluid accumulation. Physical signs and symptoms are then

TABLE 18-1	Categorization of Severity of Weight Loss by Percentage of Weight Lost Over Time	
Time Period	**Significant Weight Loss (%)**	**Severe Weight Loss (%)**
1 week	1-2	>2
1 month	5	>5
3 months	7.5	>7.5
6 months	10	>10

Modified from the American Society for Parenteral and Enteral Nutrition (A.S.P.E.N.): Nutritional and metabolic assessment of the hospitalized patient, *JPEN J Parenter Enteral Nutr* 1(1):11, 1977. A.S.P.E.N. does not endorse the use of this material in any other form than its entirety.

enteral A feeding modality that provides nutrients, either orally or by tube feeding through the gastrointestinal tract.

parenteral A feeding modality that provides nutrient solutions intravenously rather than through the gastrointestinal tract.

correlated to the patient's disease process and current medical condition.

Basal Energy Expenditure

An estimate of an adult patient's energy or kilocalorie (kcalorie or kcal) needs can be performed using more than 200 different calculations. The Harris-Benedict equations (HBE) were originally published in 1919 and are the most commonly used regression formulas for estimating basal energy expenditure.[13] Daily energy requirements are estimated by combining basal energy expenditures (BEE), disease/injury energy needs, and physical activity (see Chapter 5). A healthy person's energy requirements will not include a factor for disease/injury. The hospitalized patient's increased disease/injury energy requirement is often offset by decreased physical activity.

HBE uses measures of weight in kilograms, height in centimeters, and age in years, as follows[13]:

Women: BEE = 655 + [9.6 × Weight (kg)] +
$$[1.8 \times \text{Height (cm)}] - [4.7 \times \text{Age (yr)}]$$

Men: BEE = 66.5 + [13.8 × Weight (kg)] +
$$[5.0 \times \text{Height (cm)}] - [6.8 \times \text{Age (yr)}]$$

For example, for a 35-year-old woman weighing 60 kg (132 pounds) who is 165 cm (5 ft 5 in) tall, the formula would appear as follows:

$$655 + (9.6 \times 60) + (1.8 \times 165) - (4.7 \times 35) =$$
$$655 + 576 + 297 - 165 = 1364 \text{ kcal/day}$$

The HBE has been found to overestimate energy needs by 5% to 15%. The Mifflin-St Jeor (MSJ) equations were published in 1990 and have a greater accuracy than HBE in normal weight and obese patients.[14,15] In addition, the MSJ equation development included obese patients. The MSJ equation uses measures of weight in kilograms, height in centimeters, and age in years to calculate resting energy expenditure (REE):

Women: REE = (10 × Wt) + (6.25 × Ht) −
$$(5 \times \text{Age}) - 161$$

Men: REE = (10 × Wt) + (6.25 × Ht) − (5 × Age) + 5

For example, for a 35-year-old woman, 60 kg (132 pounds), 165 cm (5 ft 5 in):

$$(10 \times 60) + (6.25 \times 165) - (5 \times 35) - 161 = 600 +$$
$$1031 - 175 - 161 = 1295 \text{ kcal/day}$$

The term *resting energy expenditure (REE)* is often used interchangeably with BEE in discussing basal energy needs. In general, energy provision to critically ill patients should not exceed 20% above BEE/REE. However, there are metabolic conditions such as severe burns or head injury that create energy needs up to 50% to 100% above BEE.

Energy requirements for hospitalized patients on nutrition support vary with degree of metabolic stress, but generally range from 20 to 35 kcal/kg. Regardless of the calculation used to estimate energy expenditure, it is important to monitor the impact of nutrients provided to determine changes needed to maintain or replete the patient. Energy and nutrients are adjusted based on patient tolerance and desired versus actual response to nutrient provision.

The more malnourished a patient is, the more carefully resumption of nutrition should be done. Refeeding syndrome is a life-threatening response to overaggressive provision of energy to a patient who has been chronically starved. Hallmark symptoms of refeeding are a shift of electrolytes from blood into the cell resulting in decreased blood levels of potassium, phosphorus, and magnesium along with increased blood glucose levels and fluid retention.[16] The end result can be cardiac collapse and death.

Critically ill patients with major trauma, sepsis, and inflammation demonstrate catabolism (breakdown of body tissue) resulting in a net loss of body mass. When protein is broken down, the nitrogen component of amino acids is released and excreted in urine. Nitrogen lost in urine can be as high as 15 to 30 g over 24 hours. This can result in a negative nitrogen balance if the patient is losing more nitrogen in urine than is provided from protein in the diet. Catabolic periods with losses of lean body mass are inevitable after trauma and extensive surgery. The catabolic process increases nutrient demand and requirements. Initiating nutrition support in these patients reduces, but does not eliminate, negative nitrogen balance that occurs after traumatic injury or critical illness.

Nitrogen Balance

Nitrogen balance studies are calculations that estimate of the degree of catabolism. The patient's intake of protein (nitrogen) is subtracted from nitrogen output through urinary and insensible losses:

$$N_2 \text{ Balance} = N_2 \text{ Intake} - N_2 \text{ Loss}$$

$$N_2 \text{ Intake} = \text{Protein intake} \div 6.25*$$

$$N_2 \text{ Loss} = \text{Urinary urea nitrogen} + 4\dagger$$

For example, a patient receiving 50 g of protein per day in an enteral tube feeding is getting 8 g of nitrogen per day (50 g ÷ 6.25 = 8 g). If that individual's nitrogen losses are 10 g per 24 hours (6 g in urine per nitrogen balance study + 4 g of insensible losses), the patient's nitrogen balance is −2 g/24 hr. Increasing protein in the enteral tube feeding to more than 62.5 g protein per day will result in a positive nitrogen balance.

---

*6.25 g of protein yields 1 g N_2.
†Estimated insensible losses of N_2.

However, nitrogen balance calculation is not accurate with renal failure or retained nitrogen such as elevated blood urea nitrogen (BUN). Other sources of nitrogen such as blood products, as well as losses of nitrogen from wounds, stool, nasogastric suction, and bleeding, must also be taken into account when calculating nitrogen balance. The 4 g of insensible nitrogen loss may not be an accurate estimate and could affect accuracy of the results. Measurement of urinary urea nitrogen requires an accurate 24-hour urine collection. Nitrogen balance should be performed serially (e.g., weekly) to monitor changes in status because the patient's condition does not remain constant.

Hepatic Proteins as Nutrition Indicators

Hepatic proteins, albumin, transferrin, and prealbumin are often used to determine the patient's nutritional status. During critical illness, hepatic production of constitutive proteins—albumin, transferrin, and prealbumin—is decreased in favor of increased production of acute phase reactants required for survival.[12,17] A decreased serum value of albumin, prealbumin, or transferrin therefore signifies an inflammatory process or how sick the patient is and does not provide information about the patient's nutritional status or response to nutrition therapy. These proteins are better used as prognostic indicators of the patient's risk of complications (morbidity) and death (mortality).

Management of Nutrition Support Patients

Management of nutrition support is ideally performed by an official interdisciplinary nutrition support committee or team composed of designated members from the departments of medicine, surgery, nutrition, nursing, and pharmacy.[18] Each team member should be certified in nutrition support by an accrediting body such as the National Board of Nutrition Support Certification and the Board of Pharmaceutical Specialties. The American Society for Parenteral and Enteral Nutrition (A.S.P.E.N.) has developed standards of practice for nutrition support professionals and interdisciplinary nutrition support competencies.[19-23] However, in many facilities, nutrition support management is overseen by an informal collection of interested clinicians, a sole nutrition support practitioner, or no one person in particular. Standards of the Joint Commission on Accreditation of Healthcare Organizations (JCAHO) and the Accreditation Manual for Hospitals (AMH) have focused on key multidisciplinary processes that ensure performance of nutrition screening and assessment to promote quality patient outcomes.[24] (See the *Focus on Culture* box, "What's Religion Got to Do With It?" for additional considerations surrounding nutrition support.)

Baseline nutrition data obtained before starting nutrition support provide a means of measuring effectiveness of treatment. At designated periods during therapy, certain tests are repeated to monitor the patient's course and reduce metabolic complications. Specific protocols vary in different medical centers. However, a general guide for standard monitoring data is summarized in Box 18-2.[25]

Generally, clinicians give primary importance to the following three major monitoring parameters: (1) serial weights to determine adequacy of total energy provision and to monitor fluid status, (2) physical examination for micronutrient adequacy and changes in body fat and muscle mass, and, ultimately (3) improvement in functional status.

All baseline and monitoring data are recorded in the patient's chart, along with all enteral and parenteral solution orders.

There are no evidence-based "rules" for the time to start nutrition support with either enteral or parenteral nutrition. Determination of when to initiate nutrition support depends on the patient's nutritional status and the anticipated time period before oral diet can be resumed and tolerated. A.S.P.E.N. guidelines recommend that nutrition support should be considered when patients have had an inadequate oral intake for 7 to 14 days or the patient's oral intake is anticipated to remain inadequate for 7 to 14 days.[7] A 5- to 10-day timeline is recommended

---

BOX 18-2	Clinical Parameters to Monitor During Nutrition Support

Daily intake and output (I/O)
Daily weights
Physical examination
Temperature, pulse, respirations
Laboratory parameters:
- Acid-base status
- Blood urea nitrogen (BUN)
- Complete blood cell count (CBC)
- Creatinine
- Electrolytes
- Glucose
- International Normalized Ratio (INR)
- Liver function tests
- Osmolarity, serum and urine
- Platelet count
- Prothrombin time (PT)
- Triglyceride level
- Urinary urea nitrogen
- Urine specific gravity
- Vitamins and minerals

---

constitutive proteins Albumin, prealbumin, transferrin. Plasma proteins often used to assess the response to nutrition support. Serum levels are nonspecific and nonsensitive to nutritional status or requirements.

FOCUS ON CULTURE

What's Religion Got to Do With It?

"That was not a natural death. It was an imposed death." said Cardinal Renato Martino, a top Vatican official. "When you deprive somebody of food and water, what else is it? Nothing else but murder." In this impassioned statement the Cardinal was referring to the landmark battle over the life of Terri Schiavo following her death after nearly 2 weeks without any nutrition support. Over 15 years had passed since Terri Schiavo had suffered severe brain damage stemming from heart failure and had relied on enteral nutrition for survival ever since. The legal decision to remove her tube feeding created a national uproar and sparked many debates over end-of-life issues, including nutrition support. The Catholic Church fervently opposed the legal action taken and was especially vocal in the events surrounding Terri Schiavo's death because she was Catholic.

What role does religion have in issues such as nutrition support? In this section we will encapsulate beliefs of three religions, focusing on end-of-life issues, particularly nutrition support.

Catholicism

Because Catholics believe they are stewards of their bodies and life is to be respected, the act of withholding nutrition support is not something to be taken lightly. However, bodily life is not to be maintained at all costs. The late John Paul II wrote: "Certainly there is a moral obligation to care for oneself and allow oneself to be cared for, but this duty must take account for concrete circumstances. It needs to be determined whether the means of treatment available are objectively proportionate to the prospects for improvement."

In short, withdrawal of nutrition support is not condemned, but rather only recommended when quality of life is so low nutrition is of absolutely no benefit. Although it is hard to know where the point of "no benefit" is, it is the duty of a Catholic to promote a social order in which there is a certain level of responsibility to those who are marginalized or in a vegetative state. Each case merits special consideration, and in most cases nutrition is considered a basic form of care likened to warmth and cleanliness.

Judaism

According to Judaism, life possesses an intrinsic value as a divine gift of creation. As in Catholicism, humans are thought to be only a temporary steward of the body and therefore must treat the body with utmost respect and sensitivity. Jewish law mandates humans must do everything in their power to heal themselves when ill and must also strive to save the lives of others. This obligation, however, applies only to those therapies that have a reasonable chance of success, and although some believe tube feeding is equivalent to medical treatments, Jewish tradition disagrees with this opinion. According to Jewish authorities, nutrition in any form is a basic human need and should be provided to all patients unless feeding itself causes suffering. Consequently, Jewish law further accentuates feeding must be done in a kind and compassionate manner, emphasizing the importance this religion places on nourishment.

Islam

Not unlike the other religions mentioned in this section, in Islam humans are thought of as stewards of their bodies, which are viewed as a "gift" from God. Sanctity of life is a monumental principle, and every moment of life is deemed precious and must be preserved. Even so, death is believed to be a natural part of life, and treatment does not have to be provided if it merely prolongs the final stages of a terminal illness. Nutrition support—especially enteral—is considered part of basic care rather than a treatment; therefore it is a religious obligation to provide nourishment unless such an act shortens life.

Religion and end-of-life issues like nutrition support are complicated and sensitive matters that must be approached with understanding and tolerance. People from different religious backgrounds can have varying views on this subject that can drastically affect the choice of care provided. The Terri Schiavo case brought to life a plethora of issues that will not likely be resolved any time soon; however, when dealing with nutrition support cases, it is important to consider the implications that the patient's religion can have for your decisions and actions.

References

Associated Press: Vatican: Schiavo's death "cruel," *Fox News,* March 31, 2005.

Clarfiels A et al: Ethical issues in end-of-life geriatric care: the approach of three monotheistic religions—Judaism, Catholicism, and Islam, *J Am Geriatr Soc* 51:1149, 2003.

Cooley M: Faith, ethics help many in agonizing dilemma, *The Spokesman-Review,* March 27, 2005, ProQuest Information and Learning Company.

Huggins C: *Survey finds physicians willing to allow patients' religion to trump medical advice* [news release, Professional Medical News], New York, 2005 (August 9), Reuters Health Information.

Jotkowitz A, Clarfield A, Slick S: The care of patients with dementia: a modern Jewish ethical perspective, *J Am Geriatr Soc* 53:881, 2005.

Sunshine E: Truncating Catholic tradition: Florida bishops avoid full consideration of ethical issues in Schiavo case, *National Catholic Reporter* 2005 (April 8). Retrieved December 22, 2005, from *http:// ncronline.org/NCR_Online/archives2/2005b/040805/040805k.php.*

for critically ill patients. Other guidelines available to identify when to feed are the "rule of five" and degree of weight loss. The "rule of five" states that if a patient has had no food for 5 days and is unable to tolerate an oral diet for an additional 5 days, nutrition support should be considered to reduce the risk of developing malnutrition. The weight loss rule stratifies patients according to percentage of weight loss of their usual body weight over a designated period (see Table 18-1). Patients who have undergone severe weight loss and are unable to tolerate oral nutrition for 5 to 7 days or longer are candidates for nutrition support.

ENTERAL NUTRITION VERSUS PARENTERAL NUTRITION

There is ongoing debate concerning evidence-based effectiveness of parenteral and enteral nutrition support. Questions focus on what constitutes early enteral nutrition, how to select the most appropriate enteral tube feeding formula according to each patient's specific disease state, what is the preferred method of formula delivery, and which factors contribute to enteral tube feeding–related complications, such as diarrhea or respiratory problems.[26,27] In all

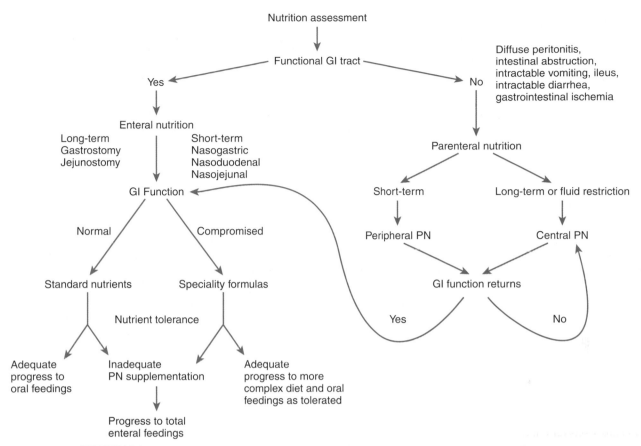

FIGURE 18-1 Route of administration of specialized nutrition support. *(Redrawn from A.S.P.E.N. Board of Directors:* Clinical pathways and algorithms for delivery of parenteral and enteral nutrition support in adults, *Silver Spring, Md,* *1998, A.S.P.E.N.)* A.S.P.E.N. does not endorse the use of this material in any form other than its entirety.

cases when the gastrointestinal tract is functioning, enteral nutrition support should be used to restore or maintain an optimal state of nutrition. PN should be reserved for patients with a nonfunctional gastrointestinal tract or an inadequately functional gastrointestinal tract that prevents the patient from meeting nutrient needs enterally. In some cases the patient can take some enteral feeding but impairment in either digestive or absorptive capacity requires supplementation with parenteral therapy. The Veterans Affairs (VA) Cooperative Study showed perioperative nutrition support was beneficial for severely malnourished patients but contributed to increased complications in mild to moderately malnourished patients.[28] The gastrointestinal tract should always be the first choice for nutrition support. Figure 18-1 provides an algorithm for determining the route of nutrition support.[7]

PN is associated with serious complications, as shown in Box 18-3. Reliance on PN when the gastrointestinal tract is functional can contribute to disuse of the gastrointestinal tract with subsequent bacterial overgrowth, hepatic abnormalities, deterioration of gastrointestinal integrity with subsequent migration of intestinal bacteria into the systemic circulation, and sepsis. Patients reliant solely on PN are at risk for septic and hepatic

---

BOX 18-3	**Complications Associated With Parenteral Nutrition**

Catheter-Related

Air embolism
Catheter embolization
Catheter occlusion
Improper tip location
Phlebitis
Pneumothorax
Sepsis
Venous thrombosis

Gastrointestinal

Fatty liver
Gastric hyperacidity
Gastrointestinal atrophy
Hepatic cholestasis

Metabolic

Acid-base imbalance
Electrolyte abnormalities
Essential fatty acid
  deficiency
Fluid imbalance
Glucose intolerance
Metabolic bone disease
Mineral abnormalities
Overfeeding
Refeeding syndrome
Triglyceride elevation

---

complications that can contribute to morbidity and mortality. The gastrointestinal tract is the body's largest immune organ. Gastrointestinal disease that prevents or reduces use of the gastrointestinal tract may itself contribute to adverse effects often associated with PN. Therefore it may not be the route of feeding, but rather the inability to use the gut that increases infectious and metabolic complications.[29] Some adverse effects of PN may be related to inability to provide all necessary nutrients parenterally. Parenteral solutions are not as "complete" (i.e., do not contain the wide variety of nutrients) as enteral formulas or oral diet because of the complexity of adding all nutrients found in nature to an intravenous solution.

ENTERAL TUBE FEEDING IN CLINICAL NUTRITION

Modes of Enteral Nutrition Support

Many patients with a functioning gastrointestinal tract do not or cannot eat a sufficient amount of nutrients by mouth to restore, repair, or maintain physiologic systems or body tissues. The first option for providing adequate nutrition should be to deliver nutrients orally. The patient can be given small, frequent nutrient-dense meals with an oral liquid nutritional supplement. If oral intake remains suboptimal despite attempts to increase nutrient intake with nutritional supplements and diet changes, enteral tube feeding can be initiated to meet nutrient and energy requirements. If it is not feasible to use the gastrointestinal tract for feeding or if the gastrointestinal tract cannot effectively provide consistent and adequate nutrition, PN may be an appropriate feeding modality. Therefore the following questions must be answered:

- Does the patient require nutrition support?
- What is the optimal route of feeding: oral, tube feeding, parenteral?
- Will the enteral route alone be sufficient to meet nutrient and energy requirements?
- What type of formula is needed, and how should it be provided?
- Does the patient require long-term nutrition support?

Oral Diet

When a patient does not consume a nutritionally complete diet, the energy value of foods in the oral diet can be increased according to patient tolerance and preference with added sauces, seasonings, and dressings. Frequent, less bulky, concentrated small meals may be helpful so the patient is not overwhelmed or discouraged by a tray full of food. If a patient is on a modified diet (such as a low-fat, low-sodium, or diabetic diet), liberalization of the diet as much as medically feasible can help improve oral intake. For example, changing from a regimented 1800-kcal diabetic diet to a carbohydrate-counting diet allows the patient more flexibility in food selection. In some cases, it may be necessary to liberalize to an unrestricted or regular diet in order to increase oral intake. Depending on the patient's condition and food preferences, an oral liquid nutritional supplement, commercially available or made in-house, can be provided with or between meals. However, taste fatigue

can happen fairly rapidly when patients are receiving two to six cans of an oral nutritional supplement per day. Patients may use their nutritional supplements as meal replacements, therefore not increasing overall energy and nutrient intake. It is important to offer nutritional supplements in a variety of flavors and textures to maintain adequate consumption. Some facilities, particularly those specializing in long-term care, have found that dispensing oral nutritional supplements in small amounts of 30 to 60 ml during times when medications are administered improved oral nutritional supplement intake and nutrient delivery.[30,31]

Enteral Tube Feeding

If a sufficient oral intake of nutrients and energy is not possible, then the next option is enteral nutrition by tube feeding, either as a supplement to oral dietary intake or as the sole source of nutrition.

Indications for Enteral Tube Feeding

A.S.P.E.N. has published guidelines for indications for nutrition support.[7] Enteral tube feeding is indicated for patients who are or who are likely to become malnourished and unable or unwilling to consume adequate nutrition by mouth. Factors that affect the decision to provide enteral tube feeding include the patient's preadmission nutritional status, risk for malnutrition based on current disease/condition, ability to consume a nutritionally complete oral diet, and functional status of the gastrointestinal tract. Research found no benefit of aggressive early enteral tube feeding for patients who were not malnourished versus those who waited 6 days to begin an oral diet.[32]

ENTERAL TUBE FEEDING FORMULAS

Complete Enteral Tube Feeding Formulas

Blenderized or Commercial

Our current age of advanced nutrition science and technology has brought a variety of commercial enteral formulas and smaller, safer, more comfortable feeding tubes. The majority of enteral tube feedings in healthcare facilities are given with a defined, commercially prepared enteral tube feeding formula. However, financial or personal reasons may motivate a patient or family to use blenderized formulas for home enteral tube feeding. Although there may be emotional comfort in the use of home-prepared food, there are problems involved (see the *Complementary and Alternative Medicine {CAM}* box, "Home-made Enteral Formulas: A Recipe for Trouble?"). These problems involve its physical form that could cause tube clogging, an increased risk of bacterial contamination, and inconsistent nutrient adequacy based on foods used and preparation techniques. The blenderized formula must be given into the stomach and requires a normal

COMPLEMENTARY AND ALTERNATIVE MEDICINE (CAM)
Homemade Enteral Formulas: A Recipe for Trouble?

Home-based enteral nutrition support is a common and safe practice that has been in existence for decades. Many people have benefited from the freedom and medical support it provides and can maintain a healthy nutritional status in spite of the fact they cannot consume an oral diet. Advancements in pumps, tubes, and placement of tubes are all contributing factors to the success rate of home tube feeding, but another major improvement of note are enteral feeding solutions themselves. Over the years, commercial enteral feeding solutions have grown to encompass many brands and formulas specialized for nutrient needs or even a particular disease state. Most formulas can supply total nutrition to the recipient of enteral nutrition support and cause few side effects if administered and calculated correctly. So with all of the options commercially available, why would someone want to make their own "homemade" enteral solutions, and is it safe to do so?

In the past, homemade enteral solutions were a widely used and accepted entity for enteral nutrition support at home and even in hospitals. Many people, particularly home caretakers, considered homemade solutions a more economical and personally fulfilling method. Home caretakers such as mothers, fathers, or spouses believed making the solutions was a more affectionate and devoted method as apposed to simply opening a can. Even so, current consensus directs the consumer away from these homemade solutions not only because of the advancements in commercial formulas, but also because of potential problems with homemade solutions.

As mentioned above, commercial formulas are nutritionally complete and specialized for a wide array of nutritional and disease states. These commercial feedings are also consistent in their formulation and, as such, are easily quantifiable to readily meet the recipient's needs. Conversely, homemade solutions of varying composition have no exact method of quantification or verification of nutritional content. Furthermore, these solutions are not tested for digestive and absorptive properties like commercial solutions, which can lead to a host of problems such as dehydration, constipation, vitamin deficiency, and even severe malnourishment.

Sanitation is a critical variable to consider when dealing with nutrition support and choosing an enteral feeding solution. Its importance cannot be overstated. Although there is no way to totally avoid contamination of enteral feeding, use of commercially prepared solutions can considerably limit the chance of a health risk. Points of potential contamination such as preparation, cooking, and blenderizing are all omitted, leaving the caretaker with less of a chance of exposing the recipient to a potentially serious bacterial or viral infection—this can be especially important for those who have an altered immune system. In addition, commercially available formulas lessen the workload of the administer and guard the recipient from clogs associated with underblenderized feedings.

For the vast majority of those receiving enteral nutrition support, commercially available tube feeding solutions are the appropriate choice. The advantages of being easily quantifiable and safe from foodborne illness and providing complete nutritional content far outweigh any advantages of a homemade solution. Guiding those who might otherwise use homemade tube feedings can simplify nutrition support and protect them from potential complications.

References

Duperret E, Trautlein J: *Homemade tube feeding formula . . . Two dietitians' perspective,* Tucson, Ariz, 2003 (November 20), Mealtime Notions. Retrieved December 22, 2005, from *www.marshadunnklein.com/Guest.htm.*

Malone A: Enteral formula selection: a review of selected categories, *Pract Gastroenterol* June(Series 28):44, 2005.

Mokhalalati J et al: Microbial, nutritional and physical quality of commercial and hospital prepared tube feedings in Saudi Arabia, *Saudi Med J* 25(3):331, 2004.

Stanley D: Forward, *JPEN J Parenter Enter Nutr* 25(5 suppl):S2, 2002 (10 September) (ProQuest Information and Learning Company).

Sullivan M et al: Nutritional analysis of blenderized enteral diets in the Philippines, *Asia Pac J Clin Nutr* 13(4):385, 2004.

gastrointestinal tract to digest and absorb the nutrients contained in the formula. Use of blenderized formulas has decreased over the past 20 years with the proliferation of commercially available enteral tube feeding formulas.

Commercial Enteral Tube Feeding Formulas

In contrast, commercial enteral tube feeding formulas provide sterile, nutritionally complete, homogenized solutions suitable for small-bore enteral feeding tubes. Enteral tube feeding formulas are available as polymeric, semielemental or oligomeric, and elemental or monomeric[33] (Table 18-2). It is important to keep abreast of products currently available because new formulations and enteral tube feeding products are constantly being developed. Polymeric enteral tube feeding formulas require digestion and are available with and without fiber. Macronutrients and micronutrients of a polymeric tube feeding formula can be modified for specific needs of

patients with various disease states. Semielemental or oligomeric tube feeding formulas are partially digested or hydrolyzed. Smaller molecules increase the osmolality of the formula. Elemental or monomeric tube feeding formulas are completely predigested and require only absorption for assimilation into the body. These formulas have the highest osmolality, lowest viscosity, and worst taste of all enteral tube feeding formulas. Tube feeding formulas will also vary according to nutrient density

> osmolality The ability of a solution to create osmotic pressure and determine the movement of water between fluid compartments; determined by the number of osmotically active particles per kilogram of solvent; serum osmolality is 280 to 300 mOsm/kg.

| TABLE 18-2 | Categories and Macronutrient Sources for Various Types of Enteral Formulas |

Type of Formula	Protein Sources	Carbohydrate Sources	Fat Sources	Kcal/ml	Protein Content	Nonprotein Calorie-to-Nitrogen Ratio	Examples
Intact (Polymeric)	Calcium and magnesium caseinates Sodium and calcium caseinates Soy protein isolate Calcium-potassium caseinate Delactosed lactalbumin Egg white solids Beef Nonfat milk	Maltodextrin Corn syrup solids Sucrose Cornstarch Glucose polymers Sugar Vegetables Fruits Nonfat milk	Medium-chain triglycerides Canola oil Corn oil Lecithin Soybean oil Partially hydrogenated soybean oil High-oleic safflower oil Beef fat	1-2	30-84 g/L	75-177:1	Boost (No) Compleat (No) Fibersource (No) Isocal (No) Isosource (No) Jevity (R) Nutren (Ne) Osmolite (R) Resource (No) TwoCal HN (R) Ultracal (No)
Hydrolyzed (Oligomeric or Monomeric)	Enzymatically hydrolyzed whey or Casein Soybean or lactalbumin hydrolysate Whey protein Free amino acids Soy protein hydrolysate	Hydrolyzed cornstarch Sucrose Fructose Maltodextrin Tapioca starch Glucose oligosaccharides	Medium-chain triglycerides Sunflower oil Lecithin Soybean oil Safflower oil Corn oil Coconut oil Canola oil Sardine oil	1-1.33	21-52.5 g/L	67-282:1	Advera (R) AlitraQ (R) Criticare HN (No) Crucial (Ne) Peptamen (Ne) Perative (R) Tolerex (No) Vital HN (R) Vivonex Plus (No)
Modular							
Protein	Low-lactose whey and casein Calcium caseinate Free amino acids	—	—	**Per 100 g** 370-424	**Per 100 g** 75-88.5	—	Casec (No) ProMod (R) Resource Protein Powder (No)
Carbohydrate	—	Maltodextrin Hydrolyzed cornstarch	—	**Per 100 g** 380-386	—	—	Moducal (No) Polycose (R)
Fat	—	—	Safflower oil Polyglycerol esters of fatty acids Soybean oil Lecithin Medium-chain triglycerides Fish oil	**Per 1 Tbsp** 67.5-115	—	—	MCT Oil (No) Microlipid (No)

Modified from Gottschlich MM, Shronts EP, Hutchins AM: Defined formula diets. In Rombeau JL, Rolandelli RH, eds: *Clinical nutrition: enteral and tube feeding*, ed 3, Philadelphia, 1997, WB Saunders. *No*, Novartis; *R*, Ross; *Ne*, Nestle.

from 1 to 2 kcal/ml. More concentrated formulas are designed for patients with fluid intolerance, such as those with renal, hepatic, or cardiac failure, as well as for patients who desire less volume or fewer feedings per day. However, it is imperative to provide adequate water for patients without a fluid restriction receiving a concentrated enteral tube feeding formula so they do not become dehydrated.

Nutrient Components

Carbohydrates

Approximately 50% to 60% of the energy in the American diet comes from carbohydrates, starches, and sugars. Carbohydrates are the body's primary energy source (see Chapter 2). Although large starch molecules are well tolerated and easily digested by most patients, their relative insolubility creates problems in enteral tube feeding formulas. Thus smaller sugars formed by partial or complete breakdown of cornstarch as well as other glucose polymers are common tube feeding formula components[33] (see Table 18-2). Very few enteral tube feeding formulas contain lactose because lactose intolerance is common among hospitalized patients. Tube feeding formulas can also contain soluble and insoluble fiber. There is considerable controversy as to the benefit of providing fiber in enteral tube feeding formulations.[26,33] Insoluble fiber increases stool volume and thus is used to treat problems with gastric motility: constipation and diarrhea. Soluble fiber has been promoted to improve blood sugar control, reduce serum cholesterol levels, and maintain colon health. The focus on maintaining normal intestinal bacteria has resulted in increased research and availability of prebiotics and probiotics given with or in enteral tube feeding formulas. Prebiotics, nondigestible food components, provide fuels to enhance repletion of normal bacterial found in the gastrointestinal tract, whereas probiotics, live nonpathogenic microbes, are designed to repopulate by providing "good" bacteria directly to the gastrointestinal tract.[34] The strain of probiotic and combination of strains most effective depends upon the therapeutic intent.

Protein

Protein content of standard enteral tube feeding formulas is designed to maintain body cell mass and promote tissue synthesis and repair (see Chapter 4). Biologic quality of dietary protein depends on its amino acid profile, especially its relative proportions of essential amino acids. To supply these needs, the following three major forms of protein are used in nutrition support enteral tube feeding formulas: (1) intact proteins, (2) hydrolyzed proteins, and (3) crystalline amino acids[33] (see Table 18-2).

1. *Intact proteins:* Intact proteins are the complete and original forms as found in foods, although protein isolates such as lactalbumin and casein from milk are intact proteins that have been separated from their original food source. These larger polypeptides and proteins must be broken down further (digested) before they can be absorbed.

2. *Hydrolyzed proteins:* Hydrolyzed proteins are protein sources that have been broken down by enzymes into smaller protein fragments and amino acids. These smaller products—tripeptides, dipeptides, and free amino acids—are absorbed more readily into the blood circulation.

3. *Crystalline amino acids:* Pure crystalline amino acids are easily absorbed. Small size of the amino acid results in an increase in osmolality of the formula. Amino acids result in a bitter-tasting formula. If an elemental tube feeding formula is used as an oral supplement, it requires flavoring aids or special preparation methods to improve taste, for example, pudding, frozen slush, or Popsicle. However, despite flavorings, the taste can still be unacceptable to a sick patient or can quickly lead to taste fatigue and refusal by the patient.

Fat

Major roles of fat in an enteral tube feeding formula are to supply a concentrated energy source, essential fatty acids, and a transport mechanism for fat-soluble vitamins. Major forms of fat used in standard formulas are butterfat in milk-based mixtures; vegetable oils from corn, soy, safflower, or sunflower; medium-chain triglycerides (MCT); and lecithin[33] (see Table 18-2). Vegetable oils supply a rich source of the essential fatty acids—linoleic and linolenic acids. Researchers continue to examine outcomes related to enteral tube feeding formulas containing various combinations of short-chain fatty acids, medium-chain fatty acids, and omega-3 fatty acids (see Chapter 3).[35,36]

Vitamins and Minerals

Standard whole diet commercial tube feeding formulas provide 100% of the Recommended Dietary Allowance (RDA) and Dietary Reference Intake (DRI) for vitamins and minerals when the formula is provided at a specific volume per day. The volume required to provide the RDA/DRI varies with each tube feeding formula and the nutrient requirements of the patient. Delivery of a reduced volume and use of diluted formulas may require supplementation with vitamin and mineral preparations. Patients with nutrient deficiencies may require supplementation of specific vitamins and minerals in addition to the standard vitamin and mineral composition of the enteral tube feeding formula. Several enteral tube feeding formulas are designed for specific patient populations and contain micronutrients designed to meet the requirements of the particular disease state or condition.

Physical Properties

After selecting a tube feeding formula according to the patient's nutritional requirements and gastrointestinal function, the clinician must consider physical properties of the formula that can affect tolerance. Individual intolerance is reflected in delayed gastric emptying, abdominal distention, cramping and pain, diarrhea, or constipation. A factor often evaluated when a patient demonstrates intolerance is osmolality of the enteral tube feeding formula. Osmolality is based on concentration of the formula and defined as number of osmotic particles per kilogram of solvent (water), energy-nutrient density, and residue content. However, there is no evidence that enteral tube feeding formula osmolality is the primary contributor to formula intolerance. Enteral tube feeding formulas can approximate 700 mOsm, whereas some medications are 4000 mOsm or greater. Signs and symptoms of enteral tube feeding intolerance, of which diarrhea is the most common, are more often related to inappropriate tube feeding techniques or drug interactions.

Medical Foods for Special Needs

Certain tube feeding formulas designed for special nutrition therapy are called medical foods. The Food and Drug Administration (FDA) first recognized the concept of medical foods as distinct from drugs in 1972, when the first special formula was developed for treatment of the genetic disease phenylketonuria (PKU) in newborns (see Chapter 11). The definition of medical foods remained rather murky as medical research developed an increasing number of special formulas. In 1988 Congress amended the Orphan Drug Act to include medical foods, defining them as food specifically formulated for use under medical supervision for primary treatment of metabolic-genetic diseases having distinctive nutritional requirements based on recognized scientific principles.[37] The Orphan Drug Act Amendment was subsequently incorporated into the reformed Nutrition Labeling and Education Act of 1990.

There has been an explosion of specialty enteral tube feeding formulas developed over the past 10 years. There are several products available in each category of disease- or condition-specific formulation: (1) end-stage renal disease, (2) hepatic disease, (3) pulmonary disease, (4) diabetes mellitus, (5) malabsorption syndromes, (6) immunoincompetence, (7) oncology, and (8) metabolic stress. Every patient with one of the above diagnoses does not need a specialty tube feeding formula. Indications for specialty tube feeding formulas are limited to a small subset of patients within each disease state classification for which a specialty formula is designed. There is considerable discussion on the treatment- and cost-effectiveness of specialty tube feeding formulas with continued need for scientific evidence to support their use.[26]

Modular Enteral Tube Feeding Formulas

Commercially available nutritionally complete enteral formula products for tube feeding are designed with a fixed ratio of nutrients to meet general standards for nutritional needs. However, some patients' particular needs are not met by these standard fixed-ratio tube feeding formulas, and they require an individualized modular formula. An individual formula, composed completely of modular components, is planned, calculated, prepared, and administered with the expertise of the RD. Modular enteral components are listed in Table 18-2. However, the more common use of modular components is the addition of carbohydrate, fat, or protein to a commercial formula to individualize the calorie and protein content of the formula for the patient. For example, additional protein powder can be added to increase the amount of protein per liter, or more carbohydrate or fat can be added to increase energy concentration. Other modular nutrients such as fiber and probiotics or prebiotics can also be added to the feeding regimen but should be given separately through the feeding tube and not added directly to the commercial tube feeding formulation. Every component added to an enteral tube feeding formula can increase the osmolality and viscosity of the formula and contribute to feeding intolerance, bacterial contamination, or clogging of the feeding tube.

Blue food dye is often added to tube feeding formulas to detect aspiration of formula into the trachea and lungs. There is concern as to safety, specificity, and sensitivity of blue dye in identifying aspiration in tube-fed patients.[38-40] Addition of blue food dye increases risk of bacterial contamination, false-positive occult stool test, discoloration of the skin and body fluids, and death. There also is no standardization for how much food dye to add per liter of tube feeding formula, with formula hues ranging from pale to cobalt blue. Methylene blue should not be added to tube feeding formulas because it can adversely affect cellular function.[41] Colored dyes are not diagnostic for aspiration, are potentially harmful, and should not be added to tube feedings.[40] Nonrecumbent positioning (elevating the head of the bed 30 to 40 degrees) is an evidence-based method for aspiration prevention and should be emphasized in all tube-fed patients.[40]

ENTERAL TUBE FEEDING DELIVERY SYSTEMS

Tube Feeding Equipment

Nasoenteric Feeding Tubes

Small-bore nasoenteric feeding tubes, generally from 8 to 12 French, made of softer, more flexible polyurethane and silicone materials have replaced former large-bore stiff tubing. Small-bore feeding tubes are more comfortable for patients and permit the infusion of commercially available

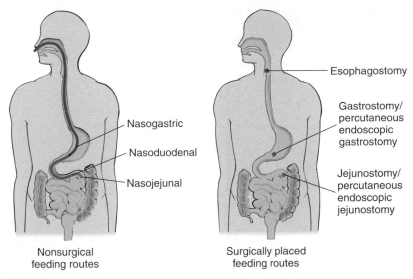

Nasogastric

Nasoduodenal

Nasojejunal

Nonsurgical
feeding routes

Esophagostomy

Gastrostomy/
percutaneous
endoscopic
gastrostomy

Jejunostomy/
percutaneous
endoscopic
jejunostomy

Surgically placed
feeding routes

FIGURE 18-2   Types of enteral feeding routes. *(From Rolin Graphics in Grodner M, Anderson SL, DeYoung S: Founda-*tions and clinical applications of nutrition: a nursing approach, *ed 2, St. Louis, 2000, Mosby.)*

enteral tube feeding formulas. Nasoenteric tubes can be inserted into either the stomach or beyond the pyloric valve into the small intestine: duodenum or jejunum[42] (Figure 18-2). Distal placement of a feeding tube beyond the ligament of Treitz into the jejunum is often preferred for patients with a history or risk of aspiration, impaired gastric emptying, depressed gag reflex, neurologic impairment, and critical illness.[27] Feeding tube insertion can be done blindly at the bedside or using radiographic visualization. Placement of a feeding tube should be performed by experienced, trained personnel. Feeding tube placement is an invasive procedure and carries the risk of misplacement into the lungs or brain, as well as perforation of the gastrointestinal tract. During placement, aspirates of gastrointestinal contents can be checked for pH and enzyme concentration, as well as visually inspected to reduce the number of radiographs required to determine when the desired location has been reached.[43] However, no tube feeding should be infused until feeding tube placement is confirmed by radiography.

Tube Feeding Enterostomies

Nasoenteric tube placement is usually indicated for short-term therapy. However, for enteral feeding anticipated more than 3 to 4 weeks, surgically or endoscopically placed enterostomies are preferred[42] (see Figure 18-2), as follows:

- *Esophagostomy:* A cervical esophagostomy can be placed at the level of the cervical spine to the side of the neck after head and neck surgeries for cancer or traumatic injury. This removes the discomfort of a nasoenteric tube, and the entry point can be concealed under clothing.

- *Gastrostomy:* A gastrostomy tube is surgically or endoscopically placed in the stomach if the patient is not at risk for aspiration and has normal gastric motility.

- *Jejunostomy:* A jejunostomy tube is surgically or endoscopically placed after the ligament of Treitz in the jejunum, the middle section of the small intestine. This procedure is indicated for patients with neurologic impairment, a risk or history of aspiration, an incompetent gag reflex, or gastric dysfunction. Gastric dysfunction can be related to gastric atony, gastroparesis, gastric cancer, gastric outlet obstruction, or gastric ulcerative disease.

Care and Maintenance of Enteral Feeding Tubes

Enteral feeding tubes should be flushed routinely with water to maintain patency and prevent clogging. Tap water is generally sufficient. If there is concern about safety of the water source or if the patient is immunosuppressed, sterile water should be used to flush the feeding tube. Standard flushing volumes are 30 ml of water every 4 hours during continuous feedings. Water flushes for intermittent and bolus enteral feedings are a minimum of 30 ml immediately after each feeding. The amount of water flushed through the tube is adjusted according to the patient's fluid requirements and tolerance. Larger fluid volumes will be needed for patients who cannot

medical foods Specially formulated nutrient mixtures for use under medical supervision to treat various metabolic diseases.

> ### General Comfort Tips for Patients on Nasoenteric Tube Feedings
>
> - *Thirst, oral dryness:* Lubricate lips, chew sugarless gum, brush teeth, rinse mouth frequently with water, suck lemon drops occasionally. If small amount of water by mouth is permitted, let ice cubes melt in mouth to soothe mouth and esophagus.
> - *Tube discomfort:* Gargle with a mixture of warm water and mouthwash, gently blow nose, and clean tube regularly with water-soluble lubricant. If persistent, pull tube out gently, clean it, and reinsert a new tube. (Many long-term users of tube feeding have learned to pass their own nasogastric tubes.)
> - *Tension, fullness:* Relax and breathe deeply after each tube feeding infusion.
> - *Loud stomach noises:* Take feedings in private.
> - *Limited mobility:* Change positions in bed or chair, and walk around the house or hospital corridor. Perform range-of-motion exercises while confined to bed.
> - *General gustatory distress with feeding:* Warm or chill tube feeding formula, but avoid having formula too cold because that increases risk of diarrhea.
> - *Persistent hunger:* Chew a favorite food, then spit it out; chew gum; or suck lemon drops.
> - *Inability to drink:* Rinse mouth frequently with water or other liquids.

drink water for hydration; smaller fluid volumes are needed for patients on fluid restrictions.

Ideally no medications should be put down small-bore feeding tubes because medications are a primary contributor to feeding tube clogs. However, the reality of life often requires administration of medications via feeding tubes. Flush with 30 ml water before and after medication administration. Each medication should be administered separately with 5 ml water flushed through the tube between each medication. Check with a pharmacist when determining which medications are compatible with administration through a feeding tube (see the *Diet-Medications Interactions* box, "Drug-Nutrient 'Enteralactions'"). Medications should never be added directly to the tube feeding formula because of the risk of drug-nutrient interactions. Warm water, a 30- to 60-ml syringe, and a pumping action can be used to dislodge a clog within the feeding tube. No evidence supports the use of other liquids such as soft drinks or juices to declog feeding tubes.[44] A pancreatic enzyme and bicarbonate mixture may be effective against formula clogs but will not dissolve medication clogs.[45]

Tube Feeding Containers and Pumps

The enteric tube feeding system includes the formula container, connection tubing, and often an infusion pump. A variety of tube feeding containers and feeding sets are available. Tube feeding formulas can be administered by syringe, gravity drip, or a volumetric pump. A pump may be needed for more accurate control, which is essential for tube feedings given directly into the small intestine, tube feedings infused at slow rates, and tube feedings using more viscous formulas. Critically ill patients should also be tube fed by volumetric pump to increase tolerance to enteral nutrition support.

Tube feeding delivery systems are categorized as either open or closed. An open delivery system involves pouring a volume of formula from a can or mixing bowl/container into an empty tube feeding bag, syringe, or infusion container. The infusion bag/container is reopened and refilled periodically with more formula. Clean technique is required when decanting the tube feeding formula into the bag and when handling the tubing connections. Formula hang time is limited to 8 hours or less.[24,46] Hang time is further reduced if additives such as protein powder are placed into the formula. The tube feeding infusion bag should be rinsed with sterile water before initial filling and subsequent refilling with formula.[24] The tube feeding administration set, tubing and infusion bag, should be changed every 24 hours. The primary benefit of the open system is ability to modulate the tube feeding formula.

The closed system is composed of a sterile vessel that is purchased prefilled with tube feeding formula. The container is spiked and connected to an infusion pump. Hang time is expanded to 24 to 48 hours (refer to manufacturer's guidelines for hang time of product being used). Benefits of the closed system are a reduction of time, labor, and contamination risk.[47,48] Caveats of the closed system are its higher cost and inability to modulate the formula. Regardless of the system used, good hand washing is essential for reduction in bacterial contamination. Clinicians working with patients on tube feedings need to be familiar with different delivery systems, types of enteral feeding tubes, and features of enteral feeding pumps to determine which products are preferable for their facility and patient population.

Infusion of Enteral Tube Feeding

Tube feedings can be provided via bolus, intermittent, or continuous infusion through a feeding tube. Patients can progress from one infusion modality to another as their medical condition changes. All enteral tube feedings should be initiated at full strength. Tolerance to tube feeding has not been shown to be improved with dilution of the formula.[49] Enteral tube feedings should be introduced gradually and progressed per patient tolerance. Gastric tube feedings can be given as bolus, intermittent, or continuous feedings. Small bowel tube feedings are given as continuous feedings.

Bolus tube feeding is generally initiated with 120 to 240 ml of formula every 3 to 4 hours and increased by 60 to 240 ml every 8 to 12 hours depending on degree of illness and tolerance. The infusion period is relatively short, 10 to 20 minutes, and is infused through a syringe or from a bag by the flow of gravity.[50] The infusion should not exceed 40 to 60 ml/min. Gravity infusion is con-

DIET-MEDICATIONS INTERACTIONS

Drug Nutrient 'Enteralactions'

Even though enteral nutrition support is becoming rather ordinary, there are relatively few clinical studies available documenting drug-nutrient interactions associated with enteral feeding solutions. This relates to the fact that administration of drugs through a feeding tube should be considered a last resort, but it can also be linked to the theory that interactions are so common and varied they are simply not reported. However, potential consequences of interactions should not be taken lightly. Use of enteral nutrition support poses many pharmaceutical and dietary complications that can physically interfere with administration of nutrition, alter bioavailability of a given drug, or cause long-term vitamin and mineral deficiencies.

Physical interferences with nutrition support are problems related to manipulation of the delivery system of nutrition support or the drug before it enters the body. Physical interferences are the most commonly reported problems and include but are not limited to occlusion of the feeding tube related to medication administration, manipulation of solid dosage forms of drugs, and exposure of photosensitive drugs to light for extended periods of time. No medication is formulated to be administered in combination with enteral nutrition support; therefore the composition can sometimes alter viscosity of enteral feeding solutions and cause occlusion of the feeding tube. Furthermore, when crushing a solid dose pill for administration through a feeding tube, occlusion is not only risked, but also bioavailability of the medication and timed-release properties will be altered considerably. Any type of drug added to a feeding solution will have longer exposure to ultraviolet light than if taken orally, which in some cases can compromise therapeutic effects.

The recipient of enteral nutrition support is able to obtain total nutrition from his or her enteral feeding solutions; however, composition of these enteral feeds differ considerably from orally fed diets. Enteral feeds contain higher concentrations of proteins, vitamins, and minerals, which can bind drugs or alter the mechanism by which they are metabolized. Closely related, but resulting in a more long-term effect are vitamin and mineral binding. Chronic problems such as osteoporosis can develop over time as a result of an interaction that goes unnoticed. The following is a brief list of some classically noted drug-nutrient interactions related to enteral nutrition support.

Drug	Interaction	Possible Remedy
Phenytoin	Probable cause of interaction is the binding of phenytoin to caseinate proteins found in enteral feeds, preventing its absorption from the gastrointestinal tract.	Withhold feedings for 2 hours after administration of phenytoin. Increased dosage might be in order.
Quinolones	Concurrent administration of a quinolone and enteral feed could compromise antimicrobial efficiency. This is related to the divalent cations found in enteral nutrition formulas.	Withhold feedings 1 hour before and 1 hour after administration of quinolones. Increase dosage when converting from intravenous to oral form.
Warfarin	Decreased bioavailability of this drug results from high binding of warfarin to proteins found in enteral nutrition. In addition, vitamin K was formerly found to reverse anticoagulant effects of warfarin, but most current enteral feeds contain little or no vitamin K.	Avoid concurrent administration of warfarin and enteral nutrition solutions. Chose enteral nutritional supplements that contain limited vitamin K content.

Working as a team with physicians, nurses, speech pathologists, and pharmacists can substantially reduce interactions stemming from enteral nutrition support. By educating those who administer and prescribe medications, risks involved can be controlled and monitored correctly.

References

A.S.P.E.N. Board of Directors: Section IX: drug nutrient interactions, *JPEN J Parenter Enter Nutr* 26:1, 2002.

British Association for Parenteral and Enteral Nutrition, The British Pharmaceutical Nutrition Group: *Drug administration via enteral feeding tubes: a guide for general practitioners and community pharmacists*, Redditch, UK, 2001, Author [*www.bpng.org.uk*].

Finch C, Self T: Medication and enteral tube feedings: clinically significant interactions, *J Crit Illness* 16:20-21, 2001.

Fitzgerald M: What do I need to know about drug interactions with enteral feeding? *Medscape Nurs* 7:1, 2005.

trolled by a roller clamp, raising or lowering the formula container, or advancing the plunger into the syringe.

Intermittent tube feedings are similar to bolus feedings but are given over a longer time period of 30 to 60 minutes every 3 to 6 hours. The enteral tube feeding formula is placed in a bag with rate controlled by a roller clamp. This method is used to provide periodic gastric feedings to patients who do not tolerate the more rapid infusion of a bolus feeding. Maximum amount of formula given by bolus or intermittent feedings varies from 240 to 500 ml per feeding and is based on patient tolerance and requirements.

Continuous tube feedings are provided over a defined period with the formula infused by gravity or pump. Continuous feedings can be given over 24 hours or cycled over a shorter period, such as 8 to 20 hours per day. Enteral tube feeding tolerance is generally better in critically ill

> **viscous** Physical property of a substance dependent on the friction of its component molecules as they slide by one another; viscosity.

patients who are fed continuously regardless of whether fed into the stomach or small bowel.

All patients fed through a feeding tube should have the head of the bed elevated 30 to 45 degrees to reduce the risk of aspiration.[51] Patients fed with a tube into the small bowel can still aspirate gastric contents and may require concomitant gastric decompression during small bowel feeding.[52] Patients who must lie flat or in Trendelenburg's position should have enteral feedings stopped.

MONITORING THE TUBE-FED PATIENT

Monitoring of the tube-fed patient should focus on transitioning to an oral diet and reducing or eliminating dependency on tube feeding. All patients being nourished by tube feeding should be carefully monitored for signs and symptoms of enteral tube feeding intolerance. Tolerance to enteral tube feeding is determined by gastrointestinal signs of vomiting, abdominal distention or bloating, and frequency and consistency of bowel movements. If problems occur, the tube feeding formula may need to be changed or infusion rate adjusted or method of administration changed until tolerance improves and symptoms subside. In most instances the tube feeding formula itself is not the causative agent for the intolerance. Two parameters—residual volume and diarrhea—are often used to determine tolerance to tube feeding. Both are terms that have no standardized definition within each institution, much less nationwide standard definitions.

Diarrhea is generally defined by the person cleaning it up and can be based on volume, frequency, and/or consistency of the stools. There are 14 definitions of diarrhea in the literature.[53] Commonly used definitions are greater than three stools per day or more than 500 ml of stool per day for 2 consecutive days.[54] Each healthcare facility should define diarrhea and then create an algorithm or protocol for treatment to reduce unnecessary interruptions of enteral feeding.[54] The most common cause of diarrhea in the tube-fed patient is medications, primarily antibiotics and medications containing sorbitol (see the discussion later in this chapter under the heading "Health Promotion").

Residual volume interpretation is also often determined by caregiver experience and not evidence-based guidelines. Enteral feeds are interrupted for gastric residual volumes ranging from 50 to 200 ml.[55] A research study defined acceptable residual volume as less than 200 ml with a nasogastric tube and less than 100 ml with a gastrostomy tube.[56] The authors suggested high residual volumes be correlated with the presence of physical signs of intolerance before stopping enteral feeding. Another study found that if patients were given a prophylactic prokinetic agent, a residual volume of 250 ml was tolerated.[57] The A.S.P.E.N. Guidelines[7] and the Canadian Clinical Practice Guidelines[58] state a high residual volume is greater than 200 ml for two consecutive checks and greater than 250 ml, respectively. In contrast, according to a survey of intensive care unit (ICU) nurses, the nurses believed a residual volume greater than 100 ml was excessive.[59] A patient with a history of aspiration or reflux is at risk of aspiration even with low gastric residuals; therefore residual volumes do not always correlate with risk of aspiration.

Gastrointestinal aspirates containing gastric enzymes and hydrochloric acid required for digestion, electrolytes, enteral formula, and fluid should be returned to the patient after determining the volume. However, if doing so would make the patient uncomfortable or if the volume removed exceeds 300 ml, discard the residuals and recheck in 1 to 2 hours. The feeding tube should be flushed with 30 ml water after checking and returning residuals to be sure gastric contents with digestive enzymes are no longer within the lumen of the feeding tube. Patient tolerance of tube feeding formula, state of hydration, and nutritional response to tube feeding should be monitored using data collected from a variety of sources, including laboratory, anthropometric, physical and clinical assessment, and nursing records. Protocols for enteral tube feeding can provide guidelines for troubleshooting problems and improve nutrient delivery.[60,61]

Clinical and Laboratory Parameters to Monitor

Daily blood and urine tests for glucose during the first week or so, according to protocol, reflect carbohydrate tolerance. Patients who have diabetes or those who are severely stressed or septic may have difficulty metabolizing carbohydrate and are monitored closely. It is important not to overfeed patients on nutrition support. Historically insulin has been provided as needed to maintain serum glucose level at less than 200 mg/dl. However, there is a growing body of evidence that glycemic control less than 110 mg/dl[62] and less than 140 mg/dl[63] can significantly reduce mortality and morbidity in ICU patients.

Daily weights, compared with a baseline weight before start of the tube feeding, along with daily input and output measures are essential for an accurate assessment of patient tolerance and nutrient adequacy. Routine monitoring also includes serum tests for potassium, sodium, chloride, carbon dioxide, creatinine, and blood urea nitrogen and complete blood cell counts along with periodic tests for urine specific gravity. Sudden weight changes can indicate fluid imbalance and need to be investigated. (See Box 18-2 for a list of nutrition support monitoring parameters.)

Hydration Status

Signs of volume deficit or dehydration include weight loss, poor skin turgor, dry mucous membranes, and low blood pressure from decreased blood volume. Patients also demonstrate increased serum levels of sodium, albumin, hematocrit, and blood urea nitrogen, as well as elevated urine specific gravity levels. Severe dehydration is critical and life threatening. Fluid requirements can be estimated by several available formulas, such as

1 ml water per kcalorie or 30 to 35 ml/kg. Water content of the enteral tube feeding formula and the amount of water given with medications and routine flushing of the feeding tube, as well as the patient's medical condition, are taken into consideration when determining the patient's fluid requirements. Fluids must be monitored for adequacy and adjusted as necessary to attain and maintain adequate hydration. Patients with large fluid losses from fistulas, ostomies, and drains may require intravenous hydration in conjunction with enteral tube feeding nutrition.

Signs of volume excess or overhydration include weight gain, edema, jugular vein distention, elevated blood pressure, and decreased serum levels of sodium, albumin, blood urea nitrogen, and hematocrit. Patients with renal, cardiac, and hepatic impairment may require less fluid than do other patients.

Documentation of the Enteral Nutrition Tube Feeding

The patient's medical record is an essential means of communication among members of the healthcare team. The healthcare team is involved in actions and documentation related to (1) all ongoing nutritional analyses of actual tube feeding formula intake, (2) tolerance of the formula and any complications, (3) desired versus actual outcomes, (4) recommendations for adjustments in tube feeding formula, routine tube flushing, and method and rate of delivery, and (5) education of patient and family.

BOX 18-4	Indications and Contraindications for Parenteral Nutrition

Indications

1. Nonfunctional gastrointestinal (GI) tract
   a. Obstruction
   b. Intractable vomiting or diarrhea
   c. Short-bowel syndrome
   d. Paralytic ileus
2. Inability to adequately utilize GI tract
   a. Slow progression of enteral nutrition
   b. Limited tolerance of enteral nutrition
3. Perioperative
   a. Severely malnourished
   b. Nothing by mouth (NPO) for at least 1 week before surgery

Contraindications

1. No central venous access
2. Grim prognosis when parenteral nutrition (PN) will be of no benefit
3. Enteral nutrition is an alternative means of support

Conditions Previously Treated With PN That Benefit From Enteral Feeding

1. Inflammatory bowel disease
2. Pancreatitis

Modified from Fuhrman MP: Parenteral nutrition, *Dietitian's Edge* 2(1):53, 2001.

PARENTERAL FEEDING IN CLINICAL NUTRITION

PN should be reserved for patients unable to receive adequate nutrition via the enteral route. A.S.P.E.N. has published general guidelines to determine when PN support is appropriate.[7] Indications and contraindications for PN are listed in Box 18-4.

Basic Technique

Guidelines for ordering PN are given in Box 18-5, and an example of a basic PN solution is given in Box 18-6.

BOX 18-5	Guidelines for Ordering Parenteral Nutrition

1. Determine that the patient has central intravenous access.
2. Identify amount of energy, protein, and fluid desired.
3. Determine desired distribution of dextrose and lipids.
4. Indicate additives desired.
   a. Vitamins
   b. Minerals
   c. Electrolytes
   d. Medications
   e. Sterile water
5. Determine infusion rate based on compounded volume and time of infusion.

BOX 18-6	Example of a Basic PN Formula for a 65-kg Patient Providing Approximately 25 kcal/kg and 1.2 g Protein per Kilogram

Base Solution

70% Dextrose	350 ml	245 g	833 kcal
10% Amino acids	800 ml	80 g	320 kcal
20% Lipid	250 ml	50 g	500 kcal
TOTAL	1400 ml		1653 kcal

Additives

Standard Electrolytes	Amount per Day
Sodium chloride	20 mEq
Sodium acetate	50 mEq
Potassium chloride	30 mEq
Potassium phosphate	30 mEq (20 mmol phosphorus)
Calcium gluconate	10 mEq
Magnesium sulfate	10 mEq
Multivitamin preparation	10 ml
Trace element preparation	1 ml
Medications	
Regular insulin	Only with hyperglycemia
H$_2$-antagonists	Dose depends on
Famotidine 40 mg	H$_2$-antagonist and renal functions

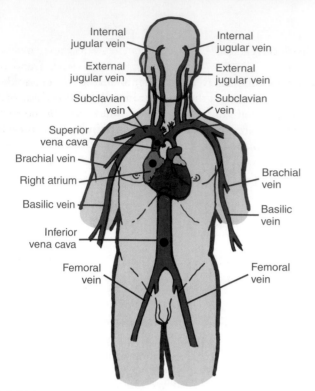

Internal jugular vein
Internal jugular vein
External jugular vein
External jugular vein
Subclavian vein
Subclavian vein
Superior vena cava
Brachial vein
Right atrium
Basilic vein
Brachial vein
Basilic vein
Inferior vena cava
Femoral vein
Femoral vein

FIGURE 18-3 Sites of central venous access for parenteral nutrition. *(From Fuhrman MP: Management of complications of parenteral nutrition. In Matarese LE, Gottschlich MM, eds: Contemporary nutrition support practice: a clinical guide, Philadelphia, 1998, WB Saunders.)*

PN refers to any intravenous feeding method. Nutrients are infused directly into the blood when the gastrointestinal tract cannot or should not be used. The following two parenteral routes are available[64] (Figure 18-3):

1. *Central parenteral nutrition (CPN):* A large central vein is used to deliver concentrated solutions for nutrition support. Osmolarity of central vein parenteral formulas can be as high as 1700 to 1900 mOsm/L. High formula osmolarity requires infusion of the formula into a large vessel with rapid blood flow. A central line generally originates from the subclavian, internal jugular, or femoral vein with the tip in the superior vena cava, right atrium of the heart, or inferior vena cava. Central line access can also be achieved with a peripherally inserted central catheter (PICC) that is inserted in the basilic vein with the tip in the superior vena cava or right atrium.

2. *Peripheral parenteral nutrition (PPN):* A smaller peripheral vein, usually in the distal arm or hand, is used to deliver less-concentrated solutions for periods less than 14 days. Osmolarity of PPN is limited to 900 mOsm/L or less to reduce risk of thrombophlebitis in smaller vessels of the upper distal extremities.[65]

Parenteral Nutrition Development

The pioneering work of American surgeons such as Jonathan Rhodes and Stanley Dudrick in the late 1960s propelled PN from theory into reality.[66] In the following years, development of the surgical technique, equipment, and solutions to meet nutritional requirements of catabolic illness and injury and development of antibiotics and diuretics led to its current widespread use and future directions.[26,67] PN was preferentially used to treat critically ill patients until a resurgence in enteral nutrition in the 1990s as more was learned about the importance of maintaining gastrointestinal integrity. PN is associated with potentially serious mechanical, metabolic, and gastrointestinal complications (see Box 18-3). PN should be used judiciously to minimize the risks involved. PPN can be used in many cases as a viable alternative for brief periods for patients without central vein access.[68]

Basic factors govern decisions about use of PN: availability and functional capacity of the gastrointestinal tract, prognosis, and availability of central intravenous access.[7] The cost of PN is generally greater than that of enteral feeding, and institutions have demonstrated cost savings when inappropriate use of PN has been decreased.[69,70] Patients must have central intravenous access to receive PN with one port designated exclusively for PN. Thus careful assessment of each situation should weigh benefits and burdens of providing PN for nutrition support.

Indications for PN include inability to access or malfunction of the gastrointestinal tract. Patients may have inadequate absorption of nutrients in the gastrointestinal tract because of reduced bowel length or inflammation. Examples of indications for PN are obstruction, fistula, severe inflammation, intractable vomiting or diarrhea, or gastrointestinal bleeding (see Box 18-4). If the gastrointestinal tract is functional but the patient cannot or will not consume sufficient nutrients orally, enteral tube feeding should be considered. Many conditions that had been previously thought to be an indication for PN are treated with enteral tube feeding, such as pancreatitis, severe malnutrition, ileus, and coma.

Candidates for Parenteral Nutrition

Parenteral nutrition should be reserved for patients unable to receive or tolerate adequate nutrients via the enteral route. On the basis of these general considerations, a number of clinical situations suggest a need for aggressive PN support, as follows:

- *Preoperative nutrition intervention:* This measure may benefit moderately to severely malnourished patients who can receive nutrition support for a minimum of 7 to 14 days preoperatively.[7] PN should be given only if enteral nutrition support is not feasible or tolerated. The VA Cooperative Study demonstrated the greatest benefit of perioperative PN was experienced by severely malnourished patients.[28]

- *Postoperative surgical complications:* Complications that often result in initiation of PN are prolonged paralytic ileus and obstruction; stomal dysfunction; short-bowel syndrome; enterocutaneous, biliary, or pancreatic fistula; chylothorax; chylous ascites; and peritonitis. However, there are reports of successful enteral feeding with short-bowel syndrome, fistula, and chylous leaks when patients are given an elemental or semielemental, low-fat enteral formula.[71-73] PN is not indicated in patients who can resume enteral nutrition within 7 to 10 days postoperatively.[7]
- *Bowel inflammation:* Intractable gastroenteritis, regional enteritis, ulcerative colitis, extensive diverticulitis, and radiation enteritis may require PN if the gastrointestinal inflammation is severe and prolonged.[7] Studies have shown that in some cases enteral feeding can be feasible and beneficial in diseases with bowel inflammation.[74]
- *Malabsorption:* Nutrient losses and interference with nutrient absorption occur with chemotherapy and radiation therapy. The malabsorption that is associated with severe gastrointestinal inflammation, acute severe pancreatitis, and massive burns can exceed the ability to meet nutrient requirements enterally.

Peripheral Parenteral Nutrition

Generally, decisions to use PPN instead of CPN are based on energy demands, anticipated time of use, and availability of intravenous access. Characteristics of PPN include caloric value generally less than 2000 kcal/day, of which 50% to 60% is provided by lipids; infusion volume of 2 to 3 L (dilution of the formula is required for peripheral vein tolerance); and use of infusion for less than 14 days.[68] PPN cannot be used when the patient has problems with fluid retention or hyperlipidemia.

PARENTERAL SOLUTIONS

The Parenteral Nutrition Prescription

The PN prescription and plan of care are based on the calculation of basic nutritional requirements plus additional needs resulting from the patient's degree of illness or injury, malnutrition, and physical activity. An example of a basic PN formula is shown in Box 18-6. The same principles of nutrition therapy are applied whether the patient is fed enterally or parenterally. Nutritional needs are fundamental—energy, protein, electrolytes, minerals, and vitamins. Guidelines are available that address PN labeling, compounding, formulations, stability, and filtering.[75] The guidelines are designed to reduce errors and complications in prescribing, preparing, labeling, and infusing parenteral solutions.

Preparation of the Parenteral Nutrition Solution

There are a variety of PN component solutions with varying concentrations and nutrient compositions. Standard components of PN can include dextrose, lipids, amino acids, electrolytes, vitamins, minerals, and medications. Although PN is compounded with modular components and hence an ability to adjust dextrose, lipid, and protein independent of each other, the energy provided to meet estimated or measured energy needs should include total energy (kcalories) from carbohydrate, fat, and protein (Table 18-3). Estimated as well as measured energy equations are based on total energy (kcalories) requirements.

Protein-Nitrogen Source

Nitrogen is supplied by essential and nonessential crystalline amino acids in the PN solution. Standard commercial amino acid solutions range in concentration from 3% to 20%. Standard amino acid solutions are appropriate for almost all adult patients receiving PN. Protein has an energy value of 4 kcal/g (see Table 18-3) and usually provides 10% to 20% of the total energy provided in PN.

In addition to standard amino acid solutions, three types of specialized amino acid solutions have been formulated for specific disease states. The two disease-specific formulas are more expensive than standard solutions, and

TABLE 18-3	Caloric Value per Milliliter of Parenteral Components	
Nutrient	**Concentration (%)**	**Kcal/ml**
Dextrose	70	2.38
	50	1.85
Lipids	30	3.0
	20	2.0
	10	1.1
Amino acids	15	0.6
	10	0.4
	8.5	0.34

osmolarity The number of millimoles of liquid or solid in a liter of solution; parenteral nutrition solutions given by central vein have an osmolarity around 1800 mOsm/L; peripheral parenteral solutions are limited to 600 to 900 mOsm/L (dextrose and amino acids have the greatest impact on a solution's osmolarity).

fistula Abnormal connection between two internal organs, an internal organ and the skin, or an internal organ and a body cavity.

their effectiveness has not been demonstrated. One type is enriched with the branched-chain amino acids (BCAAs) isoleucine, leucine, and valine and is designed for patients with liver failure. A renal failure formula contains only essential amino acids to prevent the development of hyperuremia. Neither disease-specific formula has been found to improve outcomes in these patient populations.[7] Infusion of BCAA may be beneficial in a very small population of patients with chronic hepatic encephalopathy that is unresponsive to drug therapy.[7] The third type of specialized amino acid formula is designed specifically for the needs of pediatric patients and is selected based on the age and nutrient requirements of the child.

Carbohydrate-Dextrose

Dextrose is the most common and least expensive source of energy used for PN support. Dextrose is available in concentrations ranging from 2.5% to 70%. Hypertonic solutions of 50% to 70% dextrose are often used in PN formulations and provide 50 or 70 g of dextrose per 100 ml, respectively. Glucose used in PN support is commercially available as dextrose monohydrate ($C_6H_{12}O_6H_2O$), which has an energy value of 3.4 kcal/g versus the energy value of 4 kcal/g of dietary glucose ($C_6H_{12}O_6$). The caloric values of dextrose solutions are given in Table 18-3. Initial dextrose content of PN should not exceed 200 g. Gradual introduction of dextrose enables the clinician to evaluate blood sugar response and, if necessary, institute insulin therapy. The amount of dextrose provided is increased to goal according to patient tolerance and should not exceed 5 mg/kg/min.

Glycerol is another form of carbohydrate used in parenteral solutions. It provides 4.3 kcal/g and is available as a component along with amino acids in a commercially available PPN solution.

Fat-Lipids

Lipid emulsions provide a concentrated energy source, 9 kcal/g, as well as the essential fatty acids linoleic and linolenic acid. A minimum of 4% to 10% of the daily energy intake should consist of fat to prevent essential fatty acid deficiency. Lipids are available in 10% (1.1 kcal/ml), 20% (2 kcal/ml), and 30% (3 kcal/ml) products (see Table 18-3). A 500-ml bottle of 10%, 20%, or 30% fat emulsion provides 550, 1000, and 1500 kcal, respectively. Commercial lipid emulsion products consist of soybean and safflower oils combined or soybean oil alone. Content of lipid in a parenteral solution is usually limited to 20% to 30% of total energy because lipids have been reported to adversely affect the immune system.[76] However, infusion of lipids over 24 hours may limit this adverse effect. Research on alternative lipid sources includes forms such as short-chain fatty acids, medium-chain fatty acids, omega-3 fatty acids, and blended or structured lipids. However, these alternatives are not available for commercial use in the United States. Lipid

emulsions can be infused separately through the Y-port of the intravenous catheter (piggybacked) or combined with the dextrose and amino acid base in what is called a total nutrient admixture (TNA) or 3-in-1.[75]

Electrolytes

The body maintains a balance of fluid and electrolytes in intracellular and extracellular spaces of all tissues to maintain homeostasis (see Chapter 7). Electrolyte status is affected by disease state and metabolic condition of the patient. Electrolytes in PN formulas are based on normal electrolyte balance with adjustments according to individual patient requirements. Electrolytes should be routinely monitored to determine electrolyte requirements in PN.

In general, basic electrolyte recommendations are as shown in Table 18-4, with chloride and acetate balanced among the salts. Commercial amino acid formulations are available with or without added electrolytes. Amounts of electrolytes present in the amino acid solution must be taken into account when calculating additions of electrolytes for a specific patient. Guidelines for electrolyte management include (1) identify and correct any preexisting deficits before initiating PN, (2) determine the cause of electrolyte abnormalities, (3) replace excessive fluid and electrolyte losses, and (4) monitor and assess electrolyte status daily. Depending on requirements for electrolyte replacement, it may be necessary to give additional electrolytes outside the PN because there are limitations on what can be added to a parenteral solution based on solution stability and compatibility.[72] Selected electrolytes can be omitted from the parenteral solution when serum levels exceed normal values, such as potassium and phosphorus with renal failure. Electrolyte levels should be checked in all patients before starting PN and routinely throughout PN therapy.

Vitamins

Vitamin requirements are based on normal standards (see Chapter 6), with adjustments made according to metabolic states that require either more or less of a specific vitamin. All patients on PN should receive vitamins daily. Serum levels of vitamins should be monitored in patients requiring long-term PN or when deficiencies or excesses are suspected.

The Nutrition Advisory Group of the American Medical Association has established guidelines for parenteral administration of 12 vitamins: A, D, E, thiamin, riboflavin, niacin, pantothenic acid, pyridoxine, folic acid, biotin, cyanocobalamin, and ascorbic acid (see Table 18-4).[77] Multivitamin infusion preparations based on these guidelines are commercially available. Vitamin K has not historically been a component of any injectable vitamin formulation for adults. The FDA mandated changes in parenteral vitamin formulations that included addition of 150 μg of vitamin K to injectable multivitamin preparations.[78] It will be important to monitor International Normalized Ratio (INR) levels, particularly for patients on anticoagulation therapy started or stopped on PN containing vitamin K. An injectable multivitamin preparation without vitamin K is also available.

Trace Elements

The American Medical Association has set guidelines for addition of four trace elements in PN solutions: zinc, copper, manganese, and chromium (see Table 18.4).[79] Trace element preparations are available with combinations of the aforementioned four trace elements only, the standard four plus selenium, or the standard four plus selenium, molybdenum, and iodine. Each trace element is also available as a single injectable mineral product. There is a growing amount of literature as to the importance of providing selenium to PN patients who are critically ill[80,81] and those who require long-term PN.[82] Iron is not routinely added to PN because of incompatibility with intravenous lipids, as well as the potential adverse effects of iron dextran. Other forms of intravenous iron have less adverse effects but are not approved for addition to the PN solution. Intravenous iron should only be given to patients with iron deficiency anemia and administered apart from the PN admixture or added to a 2-in-1 PN solution.[75] A dose of 25 to 50 mg of iron dextran once a month should be sufficient to meet iron needs in a patient without blood loss.[75]

Patients on long-term PN without trace element supplementation are at risk for micronutrient deficiencies.[82,83] There have also been reports of excess trace element levels with infusion of standard trace element preparations.[84] Patients requiring long-term PN should be routinely monitored for potential trace element deficiencies and toxicities.

Medications

Medications often added to PN include insulin, H_2-antagonists, heparin, metoclopramide, and octreotide. Inclusion of these medications and others will depend on each institution's guidelines and protocols for addition of medications to PN solutions. There are many issues concerning compatibility, bioavailability, efficacy, interactions, and safety when including medications in PN solutions. Consult a pharmacist whenever considering the addition of a medication to PN solutions.

> admixture A mixture of ingredients that each retain their own physical properties; a combination of two or more substances that are not chemically united or that exist in no fixed proportion to each other.

TABLE 18-4	Micronutrients and Parenteral Nutrition for Adults
Micronutrients	**Standard Daily Amounts**
Electrolytes	
Potassium (K)	1-2 mEq/kg
Sodium (Na)	1-2 mEq/kg
Phosphate (HPO_4)	20-40 mmol
Magnesium (Mg)	8-20 mEq
Calcium (Ca)	10-15 mEq
Acetate	Balance with chloride to maintain acid-base balance
Chloride	Balance with acetate to maintain acid-base balance
Vitamins	
Vitamin A	3300 IU
Vitamin D	200 IU
Vitamin E	10 IU
Vitamin K	150 μg
Thiamin (B_1)	6 mg
Riboflavin (B_2)	3.6 mg
Niacin (B_3)	40 mg
Folic acid	600 μg
Pantothenic acid	15 mg
Pyridoxine (B_6)	6 mg
Cyanocobalamin (B_{12})	5 μg
Biotin	60 μg
Ascorbic acid (Vitamin C)	200 μg
Trace Elements	
Chromium	10-15 μg
Copper	0.3-0.5 μg
Iodine	Not routinely provided 50 μg for pregnant women
Iron	Not routinely provided 25-50 mg per month without blood loss
Manganese	60-100 μg
Selenium	20-60 μg
Zinc	2.5-5 mg
Molybdenum	Not routinely provided

Data from Fuhrman MP: Complication management in parenteral nutrition. In Matarese LE, Gottschlich MM, eds: *Contemporary nutrition support practice: a clinical guide,* ed 2, Philadelphia, 2003, Saunders; Task force for the revision of safe practices for parenteral nutrition et al: Safe practices for parenteral nutrition, *JPEN J Parenter Enteral Nutr* 28(suppl): S39, 2004; American Medical Association, AMA Department of Foods and Nutrition: Multivitamin preparations for parenteral use: a statement by the Nutrition Advisory Group, *JPEN J Parenter Enteral Nutr* 3:258, 1979; Parenteral multivitamin products; drugs for human use; drug efficacy study implementation; amendment (21 CFR 5.70), *Fed Register* 65:21200, 2000; and Expert Panel for Nutrition Advisory Group, AMA Department of Foods and Nutrition: Guidelines for essential trace element preparations for parenteral use, *JAMA* 241:2051, 1979.

PARENTERAL NUTRITION DELIVERY SYSTEM

Equipment

Strict aseptic technique throughout PN administration by all healthcare personnel is absolutely essential. This includes (1) solution preparation by the pharmacist, (2) surgical placement of the venous catheter by the physician, (3) care of the catheter site and all external equipment, and (4) administration of the solution by the nurse. At every step of the PN process, strict infection control is a primary responsibility of all healthcare professionals.

Venous Access

Surgical placement of the venous catheter is done by the physician at the bedside or in a surgical suite, using local or general anesthesia. Intravenous catheters are available with single, double, triple, or quadruple lumens. There is inconsistent data as to whether the number of lumens contributes to the risk of catheter-related infection.[85-87] Catheters are also categorized as either temporary or permanent. Temporary catheters involve a direct percutaneous puncture into a major vessel and are used short-term during hospitalization. Permanent catheters are designed for long-term use and are available as implanted ports, tunneled catheters, and PICCs. The tip of a central venous catheter is located in the inferior or superior vena cava, which leads directly into the heart[64] (see Figure 18-3). Placement of the catheter tip in the vena cava allows infusion of concentrated solutions, five times the concentration of blood plasma, to be infused at a rate of 2 to 3 ml/min. Hypertonic solutions are immediately diluted by the large blood flow of 2 to 5 L/min in the vena cava.

Catheter-related sepsis is a serious complication, particularly with the increase in colonization of resistant strains of microorganisms that limit available treatment options. Antibiotic-impregnated catheters and dressings are available and are associated with reduced catheter-related septic complications.[88-90] Filters (0.22 μm) on intravenous catheter tubing prevent infusion of not only particulate matter but also certain microorganisms.[75] However, a larger filter (2.1 μm) that is less effective against microorganisms must be used with PN containing lipids. Clinicians must use aseptic technique when inserting and caring for intravenous catheters.

Solution Infusion and Administration

Volumetric infusion pumps should be used to deliver the parenteral solution at a constant rate to prevent metabolic complications. Protocols for external delivery system tubing changes are provided by infection control guidelines. Routine flushing of intravenous catheters is recommended to maintain catheter patency. Needleless intravenous access devices reduce risk of needlestick injuries but can increase risk of catheter-related infections. According to the Intravenous Nurses Society standards of practice, needleless devices should be changed every 24 hours, the injection port should be disinfected with alcohol before accessing, and all junctions should be secured with Luer-locks, clasps, or threaded devices.[91]

Infusion of PN is generally over 24 hours, particularly in the critically ill. PN is usually cycled for patients at home or who need "time off" during hospitalization for physical therapy or other routine activities. PN can be cycled over 10 to 12 hours if desired and if the patient can tolerate the larger volume over a shorter period. Rate of infusion is based on the final compounded volume and length of time the infusion is to be given. Administration of PN should be adjusted based on the patient's response and tolerance to the regimen (see the *Perspectives in Practice* box, "Parenteral Nutrition Administration"). When PN is being discontinued, the infusion rate should be cut by one half for an hour and then stopped. Abrupt interruption of PN infusion may require hanging 10% dextrose to prevent possible rebound hypoglycemia.[75]

Monitoring

Complications of PN include catheter, gastrointestinal, and metabolic problems (see Box 18-3). In the hands of well-trained PN clinicians, risks can be minimized and complications controlled.[92] Specific evidence-based protocols, updated periodically, guide continuing assessment and monitoring.[93] Every patient on PN should undergo a routine nutrition reassessment with adjustments made in the feeding regimen according to the patient's metabolic and nutritional needs. Every effort should be made to transition the patient from PN to enteral tube feeding or oral diet whenever feasible or appropriate. Providing at least a portion of energy via the gastrointestinal tract may help reduce the adverse effects associated with PN.[64]

HOME NUTRITION SUPPORT

Patients being discharged with home nutrition support and those started on nutrition support while in the home require special consideration. Several factors must be evaluated to ensure that the home environment is safe and the patient and family are able and willing to accept the responsibility of home infusion therapy. The home should have refrigeration, running water, electricity, and adequate storage for supplies. The patient and family must be capable of and willing to learn techniques required to administer the feeding as well as manage the feeding access. It is also important that the patient and family accept responsibility to comply with the infusion regimen so the patient receives nutrients as prescribed. There is ongoing communication among the patient, physician, and home infusion provider, but ultimately

PERSPECTIVES IN PRACTICE
Parenteral Nutrition Administration

Of all the various ways of nourishing the human body—normal eating, liquid diets, enteral nutrition, and parenteral nutrition (PN)—PN requires the highest degree of skilled and precise administration. There is always a risk of potentially life-threatening complication and infection. Roles of trained nutrition support clinicians are central to the success of PN. The nutrition support nurse administers the PN solution according to the nutrition support team protocol, monitoring the entire PN system frequently to see that it is operating accurately.

Specific clinical protocols will vary somewhat, but they usually include the following points:

- *Start slowly:* Give the patient time to adapt to the glucose and electrolyte concentration of the solution.
- *Schedule carefully:* PN volume can vary from 1 to 3 L and should be infused with an infusion pump. The infusion rate is based on the total volume of the compounded solution.
- *Monitor closely:* Note metabolic effects of glucose and electrolytes. Blood glucose levels should not exceed 200 mg/dl

during initiation of PN and should not exceed 110 to 150 mg/dl when the patient is stable on the formula. First-day formulas generally contain no more than 200 g dextrose. Monitor glycemic tolerance closely, particularly the first couple of days, as the feeding is advanced. Electrolyte status and glucose levels should be determined before and throughout PN administration. Increase energy provision only as patient tolerates macronutrient content.
- *Make changes cautiously:* Monitor and report the effect of all changes, and proceed slowly.
- *Maintain a constant rate:* Keep to the correct hourly infusion rate, with no "catch-up" or "slow-down" effort to meet the original volume order.
- *Discontinue PN:* Reduce the rate by one half for 1 hour before discontinuing. If patient has had insulin added to PN and is not receiving enteral tube feeding, monitor for rebound hypoglycemia (check serum glucose 2 hours after stopping PN infusion).

---

the patient must self-manage the therapy and work closely with the home nutrition support team. The Oley Foundation provides a network of support for patients on chronic, long-term home enteral and parenteral therapies. (Refer to the *Websites of Interest* section at the end of this chapter for the website of the Oley Foundation.) Reimbursement for services must be confirmed before sending a patient home on nutrition support. The process can require additional diagnostic testing and documentation in order for the patient to qualify, particularly when Medicare is the source of reimbursement.

Home Enteral Tube Feeding

Patient Selection

Developments in enteral tube feeding formulas and portable, lightweight infusion equipment have simplified home tube feeding and made it easier to manage. As a result, the number of patients receiving home tube feeding continues to grow as a means of cutting hospital costs and allowing earlier family support at home. Success of home infusion of enteral tube feeding relies on the education and training of both patient and family.[94]

Teaching Plan

Educating the patient and family for home infusion of enteral tube feeding is a team responsibility. This team may be hospital based or affiliated with the home infusion company that will manage the patient's care after discharge. The RD, nurse, and pharmacist develop and carry out a teaching plan, which includes topics and related tasks in preparing patients and families for discharge on home enteral feeding[89] (Box 18-7). The goal is to promote self-care and monitoring.

BOX 18-7	Home Enteral Tube Feeding Education Topics and Tasks

- Which enteral formulation is used and why
- How to prepare the tube feeding formula for infusion
- How to infuse the formula through the feeding tube
- How to correctly use and troubleshoot problems with the equipment
- How much water and how often to flush the feeding tube
- How to care for the tube site
- How to recognize tube feeding formula intolerance
- How to avoid and treat complications
- How to give medications and other separate nutrients through the feeding tube
- When to call the physician or home infusion provider

The hospital or home infusion company should provide a teaching manual with illustrations to guide the teaching-learning process and to be used as a reference at home. The teaching plan should start as soon as the decision for home tube feeding is made. A social worker identifies and if possible resolves any personal, psychosocial, safety, or economic issues with home infusion.

Finally, the teaching plan should allow sufficient time before discharge for the patient and family to demonstrate competency in (1) administering the tube feeding formula and (2) recording all necessary information about formula and fluid intake, formula tolerance, and complications. Directions for recording information are included in the home infusion manual. Records are reviewed regularly by the home nutrition support team and the patient's physician.

Follow-Up Monitoring

The plan for follow-up monitoring should be guided by specific protocols developed by the home infusion provider for laboratory, clinical, and home nutrition assessments. The home nutrition support team checks the patient's progress and works with the patient and family to troubleshoot any problems that arise and make required adjustments in the formula or tube feeding plan. Whenever feasible and appropriate the RD works closely with the patient and family to transition from tube feeding to oral intake. A study by Silver et al reported older adults receiving home enteral tube feeding with no consistent clinical follow-up experienced complications associated with unscheduled healthcare visits and readmissions to the hospital.[95] This study demonstrated the potential for improving outcomes with more frequent monitoring, reassessment, and intervention by a home nutrition support team that includes an RD.

Home Parenteral Nutrition

The patient sent home with PN requires education and training on the provision of PN in the outpatient setting. In the hands of knowledgeable and capable patients and their families, home PN allows mobility and independence. Equipment used in the home is small and portable—fitting in a backpack to allow patients to resume normal activities. The patient and family must be trained to use aseptic technique for adding micronutrients and medications to the solution and for accessing the intravenous catheter or port. Special equipment, solutions, and guidelines for training and supervising patients and families have been developed and are successfully used by hundreds of patients. Ongoing assessment of gastrointestinal function must be performed to determine if the patient is ready to transition to enteral feedings either oral or via feeding tube. Patients are also monitored closely for the development of complications associated with long-term PN infusion.

A study in complex inflammatory bowel disease patients demonstrated home PN could be successfully used to delay or avoid surgery.[96] The study also found anxiety about managing PN at home decreased for most of the patients after 1 week at home.

Health Promotion

Troubleshooting Diarrhea in Tube-Fed Patients

Diarrhea is one of the most common complications associated with tube feeding, yet the reported incidence ranges widely from as little as 2% to as much as 70% in general patient populations and as high as 80% in intensive care patients. Questions that relate to this wide variance and that plague investigators apparently center on definition and cause. But the ultimate bottom line for patient and family and their health insurers is the price of clinical search for the cause and appropriate method of treatment. Although clinicians search for an effective treatment, diarrhea results in reduced energy intake, dehydration, electrolyte abnormalities, and skin breakdown. Diarrhea also causes the patient discomfort, embarrassment, and frustration.

Problem of Definition

If we are ever going to determine an accurate occurrence rate, etiology, and treatment of diarrhea, there must be a precise operational definition on which to establish a research design and evaluate results. There are at least 14 definitions for diarrhea in the literature. However, there is little agreement on which definition most accurately reflects diarrhea that requires intervention. Common definitions include output of more than 500 ml on 2 consecutive days or more than three stools per day. From a nursing standpoint, collection and measurement of stool outputs are much less desirable than tracking number of occurrences. However, the true definition of diarrhea may need to reflect consistency and volume and not just number of stools per 24 hours. Most institutions do not have a standard definition for diarrhea; therefore, in most cases, diarrhea is defined by the person cleaning it up. Diagnosis of the cause of diarrhea and subsequent treatment consume time and healthcare resources. Meanwhile the patient is losing fluid, electrolytes, and nutrients through uncontrolled stool output. This can further exacerbate impaired nutritional status. Diarrhea not only takes a physical and nutritional toll on the patient but also has a psychologic effect of embarrassment and humiliation from an inability to control bodily functions and the loss of privacy.

A recently reported case of unexplained diarrhea in a tube-fed patient illustrates the difficult—and often costly—search for the cause (see the *Case Study* box, "The Case of the Costly Chase").

Factors Contributing to Diarrhea

Reported causes of diarrhea in tube-fed patients also vary. The finger of blame for diarrhea usually is aimed at the tube feeding formula. This results in manipulation of the formula—selection and concentration and infusion methods—usually to no avail because feeding intolerance is generally a manifestation, not the cause, of diarrhea. A variety of causes for diarrhea have been reported. The most common contributors to diarrhea in tube-fed patients are medications or some aspect of the patient's condition. However, many times there is not one single contributor but rather a combination of events or therapies that result in diarrhea.[53,54,87-100]

CASE STUDY

The Case of the Costly Chase

A reported case of unexplained diarrhea in a tube-fed patient illustrates the difficult, and often costly, search for the cause. Max was a 55-year-old man who had had an aortic aneurysm and underwent emergency surgery to repair it. In the intensive care unit, the postoperative course was complicated by respiratory problems requiring ventilator assistance. He was administered a bronchodilator drug, theophylline, in tablet form, crushed and administered by nasogastric tube with water. When Max was started on an enteral tube feeding with an isotonic formula, crushed theophylline tablets were changed to a sugar-free theophylline solution. Within a day Max began to have progressive abdominal distention and continuous liquid diarrhea. To rule out an abdominal catastrophe related to the aneurysm or surgery, a computed abdominal tomography scan, an aortogram, and colonoscopy were performed, but all of these studies were normal.

Despite stopping the enteral tube feeding, the distention and diarrhea continued. Stool specimens were tested for fecal leukocytes, parasites, and *Clostridium difficile* toxin, and an enteric pathogen culture was prepared. All were nondiagnostic. Extensive additional serum and urine tests, as well as a sigmoidoscopy with rectal biopsy, gave no clue. Then stool electrolytes and osmolality measures suggested an osmotic diarrhea. Because Max was not receiving enteral tube feedings, his physicians thought a secretory bacterial toxin was probably causing continuing diarrhea, so the previous studies were repeated to confirm the osmotic nature of the diarrhea. In addition, all medications were reviewed, but none appeared to be the cause.

Because the continued diarrhea prohibited enteral tube feeding and Max needed to be fed, parenteral nutrition was ordered. This move immediately brought an automatic nutrition support service consultation, which included assessment of medications. This evaluation revealed that the sugar-free theophylline solution was 65% sorbitol.

Sorbitol is a polyhydric alcohol used as a sweetener in many sugar-free products such as dietetic foods and chewing gum. There was no information about sorbitol on the label or package insert of the drug because sorbitol is considered an "inactive" ingredient. Sorbitol content was obtained by contacting the manufacturer.

Fortunately for Max, however, the nutrition support team did know the components of the medication and found the hidden culprit. The registered dietitian knew sorbitol in larger doses is a laxative! Calculations of the regular daily amount of theophylline Max was taking showed he was receiving nearly 300 g of sorbitol daily when the usual laxative dose was only 20 to 50 g. The nutrition support team immediately recommended that this sorbitol-sweetened solution of theophylline be discontinued and a sorbitol-free form of the medication be used instead. Almost immediately the diarrhea began to decrease, and in 3 days it was gone.

The extent of this costly chase was revealed in Max's hospital bill. He had continued to receive the faulty drug for almost half of his 3-month hospital stay, during which time the diarrhea prevented enteral tube feeding and he had to have the more expensive parenteral nutrition. The parenteral nutrition cost $5000 more than enteral feedings would have cost for the same period. In addition, all the extensive investigations to find the cause of the diarrhea cost $5300, which together with the indirect costs for extra days of care and supplies made a total hospital bill of about $200,000.

Causes of diarrhea in tube-fed patients are many, but in the hands of a skilled nutrition support team, the formula is seldom one of them. It is often found in the medications. Just remember what this medication's hidden ingredient—sorbitol—cost Max.

Data from Wong K: The role of fiber in diarrhea management, *SupportLine* 20:16, 1998.

Formula

Tube feeding formula osmolality or concentration and rate of delivery are often blamed for instigating diarrhea. However, reports have shown no increase in incidence of diarrhea when the formula concentration varied widely from 145 to 430 mOm/L, and no significant association has been made between malabsorption and formula osmolality or rate of delivery. Formulas providing more than 30% of total kcalories as fat have been associated with a higher incidence of diarrhea, whereas those providing 20% fat rarely were involved. Further study of fat composition is needed, specifically comparing medium-chain versus long-chain triglycerides and omega-3 versus omega-6 fatty acids. Studies of the role of fiber in tube feedings have had conflicting results. There is no consistency in the types and amount of fiber in enteral tube feeding formulas. Soluble fiber can increase colonic absorption of water. However, when the fiber given to a patient is increased rapidly, the patient will experience flatulence, abdominal distention, and constipation. Reviewers have found the studies thus far have been few, models used variable, limitations substantial, and conclusions of investigators mixed. In general, amount and type of fiber in enteral formulas are not significant enough to prevent or contribute to diarrhea.[53,54,97-100]

Bacterial Contamination

There are studies that have shown the more manipulation and additives, such as modular components, added to an enteral formula, the more likely the formula will become contaminated. Tube feeding formula hang time, open versus closed delivery systems, and preparation technique can affect the risk of bacterial contamination of the enteral tube feeding formula. Formula added to open delivery systems should hang no longer than 8 hours (even shorter periods of time if additives are combined with the formula). Closed systems that use containers prefilled with formula can hang 24 to 48 hours. The fewer times any system is handled and opened, the less chance there is for contamination. Commercial formula manufacturers are making formulas now that contain microbial inhibitors to reduce the risk of bacterial contamination of the enteral formula itself.[53,54,97,100]

Infusion Method

Intragastric feedings are associated with an increased incidence of diarrhea. Infusion of a large amount of energy into the stomach stimulates the colon to secret water, sodium, and chloride with resulting inability of the colon to absorb nutrients.[53,54,97-100]

Patient's Condition

Malnourished or critically ill patients are more susceptible to mucosal tissue breakdown and malabsorption leading to diarrhea. Hypoalbuminemia has also been reported to be a potential cause of diarrhea because of its effect on reducing colloidal osmotic pressure within blood vessels, which could lead to edema of the intestinal mucosa, malabsorption, and diarrhea. However, there has been no correlation between patients with hypoalbuminemia and incidence of diarrhea. Patients with pancreatic insufficiency, celiac disease, small bowel syndrome, fecal impaction, diabetes mellitus, or gastrointestinal inflammation are at greater risk for diarrhea.[53,54,97-100]

Medications

Multiple medications routinely given to hospitalized patients have been related to diarrhea. Antibiotics are most often associated with gastrointestinal side effects. However, patients more susceptible to developing diarrhea are those who are critically ill and on multiple medications. Extensive treatment with antibiotics and disuse of the gastrointestinal tract contribute to a change in the bacterial milieu of the intestine with proliferation of the enteric pathogen *Clostridium difficile*. Other medications associated with development of diarrhea are H_2-blockers, lactulose or laxatives, magnesium-containing antacids, potassium and phosphorus supplements, antineoplastic agents, and quinidine. Medications are often hyperosmolar and require dilution before infusion through a feeding tube. In general, drug reactions may relate to the metabolically active agent or to another ingredient added for its physical properties in the form of the drug, such as tablet or liquid, as the case in the *Case Study* box illustrates. Probiotics, nonpathogenic lactic acid bacteria, are receiving more attention as a potential treatment of diarrhea and as a means of preventing bacterial overgrowth and *C. difficile* infections.[53,54,97-100]

TO SUM UP

For patients with functioning gastrointestinal tracts, enteral nutrition support has proved to be a potent tool against present or potential malnutrition. Enteral nutrition support is achieved by an oral diet with nutrient-dense supplementation or alternately by tube feeding when the patient cannot, will not, or should not eat. Commercial tube feeding formulas with or without modular enhancement provide complete nutrition when provided in adequate amounts. Enteral tube feeding can be provided through nasoenteric or enterostomy feeding tubes with an open or closed delivery system. Tubing and container adaptations and development of small, mobile infusion pumps, together with a comprehensive teaching plan for patient and family and follow-up monitoring by a clinical team, allow many patients the option of home tube feeding.

For patients with a dysfunctional gastrointestinal tract, PN is a life-sustaining therapy. This feeding method depends heavily on biomedical technology for the development of tubes, bags, pumps, and other equipment for feeding nutrients directly into the vein. Route of entry may be a large central vein for intravenous feeding over a long period or a smaller peripheral vein for feeding less-concentrated solutions for a shorter period. Home PN is successfully used by many patients with the support of family, friends, and a home nutrition support team.

QUESTIONS FOR REVIEW

1. Describe several types of patient situations in which enteral tube feeding may be indicated. What nutrition assessment procedures may help to identify these individuals?

2. Describe nutrient components of a typical complete polymeric enteral formula. How does it differ from a modular formula? How does it differ from a semielemental and an elemental formula?

3. Define PN, and identify examples of conditions in which it would be used.

   The following questions apply to the case of a man referred to nutrition support services. Imagine you are caring for this patient.

   A previously healthy 45-year-old man, while on a long transport haul as a truck driver, was in an accident in which he sustained a severe abdominal injury requiring extensive surgical repair and leaving the gastrointestinal tract unavailable for use for an undetermined period. He is referred to the nutrition support team for PN. Early in this care he asks you how this feeding works.

4. How would you describe and explain the PN feeding process?

5. What nutrition assessment parameters would be beneficial in identifying his risk of developing malnutrition and his tolerance of parenteral therapy?

6. List typical components of a basic PN formula he may require, and describe the purpose of each to help reassure him of its adequacy and importance.

7. Sufficient energy (kcalorie) intake is essential to immediately meet his metabolic needs after surgery. Assume a normal preinjury weight (175 lb) and height (70 inches) and an added stress factor of 1.2 times his BEE. Calculate his total energy requirement, using the HBE and the MSJ equation. Compare the results.

8. Define hepatic proteins, and describe why they are not appropriate indicators of nutritional status. How can you monitor the effectiveness of the PN formula in meeting his nutrition support needs for recovery?

REFERENCES

1. Borum PR: Nutrient metabolism. In Gottschlich MM et al, eds: *The science and practice of nutrition support: a case-based core curriculum,* Dubuque, Iowa, 2001, Kendall/Hunt Publishing.

2. Butterworth CE: The skeleton in the hospital closet, *Nutr Today* 9:4, 1974.

3. Bistrian BR et al: Protein status of general surgical patients, *JAMA* 230:858, 1974.

4. Naber T et al: Prevalence of malnutrition in nonsurgical hospitalized patients and its association with disease complications, *Am J Clin Nutr* 66:1232, 1997.

5. Detsky AS et al: What is subjective global assessment of nutritional status? *JPEN J Parenter Enteral Nutr* 11(1):8, 1987.

6. Braunschweig C et al: Impact of declines in nutritional status on outcomes in adult patients hospitalized for more than seven days, *J Am Diet Assoc* 100:1316, 2000.

7. A.S.P.E.N. Board of Directors and The Clinical Guidelines Task Force: Guidelines for the use of parenteral and enteral nutrition in adult and pediatric patients, *JPEN J Parenter Enteral Nutr* 26:1SA, 2002.

8. Moore FA et al: Early enteral feeding, compared with parenteral, reduces postoperative septic complications: the results of a meta-analysis, *Ann Surg* 216:172, 1992.

9. Lipman TO: Grains or veins: is enteral nutrition really better than parenteral nutrition? A look at the evidence, *JPEN J Parenter Enteral Nutr* 22:167, 1998.

10. Shopbell JM et al: Nutrition screening and assessment. In Gottschlich MM et al, eds: *The science and practice of nutrition support: a case-based core curriculum,* Dubuque, Iowa, 2001, Kendall/Hunt Publishing.

11. Lacey K, Pritchett E: Nutrition care process and model: ADA adopts road map to quality care and outcomes management, *J Am Diet Assoc* 103:1061, 2003.

12. Fuhrman MP et al: Hepatic proteins and nutrition assessment, *J Am Diet Assoc* 104:1258, 2004.

13. Harris JA, Benedict FG: *A biometric study of basal metabolism,* Washington, DC, 1919, Carnegie Institution of Washington.

14. Mifflin MD et al: A new predictive equation for resting energy expenditure in healthy individuals, *Am J Clin Nutr* 51(2):241, 1990.

15. Frankenfield D et al: Validation of several established equations for resting metabolic rate in obese and nonobese people, *J Am Diet Assoc* 103:1152, 2003.

16. Crook MA et al: The importance of the refeeding syndrome, *Nutrition* 17:632, 2001.

17. Vanek VW: The use of serum albumin as a prognostic or nutritional marker and the pros and cons of IV albumin therapy, *Nutr Clin Pract* 13:110, 1998.

18. Meyer J et al: Benefits of a nutrition support service in an HMO setting, *Nutr Clin Pract* 16:25, 2001.

19. American Society for Parenteral and Enteral Nutrition Board of Directors: Standards of practice for nutrition support nurses, *Nutr Clin Pract* 16:56, 2001.

20. American Society for Parenteral and Enteral Nutrition Board of Directors: Standards of practice for nutrition support pharmacists, *Nutr Clin Pract* 14:275, 1999.

21. American Society for Parenteral and Enteral Nutrition Board of Directors: Standards of practice for nutrition support physicians, *Nutr Clin Pract* 18:270, 2003.

22. American Society for Parenteral and Enteral Nutrition Board of Directors: Standards of practice for nutrition support dietitians, *Nutr Clin Pract* 15:53, 2000.

23. Board of Directors, American Society for Parenteral and Enteral Nutrition: Interdisciplinary nutrition support core competencies, *Nutr Clin Pract* 14:331, 1999.

24. JCAHO Board of Directors: *Comprehensive accreditation manual for hospitals,* Oakbrook Terrace, Ill, 2000, Joint Commission on Accreditation of Healthcare Organizations.

25. Fuhrman MP: Parenteral nutrition: a clinician's perspective, *Dietitians Edge* 2(1):53, 2001.

26. Charney P: Enteral nutrition: indications, options and formulations. In Gottschlich MM et al, eds: *The science and practice of nutrition support: a case-based core curriculum,* Dubuque, Iowa, 2001, Kendall/Hunt Publishing.

27. Roth JL, Clohessy S: Administration of enteral nutrition: initiation, progression, and transition. In Rolandelli RH, ed: *Clinical nutrition: enteral and tube feeding,* ed 4, Philadelphia, 2005, Elsevier Saunders.

28. Veterans Affairs Total Parenteral Nutrition Cooperative Study Group: Perioperative total parenteral nutrition in surgical patients, *N Engl J Med* 325:525, 1992.

29. Jeejeebhoy KN: Total parenteral nutrition: potion or poison? *Am J Clin Nutr* 74:160, 2001.

30. Lewis DA, Boyle K: Nutritional supplement use during medication administration: selected case studies, *J Nutr Elder* 17(4):53, 1998.

31. Turic A et al: Nutrition supplementation enables elderly residents in long-term care facilities to meet or exceed RDAs without displacing energy or nutrient intakes from meals, *J Am Diet Assoc* 98:1457, 1998.

32. Watters JM et al: Immediate postoperative enteral feeding results in impaired respiratory mechanics and decreased mobility, *Ann Surg* 266:369, 1997.

33. Charney P, Russell M: Enteral formulations: standard. In Rolandelli RH, ed: *Clinical nutrition: enteral and tube feeding,* ed 4, Philadelphia, 2005, Elsevier Saunders.

34. Matarese LE et al: The role of probiotics in gastrointestinal disease, *Nutr Clin Pract* 18:507, 2003.

35. Gadek JE et al: Effect of enteral feeding with eicosapentaenoic acid, a-linolenic acid, and antioxidants in patients with acute respiratory distress syndrome, *Crit Care Med* 27:1409, 1999.

36. Consensus recommendations from the U.S. Summit on Immune-Enhancing Enteral Therapy, *JPEN J Parenter Enteral Nutr* 25:S61, 2001.

37. Talbot JM: Guidelines for the scientific review of enteral food products for special medical purposes, *JPEN J Parenter Enteral Nutr* 15(suppl 3):100S, 1991.

38. Metheny NA, Clouse RE: Bedside methods for detecting aspiration in tube-fed patients, *Chest* 111:724, 1997.

39. Maloney JP et al: Systemic absorption of food dye in patients with sepsis [letter], *N Engl J Med* 343:1047, 2000.

40. Maloney JP, Ryan TA: Detection of aspiration in enterally fed patients: a requiem for bedside monitors of aspiration, *JPEN J Parenter Enteral Nutr* 26:S34, 2002.

41. Cannon R et al: *Methods and tubes for establishing enteral access: discussion. Enteral nutrition support for the 1990s: innovations in nutrition, technology, and techniques.* Report of the 12th Ross Roundtable on Medical Issues. Columbus, Ohio, 1992, Ross Products Division, Abbott Laboratories.

42. Moore MC, ed: Enteral nutrition. In *Mosby's pocket guide series: nutritional care,* ed 4, St. Louis, 2001, Mosby.

43. Metheny NA et al: pH and concentration of bilirubin in feeding tube aspirates as predictors of tube placement, *Nurs Res* 48(4):189, 1999.

44. Metheny N et al: Effect of feeding tube properties and three irrigants on clogging rates, *Nurs Res* 37:165, 1988.

45. Sriram K et al: Prophylactic locking of enteral feeding tubes with pancreatic enzymes, *JPEN J Parenter Enteral Nutr* 21(6):353, 1997.

46. Orlee K et al: Enteral formulations. In A.S.P.E.N. Board of Directors, ed: *A.S.P.E.N. nutrition support practice manual,* Silver Spring, Md, 1998, American Society for Parenteral and Enteral Nutrition.

47. Vanek VW: Closed versus open enteral delivery systems: a quality improvement study, *Nutr Clin Pract* 15:234, 2000.

48. Herlick SJ et al: Comparison of open versus closed systems of intermittent enteral feeding in two long-term care facilities, *Nutr Clin Pract* 15:287, 2000.

49. Keohane PP et al: Relation between osmolarity of the diet and gastrointestinal side effects in enteral nutrition, *BJM* 288:678, 1984.

50. Lysen LK: Enteral equipment. In Matarese LE, Gottschlich MM, eds: *Contemporary nutrition support practice: a clinical guide,* ed 2, Philadelphia, 2003, Saunders.

51. Ibanaez J et al: Gastroesophageal reflux in intubated patients receiving enteral nutrition: effect of supine and semirecumbent positions, *JPEN J Parenter Enteral Nutr* 16:419, 1992.

52. Cogen R et al: Complications of jejunostomy tube feeding in nursing facility patients, *Am J Gastroenterol* 86:1610, 1991.

53. Mobarhan S, Demeo M: Diarrhea induced by enteral feeding, *Nutr Rev* 53:67, 1995.

54. Fuhrman MP: Diarrhea and tube feeding, *Nutr Clin Pract* 14:83, 1999.

55. Kirby DF et al: American Gastroenterological Association technical review on tube feeding for enteral nutrition, *Gastroenterology* 108:1282, 1995.

56. McClave SA et al: Use of residual volume as a marker for enteral feeding tolerance: prospective, blinded comparison with physical examination and radiographic findings, *JPEN J Parenter Enteral Nutr* 16(2):99, 1992.

57. Pinilla JC et al: Comparison of gastrointestinal tolerance to two enteral feeding protocols in critically ill patients: a prospective, randomized trial, *JPEN J Parenter Enteral Nutr* 25:81, 2001.

58. Heyland DK et al: Canadian clinical practice guidelines for nutrition support in mechanically ventilated, critically ill adult patients, *JPEN J Parenter Enteral Nutr* 27:355, 2003.

59. Mateo MA: Nursing management of enteral tube feeding, *Heart Lung* 25:318, 1996.

60. Spain DA et al: Infusion protocol improves delivery of enteral tube feeding in the critical care unit, *JPEN J Parenter Enteral Nutr* 23:288, 1999.

61. Heyland DK et al: Validation of the Canadian clinical practice guidelines for nutrition support in mechanically ventilated, critically ill adult patients: results of a prospective observational study, *Crit Care Med* 32:2260, 2004.

62. van den Berghe G et al: Intensive insulin therapy in critically ill patients, *N Engl J Med* 345:1359, 2001.

63. Krinsley JS: Effect of an intensive glucose management protocol on the mortality of critically ill adult patients, *Mayo Clin Proc* 79:992, 2004.

64. Fuhrman MP: Complication management in parenteral nutrition. In Matarese LE, Gottschlich MM, eds: *Contemporary nutrition support practice: a clinical guide,* ed 2, Philadelphia, 2003, Saunders.

65. Mirtallo JM: Introduction to parenteral nutrition. In Gottschlich MM et al, eds: *The science and practice of nutrition support: a case-based core curriculum,* Dubuque, Iowa, 2001, Kendall/Hunt Publishing.

66. Dudrick SJ et al: Can intravenous feeding as the sole means of nutrition support growth in the child and restore weight loss in an adult? *Ann Surg* 169:974, 1969.

67. Klein S et al: Nutrition support in clinical practice: review of published data on recommendations for future directions, *JPEN J Parenter Enter Nutr* 21(3):133, 1997.

68. Stokes MA, Hill GL: Peripheral parenteral nutrition: a preliminary report on its efficacy and safety, *JPEN J Parenter Enteral Nutr* 17(2):145, 1993.

69. Trujillo ED et al: Metabolic and monetary costs of avoidable parenteral nutrition use, *JPEN J Parenter Enteral Nutr* 23:109, 1999.

70. Speerhas RA et al: Five year follow-up of a program to minimize inappropriate use of parenteral nutrition [abstract], *JPEN J Parenter Enteral Nutr* 25:S4, 2001.

71. Tulsyan N et al: Enterocutaneous fistulas, *Nutr Clin Pract* 16:74, 2001.

72. Byrne TA et al: Beyond the prescription: optimizing the diet of patients with short bowel syndrome, *Nutr Clin Pract* 15:306, 2000.

73. Spain DA, McClave SA: Chylothorax and chylous ascites. In Gottschlich MM et al, eds: *The science and practice of nutrition support: a case-based core curriculum,* Dubuque, Iowa, 2001, Kendall/Hunt Publishing.

74. Kelly DG, Nehra V: Gastrointestinal disease. In Gottschlich MM et al, eds: *The science and practice of nutrition support: a case-based core curriculum,* Dubuque, Iowa, 2001, Kendall/ Hunt Publishing.

75. Task force for the revision of safe practices for parenteral nutrition et al: Safe practices for parenteral nutrition, *JPEN J Parenter Enteral Nutr* 28(suppl): S39, 2004.

76. Seidner DL et al: Effect of long-chain triglyceride emulsions on reticuloendothelial system function in humans, *JPEN J Parenter Enteral Nutr* 13:614, 1989.

77. American Medical Association, AMA Department of Foods and Nutrition: Multivitamin preparations for parenteral use: a statement by the Nutrition Advisory Group, *JPEN J Parenter Enteral Nutr* 3:258, 1979.

78. Parenteral multivitamin products; drugs for human use; drug efficacy study implementation; amendment (21 CFR 5.70), *Fed Register* 65:21200, 2000.

79. Expert Panel for Nutrition Advisory Group, AMA Department of Foods and Nutrition: Guidelines for essential trace element preparations for parenteral use, *JAMA* 241:2051, 1979.

80. Forceville F et al: Selenium, systemic immune response syndrome, sepsis, and outcome in critically ill patients, *Crit Care Med* 26:1536, 1998.

81. Angstwurm MAW et al: Selenium replacement in patients with severe systemic inflammatory response syndrome improves clinical outcome, *Crit Care Med* 27:1807, 1999.

82. Cohen HJ et al: Glutathione peroxidase and selenium deficiency in patients receiving home parenteral nutrition: time course for development of deficiency and repletion of the enzyme activity in plasma and blood cells, *Am J Clin Nutr* 49:132, 1989.

83. Fuhrman MP et al: Pancytopenia following removal of copper from TPN, *JPEN J Parenter Enteral Nutr* 24:361, 2000.

84. Masumoto K et al: Manganese intoxication during intermittent parenteral nutrition: report of two cases, *JPEN J Parenter Enteral Nutr* 25:95, 2001.

85. Pemberton L et al: Sepsis from triple- vs single-lumen catheters during total parenteral nutrition in surgical or critically ill patients, *Arch Surg* 121:591, 1986.

86. Farkas J et al: Single- versus triple-lumen central catheter-related sepsis: a prospective randomized study in a critically ill population, *Am J Med* 93:277, 1992.

87. Savage AP et al: Complications and survival of multilumen central venous catheters used for total parenteral nutrition, *Br J Surg* 80:1287, 1993.

88. Maki DG et al: Prevention of central venous catheter-related bloodstream infection by use of an antiseptic-impregnated catheter: a randomized, controlled trial, *Ann Intern Med* 127:257, 1997.

89. Veenstra DL et al: Cost-effectiveness of antiseptic-impregnated central venous catheters for the prevention of catheter-related bloodstream infection, *J Am Med Assoc* 282:554, 1999.

90. Centers for Disease Control and Prevention: Guidelines for the prevention of intravascular catheter-related infections, *MMWR Morb Mortal Wkly Rep* 51(RR-10):1-26, 2002.

91. Intravenous Nurses Society: Infusion nursing standards of practice, *J Intraven Nurs* 23(6 suppl):S1-S85, 2000.

92. Dodds ES et al: Metabolic occurrences in total parenteral nutrition patients managed by a nutrition support team, *Nutr Clin Pract* 16:78, 2001.

93. Klein CJ et al: Nutrition support care map targets monitoring and reassessment to improve outcomes in trauma patients, *Nutr Clin Pract* 16:85, 2001.

94. American Society for Parenteral and Enteral Nutrition Board of Directors: Standards for home nutrition support, *Nutr Clin Pract* 14:151, 1998.

95. Silver HJ et al: Older adults receiving home enteral nutrition: enteral regimen, provider involvement, and health care outcomes. *JPEN J Parenter Enteral Nutr* 28:92, 2004.

96. Evans JP et al: Home total parenteral nutrition: an alternative to early surgery for complicated inflammatory bowel disease. *J Gastrointest Surg* 7:562, 2003.

97. Bowling TE: Enteral-feeding-related diarrhea: proposed causes and possible solutions, *Proc Nutr Soc* 54:579, 1995.

98. Ringel AF, Jameson GL, Foster ES: Diarrhea in the intensive care patient, *Crit Care Clin North Am* 11:465, 1995.

99. Wong K: The role of fiber in diarrhea management, *Support Line* 20:16, 1998.

100. Williams MS et al: Diarrhea management in enterally fed patient, *Nutr Clin Pract* 13:225, 1998.

FURTHER READINGS AND RESOURCES

Readings

American Society for Parenteral and Enteral Nutrition Board of Directors and Task Force on Standards for Specialized Nutrition Support of Hospitalized Adult Patients, Standards for Specialized Nutrition Support: Adult hospitalized patients, *Nutr Clin Pract* 17: 384, 2002.

A.S.P.E.N. Board of Directors and the Clinical Guidelines Task Force: Guidelines for the use of parenteral and enteral nutrition in adult and pediatric patients, *JPEN J Parenter Enteral Nutr* 26(suppl):1SA, 2002.

Heyland DK et al: Canadian clinical practice guidelines for nutrition support in mechanically ventilated, critically ill adult patients, *JPEN J Parenter Enteral Nutr* 27:355, 2003.

Task Force for the Revision of Safe Practices for Parenteral Nutrition and the A.S.P.E.N. Board of Directors: Safe practices for parenteral nutrition, *JPEN J Parenter Enteral Nutr* 28(suppl):S30, 2004.

Websites of Interest

- The American Society for Parenteral and Enteral Nutrition (A.S.P.E.N.): *www.nutritioncare.org*.
- American Dietetic Association: *www.eatright.org*.
- Dietitians in Nutrition Support: *www.dnsdpg.org*.
- The Oley Foundation: *www.oley.org*.
- CIGNA Medicare; this website offers free Medicare training for clinicians regarding Medicare qualifications for home enteral and parenteral nutrition: *www.cignamedicare.com/webtraining*.

CHAPTER 19

Gastrointestinal Diseases

Sara Long

In this chapter we consider diseases of the gastrointestinal (GI) tract and surrounding accessory organs—liver, gallbladder, and pancreas. In health, digestion and absorption of food are accomplished through a series of intimately interrelated actions among and within these organ systems. To the extent disease or malfunction at any point interferes with this finely interwoven process, adequate nutrition is provided either through quantitative or qualitative modifications to food.

The GI tract is a sensitive mirror of the individual human condition. Its physiologic function often reflects physical and psychologic conditioning. In this chapter these basic functions, healing process, nutrition therapy indicated, and individuals' personal needs will be discussed. The Complementary and Alternative Medicine box, "Alternative Treatments for Diseases of the Gastrointestinal Tract" outlines the effectiveness of alternative treatments for diseases of the GI tract.

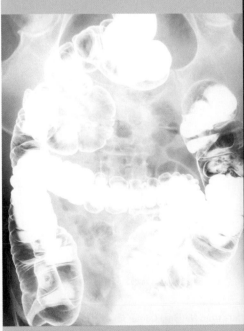

COMPLEMENTARY AND ALTERNATIVE MEDICINE (CAM)
Alternative Treatments for Diseases of the Gastrointestinal Tract

What Is Known From the Scientific Evidence About CAM Modalities for Gastrointestinal Disorders?
There are no well-documented herbal treatments for gastrointestinal (GI) disorders, although use of probiotics to treat Crohn's disease shows some promise.

What CAM Therapies Might Be Used to Treat Gastrointestinal Disorders?

Gastrointestinal Disorder	Herb	Scientific Name	Active Ingredient	Efficacy	Side Effects and/or Risks
Cirrhosis	Milk thistle (plant)	*Silybum marianum*	Silymarin (found in the fruit)	Inconsistent results	Generally well-tolerated, can cause laxative effect, allergic reactions in people allergic to ragweed, chrysanthemum, marigold, and daisy.
Crohn's disease	Fish oil	Docosahexaenoic acid (DHA), eicosapentaenoic acid (EPA), omega-3 fatty acids, omega-3 oils		Mixed results as to whether or not fish oil helped keep the disease controlled in patients who were in remission.	Possible risk of bleeding complications.
Dyspepsia	Curcumin	*Curcuma longa*	Polyphenol	Stimulates contraction of the gallbladder; provides full or partial relief of symptoms	Could present risks in individuals with gallbladder disease; maximum safe doses in individuals with severe hepatic or renal disease not known.
Hepatitis C	Milk thistle (plant)	*Silybum marianum*	Silymarin (found in the fruit)	*May* be some benefits, but none definitively beneficial in treating hepatitis C	See above.
	Licorice root (plant)	*Glycyrrhiza glabra*	Glycyrrhizin	*May* have antiviral properties in vitro, has potential for reducing long-term complications of chronic hepatitis C in patients who do not respond to interferon; does not reduce amount of hepatitis C virus (HCV) in patients' blood	Licorice intake over a long period of time can lead to hypertension, salt and water retention, swelling, depletion of potassium, headache, and/or sluggishness; can worsen ascites; can interact with certain drugs (diuretics, digitalis, antiarrhythmic agents, and corticosteroids) (see Chapter 17).

Data from National Center for Complementary and Alternative Medicine: *Research report: hepatitis C and complementary and alternative medicine—2003 update*, Bethesda, Md, 2003, Author. Retrieved December 15, 2005, from *http://nccam.nih.gov/health/hepatitisc/*; and Bratman S, Girman AM: *Mosby's handbook of herbs and supplements and their therapeutic use*, St. Louis, 2003, Mosby/Elsevier Science.

NSAID, Nonsteroidal antiinflammatory drug; *GLA,* gamma-linolenic acid.

COMPLEMENTARY AND ALTERNATIVE MEDICINE (CAM)—cont'd
Alternative Treatments for Diseases of the Gastrointestinal Tract

Gastrointestinal Disorder	Herb	Scientific Name	Active Ingredient	Efficacy	Side Effects and/or Risks
Hepatitis C— cont'd	Thymus extract (gland)	(Should not be confused with the prescription drug thymosin alpha-1)	Peptides from thymus glands of cows or calves sold as dietary supplements	Very little research, but none found the product beneficial for patients with hepatitis C	Thrombocytopenia (drop in number of platelet cells in blood); concern about possible contamination from diseased animal parts (people on immunosuppressive drugs should use caution).
	Schisandra (plant)	*Schisandra chinensis, Schisandra sphenanthera*	Extracts from its fruits	Some antioxidant effect, no reports on safety and effectiveness using schisandra alone to treat hepatitis C in humans	Found as an ingredient in herbal formulas; considered generally safe; in some it may cause heartburn, acid indigestion, decreased appetite, stomach pain, or allergic skin rashes.
	Colloidal silver	Silver	Metallic element	Silver has no known function in the human body, not an essential mineral supplement, claims of silver "deficiency" in the body are unfounded	Silver builds up in body tissues: argyria—a bluish gray discoloration of the body, especially skin, other organs, deep tissues, nails, and gums. Argyria is not treatable or reversible. Other possible problems include neurologic (such as seizures), kidney damage, stomach distress, headaches, fatigue, and skin irritation. May interfere with absorption of the following drugs: penicillamine, quinolones, tetracyclines, and thyroxine.

Continued

COMPLEMENTARY AND ALTERNATIVE MEDICINE (CAM)—cont'd
Alternative Treatments for Diseases of the Gastrointestinal Tract

Gastrointestinal Disorder	Herb	Scientific Name	Active Ingredient	Efficacy	Side Effects and/or Risks
Irritable bowel syndrome (IBS)	Peppermint oil	*Menthe piperita*	Menthol	Provides anti-spasmodic properties; *may* provide some relief from crampy abdominal pain	Enteric-coated peppermint believed to be reasonably safe in healthy adults; non–enteric-coated peppermint oil can cause heartburn; maximum dosages in individuals with severe hepatic or renal disease not known.
	Probiotics	*Lactobacillus plantarum*	Acidophilus	Evidence of efficacy is mixed; may reduce intestinal gas and pain	No known safety issues.
	Flaxseed	*Linum usitatissimum*	Lignans, alpha-linolenic acid	Helps relieve constipation, abdominal pain, and bloating	Not associated with any significant adverse effects.
Nausea	Ginger	*Zingiber officinale*		As effective for motion sickness as standard pharmaceutical agents; also effective in reducing nausea in pregnancy	No drug interactions are known; ginger should be used with care in patients using anticoagulants or antiplatelet agents.
Peptic ulcer disease	Licorice, deglycyrrhizinated (DGL)	*Glycyrrhiza glabra*	DGL is a specially processed form of licorice that does not produce pseudohyperaldosteronemia.	No evidence that DGL eradicates *Helicobacter pylori;* it may protect gastric lining from NSAID-induced gastritis; no more effective than antacids in providing relief	May reduce testosterone levels in men; maximum safe doses in those with severe hepatic or renal disease not known; licorice appears to potentiate topical and oral corticosteroids; should be used with caution in patients taking thiazide or loop diuretics, or digitalis.
	Probiotics	*Lactobacillus plantarum*	Acidophilus	Exerts inhibitory action on *H. pylori,* but not enough to eradicate it; may be useful adjunct to standard antibiotic therapy	See above.

COMPLEMENTARY AND ALTERNATIVE MEDICINE (CAM)—cont'd
Alternative Treatments for Diseases of the Gastrointestinal Tract

Gastrointestinal Disorder	Herb	Scientific Name	Active Ingredient	Efficacy	Side Effects and/or Risks
Ulcerative colitis (UC)	Probiotics	*Escherichia coli* spp	Nonpathogenic strain of *E. coli*	Can prevent acute attacks of UC as effectively as mesalazine	See above.
	Essential fatty acids	DHA, EPA, omega-3 fatty acids, omega-3 oils	Fish oils	Might be helpful for reducing symptoms of UC; regular use does not appear to help prevent disease flare-ups	See above.
	Essential fatty acids	Omega-6 fatty acid GLA	Evening primrose oil	Somewhat beneficial in preventing flare-ups	See above.

DIGESTIVE PROCESS

When food is taken into the mouth, the act of eating stimulates the GI tract into accelerated action. Throughout the digestive process, highly coordinated systems and interactive functions respond (Figure 19-1). Secretory functions provide the necessary environment and agents for chemical digestion. *Peristalsis* and gravity move the food mass along. Nutrients are absorbed into circulation and carried to cells that take up what is needed to nourish the body. Emotional factors influence overall individual response pattern. This highly individual and interrelated functional network forms the basis for nutrition therapy in disease.

After food is taken into the mouth and masticated (forming a bolus), swallowing occurs, allowing the bolus to pass from the laryngopharynx into the esophagus entrance at the upper esophageal sphincter (Figure 19-2). Food is pushed through the esophagus by gravity and involuntary muscular movements, called *peristalsis,* controlled by the medulla oblongata. Circular muscle fibers contract, constricting the esophageal wall and squeezing the bolus toward the stomach. The lower esophageal sphincter muscle at the entry to the stomach forms a controlling valve, relaxing to receive the bolus and then closing to hold each bolus for some initial digestive action of enzymes. Stomach cells produce enzymes to break down food particles and protect themselves from being broken down. Passage of food from mouth to stomach takes about 4 to 8 seconds.

Chyme (semiliquid mass) is released by the stomach through the pyloric sphincter into the duodenum, the first section of the small intestine, where most digestion occurs. A number of small intestine and accessory organ conditions may interfere with normal food passage and create malabsorption problems. These overall conditions vary widely from brief periods of functional discomfort to serious disease and complete obstruction. In making nutrition therapy recommendations for food choices and feeding mode, the dietetics practitioner will take into account the degree of dysfunction.

PROBLEMS OF THE MOUTH AND ESOPHAGUS

Mouth Problems

Teeth and jaw muscles in the mouth work together to break down food into a form that can be easily swallowed. Conditions that interfere with this process interfere with nutritional intake.

Tissue Inflammation

Tissues of the mouth often reflect a person's basic nutritional status. In malnutrition, tissues of the mouth deteriorate and become inflamed and are more vulnerable to local infection or injury, causing pain and difficulty with eating. These conditions (Figure 19-3) in the oral cavity include (1) *gingivitis,* inflammation of the gums, involving the mucous membrane with its supporting fibrous tissue circling the base of the teeth (see Figure 19-3, *A*); (2) *stomatitis,* inflammation of the oral mucosa lining the mouth (see Figure 19-3, *B*); (3) *glossitis,* inflammation of the tongue (see Figure 19-3, *C*); and (4) *cheilosis,* a cracking and dry scaling process at the corners of the mouth affecting the lips and corner angles, making opening the mouth to receive food difficult (see Figure 19-3, *D*).

These oral tissue problems may also be nonspecific and unrelated to nutritional factors. In some cases, gingivitis and stomatitis occur in mild form in relation to another disease or stress. Occasionally a severe form of acute necrotizing ulcerative gingivitis occurs. It is caused by a

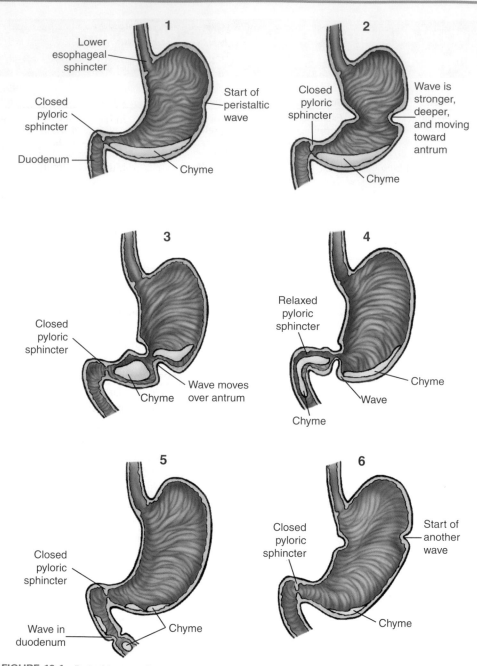

FIGURE 19-1   Peristaltic waves force chyme toward the pyloric sphincter. Meanwhile, a small amount of chyme is squirted into the duodenum, and the remainder is forced back into the stomach, where further mixing occurs. *(From Monahan FD, Neighbors M:* Medical-surgical nursing: foundations for clinical practice, *ed 2, Philadelphia, 1998, WB Saunders.)*

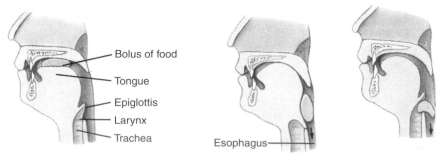

FIGURE 19-2   Parts of the mouth, pharynx, and esophagus involved in the swallowing process. *(From Wordlaw GM, Insel PM:* Perspectives in nutrition, *ed 2, New York, 1993, McGraw-Hill.)*

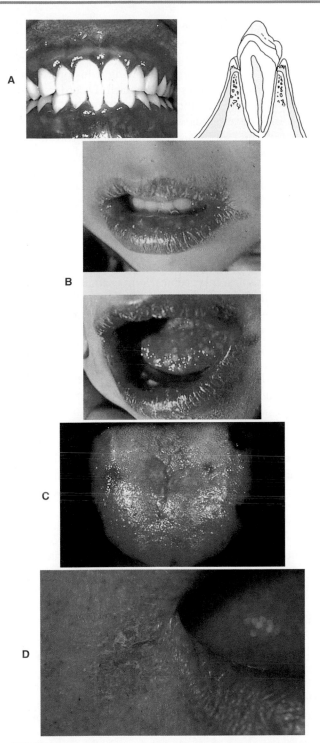

FIGURE 19-3 Tissue inflammation of the mouth. **A,** Gingivitis. **B,** Stomatitis. **C,** Glossitis. **D,** Cheilosis. (*A from Murray PR et al: Medical microbiology, ed 2, St. Louis, 1994, Mosby; B from Doughty DB, Broadwell-Jackson D: Gastrointestinal disorders, St. Louis, 1993, Mosby; C courtesy Hoffbrand AV, Pettit JE, eds: Sandoz atlas of clinical hematology, London, 1988, Gower Medical; D from Lemmi FO, Lemmi CAE: Physical assessment findings CD-ROM, Philadelphia, 2000, WB Saunders.*)

specific infectious bacterium, *Fusobacterium nucleatum,* often in conjunction with the spirochete *Treponema vincentii;* it is also known as Vincent's disease, from the Paris physician Henri Vincent (1862-1950), who first identified the disease process. Gums around the bases of teeth become

puffy, shiny, and tender overlapping the teeth margins. Affected gums often bleed, especially during tooth brushing. This serious condition destroys gum tissue and supporting tissues of the teeth and requires a course of antibiotic treatment.

Mouth pain in these conditions often causes decreased food intake. Maintaining adequate nutritional intake then becomes a major problem. Generally patients are given high-protein, high-kilocaloric (kcaloric) liquids and then soft foods, usually nonacidic and without strong spices to avoid irritation. Temperature extremes may also be avoided if they cause pain. Gradually foods are increased according to toleration, and foods are often supplemented with vitamins and minerals. In severe disease, use of a mouthwash containing a mild topical local anesthetic before meals helps relieve the pain of eating.

Dental Problems

Incidence of dental caries has recently been reduced in children and young adults. However, it is still present in many older adults, especially those unable to afford regular dental care, and causes tooth loss and chewing problems. In older adults, some 65 million in the United States alone, periodontal disease is a major cause of tooth loss. Especially if dental caries is untreated or if dental hygiene is poor, gum tissue at the base of the teeth becomes damaged and pockets form between the gums and the teeth. Dental plaque forms from a sticky deposit of mucus, food particles, and bacteria. Plaque hardens into *calculus,* a mineralized coating developed from plaque and saliva. These hardened particles then collect in pocket openings at the base of the teeth where bacteria attack periodontal tissue. The result is bacterial erosion of bone tissue surrounding affected teeth and subsequent tooth loss. Preventive care through daily dental care with fluoridated toothpaste, careful flossing, and periodic plaque removal by the dental hygienist forms the best approach. Extensive tooth loss leads to the need for tooth replacement with dentures. In many older adults these dentures become ill fitting, especially when weight loss occurs, and hinder adequate chewing. All of these dental problems need to be reviewed as part of the physical assessment in any patient's nutrition history so that food textures and forms can be adjusted to individual needs.

Salivary Glands and Salivation

Disorders of the salivary glands affect eating because saliva carries an *amylase* that begins starch breakdown and is vital in moistening food to facilitate chewing. Problems may arise from infection, such as infection with the mumps virus that attacks the parotid gland. Other problems come from excessive salivation, which occurs in numerous disorders affecting the nervous system, such as Parkinson's disease, and from local disorders such as mouth infections or injury. Problems may arise from any disease or drug that causes overactivity of the parasympathetic division of the autonomic nervous system, which controls the salivary glands.

Conversely, lack of salivation, which causes *xerostomia* (dry mouth), may be a temporary condition caused by fear, salivary gland infection, or action of anticholinergic drugs that hinder the normal action of neurotransmitters. Clients with dry mouth best tolerate moist, soft foods with added gravies and sauces. Permanent xerostomia is rare but does occur in Sjögren's syndrome, a symptom complex of unknown cause thought to be an abnormal immune response. It occurs in middle-age or older women and is marked by dry mouth and enlargement of parotid glands; it is often associated with rheumatoid arthritis or radiation therapy. There is difficulty in swallowing and speaking, interference with taste, and tooth decay. Salty foods dry the mouth and should be avoided. Chewing gum or sucking on sugarless candy can increase salivary secretions. Extreme mouth dryness may be partially relieved by spraying the inside of the mouth with an artificial saliva solution.

Swallowing Disorders

Most people take swallowing for granted. Each day we eat, chew, and swallow without giving it a second thought. However, the process of swallowing involves highly integrated actions of mouth, pharynx, and esophagus (see Figure 19-2). Swallowing difficulty, known medically as *dysphagia,* is a fairly common problem arising from many causes, including stroke, aging, developmental disabilities, and nervous system diseases. It may be only temporary, such as a piece of food lodged in the back of the throat, for which the Heimlich maneuver is appropriate first aid, or it may be involved with insufficient production of saliva and xerostomia. Such dysfunctional swallowing often causes children and adults alike to aspirate food particles, in turn causing coughing and choking episodes. Dysphagia is of concern for many reasons. Foods may enter the trachea and aspirate into the lungs, allowing bacteria to multiply, leading to pneumonia. Clients with dysphagia are usually referred to a special interdisciplinary team that includes a physician, speech pathologist, nurse, clinical dietitian, physical therapist, and an occupational therapist, with special training in swallowing problems. Thin liquids are the most difficult food form to swallow. Depending on the level of dysphagia, liquids may need to be thickened. Thickening agents include baby rice, commercially prepared thickeners, potato flakes, or mashed potatoes. Levels of thickness include thick (yogurt or pudding consistency) and medium thick (nectar consistency).

Esophageal Problems

Central Problems

The esophagus is a long, muscular tube lined with mucous membranes that extends from the pharynx, or throat, to the stomach (see Figure 19-2). It is bounded on both ends by circular muscles, or sphincters, that act as valves to control food passage. The upper sphincter remains closed except during swallowing, thus preventing airflow into the esophagus and stomach. Disorders along the tube that may disrupt normal swallowing and food passage include esophageal spasm (uncoordinated contractions of the esophagus), esophageal stricture (a narrowing caused by a scar from previous inflammation, ingestion of caustic chemicals, or a tumor), and esophagitis (an inflammation). These problems hinder eating and require medical attention through dilation, stretching procedures, or surgery to widen the tube or drug therapy.

Lower Esophageal Sphincter Problems

Defects in the operation of the lower esophageal sphincter (LES) muscles may come from changes in smooth muscle itself or from nerve-muscle hormonal control. In general, these LES problems arise from spasm, stricture, or incompetence.

Achalasia

If the LES does not relax normally when presented with food during swallowing, the uncommon condition of achalasia (a meaning "without" and *chalasia* meaning "relaxation") occurs. A primary esophageal motility ailment, achalasia is characterized by absence of esophageal peristalsis and failure of the LES to relax upon swallowing. These aberrations bring about a functional obstruction at the gastroesophageal junction. Signs and symptoms characterizing achalasia are dysphagia (most common), regurgitation, chest pain, heartburn, and weight loss.[1,2]

Exact etiology of achalasia is unknown, but it is thought to be either an autoimmune disorder, infectious agent, or both.[2] Medical intervention and treatments are outlined in Table 19-1. Nutritional requirements of patients with achalasia vary with severity of the disease and approach to treatment. Generally, nutrient-dense liquids and semisolid foods, taken at moderate temperatures, in small quantities, and at frequent intervals are usually tolerated by patients with achalasia.[3]

Gastroesophageal Reflux Disease

Gastroesophageal reflux disease (GERD), backflow or regurgitation of gastric contents from the stomach into the esophagus, is a very common disease. Regurgitation of acid gastric contents into the lower part of the esophagus creates constant tissue irritation because the wall of the esophagus is not protected from the acid of the stomach. During reflux, many patients feel a burning sensation behind the sternum that radiates toward the mouth, producing the most common symptom of GERD: heartburn (pyrosis), which is unrelated to disease of the heart (see the Diet-Medications Interactions box, "Potential Food Interactions With Drugs Used to Treat Heartburn"). Additional symptoms of GERD include acid indigestion

TABLE 19-1	Medical Interventions and Treatment of Achalasia

Type	Description and Efficacy
Pharmacologic: calcium channel blockers, nitrates, anticholinergic agents, opioids	Drugs relax smooth muscle of distal esophagus and LES. Approximately 10% benefit; effectiveness may be transient because these drugs frequently fail to relieve symptoms or are associated with significant adverse effects.
Mechanical: dilation by pneumatic balloons	Esophageal dilation that decreases LES pressure. Successful in decreasing LES pressure in 60% to 80% of patients, but may not relieve or improve symptoms.
Botulism toxin: Botox	Intrasphincteric LES injection to block release of acetylcholine. Only 30% of patients will have relief of dysphagia 1 year after treatment.
Surgical: esophageal myotomy	Considered to be the primary treatment, controlled division of muscle fibers of the lower esophagus and proximal stomach, followed by a partial fundoplication to prevent reflux. Relieves symptoms in 80% to 95% of patients.

Data from Patti M et al: *Achalasia,* Omaha, Neb, 2004 (updated February 21), eMedicine.com, Inc. Available at *www.emedcine.com.* Accessed March 27, 2005; and Sawyer MAJ et al: *Achalasia,* Omaha, Neb, 2003 (updated March 28), eMedicine.com, Inc. Available at *www.emedicine.com.* Accessed March 27, 2005.
   LES, Lower esophageal sphincter.

 DIET-MEDICATIONS INTERACTIONS

Potential Food Interactions With Drugs Used to Treat Heartburn

Drugs and nutrients share related characteristics in the body. They are most often absorbed from the same sites in the intestine. Both can alter physiologic processes, and both can be toxic in high doses. Drugs used to treat heartburn, gastroesophageal reflux disease (GERD), and peptic ulcer disease (PUD) are commonly used. Many are available without prescription. Let's look at common drug-nutrient and herb-drug interactions.

Antacids and Alginates

Antacids may have an effect on absorption of vitamins and iron. Antacids should be taken at least 2 hours before or after iron preparations. The effect of aluminum-containing antacids may be decreased by high-protein meals. Prolonged antacid use along with excessive consumption of calcium may cause high calcium levels and result in serious metabolic disease. Folate absorption or utilization may be impaired by antacids, which may increase risk of neural tube defects as well as congenital anomalies of heart, palate, and urinary tract. Folate supplementation may offset this increased risk. Concurrent ingestion of antacids and manganese may reduce manganese absorption.

H₂-Receptor Antagonists

The H₂-blocker cimetidine reacts with many drugs, including caffeine and alcohol. Cimetidine may also increase the likelihood of alcohol intoxication. H₂-blockers decrease the body's ability to excrete caffeine; consequently, large quantities of caffeine may cause tremors, insomnia, or heart palpitations. Folate absorption or utilization may be impaired by H₂-blockers, which may increase risk of neural tube defects as well as congenital anomalies of heart, palate, and urinary tract. Folate supplementation may offset this increased risk.

H₂-blockers may impair iron absorption through effects on the pH of the digestive tract. H₂-blockers may also impair absorption of selenium. Vitamin B_{12} from food is impaired by H₂-blockers, but absorption of B_{12} supplements is not affected. Magnesium supplements can interfere with absorption of H₂-blockers. Magnesium supplements should be taken at least 2 hours before or after this medication.

Proton Pump Inhibitors

Proton pump inhibitors (PPIs) may hinder absorption of iron products, thus lessening their effectiveness. PPIs may also impair absorption of selenium. Vitamin B_{12} from food is impaired by PPIs but absorption of B_{12} supplements is not affected. PPIs may potentiate phototoxic effects of *Hypericum* (St. John's wort).

Data from Windle ML: *Understanding heartburn/GERD medications,* Omaha, Neb, 2005 (updated September 22), eMedicineHealth. Retrieved December 15, 2005, from *http://www.emedicinehealth.com/Articles/43286-1.asp;* and Bratman S, Girman AM: *Mosby's handbook of herbs and supplements and their therapeutic use,* St. Louis, 2003, Mosby/Elsevier Science.

Heimlich maneuver A first-aid maneuver to relieve a person who is choking from blockage of the breathing passageway by a swallowed foreign object or food particle. Standing behind the person, clasp the victim around the waist, placing one fist under the sternum (breastbone) and grasping the fist with the other hand. Then make a quick, hard, thrusting movement inward and upward.

achalasia Failure to relax the smooth muscle fibers of the gastrointestinal tract at any point of juncture of its parts; especially failure of the esophagogastric sphincter to relax when swallowing, as a result of degeneration of ganglion cells in the wall of the organ. The lower esophagus also loses its normal peristaltic activity. Also called cardiospasm.

pyrosis Heartburn.

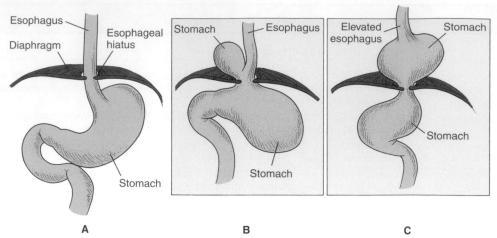

FIGURE 19-4   Hiatal hernia compared with normal stomach placement. **A,** Normal stomach. **B,** Paraesophageal hernia (esophagus in normal position). **C,** Esophageal hiatal hernia (elevated esophagus).

TABLE 19-2	Treatment of Gastroesophageal Reflux Disease Stages

Category	Recommended Treatments
Mild heartburn only (occasional bouts for ≥1 week)	Early low-fat dinners
	Elevation of head of bed
	H_2-antagonist × 6 weeks and alkali antacids prn
Moderately severe heartburn (months of daily symptoms of heartburn/chest pressure) or poor response to H_2-receptor antagonist	Proton pump inhibitors (PPIs) single dosage × 6 weeks
Recurrence and persistence of moderately severe GERD symptoms (rapid recurrence of symptoms after course of PPI therapy; occasional odynophagia/dysphagia)	Gastroenterology consultation; endoscopy and biopsy of esophageal-gastric junction for Barrett's metaplasia
	Recurrent courses of PPI therapy
Severe, persistent GERD symptoms (daily symptoms, often with odynophagia; dysphagia)	Continuous PPI therapy (often two capsules per day)
	Add cisapride
	Consider referral for laparoscopic fundal placation
Recalcitrant GERD symptoms (persistent daily/nightly symptoms with regurgitation; odynophagia, dysphagia, poor response to full drug therapy)	Maximal PPI therapy and cisapride
	Laparoscopic fundal placation

Data from Gray GM: Gastro-esophageal reflux disease (GERD): The spectrum of esophagitis, Barrett's, dysphagia, and cancer, *Gastroenterology: Gastro-esophageal reflux disease (GERD)*, New York, 1996-2005, interMD-net Corporation. Available at www.cyberounds.com. Accessed January 4, 2000.

prn, As needed.

and/or regurgitation, which often have a negative effect on quality of life.[4,5]

Other less common symptoms include iron deficiency anemia with chronic bleeding and aspiration, which may cause cough, dyspnea, or pneumonitis. Sometimes substernal pain radiates into the neck and jaw or down the arms. Acid reflux may be caused by a hiatal hernia, pregnancy (estrogen and progesterone have been shown to reduce LES pressure), obesity, pernicious vomiting, or nasogastric tubes. A number of drugs also lower LES pressure, causing GERD and heartburn to be a side effect of drugs used in the treatment of other conditions.

Acid and pepsin cause tissue erosion with symptoms of substernal burning, cramping, pressure sensation, or severe pain.[6] Symptoms are aggravated by lying down or any increase of abdominal pressure, such as that caused by tight clothing. The condition is related to (1) a nonfunctioning gastroesophageal sphincter, (2) frequency and duration of the acid reflux, and (3) inability of the esophagus to produce normal secondary peristaltic waves to prevent prolonged contact of the mucosa with the acid pepsin. A hiatal hernia (Figure 19-4) may or may not be present. The most common complications of GERD are stenosis and esophageal ulcer.

Treatment of GERD is aimed at one or more aspects that cause or continue symptoms (Table 19-2).[7] Nutrition therapy plays only a minor role in the management (Box 19-1) of GERD, and none of the dietary measures can be classified as evidence-based treatment.[8]

Hiatal Hernia

The esophagus normally enters the chest cavity at the *hiatus,* an opening in the diaphragm membrane, and immediately joins the upper portion of the stomach. A hiatal hernia occurs when a portion of the upper part of the stomach at this entry point of the esophagus protrudes through the hiatus alongside the lower portion of the

Modified from Cummings JH: Nutritional management of diseases of the gut. In Garrow JS, James WPT, Ralph A, eds: *Human nutrition and dietetics,* ed 10, Edinburgh, 2001, Churchill Livingstone.

BOX 19-1	Management of Gastroesophageal Reflux Disease

Lifestyle

Stop smoking
Avoid alcohol, chocolate, fatty foods, large meals at night

Mechanical

Reduce weight
Avoid bending
Avoid tight, constrictive clothing
Elevate head of bed or use pillows

Pharmacologic

Review current medication use
Combat gastric acid
- Simple antacids and alginates
- H_2-receptor antagonists:
  - Cimetidine
  - Ranitidine
  - Famotidine
  - Nizatidine
- Proton pump inhibitors (PPIs)
  - Omeprazole
  - Lansoprazole
- Prokinetic agents
  - Metoclopramide
  - Cisapride

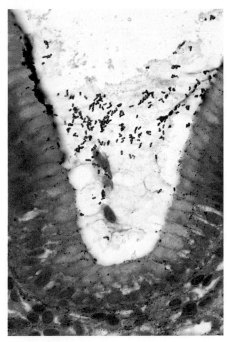

FIGURE 19-5   *Helicobacter pylori. (From Kumar V, Abbas AK, Fausto N:* Robbins and Cotran pathologic basis of disease, *ed 7, Philadelphia, 2005, Elsevier/Saunders.)*

esophagus (see Figure 19-4). Food is easily held in this herniated area of the stomach and mixed with acid and pepsin; then it is regurgitated back up into the lower part of the esophagus. Gastritis can occur in this herniated portion of the stomach and cause bleeding and anemia. Reflux of gastric acid contents causes symptoms similar to those described earlier.

A regular diet of choice using frequent small feedings for comfort is usually tolerated. Also, because obesity is often associated with hiatal hernia, weight reduction is a primary goal. Avoiding tight clothing helps relieve discomfort. Patients will need to avoid leaning over or lying down immediately after meals and should sleep with the head of the bed elevated. Antacids help relieve the burning sensation. Large hiatal hernias or smaller sliding hernias may require surgical repair.

PROBLEMS OF THE STOMACH AND DUODENUM

Peptic Ulcer Disease

One in 10 Americans will be affected by peptic ulcer disease (PUD) sometime during their lives,[9,10] and approximately 10% of patients seen in emergency departments with abdominal pain are diagnosed with PUD.[9] Prevalence of PUD has decreased in the United States over the past 30 years as in other developed countries, but is increasing in developing countries.[9]

An *ulcer* is the loss of tissue on the surface of the mucosa. In the GI tract, an ulcer extends through mucosa, submucosa, and often into the muscle layer. *Peptic ulcer* is the general term for an eroded mucosal lesion in the central portion of the GI tract. A peptic ulcer can occur in any area of the stomach exposed to pepsin. Areas affected include the lower portion of the esophagus, stomach, and first portion of the duodenum, called the *duodenal bulb.* Esophageal and gastric ulcers are less common. Most ulcers occur in the duodenal bulb, where gastric contents emptying into the duodenum through the pyloric valve are most concentrated. Gastric ulcers occur usually along the lesser curvature of the stomach. PUD itself is a benign disease, but ulcers do tend to recur. Gastric ulcers are more prone to develop into malignant disease. Weight loss is common in patients with gastric ulcers. Patients with duodenal ulcers may gain weight from frequent eating to counteract pain.

Peptic ulcer is caused by *Helicobacter pylori* in the stomach or intake of nonsteroidal antiinflammatory drugs (NSAIDs).[8] Nutrition or diet is not thought to play a significant role in the cause. *H. pylori* is a short, spiral-shaped, microaerophilic gram-negative bacillus (Figure 19-5) that

---

gastritis Inflammation of the stomach.

attaches itself to gastric mucosa.[8,9] It is able to survive the acidic environment of the stomach by secreting enzymes to neutralize the acid. This allows *H. pylori* to find its way to the protective mucous lining of the stomach, and its spiral shape facilitates burrowing through the lining.[10]

Intake of aspirin or other NSAIDs such as ibuprofen (Motrin), naproxen (Naprosyn), and etodolac (Lodine) induce ulcer formation by interfering with formation of prostaglandins, the chemicals that help the mucosal lining resist caustic acid damage.[9] They irritate gastric mucosa and cause bleeding, erosion, and ulceration, especially with prolonged or excessive use. The NSAID group of drugs is so named to distinguish them from the corticosteroids, synthetic variants of the natural adrenal hormones. The NSAIDs include a dozen antiinflammatory drugs.

Clinical Symptoms

Basic symptoms of peptic ulcer are increased gastric tone and painful hunger contractions when the stomach is empty. In duodenal ulcer, amount and concentration of hydrochloric acid are increased. In gastric ulcer, amount and concentration of hydrochloric acid may be normal. Nutritional deficiencies are evident in low plasma protein levels, anemia, and loss of weight. Hemorrhage may be the first sign in some patients. Diagnosis is based on clinical findings, radiographs, or visualization by fiberoptic gastroscopy.

The primary goal of medical management for PUD is control of *H. pylori*. Additional supportive goals are to (1) alleviate symptoms, (2) promote healing, (3) prevent recurrences, and (4) prevent complications. In addition to general traditional measures, the rapidly expanding knowledge base and development of a number of new drugs have increased the physician's available management tools.

General Therapeutic Measures

Adequate rest, relaxation, and sleep have long been a foundation for general care of PUD to enhance the body's natural healing process. Positive stress coping and relaxation skills, which help patients deal with personal psychosocial stressors, can be learned and practiced. Simple encouragement to talk about anxieties, anger, and frustrations helps to make patients feel better, and as soon as they are able, appropriate physical activity helps work out tensions. Habits that contribute to ulcer development, such as smoking and alcohol use, should be eliminated. Common drugs such as aspirin and NSAIDs should be avoided.

Pharmacologic Management

Current pharmacologic management of PUD has a wider choice of drugs to control underlying physiologic cause and clinical symptoms and to support healing. In various ways the following five types of drugs now suppress gastric acid and pepsin secretion, protect mucosal tissue, buffer acid, and eliminate infection:

1. *Histamine H2-receptor antagonists:* These agents, commonly called H2-blockers, are popular drugs for controlling gastric acid secretion. They decrease hydrochloric acid production by competing with histamine for receptor sites on parietal cells. Normally histamine attaches to its specific cellular receptors (type H2) on acid-producing parietal cells of gastric mucosa and mediates secretion of hydrochloric acid. Thus the blocking action of these agents effectively controls acid and pepsin because inactive pepsinogen requires acid for activation. The four drugs in this classification have now been reclassified for over-the-counter purchase: (1) cimetidine (Tagamet), (2) ranitidine (Zantac), (3) famotidine (Pepcid), and (4) nizatidine (Axid).

2. *Proton pump inhibitors:* This newer class of drugs, more potent than H2-blockers, also suppresses gastric acid, but by a different action. Without competition, in parietal cells they irreversibly prevent action of a key enzyme that actively secretes hydrogen ions needed for hydrochloric acid (HCl) production. Without available H+ ions, HCl cannot be made. Then without acid, ulcers heal rapidly. There are five drugs in this category that have been approved by the Food and Drug Administration (FDA): (1) lansoprazole (Prevacid), (2) omeprazole (Prilosec), (3) esomeprazole (Nexium), (4) rabeprazole (Aciphex), and (5) pantoprazole (Protonix). Proton pump inhibitors may interfere with liver metabolism of anticoagulants, diazepam (Valium), or phenytoin (Dilantin). Serum levels of these drugs should be monitored during concurrent therapy.

3. *Mucosal protectors:* Drugs of this type act as cytoprotective agents by helping the stomach heal itself. They produce a gel-like suspension that binds to the ulcer base and covers it and surrounding normal mucosal tissue to protect involved tissue from harm while it heals. This drug also forms complexes with pepsin that inactivates pepsin. An example of this type of drug is sucralfate (Carafate). These drugs are not as effective as the other options.

4. *Antacids:* These well-known substances counteract or neutralize acidity. They are safe and inexpensive to use. Two main types are (1) magnesium-aluminum compounds (Maalox, Mylanta) and (2) aluminum hydroxide (Basaljel, Amphojel). Aluminum-based preparations may cause constipation; magnesium-based preparations may cause diarrhea.

5. *Antibiotics:* Drugs of this type are used to control the *H. pylori* infection associated with PUD. Treatment using one or two antibiotics such as amoxicillin, tetracycline (not to be used for children less than 12 years of age), metronidazole, or clarithromycin is recom-

mended for 10 days to 2 weeks, in conjunction with either ranitidine bismuth citrate, bismuth subsalicylate, or a proton pump inhibitor. The combination of acid suppression by the H_2-blocker or proton pump inhibitor with antibiotics helps alleviate ulcer-related symptoms such as abdominal pain and nausea, heal inflammation, and may enhance efficacy of the antibiotics.[11] Currently eight *H. pylori* treatment regimens are approved by the FDA (Box 19-2), although other combinations have been used effectively. Better eradication rates have been demonstrated using triple-therapy regimens rather than dual therapy and/or longer length of treatment (14 days instead of 10 days). Major reasons for treatment failure are antibiotic resistance and patient noncompliance.[11]

BOX 19-2 | Food and Drug Administration–Approved Treatment Options for Peptic Ulcer Disease

Omeprazole 40 mg every day + clarithromycin 500 mg three times a day × 2 wks, then omeprazole 20 mg every day × 2 wks

-OR-

Ranitidine bismuth citrate (RBC) 400 mg twice daily + clarithromycin 500 mg three times a day × 2 wks, then RBC 400 mg twice daily × 2 wks

-OR-

Bismuth subsalicylate (Pepto Bismol) 525 mg four times a day + metronidazole 250 mg four times a day + tetracycline 500 mg four times a day* × 2 wks + H_2-receptor antagonist therapy as directed × 4 wks

-OR-

Lansoprazole 30 mg twice daily + amoxicillin 1 g twice daily + clarithromycin 500 mg three times a day × 10 days

-OR-

Lansoprazole 30 mg three times a day + amoxicillin 1 g three times a day × 2 wks†

-OR-

Ranitidine bismuth citrate 400 mg twice daily + clarithromycin 500 mg twice daily × 2 wks, then RBC 400 mg twice daily × 2 wks

-OR-

Omeprazole 20 mg twice daily + clarithromycin 500 mg twice daily + amoxicillin 1 g twice daily × 10 days

-OR-

Lansoprazole 30 mg twice daily + clarithromycin 500 mg twice daily + amoxicillin 1 g twice daily × 10 days

From Division of Bacterial and Mycotic Diseases, Centers for Disease Control and Prevention: Helicobacter pylori *and peptic ulcer disease:* H. pylori *fact sheet for health care providers,* Atlanta, 2001 (last updated), Author. Retrieved December 15, 2005, from *www.cdc.gov/ulcer/md.htm.*
FDA, Food and Drug Administration.
*Although not FDA approved, amoxicillin has been substituted for tetracycline for patients for whom tetracycline is not recommended.
†This dual therapy regimen has restrictive labeling. It is indicated for patients who are either allergic or intolerant to clarithromycin or for infections with known or suspected resistance to clarithromycin.

Nutritional Management

Pharmacologic therapy is the treatment of choice for peptic ulcer disease. There is no evidence diet plays a significant role in treatment when compared with pharmacologic regimens.[12,13] Dietary recommendations are formed from individual tolerance and should be considered supplemental to pharmacologic therapy. No conclusive evidence supports use of a traditional "bland" diet to decrease gastric acid secretion or increase the time it takes to heal ulcers.[14] Likewise, milk (a historical mainstay of PUD therapy) does not aid in ulcer healing and actually promotes gastric acid secretion.[13] In short, individuals with PUD should be encouraged to eat what they want.[15]

General therapeutic recommendations include the following[13-16]:

- Emphasize a balanced, nutritious diet.
- Limit the following foods and seasonings, and encourage avoidance of lifestyle habits known to increase acid secretion and/or inhibit healing:
  - Caffeine (including coffee, tea, or decaffeinated coffee), black pepper, chocolate
  - Foods that are irritating or not well tolerated
  - Alcohol, cigarette smoking, salicylates (aspirin) and other NSAIDs
  - Eating less than 2 hours before bedtime
- Minimize stress.
- Take medicine regularly as prescribed (e.g., do not stop taking medication).

Personal Focus

Sound nutritional management plays an important supportive role in total medical care of persons with PUD. The individual must be the focus of treatment. The patient is not "an ulcer," but a person with an ulcer. Course of the disease is conditioned by the individuality of the patient and his or her life situation. Presence of the ulcer affects the patient's life and quality of life. In the long run a wide range of foods, attractive to the eye and the taste, and regular, unhurried eating habits provide the best course of action (see the *Case Study* box, "The Patient With Peptic Ulcer Disease").

DISORDERS OF THE SMALL INTESTINE

Diarrhea and Malabsorption

Diarrhea

Diarrhea is not a disease, but a symptom that can be attributed to many medical conditions (see the *Perspectives in Practice* box, "Nutritional Aspects of Diarrhea"). *Diarrhea* is defined as an increase in frequency of bowel movements compared with the usual pattern or excess water content of stools affecting consistency or volume, or both. Diarrhea most directly involves the large intestine

CASE STUDY

The Patient With Peptic Ulcer Disease

Lowell is a 40-year-old businessman who was admitted to the city hospital 3 weeks ago after an incidence of vomiting bright-red blood. A medical history revealed that a dull, gnawing pain in the upper abdomen began several months ago and has increased in severity during that time. It became more severe after his most recent out-of-state trip to one of his stores. Because the pain was usually accompanied by headaches, he took aspirin to help relieve it.

Initial hospital treatment consisted of blood transfusions, intravenous fluids and electrolytes, and vitamin C. Lowell continued to feel nauseous and weak, but he stopped vomiting. However, he passed several large, tarry stools during the first 24 hours. His initial nutrition assessment results included weight 68 kg (150 lb), height 175 cm (5 ft 9 in), albumin 2.8 g/dl, prealbumin 14 mg/dl, transferrin 18% saturation value, hemoglobin 11 g/dl, and hematocrit 35%. His medications included cimetidine, sucralfate, magnesium-aluminum hydroxide, and triple antibiotic therapy.

The patient began slowly to tolerate sips of clear liquids and then advanced to a regular diet as tolerated, showing continued improvement. Before he was discharged at the end of the second week, the registered dietitian discussed general nutritional needs with Lowell and his wife. He was advised to eat his meals regularly in as relaxed a setting and manner as possible, eliminate his frequent between-meal snacks, and take his multivitamin supplement daily with his meals. Also, general guidelines and a list of a few food-related items or habits to avoid were reviewed. He was also advised to stop smoking and to rest as much as possible before returning to work. His physician had also advised him to reduce his workload and scheduled a follow-up appointment in 1 week.

Lowell's wife accompanied him to the next appointment and reported she was pleased with his ability to put aside business duties and take more time to enjoy his family. Lowell stated his two teenage sons had been surprisingly supportive in assisting him in following the prescribed regimen, and he plans to make it his general habit.

Questions for Analysis

1. The radiographic diagnosis of Lowell's illness was a gastric ulcer in the antrum lesser curvature. What does this mean? Where do most ulcers occur? Why?
2. What factors contributed to Lowell's ulcer? What effect did each of them have?
3. Evaluate the results of Lowell's initial nutrition assessment data. How would you use this information in nutrition counseling?
4. Identify Lowell's basic nutritional needs. Outline a teaching plan based on these needs that you would use to help him with his new diet plan. How would you include his wife in formulating and implementing his nutrition care plan?
5. What role does vitamin C play in Lowell's therapy? What other vitamins and minerals play a significant role in his care? Describe each role.
6. Why should Lowell give up coffee, cigarettes, and alcohol? What problems do you think he may encounter in trying to change these habits?

---

but may be caused by disease of the small intestine, pancreas, or gallbladder. General diarrhea may result from basic dietary excesses. There may be fermentation of sugars involved or excess fiber stimulation of intestinal muscle function.

Chronic diarrhea may occur as a result of GI tract motility dysfunction such as irritable bowel syndrome (IBS), malabsorption, metabolic disorders, food intolerances (e.g., lactose intolerance), food poisoning, infections, and human immunodeficiency virus (HIV) infection. In the case of lactose intolerance, accumulated concentration of undigested lactose in the intestine, resulting from the lack of the enzyme lactase, creates increased osmotic pressure. This pressure effectively draws water into the gut and stimulates hypermotility, abdominal cramping, and diarrhea. Milk treated with lactase enzyme is tolerated by these persons without the difficulty encountered with regular milk. Secretory, osmotic, and inflammatory processes in the intestine result in increased losses of fluid and electrolytes from diarrhea.[14,15]

Malabsorption

In a normally functioning body, foods are digested and then nutrients are absorbed into the bloodstream, mostly from the small intestine. Malabsorption occurs either because a disorder interferes with how food is digested or because a disorder interferes with how nutrients are absorbed. There are multiple causes of a malabsorption condition.[14,15] Symptoms of malabsorption include a change in bowel habits, apathy, fatigue, and a smooth surface on the lateral tongue. Some of these causes include the following:

- *Maldigestion problems:* pancreatic disorders, biliary disease, bacterial overgrowth, ileal disease (inflammatory bowel disease [IBD])
- *Intestinal mucosal changes:* mucosal surface alterations, intestinal surgery such as resections that shorten the bowel, lymphatic obstruction, intestinal stasis
- *Genetic disease:* cystic fibrosis with its complications of pancreatic insufficiency and lack of the pancreatic enzymes lipase, trypsin, and amylase
- *Intestinal enzyme deficiency:* lactose intolerance caused by lactase deficiency
- *Cancer and its treatment:* absorbing surface effect of radiation and chemotherapy
- *Metabolic biochemical defects:* absorbing surface effects of pernicious anemia or gluten-induced enteropathy (celiac sprue)

Here we briefly review four of these malabsorptive conditions: (1) celiac sprue, (2) cystic fibrosis, (3) IBD, and (4) short-bowel syndrome (SBS).

Celiac Disease

Metabolic Defect

In 1889 a London physician named Gee observed a number of malnourished children having steatorrhea and distended abdomens. He gave the name *celiac* to the general clinical condition from the Greek word *kolia*,

PERSPECTIVES IN PRACTICE
Nutritional Aspects of Diarrhea

Gastrointestinal (GI) disease so often presents barriers to efficient nutrient absorption that nutritional deficiencies are planned for automatically. Ironically many of these conditions also frequently lead to diarrhea, which results in further loss of fluids and electrolytes. As expected, their replacement is the initial and primary concern of therapy. However, different types of diarrhea also present other differences; control of type-specific problems requires different modes of treatment coordinated with treatment of the disease it accompanies. Before looking into possible treatment modes, examine first three of the most common types of diarrhea: watery, fatty, and small volume.

Watery diarrhea occurs when the amount of water and electrolytes moving into intestinal mucosa exceeds that amount absorbed into the bloodstream. This movement of water and electrolytes into the mucosa may be secretive or osmotic. If this movement of water and electrolytes into the mucosa is secretive, it may be active or passive. Active movement occurs with excessive gastric hydrochloric acid secretion or enterotoxin-induced infections such as cholera. Passive movement occurs with a rise in hydrostatic pressure that accompanies such infectious diseases as salmonellosis or tuberculosis, nonbacterial infections, fungal infections, renal failure, irradiation enteritis, and inflammatory bowel disease (IBD). Other conditions associated with watery diarrhea include hyperthyroidism, thyroid carcinoma, and hypermotility of the GI tract.

If this movement of water and electrolytes into the mucosa is osmotic, it will occur when nutrients are not absorbed because of intolerable levels of nonabsorbable particles present in intestinal chyme. Such particles include lactose (milk sugar) in individuals with lactase deficiency or gluten (a cereal protein found in wheat and rye and to a lesser degree in barley and oats) in persons with a reduced GI transit time caused by the removal of part of the intestinal tract.

Fatty diarrhea, or *steatorrhea,* occurs with maldigestion or malabsorption. Maldigestion involves a lack of enzymatic activity required to completely digest food, such as reduced pancreatic exocrine activity (release of intestinal enzymes from the pancreas) caused by pancreatic insufficiency. Malabsorption means digested materials do not make it across the intestinal mucosa to enter the bloodstream. This failure occurs in conditions in which the intestinal villi are destroyed, such as celiac disease.

Small-volume diarrhea occurs mainly when the rectosigmoid area of the colon is irritated, such as in IBD (Crohn's disease or ulcerative colitis). It also occurs when inflammatory conditions affect areas adjacent to the colon, as in pelvic inflammatory disease, diverticulitis, appendicitis, or hemorrhagic ovarian cysts.

Metabolic consequences of each type of diarrhea are similar. Uncontrolled, they result in syncope, hypokalemia, acid-base imbalances, and hypovolemia, with resulting renal failure. They may also be accompanied by low levels of fat-soluble vitamins, vitamin B_{12}, or folic acid or eventually lead to protein-energy malnutrition. In addition to these conditions, each type also manifests problems associated with the disorder they accompany. Workers with the Memorial Sloan-Kettering Cancer Center in New York and the Department of Medicine at Brooke Army Medical Center in Texas have developed recommendations for treating GI diseases associated with each type of diarrhea. These are summarized as follows, with the focus on the diarrheal aspects of disease:

- Watery diarrhea often accompanies inflammatory bowel conditions, such as Crohn's disease, for which nutrition therapy involves (1) increased protein and kcalories, (2) low fats and lactose, and (3) avoidance of foods that stimulate peristalsis. Thus, secretive diarrhea is reduced by eliminating foods that may stimulate gastric acid secretion, and all types of watery diarrhea are avoided by reducing the motility of the GI tract. In other conditions in which osmotic diarrhea occurs, such as dumping syndrome, this problem is avoided by giving fluids between meals to avoid any extreme difference in osmotic pressures on either side of the intestinal wall. Small, frequent meals also help prevent this problem, as well as painful distention.

- Steatorrhea frequently accompanies conditions associated with maldigestion such as chronic pancreatitis. Nutritional management of this disease involves (1) frequent meals high in protein and carbohydrates and low in fat; (2) use of medium-chain triglycerides, which are more easily absorbed under adverse conditions; and (3) avoiding gastric stimulants, especially caffeine and alcohol. Steatorrhea also accompanies conditions of malabsorption, such as gluten-sensitive enteropathy. In addition to nutritional management strategies listed, treating this type of diarrhea requires removal of products that damage the mucosal villi, including lactose and gluten, which is found in wheat, rye, barley, and oats, and food products and fillers such as hydrolyzed vegetable protein products. It sometimes requires restricting fat as well. In both cases, the primary concern is to monitor fats that would otherwise appear in the feces. As therapy progresses, fat content of the meal can be increased as tolerated to normal levels to improve palatability.

- Small-volume diarrhea may accompany diverticulosis of the colon. A high-residue diet is recommended to increase fecal bulk, thereby preventing diarrhea. To prevent flatulence and distention, fiber should be added to the diet gradually.

All types of diarrhea can result in malnutrition, primarily because of electrolyte and fluid losses. It is important to identify the type of diarrhea occurring with each patient; only then can an effective nutritional management strategy be designed to replace those losses, as well as to eliminate or prevent other nutrition-related problems that are possible for each case.

References

Banwell JG: Pathophysiology of diarrheal disorders, *Rev Infect Dis* 12(suppl 1):30, 1990.

Barrett KE, Dharmsathaphorn K: Secretion and absorption: small intestine and colon. In Yamada T, ed: *Textbook of gastroenterology,* Philadelphia, 1991, JB Lippincott.

Gorbach SL: Efficacy of lactobacillus in treatment of acute diarrhea, *Nutr Today* 31(suppl 6):19S, 1996.

Kaaila M, Isolauri E: Nutritional management of acute diarrhea, *Nutr Today* 31(suppl 6):16S, 1996.

meaning "belly" or "abdomen." It was not until the mid-1950s that the Dutch pediatrician Willem-Karel Dicke and his associates discovered the causative agent. Their tissue studies confirmed that the gliadin fraction of the protein gluten in wheat produced the fat malabsorption and further that what had been called celiac disease in children and nontropical sprue in adults was a single disease, which came to be called *celiac sprue.*[16] As currently used, the alternative terms *celiac disease* (CD) and *gluten-sensitive enteropathy* are synonymous with celiac sprue. In

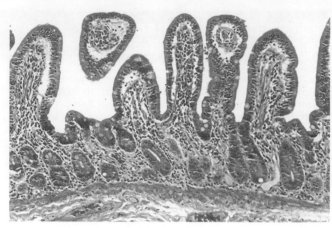

FIGURE 19-6   Comparison of normal intestinal villi and those in an individual with celiac disease. **A,** A biopsy specimen of diseased mucosa shows diffuse severe atrophy and blunting of villi. **B,** A normal mucosal biopsy specimen. *(From Kumar V, Abbas AK, Fausto N : Robbins and Cotran pathologic basis of disease, ed 7, Philadelphia, 2005, Elsevier/Saunders.)*

◆ FOCUS ON CULTURE

Did Your Ancestors Herd Dairy Cattle?

Do you or any one you know experience these symptoms—cramps, bloating, gas, diarrhea, and/or nausea—anywhere from 30 minutes to 2 hours after consuming a food or beverage containing lactose? As you learned in a previous chapter, lactose is found in milk and some dairy products, and the enzyme lactase is necessary for us to digest lactose. Lack of this enzyme, lactase, results in a condition called *lactose intolerance*.

Humans are the only mammals that continue to drink milk past weaning. Most mammals produce lactase until they are weaned and stop drinking milk. Cessation of milk drinking and lactase production characterizes most of the world's population, especially those of Asian and African ancestry. For children over the age of 5 years, 90% to 95% of people of color (blacks, Asians, Hispanics) are lactose intolerant, whereas only 20% to 25% of those of northern European descent do not tolerate dairy products. Lactose intolerance is usually referred to as a disease or disorder. Does this seem logical? Why is a trait found in 90% to 95% of the world's population abnormal? Shouldn't lactose intolerance be considered a normal adult condition?

Researchers from Cornell believe lactose tolerance is the outcome of a genetic mutation that sustains the functionality of lactase production into adulthood; allowing consumption of milk throughout life. This mutation occurs commonly among populations from northern Europe, where raising cattle and other ruminant animals was/is customarily practiced. Why does/did this population raise cattle? It appears that environmental circumstances allow dairy cattle to be safely and economically raised in the northern European region of the world. Ability to produce lactase and absorb lactose is nutritionally beneficial for adults only if milk is consistently available.

Data were collected on adult lactose absorption and malabsorption from 270 indigenous African and Eurasian populations. Adult lactose malabsorption was found to be associated with extreme hot or cold climates (high and low latitudes). Not only do the geography and climates of these regions preclude the maintaining of dairy herds, but also they are regions of the world where there is historical (pre-1900) occurrence of nine deadly communicable cattle diseases. The researchers conclude that areas of the world where adult lactose malabsorption predominates are those areas where it is/was impossible or dangerous to sustain dairy herds.

Thus the ability to digest lactose appears for the most part to be a genetic mutation.

Data from Bloom G, Sherman PW: Dairying barriers affect the distribution of lactose malabsorption, *Evol Hum Behav* 26(4):301, 2005.

---

all cases, such diseased tissues consistently show an eroded mucosal surface lacking the number and form of normal villi and having few microvilli, resulting in malabsorption of most nutrients (Figure 19-6). (See the *To Probe Further* box, "Food Intolerances With Genetic-Metabolic Disease," and the *Focus on Culture* box, "Did Your Ancestors Herd Dairy Cattle?," for more information regarding genetic malabsorption diseases.)

Gluten molecules combine with antibodies in the small intestine, causing the usually brushlike lining of the intestine to flatten, thereby being much less able to digest and absorb foods. Damage is reversed when gluten is removed from the diet. It is unclear whether these effects take place due to an immunologic response when gluten is ingested by genetically predisposed persons.[17] Resulting malabsorption promotes malnutrition and severe debilitation.[14] Gluten is a protein present in some grains such as wheat, rye, and barley but not oats, rice, or corn.[18]

CD occurs in roughly 1 in 133 persons in the United States, but only a small percentage of people living with it have been diagnosed. CD, as a rule, commonly occurs in women, whites and others of European ancestry, and

FOOD INTOLERANCES FROM GENETIC-METABOLIC DISEASE

Certain food intolerances may stem from underlying genetic disease that affects metabolism of one or more specific nutrients. Genetic disease results from the individual's specific gene inheritance. Genes in each cell control the metabolic functions of the cell. They regulate synthesis of some 1000 or more specific cell enzymes that control metabolism within the cell. When a specific gene is abnormal *(mutant)*, the enzyme whose synthesis that gene controls cannot be made. In turn, specific metabolic reaction controlled by that specific missing enzyme cannot take place. Specific genetic disease caused by this metabolic block then manifests clinical symptoms connected with resulting abnormal metabolic products. As primary examples here, we look briefly at two such genetic diseases affecting food-nutrient intolerances: (1) phenylketonuria (PKU), which affects amino acid metabolism and hence protein foods; and (2) galactosemia, which affects carbohydrate metabolism, specifically food sources of lactose. Both are detected by newborn screening procedures that are mandatory by law.

Phenylketonuria

PKU results from the missing cell enzyme phenylalanine hydroxylase, which metabolizes one of the essential amino acids, phenylalanine, to tyrosine, another nonessential amino acid. Phenylalanine then accumulates in the blood, and its alternate metabolites, the phenyl acids, are excreted in the urine. One of these urinary acids, phenylpyruvic acid, is a phenylketone; hence the name of the disease. Untreated, PKU can produce devastating effects, but present nutrition therapy can avoid these results. In past years, before current newborn screening laws and dietary treatment practices from birth, the most profound effect observed in persons with untreated PKU was severe mental retardation. The intelligence quotient (IQ) of affected persons was usually below 50 and often less than 20. Central nervous system damage caused irritability, hyperactivity, convulsive seizures, and bizarre behavior.

PKU can now be well controlled by special nutrition therapy. After screening at birth, a special low-phenylalanine diet effectively controls serum phenylalanine levels so they are maintained at appropriate amounts to prevent clinical symptoms and promote normal growth and development. Because phenylalanine is an essential amino acid necessary for growth, it cannot be totally removed from the diet. Blood levels of phenylalanine are constantly monitored, and the metabolic team nutritionist calculates the special diet for each infant and child to allow only limited amount of phenylalanine tolerated. Based on extensive studies, guidelines for nutritional management of PKU are currently being used effectively to build lifetime habits; research now indicates there is no safe age at which a child may discontinue the diet. This dietary management is built on two basic components: (1) a substitute for milk, a special medical food continued past infancy and childhood into adolescence and adulthood; and (2) guidelines for adding solid foods, both regular and special low-protein products, and then building continuing food habits.

Initial education and continuing support of parents is essential because dietary management of PKU is the only known effective method of treatment and because maintaining the diet becomes more difficult as the child grows older. Parents must understand and accept the necessity of the diet, and this requires patience, understanding, and continued reinforcement. The PKU team, together with parents, provides initial and continuing care so the child with PKU will grow and develop normally. When PKU is diagnosed at birth, as a result of widespread screening programs, a child can have a healthy and happy life, instead of the profound disease consequences experienced in the past. Current practice of long-term nutritional management is especially critical for young women with PKU who are considering pregnancy. At least 6 months before becoming pregnant, women with PKU should meet with a metabolic team to discuss treatment and follow-up. It is possible for women with PKU to have normal children. However, maternal PKU presents possibility of a potentially high-risk pregnancy if a low-phenylalanine diet is not strictly followed.

Galactosemia

This genetic disease affects carbohydrate metabolism so the body cannot use the monosaccharide galactose. Three enzymes are responsibly for conversion of galactose to glucose, and in galactosemia at least one of the enzymes is defective or missing. Milk, infants' first food, contains a large amount of the precursor lactose (milk sugar). When infants with galactosemia are given breast milk or regular infant formula, they vomit and have diarrhea. After galactose is initially combined with phosphate to begin metabolic conversion to glucose, it cannot proceed further in the infant with galactosemia. Galactose rapidly accumulates in the blood and in various body tissues. In the past, excess tissue accumulations of galactose caused rapid damage in the untreated infant. Clinical symptoms appeared soon after birth, and the child failed to thrive. Continued liver damage brought jaundice, an enlarged liver with cirrhosis, enlarged spleen, and ascites. Without treatment, death usually resulted from liver failure. If the infant survived, continuing tissue damage and hypoglycemia in the optic lens and the brain caused cataracts and mental retardation. Now, however, with newborn screening programs, infants with galactosemia are diagnosed at birth and started on special dietary management. With this vital nutrition therapy, children can grow and develop normally.

The main indirect source of dietary galactose is the lactose in milk. A galactose-free diet (free of all forms of milk and lactose) is followed, and the infant is fed a soy-based formula. Breast-feeding is not an option when this genetic condition is present. The body synthesizes the amount of galactose needed for body structures. As solid foods are added to the infant's diet at about 6 months of age, careful attention must be given to avoiding lactose from other food sources. Parents quickly learn to check labels carefully on all commercial products to detect any lactose or lactose-containing substances.

Websites of Interest

GALACTOSEMIA

Parents of Galactosemic Children, Inc.: *www.galactosemia.org.*
National Organization for Rare Disorders: *www.rarediseases.org.*

PHENYLKETONURIA (PKU)

National PKU News: *www.pkunews.org.*
The Arc: *Q & A on PKU: www.thearc.org/faqs/pku.html.*
National Coalition for PKU and Allied Disorders: *www.pku-allieddisorders. org.*
Children's PKU Network: *www.pkunetwork.org.*

Data from Elsas LJ II, Acosta PB: Nutritional support of inherited metabolic disease. In Shils ME, Olson JA, Shike M, eds: *Modern nutrition in health and disease,* ed 8, vol 2, Philadelphia, 1994, Lea & Febiger.

TABLE 19-3	Gastrointestinal Symptoms Associated With Celiac Disease

Symptom	Comments
Abdominal pain	
Abdominal distention	Bloating, gas, indigestion
Constipation	
Decreased appetite	May also be increased or unchanged
Diarrhea	Chronic or occasional
Lactose intolerance	Common upon diagnosis; usually resolves following treatment
Nausea and vomiting	
Steatorrhea	Stools that float, are foul smelling, bloody, or "fatty"
Weight loss	Unexplained (people can be overweight or normal weight upon diagnosis)

Data from U.S. National Library of Medicine, National Institutes of Health: *Medline Plus A.D.A.M. medical encyclopedia: celiac disease—sprue*, Atlanta, 2005 (updated October 27), A.D.A.M. Inc. Retrieved December 15, 2005, from *www.nlm.nih.gov/medlineplus/ency/article/000233.htm.*

first-degree relatives. It can occur at any age from infancy to late adulthood.[14,15,17,19]

Clinical Symptoms

Symptoms vary significantly from person to person. They may be intestinal or nonintestinal in nature, which makes diagnosis difficult. One person may present with diarrhea, another with constipation, and yet another with no stool elimination problems.[18] Children with CD most often display failure to thrive, with or without malabsorption. Adults most frequently present with anemia caused by iron and/or folate deficiency.[15] A partial listing of GI symptoms is summarized in Table 19-3.

Diagnosis

Antigliadin antibodies IgG and IgA are present in over 90% of patients with CD; therefore both tests should be obtained to verify diagnosis.[18] Intestinal biopsy is then used to confirm diagnosis in patients with positive serologic tests.[18] Depending on the degree of intestinal involvement, a complete blood count (CBC); levels of serum iron or ferritin, red cell folate, vitamin B_{12}, serum calcium, alkaline phosphatase, albumin, and beta carotene; and prothrombin time should be obtained in patients suspected of malabsorbing.[15,18]

Nutritional Management

The goal of nutritional management is to control intake of dietary gluten and prevent malnutrition. The diet is better defined as low gluten rather than gluten free because it is impossible to remove completely all gluten. Usually a small amount is tolerated by most patients, except in prolonged use of newer products labeled "gluten free" but

containing wheat starch as a thickening agent, which cannot be recommended.[19] Wheat and rye are the main sources of gluten; it is also present in oats and barley. Thus these four grains have always been eliminated from the diet. However, a growing body of evidence now suggests that moderate amounts of oats may be safely used in diets of most adults with CD.[20] Corn and rice are usually the substitute grains used. Parents of children with celiac sprue need special instructions about food products to avoid, what constitutes a basic meal pattern, and recipes for food preparation. Careful label reading must be discussed because many commercial products use the offending grains as thickeners or fillers, and parents' knowledge of gluten-containing food products is highly variable and influences the child's attitudes toward dietary compliance. With an increasing number of processed foods being marketed, as well as increasing use of ethnic foods in Western society, it is difficult to detect all foods containing gluten; therefore a home test kit for gluten has been developed.[21] Good dietary management varies according to the child's age, pathologic conditions, and clinical status. Generally, a dietary program based on the low-gluten diet may be followed. In a small subgroup of patients, symptoms persist despite strict adherence to the diet. In rare instances, persons with such a refractory form of the disease respond only to parenteral nutrition support.[16]

Cystic Fibrosis

Genetic-Metabolic Defect

Cystic fibrosis (CF) is inherited as an autosomal recessive trait in about 3% of the white population. It is the most common fatal genetic disease among whites, occurring in about 1 in 3300 live white births, 1 in 15,300 black births, and 1 in 32,000 Asian American births.[22] Approximately one third of CF cases in the United States involve adults. The leading characteristic of CF is hypersecretion of abnormal, thick mucus that obstructs exocrine glands and ducts.[22-24] Therefore it can be classified as a respiratory disease or GI disorder.

The CF gene (found on chromosome 7q) is very large, and over 600 mutations causing CF have been described.[22,25] The gene product is the CF transmembrane regulator (CFTR) protein, which regulates chloride transport and water flux across epithelial cells.[22,24,25] This results in an abnormally high concentration of sodium in perspiration and low water content in mucus.[22,24,25] CF primarily affects the pancreas, intestinal tract, sweat glands, and lungs and in males causes infertility[22,24] (Figure 19-7).

Clinical Symptoms

Classic clinical symptoms of CF include the following effects in body organ systems[22,24,25]:

- Thick mucus in the lungs that accumulates and clogs air passages, damages epithelial tissue of these

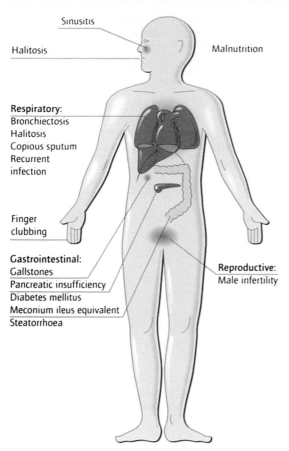

FIGURE 19-7 Cystic fibrosis. *(From Axford JS, O'Callaghan CA: Medicine, ed 2, Malden, Mass, 2004, Blackwell Science.)*

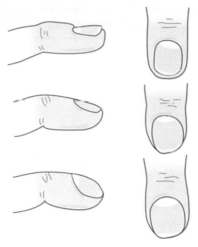

FIGURE 19-8 Clubbing of the fingers. *(From Axford JS, O'Callaghan CA: Medicine, ed 2, Malden, Mass, 2004, Blackwell Science.)*

airways, and leads to chronic obstructive pulmonary disease (COPD) and frequent respiratory infections, both contributing to increased metabolism and increased energy-nutrient needs.

- Pancreatic insufficiency caused by progressive clogging of pancreatic ducts and functional tissue degeneration, resulting in lack of normal pancreatic enzymes leading to bulky, foul-smelling, oily stools (steatorrhea); progressive loss of functional insulin-producing beta cells in the islets of Langerhans, resulting in type 1 diabetes mellitus (T1DM).
- Malabsorption of undigested food nutrients and extensive malnutrition and stunted growth.
- Excessive sweating in hot weather that may lead to dehydration and circulatory failure.
- Biliary cirrhosis caused by progressive clogging of bile ducts producing biliary obstruction and functional liver tissue degeneration.
- Inflammatory complications may include arthritis, finger clubbing (Figure 19-8), or vasculitis.
- Gallbladder disease, peptic ulcer disease, GERD, or episodes of partial intestinal obstruction.
- Delayed puberty and maturity probably due to chronic malnutrition. Males are typically infertile because the vas deferens fails to develop.

Nutritional Management

Current nutritional management of CF follows guidelines developed by a consensus committee of the U.S. Cystic Fibrosis Foundation (CFF).[26] This more aggressive nutritional management program, used in all CFF centers throughout the United States, results from three factors: (1) increased knowledge of disease process, (2) early diagnosis and intervention, and (3) improved therapeutic products such as replacement pancreatic enzymes in the form of capsule-encased enteric-coated microspheres—"beads"—that correct maldigestion and help support energy-nutrient growth needs.[27] With this pancreatic enzyme replacement therapy, commonly called "PERT," it is now recommended that persons with cystic fibrosis consume a high-energy, high-protein diet with no fat restriction. However, some persons continue to follow the low-fat advice given to them before the development of the enteric-coated enzyme preparations.[28] Treatment with PERT is very individualized. Even with maximum use, 10% to 20% of the ingested energy will usually be malabsorbed. The overall goal is to support normal nutrition and growth for all ages.

This PERT management program is based on an initial and ongoing schedule for assessment, including anthropometrics, laboratory studies, and nutrition evaluation (Table 19-4). Related therapy is then outlined in five levels according to individual assessment results and nutrition care needs and actions (Table 19-5).

cirrhosis Chronic liver disease, characterized by loss of functional cells, with fibrous and nodular regeneration.

TABLE 19-4	Basic Nutrition Assessment for Nutritional Management of Cystic Fibrosis

Key Assessments		Monitoring Schedule and Indications	
Anthropometry		**Biochemical Data**	
Weight	Every 3 months or as needed for growth evaluation.	CBC	Yearly routine care, interim as needed to detect deficiencies, iron status
Height (length)		TIBC, serum iron, ferritin	
BMI (adults)			
Head circumference (until age 2 yr)		Plasma/serum retinol, alpha-tocopherol	As indicated, weight loss, growth failure, clinical deterioration
Midarm circumference		Albumin, prealbumin	
Triceps skinfold		Electrolytes, acid-base balance	Summer heat, prolonged fever
Midarm muscle circumference (derived)*		Random glucose	Annually to detect CF-related DM (CFDM)
		Dietary Evaluation	
		Dietary intake	As indicated, history and food records, full energy-nutrient analysis
		3-day fat balance study†	As indicated, weight loss, growth failure, clinical deterioration
		Anticipatory guidance	Yearly, interim as needed according to growth or situational needs

Data from Hollander FM et al: Assessment of nutritional status in adult patients with cystic fibrosis: whole-body bioimpedance vs body mass index, skinfolds, and leg-to-leg bioimpedance, *J Am Diet Assoc* 105(4):549, 2005; Ramsey BW, Farrell PM, Pencharz P: Nutritional assessment and management in cystic fibrosis: a consensus report—The Consensus Committee, *Am J Clin Nutr* 55:108, 1992; and Yankaskas JR: Cystic fibrosis adult care: consensus conference report, *Chest* 125:1S, 2004.

CBC, Complete blood count; *TIBC,* total iron-binding capacity; *BMI,* body mass index; *CF,* cystic fibrosis; *DM,* diabetes mellitus.
*See Chapter 16 for equations.
†Three-day food records for analysis of fat intake; stool collections for analysis of fat content and degree of malabsorption.

TABLE 19-5	Levels of Nutrition Care for Management of Cystic Fibrosis

Levels of Care	Patient Groups	Nutrition Actions
Level I—Routine care	All	Diet counseling, food plans, enzyme replacement, vitamin supplements, nutrition education, exploration of problems
Level II—Anticipatory guidance	Above 90% ideal weight-height index, but at risk of energy imbalance; severe pancreatic insufficiency, frequent pulmonary infections, normal periods of rapid growth	Increased monitoring of dietary intake, complete energy-nutrient analysis, increased kcaloric density as needed; assess behavioral needs; provide counseling, nutrition education
Level III—Supportive intervention	85%-90% ideal weight-height index, decreased weight-growth velocity	Reinforce all the above actions, add energy-nutrient–dense oral supplements
Level IV—Rehabilitative care	Consistently below 85% ideal weight-height index, nutritional and growth failure	All of the above plus enteral nutrition support by nasoenteric or enterostomy tube feeding (see Chapter 18)
Level V—Resuscitative or palliative care	Below 75% ideal weight-height index, progressive nutritional failure	All of the above plus continuous enteral tube feedings or TPN (see Chapter 18)

Modified from Ramsey BW, Farrell PM, Pencharz P: Nutritional assessment and management in cystic fibrosis: a consensus report—The Consensus Committee, *Am J Clin Nutr* 55:108, 1992.
TPN, Total parenteral nutrition.

Inflammatory Bowel Diseases

Nature and Incidence

The general term *inflammatory bowel disease (IBD)* is now used to apply to two intestinal conditions with similar symptoms but different underlying clinical problems— Crohn's disease and ulcerative colitis (UC).[14,15,18] Both conditions produce extended mucosal tissue lesions, although these lesions differ in extent and nature (Figure 19-9). However, they have been classified medically in a single group because they are similar in their clinical symptoms and management. Their causes remain unknown, although heredity, environment, and immune functions are thought to be contributing factors.[29] Incidence of these diseases, especially Crohn's disease, has increased worldwide. Crohn's disease is particularly prevalent in industrialized areas of the world. It also appears among otherwise low-risk persons who move from rural to urban centers, with incidence being highest in people from 20 to 40 years of age and in Jews.

Clinical Manifestations

Also called *regional enteritis* and *granulomatous colitis,* inflammation produced by Crohn's disease extends through all layers of the intestinal wall, most commonly in the proximal portion of the colon and less often the terminal ileum.[14] UC is an inflammatory disease of mucosal layers of the rectum and colon. Similarities and differences between the two diseases are summarized in Table 19-6.

Medical Management

Because the cause of IBD is unknown, treatment is focused on alleviating and reducing inflammation. Similar drug therapies are used for Crohn's disease and UC. Crohn's disease affecting the colon is often treated with the antibiotic metronidazole.[14] Newer treatments include the antitumor necrosis factor agent infliximab.[15] Corticosteroids are commonly used to treat acute exacerbations of Crohn's disease and UC, but side effects limit long-term use. Sulfasalazine and immunomodulating agents such as azathioprine and mercaptopurine are occasionally used for their corticosteroid-sparing effects. Methotrexate can be given in low doses as an alternative to azathioprine in patients with Crohn's disease who are unresponsive or intolerant of azathioprine.[14,15,18]

A small percentage of patients with UC require surgery. Most common surgical procedures include total colectomy or ileostomy (Figure 19-10).[15] Approximately 80% of patients with Crohn's disease will eventually require surgery. Fifty percent of these patients will require a second surgery within 10 years as a result of disease recurrence. Strictures often require minimal resection; colitis may require colectomy with ileorectal anastomosis or ileostomy. Abscesses are drained, and enteric fistulae are resected.[15,18]

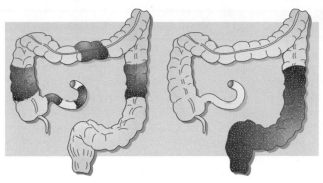

FIGURE 19-9 Crohn's disease *(left)* and ulcerative colitis *(right)*. Crohn's disease typically involves the small and large intestine in a segmental manner; ulcerative colitis generally starts in the rectum and progresses to involvement of varying lengths of the colon. *(Modified from Cotran CS, Kumar V, Robbins SJ: Robbins' pathologic basis of disease, ed 4, Philadelphia, 1989, WB Saunders.)*

Nutrition Therapy

Nutrition therapy centers on supporting the healing process and avoiding nutritional deficiency states and will be contingent upon functional condition of the GI tract. For the duration of acute exacerbations of Crohn's disease and UC, these aspects will guide the nutrition therapy: (1) amount of diarrheal output and (2) bleeding.[30] Nutrition therapy is provided during periods of exacerbation, as follows[30,31]:

- Hydrolyzed enteral feedings or total parenteral nutrition (TPN)
- Progression to low-fat, low-residue, high-protein, high-calorie, small, frequent meals
- Supplements
- Vitamins A, E, C , B_{12}, folate
- Iron

Nutrition Therapy During Remission

Nutrition therapy in remission includes the following[30,31]:

- Tailor (for patient's current GI function) energy (kilocalories [kcalories or kcal]) and protein at levels to maintain weight and replenish nutrient stores.
- Avoid foods high in oxalate (Appendix G).
- Increase antioxidant intake (see Chapter 6).
- Use probiotics and prebiotics.

---

probiotics Microbial foods or supplements that can be used to modify or reestablish intestinal flora and improve health of the host.

prebiotics Nondigestible food products that promote growth of symbiotic bacterial species already present in the colon.

TABLE 19-6	Similarities and Differences Between Crohn's Disease and Ulcerative Colitis

Manifestation	Crohn's Disease	Ulcerative Colitis
Cause	Unknown	Unknown
Genetics	Increased prevalence in first-degree relatives. NOD2 gene mutation on chromosome 16	Increased prevalence in first-degree relatives. Susceptibility loci on chromosomes 2 and 6.
Site of inflammation	Any part of the GI tract	Rectum, and spreads proximally
Mucosal layers affected		Epithelial
Abdominal pain	Common	Common
Diarrhea	Common	Common
Rectal bleeding	Sometimes	Common
Perforations	Common	Yes
Fibrosis, stricture, and fistulas	Common	No
Toxic megacolon	Rare	Common
Weight loss	Common	Common
Steatorrhea	Sometimes	No
Perianal disease	Common	No
Fever	Yes	No
Epidemiology	Developed countries, major age peak at 20-40 years of age, more common in women	Developed countries, major age peak at 20-40 years of age, more common in women
Relapses and remissions	Chronic	Usually no symptoms between attacks
Complications	Abscess, obstruction, fistulas, perianal disease, increased risk of colon cancer, malabsorption, kidney stones (oxalate and uric acid), gallstones	Many and varied including joint disorders, fatty liver, disorders of the eyes and skin
Prophylactic therapy	Not well established	Colonoscopy with multiple biopsies every 1-3 years
Prognosis	Recurrent morbidity throughout lives; risk of death approximately twice the general population	Mortality rate similar to general population

Data from Sartin JS: Gastrointestinal disorders. In Copstead LC, Banasik JL: *Pathophysiology,* ed 3, St. Louis, 2005, Elsevier/Saunders; and Axford JS, O'Callaghan CA: *Medicine,* ed 2, Oxford, 2004, Blackwell Science.

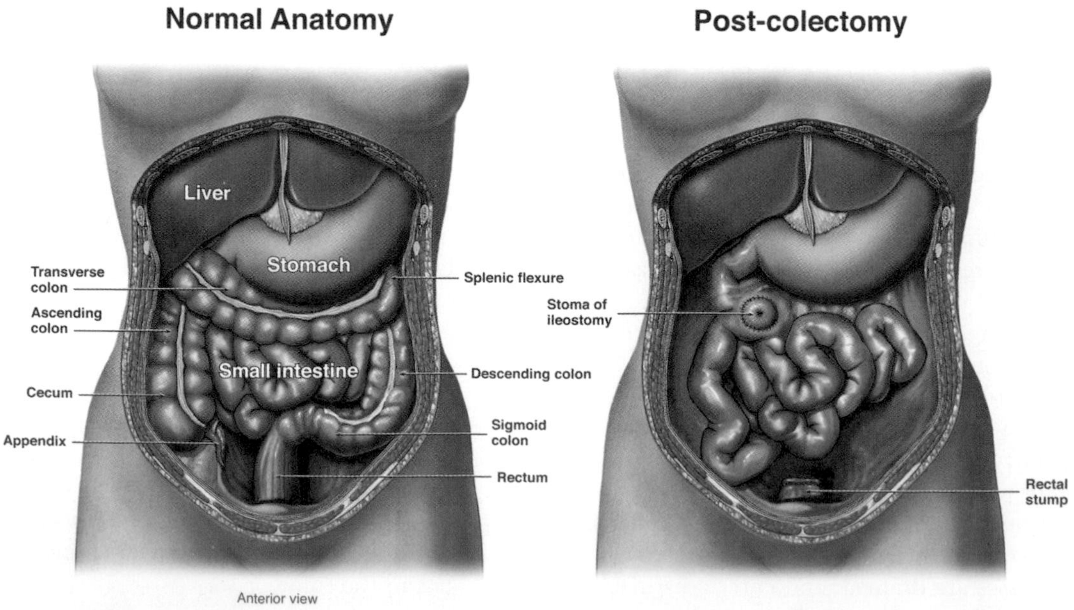

Normal Anatomy

Liver
Stomach
Transverse colon
Ascending colon
Cecum
Appendix
Small intestine
Splenic flexure
Descending colon
Sigmoid colon
Rectum

Anterior view

Post-colectomy

Stoma of ileostomy
Rectal stump

FIGURE 19-10 Colectomy (colon removal) with ileostomy. *(Medical Illustration Copyright © 2006 Nucleus Medical Art, All rights reserved. www.nucleusinc.com.)*

TABLE 19-7	Guidelines for Initiating Enteral Nutrition in Intestine Transplant Recipients	
Nutrient	**Guideline**	**Comment**
Carbohydrates	Concentrated sweets and hyperosmolar fruit juice may cause osmotic diarrhea.	Carbohydrate malabsorption and secondary lactase deficiency may increase luminal osmolarity and increase stomal output.
Fat	MCT or IV lipids short term. Long-chain fatty acid absorption may improve within 2-6 weeks as lacteals and lymphatics are regenerated.	Lacteals and lymphatics of small intestine are severed during organ retrieval causing fat malabsorption initially.
Glutamine	An enteral formula enriched with glutamine may theoretically improve absorptive function and mucosal structure after transplantation.	Glutamine is a conditionally essential amino acid and fuel for enterocytes.
Bicarbonate	Supplement.	Bicarbonate losses from the ostomy are often increased.
Fluid	Rehydration solutions may be helpful.	High intestinal losses are common.

Modified from Hasse JM: Nutrition assessment and support of organ transplant recipients, *JPEN J Parenter Enteral Nutr* 25:120, 2001, with permission from the American Society for Enteral and Parenteral Nutrition (A.S.P.E.N.). A.S.P.E.N. does not endorse the use of this material in any form other than its entirety.
MCT, Medium-chain triglycerides; *IV,* intravenous.

Short-Bowel Syndrome

Etiology

SBS is a malabsorptive condition secondary to surgical removal of parts of the small intestine with extensive dysfunction of the remaining portion of the organ.[14,15,18] Severity of malabsorption is contingent on amount and location of bowel resection.[14,15,18] Removal of the distal two thirds of ileum and ileocecal valve often results in severe malnutrition because the ileocecal valve controls transit time of intestinal contents. Removal often promotes a transit time too rapid for sufficient absorption of nutrients. Absorption of water, electrolytes, protein, fat, carbohydrates, vitamins, and minerals is significantly reduced when large portions of the small intestine are lost.[14,15]

Typically, in an adult the small intestine is 20 feet long and the large intestine is 7 feet long. A general definition for SBS is a resection of more than 50% of the small intestine. Resections result from inherent conditions such as Crohn's disease or radiation enteritis, surgical bypass, or massive abdominal injury and trauma. They may also be required for vascular problems such as blood clots causing death of involved tissue or for extensive fistula formation, radiation injury, congenital abnormalities, or cancer. After resection, the remaining small intestine has remarkable ability to adapt.[18] Remaining villi may enlarge and lengthen, consequently increasing absorptive surface area of the remaining intestine. Nutrients must be ingested orally for this adaptive sequence to take place, and gradual increase in oral intake after resection could promote gradual recovery in absorptive capability.[14] Parenteral nutrition support may be necessary for the short term or indefinitely following surgical shortening of the gut.[14,15]

Nutritional Management

Degrees of surgical resection create different problems, and nutrition therapy must be tailored to individual functional capacity remaining. Initial nutritional needs are usually supplied by early enteral or parenteral nutrition support (see Chapter 18). Frequent monitoring of responses to nutrition support, especially fluid and electrolyte balances and malnutrition signs, is essential. The patient is weaned from nutrition support to an oral diet as tolerated, accompanied by vitamin and mineral supplementation. Nutritional status should continue to be monitored. As adaptation progresses, early restriction of fat may be liberalized somewhat with moderate use of the more easily absorbed medium-chain triglycerides (MCT oil) to obtain needed kcalories.

Bowel Transplantation

A specialized procedure, intestinal transplants are performed in 48 Intestine Transplant Centers located in 25 states. Patients with complications from or failure of TPN such as recurrent sepsis, thrombosis of access sites, metabolic disorders, cholestasis, and hepatic dysfunction may be considered candidates for intestine transplant, which may involve the entire small intestine or just a segment of it. Most intestine transplants are whole organ transplants and are often performed in combination with a liver transplant. Cadaver transplants are more common than live donor transplants.[32,33]

Patients undergoing small-bowel transplantation can have problems transitioning to oral nutrition. Furthermore, special feeding considerations should be taken into consideration during the initial posttransplant phase when the graft begins to function (Table 19-7).[30] Large amounts of fluids lost after surgery must be replaced to prevent dehydration. Oral rehydration solutions may be used, although intravenous (IV) fluids may be required to replace not only lost fluids, but magnesium, zinc, bicarbonate, potassium, and sodium as well. Fiber, pectin, paregoric, and loperamide may enhance intestinal absorption by slowing transit time.[19,34]

DISORDERS OF THE LARGE INTESTINE

Flatulence

Everyone has it. Most believe they have too much. And everyone is embarrassed if they pass gas in the wrong place at the wrong time. History views flatulence with mixed reviews. Hippocrates professed, "Passing gas is necessary to well-being." The Roman Emperor Claudius decreed, "All Roman citizens shall be allowed to pass gas whenever necessary." Regrettably for flatulent Romans, Emperor Constantine later overturned this pronouncement in a 315 BC edict.[35]

Etiology

Flatulence is the condition of having excessive stomach or intestinal gas. Gas in the gut is the result of swallowed air or production in the intestines. Air swallowing (aerophagia) is a common cause of gas in the stomach. Small amounts of air are swallowed when eating and drinking. Some people swallow additional air while they eat or drink rapidly, chew gum, smoke, or wear dentures that are too loose. Most swallowed air is expelled from the stomach by burping or belching. Residual gas moves into the small intestine and is partially absorbed. A small quantity of gas travels to the large intestine and is expelled through the rectum.

Gas is produced in the intestines when normal, harmless bacteria in the large intestine break down undigested foods humans cannot due to a lack of specific digestive enzymes. Gas in the intestines is made of primarily odorless vapors—carbon dioxide (CO_2), oxygen (O_2), nitrogen (N), hydrogen (H_2), and sometimes methane (CH_4). The unpleasant odor of flatulence is produced by bacteria in the large intestine that release small amounts of gases that contain sulfur (S). These gases eventually exit the body through the rectum. H_2 and CO_2 are produced after ingestion of certain fruits and vegetables containing indigestible carbohydrates and in those with malabsorption syndromes (CF, CD, pancreatic insufficiency). Large amounts of disaccharides pass into the colon and are fermented to H_2 in those with lactose deficiency. CH_4 is produced in approximately one third of the population and is influenced minimally by food ingestion. Tendency to produce CH_4 appears to be a familial trait.[34] Foods that produce gas in one person may not produce gas in another. Most foods that produce gas contain carbohydrates (Table 19-8); fats and proteins cause little gas.

Medical Management

The most common ways to reduce production of gas are changing diet, taking medications, and reducing amount of air swallowed. The difficulty in suggesting dietary modification is individual tolerances. The quantity of gas produced by particular foods varies from person to person. Effective dietary change is typically the result of learning by way of trial and error.

TABLE 19-8 | **Foods That May Cause Gas**

Category		Food Sources
Sugars	Raffinose	Beans, cabbage, brussels sprouts, broccoli, asparagus, other vegetables, whole grains
	Lactose	Milk, milk products (cheese, ice cream, processed foods)
	Fructose	Onions, artichokes, peas, wheat, also used as a sweetener in some soft drinks and fruit drinks
	Sorbitol	Fruits (apples, pears, peaches, prunes), also used as an artificial sweetener in many dietetic foods and sugar-free candies and gums
Starches		Potatoes, corn, noodles, wheat products (rice is the only starch that does not produce gas)
Fiber	Soluble	Oat bran, beans, peas, most fruits
	Insoluble	Wheat bran, some vegetables

Modified from National Digestive Disease Information Clearinghouse (NDDIC), National Institute of Diabetes and Digestive and Kidney Diseases (NIDDK), National Institutes of Health (NIH): *Gas in the digestive tract*, NIH Publication No. 04-883, Bethesda, Md, 2004 (March), Author. Retrieved December 15, 2005, from *http://digestive.niddk.nih.gov/ddiseases/pubs/gas/*.

Few well-controlled studies have demonstrated clear-cut benefit from any drug.[35] Some over-the-counter (OTC) medicines are available to help reduce symptoms (Table 19-9). Although gas may be unpleasant and embarrassing, it is not life-threatening. Education concerning causes, ways to reduce symptoms, and treatment help most people find relief.[36]

Irritable Bowel Syndrome

Etiology

Sometimes called *spastic colon*, IBS is a recurring functional disorder typified by abdominal pain or discomfort with alternating diarrhea and constipation for which there is no organic explanation.[14,15,18] For those with IBS, quantity of symptoms is not as important as quality of life. Work, social life, and even sexual intercourse can be disrupted by IBS.[14] IBS is an extremely common disorder, affecting up to 20% of the U.S. population, but most never seek medical attention.[14,18]

Clinical Symptoms

Manifestation of IBS may differ to a great extent from person to person. Some experience only diarrhea or constipation, whereas others experience an alternating pattern of both.[14] Some symptoms may be more marked than others.[37] There are no physical findings or diagnostic tests that confirm the diagnosis of IBS.[37] Diagnosis is determined in the presence of congruent symptoms and

TABLE 19-9	Nonprescription Medications Used to Treat Flatulence

Medication	Classification	Action
Simethicone Mylanta II Maalox II Di-Gel	Antacid	Foaming agent that joins gas bubbles in the stomach, making gas more easily belched away; no effect on intestinal gas
Lactase Lactaid Lactrase	Enzyme	Aids lactose digestion
Beano	Enzyme supplement	Contains sugar-digesting enzyme the body lacks to digest sugar in beans and many vegetables; has no effect on gas caused by lactose or fiber
Charcocaps	Activated charcoal	May produce relief from gas produced in colon

Data from National Digestive Disease Information Clearinghouse (NDDIC), National Institute of Diabetes and Digestive and Kidney Diseases (NIDDK), National Institutes of Health (NIH): *Gas in the digestive tract,* NIH Publication No. 04-883, Bethesda, Md, 2004 (March), Author. Retrieved December 15, 2005, from *http://digestive.niddk.nih.gov/ddiseases/pubs/gas/*; and Maslar J, Kreplick LW: *Flatulence (gas),* Omaha, Neb, 2005 (updated October 21), eMedicine Consumer Health. Retrieved December 15, 2005, from *www.emedicinehealth.com/Articles/5940-1.asp.*

after ruling out organic diseases.[18,37] More than half of those diagnosed with IBS are female.

The symptom-based Rome II diagnostic criteria for IBS emphasize a clear-cut diagnosis instead of excluding other medical conditions.[37] These criteria are based on a detailed history, physical examination, and limited diagnostic tests, as well as presentation of a particular set of symptoms, as follows[38]:

- At least 12 weeks or more (consecutive or nonconsecutive) in the preceding 12 months of abdominal discomfort or pain accompanied by at least two of the following features:
  - It is relieved with defecation and/or
  - Onset is associated with a change in frequency or stool, and/or
  - Onset is associated with a change in form (appearance) of stool
- The following other symptoms support, but are not essential, to the diagnosis of IBS:
  - More than three bowel movements per day or fewer than three bowel movements per week
  - Lumpy/hard or loose/watery stool form
  - Abnormal stool passage (straining, urgency, or feeling of incomplete evacuation)
  - Passage of mucus
  - Bloating or feeling of abdominal distension

Medical Management

Possibly the most helpful treatment intervention is to proffer assurance and a straightforward explanation of the functional nature of symptoms.[18] Patients should be assured that their symptoms are real, not caused by stress or a psychologic or psychiatric disorder,[18,37] although in some individuals stress can trigger or exacerbate symptoms of IBS.[37]

A chronic disorder, IBS can be treated but not cured. Although no study has shown a clearly demonstrable benefit for a specific drug,[39] patients with more severe symptoms that do not respond to conservative treatment (education, reassurance, and nutrition therapy) may respond to drug therapy, as follows[18,39]:

- *Antispasmodic (anticholinergic) agents:* acute episodes of pain or bloating
- *Antidiarrheal agents:* agents that may be best used prophylactically in situations in which diarrhea is anticipated (stressful situations) or inconvenient (social engagements)
- *Anticonstipation agents:* fiber supplementation with bran, psyllium, methylcellulose, or polycarbophil can be beneficial in most cases; those unresponsive to fiber may benefit from osmotic laxatives (e.g., milk of magnesia)

Nutritional Management

Dietary triggers of IBS have not been established; however, dietary modification may well provide symptomatic benefit. For some, a food diary in which food intake, symptoms, and activities are recorded may uncover dietary or psychosocial aspects that predispose symptoms. Malabsorption of lactose, fructose, and sorbitol can cause bloating, distention, flatulence, and diarrhea. An assortment of foods can trigger flatulence (see Table 19-8), which may cause pain and distention in some patients.[18]

For patients presenting primarily with constipation, a high-fiber diet (20 to 30 g/day) may ease symptoms. One tablespoon of bran powder 2 to 3 times daily with food or in 8 oz or more of liquid provides the recommended amount. Some patients may describe increased gas and distention from fiber supplementation with bran; therefore psyllium, methylcellulose, or polycarbophil are often better tolerated.[18]

Diverticular Disease

Nature and Etiology

A *diverticulum* is a small tubular sac that protrudes from a main canal or cavity in the body (Figure 19-11). Formation and presence of small diverticula protruding from the intestinal lumen, usually the colon, produce the condition diverticulosis. More often diverticulosis occurs in older adults. It develops at points of weakened musculature in

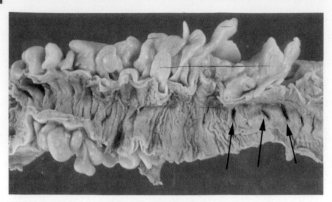

FIGURE 19-11 Diverticula. *(From Lewis SM, Heitkemper M, Dirksen S: Medical-surgical nursing: assessment and management of clinical problems, ed 6, St. Louis, 2004, Elsevier/Mosby.)*

the bowel wall, along the track of blood vessels entering the bowel from within. Direct cause is a progressive increase in pressure within the bowel from segmental circular muscle contractions that normally move the remaining food mass along and form the feces for elimination. When pressures become sufficiently high in one of these segments and dietary fiber is insufficient to maintain the necessary bulk for preventing high internal pressures within the colon, diverticula, small protrusions of the muscle layer, develop at that point. The condition causes no problem unless small diverticula become infected and inflamed from fecal irritation and colon bacteria. This diseased state is called *diverticulitis.* The commonly used collective term covering diverticulosis and diverticulitis is *diverticular disease.*

Clinical Symptoms

As the inflammatory process grows, increased hypermotility and pressures from luminal segmentation cause pain. Pain and tenderness are usually localized in the lower left side of the abdomen and are accompanied by nausea, vomiting, distention, diarrhea, intestinal spasm, and fever. If the process continues, intestinal obstruction or perforation may necessitate surgical intervention.

Nutritional Management

Diverticular disease is a common GI disorder among middle-age persons and older adults. It may often be accompanied by malnutrition. Aggressive nutrition therapy hastens recovery from an attack, shortens hospital stay, and reduces costs. Numerous studies and extensive clinical practice have demonstrated better management of chronic diverticular disease with an increased amount of dietary fiber than with old practices of restricting fiber. In acute episodes of active disease, however, the amount of dietary fiber should be reduced. The relationship of dietary fiber and diverticular disease has been further reinforced by studies of populations, such as those in Japan, that have recently experienced the westernization of their

culture. Chapter 2 provides an extended discussion of dietary fiber and its relation to health and disease.

Constipation

A common disorder, usually of short duration, constipation is characterized by retention of feces in the colon beyond normal emptying time. It is a problem for which Americans spend a quarter of a billion dollars each year on laxatives. However, "regularity" of elimination is highly individual, and it is not necessary to have a bowel movement every day to be healthy. Usually this common, short-term problem results from various sources of nervous tension, worry, and changes in social setting. Such situations include vacations and travel with alterations in usual routines. Also, it may be caused by prolonged use of laxatives or cathartics, low-fiber diets, inadequate fluid intake, or lack of exercise, all of which can contribute to a decreased intestinal muscle tone. Increasing activity and improving dietary intake to include adequate fiber (goal of 25 to 35 g/day) and fluid are usually sufficient strategies to remedy the situation. If chronic constipation persists, however, agents that increase stool bulk may be necessary. These bulking agents include bran or more soluble forms of fiber. Taking laxatives or enemas on a regular basis should be avoided. The problem of constipation occurs in all age-groups but is almost epidemic in older adults. In all cases, a personalized approach to management of constipation is fundamental.

DISEASES OF THE GASTROINTESTINAL ACCESSORY ORGANS

Three major accessory organs—(1) the liver, (2) the gallbladder, and (3) the pancreas (Figure 19-12)—lie adjacent to the GI tract and produce important digestive agents that enter the intestine and aid in processing of food substances. Specific enzymes are produced for each of the major nutrients, and bile is added to assist in enzymatic digestion of fats. Diseases of these organs can easily affect GI function and cause problems in the normal handling of specific types of food.

Viral Hepatitis

Etiology

Viral hepatitis (inflammation of the liver) is a major public health problem throughout the world, affecting hundreds of millions of people. It causes considerable illness and death in human populations from acute infection or its effects, which may include chronic active hepatitis, cirrhosis, and primary liver cancer. During the past few years, knowledge of viruses causing different types of hepatitis has grown rapidly. Currently, six unrelated human hepatitis viruses, A, B, C, D, E, and the newly discovered

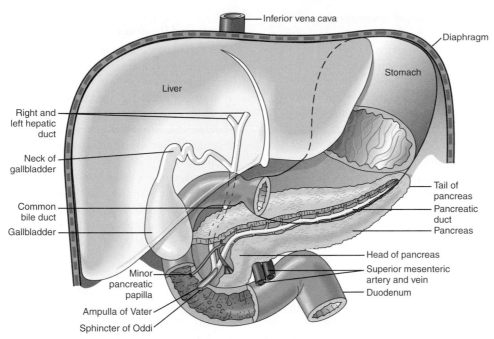

FIGURE 19-12 Liver, pancreas, and gallbladder. *(From Copstead-Kirkhorn L-E, Banasik JL:* Pathophysiology, *ed 3, Philadelphia, 2005, Elsevier/Saunders.)*

hepatitis virus G, have been isolated and described.[40] The two most common and well known are A and B, which serve as examples, as follows:

1. *Hepatitis A virus (HAV):* HAV is transmitted via the classic oral-fecal route through contaminated food and water. It is a prevalent infection worldwide, especially where there is overcrowding and poor hygiene or sanitation. An HAV vaccine has been developed that is far more effective than the former large and painful injection of gamma globulins, antibodies isolated from the blood. This vaccine protects travelers to developing countries, where the virus is endemic and may easily contaminate water and food.[40,41]

2. *Hepatitis B virus (HBV):* HBV is mainly spread via parenteral contact with infected blood or blood products, including contaminated needles, and sexual contact.[41] It has now been implicated worldwide as the major causative factor in chronic liver disease and associated liver cancer. HBV infection is closely related to the body's immune system. Approximately 10% to 20% of those who become infected with HBV become chronic carriers. Of this number, approximately 20% acquire chronic hepatitis eventually progressing to cirrhosis and, later in some, liver cancer.[40] Universal immunization is recommended for persons of any age, but particularly for the following high-risk groups: male homosexuals, Alaska Natives, immigrants from highly endemic areas, illicit drugs users, domestic associates of HBV carriers, hemodialysis patients, residents of institutions, medical and dental personnel, patients needing frequent transfusions, and those planning to reside in high-risk areas (e.g., Far East and sub-Saharan Africa).[41,42]

Clinical Symptoms

Viral agents of hepatitis produce diffuse injury to liver cells, especially parenchymal cells. In milder cases, liver injury is largely reversible, but with increasing severity, more extensive necrosis occurs. In some cases, massive necrosis may lead to liver failure and death. A cardinal symptom of hepatitis is anorexia, contributing to risk of malnutrition. Varying clinical symptoms appear depending on the degree of liver injury. Jaundice, a major symptom, may or may not be obvious, depending on severity of the disease, and can have both nutritional and psychologic effects. In an outbreak of hepatitis, many infected persons

---

endemic Characterizing a disease of low morbidity that remains constantly in a human community but is clinically recognizable in only a few.

parenchymal cells Functional cells of an organ, as distinguished from the cells constituting its structure or framework.

necrosis Cell death caused by progressive enzyme breakdown.

jaundice A syndrome characterized by hyperbilirubinemia and deposits of bile pigment in the skin, mucous membranes, and sclera, giving a yellow appearance to the patient.

may be nonicteric and thus go undiagnosed and untreated because jaundice has not developed sufficiently to be seen. Malnutrition and impaired immunocompetence contribute to spontaneous infections and continuing liver disease. General symptoms, in addition to anorexia, include malaise, weakness, nausea and vomiting, diarrhea, headache, fever, enlarged and tender liver, and enlarged spleen. When jaundice develops, it usually occurs for a preicteric period of 5 to 10 days, deepens for 1 to 2 weeks, then levels off and decreases. After this crisis point, there is a sufficient recovery of injured cells, and a convalescence of 3 weeks to 3 months follows. Optimal care during this time is essential to avoid relapse.

General Treatment

Bed rest is essential. Physical activity and exercise increases both severity and duration of the disease. A daily intake of 3000 to 3500 ml of fluid guards against dehydration and gives a general sense of well-being and improved appetite. However, optimal nutrition is the major therapy. It provides the essential foundation for recovery of the injured liver cells and overall return of strength.

Nutrition Therapy

A complete nutrition assessment and initial personal history provide the basis for planning care. Nutrition therapy principles relate to the liver's function in metabolizing each of the nutrients, as follows:

- *Adequate protein:* Protein is essential for liver cell regeneration, as well as for maintaining all essential bodily functions. It also provides lipotropic agents such as methionine and choline for conversion of fats to lipoproteins and removal from the liver, thus preventing fatty infiltration. The daily diet should supply 1.0 to 1.2 g/kg of actual body weight of high-quality protein.[30] This amount is usually enough to achieve a positive nitrogen balance.
- *High carbohydrate:* Sufficient available glucose must be provided to restore protective glycogen reserves and meet the energy demands of the disease process. Also, adequate glucose for energy ensures the use of protein for vital tissue regeneration. Diet should supply approximately 50% to 55% of the total kcalories as carbohydrates, or 300 to 400 g/day.
- *Low fat:* Less than 30% of calories should come from fat in case of steatorrhea.[30]
- *Four to six small feedings:* To promote adequate intake and minimize loss of muscle, at least three meals and a bedtime snack are recommended.[30]
- *Sodium:* If fluid retention is present, limit sodium to 90 mEq/day (approximately 2000 mg).[30]
- *Micronutrients:* Fat-soluble vitamins should be provided in water-soluble form. Other water-soluble vitamins also require supplementation.

Meals and Feedings

The problem of supplying a diet adequate to meet increased nutritional demands of a patient with an illness that makes food almost repellent calls for creativity and supportive encouragement. As the patient improves, appetizing and attractive food is needed. Because nutrition therapy is key to recovery, a major nutrition and nursing responsibility requires devising ways to encourage the increased amounts of food intake needed. The clinical dietitian and nursing staff should work together to achieve mutual goals planned for the patient. All staff attendants must follow appropriate precautions in handling patient trays to prevent spread of the infection.

Cirrhosis

Cirrhosis is the general term used for advanced stages of liver disease, regardless of the initial cause of the disease. Among all digestive diseases, cirrhosis of the liver, caused by chronic alcohol abuse, is the leading nonmalignant cause of death in the United States and most of the developed world. The majority of deaths occur among young and middle-age adults. The French physician René Laënnec (1781-1826) first used the term *cirrhosis* (from the Greek work *kirrhos,* meaning "orange yellow") to describe the abnormal color and rough surface of the diseased liver. The cirrhotic liver is a firm, fibrous, dull yellowish mass with orange nodules projecting from its surface (Figure 19-13).

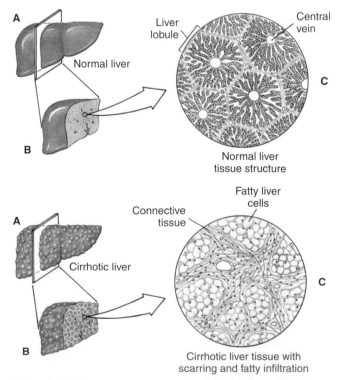

FIGURE 19-13 Comparison of normal liver and liver with cirrhotic changes. **A,** Anterior view of organ. **B,** Cross-section. **C,** Tissue structure. (*Medical and Scientific Illustration.*)

Etiology

Some forms of cirrhosis result from biliary obstruction, with blockage of the biliary ducts and accumulation of bile in the liver.[40,42] Other cases may result from liver necrosis from undetermined causes or, in some cases, from previous viral hepatitis. A common problem is fatty cirrhosis, associated with the complicating factor of malnutrition. Continuing fatty infiltration causes cellular destruction and fibrotic tissue changes.

Clinical Symptoms

Early signs of cirrhosis include GI disturbances such as nausea, vomiting, loss of appetite, distention, and epigastric pain. In time, jaundice may appear, with increasing weakness, edema, ascites, and anemia from GI bleeding, iron deficiency, or hemorrhage. A specific macrocytic anemia from folic acid deficiency is also frequently observed. Steatorrhea is a common symptom. Major symptoms are caused by a basic protein deficiency and its multiple metabolic problems: (1) plasma protein levels fall, leading to failure of the capillary fluid shift mechanism (see Chapter 8), causing ascites; (2) lipotropic agents are not supplied for fat conversion to lipoproteins, and damaging fat accumulates in the liver tissue; (3) blood-clotting mechanisms are impaired because factors such as prothrombin and fibrinogen are not adequately produced; and (4) general tissue catabolism and negative nitrogen balance continue the overall degenerative process.

As the disease progresses, increasing fibrotic scar tissue impairs blood circulation through the liver, and portal hypertension follows.[40] Contributing further to the problem is continuing ascites. Impaired portal circulation with increasing venous pressure may lead to esophageal varices, with danger of rupture and fatal massive hemorrhage.

Drug therapy includes use of broad-spectrum antibiotics to limit growth of intestinal bacteria and laxatives to speed intestinal transit time, limiting the amount of time available for bacteria to produce ammonia in the GI tract. Lactulose, a synthetic derivative of lactose consisting of one molecule of galactose and one molecule of fructose, is a laxative that is used in the treatment of hepatic encephalopathy. Lactulose is ionized, cannot diffuse across the colon membrane, and is excreted in the stool. Lactulose can reduce blood ammonia levels by 25% to 50%. Diuretics may be given to reduce fluid retention and prevent ascites.

Nutrition Therapy

When alcoholism is an added underlying problem, treatment is difficult. Each patient requires supportive care. Therapy is usually aimed at correcting fluid and electrolyte problems and providing as much nutrition support as possible for hepatic repair. In any case, guidelines for nutrition therapy for cirrhosis of the liver should include the following principles:

- *Energy:* 30 to 35 kcal/kg body weight. Fluid retention, if present, will affect the accuracy of estimating kcalorie needs. As muscle tissue is wasted, it is often replaced by fluid weight. An estimated dry weight (post paracentesis of ascites or well diuresed) should be used when feasible to estimate kcalories needs.[30]

- *Protein intake:* 1 to 2 g/kg body weight. Intake should be adequate to regenerate liver cells and prevent infections but not excessive to the point of aggravating ammonia buildup and inducing hepatic coma. Protein estimations should be based on dry weight whenever possible.[30]

- *Sodium:* Intake is usually restricted to less than 2000 mg/day to help reduce fluid retention.[30] A sodium intake level of less than 2000 mg/day is considered quite restrictive, and palatability of food is usually a problem. It may be necessary to liberalize the sodium restriction to improve intake.

- *Texture:* If esophageal varices develop, it may be necessary to give soft foods that are smooth in texture to prevent the danger of rupture and hemorrhage.

- *Carbohydrate:* Adequate intake is needed to prevent catabolism of body protein for energy, which would further increase blood ammonia. Intestinal bacteria make ammonia from undigested proteins (proteins from shed mucosal cells, protein from GI tract bleed, and dietary proteins).

- *Fat:* Moderate fat intake helps make food more appealing and increases kcalorie content, making it important in the diet of a person with cirrhosis. Fat intake only needs to be restricted when there is steatorrhea, and even then MCT oil can be used.[30]

- *Vitamins and minerals:* The central role of the liver is to metabolize and store vitamins and minerals. Usually all people with advanced liver disease require supplementation of some vitamins, minerals, and trace elements. Nutrient supplementation is determined by monitoring serum levels and checking for clinical signs of deficiencies.

- *Alcohol:* To protect the liver from further injury abstinence from alcohol is mandatory.

- *Personalized food plan:* Adequate intake is more likely, thus hastening recovery, if the food plan is structured

---

icteric Alternative term for jaundice: nonicteric indicates absence of jaundice; preicteric indicates a state before development of icterus, or jaundice.

immunocompetence The ability or capacity to develop an immune response, that is, antibody production and/or cell-mediated immunity, after exposure to antigen.

to include likes/dislikes and real-life schedule of the patient. If appetite is a problem, several small meals per day instead of full meals may be required.[30]

- *Fluids:* Fluids should be encouraged unless ascites or edema is present. Water is the fluid of choice.[30] Calorie-dense beverages such as juicelike drinks and soft drinks provide excess calories with little nutrient, often taking the place of nutrient-dense foods.

Hepatic Encephalopathy

The term *encephalopathy* refers to any disease or disorder that affects the brain, especially chronic degenerative conditions. Effect on the brain in hepatic encephalopathy is a major serious complication of end-stage liver disease. Accumulation of toxic substances in the blood as a result of liver failure impairs consciousness and contributes to memory loss, personality change, tremors, seizures, stupor, and coma.

Etiology

As cirrhotic changes continue in the liver, portal blood circulation diminishes and liver functions begin to fail. The normal liver has a major function of removing ammonia from blood by converting it to urea for excretion. The failing liver can no longer inactivate or detoxify substances or metabolize others. A key factor involved in the progressive disease process is an elevated blood level of ammonia, although it is by no means the sole agent. Resulting hepatic encephalopathy brings changes in consciousness, behavior, and neurologic status.

Clinical Symptoms

Typical response involves disorders of consciousness and alterations in motor function. There is apathy, confusion, inappropriate behavior, and drowsiness, progressing to coma. Speech may be slurred or monotonous. A coarse, flapping tremor known as *asterixis* is observed in the outstretched hands, caused by a sustained contraction of a group of muscles. Breath may have a fecal odor, *fetor hepaticus.*

Basic Treatment Objectives

Fundamental objectives of treatment are twofold: (1) removal of sources of excess ammonia and (2) provision of nutrition support. Parenteral fluid and electrolytes are used to restore normal balances. Lactulose and neomycin may be used to control ammonia levels. Neomycin is an antibiotic that reduces the population of urea-splitting organisms within the bowel that produce ammonia.

Nutrition Therapy

General nutrition support for hepatic encephalopathy is based on the following three principles of dietary management:

1. *Low protein:* 0.5 g protein per kilogram of body weight. General protein intake is reduced individually as necessary to restrict the dietary sources of nitrogen in amino acids. Dietary protein should be of high biologic value and spaced throughout the day.[30]
2. *Kcalories and vitamins:* Adequate energy intake is crucial to the patient's recovery, especially through impact of kcaloric intake on liver glycogen reserves and their protective role in the healing process. Amounts of kcalories and vitamins are prescribed according to need, with sufficient carbohydrate as the primary energy source and some fat as tolerated. Vitamin K is usually given parenterally, along with other vitamins and minerals, especially zinc, in which the patient may be deficient.
3. *Fluid intake:* Fluid intake-output balance is carefully controlled.

Liver Transplantation

Liver transplantation is the treatment of choice for patients with end-stage liver disease who have not responded to conventional treatment.[40,41] Patients being considered for liver transplantation undergo extensive physiologic and psychologic evaluations to detect possible contraindications to the procedure.[41]

As with all major surgery, aggressive nutrition support reduces risks. Careful pretransplantation nutrition assessment and support helps prepare the patient for the surgery. Enteral or parenteral nutrition support may be required for optimal postoperative nutritional status.

Gallbladder Disease

Metabolic Function

Basic function of the gallbladder is to concentrate and store the bile produced in its initial watery solution by the liver. The liver secretes about 600 to 800 ml of bile per day, which the gallbladder normally concentrates fivefold to tenfold to accommodate this daily bile production in its small capacity of 40 to 70 ml. Through the cholecystokinin (CCK) mechanism, presence of fat in the duodenum stimulates contraction of the gallbladder with release of concentrated bile into the common duct and then into the small intestine.

Cholecystitis and Cholelithiasis

The prefix *chole* of the two terms *cholecystitis* and *cholelithiasis* comes from the Greek word *chole,* which means "bile." Thus cholecystitis is an inflammation of the gallbladder, and cholelithiasis is the formation of gallstones. Incidence of gallstones is associated with age, gender, and an assortment of medical factors (Box 19-3).

Inflammation of the gallbladder usually results from a low-grade chronic infection and may occur with or without gallstones. However, in 90% to 95% of patients, acute cholecystitis is associated with gallstones and is caused by the obstruction of the cystic duct by stones, resulting in acute inflammation of the organ. Gallstones can be classified into the following two main groups: (1) cholesterol stones and (2) pigment stones[43]:

1. *Cholesterol stones:* In the United States and most Western countries, more than 75% of gallstones are cholesterol stones. The infectious process produces changes in gallbladder mucosa, which affects its absorptive powers. The main ingredient of bile is cholesterol, which is insoluble in water. Normally, cholesterol is kept in solution by other ingredients in bile. However, when the absorbing mucosal tissue of the gallbladder is inflamed or infected, changes occur in the tissue. Absorptive powers of the gallbladder may be altered, affecting solubility of the bile ingredients. Excess water or excess bile acid may be absorbed. Under these abnormal absorptive conditions cholesterol may precipitate, forming gallstones of almost pure cholesterol.

2. *Pigment stones:* Both black and brown pigment gallstones, although they differ in chemical composition and clinical features, are colored by the presence of *bilirubin,* the pigment in red blood cells. They are associated with chronic hemolysis in conditions such as sickle cell disease, thalassemia, cirrhosis, long-term TPN, and advancing age. Pigment stones are often found in bile ducts and may be related to a bacterial infection with *Escherichia coli.*

Clinical Symptoms

When inflammation, stones, or both are present in the gallbladder, contraction from the cholecystokinin-pancreozymin (CCK-PZ) mechanism causes pain. Sometimes the pain is severe. There is fullness and distention after eating and particular difficulty with fatty foods.

General Treatment

Surgical removal of the gallbladder, a cholecystectomy (Figure 19-14), is usually indicated. If the patient is obese, some weight loss before surgery is advisable if surgery can be delayed. Supportive therapy is largely nutritional. Several nonsurgical treatments for removing the stones, using chemical dissolution or mechanical stone fragmentation, have been developed. These methods provide effective alternatives to surgery in some cases.[43]

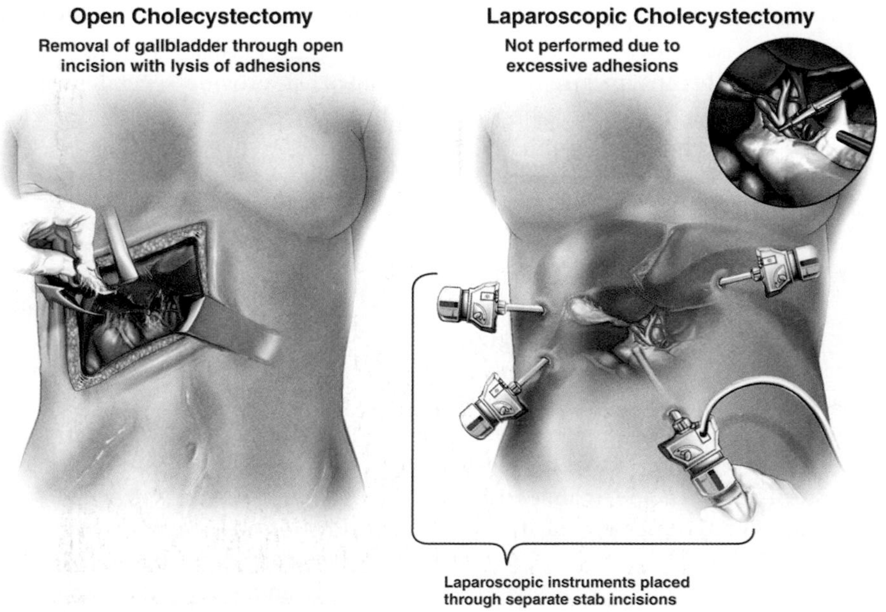

BOX 19-3	Risk Factors for Gallbladder Disease

Female gender
Ethnicity: Native American, particularly Pima Indians of North America
High cholesterol diet
Use of oral contraceptives
Obesity (BMI >30)
Ileal resection or disease
Diabetes mellitus
Rapid weight loss (in obese persons)
Positive family history
Some medications (e.g., lipid-lowering agents)
Gallbladder hypomobility

Data from Axford JS, O'Callaghan CA: *Medicine,* ed 2, Oxford, 2004, Blackwell Science; and Sartin JS: Alterations in function of the gallbladder and exocrine pancreas. In Copstead LC, Banasik JL: *Pathophysiology,* ed 3, St. Louis, 2005, Elsevier.

Open Cholecystectomy
Removal of gallbladder through open incision with lysis of adhesions

Laparoscopic Cholecystectomy
Not performed due to excessive adhesions

Laparoscopic instruments placed through separate stab incisions

FIGURE 19-14 Open and laparoscopic cholecystectomy. *(Medical Illustration Copyright © 2006 Nucleus Medical Art, All rights reserved.* www.nucleusinc.com.*)*

Nutrition Therapy

Basic principles of nutrition therapy for gallbladder disease include the following:

- *Fat:* Because dietary fat is the principal cause of contraction of the diseased organ and subsequent pain, it is poorly tolerated. Energy should come primarily from carbohydrate foods, especially during acute phases. Control of fat will also contribute to weight control, a primary goal because obesity and excess food intake have been repeatedly associated with the development of gallstones.
- *Kcalories:* If weight loss is indicated, kcalories will be reduced according to need. Principles of weight management are discussed in Chapter 6. Usually such a diet will have a relatively low percentage of calories from fat, meeting the needs of the patient for fat moderation.
- *Cholesterol and "gas formers":* Two additional modifications usually found in traditional diets for gallbladder disease concern restriction of foods containing cholesterol and foods labeled "gas formers." Neither modification has a valid rationale. The body daily synthesizes more cholesterol than is present in an average diet. Thus restriction of dietary cholesterol has little effect in reducing gallstone formation. Total dietary fat reduction is more important. As for the use of "gas formers," such as legumes, cabbage, or fiber, blanket restriction seems unwarranted because food tolerances in any circumstances are highly individual.

Diseases of the Pancreas

Pancreatitis

Acute inflammation of the pancreas (pancreatitis) is caused by digestion of the organ tissues by enzymes it produces, principally *trypsin.* Normally, enzymes remain in inactive form until pancreatic secretions reach the duodenum through the common duct. However, gallbladder disease may cause a gallstone to enter the common bile duct and obstruct flow from the pancreas or cause a reflux of these secretions and bile from the common duct back into the pancreatic duct. This mixing of digestive materials activates powerful pancreatic enzymes within the gland. In such activated form, they begin their damaging effects on pancreatic tissue itself, causing acute pain. Sometimes infectious pancreatitis may occur as a complication of mumps or a bacterial disease. Mild or moderate pancreatitis may subside completely, but it has a tendency to recur. Alcohol in Western societies and malnutrition worldwide are the major causes of chronic pancreatitis.

General Treatment

Initial care consists of measures recommended for acute disease involving shock. These measures include IV feeding at first, replacement therapy of fluid and electrolytes, blood transfusions, antibiotics and pain medications, and gastric suction.

Nutrition Therapy

In early stages (acute pancreatitis), oral feedings are withheld because entry of food into the intestines stimulates pancreatic secretions and usually causes pain. Nutritional status is maintained by IV fluids or jejunal enteral feeding with peptide-based or elemental enteral nutrition formulas. Most patients with pancreatitis are able to resume oral feeding in 2 days.[44,45]

Parenteral nutrition is generally not recommended in pancreatitis unless a patient fails an enteral feeding trial.[44,45] Pseudocysts, intestinal and pancreatic fistulas, pancreatic abscesses, and pancreatic ascites may make enteral feeding impossible.

Health Promotion

A single layer of cells maintains a barrier between toxins and infections in the GI tract. At the same time, this same layer of cells absorbs macronutrients, micronutrients, and water and puts them into circulation. If that is not enough, these cells also regulate bodily functions via hormonal and immunologic mechanisms. It is plain to see why we would want to keep this remarkable organ healthy!

Keeping the GI tract healthy begins at an early age. Breast-feeding reduces risk of GI tract infections in infants.[46] Exposure to cigarette smoke and its metabolites (either through maternal smoking habits or second-hand smoke) appears to be linked to infantile colic. For that reason it seems reasonable that decreased exposure to tobacco smoke can provide long-term health benefits to both mothers and their children.[47]

In 1998 Hasler[48] summarized research that identified foods that provide several physiologic benefits. Among the findings are the following:

- People consuming diets high in fruits and vegetables have only one half the cancer risk of those who consume very little of these foods.
- Intake of lycopene, the primary carotenoid found in tomatoes, is inversely associated with reduced risk of digestive tract cancer, among other cancers.
- Garlic and onions *may* offer a protective effect on cancers of the GI tract.
- Probiotics (fermented dairy products, such as yogurt) reduce risk of various cancers, particularly colon cancer.
- Prebiotics (fermentable carbohydrates, such as starches, dietary fibers, other nonabsorbable sugars, sugar alcohols, and oligosaccharides) stimulate growth and/or activity of one or more of the "friendly" bacteria that live in the gut.

In addition to how we eat, how we live plays an important role in GI health. There is strong evidence that physical activity reduces risk of colon cancer by half. Physical activity *may* also reduce risk of cholelithiasis, constipation, diverticulosis, GI hemorrhage, and inflammatory bowel disease.[49] Hand washing for a minimum of 20 seconds (the amount of time it takes to sing "Happy Birthday" twice) with hot, soapy water will reduce risk of oral-fecal contamination that could cause foodborne illnesses and certain types of hepatitis.

This information can be summed up very simply: Mom was right when she asked you to do the following:

- Eat your fruits and vegetables.
- Go out and play (get plenty of physical activity).
- Wash your hands before eating.

TO SUM UP

Nutrition therapy for GI disease is based on careful consideration of the following four major factors:

1. Secretory functions, providing chemical agents and environment necessary for digestion to occur
2. Neuromuscular functions required for motility and mechanical digestion
3. Absorptive functions, enhancing entry of nutrients into the circulatory system
4. Psychologic factors reflected by changes in GI function

Esophageal problems vary widely from simple dysphagia to serious diseases or obstruction. Nutrition therapy and mode of intake vary according to degree of dysfunction.

PUD is a common GI problem affecting millions of Americans. It is an erosion of the mucosal lining, mainly in the duodenal bulb and less commonly in the lower antrum portion of the stomach. It results in increased gastric tone and painful hunger contractions on an empty stomach, as well as nutrition problems such as low plasma protein levels, anemia, and weight loss. Current medical management consists of acid and infection control with a coordinated system of drugs, rest, and a regular diet with few food and drink considerations to supply essential nutrition support for tissue healing.

Intestinal diseases are classified as (1) anatomic changes, such as development of small tubular sacs branching off the main alimentary canal in diverticular disease; (2) malabsorption, from multiple maldigestive and malabsorptive conditions; (3) IBD, resulting from mucosal changes and infectious processes, as seen in ulcerative colitis and Crohn's disease; or (4) SBS, resulting from surgical resection of parts of the intestine. Nutrition therapy involves fluid and electrolyte replacement, modifications in the diet's protein and energy content and food texture, and increased vitamins and minerals, with continuous adjustment of the diet according to changes in toleration for specific foods. Allergic responses to common food allergens, as well as missing cell enzymes in genetic disease, may also contribute to GI and metabolic problems from related food intolerances.

Accessory organs to the GI tract—liver, gallbladder, and pancreas—have important functions related to nutrient digestion, absorption, and metabolism, and their diseases interfere with these normal functions. Common liver disorders include hepatitis, usually caused by viral infection, and cirrhosis, an advanced liver disease leading to hepatic encephalopathy and progressive liver failure. Nutrient and energy levels required vary with each condition.

Diseases of the gallbladder include cholecystitis, inflammation that interferes with the absorption of water and bile acids, and cholelithiasis, or gallstone formation. Treatment involves a generally reduced-fat diet and surgical removal of the gallbladder. Diseases of the pancreas include acute and chronic forms of pancreatitis, in which alcohol abuse can be a primary cause. Other causes include biliary disease, malnutrition, drug reactions, abdominal injury, and genetic predisposition. In acute pancreatitis, pain is severe because of pancreatic enzyme reflux with self-digestion of pancreatic tissue by its own enzymes. Parenteral nutrition support is used to avoid enzyme stimulus, with gradual return to small, frequent meals as the attack subsides. In chronic pancreatitis, which is caused by alcoholism in Western societies and malnutrition worldwide, maldigestion from lack of enzymes because of pancreatic insufficiency creates nutrition problems. Nutrition care focuses on a nourishing diet with enzyme replacement and vitamin-mineral supplementation.

QUESTIONS FOR REVIEW

1. What is the basic principle of diet planning for patients with esophageal problems? Outline a general nutrition care plan for a patient with GERD complicated by a hiatal hernia.

2. In current practice what are the basic principles of diet planning for patients with PUD? How do these principles differ from former traditional therapy?

3. Outline a course of nutritional management for a person with PUD, based on the current approaches to medical management. How would you plan nutrition education for continuing self-care and avoidance of recurrence?

4. Describe the etiology, clinical signs, and treatment of each of the following intestinal diseases: malabsorption and diarrhea, IBD, diverticular disease, IBS, and constipation.

5. Compare the basis of food intolerances resulting from food allergy and a specific genetic disease such as cystic fibrosis.

6. How are the major metabolic functions of the liver affected in liver disease? Give some examples.

7. What is the rationale for treatment in the spectrum of liver disease—hepatitis, cirrhosis, and hepatic encephalopathy?

8. Develop a 1-day food plan for a 45-year-old man, 183 cm (6 ft 1 in) tall, weighing 90 kg (200 lb), with infectious hepatitis. Develop another plan for a similar patient with cirrhosis of the liver. What principles of diet therapy apply for each?

9. What are the principles of nutrition therapy for gallbladder disease? Write a 1-day meal plan for a 30-year-old woman, 165 cm (5 ft 6 in) tall, weighing 81 kg (180 lb), who has an inflamed gallbladder with stones and is awaiting a cholecystectomy.

10. Compare acute and chronic forms of pancreatitis in terms of etiology, symptoms, and nutrition therapy. What role does special enteral and parenteral nutrition support play in this therapy?

REFERENCES

1. Patti M et al: *Achalasia,* Omaha, Neb, 2004 (updated February 21), eMedicine.com, Inc. Available at *www.emedcine.com.* Accessed March 27, 2005.

2. Sawyer MAJ et al: *Achalasia,* Omaha, Neb, 2003 (updated March 28), eMedicine.com, Inc. Available at *www.emedicine.com.* Accessed March 27, 2005.

3. Nelms MN, Sucher K, Long S: *Understanding nutrition therapy and pathophysiology,* Belmont, Calif, 2007, Wadsworth/Thomson Learning.

4. Fass R, Ofman JJ: Gastroesophageal reflux disease—Should we adopt a new conceptual framework? *Am J Gastroenterol* 97(8):1901, 2002.

5. Revicki DA et al: The impact of gastroesophageal reflux disease on health-related quality of life, *Am J Med* 104(3):252, 1998.

6. Lagergren J et al: Symptomatic gastroesophageal reflux as a risk factor for esophageal adenocarcinoma, *N Engl J Med* 340(11):825, 1999.

7. Meining A, Classen M: The role of diet and lifestyle measures in the pathogenesis and treatment of gastroesophageal reflux disease, *Am J Gastroenterol* 95(10):2692, 2000.

8. Marshall BJ, Warren JR: Unidentified curved bacilli in the stomach of patients with gastritis and peptic ulcerations, *Lancet* 8390:1311, 1984.

9. Blaser MJ: The bacteria behind ulcers, *Sci Am* 274(2):104, 1996.

10. Marchetti M et al: Development of a mouse model of *Helicobacter pylori* infection that mimics human disease, *Science* 267(5204):1655, 1995.

11. Division of Bacterial and Mycotic Disease, Centers for Disease Control and Prevention: Helicobacter pylori *and peptic ulcer disease,* Atlanta, 2001 (last updated), Author. Retrieved December 15, 2005, from *www.cdc.gov/ulcer/.*

12. National Institutes of Health, NIH Consensus Development Program: Helicobacter pylori *in peptic ulcer disease,* NIH Consensus Development Conference Statement, Bethesda, Md, 1994, Author. Retrieved December 15, 2005, from *http://consensus.nih.gov/1994/1994HelicobacterPyloriUlcer094html.htm.*

13. Merck & Co, Inc: *The Merck manual of diagnosis and therapy: peptic ulcer disease,* Whitehouse Station, NJ, 1995-2005, Author. Available at *www.merck.com.* Accessed June 7, 2005.

14. Sartin JS: Gastrointestinal disorders. In Copstead LC, Banasik JL: *Pathophysiology,* ed 3, Philadelphia, 2005, Elsevier/Saunders.

15. Davies GR, Rampton D: Gastrointestinal disease. In Axfdord J, O'Callaghan C, eds: *Medicine,* ed 2, London, 2004, Blackwell Science.

16. Trier JS: Celiac sprue, *N Engl J Med* 325(24):1709, 1991.

17. Beyer P: Medical nutrition therapy for lower gastrointestinal tract disorders. In Mahan LK, Escott-Stump S, eds: *Krause's food, nutrition, and diet therapy,* ed 11, Philadelphia, 2004, Elsevier/Saunders.

18. McQuaid KR: Alimentary tract. In Tierney LM, McPhee SJ, Papadakis MA, eds: *Current medical diagnosis and treatment CMDT 2003,* ed 42, New York, 2003, McGraw-Hill.

19. U.S. National Library of Medicine, National Institutes of Health: *Medline Plus medical encyclopedia: celiac disease—Sprue,* Bethesda, Md, 2005 (updated December 13), Author. Retrieved December 15, 2005, from *www.nlm.nih.gov/medlineplus/ency/article/000233.htm.*

20. Thompson T: Do oats belong in a gluten-free diet? *J Am Diet Assoc* 97(12):1513, 1997.

21. Skerritt JH, Hill AS: Self-management of dietary compliance in celiac disease by means of ELISA "home test" to detect gluten, *Lancet* 337:379, 1991.

22. Merck & Co, Inc: *The Merck manual of diagnosis and therapy: cystic fibrosis,* Whitehouse Station, NJ, 1995-2005, Author. Available at *www.merck.com.* Accessed June 7, 2005.

23. Schumann L: Obstructive pulmonary disorders. In Copstead LC, Banasik JL: *Pathophysiology,* ed 3, Philadelphia, 2005, Elsevier/Saunders.

24. Chesnutt MS, Prendergast TJ: Lung. In Tierney LM, McPhee SJ, Papadakis MA, eds: *Current medical diagnosis and treatment CMDT 2003,* ed 42, New York, 2003, McGraw-Hill.

25. Clark E, Tobias J: Chest disease. In Axfdord J, O'Callaghan C, eds: *Medicine,* ed 2, London, 2004, Blackwell Science.

26. Cystic Fibrosis Foundation: Guidelines for patient services, evaluation, and monitoring in cystic fibrosis centers, *Am J Dis Child* 144:1311, 1990.

27. Brady MS et al: Effectiveness of enteric coated pancreatic enzymes given before meals in reducing steatorrhea in children with cystic fibrosis, *J Am Diet Assoc* 92(7):813, 1992.

28. Dowsett J: Nutrition in the management of cystic fibrosis, *Nutr Rev* 54(1):31, 1996.

29. Podolsky DK: Inflammatory bowel disease, *N Engl J Med* 347(6):417, 2002.

30. American Dietetic Association: *ADA nutrition care manual,* Chicago, 2005, Author. Available at *http://nutritioncaremanual.org.* Accessed June 9, 2005.

31. Campos FG et al: Pharmacological nutrition in inflammatory bowel disease, *Nutr Hosp* 18(2):57, 2003.

32. Organ Procurement and Transplantation Network: *Organ datasource,* Richmond, Va, 2003, United Network for Organ Sharing. Available at *www.optn.org.* Accessed June 9, 2005.

33. Greenstein SM, Prowse O: *Intestinal transplantation,* Omaha, Neb, 2004 (updated August 12), eMedicine.com, Inc.. Available at *www.emedicine.com.* Accessed June 9, 2005.

34. Weseman RA: Adult small bowel transplantation. In Hasse JM, Blue LS, eds: *Comprehensive guide to transplant nutrition,* Chicago, 2002, American Dietetic Association.

35. Merck & Co, Inc: *The Merck manual of diagnosis and therapy: gas,* Whitehouse Station, NJ, 1995-2005, Author. Available at *www.merck.com.* Accessed June 11, 2005.

36. Maslar J, Kreplick LW: *Flatulence (gas),* Omaha, Neb, 2003-2005, eMedicineHealth.com. Available at *www.emedicinehealth.com.* Accessed June 11, 2005.

37. Drossman DA: The functional gastrointestinal disorders and the Rome II process, *Gut* 45:1, 1999.

38. International Foundation for Functional Gastrointestinal Disorders: *About irritable bowel syndrome (IBS),* Milwaukee, 1999-2005, Author. Retrieved December 15, 2005, from *www.aboutibs.org.*

39. Camilleri M. Management of the irritable bowel syndrome, *Gastroenterol 2001* 120(3), 2001.

40. Neuberger J: Liver, biliary tract, and pancreatic disease. In Axfdord J, O'Callaghan C (eds): *Medicine,* ed 2, London, 2004, Blackwell Science.

41. Sartin JS: Liver diseases. In Copstead LC, Banasik JL: *Pathophysiology,* ed 3, Philadelphia, 2005, Elsevier/Saunders.

42. General recommendations in immunization: recommendations of the Advisory Committees on Immunization Practices (ACIP) and the American Academy of Family Physicians (AAFP), *MMWR Morb Mortal Wkly Rep* 51(RR02):1, 2002.

43. Sartin JS: Alterations in function of the gallbladder and exocrine pancreas. In Copstead LC, Banasik JL: *Pathophysiology,* ed 3, Philadelphia, 2005, Elsevier.

44. Abou-Assi S et al: Hypocaloric jejunal feeding is better than total parenteral nutrition in acute pancreatitis: results of a randomized comparative study, *Am J Gastroenterol* 97:2255, 2002.

45. Kalfarentzos F et al: Enteral nutrition is superior to parenteral nutrition in severe acute pancreatitis: results of a randomized prospective trial, *Br J Surg* 84:1665, 1997.

46. Kramer MS et al: Promotion of Breastfeeding Intervention Trial (PROBIT): a randomized trial in the Republic of Belarus, *JAMA* 285(4):413, 2001.

47. Shenassa ED, Brown M: Maternal smoking and infantile gastrointestinal dysregualation: the case of colic, *Pediatrics* 114(4):497, 2004.

48. Hasler CM: Scientific status summary: functional foods—their role in disease prevention and health promotion, *Food Technol* 52(11):63, 1998.

49. Peters HPF et al: Potential benefits and hazards of physical activity and exercise on the gastrointestinal tract, *Gut* 48:435, 2001.

FURTHER READINGS AND RESOURCES

Readings

Chartrand LJ et al: Wheat starch intolerance in patients with celiac disease, *J Am Diet Assoc* 97(6):612, 1997.

Thompson T: Do oats belong in a gluten-free diet? *J Am Diet Assoc* 97(12):1413, 1997.

These two articles provide a helpful resource for practical ways of providing food for special diets.

Dalton CB, Drossman DA: Diagnosis and treatment of irritable bowel syndrome, *Am Fam Physician* 55(3):875, 1997.

The authors present a sensitive article about this common but frustrating condition in older adults, providing helpful background for all those who care for these patients.

Mann LL, Wong K: Development of an objective method for assessing viscosity of formulated foods and beverages for the dysphagic diet, *J Am Diet Assoc* 96(6):585, 1996.

Here are practical ways of providing soft foods for persons with a range of swallowing disorders, a real need especially when the disorder is long term or permanent and economy is a problem.

Websites of Interest

Celiac Sprue
- Celiac Sprue Association: *www.csaceliacs.org.*
- Celiac Disease Foundation: *www.celiac.org.*
- Colorado Center for Digestive Disorders: *www.gastromd.com.*
- Ask the Dietitian: *Gluten and celiac sprue: www.dietitian.com/gluten.html.*

Cirrhosis
- National Institute of Diabetes and Digestive and Kidney Diseases: *www.niddk.nih.gov.*
- American Gastroenterological Association: *Cirrhosis of the liver: www.gastro.org/wmspage.cfm?parm1=681.*
- American Liver Foundation: *www.liverfoundation.org.*

Dysphagia
- Dysphagia Resource Center: *www.dysphagia.com.*
- Dysphagia-Diet.com: *www.dysphagia-diet.com.*
- Dysphagiaonline.com: *www.dysphagiaonline.com.*

Gastroesophageal Reflux Disease (GERD)
- GERD Information Resource Center: *www.gerd.com.*
- About GERD: *www.aboutgerd.org.*
- American Gastroenterological Association: *www.gastro.org.*

Celiac Disease
- Celiac Disease Foundation: *www.celiac.org.*
- Medline Plus: *Celiac disease: www.nlm.nih.gov/medlineplus/celiacdisease.htm.l*
- National Digestive Diseases Information Clearinghouse: *Celiac disease: http://digestive.niddk.nih.gov/ddiseases/pubs/celiac/.*

Cystic Fibrosis (CF)
- Cystic Fibrosis Foundation: *www.cff.org/home/.*
- CysticFibrosis.com: *www.cysticfibrosis.com.*
- Canadian Cystic Fibrosis Foundation: *www.ccff.ca.*

Irritable Bowel Syndrome (IBS)
- About IBS: *www.aboutibs.org.*
- Irritable Bowel Syndrome (IBS) Self Help and Support Group: *www.ibsgroup.org.*

Pancreatitis
- National Institute of Diabetes and Digestive and Kidney Diseases: *www.niddk.nih.gov.*
- eMedicine; search for *pancreatitis* for a number of resources: *www.emedicine.com.*
- Tummyhealth.com: *www.tummyhealth.com.*

Peptic Ulcer Disease
- National Library of Medicine: Helicobacter pylori in Peptic Ulcer Disease: www.nlm.nih.gov/archive/20040830/pubs/cbm/pepulcer.html.
- National Institute of Diabetes and Digestive and Kidney Diseases: www.niddk.nih.gov.

CHAPTER 20

Diseases of the Heart, Blood Vessels, and Lungs

Sara Long

In this chapter, we consider interrelated diseases of the circulatory system—heart, blood vessels, and lungs. In recent decades, these diseases of modern civilization have become the major causes of death in the United States and most other Western societies. The magnitude of this overall healthcare problem is enormous.

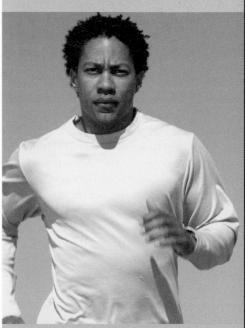

CORONARY HEART DISEASE: THE PROBLEM OF ATHEROSCLEROSIS

The Underlying Disease Process

Atherosclerosis, the major arteriosclerosis disease and underlying pathologic process in coronary heart disease (CHD), is paramount in ongoing study in modern medicine. The characteristic lesions involved are raised fibrous plaques (Figure 20-1). They appear on the interior surface, the intima, of blood vessel as discrete lumps elevated above unaffected surrounding tissue and ranging in color from pearly gray to yellowish gray. The main cellular component of plaque is a smooth muscle cell similar to the major cell of the normal artery wall. Plaque usually contains fatty material, such as lipoproteins, that carry cholesterol in the blood. Deep in the lesions are debris from dead and dying cells and varying amounts of lipids. Crystals of cholesterol can be seen with the unaided eye in the softened cheesy debris of advanced lesions.

It is this fatty debris that suggested the original name *atherosclerosis,* from the Greek words *athera* ("gruel") and *sclerosis* ("hardening"). This fatty degeneration and thickening narrow the vessel lumen and may allow a blood clot, an embolus, to develop from its irritating presence. Eventually the clot may cut off blood flow in the involved artery. If the artery is a critical one, such as a major coronary vessel, a heart attack occurs. Tissue area serviced by the involved artery is deprived of its vital oxygen (O_2) and nutrient supply, a condition called ischemia, and the cells die. The localized area of dying or dead tissue is called an infarct. Because the artery involved supplies cardiac muscle, the *myocardium,* the result is called an acute myocardial infarction (AMI). The two major coronary arteries, with their many branches, are so named because they lie across the brow of the heart muscle and resemble a crown (Figure 20-2). Figure 20-3 shows the anterior internal view of the normal human heart.

Thus the focus of the problem in CHD is development of these characteristic fatty plaques called atheromas. Injury to the important inner endothelial lining of the blood vessel wall leads to a thickening thrombosis and lipid deposits, with the development of atherosclerosis. According to the American Heart Association, three proven causes of damage to arterial walls are (1) elevated levels of serum cholesterol and triglycerides, (2) high blood pressure, and (3) tobacco smoke.[1] The major risk factor for plaque development is a lipoprotein, low-density lipoprotein (LDL) cholesterol, that carries cholesterol in the blood.[2] Additional risk factors are shown in Box 20-1 (see also the *Focus on Culture* box, "Is Cardiovascular Disease an Equal Opportunity Disease?").

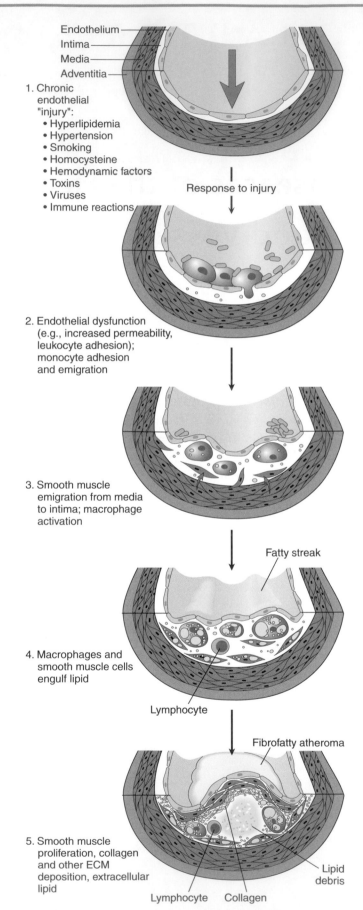

1. Chronic endothelial "injury":
   - Hyperlipidemia
   - Hypertension
   - Smoking
   - Homocysteine
   - Hemodynamic factors
   - Toxins
   - Viruses
   - Immune reactions

Endothelium
Intima
Media
Adventitia

Response to injury

2. Endothelial dysfunction (e.g., increased permeability, leukocyte adhesion); monocyte adhesion and emigration

3. Smooth muscle emigration from media to intima; macrophage activation

Fatty streak

4. Macrophages and smooth muscle cells engulf lipid

Lymphocyte

Fibrofatty atheroma

5. Smooth muscle proliferation, collagen and other ECM deposition, extracellular lipid

Lipid debris

Lymphocyte   Collagen

FIGURE 20-1 Raised fibrous plaques. (*From Kumar V, Cotran R, Robbins S: Robbins basic pathology, ed 7, Philadelphia, 2003, Saunders/Elsevier.*)

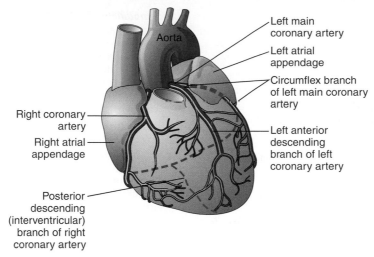

FIGURE 20-2   Coronary blood circulation. *(From Copstead-Kirkhorn LE, Banasik JL, eds:* Pathophysiology, *ed 3, Philadelphia, 2005, Elsevier/Saunders.)*

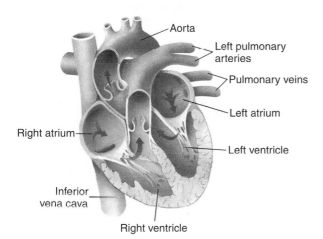

FIGURE 20-3   The normal human heart. Anterior internal view showing cardiac circulation. *(From Seeley RR, Stephens TD, Tate P:* Anatomy and physiology, *ed 2, New York, 1992, McGraw-Hill.)*

Cholesterol, Lipoproteins, and Lipids

Cholesterol is a soft, fatlike substance found in all cell membranes and blood and is a precursor of bile acids and steroid hormones. Cholesterol and triglycerides (TG) cannot dissolve in blood and must be transported to and from cells by individual components containing both lipid and proteins (lipoproteins). The following five types of lipoproteins (Figure 20-4) are classified according to fat content and thus their density, with those having the highest fat content possessing the lowest density[3]:

1. *Chylomicrons* have the highest lipid content and lowest density and are composed mostly of dietary TG, with a small amount of carrier protein. They accumulate in portal blood after a meal and are efficiently cleared from the blood by the specific enzyme lipoprotein lipase.

2. *Very low-density lipoproteins (VLDLs)* still carry a large lipid (TG) content but include about 20% cholesterol. These lipoproteins are formed in the liver from endogenous fat sources.

---

atherosclerosis Common form of arteriosclerosis, characterized by the gradual formation—beginning in childhood in genetically predisposed individuals—of yellow cheeselike streaks of cholesterol and fatty material that develop into hardened plaques in the intima or inner lining of major blood vessels, such as coronary arteries, eventually in adulthood cutting off blood supply to the tissue served by the vessels; the underlying pathologic process of coronary heart disease.

arteriosclerosis Blood vessel disease characterized by thickening and hardening of artery walls, with loss of functional elasticity, mainly affecting the intima (inner lining) of the arteries.

intima General term indicating an innermost part of a structure or vessel; inner layer of the blood vessel wall.

plaque Thickened deposits of fatty material, largely cholesterol, within the arterial wall that eventually may fill the lumen and cut off blood supply to the tissue served by the damaged vessel.

ischemia Deficiency of blood to a particular tissue, resulting from functional blood vessel constriction or actual obstruction walls in atherosclerosis.

infarct An area of tissue necrosis caused by local ischemia, resulting from obstruction of blood circulation to that area.

atheroma A mass of fatty plaque formed in inner arterial walls in atherosclerosis.

BOX 20-1 | **Major Risk Factors in Cardiovascular Disease**

Lipid Risk Factors
- LDL cholesterol >130 mg/dl
- HDL cholesterol <40 mg/dl
- Total cholesterol >200 mg/dl
- Triglycerides >150 mg/dl

Nonlipid Risk Factors

Modifiable
- Tobacco smoke and exposure to tobacco smoke
- Hypertension (>140/90 mm Hg)
- Physical inactivity
- Obesity (BMI >30 kg/m^2) and overweight (BMI 25 to 29.9 kg/m^2)
- Diabetes mellitus
- Atherogenic diet (↑ intakes of saturated fats and cholesterol)
- Thrombogenic state
- Excessive alcohol consumption (>1 drink per day for women and >2 drinks per day for men)
- Individual response to stress and coping
- Some illegal drugs (cocaine and IV drug abuse)

Nonmodifiable
- Male gender
- Age (males >45 years, females >55 years)
- Heredity (including race)
- Family history of premature CHD (MI or sudden death <55 years of age in father or other male first-degree relative, or <65 years of age in mother or other female first-degree relative)

Probable Risk Factors (Emerging)
- Lipoprotein (a)
- Small LDL particles (pattern B)
- HDL subtypes
- Apolipoprotein B
- Homocysteine
- Fibrinogen
- High-sensitivity C-reactive protein
- Impaired fasting glucose (100-125 mg/dl)

Data from *National Cholesterol Education Program (NCEP): Third report of the NCEP Expert Panel on Detection, Evaluation, and Treatment of High Blood Cholesterol in Adults (Adult Treatment Panel III), full report,* Washington, DC, 2002, National Institutes of Health, National Heart, Lung, and Blood Institute. Retrieved December 20, 2005, from *http://www.nhlbi.nih.gov/guidelines/cholesterol/atp3_rpt.htm;* and Banasik JL: Alterations in cardiac function. In Copstead LC, Banasik JL, eds: *Pathophysiology,* ed 3, St. Louis, 2005, Elsevier/Saunders.

LDL, Low-density lipoprotein; *HDL,* high-density lipoprotein; *BMI,* body mass index; *CHD,* coronary heart disease; *MI,* myocardial infarction.

 FOCUS ON CULTURE

Is Cardiovascular Disease an Equal Opportunity Disease?

"Race and ethnicity in the United States are associated with health status."

Marian E. Gornick, *Health Care Financing Reviews,* Summer 2000.

The Pfizer Journal Panel[1] states the following:

The system of healthcare that exists in this country was developed at a time when life expectancy was short, diseases generally came on quickly and were all too frequently fatal, and patients needed lifesaving interventions at a relatively young age. The system hasn't changed, yet the individuals who need healthcare now live a very long life, develop diseases that are chronic and disabling, and need prevention over a longer lifespan. One hundred million Americans have at least one chronic condition, and half of them have more. Among Americans older than 65, 88% have one or more chronic illnesses, and one-quarter of them have at least four conditions that should be treated.

After controlling for differences in age, health insurance status, disease severity, and other health problems, the following research findings might not be surprising, but nonetheless are disheartening:

- Blacks, Hispanics, and other minorities on average have more underlying risk factors for cardiovascular disease (CVD), including hypertension, obesity, smoking, physical inactivity, higher level of body mass index (BMI), and non–high-density lipoprotein (HDL) cholesterol.
- After minority patients develop CVD, they are less likely to receive higher-quality care and as a result are more likely to die.
- Blacks receive clot-reducing drugs after a heart attack at about 50% the rate of whites.
- Approximately 18% of black patients have angioplasty surgery within 48 hours of a heart attack or stroke, compared with almost 30% of white patients.
- Black women are "less familiar" with early warning signs of CVD.
- CVD deaths are highest among blacks at all ages.
- All low-income and less-educated U.S. residents have higher mortality rates for heart disease and stroke than other residents.

Over the past 30 years CVD mortality rates have been decreasing across all racial and ethnic groups, but decline has been much greater for white Americans. Black Americans have mortality rates for CVD about 50% higher than those of white Americans. Hispanic Americans are substantially more likely to be uninsured than white Americans, and Hispanic Americans are far more likely to lack a usual source of healthcare than any other group. Research has also found some immigrant families who assimilate into the United States, many of whom are Hispanic, experience deteriorating health status over subsequent generations.

So there is more to CVD than just risk factors. It may not be enough to teach prevention to the masses. Different life experiences attributed to different ethnic groups, as well as economic, time, and residential constraints, may compete with heart-healthy behaviors to increase risk of CVD. So if you are a college student reading this information, be thankful. You have just decreased your risk of CVD simply by being educated.

Reference

1. Pfizer Journal Panel: The quality of health care in the United States: building quality into the health care system, *Pfizer Journal* 9(9):1, 2005. Retrieved December 20, 2005, from *www.thepfizerjournal.com/default.asp?a=journal&n=tpj41.*

Bibliography

De Lew N, Weinick RM: An overview: eliminating racial, ethnic, and SES disparities in health care, *Health Care Financ Rev* 21(4):1, 2000.

Gornick ME: Disparities in Medicare services: potential causes, plausible explanations, and recommendations, *Health Care Financ Rev* 21(4):23, 2000.

The Henry J. Kaiser Family Foundation: Racial/ethnic differences in cardiac care: the weight of the evidence, *Highlights,* October 2002.

Winkleby MA et al: Ethnic and socioeconomic differences in cardiovascular disease risk factors: findings for women from the Third National Health and Nutrition Examination Survey, 1980-1994, *JAMA* 280(4):356, 1998.

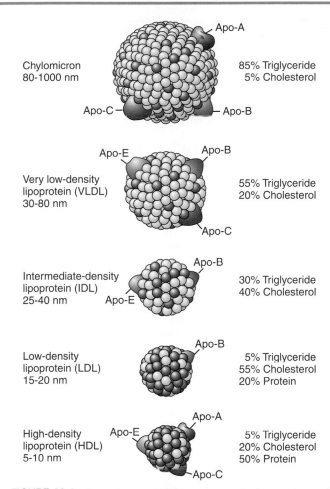

Chylomicron
80-1000 nm

Apo-A

85% Triglyceride
5% Cholesterol

Apo-C

Apo-B

Very low-density
lipoprotein (VLDL)
30-80 nm

Apo-E

Apo-B

55% Triglyceride
20% Cholesterol

Apo-C

Intermediate-density
lipoprotein (IDL)
25-40 nm

Apo-B

Apo-E

30% Triglyceride
40% Cholesterol

Low-density
lipoprotein (LDL)
15-20 nm

Apo-B

5% Triglyceride
55% Cholesterol
20% Protein

High-density
lipoprotein (HDL)
5-10 nm

Apo-E

Apo-A

5% Triglyceride
20% Cholesterol
50% Protein

Apo-C

FIGURE 20-4   Serum lipoprotein factions showing lipid composition and apoprotein components. *(From Copstead-Kirkhorn L-E, Banasik JL: Pathophysiology, ed 3, Philadelphia, 2005, Elsevier/Saunders.)*

Functional Classification of Lipid Disorders

Current clinical practice is based on a useful functional classification that reveals two important factors: (1) recognition of genetic factors involved and (2) focus on the role of apolipoproteins in the course of lipoprotein formation, transport, or destruction. Both factors will be encountered in readings and in clinical work with patients. Thus the outline provided in this discussion is useful in understanding clinical problems involved and in counseling patients.

Apolipoproteins

The term *apolipoprotein* refers to a major protein part of a combined metabolic product, in this case a specific protein part of a combined lipid-protein molecule. For example, apolipoprotein B is a common attachment to LDL and serves two basic functions: (1) aids transport of lipids in a water medium, blood, and (2) transports lipids into cells for metabolic purposes. When apolipoprotein B-100, a single large protein molecule, attaches to one pole of the LDL, it provides a recognition site for LDL receptors on the cell, causing the entire LDL to be transported by pinocytosis into the cell for use in cell metabolism.[3] Various types of LDL have specific receptor sites for particular apolipoproteins to which the apolipoprotein is attracted and which in large measure determine function.

Function

When lipoproteins are synthesized in the intestinal wall, liver, and blood serum, the protein component is made up of varying kinds of apolipoprotein parts. These genetically determined components influence the structure, receptor binding, and metabolism of lipoproteins. It is an apolipoprotein component that helps form special spherical droplets of lipid material for transport in the bloodstream (see Chapter 3). Apolipoprotein determination is currently a useful laboratory tool for identifying persons at high risk for CHD.[2]

Defects in Synthesis of Apolipoproteins

Current functional approach classifies lipid disorders into four major groups based on the underlying functional problem: (1) defects in apolipoprotein synthesis, (2) enzyme deficiencies, (3) LDL-receptor deficiency, and (4) other inherited hyperlipidemias.[2]

3. *Intermediate-density lipoproteins (IDLs)* continue the delivery of endogenous TG to cells and carry about 40% cholesterol.
4. *Low-density lipoproteins (LDLs)* carry, in addition to other lipids, about two thirds or more of total plasma cholesterol formed in blood serum from catabolism of VLDL. Because LDL carries cholesterol to cells for deposit in tissues, it is considered the main agent in elevated serum cholesterol levels, or the "bad" cholesterol.
5. *High-density lipoproteins (HDLs)* carry less total lipid and more carrier protein. They are formed in the liver from endogenous fat sources. Because HDL carries cholesterol from tissues to the liver for catabolism and excretion, higher serum levels of this "good" cholesterol form are considered protective against cardiovascular disease. A value of 60 mg/dl or above contributes definite protection and decreased risk.

Characteristics of these classes of lipoproteins are summarized in Table 20-1.

> apolipoprotein A separate protein compound that attaches to its specific receptor site on a particular lipoprotein and activates certain functions, such as protein synthesis of a related enzyme. For example, apolipoprotein C-II is an apolipoprotein of HDL and VLDL that functions to activate the enzyme lipoprotein lipase.

TABLE 20-1	Characteristics of the Classes of Lipoproteins

Characteristic	Chylomicrons	Very Low-Density (VLDL)	Intermediate-Density (IDL)	Low-Density (LDL)	High-Density (HDL)
Composition					
Triglycerides (TG)	85%; diet, exogenous	55%; endogenous	30%; endogenous	5%; endogenous	5%; endogenous
Cholesterol	5%	20%	40%	55%	20%
Phospholipid	3%-6%	15%-20%	20%	15%-22%	25%-30%
Protein	1%-2%	5%-10%	10%	20%	50%
Function	Transport dietary TG to plasma and tissues, cells	Transport endogenous TG to cells	Continue transport of endogenous TG to cells	Transport cholesterol to peripheral cells	Transport free cholesterol from membranes to liver for catabolism
Place of synthesis	Intestinal wall	Liver	Liver	Liver	Liver
Size, density					
Description	Largest, lightest	Next largest, next lightest	Intermediate size, lighter	Smaller, heavier	Smaller, densest, heaviest
Density	0.095	0.095-1.006	1.00-1.03	1.019-1.063	1.063-1.210
Size in nanometers (nm)	80-1000	30-80	25-40	15-20	5-10

General Principles of Nutrition Therapy

Basic Guidelines

The National Cholesterol Education Program (NCEP) periodically publishes revised guidelines for clinical management of high serum cholesterol. The Adult Treatment Panel I (ATP I) delineated strategy for primary prevention of CHD in persons with high levels of LDL cholesterol (160 mg/dl) or those with borderline-high LDL cholesterol (130 to 159 mg/dl) and two or more risk factors. The Adult Treatment Panel II (ATP II) substantiated these strategies and made further recommendations for intensive management of LDL cholesterol in persons with established CHD. A new, lower LDL cholesterol of 100 mg/dl was established. The Adult Treatment Panel III (ATP III) report identified more intensive LDL-lowering therapy. The ATP III[2] suggests a comprehensive lifestyle approach to reducing risk for CHD called therapeutic lifestyle changes (TLC) and incorporates the following components[2,3]:

- Reduced intake of saturated fats and cholesterol
- Therapeutic dietary options for enhancing LDL lowering (plant stanols/sterols and increased soluble fiber)
- Weight reduction
- Increased regular physical activity

Components of TLC are outlined in Table 20-2. The ATP III also suggests ranges for other macronutrients in the TLC Diet (Table 20-3).

Components of the Therapeutic Lifestyle Changes Diet

Saturated Fat and Cholesterol. In view of the fact that the major LDL-raising nutrient components are saturated fat and cholesterol, reducing saturated fat (less than 7% of

total energy intake) and cholesterol (less than 200 mg/day) in the diet is the foundation of the TLC Diet.[2] The strongest nutritional influence on serum LDL cholesterol levels is saturated fats.[4] In fact, there is a "dose-response relationship" between saturated fats and LDL cholesterol levels. For every 1% increase in kilocalories (kcalories or kcal) from saturated fats as a percentage of total energy, serum LDL cholesterol increases approximately 2%. On the other hand, a 1% decrease in saturated fats will lower serum cholesterol by approximately 2%.[5,6] Although weight reduction by itself, even of a few pounds, will reduce LDL cholesterol levels,[5,7] weight reduction attained using a kcalorie-controlled diet low in saturated fats and cholesterol will improve and maintain LDL cholesterol lowering.[2,8,9] Although dietary cholesterol does not have the same influence as saturated fat on serum LDL cholesterol levels, high cholesterol intakes raise LDL cholesterol levels.[2,10,11] Therefore reducing dietary cholesterol to less than 200 mg/day decreases serum LDL cholesterol in most persons.[2]

Monounsaturated Fat. The TLC Diet recommends substitution of monounsaturated fat for saturated fats at an intake level of up to 20% of total energy intake[2] because monounsaturated fats lower LDL cholesterol levels relative to saturated fats[2,5] without decreasing HDL cholesterol or TG levels.[2,5,12,13] It is recommended that plant oils and nuts be used because they are the best sources of monounsaturated fats.[2]

Polyunsaturated Fats. Polyunsaturated fats, in particular linoleic acid, reduce LDL cholesterol levels when used instead of saturated fats. However, they can also bring about small reductions in HDL cholesterol when

TABLE 20-2	Essential Components of Therapeutic Lifestyle Changes (TLC)

Component	Recommendation
LDL-raising nutrients	
Saturated fats	<7% of total energy intake
Dietary cholesterol	<200 mg/day
Therapeutic options for LDL lowering	
Plant stanols/sterols	2 g/day
Soluble fiber	10-25 g/day
Total energy (kcalories)	Adjust total energy intake to maintain desirable body weight/prevent weight gain
Physical activity	Include enough moderate exercise to expend at least 200 kcal/day
Trans fats	Avoid
Limit sodium to 2400 mg per day	When indicated

Data from National Cholesterol Education Program (NCEP): *Third report of the NCEP expert panel on detection, evaluation, and treatment of high blood cholesterol in adults (Adult Treatment Panel III), full report,* Washington, DC, 2002, National Institutes of Health, National Heart, Lung, and Blood Institute. Retrieved December 20, 2005, from *www.nhlbi.nih.gov/guidelines/cholesterol/atp3_rpt.pdf;* and American Dietetic Association: *Nutrition care manual,* Chicago, 2005 (updated as necessary), Author. Available at *http://nutritioncaremanual.org.* Accessed July 18, 2005 via password.

LDL, Low-density lipoprotein.

TABLE 20-3	Nutrient Composition of the Therapeutic Lifestyle Changes (TLC) Diet

Component	Recommendation
Polyunsaturated fat, including omega-3 fatty acids	Up to 10% total energy intake
Monounsaturated fat	Up to 20% total energy intake
Total fat	25%-35% total energy intake*
Carbohydrate†	50%-60% total energy intake
Dietary fiber	20-30 g/day
Protein	Approximately 15% total energy intake

Data from National Cholesterol Education Program (NCEP): *Third report of the NCEP Expert Panel on Detection, Evaluation, and Treatment of High Blood Cholesterol in Adults (Adult Treatment Panel III,) executive summary,* NIH Publication No 01-3670, Washington, DC, 2001, National Institutes of Health, National Heart, Lung, and Blood Institute. Retrieved December 20, 2005, from *www.nhlbi.nih.gov/guidelines/cholesterol/atp3xsum.pdf;* and American Dietetic Association: *Nutrition care manual,* Chicago, 2005 (updated as necessary), Author. Available at *http://nutritioncaremanual.org.* Accessed July 18, 2005 via password.

*Adult Treatment Panel III allows for increase of total fat to 35% total energy intake and reduction in carbohydrate to 50% for persons with the metabolic syndrome. Any increase in fat intake should be in the form of either polyunsaturated or monounsaturated fat.

†Carbohydrates should come primarily from foods rich in complex carbohydrates, including grains—especially whole grains—fruits, and vegetables.

compared side by side with monounsaturated fats.[2,5] The TLC Diet recommends liquid vegetables oils, semiliquid margarines (soft, tub margarines), and other margarines low in *trans* fatty acids be used because they are the best sources of polyunsaturated fats; intakes can range up to 10% of total energy intake.[2]

Total Fat. In view of the fact that only saturated fats and trans fatty acids increase LDL cholesterol levels,[14] serum levels of LDL cholesterol are unrelated to total fat intake per se.[2] For that reason, the ATP III suggests it is not crucial to limit total fat intake for the specific goal of reducing LDL cholesterol levels, provided saturated fats are decreased to goal levels.[2]

Carbohydrate. When saturated fats are replaced with carbohydrates, LDL cholesterol levels are reduced. On the other hand, very high intakes of carbohydrates (greater than 60% of total energy intake) are associated with a reduction in HDL cholesterol and a increase in serum TG.[2,5,12,15,16] Increasing soluble fiber intake can sometimes reduce these responses.[2,16-18] On average, increasing soluble fiber to 10 to 25 g/day is accompanied by an approximately 5% reduction in LDL cholesterol.[19,20]

Protein. Despite the fact that dietary protein as a rule has an insignificant effect on serum LDL cholesterol level, replacing animal protein with plant-based protein has been reported to decrease LDL cholesterol.[2,21] This may be due to plant-based foods' providing good sources of proteins (legumes, dry beans, nuts, whole grains, and vegetables) containing less saturated fat than many animal proteins and no cholesterol. This is not to say animal proteins cannot be low in saturated fat and cholesterol. Fat-free and low-fat dairy products, egg whites, fish, skinless poultry, and lean cuts of beef and pork are also low in saturated fat and cholesterol. All foods of animal origin will contain cholesterol.

Further Dietary Options for Reducing LDL Cholesterol. Adding 5 to 10 g of soluble fiber (oats, barley, psyllium, pectin-rich fruit, and beans) per day is associated with approximately a 5% reduction in LDL cholesterol[19,20] and is regarded as a therapeutic option to enhance reduction of LDL cholesterol.[2] Plant sterols present an additional therapeutic option.[2] Daily intakes of 2 to 3 g plant stanol/sterol esters (isolated from soybean and tall pine-tree oils) have been shown to lower LDL cholesterol by 6% to 15%.[22-28]

> *trans* fatty acids Fatty acids that have been hydrogenated to be used in margarine and in the food industry; have been shown to increase LDL cholesterol and lower HDL cholesterol.

General Approach to Therapeutic Lifestyle Changes

The ATP III[2] suggests patients at risk for CHD or with CHD be referred to registered dietitians or other qualified nutritionists for the duration of all stages of nutrition therapy (NT). After 6 weeks of TLC, LDL cholesterol should be measured to evaluate response to TLC. If the LDL cholesterol target has been realized or an improvement in LDL lowering has occurred, NT should be uninterrupted. If the goal has not been attained, there are a number of alternatives from which the physician can select. First, NT can be reexplained and reinforced. Next, therapeutic dietary options can be integrated into TLC. Response to NT should be assessed in an additional 6 weeks. If the LDL cholesterol target is achieved, the current intensity of nutrition therapy should be continued indefinitely. If there is downward movement in LDL cholesterol measures, thought should be given to continuing NT before adding LDL-lowering medications. If it looks unlikely the LDL target will be realized with NT, medications should be considered.[2] The "Guide to Therapeutic Lifestyle Changes (TLC) Healthy Lifestyle Recommendations for a Healthy Heart" is shown in Box 20-2.

Drug Therapy

Although use of TLC will attain LDL cholesterol target goal for many, a segment of the population will need LDL-lowering medications to achieve the prescribed goal for LDL cholesterol.[2,29] If treatment with TLC alone is unsuccessful after 3 months, the ATP III recommends initiation of drug treatment. When drugs are used, however, TLC also should continue to be used concomitantly. NT affords further CHD risk reduction beyond drug efficacy.[2] Actions of combined use of TLC and LDL cholesterol–lowering medications may include the following[3]:

- Intensive LDL lowering with TLC, including therapeutic dietary options
  - May prevent need for drugs
  - Can augment LDL-lowering medications
  - May allow for lower doses of medications
- Weight control plus increased physical activity
  - Reduces risk beyond LDL cholesterol lowering
  - Constitutes principal management of metabolic syndrome
  - Raises HDL cholesterol
- Initiating TLC before medication consideration
  - For most people, a trial of NT of about 3 months is advised before initiating drug therapy
  - Ineffective trials of NT exclusive of medications should not be protracted for an indefinite period if goals of therapy are not approached in a reasonable period; medication should not be withheld if it is needed to reach targets in persons with a short-term and/or long-term CHD risk that is high
- Initiating drug therapy simultaneously with TLC
  - For severe hypercholesterolemia in which NT alone cannot attain LDL cholesterol targets
  - For those with CHD or CHD risk equivalents in whom NT alone will not attain LDL cholesterol targets

The general strategy for initiation and progression of drug therapy is outlined in Figure 20-5. (See also the *Complementary and Alternative Medicine {CAM}* box, "It Does a Heart Good. Or Does It?," and the *Diet-Medications Interactions* box, "Possible Interactions Between Cardiovascular Diseases and Natural Therapies," for information about particular herbs and supplements that affect the cardiovascular system.)

Acute Cardiovascular Disease: Myocardial Infarction

Medical Management

Initial medical treatment of myocardial infarction (MI), or heart attack, usually includes strong analgesics (usually morphine sulfate) for severe unremitting pain, O_2 therapy, intravenous nitroglycerine for ischemic discomfort, control of hypertension, or management of pulmonary congestion, and aspirin to produce a rapid antithrombotic effect.[30] This protocol is sometimes referred to as MONA (morphine, oxygen, nitroglycerine, and aspirin).

Nutritional Management

In the initial acute phase of cardiovascular disease, an MI requires close attention to dietary modifications. The basic clinical objective is cardiac rest to allow the healing process to begin. All care is directed toward this basic need for cardiac rest so the damaged heart can be restored to normal functioning. In addition to TLC (see Table 20-3), sodium may be restricted to 2 to 4 g for hypertension or to control edema[2,31] (see the *Case Study* box, "The Patient With Myocardial Infarction").

---

metabolic syndrome Multiple metabolic risk factors in one individual: waist circumference greater than 102 cm in men, greater than 88 cm in women; serum triglycerides greater than 150 mg/dL; HDL cholesterol less than 40 mg/dl in men, less than 50 mg/dl in women; blood pressure greater than 130/85 mm Hg; fasting blood glucose greater than 110 mg/dl.

Food Items to Choose More Often

Breads and Cereals

6 servings per day, adjusted to caloric needs
Breads, cereals, especially whole grains; pasta; rice; potatoes; dry beans and peas; low-fat crackers and cookies

Vegetables

3-5 servings per day fresh, frozen, or canned without added fat, sauce, or salt

Fruits

2-4 servings per day fresh, frozen, canned, dried

Dairy Products

2-3 servings per day fat-free, ½%, 1% milk, buttermilk, yogurt, cottage cheese, fat-free and low-fat cheese

Eggs

<2 egg yolks per week; egg whites or egg substitute

Meat, Poultry, Fish

5 oz per day
Lean cuts loin, leg, round, extra lean hamburger; cold cuts made with lean meat or soy protein; skinless poultry; fish

Fats and Oils

Amount adjusted to caloric level: unsaturated oils; soft or liquid margarines and vegetable oil spreads; salad dressings, seeds, and nuts

TLC Diet Options

Stanol/sterol-containing margarines; soluble fiber food sources: barley, oats, psyllium, apples, bananas, berries, citrus fruits, nectarines, peaches, pears, plums, prunes, broccoli, brussels sprouts, carrots, dry beans, soy products (tofu, miso)

Food Items to Choose Less Often

Breads and Cereals

- Many baked products, including doughnuts, biscuits, butter rolls, muffins, croissants, sweet rolls, Danish, cakes, pies, coffee cakes, cookies
- Many grain-based snacks, including chips, cheese puffs, snack mix, regular crackers, buttered popcorn

Vegetables

Vegetables fried or prepared with butter, cheese, or cream sauce

Fruits

Fruits fried or served with butter or cream

Dairy Products

Whole milk, 2% milk, whole-milk yogurt, ice cream, cream, cheese

Eggs

Egg yolk, whole eggs

Meat, Poultry, Fish

Higher-fat meat cuts: ribs, t-bone steak, regular hamburger, bacon, sausage; cold cuts: salami, bologna, hot dogs; organ meats: liver, brains, sweetbreads; poultry with skin; fried meat; fried poultry; fried fish

Fats and Oils

Butter, shortening, stick margarine, chocolate, coconut

Recommendations for Weight Reduction

Weigh Regularly

Record weight, body mass index, and waist circumferences

Lose Weight Gradually

Goal: lose 10% of body weight in 6 months; lose ½-1 lb per week

Develop Healthy Eating Patterns

- Choose healthy foods (see "Food Items to Choose More Often")
- Reduce intake of foods in "Food Items to Choose Less Often"
- Limit number of eating occasions
- Avoid second helpings
- Identify and reduce hidden fat by reading food labels to choose products lower in saturated fat and calories, and ask about ingredients in ready-to-eat foods prepared away from home
- Identify and reduce sources of excess carbohydrates such as fat-free and regular crackers; cookies and other desserts; snacks; and sugar-containing beverages

Recommendations for Increased Physical Activity

Make Physical Activity Part of Daily Routines

- Reduce sedentary time
- Walk, wheel, or bike ride more, drive less; take the stairs instead of an elevator; get off the bus a few stops early and walk the remaining distance; mow the lawn with a push mower; rake leaves; garden; push a stroller; clean the house; do exercises or pedal a stationary bike while watching television; play actively with children; take a brisk 10-minute walk or wheel before work, during your work break, and after dinner

Make Physical Activity Part of Exercise or Recreational Activities

Walk, wheel, or jog; bicycle or use an arm pedal bicycle; swim or do water aerobics; play basketball; join a sport team; play wheelchair sports; golf (pull cart or carry clubs); canoe; cross-country ski; dance; take part in an exercise program at work, home, school, or gym

Data from U.S. Department of Health and Human Services, Public Health Service, National Institutes of Health, National Heart, Lung, and Blood Institute: *The DASH eating plan*, NIH Publication No. 03-4082, Bethesda, Md, 2003 (May, revised), Author. Available at *www.nhlbi.nih.gov.* Accessed July 18, 2005.

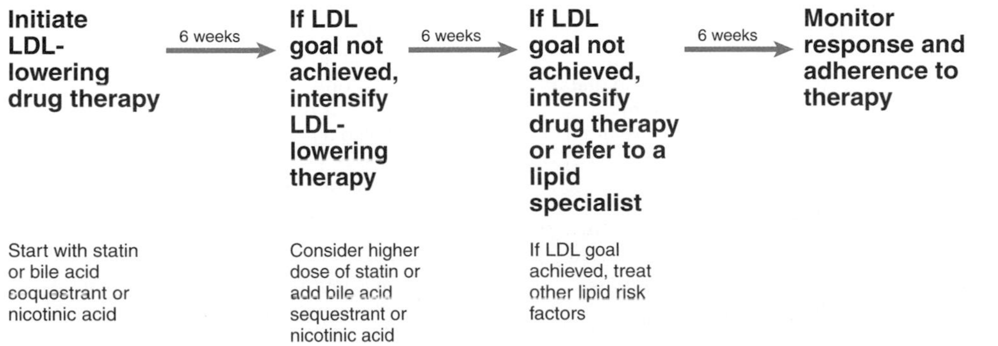

Initiate LDL-lowering drug therapy —6 weeks→ **If LDL goal not achieved, intensify LDL-lowering therapy** —6 weeks→ **If LDL goal not achieved, intensify drug therapy or refer to a lipid specialist** —6 weeks→ **Monitor response and adherence to therapy**

Start with statin or bile acid coquestrant or nicotinic acid

Consider higher dose of statin or add bile acid sequestrant or nicotinic acid

If LDL goal achieved, treat other lipid risk factors

FIGURE 20-5 Progression of drug therapy. *(From the National Cholesterol Education Program {NCEP}: Third report of the NCEP Expert Panel on Detection, Evaluation, and Treatment of High Blood Cholesterol in Adults [Adult Treatment Panel III], full report, Washington, DC, 2001, National Institutes of Health, National Heart, Lung, and Blood Institute.)*

Herbs are used by many to treat "what ails them." Although research is constantly being undertaken to test the efficacy of herbs, there remains a paucity of information available. The following table reviews herbal medicines that affect the cardiovascular system in terms of both efficacy and safety. In an effort to simplify the information, herbs are classified under the primary diseases they treat. But please keep in mind most herbal medicines have multiple cardiovascular effects that overlap. It is also important to remember herbs sold in the United States are not standardized doses or preparations; therefore there is no regulation regarding the safety of herbal products.

Cardiovascular Disorder	Herb/Supplement Commonly Used	Efficacy of Herb/Supplement
Congestive heart failure (CHF)	Coenzyme Q$_{10}$ (CoQ$_{10}$) (Mitoquinon, ubidecarenone, ubiquinone)	Reasonably good evidence supports use of CoQ$_{10}$ as adjunct therapy; thought to work by improving efficiency of cardiac muscle
	Hawthorn (Crataegus laevigata, C. monogyna, C. oxyacantha, C. pentagyna)	No evidence hawthorn reduces CHF morbidity or mortality
	Carnitine	Improves myocardial contractility and relaxation and cardiac pump function in patients with ventricular dysfunction
	Taurine	May be useful in adjuvant therapy in class II, III, and IV CHF
	Arginine	May improve some CHF symptoms
	Creatine	May improve skeletal muscle exercise tolerance in patients with CHF
	Vitamin B$_1$ (Thiamin)	Slight evidence that intravenous thiamin followed by oral supplementation could improve heart function in patients with CHF
	Vitamin E (Alpha-tocopherol)	Ineffective for treatment of CHF
	Garlic (Allium spp, including Allium sativum)	May mildly reduce blood pressure approximately 10 mm Hg systolic and 5 mm Hg diastolic
Blood pressure	Coenzyme Q$_{10}$ (CoQ$_{10}$)	Adjunctive treatment with 120 mg CoQ$_{10}$ daily has been shown to reduce average blood pressure by about 9%; may prolong hypotensive effects of enalapril and nitrendipine without changing their maximal effect
	Fish oils (Alternative names/supplement forms: docosahexaenoic acid [DHA], eicosapentaenoic acid [EPA], omega-3 fatty acids, omega-3 oils)	May be slight antihypertensive effect
	Hawthorn	May increase exercise tolerance
	Carnitine	May increase exercise tolerance; decrease number of premature ventricular contractions (PVCs); may decrease need for some medications such as nitroglycerides, beta-blockers, antihypertensives, diuretics, anticoagulants, antiarrhythmics, and hypolipidemics
	Inositol hexaniacinate (a form of niacin)	May improve walking distance
	L-carnitine	Improves muscle energy utilization
	Mesoglycans	May improve walking distance
	Policosanol	Improves walking distance
	Oxerutins	In combination with compression stockings, effective in reducing leg edema
	Diosmin/hesperidin (citrus bioflavonoids)	Significantly improves symptoms
	Butcher's broom (Ruscus aculeatus)	Improves symptoms of venous insufficiency
	Grape leaf	Dose-dependent improvements in symptoms
	Oligomeric proanthocyanidin complexes (OPCs)	Provide significant benefit in chronic venous insufficiency
	Gotu kola (Centella asiatica)	Dose-dependent improvements in symptoms
Angina pectoris	N-acetyl cysteine (NAC) (modified form of the dietary amino acid cysteine)	Given in combination with nitroglycerine is more effective than either drug alone in preventing death, myocardial infarction (MI), or need for revascularization; unfortunately, combined treatment also associated with high rate of severe headache
Hypertension	Stevia	May posses antihypertensive effects; considered safe when used at recommended doses
Peripheral vascular disease (intermittent claudication)	Ginkgo (Ginkgo biloba)	Modest improvement in pain-free walking
Venous insufficiency	Horse chestnut (Aesculus hippocastanum)	Used in combination with compression stockings, useful treatment for pain, itching, leg fatigue, and feelings of tension in the legs

References

Bratman S, Girman AM: *Mosby's handbook of herbs and supplements and their therapeutic uses,* St. Louis, 2003, Mosby/Elsevier Science.

Kuhn MA, Winston D: *Herbal therapy and supplements: a scientific and traditional approach,* Philadelphia, 2001, Lippincott.

Springhouse Corporation: *Professional guide to complementary and alternative therapies,* Baltimore, 2001, Springhouse.

 ## DIET-MEDICATIONS INTERACTIONS

Possible Interactions Between Cardiovascular Diseases and Natural Therapies

Pharmaceutical Class	Natural Therapy	Interaction
Warfarin	Coenzyme Q_{10}	Concurrent use may reduce effectiveness of drug; may increase excretion or metabolism of warfarin
ACE inhibitors	Arginine, potassium	Possible hyperkalemia
	Dong quai (*Angelica polymorpha sinensis*), St. John's wort (*Hypericum perforatum*)	Possible increased risk of photosensitivity
	Iron	Mutual absorption interference; possible reduction of ACE inhibitor–induced cough
	Licorice (natural)	Antagonism of drug action
	Zinc	Correction of possible drug-induced depletion
Digitoxin, digoxin	*Eleutherococcus* (Siberian ginseng)	Interference with laboratory measurement of digoxin levels
	Hawthorn (*Crataegus laevigata, C. monogyna, C. oxyacantha, C. pentagyna*)	May interfere with effects of digoxin or serum monitoring
	Horsetail, licorice (natural)	Possible hypokalemia leading to increased drug toxicity
	Magnesium	Absorption interference
	St. John's wort	Decreased serum levels of drug with possible rebound toxicity if herb is stopped
Loop diuretics	Dong quai, St. John's wort	Possible increased risk of photosensitivity
	Licorice (natural)	Potentiation of hypokalemic action of drug
Potassium-sparing diuretics	Arginine	Possible increased risk of hyperkalemia
	Licorice (natural)	Antagonism of drug action
	Magnesium	Risk of hypermagnesemia
	White willow (*Salix alba*)	Possible interference of salicylate content with spironolactone action
	Zinc	Excessive zinc levels with spironolactone
Thiazide diuretics	Calcium	Potential risk of hypercalcemia
	Dong quai, St. John's wort	Possible increased risk of photosensitivity
	Licorice (natural)	Potentiation of hypokalemic action of drug
Fluoroquinolones, tetracyclines	Calcium	Mutual absorption interference
Levothyroxine	Calcium	Possible absorption interference
Calcium channel blockers	Combined high-dose calcium and vitamin D, grapefruit juice	Possible antagonism of drug action
Anticoagulant and antiplatelet agents	Fish oil	Possible increased risk of bleeding complications
	Vitamin C	Possible antagonism of drug action
	Garlic, ginkgo, high-dose vitamin E, policosanol	Possible increased risk of bleeding complications
	Horse chestnut, OPCs	Possible increased risk of bleeding complications
Amiloride	Magnesium	Possible hypermagnesemia
Beta-blockers	Calcium	Absorption interference
	Chromium	Increased HDL levels
Nitrates	NAC	Increase of headache side effects

References

Bratman S, Girman AM: *Mosby's handbook of herbs and supplements and their therapeutic uses,* St. Louis, 2003, Mosby.

Kuhn MA, Winston D: *Herbal therapy and supplements: a scientific and traditional approach,* Philadelphia, 2001, Lippincott.

Springhouse Corporation: *Professional guide to complementary and alternative therapies,* Baltimore, 2001, Springhouse.

ACE, Angiotensin-converting enzyme; *OPCs,* oligomeric proanthocyanidin complexes; *HDL,* high-density lipoprotein; *NAC,* N-acetyl cysteine.

The Patient With Myocardial Infarction

Edward is a 37-year-old sedentary executive who was seen for an annual physical examination 6 months ago. He had no complaints other than feeling the "everyday pressures" of his job as a corporate attorney and head of the legal division. He admitted smoking two packs of cigarettes a day as a means of relieving stress.

Edward is 175 cm (5 ft 9 in) tall and at the time of his examination weighed 83 kg (185 lb). His blood pressure was 148/90 mm Hg, and his serum cholesterol level was 285 mg/dl. He was advised to quit smoking, exercise daily at a moderate pace, and lose 9 kg (20 lb).

He arrived in the hospital emergency department 3 months later complaining of severe chest pains and difficulty breathing. His wife reported he had appeared pale that evening, had broken out into a cold sweat, and had vomited shortly after arriving home from work. Once regular breathing was restored by the emergency medical team and his pain subsided, a number of laboratory tests were ordered. These tests included serum glutamic-oxaloacetic transaminase (SGOT), lactate dehydrogenase (LDH), prothrombin time, lipid panel plus high-density lipoprotein (HDL) cholesterol, sedimentation rate, coagulation times, fasting plasma glucose (FPG), blood urea nitrogen (BUN), and complete blood count (CBC). An electrocardiogram (ECG) was also ordered. The patient was then transferred to the coronary care unit for closer monitoring.

The following tests results were elevated: SGOT, LDH, LDL, and total cholesterol, triclycerides, glucose, prothrombin time, white blood cell count, and sedimentation rate. HDL level was low. The ECG revealed an infarction of the posterior wall of the myocardium. The diagnosis was myocardial infarction (MI), with underlying familial hypercholesterolemia.

In consultation with the clinical dietitian (RD) the cardiologist ordered a liquid diet, increasing it to a soft diet with low saturated fats 2 days later. The RD noted continued improvement in the patient's appetite accompanying recovery and recommended changing the diet order to the therapeutic lifestyle changes (TLC) diet.

A week later Edward was discharged. During convalescence the RD and nurse met with him and his wife several times to discuss his continuing care at home. At each follow-up clinic visit with the physician and nutritionist, Edward showed good general recovery and enjoyment of his new modified fat and cholesterol food habits.

Questions for Analysis

1. What predisposing factors in Edward's lifestyle place him in the high-risk category for coronary heart disease (CHD)?
2. Why was moderate, consistent exercise originally recommended?
3. Explain the causes for Edward's initial symptoms.
4. How does each laboratory test ordered in the emergency department relate to cell metabolism? Why were results elevated?
5. Explain the association between the final diet order and his lipid disorder.
6. Outline a 1-day menu for Edward that complies with the final hospital diet order.
7. What nondietary needs might Edward have while convalescing at home? What community agencies might be of assistance?

Metabolic Syndrome

If the patient has metabolic syndrome, further attention must be given to the following[30]:

- Weight management
- Gradual increase in physical activity under physician's supervision
- Limiting alcohol intake

Chronic Coronary Heart Disease: Congestive Heart Failure

In chronic CHD a condition of congestive heart failure (CHF) may develop over time. Each year over 550,000 new cases are diagnosed.[1] The progressively weakened heart muscle, the *myocardium,* is unable to maintain an adequate cardiac output to sustain normal blood circulation. Resulting fluid imbalances cause edema, especially pulmonary edema, to develop. This condition brings added problems in breathing called respiratory distress or dyspnea, which places added stress on the laboring heart. The most common cause of CHF is myocardial ischemia from coronary artery disease, hypertension, and cardiomyopathy. About half of CHF patients suffer diastolic dysfunction while systolic function is preserved. This is more likely to develop in older adults, women, and those without history of MI.[1]

Etiology: Relationship to Sodium and Water

Fluid congestion of chronic heart disease relates to imbalances in the body's capillary fluid shift mechanism and its resulting hormonal effects, as follows:

- *Imbalance in capillary fluid shift mechanism:* As the heart fails to pump out returning blood fast enough, venous return is delayed. This causes a disproportionate amount of blood to accumulate in the vascular system working with the right side of the heart. Venous pressure rises, a sort of "backup" pressure effect, and overcomes the balance of filtration pressures necessary to maintain the normal capillary fluid shift mechanism (see Chapter 7). Fluid that would normally flow between interstitial spaces and blood vessels is held in the tissue spaces rather than recirculated.
- *Hormonal mechanisms:* Two hormonal mechanisms are involved in fluid balance in normal circulation. In this instance, both of the following contribute to cardiac edema:
  1. *Aldosterone mechanism:* This mechanism, described more completely by its full name of the renin-angiotensin-aldosterone mechanism, is normally a lifesaving sodium- and water-conserving mechanism to ensure essential fluid balances. In this case, however, it only compounds the edema problem. As the heart fails to propel blood circulation forward, deficient cardiac output effectively reduces blood flow through kidney nephrons. Decreased renal blood pressure triggers the renin-angiotensin system. Renin is an enzyme from the renal cortex that combines in blood with its substrate, angiotensinogen, which is produced in the liver, to produce in turn angiotensin I and II. Angiotensin II acts as a stimulant to the adrenal glands to produce aldosterone. This hormone in turn effects a reabsorption of sodium in an ion exchange with potassium in the distal tubules

of the nephrons, and water reabsorption follows. Ordinarily this is a lifesaving mechanism to protect the body's vital water supply. In congestive heart failure, however, it only adds to the edema problem. The mechanism reacts as if the body's total fluid volume is reduced, when in truth the fluid is excessive; it is just that it is not in normal circulation but is being retained in the body's tissues.

2. *Antidiuretic hormone mechanism:* This water-conserving hormonal mechanism also adds to edema. Cardiac stress and reduced renal flow cause the release of antidiuretic hormone (ADH), also known as vasopressin, from the pituitary gland. ADH then stimulates still more water reabsorption in nephrons of the kidney, further increasing the problem of edema.

Increased Cellular Free Potassium

As reduced blood circulation depresses cell metabolism, cell protein is broken down and releases its bound potassium in the cell. As a result, the amount of free potassium inside the cell is increased, which increases intracellular osmotic pressure. Sodium ions in fluid surrounding the cell then also increase in number to balance increased osmotic pressure within the cell and to prevent cell dehydration. In time, the increased sodium outside the cell causes still more water retention.

Nutritional Management

Basis for all care of the person with congestive heart disease is improving cardiac output while reducing workload of the heart and minimizing congestive symptoms. Medical treatment involves O_2 therapy, decreased physical activity, and drug therapy with (1) diuretic and venodilator agents to control fluid congestion in the lungs, (2) digitalis drugs to strengthen contractions of the heart muscle, (3) sympathetic antagonists, angiotensin-converting enzyme (ACE) inhibitors, nitrate, and vasodilators to decrease workload of the heart.[32] Nutrition support involves the following[30]:

- *Sodium* is usually restricted to 2 g/day and may be adjusted upwards to 3 g/day if necessary to promote dietary intake.
- *Fluids* may be restricted to 1500 ml per day if needed.
- *Texture* may be modified to soft foods so little physical effort is needed.
- *Meals* may be divided into smaller feedings to also decrease effort necessary for eating.
- *Alcohol* is generally limited to one drink per day. If alcohol is thought to be a causative factor in the heart disease, abstinence is mandatory.

Cardiac Cachexia

Etiology

Sometimes with prolonged myocardial insufficiency and heart failure an extreme clinical condition of cardiac cachexia develops. Progressive, profound malnutrition results from an insufficient O_2 supply that cannot meet demands of red blood cell formation by bone marrow or energy needs for basic breathing. The enlarged, laboring heart is unable to maintain a sufficient blood supply to the body tissues, and nutrient delivery to cells is impaired. Edema, unpalatable sodium-restricted diets, drug reactions, and postoperative complications of cardiac surgery all worsen the anorexia and reduce food intake. In addition, the individual has probably become hypermetabolic and hypercatabolic. It should be no surprise the incidence of nosocomial (hospital-induced) cardiac cachexia is a common occurrence.

Nutrition Therapy

The goal is to help restore heart-lung function as much as possible and to rebuild body tissue. Team care involving the physician, clinical dietitian, nurse, patient, and family is essential. Nutrition support focuses on energy, nutrients, supplements, and feeding plan, as follows[33]:

- *Energy:* Sufficient kcalories are needed to cover basal energy needs, as well as energy for minimal activity and the hypermetabolism of severe congestive heart failure; more kcalories may be needed if major surgery is planned. Depending on the extent of malnutrition indicated by nutrition assessment, an increase of 30% to 50% of basal needs may be indicated.
- *Fluids:* Sufficient but not excessive fluid intake is needed, at a rate of about 0.5 ml/kcal/day or 1000 to 1500 ml/day.
- *Protein:* Approximately 1.0 to 1.5 g/kg body weight is needed to replace tissue losses and cover malabsorption.
- *Sodium:* Sodium restriction varies with individual status, usually in a range of 1 to 2 g/day, with attention to multiple alternate seasonings to enhance palatability of food.
- *Mineral-vitamin supplementation:* May need to supplement intake with folate, magnesium, thiamine, zinc, and iron depending on serum levels. Increasing vitamins E, B_6, B_{12}, and thiamin may be beneficial.
- *Feeding plan:* Small, frequent feedings are better tolerated. Large meals add to the risk of carbon dioxide (CO_2) accumulation and respiratory failure.
- *Enteral and parenteral nutrition support:* Tube feedings or parenteral nutrition may be appropriate. Several

---

pulmonary edema Accumulation of fluid in tissues of the lung.

antidiuretic hormone (ADH) Water-conserving hormone from posterior lobe of pituitary gland; causes resorption of water by kidney nephrons according to body need.

vasopressin Alternative name of ADH.

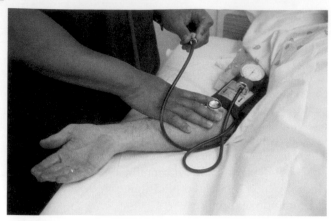

FIGURE 20-6 Monitoring blood pressure. *(From Potter PA, Perry AG:* Basic nursing: essentials for practice, *ed 5, St. Louis, 2003, Mosby/Elsevier Science.)*

enteral feeding formulas that have a low volume with a high density of kcalories are available. These are suitable for patients requiring fluid restriction.

ESSENTIAL HYPERTENSION AND VASCULAR DISEASE

Blood Pressure Controls

Arterial Pressure

As commonly measured, blood pressure is an indication of arterial pressure in vessels of the upper arm. This measure is obtained by an instrument for determining force of the pulse (Figure 20-6). This instrument is called a *sphygmomanometer,* from the Greek words *sphygmos* ("pulse"), *manos* ("thin"), and *metron* ("measure"). Pulse pressure is measured in millimeters of mercury (mm Hg) rise or in equivalent values read on gauges or digital indicators. The higher, or upper, value recorded is systolic pressure from contraction of the heart muscle. The lower value recorded is diastolic pressure, produced during the relaxation phase of the cardiac cycle.

Several factors contribute to maintaining fluid dynamics of normal blood pressure: (1) increased pressure on forward blood flow; (2) increased resistance from containing blood vessels; and (3) increased viscosity of blood itself, making movement through vessels more difficult. Of these factors, increased viscosity is a rare event. Thus in discussing high blood pressure in general terms, we are dealing with the first two factors, pumping pressure of the heart muscle propelling blood forward and resistance to this forward flow presented by blood vessel walls normally or by any abnormal added constriction or thickening.

Muscle Tone of Blood Vessel Walls

In hypertension the body's finely tuned mechanisms designed to maintain fluid dynamics are not operating effectively. Normally these systems include several agents that act to variously dilate and constrict blood vessels to meet whatever need is present at a given time. In a person with hypertension, however, dilation or constriction of blood vessels does not occur in the normal manner. If not effectively treated, uncontrolled elevated blood pressure results. Body systems that operate to help maintain normal blood pressure include (1) neuroendocrine functions of the sympathetic nervous system, mainly mediated by chemical neurotransmitters, such as norepinephrine; (2) hormonal systems such as the renin-angiotensin-aldosterone mechanism and its vasopressor effect; and (3) enzyme systems such as the kallikrein-kinin mechanism (sometimes operating with prostaglandins), which controls substances that act to dilate or constrict smooth muscle as needed.

The Problem of Hypertension

High blood pressure is one of the most prevalent vascular diseases worldwide. As the population ages, prevalence of hypertension will increase. It is a major factor in the development of stroke, heart attack, heart failure, and kidney disease.[34] At least 95% of these persons have essential hypertension, meaning its cause is unknown, although there is apparently a strong familial predisposition with its onset in young teenage years. It has often been called the "silent disease" because it carries no overt signs, but it can have serious implications if not treated and controlled.[35] The large United States study—Dietary Approaches to Stop Hypertension (DASH)—has clearly indicated that a diet rich in fruits, vegetables, and low-fat dairy foods and with reduced saturated and total fat can substantially lower blood pressure.[36] Individual treatment uses current antihypertensive drugs as needed.

Classifications of Blood Pressure

Hypertension is defined as systolic blood pressure of 140 mm Hg or higher, diastolic blood pressure of 90 mm Hg or higher, or taking antihypertensive medication. The objective of identifying and treating hypertension is to reduce morbidity and mortality. For that reason, classification of adult (greater than 18 years of age) blood pressure (Table 20-4) provides a mechanism for identifying high-risk individuals and provides guidelines for follow-up and treatment.[32]

Prevention and Treatment

The goal of prevention and management of hypertension is to reduce morbidity and mortality by the least intrusive means possible.[32] Lifestyle modifications (Table 20-5) offer potential for preventing hypertension, have been shown capable of lowering blood pressure, and can reduce cardiovascular risk factors at minimal cost and risk.[32]

TABLE 20-4	Classification of Blood Pressure for Adults

Blood Pressure (BP) Classification	Systolic (mm Hg)*	Diastolic (mm Hg)	Lifestyle Modification	Initial Drug Therapy	
				Without Compelling Indication	With Compelling Indication†
Normal‡	<120	And <80	Encourage	No antihypertensive drug indicated	Drug(s) for compelling indications§
Prehypertension	120-139	Or 80-89	Yes		
Stage 1 hypertension¶	140-159	Or 90-99	Yes	Thiazide-type diuretics for most. May consider ACEI, ARB, BB, CCB, or combinations	Drug(s) for the compelling indications§ Other antihypertensive drugs (diuretics, ACEI, ARB, BB, CCB) as needed
Stage 2 hypertension¶	≥160	Or ≥100	Yes	Two-drug combination for most§	

Data from National High Blood Pressure Program: *The seventh report of the Joint National Committee on Prevention, Detection, Evaluation, and Treatment of High Blood Pressure,* National Institutes of Health, National Heart, Lung, and Blood Institutes, NIH Publication No. 03-5233, Washington, DC, 2003, U.S. Government Printing Office.

ACEI, Angiotensin-converting enzyme inhibitor; *ARB,* adolsterone receptor blocker; *BB,* beta-blocker; *CCB,* calcium channel blocker.

*Treatment determined by highest BP category.

†Heart failure, postmyocardial infarction, high coronary disease risk, chronic kidney disease, recurrent stroke prevention.

‡Optimal blood pressure with respect to cardiovascular risk is below 120/80 mm Hg. However, unusually low readings should be evaluated for clinical significance.

§Initial combined therapy should be used cautiously in those at risk for orthostatic hypotension.

¶Based on the average of two or more readings taken at each of two or more visits after initial screening.

TABLE 20-5	Lifestyle Modifications to Manage Hypertension*†

Modification	Recommendations	Approximate SBP Reduction (Range)
Weight reduction	Maintain normal body weight (BMI 18.5-24.9 kg/m^2).	5-20 mm Hg per 10 kg weight loss
Adapt DASH eating plan	Consume a diet rich in fruits, vegetables, and lowfat dairy products with a reduced content of saturated and total fat.	8-14 mm Hg
Dietary sodium reduction	Reduce dietary sodium intake to no more than 2.4 g sodium or 6 g sodium chloride.	2-8 mm Hg
Physical activity	Engage in regular aerobic physical activity such as brisk walking (at least 30 minutes per day, most days of the week).	4-9 mm Hg
Moderation of alcohol consumption	Limit consumption to no more than 2 drinks (1 oz. or 30 ml ethanol; e.g., 24 oz beer, 10 oz wine, or 3 oz 80-proof whiskey) per day in most men and to no more than 1 drink per day in women and lighter-weight persons.	2-4 mm Hg

Data from National High Blood Pressure Program: *The seventh report of the Joint National Committee on Prevention, Detection, Evaluation, and Treatment of High Blood Pressure,* National Institutes of Health, National Heart, Lung, and Blood Institutes, NIH Publication No. 03-5233, Washington, DC, 2003, U.S. Government Printing Office.

SBP, Systolic blood pressure; *BMI,* body mass index; *DASH,* Dietary Approaches to Stop Hypertension.

*For overall cardiovascular risk reduction, stop smoking.

†The effects of implementing these modifications are dose- and time-dependent and could be greater for some individuals than others.

Nutritional Management of Hypertension

Taste for a given amount of salt with food is an acquired one, not a physiologic necessity. Sufficient sodium for the body's need is provided as a natural mineral in foods consumed. Some persons salt their foods heavily and thus form high salt taste levels. Others form lighter tastes by using smaller amounts. Common daily adult intakes of

essential hypertension An inherent form of hypertension with no specific discoverable cause and considered to be familial; also called primary hypertension.

sodium range widely from about 2 to 4 g with lighter tastes to as high as 10 to 12 g with heavier use. Salt (sodium chloride [NaCl]) intakes are about twice these amounts because sodium (Na) makes up about 40% of the NaCl molecule. The large amount of salt in the American diet, estimated to be about 6 to 15 g of sodium per day (260 to 656 mEq), is largely a result of the increased use of many processed food products. The main source of dietary sodium is food processing (about 75%). Approximately 10% to 11% occurs naturally in foods, about 15% is discretionary (half of which is contributed by table salt and half by cooking), and less than 1% comes from water.

Other nutrients that affect blood pressure are potassium and calcium. High potassium intake from food sources (see the *Perspectives in Practice* box, "Dietary Approaches to Stop Hypertension [DASH] Diet Pattern") such as fresh fruits and vegetables may protect against developing hypertension and improve blood pressure control in those who do have hypertension.[32] Calcium in the form of low-fat dairy products (which are also low in saturated and total fat) is also recommended to reduce blood pressure. Moderate consumption of alcohol (equivalent to two drinks per day for men, one drink per day for women) is also known to reduce blood pressure.[32]

Cerebrovascular Accident

Arteriosclerotic vascular injury and hypertension may also affect blood vessels in the brain. A cerebrovascular accident (CVA), or stroke, occurs when a blood vessel carrying O_2 and nutrients to the brain ruptures (*hemorrhagic stroke*) or is clogged by a blood clot (*ischemic stroke*), interrupting blood flow to an area of the brain. When any part of the brain does not receive blood and O_2, nerve cells in the affected area die, resulting in loss of control of abilities that area of the brain once controlled. During the past two decades, with the declining U.S. early death rate from heart disease, stroke stands in third place as a leading cause of death of adults ages 25 to 65 years.[37] Nearly 170,000 Americans die annually of stroke, meaning someone in the United States experiences a stroke every 45 seconds.[38] Among all U.S. population groups, the incident rate for first stroke among blacks is almost double that of European Americans.[37]

There are four main types of stroke; two are caused by blood clots, and two are caused by ruptured blood vessels. Cerebral thrombosis and cerebral embolism account for approximately 70% to 80% of all strokes. Cerebral thrombosis, the most common stroke, occurs when a thrombus forms and blocks blood flow in an artery bringing blood to part of the brain. They usually occur at night or first thing in the morning when blood pressure is low. They are often preceded by a transient ischemic attack (TIA), or "ministroke." Cerebral embolism occurs when an embolus forms away from the brain, usually in the heart. The clot is carried in the bloodstream until it lodges in an artery leading to or in the brain and blocks the flow of blood.[1] A *subarachnoid hemorrhage* occurs when a blood vessel on the brain's surface ruptures and bleeds into the space between the brain and skull. A *cerebral hemorrhage* occurs when a defective artery in the brain bursts, flooding the surrounding tissue with blood.[1]

Nutrition Therapy

Paralysis and other problems may occur, depending on the site and extent of brain damage resulting from a stroke. Patients who experience left-sided CVA most commonly experience sight and hearing losses, including ability to see where food is on plates or trays. Right-hemisphere, bilateral, or brainstem CVA causes significant problems with feeding and swallowing, in addition to speech problems.[32]

Dysphagia often occurs, and foods that cause choking or that are hard to manage should be avoided (dry or crisp foods, peanut butter, thinly pureed foods, raw vegetables, to mention a few). If the patient has problems with saliva production, foods can be moistened with small amounts of liquid (au jus or gravy). Because thin liquids are often difficult to swallow, thickeners are used to make semisolid foods from soups, beverages, and juices.[32]

Peripheral Vascular Disease

Peripheral vascular disease (PVD) is characterized by narrowing of blood vessels in the legs and sometimes the arms. Blood flow is restricted and causes pain in affected area. Contributory risk factors include hypertension and diabetes mellitus. However, the greatest risk factor is cigarette smoking, which constricts blood vessels. More than 90% of patients with PVD are or were moderate to heavy smokers.

Symptoms and Complications

As arteries gradually narrow because of atherosclerosis (the most common cause), an aching, tired feeling occurs in leg muscles when walking. Resting the leg for a few minutes relieves pain, but it recurs shortly when walking is resumed. For this reason the symptom is called intermittent claudication. Sometimes a sudden arterial blockage occurs when a blood clot develops on the top of

---

dysphagia Difficulty in swallowing, commonly associated with obstructive or motor disorders of the esophagus.

intermittent claudication A symptomatic pattern of peripheral vascular disease, characterized by the absence of pain or discomfort in a limb, usually the legs, when at rest, which is followed by pain and weakness when walking, intensifying until walking becomes impossible, and then disappearing again after a rest period; seen in occlusive arterial disease.

PERSPECTIVES IN PRACTICE
Dietary Approaches to Stop Hypertension (DASH) Diet Pattern

The following list indicates the number of recommended daily servings from each food group with examples of food choices (based on the 2000-kcal reference diet). The number of servings may increase or decrease, depending on individual calorie needs, and may be found on the DASH website (www.nhlbi.nih.gov/health/public/heart/hbp/dash/).

Food Group	Daily Serving (Except Where Noted)	Serving Sizes	Examples and Notes	Significance to the DASH Diet Pattern
Grains and grain products	7-8	1 slice bread 1 oz dry cereal* ½ cup cooked rice, pasta, or cereal	Whole wheat bread, English muffin, pita bread, bagel; cereals; grits; oatmeal	Major source of energy and fiber
Vegetables	4-5	1 cup raw, leafy vegetable ½ cup cooked vegetables 6 oz vegetable juice	Tomatoes, potatoes, carrots, peas, squash, broccoli, turnip greens, collard, kale, spinach, artichokes, beans, sweet potatoes	Rich sources of potassium, magnesium, and fiber
Fruits	4-5	6 oz fruit juice 1 medium fruit ¼ cup dried fruit ½ cup fresh, frozen, or canned fruit	Apricots, bananas, dates, grapes, oranges, orange juice, tangerines, strawberries, mangoes, melons, peaches, pineapple, prunes, raisins	Important sources of potassium, magnesium, and fiber
Low-fat or nonfat dairy foods	2-3	8 oz milk 1 cup yogurt 1½ oz cheese	Fat-free or 1% milk, fat-free or lowfat buttermilk; nonfat or low-fat yogurt; part-nonfat mozzarella cheese, nonfat cheese	Major sources of calcium and protein
Meat, poultry, and fish	<2	3 oz cooked meats, poultry, or fish	Select only lean meats; trim away visible fats; broil, roast, or boil, instead of frying; remove skin from chicken	Rich sources of protein and magnesium
Nuts, seeds, and legumes	4-5/wk	1½ oz or ½ cup nuts ½ oz or 2 tbsp seeds ½ cup cooked legumes	Almonds, filberts, mixed nuts, peanuts, walnuts, sunflower seeds, kidney beans, lentils	Rich sources of energy, magnesium, potassium, protein, and fiber
Fats and oils†	2-3	1 tsp soft margarine 1 tbsp low-fat mayonnaise or salad dressing 2 tbsp light salad dressing 1 tsp vegetable oil	Soft margarine, lowfat mayonnaise, light salad dressing, vegetable oil (such as olive, corn, canola, or safflower)	DASH has 27% of calories as fat, including that in or added to foods
Sweets	5/wk	1 tbsp sugar 1 tbsp jelly or jam ½ oz jelly beans 8 oz lemonade	Maple syrup, sugar, jelly, jam; fruit-flavored gelatin, jelly beans, fruit punch, sorbet, ices, hard candy	Sweets should be low in fat

*Equals ½ to 1¼ cup depending on cereal type. Check the product's nutrition label.

†Fat content changes serving counts for fats and oils. For example, 1 tbsp of regular salad dressing equals 1 serving; 1 tbsp of low-fat dressing equals ½ serving; 1 tbsp of fat-free dressing equals 0 servings.

Strategies for Adopting DASH

Dietary changes are best achieved through small changes in food selections. Use this list of tips as a way to initiate discussion and dietary compliance to reduce hypertension among your clients.

Tips on Eating the DASH Way

- Change gradually.
  - If you now eat one or two vegetables a day, add a serving at lunch and another at dinner.
  - If you do not eat fruit now or have only juice at breakfast, add a serving to your meals or have it as a snack.

- Gradually increase your use of fat-free and low-fat dairy products to three servings a day. For example, drink milk with lunch or dinner instead of soda, sugar-sweetened tea, or alcohol. Choose low-fat (1%) or fat-free (skim) dairy products to reduce your intake of saturated fat, total fat, cholesterol, and kcalories.
- Read food labels on margarines and salad dressings, and choose those lowest in unsaturated fat. Some margarines are now *trans* fat free.
- Treat meat as one part of the whole meal instead of the focus.
  - Limit meat to 6 oz a day (two servings)—all that is needed. Three to 4 oz is about the size of a deck of cards.

Continued

PERSPECTIVES IN PRACTICE—cont'd
Dietary Approaches to Stop Hypertension (DASH) Diet Pattern

- If you now eat large portions of meat, cut them back gradually—by one half or one third at each meal.
- Include two or more vegetarian-style (meatless) meals each week.
- Increase servings of vegetables, rice, pasta, and dry beans at meals. Try casseroles, pasta, and stir-fry dishes that have less meat and more vegetables, grains, and dry beans.
- Use fruit or other foods low in saturated fat, cholesterol, and kcalories as desserts and snacks.
  - Fruits and other low-fat foods offer great taste and variety. Use fruits canned in their own juice. Fresh fruits require little or no preparation. Dried fruits are a good choice to carry with you or to have ready in the car.
  - Try these snacks ideas: unsalted pretzels or nuts mixed with raisins, graham crackers, low-fat and fat-free yogurt and frozen yogurt, popcorn with no salt or butter added, and raw vegetables.

- Try these other tips.
  - Choose whole grain foods to get added nutrients such as minerals and fiber. For example, choose whole wheat bread and whole grain cereals.
  - If you have trouble digesting dairy products, try taking lactase enzyme pills or drops (available at drugstores and groceries) with the dairy foods, or buy lactose-free milk or milk with lactase enzyme added to it.
  - Use fresh, frozen, or no-salt-added canned vegetables.

References

U.S. Department of Health and Human Services, Public Health Service, National Institutes of Health, National Heart, Lung, and Blood Institute: *The DASH diet,* NIH Publication No. 01-4082, Bethesda, Md, 2001 (May, revised), Author. Available at *www.nhlbi.nih.gov.*

U.S. Department of Health and Human Services, Public Health Service, National Institutes of Health, National Heart, Lung, and Blood Institute: *The DASH eating plan,* NIH Publication No. 03-4082, Bethesda, Md, 2003 (May, revised), Author. Available at *www.nhlbi.nih.gov.*

---

a plaque or a clot formed in the heart is carried to a peripheral artery and blocks it. The blockage causes sudden severe pain in the affected area, which becomes cold and either pale or blue and has no pulse. Movement and sensation are lost.

Treatment

By far the most important treatment for the patient is to stop smoking. As with coronary vessels, surgery on diseased vessels is sometimes required: (1) arterial reconstructive surgery to bypass them, (2) endarterectomy to remove obstructing fatty deposits on inner linings, or (3) balloon angioplasty to widen vessels. Drug therapy may include antiplatelet or anticoagulant agents to prevent blood clotting. Nutrition therapy consists of regular fat and cholesterol modifications described for CHD. Exercise is also important. The person should walk every day with medical clearance, gradually increasing to about 1 hour—stopping whenever intermittent pain occurs and resuming when it stops. Regular inspection of feet, daily washing and stocking change, good-fitting shoes to avoid pressure, and scrupulous foot care (ideally by a podiatrist) are essential to prevent infection.

PULMONARY DISEASES

Chronic Obstructive Pulmonary Disease

Clinical Characteristics

Progressive congestive heart failure contributes to lung disease and risk of respiratory failure. Malnutrition is common with the debilitating condition of chronic obstructive pulmonary disease (COPD). This term describes a group of disorders in which airflow in the lungs is limited and respiratory failure develops. Two main interrelated COPD conditions are (1) chronic bronchitis and (2) emphysema. Malnutrition usually accompanies COPD, and its presence increases illness and death rates associated with the disease process. Anorexia and significant weight loss reflect a growing inability to maintain adequate nutritional status, which in turn severely compromises pulmonary function. Progression of the disease process, with its increasing shortness of breath, prevents the person from living a normal life, and prognosis is poor. Eventually, in progressive respiratory failure, the patient becomes dependent on a mechanical respirator and controlled O_2 supply. A poor prognosis is associated with a compromised nutritional status in these patients.

Nutritional Management

Respiratory failure is actually a failure of pulmonary exchange of O_2 and CO_2. Thus its common manifestations are hypoxemia, deficient oxygenation of blood, and hypercapnia, excess CO_2 in the blood. Patients with COPD have greater energy requirements, which will vary for each individual. Requirements for carbohydrate, protein, and fat will be determined by the underlying lung disease, oxygen therapy, medications, weight status, and any acute fluid fluctuations.[39] A balanced proportion of protein (15% to 20% total kcalories) with fat (30% to 45% total kcalories) and carbohydrate (40% to 55% total kcalories) is necessary to maintain appropriate respiratory quotient (RQ) from substrate utilization.[38] It is important not to overfeed patients with COPD. Commonly, other coexisting diseases (cardiovascular disease [CVD], diabetes mellitus [DM], renal disease, or cancer) may well be present, thereby influencing total amount and kind of carbohydrate, protein, and fat prescribed.[38]

Pneumonia

The term *pneumonia* comes from the Greek word *pneuma*, meaning "breath." It is an acute inflammation of the lung[40] caused by an infectious agent and can stem from three sources: (1) aspiration of normal bacterial flora and/or gastric contents in oropharyngeal secretions; (2) inhalation of contaminants (virus for example); or (3) contamination from systemic circulation.[41] A common disorder, community-acquired pneumonia is the most lethal infectious disease in the United States and the sixth leading cause of death.[42]

Symptoms

Generally the immune response, cough with or without sputum production, sneezing, and mucociliary clearance (pulmonary defense mechanisms) guard against pneumonia.[41] Community-acquired pneumonia is usually bacterial in origin and produces exudate that is hard to expectorate. Viral pneumonia does not produce exudate.[40,41] Hospital-acquired, or nosocomial, pneumonia develops in up to 5% of hospitalized patients.[40] Nosocomial pneumonia and community-based pneumonia are caused by different pathogens.[40] Aspiration of infected pharyngeal or gastric secretions delivers bacteria straight to the lungs. This is promoted by exogenous factors such as contamination by dirty hands and equipment, treatment with broad-spectrum antibiotics that promote emergence of drug-resistant organisms, and patient factors such as malnutrition, smoking, preexisting lung disease, advanced age, swallowing disorders, and chest or upper abdominal surgery.[40,41] Signs and symptoms are nonspecific; however, fever, purulent sputum, and leukocytosis are present in most patients.[41]

Treatment

Sputum and blood specimens are cultured before antibiotic treatment.[40] Usual treatment is with a broad-spectrum penicillin antibiotic. Erythromycin may be added if there is suspicion of an atypical organism. Oxygen therapy is often used, and in severe cases the patient may be ventilated.[40,41] Nosocomial pneumonia is treated more aggressively with broad-spectrum antibiotics and tailored to specific clinical setting due to the high mortality rate.[41]

Nutritional Management

Sufficient fluids (3 to 3.5 L) should be given daily if not contraindicated. Frequent small meals may be better tolerated. A multivitamin/mineral supplement may be beneficial, and fiber should be encouraged to avoid constipation. Adequate fruit and fruit juice intake will supply necessary potassium.[32]

Tuberculosis

Tuberculosis (TB), caused by *Mycobacterium tuberculosis*, is one of the world's more widespread and deadly diseases.[39-41]

It occurs disproportionately among disadvantaged populations such as the malnourished, the homeless, and those living in overcrowded and substandard housing.[39,41] *M. tuberculosis* is an airborne disease,[40,41] and strains resistant to one or more first-line antituberculosis drugs are increasing.[41]

Symptoms

Typical symptoms of TB are malaise, anorexia, weight loss, fever, and night sweats. Chronic cough is the most universal pulmonary symptom. It may be dry at first but becomes productive of purulent sputum as the disease progresses.[39,41] More often than not, the sputum is blood streaked. Patients appear chronically ill and malnourished.[39,41]

Treatment

The basic goals of TB treatment are as follows[39,41]:

- Administer multiple drugs to which organisms are susceptible.
- Add at least two new antitubercular agents to a regimen when treatment failure is suspected.
- Provide the safest, most effective therapy in the shortest period of time.
- Ensure adherence to therapy.

Nonadherence (due to adverse drug reaction) to treatment is a major cause of treatment failure, continued transmission of TB, and development of drug resistance.[39,41] Hospitalization for initial therapy of TB is not necessary for most patients,[41] but hospitalization has increased due to increasing resistance of the organism to treatment and an increasing number of cases.[39]

Nutritional Management

The objective of nutritional management is to maintain weight or prevent weight loss. If febrile, patients will be hypermetabolic. A well-balanced diet with liberal amounts of protein and adequate kcalories is usually necessary. Ensure the patient is consuming adequate amounts of calcium, iron, vitamin C, and B-complex vitamins.[32]

Health Promotion

Added Food Factors in Coronary Heart Disease Therapy

The primary focus of nutrition therapy for CHD is on control of lipid factors, including cholesterol and saturated

---

hypoxemia Deficient oxygenation of the blood, resulting in hypoxia, reduced O_2 supply to tissue.
hypercapnia Excess CO_2 in the blood.

fats. Two other food factors, however, play a different role. In varying ways they help to protect us from the development of CHD.[2]

Dietary Fiber

Studies indicate water-soluble types of dietary fiber have significant cholesterol-lowering effect. Soluble fiber includes gums, pectin, certain hemicelluloses, and the body's storage polysaccharide, glycogen. Foods rich in soluble fiber include oat bran and dried beans, with additional amounts in barley and fruits. Oat bran, for example, contains a primary water-soluble gum, beta-glucan, which is a lipid-lowering agent. Soluble dietary fiber has the following properties:

- Delays gastric emptying
- Slows intestinal transit time
- Slows glucose absorption
- Is fermented in colon into short-chain fatty acids that may inhibit liver cholesterol synthesis and help clear LDL cholesterol

On the other hand, insoluble dietary fiber—cellulose, lignin, and many hemicelluloses—found in vegetables, wheat, and most other grains does not have these lipid-lowering effects. Thus an increased use of soluble fiber food sources, especially oat bran and legumes, would have beneficial effects.

Omega-3 Fatty Acids

Studies indicate that omega-3 fatty acids, eicosapentaenoic acid (EPA) and docosahexaenoic acid (DHA) (see Chapter 3), found mostly in seafood and marine oils, also have protective functions. They can do the following:

- Change pattern of plasma fatty acids to alter platelet activity and reduce platelet aggregation that causes blood clotting, thus lowering the risk of coronary thrombosis
- Decrease the synthesis of VLDL
- Increase antiinflammatory effects

It would seem, then, factors in foods such as oats, dried beans, and fatty fish would provide valuable lipid-lowering additions to our diets.

TO SUM UP

CHD remains the leading cause of death in the United States. Atherosclerosis, its underlying pathologic process, involves the formation of plaque, a fatty substance that builds up along the interior surfaces of blood vessels, interfering with blood flow and damaging blood vessels. If this buildup becomes severe, it cuts off blood supplies of O_2 and nutrients to tissue cells, which in turn begin to die. When this occurs in a coronary artery, the result is an MI, or heart attack. When it occurs in a brain vessel, the result is a cerebrovascular accident, or stroke.

Risk for atherosclerosis increases with amount and type of blood lipids (lipoproteins) available. The apolipoprotein portion of lipoproteins is an important genetically determined part of the disease process. Elevated serum LDL cholesterol level is a primary factor in atherosclerosis development.

Initial dietary recommendations for acute cardiovascular disease (heart attack) include caloric restriction, soft-textured foods, and small, frequent meals to reduce the metabolic demands of digestion, absorption, and metabolism of foods and their nutrients. Maintenance of a lean body weight is important. Persons with chronic CHD (congestive heart failure) and those with essential hypertension benefit from weight management, exercise, and sodium restriction to overcome cardiac edema and to help control elevated blood pressure.

Current dietary recommendations to help prevent CHD involve maintaining a healthy weight; limiting fats to 25% to 30% of all kcalories, with the majority being unsaturated food forms; limiting sodium intake to 2 to 3 g/day; and increasing exercise.

Concerted efforts are needed to combat development of cardiac cachexia in progressive heart failure. Also, atherosclerotic plaques may occur in the extremities, usually the legs, causing PVD and the pain of intermittent claudication when walking. Progressive respiratory failure interferes with normal exchange of blood gases, O_2 and CO_2, and results in COPD, for which changed ratios of the fuel macronutrients are sometimes indicated.

QUESTIONS FOR REVIEW

1. Which types of hyperlipoproteinemia occur most often? Identify lipids that are elevated in each case, as well as predisposing factors. Describe the types of diet recommended for each.
2. Identify four dietary recommendations that should be made for the person with a heart attack. Describe how each recommendation helps recovery.
3. What dietary changes can the average American make to reduce saturated fats and to substitute polyunsaturated fats?
4. What does the term *essential hypertension* mean? Why would weight management and sodium restriction contribute to its control?
5. Outline nutrition therapy for cardiac cachexia, and discuss the rationale for each aspect of the feeding plan.
6. Discuss cause and treatment of peripheral vascular disease.
7. Outline nutrition therapy for COPD and discuss the rationale for the fuel macronutrient adjustments.

---

hyperlipoproteinemia Elevated level of lipoproteins in the blood.

REFERENCES

1. American Heart Association: *Heart disease and stroke statistics 1992-2003,* Dallas, 1999-2003, Author. Available at *www.americanheart.org.* Accessed August 8, 2005.

2. National Cholesterol Education Program (NCEP): *Third report of the NCEP Expert Panel on Detection, Evaluation, and Treatment of High Blood Cholesterol in Adults (Adult Treatment Panel III), full report,* Washington, DC, 2002, National Institutes of Health, National Heart, Lung, and Blood Institute. Retrieved December 19, 2005, from *www.nhlbi.nih.gov/guidelines/cholesterol/atp3_rpt.htm.*

3. Banasik JL: Alterations in cardiac function. In Copstead LC, Banasik JL, eds: *Pathophysiology,* ed 3, St. Louis, 2005, Elsevier/Saunders.

4. Grundy SM, Denke MA: Dietary influences on serum lipids and lipoproteins, *J Lipid Res* 31:1149, 1990.

5. Mensink RP, Katan MB: Effects of dietary fatty acids on serum lipids and lipoproteins: a meta-analysis of 27 trials, *Arterioscler Thromb* 12:911, 1992.

6. Kris-Etherton PM, Yu S: Individual fatty acids effects on plasma lipids and lipoproteins: human studies, *Am J Clin Nutr* 65(suppl 5):1628S, 1997.

7. National Institutes of Health: *Clinical guidelines on the identification, evaluation, and treatment of overweight and obesity in adults—the evidence report,* NIH Publication No. 98-4083, Bethesda, Md, 1998, National Heart, Lung, and Blood Institute. Retrieved December 19, 2005, from *www.nhlbi.nih.gov/guidelines/obesity/ob_gdlns.pdf.*

8. Caggiula AW et al: The Multiple Risk Intervention Trial (MRFIT): IV-intervention on blood lipids, *Prev Med* 10:443, 1981.

9. Stamler J et al: Relation of changes in dietary lipids and weight, trial years 1-6, to change in blood lipids in the special intervention and usual care groups in the Multiple Risk Factor Intervention Trial, *Am J Clin Nutr* 65:272S, 1997.

10. Hopkins PN: Effects of dietary cholesterol on serum cholesterol: a meta-analysis and review, *Am J Clin Nutr* 55:1060, 1992.

11. Clarke R et al: Dietary lipids and blood cholesterol: quantitative meta-analysis of metabolic ward studies, *BMJ* 314:112, 1997.

12. Garg A: High-monounsaturated-fat diets for patients with diabetes mellitus: a meta-analysis, *Am J Clin Nutr* 67(suppl 3):577S, 1998.

13. Kris-Etherton PM et al: High-monounsaturated fatty acid diets lower both plasma cholesterol and triacylglycerol concentrations, *Am J Clin Nutr* 70:1009, 1999.

14. National Research Council: *Diet and health: implications for reducing chronic disease risk,* Washington, DC, 1989, National Academies Press.

15. Knopp RH et al: Long-term cholesterol-lowering effects of 4 fat-restricted diets in hypercholesterolemic and combined hyperlipidemic men: the Dietary Alternatives Study, *JAMA* 278:1509, 1997.

16. Turely ML et al: The effect of a low-fat, high-carbohydrate diet on serum high density lipoprotein cholesterol and triglyceride, *Eur J Clin Nutr* 52:728, 1998.

17. Jenkins DJ et al: Effect on blood lipids of very high intakes of fiber in diets low in saturated fat and cholesterol, *N Engl J Med* 329:21, 1993.

18. Vuksan V et al: Beneficial effects of viscous dietary fiber from Konjac-mannan in subjects with the insulin resistance syndrome: results of a controlled metabolic trial, *Diabetes Care* 23:9, 2000.

19. U.S. Department of Health and Human Services, Food and Drug Administration: Food labeling: health claims; soluble fiber from certain foods and coronary heart disease—final rule, *Fed Reg* 28234, 1997.

20. U.S. Department of Health and Human Services, Food and Drug Administration: Food labeling: health claims; soluble fiber from certain foods and coronary heart disease—final rule, *Fed Reg* 8103, 1998.

21. Anderson JW: Dietary fibre, complex carbohydrate and coronary heart disease, *Can J Cardiol* 11(suppl G):55G, 1995.

22. Vuorio AF et al: Stanol ester margarine alone and with simvastatin lowers serum cholesterol in families with familial hypercholesterolemia caused by the FH-North Karelia Mutation, *Arterioscler Thromb Vasc Biol* 20:500, 2000.

23. Gylling H, Miettinen TA: Cholesterol reduction by different plant stanol mixtures and with variable fat intake, *Metabolism* 48:575, 1999.

24. Gylling H et al: Reduction of serum cholesterol in postmenopausal women with previous myocardial infarction and cholesterol malabsorption induced by dietary sitostanol ester margarine: women and dietary sitostanol, *Circulation* 96:4226, 1997.

25. Hallikainen MA, Uusitupa MI: Effects of 2 low-fat stanol ester-containing margarines on serum cholesterol concentrations as part of a low-fat diet in hypercholesterolemic subjects, *Am J Clin Nutr* 69:403, 1999.

26. Hendricks HF et al: Spreads enriched with three different levels of vegetable oil sterols and the degree of cholesterol lowering in normocholesterolaemic and mildly hypercholesterolaemic subjects, *Eur J Clin Nutr* 53:319, 1999.

27. Miettinen TA et al: Reduction of serum cholesterol with sitostanol ester margarine in a mildly hypercholesterolemic population, *N Engl J Med* 333:1308, 1995.

28. Vanhanen HT et al: Serum cholesterol, cholesterol, precursors, and plant sterols in hypercholesterolemic subjects with different apoE phenotypes during dietary sitostanol ester treatment, *J Lipid Res* 34:1535, 1993.

29. Sacks FM et al: The effect of pravastatin on coronary events after myocardial infarction in patients with average cholesterol levels, *N Engl J Med* 335(14), 1996.

30. Antman EM et al: ACC/AHA guidelines for the management of patients with ST-elevation myocardial infarction—executive summary: a report of the ACC/AHA Task Force on Practice Guidelines (Committee to Revise the 1999 Guidelines on the Management of Patients With Acute Myocardial Infarction), *Circulation* 110:588, 2004.

31. American Dietetic Association: *Nutrition care manual,* Chicago, 2005 (updated as necessary), Author. Available at *http://nutritioncaremanual.org.* Accessed July 18, 2005 via password.

32. Banasik JL: Heart failure and dysrhythmias: common sequelae of cardiac diseases. In Copstead LC, Banasik JL, eds: *Pathophysiology,* ed 3, St. Louis, 2005, Elsevier/Saunders.

33. Escott-Stump S: *Nutrition and diagnosis-related care,* ed 5, Philadelphia, 2002, Lippincott Williams & Wilkins.

34. National High Blood Pressure Program: *The seventh report of the Joint National Committee on Prevention, Detection, Evaluation, and Treatment of High Blood Pressure,* National Institutes of Health, National Heart, Lung, and Blood Institutes, NIH Publication No. 03-5233, Washington, DC, 2003, U.S. Government Printing Office.

35. Choka KP: Alterations in blood pressure. In Copstead LC, Banasik JL, eds: *Pathophysiology,* ed 3, St. Louis, 2005, Elsevier/Saunders.

36. Sachs FN et al: Effects on blood pressure of reduced dietary sodium and the Dietary Approaches to Stop Hypertension (DASH), *N Engl J Med* 344:3, 2001.

37. National Center for Health Statistics, Centers for Disease Control and Prevention: *Stroke/cerebrovascular disease,* Hyattsville, Md, 2005 (reviewed), Author. Retrieved December 19, 2005, from *www.cdc.gov/nchs/fastats/stroke.htm.*

38. American Heart Association: *Stroke statistics,* Dallas, 2005, Author. Available at *www.americanheart.org.* Accessed August 8, 2005.

39. Mueller DH: Medical nutrition therapy for pulmonary disease. In Mahan LK, Escott-Stump S: *Krause's food, nutrition, and diet therapy,* ed 11, Philadelphia, 2004, Elsevier/Saunders.

40. Walshaw MJ, Hind CRK. Chest disease. In Axford J, O'Callaghan C, eds: *Medicine,* ed 2, Malden, Mass, 2004, Blackwell Science.

41. Schumann L: Restrictive pulmonary disorders. In Copstead LC, Banasik JL, eds: *Pathophysiology,* ed 3, St. Louis, 2005, Elsevier/Saunders.

42. Chesnutt MS, Prendergast TJ: Lung. In Tierney LM, McPhee SJ, Papadakis MA, eds: *Current medical diagnosis and treatment 2003,* New York, 2003, Lange Medical Book/McGraw-Hill.

FURTHER READINGS AND RESOURCES

Readings

Sacks FM et al: Effects on blood pressure of reduced dietary sodium and the Dietary Approaches to Stop Hypertension (DASH) diet, *N Engl J Med* 344:3, 2001.

This article presents research methods and data that demonstrate decreased sodium intake and increased intake of fruits, vegetables, and low-fat dairy foods lower blood pressure.

Grundy SM et al: Implications of recent clinical trials for the National Cholesterol Education Program Adult Treatment Panel III Guidelines, *Circulation* 110:227, 2004.

This article reviews results of five major clinical trials of statin therapy.

U.S. Department of Health and Human Services, Public Health Service, National Institutes of Health, National Heart, Lung, and Blood Institute: *The DASH eating plan,* NIH Publication No. 03-4082, Washington, DC, 2003 (May, revised), Author. Available at *www.nhlbi.nih.gov.* Accessed July 18, 2005.

National High Blood Pressure Program: *The seventh report of the Joint National Committee on Prevention, Detection, Evaluation, and Treatment of High Blood Pressure,* National Institutes of Health, National Heart, Lung, and Blood Institutes, NIH Publication No. 03-5233, Washington, DC, 2003, U.S. Government Printing Office.

National Cholesterol Education Program (NCEP): *Third report of the NCEP Expert Panel on Detection, Evaluation, and Treatment of High Blood Cholesterol in Adults (Adult Treatment Panel III), full report,* Washington, DC, 2002, National Institutes of Health, National Heart, Lung, and Blood Institute.

These references highlight the research used as background information to develop medical and dietary recommendations for cardiovascular disease and hypertension. They are valuable references for all health professionals.

Websites of Interest

- American Heart Association: *www.americanheart.org.*
- Centers for Disease Control and Prevention, Health topic: cardiovascular disease: *www.cdc.gov/doc.do/id/0900f3ec802720b8.*
- MedlinePlus: Heart diseases: *www.nlm.nih.gov/medlineplus/heartdiseases.html.*
- Womenshealth.gov: Heart and cardiovascular disease: *www.4woman.gov/faq/heartdis.htm.*
- World Health Organization (WHO): Cardiovascular diseases: *http://www.who.int/cardiovascular_diseases/en/.*

CHAPTER 21

Diabetes Mellitus

Sara Long

In this chapter of our continuing clinical nutrition series, we look at the problem of diabetes. We seek to understand its nature and how it can be managed to maintain good health and avoid complications.

Diabetes is a serious, costly, and increasingly common chronic disease. In the United States 18.2 million (6.3%) of the population have diabetes. An estimated 13 million Americans have diagnosed diabetes, and an additional 5.2 million have undiagnosed diabetes. There are approximately 1.3 million newly diagnosed cases of diabetes each year.[1] Diabetes can be diagnosed on the basis of two fasting glucose readings of 126 mg/dl or higher or a random glucose level of 200 mg/dl or higher and symptoms such as polyuria, polydipsia, and unexplained weight loss.[2]

Although elevation of blood glucose level is the hallmark characteristic of diabetes, it is a group of metabolic disorders resulting from a defect in insulin secretion, insulin action, or both. These defects interfere with normal cellular uptake of glucose and utilization of glucose within cells. Restoring normal metabolic function is the goal in diagnosing and treating diabetes early. Restoration of normal metabolism can prevent many of the short-term complications such as hyperglycemia and hypoglycemia and the longer-term microvascular, macrovascular, and neurologic complications that affect multiple body systems.

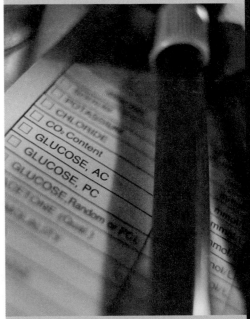

Direct and indirect health costs of diabetes are estimated to be $132 billion a year in the United States (or 1 out of every 10 healthcare dollars).[3] The death rate among middle-age people with diabetes is double the death rate of those who do not have diabetes. Diabetes causes preventable complications that can be life threatening, including heart disease. Lifestyle changes can delay the progression of diabetes, as can controlling blood glucose, lipids, and blood pressure.

NATURE OF DIABETES

History

The metabolic disease we know today as diabetes mellitus has been with us for a long time. Ancient records describe its devastating effects as observed by early healers. In the first century AD, the Greek physician Aretaeus wrote of a malady in which the body "ate its own flesh" and gave off large quantities of urine. He gave it the name *diabetes,* from the Greek word meaning "siphon" or "to pass through." Much later, in the seventeenth century, the word *mellitus,* from the Latin word for "honey," was added because of the sweet nature of the urine. This addition also distinguished it from diabetes insipidus (*insipid,* meaning "tasteless, or not sweet"), another disorder, although uncommon, in which the passage of copious amounts of urine had been observed. Today, use of the single name diabetes always means diabetes mellitus.

As medical knowledge began to grow, early clinicians—such as Rollo in England and Boushardat in France—observed that diabetes became less severe in overweight patients who lost weight. Later another French physician, Lancereaux, and his students described two kinds of diabetes: diabete gras—"fat diabetes," and diabete maigre—"thin diabetes."[4] All of these observations preceded any knowledge about insulin or any relation to the pancreas. During these times, which have aptly been called the "diabetic dark ages," persons with diabetes had short lives and were maintained on a variety of semistarvation diets.[5]

Later, evidence began to point to the pancreas as a primary organ involved in the disease process. Paul Langerhans (1847-1888), a young German medical student, found special clusters—or islets—of cells scattered throughout the human pancreas that were different from the rest of the tissue. Although their function was still unknown, these special islet cells were named for their young discoverer: the *islets of Langerhans.* Research at that time focused on the pancreas. Finally, in the years of 1921 and 1922 a University of Toronto team discovered and successfully used the controlling agent from the "island cells," naming it insulin for its source.[6]

Classification

The American Diabetes Association classifies diabetes into the following four categories[2]:

1. Type 1 diabetes (T1DM), formerly called *insulin-dependent diabetes mellitus*
2. Type 2 diabetes (T2DM), formerly called *non–insulin-dependent diabetes mellitus*
3. Gestational diabetes mellitus (GDM)
4. Impaired glucose tolerance (IGT) and impaired fasting glucose (IFG) (sometimes called *prediabetes*).

The terms *insulin-dependent diabetes mellitus* and *non–insulin-dependent diabetes mellitus* and their acronyms, *IDDM* and *NIDDM,* should no longer be used because they are confusing and have often resulted in classifying patients based on treatment rather than cause of their diabetes.[2]

T1DM is characterized by sudden, severe insulin deficiency requiring insulin therapy to prevent ketoacidosis, coma, and death. T1DM generally appears during childhood or adolescence and accounts for 5% to 10% of the cases of diabetes. However, T1DM can occur at any age, and almost half of new cases are diagnosed after 20 years of age. There are two forms of T1DM: immune-mediated diabetes and idiopathic diabetes. Immune-mediated diabetes results from a cellular-mediated autoimmune destruction of the beta cells of the pancreas.[7] Idiopathic diabetes has no known etiology.

Onset of T1DM is often rapid, accompanied by classic symptoms of weight loss and increased urination and thirst, especially if a viral infection or other stress increases the need for insulin. Onset may be less acute or there may be a "honeymoon period" of 6 to 12 months in which the diabetes may appear to be "cured" after an initial acute onset and initiation of insulin therapy. Destruction of the beta cells in the pancreas and loss of insulin production are usually gradual, accounting for the honeymoon period after insulin therapy restores normal glucose and metabolic stress is resolved.

T2DM is associated with insulin resistance and obesity combined with inadequate insulin produced in the pancreatic beta cells to compensate for the insulin resistance or an insulin secretory defect with insulin resistance.[2] T2DM accounts for 90% to 95% of all cases of diabetes, and symptoms may include poor wound healing, blurred vision, or recurrent gum or bladder infections. Many individuals are not symptomatic, and the diabetes may be detected as the result of a routine blood test. Obesity and physical inactivity are strong risk factors for T2DM.[8-10] A large waist circumference is considered to be a biomarker for insulin resistance and the metabolic syndrome associated with diabetes, hypertension, and dyslipidemia (typically low high-density cholesterol and elevated triglyceride levels).[11] Although T2DM is associated with insulin resistance and is typically diagnosed after 40 years of age, it is occurring in epidemic proportions in younger populations, including children and adolescents. Called *type 2 diabetes in the young,* the incidence and prevalence of T2DM in children have increased thirtyfold during the past 20 years.[12-18] Obesity is the most prominent clinical risk factor for T2DM,[15] and it is becoming more common among Native American/American Indian, black, and Hispanic and Latino children and adolescents.[1]

GDM is defined as carbohydrate intolerance of variable severity with onset or first recognition during pregnancy. GDM develops in 2% to 5% of all pregnancies, and 30% to 40% of women with GDM are likely to develop T2DM.[19] In both T2DM and GDM, there is a relative insulin deficiency because the pancreas fails to produce the level of insulin needed to compensate for insulin resistance.

If cross-sectional data were applied to the 2000 U.S. population, about 35 million adults (ages 40 to 74) would have IFG, 16 million would have IGT, and 41 million would have prediabetes.[1] *Prediabetes* is a term used to distinguish people at increased risk of developing diabetes. People are considered to have prediabetes if they have IFG and/or IGT. Some people have both.[1] IFG is identified through fasting blood glucose, and IGT is identified by an oral glucose tolerance test (OGTT).[12] Formerly called *borderline diabetes,* IFG, IGT, and prediabetes are associated with greater risk of heart disease and subsequent development of diabetes. Research has shown lifestyle interventions can reduce the rate of progression to T2DM.[20-22] Table 21-1 outlines criteria used to diagnose diabetes.

Contributing Causes

Genetics

For some time, early insulin assay tests developed to measure level of insulin activity in blood found insulin-like activity in diabetes to be two or three times normal insulin levels. It is now evident diabetes is a syndrome with multiple forms, resulting from (1) lack of insulin and/or (2) insulin resistance.[2]

Diabetes has long been associated with excess body weight, since the early observations of differences in "fat diabetes" and "thin diabetes."[4] Current research has reinforced the relation of overweight state to development of diabetes. Obesity can increase circulating insulin levels, which will ultimately lead to increased insulin resistance. In addition, individuals with a family history may have mutations on genes that control insulin production or may inherit insulin resistance not directly related to obesity. Thus multiple genetic mutations may interact to increase the risk of T2DM.

Diabetes has often been defined in terms of heredity, but increasing evidence indicates there is considerable genetic variation between the two main types of diabetes. Studies of T1DM have shown an autoimmune attack by

the body's insulin-producing cells is at fault, but its development is also associated with viruses such as coxsackievirus, mumps, and rubella. Insulin resistance is common in Western societies and sometimes termed *metabolic syndrome.* Insulin resistance is associated with a variety of conditions, including obesity, hypertension, hyperlipidemia, and hyperuricemia, as well as a sedentary lifestyle.[23]

Environmental Role: "Thrifty Gene"

Environmental factors apparently play a role in unmasking the underlying genetic susceptibility, a "thrifty" diabetic genotype that probably developed from primitive times for survival. This theory indicates diabetes may be associated with past genetic modifications for survival during varying periods of food availability. Gene mutations and the "thrifty" trait associated with T2DM facilitated more efficient use of limited food during times under difficult survival conditions. As food supplies became more plentiful, negative aspects of the "thrifty" trait began to appear. Such is indeed the case, for example, with the experience of Pima Indians in Arizona, as earlier studies and recent archaeological excavations there have indicated.[23-25] In earlier times this group ate a limited diet mainly of carbohydrate foods harvested through heavy physical labor in a primitive agriculture. Now, however, with the "progress" of civilization, Pimas have become obese, and half of the adults have T2DM, the highest reported rate of this type of diabetes in the world. Native Americans develop diabetes at almost three times the rate of whites. This same pattern is seen among populations of now-urbanized Pacific Islanders, South

diabetes insipidus A condition of the pituitary gland and insufficiency of one of its hormones, vasopressin (antidiuretic hormone); characterized by a copious output of a nonsweet urine, great thirst, and sometimes a large appetite. However, in diabetes insipidus these symptoms result from a specific injury to the pituitary gland, not a collection of metabolic disorders as in diabetes mellitus. The injured pituitary gland produces less vasopressin, a hormone that normally helps the kidneys reabsorb adequate water.

insulin Hormone formed in the beta cells of the islets of Langerhans in the pancreas. It is secreted when blood glucose and amino acid levels rise and assists their entry into body cells. It also promotes glycogenesis and conversion of glucose into fat and inhibits lipolysis and gluconeogenesis (protein breakdown). Commercial insulin is manufactured from pigs and cows; new "artificial" human insulin products have recently been made available.

TABLE 21-1	**Criteria for Diagnosing Diabetes**

Diabetes Type	Former Term(s)	Etiology	Criteria
Type 1 diabetes*: immune-mediated or idiopathic	Insulin-dependent diabetes mellitus (IDDM), type 1 diabetes, juvenile-onset diabetes, ketosis-prone diabetes, brittle diabetes	Beta cell destruction, usually leading to absolute insulin deficiency	Symptoms† of diabetes mellitus and casual plasma glucose ≥200 mg/dl (*Casual* is defined as any time of day without regard to last meal.) **OR**
Type 2 diabetes (adults)	Non–insulin-dependent diabetes mellitus (NIDDM), type 2 diabetes, adult-onset diabetes, maturity-onset diabetes, ketosis-resistant diabetes, stable diabetes	Insulin resistance with insulin secretory defect	Fasting plasma glucose (FPG) ≥126 mg/dl (*Fasting* is defined as no kilocaloric intake for at least 8 hr.) **OR** 2-hr postprandial plasma glucose (PPG) ≥200 mg/dl during oral glucose tolerance test (OGTT) (performed as described by the World Health Organization using glucose load containing the equivalent of 75 g anhydrous glucose dissolved in water)
Type 2 diabetes (children)			Overweight (body mass index [BMI] >85th percentile for age and gender, weight for height >85th percentile, or weight >120% of ideal for height) **PLUS** Any two of the following: • Family history of type 2 DM in first- or second-degree relative • Native American, African American, Latino, Asian American, Pacific Islander • Signs of insulin resistance or conditions associated with insulin resistance (acanthosis nigricans, hypertension [HTN], dyslipidemia, or polycystic ovary syndrome [PCOS])
Gestational diabetes (GDM)	Gestational diabetes, type 3 diabetes		*One-step approach:* Diagnostic OGTT *Two-step approach:* Initial screening to measure plasma or serum glucose concentration 1 hr after 50 g oral glucose load (glucose challenge test [GCT]) and perform diagnostic OGTT on those women exceeding glucose threshold value on GCT. Glucose threshold ≥140 mg/dl identifies ~80% of women with GDM
Impaired glucose tolerance (IGT)	Borderline diabetes, chemical diabetes		2-hr PPG ≥140 mg/dl and <200 mg/dl

Modified from American Diabetes Association: Standards of medical care for patients with diabetes mellitus, *Diabetes Care* 25(1 suppl)S33, 2002, with permission from The American Diabetes Association.

DM, Diabetes mellitus.

*Patients with any form of diabetes may require insulin treatment at some stage of their disease. Such use of insulin does not classify the patient as having type 1 diabetes.

†Symptoms include polyuria, polydipsia, and unexplained weight loss.

Asians, Asian Indians, and Creoles, although less is know about the exact numbers.[8,9] Other at-risk populations include Hispanic/Latino Americans, who are 1.5 times as likely to develop diabetes as whites, and blacks, who develop diabetes at 1.6 times the rate of whites.[1] Thus evidence suggests these groups have a genetic susceptibility to T2DM (diabetic genotype) and the disease is triggered by environmental factors, including obesity (see the *Focus on Culture* box, "Type 2 Diabetes: An Equal Opportunity Disease?"). Several specific genes involved in energy metabolism are thought to increase the risk for developing obesity and/or T2DM. As we commonly observe, lifestyle

FOCUS ON CULTURE

Type 2 Diabetes: An Equal Opportunity Disease?

Type 2 diabetes (T2DM) occurs disproportionately in people of color throughout the United States. Not only are rates of T2DM two to six times higher in Native Americans, Alaska Natives, blacks, and Hispanic Americans than in the non-Hispanic white population, but also people of color experience onset at an earlier age and complications are more harsh. Although the cause for these ethnic disparities has not been identified, it is hypothesized differences may lie in the interaction of inherent susceptibility and modifiable risk factors such as physical inactivity and poor diet.

Ethnic Group	Number With Diabetes	Prevalence (Ages 20+)	Additional Information
Non-Hispanic whites	12.5 million	8.4%	Diagnosis 2.2 times more likely than whites
Native Americans	107,775	14.5% of the population: 6.8% among Alaska Natives, 27% among Native Americans	Pima tribe has highest rate of diabetes in the world: 50% Complications of diabetes are major causes of death and health problems in most Native American populations
Blacks	2.7 million	11.4%	Diagnosis 1.6 times more likely 25% between ages 65 and 74 have diabetes 1 in 4 women over 55 years of age has diabetes
Latinos	2 million	8.2%	Diagnosis 1.5 times more likely Approximately 24% of Mexican Americans have diabetes Approximately 26% of Puerto Rican Americans have diabetes Nearly 18% of Cuban Americans have diabetes

References

American Diabetes Association: *National diabetes fact sheet,* Alexandria, Va, 2005, Author. Retrieved February 9, 2006, from *www.diabetes.org/uedocuments/NationalDiabetesFactSheetRev.pdf.*
American Diabetes Association: *Total prevalence of diabetes and prediabetes,* Alexandria, Va, Author. Retrieved January 18, 2006, from *www.diabetes.org/diabetes-statistics/prevalence.jsp.*

Brown TL: Ethnic populations. In Ross TA, Boucher JL, O'Connell BS, eds: *American Dietetic Association guide to diabetes medical nutrition therapy and education,* Chicago, 2005, American Dietetic Association.
Hosey G, Gordon S, Levine A: Type 2 diabetes in people of color, *Nurse Pract Forum* 9:108, 1998.

(dietary and physical activity habits) can interact with genetics in the development of T2DM.

Symptoms

Symptoms of T1DM in its uncontrolled state include the following:

- Increased thirst (polydipsia)
- Increased urination (polyuria)
- Increased hunger (polyphagia)
- Weight loss (more common with T1DM)
- Fruity smell to breath (symptom of ketoacidosis)
- Fatigue or weakness

These symptoms occur because in an insulin-deficient state, glucose is filtered by the kidney into urine rather than being used by cells for energy. Urine volume increases as the level of glucose excreted increases, and the body compensates for this abnormal state by breaking down fat. Ketones are formed as the result of using fat as a primary energy source.

T2DM may be asymptomatic, or symptoms may be more subtle and may include the following:

- Poor wound healing or recurrent infections
- Blurred vision (result of effects of hyperglycemia on shape of the cornea, which is returned to normal after glucose levels are stabilized)
- Skin irritation or infection
- Recurrent gum or bladder infections

Classic symptoms of diabetes are the result of short-term effects of hyperglycemia. These symptoms are reversible if blood glucose levels are returned to a normal or near-normal level.

The Metabolic Pattern of Diabetes

Overall Energy Balance and the Energy Nutrients

Because initial symptoms of glycosuria and hyperglycemia are related to excess glucose, historically diabetes was called a disease of carbohydrate metabolism. However, as more becomes known about the intimate interrelationships of carbohydrate, fat, and protein metabolism, we view it in more general terms. It is a metabolic disorder resulting from lack of insulin (absolute, partial, or unavailable) affecting more or less each basic energy nutrient. It is especially related to metabolism of the two fuels—carbohydrate and fat—in the body's overall energy system.

Normal Blood Glucose Control

Control of blood glucose level within its normal range of 70 to 120 mg/dl (3.9 to 6.7 mmol/L) is vital to normal overall fuel metabolism and other metabolic functions. A knowledge of factors involved in maintaining a normal blood glucose level is essential to understanding the impairment of these factors (see Chapters 2 and 3). An overview of these normal balancing controls is illustrated in Figure 21-1.

Sources of Blood Glucose

Two sources of blood glucose ensure a constant supply of this primary body fuel: (1) diet, energy nutrients in our food (i.e., dietary carbohydrate, protein, and fat), and (2) glycogen, backup source from constant turnover of "stored" liver glycogen by a process called glycogenolysis.

Uses of Blood Glucose

To prevent continued rise of blood glucose above normal limits, several basic uses for blood glucose are constantly available according to need. These include the following: (1) glycogenesis, conversion of glucose to glycogen for "storage" in liver and muscle; (2) lipogenesis, conversion of glucose to fat and storage in adipose tissue; and (3) glycolysis, cell oxidation of glucose for energy.

Pancreatic Hormonal Controls

The following three types of islet cells scattered in clusters throughout the pancreas (islets of Langerhans) provide hormones closely interbalanced in the regulation of blood glucose levels.

1. *Alpha cells:* Arranged around the outer rim of the islets are alpha cells, one to two cells thick, making up about 30% of the total cells. These cells synthesize glucagon.
2. *Beta cells:* The largest portion of islets is occupied by beta cells filling the central zone or about 60% of the gland. These primary cells synthesize insulin.
3. *Delta cells:* Interspersed between alpha and beta cells—or occasionally between alpha cells alone—are delta cells, the remaining 10% of total cells. These cells synthesize somatostatin.

This specific arrangement of human islet cells is illustrated in Figure 21-2.

Interrelated Hormone Functions

Juncture points of the three types of islet cells act as sensors of blood glucose concentration and its rate of change. They constantly adjust and balance the rate of secretion of insulin, glucagon, and somatostatin to match whatever conditions prevail at any time. Each of

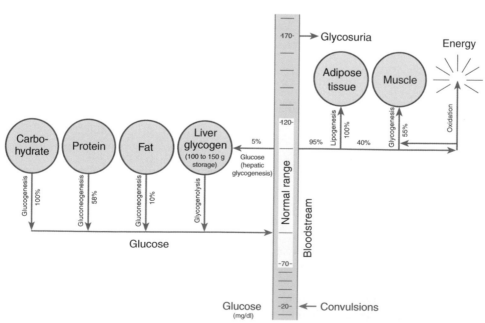

FIGURE 21-1 Sources of blood glucose (food and stored glycogen) and normal routes of control.

the following three hormones has specific interbalanced functions:

1. *Insulin:* Although precise mechanisms are not entirely clear in every case, insulin has a profound effect on glucose control. It functions extensively in the metabolism of all three energy nutrients, as follows:

   - Insulin facilitates transport of glucose through cell membranes by way of special insulin receptors. These receptors are located on the membrane of insulin-sensitive cells, including those in adipose tissue, muscle tissue, and monocytes. Researchers are reaching a better understanding of these special receptors and how to treat the disease by studying insulin receptors.[26] These insulin receptors mediate all metabolic effects of insulin. Research has shown that cells of obese persons with diabetes have fewer than the normal number of insulin receptors. Weight loss in obese individuals and physical exercise increase the number of these receptors. The insulin receptor also appears to control several metabolic steps within the cell.
   - Insulin enhances conversion of glucose to glycogen and its consequent storage in the liver (glycogenesis).
   - Insulin stimulates conversion of glucose to fat (lipogenesis) for storage as adipose tissue.
   - Insulin inhibits fat breakdown (lipolysis) and the breakdown of protein.
   - Insulin promotes uptake of amino acids by skeletal muscles, thus increasing protein synthesis.
   - Insulin influences glucose oxidation through the main glycolytic pathway.

2. *Glucagon:* The hormone glucagon functions as a balancing antagonist to insulin. It rapidly causes breakdown of liver glycogen, and—to a lesser extent—fatty acids from adipose tissue to serve as body fuel. This action raises blood glucose levels to protect the brain and other body tissues. It helps maintain normal blood glucose levels during fasting hours of sleep. A lowering of the blood glucose concentration, increased amino acid concentrations, or sympathetic nervous system stimulation triggers glucagon secretion.

3. *Somatostatin:* Although pancreatic islet delta cells are the major source of somatostatin, this hormone is also synthesized and secreted in different regions of the body, including the hypothalamus. It acts in balance with insulin and glucose to inhibit their interactions as needed to maintain normal blood glucose levels. It also helps regulate blood glucose levels by inhibiting the release of a number of other hormones as needed.

Endocrine Function of Fat Cells

Historically the primary role of body fat was considered to be stored energy, and its role in secreting peptides was largely unknown. With the discovery of leptin in the 1990s, a growing number of peptides secreted from fat have been identified. These peptides appear to have an endocrine function and may play an important role in regulating appetite, body weight, and aspects of glucose metabolism.

glycogenolysis Production of blood glucose from liver glycogen.

glycogenesis Synthesis of glycogen from blood glucose.

lipogenesis Synthesis of fat from blood glucose.

glycolysis Cell oxidation of glucose for energy.

glucagon A polypeptide hormone secreted by the alpha cells of the pancreatic islets of Langerhans in response to hypoglycemia; has an opposite balancing effect to that of insulin, raising the blood sugar, and thus is used as a quick-acting antidote for the hypoglycemic reaction of insulin. It stimulates the breakdown of glycogen (glycogenolysis) in the liver by activating the liver enzyme phosphorylase and thus raises blood sugar levels during fasting states to ensure adequate levels for normal nerve and brain function.

somatostatin A hormone formed in the delta cells of the pancreatic islets of Langerhans and the hypothalamus. It is a balancing factor in maintaining normal blood glucose levels by inhibiting insulin and glucagon production in the pancreas as needed.

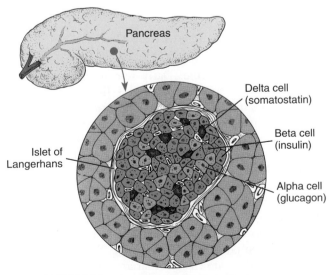

FIGURE 21-2 Islets of Langerhans, located in the pancreas.

Metabolic Changes in Diabetes

In uncontrolled diabetes, insulin is lacking to facilitate operation of normal blood glucose controls; abnormal metabolic changes occur, as follows, that affect glucose, fat, and protein and account for symptoms of diabetes:

- *Glucose:* Blood glucose cannot be oxidized properly through the main glycolytic pathway in the cell to furnish energy (see Chapter 5). Therefore it builds up in the blood (hyperglycemia).
- *Fat:* Formation of fat (lipogenesis) is curtailed, and fat breakdown (lipolysis) increases. This leads to excess formation and accumulation of ketones (ketoacidosis). Appearance of the major ketone, acetone, in urine indicates development of ketoacidosis.
- *Protein:* Tissue protein is also broken down in an effort to secure energy. This causes weight loss and nitrogen excretion in the urine.

GENERAL MANAGEMENT OF DIABETES

Treatment Goals

Basic Objectives

The diabetes healthcare team—physician, dietitian, nurse, and person with diabetes—is guided by the following three basic objectives in the care of each person with diabetes:

1. *Maintain optimal nutrition.* The first objective is to fulfill the basic nutritional requirement for health, growth and development, and a desirable body weight.
2. *Prevent hypoglycemia or hyperglycemia.* This second objective is designed to keep the person relatively free of hypoglycemia or insulin reaction, which requires immediate countermeasures, and hyperglycemia, which, if untreated, contributes to more serious ketoacidosis or diabetic coma.
3. *Prevent complications.* The third objective recognizes increased risk a person with diabetes faces for developing complicating problems that reflect damaging effects of chronic diabetes on tissues of small and large blood vessels and peripheral nerves.[27,28] These damages may occur in tissues such as eyes (retinopathy), nerves (neuropathy), and kidneys (nephropathy). In addition, coronary artery disease occurs in persons with diabetes about 4 times as often as in the general population. Peripheral vascular disease occurs about 40 times as often.

In all of these areas there is evidence consistent, well-planned food habits and exercise, balanced as needed

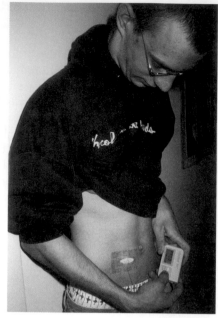

FIGURE 21-3   Insulin injecting using an insulin pump. *(From Peckenpaugh NJ: Nutrition essentials and diet therapy, ed 9, Philadelphia, 2003, Saunders.)*

with early aggressive insulin therapy, can significantly help normalize metabolism and thereby reduce risks of these potentially serious complications.[29]

This aggressive insulin therapy consists of multiple daily injections or continuous subcutaneous infusion by an insulin pump (Figure 21-3). Self-monitoring of blood glucose (SMBG) levels is used to guide decisions to improve glycemic control. The added cardiovascular risk associated with diabetes is reflected in having blood pressure and lipid goals for diabetes management that are similar to those used in treating individuals who have diagnosed cardiovascular disease (Table 21-2).

Self-Care Role of the Person With Diabetes

To effectively control diabetes, the person with diabetes must play a central role. Daily self-discipline and informed self-care, supported by a skilled and sensitive healthcare team, are required for sound diabetes management. Ultimately, all persons with diabetes must treat themselves. This is especially true with the tighter normal blood glucose control currently being used, with frequent SMBG and multiple insulin injections or an insulin infusion pump. Thus there is even greater need now for comprehensive diabetes education programs that encourage self-monitoring and self-care responsibility. Diabetes-related issues also need to be addressed as an integral component of primary care. Weight, activity, variety, and excess are themes that are relevant for assessing basic needs and providing basic recommendations.

TABLE 21-2	Metabolic Goals in Diabetes Management		

Indicator	Normal Value	Goal	Additional Action Suggested*
Plasma values (mg/dl)			
Average preprandial glucose	<110	90-130	<90/>150
Average bedtime glucose	<120	110-150	<110/>180
Whole blood values† (mg/dl)			
Average preprandial glucose	<100	80-120	<80/>140
Average bedtime glucose	<110	100-140	<100/>160
Hb_{A1c} (%)	<6	<7	>8
LDL cholesterol		<100 mg/dl	
HDL cholesterol		Men: >55 mg/dl	
		Women: >55 mg/dl	
Triglycerides		<150 mg/dl	
Blood pressure		<130/80	

Modified from American Diabetes Association: Standards of medical care for patients with diabetes mellitus, *Diabetes Care* 25(1 suppl)S33, 2002, with permission from The American Diabetes Association.
  *Depends on individual patient circumstances.
  †Measurement of capillary blood glucose.

The WAVE pocket guide (Figure 21-4) was developed to help primary care providers to briefly assess needs and provide guidance to clients with diabetes or at risk for developing diabetes.[30]

RATIONALE FOR DIABETES NUTRITION THERAPY

Nutrition therapy (NT) for diabetes is multifaceted. Physicians and nurses can no longer rely on preprinted diet sheets to assume they are providing nutrition care for patients.[31] There is no standard "ADA" or "diabetic" diet. The American Diabetes Association does not sanction any single meal plan or specific percentages of nutrients.[32] It is essential that persons with diabetes are assessed by a registered dietitian to determine an appropriate nutrition prescription and plan for self-management education.[12,32] In addition, diet orders such as "no sugar added," "no concentrated sweets," "low sugar," and "liberal diabetic" are not considered suitable because they do not reflect diabetes nutritional recommendations and pointlessly restrict sucrose. Such meal plans support the erroneous concept that simply limiting sucrose-sweetened foods will enhance blood glucose control.[32]

Nutrition therapy (NT) should be individualized, taking usual eating habits and other lifestyle factors into consideration.[33] Consistency within an eating pattern will result in better glycemic control than abiding by an arbitrary eating style.[34] Nutrition recommendations are the same for individuals with diabetes as for the general population in regard to total fat, saturated fat, cholesterol, fiber, vitamins, and minerals. Recommendations

for protein, carbohydrates, sucrose, and alcohol are modified depending on the nature of diabetes in relation to carbohydrate metabolism or effects of complications.[31]

Type 1 Diabetes Mellitus

Recognizing the need for a more comprehensive program of care of diabetes, based on the individual metabolic balance concept and designed to help delay or avoid life-

retinopathy Noninflammatory disease of the retina—the visual tissue of the eye—characterized by microaneurysms, intraretinal hemorrhages, waxy yellow exudates, "cotton wool" patches, and macular edema; a complication of diabetes that may lead to proliferation of fibrous tissue, retinal detachment, and blindness.

neuropathy General term for functional and pathologic changes in the peripheral nervous system; in diabetes, a chronic sensory condition affecting mainly the nerves of the legs, marked by numbness from sensory impairment, loss of tendon reflexes, severe pain, weakness, and wasting of muscles involved.

nephropathy Disease of the kidneys; in diabetes, renal damage associated with functional and pathologic changes in the nephrons, which can lead to glomerulosclerosis and chronic renal failure.

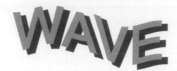

Assessment

Weight

Assess patient's Body Mass Index.*
Patient is overweight if BMI >25.

Height	Body Weight lbs.	Height	Body Weight lbs.
4'10"	≥119	5'8"	≥164
4'11"	≥124	5'9"	≥169
5'0"	≥128	5'10"	≥174
5'1"	≥132	5'11"	≥179
5'2"	≥136	6'0"	≥184
5'3"	≥141	6'1"	≥189
5'4"	≥145	6'2"	≥194
5'5"	≥150	6'3"	≥200
5'6"	≥155	6'4"	≥205
5'7"	≥159		

*Certain patients may require assessment for underweight and/or unintentional weight loss.

Activity

Ask patient about any physical activity in the past week: walking briskly, jogging, gardening, swimming, biking, dancing, golf, etc.
1. Does patient do **30 minutes** of moderate activity on **most days/wk.**?
2. Does patient do "lifestyle" activity like taking the **stairs** instead of elevators, etc.?
3. Does patient usually watch less than **2 hours of TV or videos/day**?

If patient answers **NO** to above questions, assess whether patient is willing to increase physical activity.

Variety

Is patient eating a variety of foods from important sections of the food pyramid?
  Grains (6-11 servings)
  Fruits (2-4 servings)
  Vegetables (3-5 servings)
  Protein (2-3 servings)
  Dairy (2-3 servings)

Determine **Variety** and **Excess** using one of the following methods:
• Do a quick 1-day recall.
• Ask patient to complete a self-administered eating pattern questionnaire.

Excess

Is patient eating too much:
  Fat? Saturated fat?
  Calories?
  Salt?
  Sugar?
  Alcohol?

• Ask about serving/portion sizes, preparation methods, and added fats like butter, mayonnaise, sour cream, salad dressing, etc.
• Does patient eat 4 or more meals from sit-down or take-out restaurants per week?
• Does patient indulge on the weekends?

• *What does patient think are pros/cons of his/her eating pattern?*
• *If patient needs to improve eating habits, assess willingness to make changes.*

 Nutrition Academic Award Program
Advancing nutrition, medical education, and clinical practice
Brown Medical School

FIGURE 21-4   WAVE assessment **(A)** and recommendations **(B)**. *(From Gans KM et al: REAP and WAVE: new tools to rapidly assess/discuss nutrition with patients, J Nutr 133{2 suppl} 556S, 2003, with permission from The American Society for Nutritional Sciences, on the format Textbook via the Copyright Cleareance Center.)*

threatening complications of this chronic disease, a national U.S. clinical research study supported by the National Institutes of Health was organized. The Diabetes Control and Complications Trial (DCCT)[29] involved 1441 subjects in 29 clinical centers across the country for approximately 10 years. The study was designed to compare the effects of intensive insulin therapy aimed at achieving blood glucose levels as close as possible to the normal nondiabetic range with effects of conventional therapy on early microvascular complications of T1DM.

The DCCT demonstrated that lowering Hb_{A1c} from 9% to 7% in the intensively treated group reduced the risk of the development or progression of eye, kidney, and neurologic complications by 50% to 75%.[12,35] Dietary strategies played an important role in achieving control in the intensively treated group.[36] Reduction in complications was linearly related to improvement in glycemic control, indicating risk reduction can be achieved even if intensification of treatment fails to achieve a near-normal Hb_{A1c}.[31,37] Adverse affects of intensive therapy included

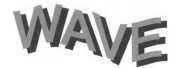 **Recommendations**

Weight	Activity

If patient is overweight:
 	
1. **State concern** for the patient, e.g., "I am concerned that your weight is affecting your health."
2. Give the patient **specific advice**, i.e.,
  a) **Make 1 or 2** changes in eating habits to reduce calorie intake as identified by diet assessment.
  b) Gradually increase activity/decrease inactivity.
  c) Enroll in a weight management program and/or consult a dietitian.
3. If patient is ready to make behavior changes, jointly **set goals** for a plan of action and arrange for follow-up.
4. **Give patient education materials/ resources.**
	Examples of moderate amounts of physical activity:
	
	• Walking 2 miles in 30 minutes
	• Stair walking for 15 minutes
	• Washing and waxing a car for 45-60 minutes
	• Gardening for 30-45 minues
	• Pushing a stroller 1½ miles in 30 minutes
	• Raking leaves for 30 minutes
	• Shoveling snow for 15 minutes
	
	1. If patient is ready to increase physical activity, jointly **set specific activity goals** and arrange for a follow-up
	2. **Give patient education materials/ resources.**

Variety	**Excess**

What is a serving?
 	
Grains (6-11 servings)
  1 slice bread or tortilla, ½ bagel, ½ roll, 1 oz. ready-to-eat cereal, ½ cup rice, pasta, or cooked cereal, 3-4 plain crackers
  Is patient eating whole grains?
Fruits (2-4 servings)
  1 medium fresh fruit, ⅓ cup chopped or canned fruit, ¾ cup fruit juice
Vegetables (3-5 servings)
  1 cup raw leafy vegetables, ½ cup cooked or chopped raw vegetables, ¾ cup vegetable juice
Protein (2-3 servings)
  2-3 oz. poultry, fish, or lean meat; 1-1½ cup cooked dry beans; 1 egg equals 1 oz. meat, 4 oz. (½ cup) tofu
Dairy (2-3 servings)
  1 cup milk or yogurt, 1½ oz. cheese
 	
See instructions 1-4 under Excess.
	How much is too much?
	
	Too much fat, saturated fat, calories
	• >6 oz/day of meat
	• Ice cream, high fat dairy products
	• Fried foods
	• High fat snacks and desserts
	• Eating out >4 meals/wk
	Too much sugar, calories
	• High sugar beverages
	• Sugary snacks/desserts
	Too much salt
	• Processed meats, canned/frozen meals, salty snacks, added salt
	1. **Discuss pros and cons** of patient's eating pattern, keeping in mind variety & excess.
	2. If patient is ready, jointly **set specific dietary goals** and arrange for follow-up.
	3. **Give patient education materials/ resources.**
	4. **Consider referral** to a dietitian for more extensive counseling and support.

B

FIGURE 21-4, cont'd See legend on p. 528.

a twofold to threefold increase in severe hypoglycemia and a weight gain of 10 lb (4.5 kg).[29] Initial weight was considerably higher, but providing consultation about overeating to prevent or treat hypoglycemia appears to attenuate the weight gain. The DCCT results indicated the strength of the expanded role of the registered dietitian, assisted as needed by the diabetes team nurse, in individualizing MNT with various diet management tools and insulin balance.[38,39]

Type 2 Diabetes Mellitus

The United Kingdom Prospective Diabetes Study (UKPDS) evaluated effects of treatments to improve glycemic control and cardiovascular risk factors in individuals with newly diagnosed diabetes. Glycemic control and cardiovascular risk reduction therapies reduced rates of both macrovascular and microvascular complications. The UKPDS confirmed DCCT findings with respect to preventing microvascular complications of diabetes and provided evidence that a comprehensive risk reduction approach could also reduce macrovascular complications.[40-43] The major cause of morbidity and mortality in persons with diabetes is cardiovascular disease. T2DM and its common coexisting conditions (e.g., hypertension and dyslipidemia) are considered to be independent risk factors for macrovascular disease.[12]

Gestational Diabetes Mellitus

For women with preexisting diabetes or GDM, risks of fetal abnormalities and mortality are increased in the presence of hyperglycemia. Maternal insulin does not cross the placenta, but glucose does, causing the fetus's pancreas to increase insulin production if the mother becomes hyperglycemic. This increased production of insulin causes macrosomia—the most typical characteristic of babies born to women with diabetes. Other problems such as hyperinsulinemia and hyperglycemia may occur.[44] Therefore every effort should be made to control blood glucose levels.[12] All women with GDM should receive counseling by a registered dietitian when possible.[45] Individualized MNT, contingent on maternal weight and height, should include provision of adequate kilocalories (kcalories or kcal) and nutrients to meet the needs of the pregnancy and be consistent with established maternal blood glucose goals.[45] At the start, SMBG should be planned 4 times a day (fasting and 1 or 2 hours postprandial).[46] Frequency can be decreased once glycemic control is established. Blood glucose goals during pregnancy are as follows[47]:

- *Fasting:* less than 95 mg/dl
- *1 Hour postprandial:* 140 mg/dl
- *2 Hours postprandial:* less than 120 mg/dl

IMPLEMENTING NUTRITION THERAPY

Nutrition intervention is governed by consideration of treatment goals and lifestyle changes the person with diabetes is ready to make, preferably to predetermined energy levels and percentages of carbohydrates, protein, and fat.[31] The objective of NT is to support and facilitate individual lifestyle and behavior changes that will lead to improved glycemic control.[31] Cultural and ethnic preferences should be taken into consideration, and persons with diabetes should be included in the decision-making process.[31]

Current nutrition principles and recommendations focus on lifestyle goals and strategies for treatment of diabetes. For the first time, the 2002 evidence-based nutrition recommendations purposely address lifestyle approaches to diabetes prevention because MNT for treating and managing diabetes may not necessarily be the same for preventing or delaying onset of diabetes.[31] Goals of NT that apply to all persons with diabetes are as follows[31]:

- Attain and maintain optimal metabolic outcomes, including the following:
  - Blood glucose levels in the normal (or near-normal) range
  - Lipid and lipoprotein profiles that reduce risk for macrovascular diseases
  - Blood pressure levels that reduce risk for vascular disease

- Prevent and treat chronic complications.
- Improve health through healthy food choices and physical activity.
- Address individual nutritional needs, taking into consideration personal and cultural preferences and lifestyle while respecting individuals' wishes and willingness to change.

Additional, more specific medical nutrition goals include the following[31]:

- *Youth with type 1 diabetes mellitus:* NT goals for children and adolescents with type 1 diabetes mellitus should ensure provision of sufficient energy for normal growth and development. Insulin regimens should be integrated into usual eating and physical activity habits.
- *Type 2 diabetes mellitus in children and adolescents:* Goals for NT for children and adolescents with T2DM should facilitate changes in eating and physical activity habits to decrease insulin resistance and enhance metabolic status.
- *Pregnant and lactating women:* NT goals for pregnant and lactating women should provide adequate energy and nutrients necessary for optimal pregnancy outcomes.
- *Older adults:* Nutritional and psychosocial needs of an aging individual should be provided in NT goals.
- *Individuals treated with insulin or insulin secretagogues:* Self-management education for treatment and prevention of hypoglycemia, acute illness, and exercise-related blood glucose problems should be included in MNT goals for individuals treated with insulin or insulin secretagogues.
- *Individuals at risk for diabetes:* For those at risk for developing diabetes, physical activity should be encouraged and food choices that facilitate moderate weight loss (or at least prevent weight gain) should be promoted.

NT recommendations for management of type 1 and type 2 diabetes mellitus are outlined in Table 21-3. In addition, any medications a person has been prescribed should be considered as well; certain foods and drinks may interfere with them (see *Diet-Medications Interactions* box, "Interactions With Diabetes Drugs").

ISSUES RELATED TO MEDICAL THERAPY

Insulin Therapy

The management goal for persons with T1DM is to maintain a normal blood glucose level as closely as possible.

---

macrosomia Unusually large size.

Nutrition principles and recommendations are classified into four categories according to levels of supporting evidence: A—those for which there is strong supporting evidence, B—some supporting evidence, C—limited supporting evidence, or D—those based on expert consensus.

Nutrition Recommendation	Grading
Carbohydrates	
Whole grains, fruits, vegetables, and low-fat milk should be included.	A
Total amount of carbohydrates in meals and snacks is more important than the source or type of carbohydrate.	A
Individuals receiving intensive insulin therapy should adjust their premeal insulin doses based on the carbohydrate content of the meal.	A
Individuals receiving fixed daily insulin doses should try to be consistent in day-to-day carbohydrate intake.	B
There is not sufficient evidence of long-term benefit to recommend or use of low-glycemic index diets as a primary strategy in food/meal planning for individuals with type 1 diabetes.	B
As for the general public, consumption of fiber should be encouraged.	B
Percentages of carbohydrates should be based on individual nutrition assessment.	B
Carbohydrate and monounsaturated fat together should provide 60%-70% of energy intake.	D
Nutritive Sweeteners	
Sucrose does not increase glycemia to a greater extent than isocaloric amounts of starch.	A
Sucrose and sucrose-containing food do not need to be restricted; however, if included in the food/meal plan, it should be substituted for other carbohydrate sources or, if added, be adequately covered with insulin or other glucose-lowering medication.	A
Fructose reduces postprandial glycemia when it replaces sucrose or starch.	B
Consumption of fructose in large amounts may have adverse effects on plasma lipids.	B
Use of sugar alcohols as sweetening agents appears to be safe.	B
Sugar alcohols may cause diarrhea, especially in children.	B
Use of added fructose as a sweetening agent is not recommended.	C
Sucrose and sucrose-containing food should be eaten in the context of a healthy diet, and the intake of other nutrients ingested with sucrose, such as fat, should be taken into account.	D
There is no reason to recommend avoidance of naturally occurring fructose in fruits, vegetables, and other food.	D
It is unlikely sugar alcohols in amounts ingested in individual food servings or meals will contribute to a significant reduction in total energy or carbohydrate intake (although no studies have been conducted to support this).	D

Nutrition Recommendation	Grading
Resistant Starches	
Resistant starches (nondigestible) have no established benefit.	C
Nonnutritive Sweeteners	
Nonnutritive sweeteners are safe when consumed within the acceptable daily intake established by the FDA.	A
It is unknown if use of nonnutritive sweeteners improves long-term glycemic control or assists in weight loss.	D
Dietary Protein	
In those with controlled type 2 diabetes, ingested protein does not increase plasma glucose concentrations, although ingested protein is just as potent a stimulant of insulin secretion as carbohydrate.	A
There is no evidence to suggest that usual protein intake (15%-20% of total daily energy) should be modified if renal function is normal.	B
Protein requirements may be greater than the RDA, but not greater than usual intake for those with less-than-optimal glycemic control.	B
Dietary protein does not slow absorption of carbohydrate and dietary protein and carbohydrate do not raise plasma glucose later than carbohydrate alone and thus do not prevent late-onset hypoglycemia.	B
It may be prudent to avoid protein intake >20% of total daily energy.	C
Long-term effects of diets high in protein and low in carbohydrate are unknown. Although such diets may produce short-term weight loss and improved glycemia, it has not been established that weight loss is maintained. Long-term effect of such diets on plasma LDL cholesterol is also a concern.	D
Dietary Fat	
In all, <10% of energy intake should be derived from saturated fats. Some (i.e., those with LDL cholesterol ≥100 mg/dl) may benefit from lowering saturated fat intake to <7% of energy intake.	A
Dietary cholesterol intake should be <300 mg/day. Some (i.e., those with LDL cholesterol ≥100 mg/dl) may benefit from lowering dietary cholesterol to <200 mg/day.	A
Intake of transunsaturated fatty acids should be minimized.	A
Current fat replacers/substitutes approved by the FDA are safe for use in food.	A
To lower plasma LDL cholesterol, energy derived from saturated fat can be reduced if concurrent weight loss is desirable or replaced with carbohydrate or monounsaturated fat if weight loss is not a goal.	A

FDA, Food and Drug Administration; *RDA,* Recommended Dietary Allowance; *LDL,* low-density lipoprotein.

Continued

TABLE 21-3 Summary of 2002 Medical Nutrition Therapy Recommendations for Diabetes Mellitus—cont'd

Nutrition Recommendation	Grading	Nutrition Recommendation	Grading
Dietary Fat—cont'd		**Micronutrients**	
Polyunsaturated fat intake should be ~10% of energy intake.	B	There is no clear evidence of benefit from vitamin and mineral supplementation for persons who do not have underlying deficiencies. Exceptions include folate for prevention of birth defects and calcium for prevention of bone disease.	B
In weight-maintaining diets, when monounsaturated fat replaces carbohydrate, it may beneficially affect postprandial glycemia and plasma triglycerides but not necessarily fasting plasma glucose of Hb_{A1c}.	B	Although difficult to ascertain, if deficiencies of vitamins and minerals are identified, supplementation can be beneficial.	B
Incorporation of 2 or 3 servings of plant stanols/sterols (~2 g) food/day, substituted for similar food, will lower total and LDL cholesterol.	B	Routine supplementation of the diet with antioxidants is not advised because of uncertainties related to long-term efficacy and safety.	B
Reduced-fat diets when maintained long term, contribute to modest loss of weight and improvement of dyslipidemia.	B	Select populations, such as elderly individuals, pregnant or lactating women, strict vegetarians, and people on kilocalorie-restricted diets, may benefit from supplementation with a multivitamin preparation.	D
Two or more servings of fish per week provide dietary n-3 polyunsaturated fat and can be recommended.	C	There is no evidence to suggest long-term benefit from herbal preparations.	D
Monounsaturated fat and carbohydrate together should provide 60%-70% of energy intake. However, increasing fat intake may result in increased energy intake.	D	**Alcohol**	
Fat intake should be individualized and designed to fit ethnic and cultural backgrounds.	D	If individuals choose to drink alcohol, daily intake should be limited to 1 drink for adult women and 2 drinks for adult men. One drink is defined as a 12-oz beer, 5-oz glass of wine, or 1.5-oz glass of distilled spirits.	A
Use of low-fat food and fat replacers/substitutes may reduce total fat and energy intake and thereby facilitate weight loss.	D	The type of alcoholic beverage consumed does not make a difference.	A
Energy Balance and Obesity		When moderate amounts of alcohol are consumed with food, blood glucose levels are not affected.	A
In insulin-resistant individuals, reduced energy intake and modest weight loss improve insulin resistance and glycemia in the short term.	A	To reduce risk of hypoglycemia, alcohol should be consumed with food.	A
Structured programs that emphasize lifestyle changes, including education, reduced fat (<30% daily energy) and energy intake, regular physical activity, and regular participant contact can produce long-term weight loss of 5%-7% of starting weight.	A	Ingestion of light-to-moderate amounts of alcohol does not raise blood pressure; excessive, chronic ingestion of alcohol raises blood pressure and may be a risk factor for stroke.	A
Exercise and behavior modification are most useful as adjuncts to other weight-loss strategies. Exercise is helpful in maintaining weight loss.	A	Pregnant women and people with medical problems such as pancreatitis, advanced neuropathy, severe hypertriglyceridemia, or alcohol abuse should be advised not to ingest alcohol.	A
Nutrition interventions, such as standard weight-reduction diets, when used alone are unlikely to produce long-term weight loss. Structured, intensive lifestyle programs are necessary.	A	There are potential benefits from ingestion of moderate amounts of alcohol, such as decreased risk of type 2 diabetes, coronary heart disease, and stroke.	B
Optimal strategies for preventing and treating obesity long term have yet to be defined.	A	Alcoholic beverages should be consumed in addition to the regular food/meal plan for all patients with diabetes. No food should be omitted.	D
Currently available weight-loss drugs have modest beneficial effects. These drugs should be used only in people with BMI >27.0 kg/m^2.	B		
Gastric reduction surgery can be considered for patients with BMI >35.0 kg/m^2. Long-term data comparing benefits and risks of gastric reduction surgery to those of medical therapy are not available.	C		

DIET-MEDICATIONS INTERACTIONS

Interactions With Diabetes Drugs

Drug Class	Drug Name(s)	Interactions
Alpha-glucosidase inhibitors	Acarbose: Precose Miglitol: Glyset	Take with first bite of main meal Limit alcohol

Biguanides	Metformin: Glucophage
	Metformin and glibenclamide:
	  Glucovance, Glucophage +
	  Glyburide
		Take with meals to decrease GI distress
		May cause anorexia
		Avoid alcohol

Insulin and related agents	Insulin mixtures, intermediate
	  acting, long-acting, rapid-
	  acting, short-acting
		May increase weight
		Use alcohol with caution and under advice from
		  physician (alcohol increases hypoglycemic effect of
		  insulin)
		Large weight gain increases insulin needs

Meglitinides (nonsulfonylurea insulin releasers)	Nateglinide: Starlix Repaglinide: Prandin	Take 15-30 minutes before meals May increase weight Tooth disorders Nausea/vomiting Diarrhea/constipation Limit alcohol May increase risk of hypoglycemia in malnutrition
Sulfonylureas	Acetohexamide: Dymelor Tolazamide: Tolinase Tolbutamide: Orinase Chlorpropamide: Diabinese	Take with first meal of the day Nausea Avoid alcohol Increased risk of hypoglycemia in geriatric or malnourished patients

Sulfonylureas—second
generation
	Glimepiride: Amaryl
	Glyburide: DiaBeta, Micronase,
	  Glynase PresTabs
		Take 30 minutes before first meal of the day
		Hyperglycemia with high doses of nicotinic acid
		May increase or decrease appetite
		Increased weight
		Dyspepsia, nausea
		Constipation/diarrhea
		Avoid alcohol
		Possible hypoglycemia in geriatric or malnourished
		  patients

Thiazolidinediones (TZDs)	Pioglitazone: Actos Rosiglitazone: Avandia	Take once a day without regard to food Increased weight

Pramlintide	Symlin	Used with insulin, an increased risk of insulin-induced
		  severe hypoglycemia, particularly in patients with
		  T1DM; seen usually within 3 hours of injection

Exenatide	Byetta	Combined with sulfonylureas, or Byetta with both
		  metformin and a sulfonylurea, hypoglycemia can
		  occur

References

American Diabetes Association: *Other diabetes medications,* Alexandria, Va, Author. Retrieved January 18, 2006, from *www.diabetes.org/type-2-diabetes/oral-medications.jsp.*

Pronsky ZM: *Food medication interactions,* ed 13, Birchrunville, Pa, 2004, Food-Medication Interactions.

RxList [website], Rancho Santa Fe, Calif, 2005, Author. Available at *www.rxlist.com.* Accessed January 18, 2005.

GI, Gastrointestinal; *T1DM,* type 1 diabetes.

Strong evidence from the DCCT, as well as accumulating practice experience, indicates that maintaining such a "normoglycemic" state helps prevent the chronic complications of long-term uncontrolled hyperglycemia.[28,48] To achieve this goal, more intensive insulin therapy with the different types of insulin now available is being used. Insulin is increasingly being used as adjunctive therapy in T2DM.

Types of Insulin

A number of insulin preparations are available for therapeutic use, and new ones are constantly being developed to meet medical care needs for individual patients and market changes. Individual responses to these insulins are highly variable. According to time of action, they are

(1) rapid-acting, (2) intermediate-acting, and (3) long-acting, as follows:

1. *Rapid-acting insulins:* These insulins have various names, depending on the manufacturer (e.g., Humulin R, Regular, Semilente, and Velosulin R). Rapid-acting insulins have their onset of action within approximately $\frac{1}{2}$ hour after injection and stay in the body for less than 5 hours. This type of insulin peaks about 2 hours after injection. A recently developed human insulin analogue, Humalog (generic name, insulin lispro), approved by the Food and Drug Administration in 1996, has the shortest time-action curve of any insulin currently available.[49,50] Short-acting insulins have their onset of action in $\frac{1}{2}$ to 1 hour and have a 6- to 8-hour duration. Short-acting insulins peak around 3 hours. A number of variables influence absorption rate, such as site of injection, physical activity, skin temperature, and any circulating antiinsulin antibodies. Effect on blood glucose can be detected in about 1 hour, peaks at 4 to 6 hours, and lasts about 12 to 16 hours.
2. *Intermediate-acting insulins:* These insulins include Humulin L, Lente, NPH, Insulatard N, and Insulatard. Effect is detected in about 2 hours, peaks at about 11 hours, and lasts about 20 to 29 hours.
3. *Long-acting insulins:* These insulins include Humulin U. Its duration is somewhat longer than that of intermediate-acting insulins. It can be difficult to use because basal insulin is difficult to predict or control when the insulin peaks. Insulin glargine rDNA, which was first released in 2001, is a recombinant deoxyribonucleic acid (DNA) insulin analogue specifically formulated to provide a long, flat response. However, insulin glargine rDNA (trade name Lantus) cannot be mixed with other insulins, and two injections are needed to combine the action with a short-acting insulin. It is a long-acting insulin that works slowly over 24 hours and may not be used in combination with another type of insulin or an oral hypoglycemic medication to keep blood glucose regulated. Treatment algorithms are developed to adjust insulin on the basis of lifestyle and SMBG.

The process of intensifying T1DM management occurs in several stages. The initial dose of insulin is usually calculated based on current body weight with 0.5 to 0.6 unit of insulin/kg/day, with approximately half being for basal needs and half being as boluses for meals. During this initial phase a consistent carbohydrate intake is needed to identify a blood glucose pattern. After mastering an understanding, the client can move on to more complex planning using monitoring results to achieve better glycemic control and a more flexible lifestyle. Bolus requirement varies widely, but the initial dose is often estimated to provide 1 unit of short-acting insulin per 15 g of carbohydrate. Gradually the client learns to adjust

insulin for changes in food or activity using a ratio of carbohydrate intake to insulin dosage. A similar approach is used for insulin therapy in other forms of diabetes. In the treatment of T2DM, insulin may be used alone or in conjunction with an oral agent.[51]

Sources of Insulin

Human insulin has replaced beef and pork insulins traditionally used to treat diabetes. These animal-derived insulins are immunogenic to humans, beef more so than pork; in time they induce antiinsulin antibodies that delay or blunt their action. Human insulin is available from two sources: (1) biosynthesis by recombinant DNA technology through rapidly reproducing bacteria that have been given the human gene and (2) chemical substitution of the terminal amino acid of the beta-chain of pork insulin. Because they carry the human insulin structure, these newer insulins are almost nonimmunogenic.

Insulin and Exercise Balance

Exercise benefits all persons with diabetes through its action in increasing the number of insulin receptors on muscle cells, thus increasing insulin efficiency.[52] However, physical activity must be regular to be effective.[53] A detailed history of personal activity and exercise habits provides information that is needed to help a client plan a wise program of regular moderate exercise. Guidelines for extra food to cover periods of heavier exercise, athletic practice, or competition can be included (Table 21-4). Gregory and colleagues[54] report the experience of a college football player with diabetes and his carefully

TABLE 21-4	Meal-Planning Guide for Active People With Type 1 Diabetes Mellitus
Exchange Needs	**Sample Menus**
Moderate Activity	
30 Minutes	
1 bread *or*	1 bran muffin *or*
1 fruit	1 small orange
1 Hour	
2 bread + 1 meat *or*	Tuna sandwich *or*
2 fruit + 1 milk	$\frac{1}{2}$ cup fruit salad + 1 cup milk
Strenuous Activity	
30 Minutes	
2 fruit *or*	1 small banana *or*
1 bread + 1 fat	$\frac{1}{2}$ bagel + 1 tsp cream cheese
1 Hour	
2 bread + 1 meat + 1 milk *or*	Meat and cheese sandwich + 1 cup milk *or*
2 bread + 2 meat + 2 fruit	Hamburger + 1 cup orange juice

planned blood sugar control during games. In general, exercise programs make persons feel better both physically and psychologically. This improved sense of well-being should not be underestimated in persons facing a chronic disease.

Insulin Delivery Systems

Intensive insulin therapy for maintaining more normal blood glucose control requires multiple injections of rapid-acting insulin, alone or in combination with basal intermediate-acting insulin. This is accomplished either by regular injection with disposal syringes or with an insulin pump. The pump is not for everyone, but for many it has made life easier to use an insulin pump to achieve a basal insulin infusion and bolus insulin for meals. It is a small device that is easily worn on the belt with a subcutaneous needle in the abdomen and buttons the wearer pushes to obtain a fixed programmed flow of insulin in balance with food intake. Frequent monitoring is needed to adjust insulin dosage with either multiple injections or the insulin pump.

Oral Antidiabetic Drugs

There are five classes of oral antidiabetic drugs used to treat hyperglycemia in T2DM: sulfonylurea, biguanide, thiazolidinedione, meglitinide, and alpha-glucosidase inhibitor. When lifestyle changes alone cannot normalize metabolism, MNT should help optimize metabolic control and reduce potential medication side effects. Table 21-5 provides a brief review of insulin and oral antidiabetic drugs (see also the *Complementary and Alternative Medicine (CAM)* box, "Herbs and Supplements Commonly Used in Diabetes Mellitus").

Insulin is often used in T2DM as adjunctive therapy when oral agents are not achieving glycemic control. A nighttime dose of insulin is commonly used to help reduce fasting glucose levels, especially if fasting levels are 13.9 mmol/L (250 mg/dl) or higher. Insulin therapy is also commonly used as adjunctive therapy when glycemic control is not achieved with oral agent monotherapy or combination therapy.

Adjunctive Therapies

Two new injectable drugs have been approved by the FDA. Exenatide (Byetta) is first in its class of drugs for treatment of T2DM for patients taking metformin, a sulfonylurea, or a combination of metformin and a sulfonylurea. This class of drugs is referred to as incretin mimetics. Isolated from the saliva of Gila monsters, exenatide works to lower blood glucose levels by increasing insulin secretion. It only has this effect in the presence of elevated blood glucose levels; therefore it does not tend to increase risk of hypoglycemia on its own.

Pramlintide (Symlin) is a synthetic form of the hormone amylin. Both amylin and insulin are produced by the beta cells in the pancreas. Amylin, insulin, and glucagon work together to maintain normal blood glucose levels. Pramlintide injections taken with meals modestly improve Hb_{A1c} levels by slowing gastric emptying rate without altering overall absorption of nutrients. In addition, pramlintide suppresses glucagon secretion from the liver and regulates food intake due to centrally mediated modulation of appetite.

Testing Methods for Monitoring Results

Frequent testing of blood glucose levels is necessary for successful "tight" control of T1DM and to reduce risk of complications.

Self-Monitoring of Blood Glucose.
For insulin doses to be administered in sufficient time intervals and amounts to maintain normal blood glucose, close monitoring of immediate blood glucose levels is mandatory.[50] Small, lightweight, easy-to-use, hand-sized meters, easily carried in pockets and handbags, are available for convenient use. A reagent test strip is inserted into the blood glucose meter, a drop of capillary blood from the finger obtained with an automatic lancer is placed on the reagent test strip, and a digital reading of the blood glucose level appears on the meter. Frequency of monitoring varies according to need for control and goal of care. More frequent self-monitoring is indicated for unstable forms of diabetes, persons using insulin pumps, and those who want close control and freedom of movement. Usually two to eight before- and after-meal tests are performed daily. During pregnancy postprandial monitoring is performed at 1 hour after meals. Glucose goals are lower during pregnancy because of the dilution effect of having a greater blood volume.

Glycated Hemoglobin.
The most common glycated hemoglobin test is the Hb_{A1c}. Glycated hemoglobins are relatively stable molecules within the red blood cell. During the 120-day life of the red blood cell, glucose molecules attach themselves to hemoglobin. This irreversible glycosylation of hemoglobin depends on the concentration of blood glucose. Glycosylation of proteins in various body systems appears to play a role in the development of diabetic complications. The higher the level of circulating glucose over the life of the red blood cells, the higher the concentration of glycohemoglobin. Thus measurement of hemoglobin A1c (Hb_{A1c}) relates to the level of blood glucose over a longer period. It provides an effective tool for evaluating the long-term management of diabetes and degree of control.[12] Because glucose attaches to hemoglobin over the life of the red blood cell, the test gives an accumulated history of glucose levels over time, providing an effective management tool for evaluating progress and making decisions about treatment changes. Obtaining a Hb_{A1c} level every 6 to 8 weeks can be used to monitor the overall glucose control.

TABLE 21-5 | **Medications Used to Treat Diabetes**

Drug Class	Drug Name(s)	Action	Target Organ(s)	Side Effects	How Taken
Alpha-glucosidase inhibitor	*Acarbose:* Precose, Glucobay, Prandese, Glucor *Miglitol:* Glyset, Miglibay, Bayglitol	Delays absorption of glucose from GI tract	Small intestine	Excess flatulence, diarrhea (particularly after high-carbohydrate meal), abdominal pain, may interfere with iron absorption	Must be taken with meals
Biguanides	*Metformin:* Glucophage *Metformin* and *glibenclamide:* Glucovance, Glucophage and Glyburide	Decrease hepatic glucose production and intestinal glucose absorption; improve insulin sensitivity	Liver, small intestine, and peripheral tissues	Less likely to gain weight; may lose weight; anorexia, nausea, diarrhea, metallic taste, may reduce absorption of vitamin B_{12} and folic acid, rarely suitable for adults >80 yr of age	Take with first main meal
Insulin and related agents	*Insulin mixtures:* Humulin 50/50, Humulin 70/30, Novolin 70/30	Exogenous insulin preparations		Hypoglycemia, fatigue, hunger, nausea, muscular weakness or trembling, headache, sweating, blurred vision, fainting, weight gain, skin irritation	Subcutaneous injection
	Intermediate-acting: Humulin L, Humulin N, Iletin II Lente, Iletin II NPH, Novolin L, Novolin N	Exogenous insulin preparations		Hypoglycemia, fatigue, hunger, nausea, muscular weakness or trembling, headache, sweating, blurred vision, fainting, weight gain, skin irritation	Subcutaneous injection
	Long-acting: Humulin U, Lantus (insulin glargine)	Exogenous insulin preparations		Hypoglycemia, fatigue, hunger, nausea, muscular weakness or trembling, headache, sweating, blurred vision, fainting, weight gain, skin irritation	Subcutaneous injection
	Rapid-acting: Humalog, insulin lispro, insulin aspart	Exogenous insulin preparations		Hypoglycemia, fatigue, hunger, nausea, muscular weakness or trembling, headache, sweating, blurred vision, fainting, weight gain, skin irritation	Subcutaneous injection, intramuscular or intravenous in special situations
	Short-acting: Humulin R, Iletin II Regular, Novolin R, Novolin BR	Exogenous insulin preparations		Hypoglycemia, fatigue, hunger, nausea, muscular weakness or trembling, headache, sweating, blurred vision, fainting, weight gain, skin irritation	Subcutaneous injection, intramuscular or intravenous in special situations
Meglitinides (nonsulfonylurea insulin releasers)	*Nateglinide:* Starlix *Repaglinide:* Prandin, Aculin	Stimulates secretion of insulin	Pancreatic beta cells	Hypoglycemia and weight gain; *repaglinide* has a lightly increased risk for cardiac events	Take with meals
Sulfonylureas	*Acetohexamide:* Dymelor *Tolazamide:* Tolinase *Tolbutamide:* Orinase *Chlorpropamide:* Diabinese *Glimepiride:* Amaryl *Glyburide:* DiaBeta, Micronase, Glynase PresTabs	Stimulates secretion of insulin	Pancreatic beta cells	Hypoglycemia and weight gain; *tolbutamide* may be associated with cardiovascular complications; *chlorpropamide* can cause hyponatremia; should not be used by women who are pregnant or nursing, or by individuals allergic to sulfa drugs; sulfonylurea interacts with many other drugs (prescription, OTC, and alternative); *Diabinese:* avoid alcohol	Take before or with meals

Data from Setter SM: New drug therapies for treatment of diabetes, *On the Cutting Edge* 19(2):3, 1998; Sharp AR: Nutritional implications of new medications to treat diabetes, *On the Cutting Edge* 19(2):1 1998; and White JR, Campbell RK: Recent developments in the pharmacological reduction of blood glucose in patients with Type 2 diabetes, *Clin Diabetes* 19:153, 2001. Retrieved January 18, 2006, from *http://clinical.diabetesjournals.org/cgi/content/full/19/4/153*

GI, Gastrointestinal; *OTC,* over-the-counter.

TABLE 21-5	Medications Used to Treat Diabetes—cont'd

Drug Class	Drug Name(s)	Action	Target Organ(s)	Side Effects	How Taken
Thiazolidine diones (TZDs)	*Pioglitazone:* Actos *Rosiglitazone:* Avandia	Improves insulin sensitivity	Activates genes involved with fat synthesis and carbo-hydrate metabolism	Possible liver damage, weight gain, mild anemia	Once or twice daily

COMPLEMENTARY AND ALTERNATIVE MEDICINE (CAM)
Herbs and Supplements Commonly Used in Diabetes Mellitus

Herb/ Supplement	Common Uses	Efficacy	Safety	Drug/Herb Interactions	Interaction
Chromium	Glycemic control	Improved glycemic control.	No adverse effects reported.	Hyperglycemic agents and any other agent used for glycemic control.	Possible risk of hypoglycemia.
Cinnamon (*Cinnamomum verum*)	Glycemic control	Increases use of endogenous insulin.	Large amounts increase heart rate and intestinal motility, followed by sleepiness and depression. As a spice, long-term use is safe.	None known.	—
Gamma-linolenic acid (GLA)					
Ginseng (*Panax ginseng*)	Glycemic control	Improved glycemic control.	Possible overstimulation and insomnia.	Hyperglycemic agents and any other agent used for glycemic control. May enhance effect of stimulants, antibiotics, MAOIs. Antagonism of warfarin. May falsely elevate digoxin levels. Increases alcohol clearance. May decrease diuretic effect of furosemide. May potentiate effects of hormones and anabolic steroid therapies.	Possible risk of hypoglycemia. Estrogenic effects of ginseng may cause vaginal bleeding and breast nodules.

MAOIs, Monamine oxidase inhibitors; *GI,* gastrointestinal; *IV,* intravenous.

Continued

COMPLEMENTARY AND ALTERNATIVE MEDICINE (CAM)—cont'd
Herbs and Supplements Commonly Used in Diabetes Mellitus

Herb/ Supplement	Common Uses	Efficacy	Safety	Drug/Herb Interactions	Interaction
Evening primrose oil *(Oenothera biennis)*	Peripheral neuropathy	May be helpful.	No adverse effects reported.	Phenothiazines.	May increase risk of seizures.
Lipoic acid	Neuropathy	Slight evidence IV lipoic acid can reduce symptoms of peripheral neuropathy in the short term. Evidence for oral lipoic acid inadequate.	No adverse reactions documented.	Some concern lipoic acid potentiates effects of insulin, but has not been documented in formal studies.	None noted.
Vanadium	Glycemic control	May improve glycemic control.	Usually well tolerated, but GI disturbances can occur. Studies suggest excess is toxic (hepatotoxicity, nephrotoxicity, teratogenicity, and developmental/ reproductive toxicity).	May cause hypoglycemia if used in conjunction with effective antidiabetic regimen.	None noted.

References

Bratman S, Girman AM: *Mosby's handbook of herbs and supplements and their therapeutic uses*, St. Louis, 2003, Mosby.
Contributors and Consultants: *Professional guide to complementary and alternative therapies*, Springhouse, Pa, 2001, Springhouse.

Kuhn MA, Winston D: *Herbal therapy and supplements: a scientific and traditional approach*, Philadelphia, 2001, Lippincott.

MAOIs, Monamine oxidase inhibitors; *GI*, gastrointestinal; *IV*, intravenous.

Physical Activity Habits

In counseling clients with diabetes, a detailed history of personal activity and physical exercise habits should be discussed. This information is then used as a basis for planning together a wise program of regular moderate exercise. Guidelines for extra food to cover periods of heavier exercise or athletic practice and competition are included[55] (see Table 21-4). Self-monitoring is a regular procedure now used by most persons with T1DM and T2DM. It is a helpful means of determining the balance needed at any point in time between exercise, insulin, and food.

Gestational Diabetes

Occasionally the stress of pregnancy may bring about GDM, which is a form of glucose intolerance that has onset during pregnancy and is resolved on parturition.[56] Risk of fetal abnormalities and mortality are increased in the presence of hyperglycemia; therefore every effort should be made to control blood glucose levels. All women with GDM should receive nutrition counseling by a registered dietitian when possible.[45]

Changes that take place during pregnancy greatly affect insulin utilization. Some hormones and enzymes produced by the placenta are antagonistic to insulin, thus reducing its effectiveness. Maternal insulin does not cross the placenta, but glucose does, causing the fetal pancreas to increase insulin production if maternal blood glucose levels get too high. Increased production of insulin causes the most predictable characteristic of infants born to women with diabetes—macrosomia, in addition to other problems such as respiratory difficulties, hypocalcemia, hypoglycemia, hypokalemia, and jaundice.[44]

Individualization of NT based on maternal weight and height is recommended.[45] MNT should include the provision of adequate kcalories and nutrients to meet pregnancy needs and should be consistent with accepted maternal blood glucose goals.[45] SMBG provides important information about the impact of food on blood glucose levels.[46] At the beginning of the pregnancy, minimal daily SMBG should be planned 4 times a day (fasting and 1 or 2 hours after each meal).[46] Blood glucose goals during pregnancy are fasting less than 95 mg/dl, 1-hour postprandial 140 mg/dl, and 2-hour postprandial less than 120 mg/dl.[32] Frequency of SMBG may be decreased once blood glucose control is established. However, some monitoring should continue throughout pregnancy.[46]

Recommended weight gains and nutrient requirements are the same as for established pregnancy guidelines, as follows[44]:

- Underweight (body mass index [BMI] less than 18.5): 28 to 40 lb
- Normal/healthy weight (BMI 18.5 to 24.9): 25 to 35 lb
- Overweight (BMI 25 to 29.9): 15 to 25 lb
- Obesity (Class 1) (BMI 30 to 34.9): greater than 15 lb
- Obesity (Class 2) (BMI 35 to 39.9): not available
- Obesity (Class 3) (BMI greater than 40): not available

No kcalorie modifications are needed for the first trimester.[31,56] During the second and third trimesters, increased energy intake of approximately 180 kcal/day is suggested.[44] High-quality protein should be increased by 25 g/day. As with any pregnancy, 600 μg/day of folic acid is recommended for prevention of neural tube defects and other congenital abnormalities.[44] Alcohol consumption is not recommended in any amount.

Kcaloric restriction must be considered with care. A minimum of 1700 to 1800 kcal/day of carefully selected foods has been shown to prevent ketosis.[57] Intakes below this level are not advised.[46] Weight gain goals are established using prepregnancy BMI. Weight gain should still occur even if patients have gained substantial weight before the onset of GDM.[46] Each patient with GDM should be evaluated individually by a registered dietitian, should have care plans fine-tuned, and should have patient education provided as required to realize weight goals.[46]

Impaired Fasting Glucose and Impaired Glucose Tolerance

The terms *impaired fasting glucose (IFG)* and *impaired glucose tolerance (IGT)* refer to a metabolic stage somewhere between normal glucose homeostasis and overt diabetes. Although not clinical entities in their own right, these conditions are risk factors for future diabetes and cardiovascular disease.[2,12] Lifestyle interventions should be consistent with current guidelines for overweight and obesity and address cardiovascular risk factors and common

concomitant conditions. The Da Qing IGT and Diabetes Study provided preliminary evidence that diet and exercise intervention can lower the conversion to overt diabetes during the 6-year period.[21] The Finnish Diabetes Prevention Study demonstrated that a lifestyle change program could reduce the risk for developing diabetes by 58% during a 3-year period.[20] In the United States, the Diabetes Prevention Program (DPP) has confirmed the findings of the Finnish trial in a highly diverse American population with IGT. The DPP addressed how an intensive diet and exercise intervention compares with metformin in a three-arm randomized clinical trial that uses placebo as the third arm.[58]

MANAGEMENT OF DIABETES NUTRITION THERAPY

Counseling Process in Nutrition Therapy for Diabetes

NT for diabetes is highly individualized. The American Diabetes Association recommendations clearly state that there is no one "diabetic" or "ADA" diet. Now the "recommended diet" is a dietary prescription based on individual nutrition assessment and treatment goals.[33] This model emphasizes actions of the diabetes team clinical dietitian in an individualized, integrated four-point approach: (1) assessment, (2) goal setting, (3) nutrition intervention, and (4) evaluation, as follows[59]:

1. *Assessment:* The first step involves a comprehensive assessment of the client's background. It includes clinical information, medical and lifestyle data such as personal self-monitoring of blood glucose, and dietary history. Interview follow-up tools such as questionnaires and food records assess general food patterns and nutrient intake.
2. *Nutrition diagnosis:* The second step identifies and labels problems the client may have.
3. *Nutrition intervention:* The third step guides the client in selecting and using the most appropriate meal-planning guide from the number that are now available, based on individual needs for knowledge and skills to change or maintain eating habits and daily living practices.
4. *Monitoring and evaluation:* Together the client and dietitian evaluate goals and nutrition intervention, as well as ongoing clinical data, to help the client succeed at the established individual program. They then make any desired adjustments, and the dietitian provides continuing counseling and education as needed.

Diabetes Meal-Planning Tools

Since the DCCT there has been growing emphasis on selecting a planning approach that meets the needs of each client from a wide array of meal-planning guides.

Regardless of the diabetes NT management tool, the first vital principle in working with persons who have diabetes is to start where they are. Any food-planning process must focus first on the unique individual rather than on the "case" or disease. Numerous planning approaches are used by skilled and sensitive clinical dietitians who tailor their actions to the person's learning needs and abilities, nutritional needs, personal needs, and lifestyle issues. Because of the widespread use of the exchange lists as a dietary management tool, they are outlined in Appendix G.

Carbohydrate Counting

Carbohydrate counting is one of the most commonly used methods of meal planning. Research shows carbohydrate is the primary nutrient affecting postprandial blood glucose level and consequently insulin requirements.[36,59] Carbohydrate quantity and distribution can affect metabolic control.[59] Carbohydrate counting can help people with diabetes become more aware of carbohydrate content of the foods they eat and consistency of food consumption at meals and snacks.[60]

At an advanced level, carbohydrate counting is a tool that allows the person with diabetes to focus on adjustment of foods, medication, and activity based on patterns from daily food intake records and blood glucose records.[59] In order to use carbohydrate counting effectively, the dietetic professional and person with diabetes must have a good understanding of intensive insulin therapy.[59]

Carbohydrate content can be measured in grams of carbohydrate or servings: one carbohydrate serving equals 15 g carbohydrate. Most people find it easier to count number of carbohydrate servings consumed rather than keeping track of grams of carbohydrate consumed.[59] Box 21-1 provides a brief outline of carbohydrate content of foods to equal one serving of carbohydrate.

Planning for Special Needs

Sick Days

When general illness occurs, food and insulin amounts must be adjusted accordingly. Texture may be modified as needed to use easily digested and absorbed liquid foods while still maintaining as much as possible glucose equivalents of the usual food plan.

Physical Activity

For any strenuous physical activity, the client with T1DM must make special plans ahead. This is particularly true of a young person with diabetes who is engaging in athletic practice or competition.[53,54] Energy demands of exercise are discussed in Chapter 14.

Travel

When a trip is planned, the clinical dietitian must confer with the client to guide food choices according to what

---

BOX 21-1	Equivalents to One 15-g Carbohydrate Serving

Grains, Breads, Cereals, Starches
1 slice bread
¾ cup dry cereal
½ cup cooked cereal
⅓ cup cooked rice or pasta

Milk and Yogurt
1 cup milk
⅓ cup (6 oz) unsweetened or sugar-free yogurt

Fruits
1 small fresh fruit
½ cup canned fruit (caned in juice)
1 cup melon or berries
¼ cup dried fruit
½ cup unsweetened fruit juice

Vegetables
½ cup cooked potatoes, peas, or corn
3 cups raw vegetables
1½ cups cooked vegetables
Small portions (½ cup) of nonstarchy vegetables are free

Sweets and Snack Foods
½ cup or ¾ oz snack food (pretzels, chips)
4-6 snack crackers
1 oz sweet snack (2 small cookies)
½ cup regular ice cream
1 tbsp sugar

From American Diabetes Association, American Dietetic Association: *Exchange lists for meal planning*, Alexandra, Va/Chicago, 2003, Authors.

---

will be available. Self-monitoring of blood glucose levels and insulin therapy equipment and making food plans are as important on vacation or a business trip as they are at home. The traveler always needs to plan ahead with the healthcare team (see the *Perspectives in Practice* box, "Travel and Illness: 'Real-Life' Situations").

Eating Out

Provide similar guidelines and suggestions for various situations when the client eats meals away from home. As a general rule, the plan must be made ahead of time; therefore accommodations for what is eaten at home before and after the meal eaten away from home reflect continuing balance needs of the day. Have the client get the menu ahead of time. Many restaurants are willing to fax their menus, or they may be available on websites.

Stress

Any form of emotional stress is reflected in variations of diabetes control.[59,61] These variations are caused by hormonal responses that act as antagonists to insulin. The clinical dietitian must help the client learn and practice a variety of useful stress reduction activities.

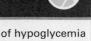

PERSPECTIVES IN PRACTICE
Travel and Illness: "Real-Life" Situations

People with diabetes do not stop living their lives just because they have diabetes. They still travel, and they still catch colds and flu and other common illnesses. Special considerations to all areas of diabetes management will enhance safe traveling, as well as the traveler's health. What kind of information does the person with diabetes need to know when traveling or if he or she becomes too ill to eat? How did the tragic events of September 11, 2001, affect airline travel for persons with diabetes? The following are a few helpful hints you may want to offer clients for these common situations.

Traveling Safely With Diabetes
General Tips
1. Ensure that you have sufficient medication (insulin or oral glucose-lowering medication) for the entire trip.
2. Carry some form of medical identification that includes type of diabetes, name, address, telephone number(s), emergency contact information, medications taken, physician's name and phone number, and additional relevant medical conditions. Preferably, this information should be worn on a necklace or bracelet (rather than carrying it in a wallet or purse).
3. Take extra snacks such as cereal bars, vanilla wafers, peanut butter crackers, or glucose tablets or gel.
4. Always keep insulin cool, especially if vacationing in the tropics or to the beach.
5. Keep some money available for food purchases if necessary. Change for a vending machine may be hard to come by.
6. Always carry blood glucose monitoring equipment. Blood glucose levels should be checked before beginning a trip, as well as every 2 hours. An extra check should be done anytime symptoms of hypoglycemia occur, even if recent blood glucose checks were acceptable.
7. Walking around and stretching every 2 to 4 hours helps stimulate circulation.
8. Whenever possible, travel with a companion.
9. Wear comfortable shoes.
10. Plan for time zone changes. Meal schedules may need to be revised to balance with insulin activity pattern.
11. If traveling abroad, learn to say the following in the local language: "I have diabetes. Please give me something sweet to drink."
12. If travel is frequent, contact a registered dietitian or diabetes educator for ideas for healthful, portable meals/snacks.

Driving Tips
1. If diabetes medication has potential to cause hypoglycemia, medications and meals will need to be timed during a long trip.
2. If diabetes medications have potential to cause hypoglycemia, food should be eaten before leaving home or snacks should be taken in the automobile. Traffic may not be conducive to stopping at a favorite store or restaurant for a quick meal or snack.
3. Keep nonperishable, carbohydrate-containing foods in the automobile in case flat tires, traffic jams, or breakdowns occur. Handy, premeasured carbohydrate amounts may be beneficial to avoid overeating or undereating. Replenish the food supply as needed to avoid running out at inopportune times.
4. Always carry blood glucose monitoring equipment when driving. Blood glucose levels should be checked before the trip begins, as well as every 2 hours while driving. An

extra check should be done if symptoms of hypoglycemia occur (even if recent blood glucose checks have been acceptable).
5. An extra glucose meter should not be kept in an automobile. Internal automobile temperatures can get very hot and very cold. Strips and meters exposed to extreme temperatures may not be accurate or function properly.
6. High blood glucose levels may cause the following symptoms that can affect driving:
   - Fatigue related to the body's inability to use glucose for energy
   - Increased urination, causing preoccupation, repeated stops, and a delay in arriving at destination
   - Blurry vision, which may impair ability to see road signs clearly; blurry vision may be especially problematic at night or while driving in rain or snow
   - Numbness or tingling in hands or feet, which may impair perception or sensation steering or when applying pressure to gas or brake pedals
7. Prompt attention to hypoglycemia and treatment is necessary to prevent mental confusion and even losing consciousness. When blood glucose is low, the first organ affected is the brain! Keep appropriate sources of carbohydrates available in the automobile.
8. If driving hours at a time, it is important to stop the automobile, get out and stretch, and walk around every 2 to 4 hours.
9. Wear medical identification. Law enforcement officers may not be familiar with diabetes or symptoms of hypoglycemia or hyperglycemia. They can mistake impaired awareness and judgment for drunkenness.
10. Whenever possible, drive with a friend.
11. If driving over several hours, set an alarm as a reminder for blood glucose checks, meals, and even times to stretch and walk.
12. Visual disturbances can occur with either hyperglycemia or hypoglycemia.
13. If driving long distances, take twice as many diabetes supplies as thought to be needed. Be aware of all medicines taken (prescription and over-the-counter).
14. Always carry money for toll booths, parking, and telephone calls. Consider keeping a cell phone to call for assistance.

Flying Tips
1. Call ahead to airlines to advise them of the diabetes and supplies needed.
2. Carry a copy of physician's prescription for insulin and/or other medications.
3. Carry a letter from the physician explaining the need to carry syringes/injection devices and insulin.
4. If problems are encountered, request to speak to a manager or supervisor.
5. Carry insulin onto the aircraft. Insulin should not be packed in luggage that will be stored in the hold of an airplane. Low temperatures can damage the insulin.
6. Notify the Transportation Security Administration (TSA) representative that you have diabetes and are carrying your supplies with you. The following are allowed through the checkpoint once screened:
   - Insulin and insulin-loaded dispensing products clearly marked and labeled
   - Unlimited number of unused syringes when accompanied by insulin or other injectable medication

Continued

PERSPECTIVES IN PRACTICE—cont'd
Travel and Illness: "Real-Life" Situations

- Lancets, blood glucose meters, blood glucose meter test strips, alcohol swabs, meter-testing solutions
- Insulin pump and supplies
- Glucagon emergency kit clearly identified and labeled
- Urine ketone test strips
- Unlimited number of used syringes when transported in sharps disposal container or other similar hard-surface container

Sick Day Survival

1. Keep taking diabetes medications even if solid foods cannot be eaten.
2. For insulin users the physician may prescribe extra doses or increased amounts of insulin during an illness.
3. Blood glucose should be tested and recorded every 4 hours.
4. Test for ketones in urine if blood glucose level stays at or over 240 mg/dl for at least 4 hours.
5. Try to use regular meal plan/diet, but if that is not possible, soft foods or liquids can be consumed to take the place of carbohydrates usually eaten. Some easily digested foods to replace one serving (15 g) of carbohydrate include the following:
   - 1/3 to 1/2 cup fruit juice
   - 1/2 cup regular soft drink
   - 1/2 cup regular gelatin
   - 1/2 cup hot cereal
   - 1/2 cup vanilla ice cream
   - 1 cup broth-based soup
6. To prevent dehydration, sip 3 to 6 oz of noncaffeinated, sugar-free beverages or water every hour. Sugar-free fluids may be alternated with liquids containing sugar to help control blood glucose levels.
7. Keep a thermometer on hand to determine body temperature.
8. When buying over-the-counter medicines, choose one that is sugar-free. In addition to the word "sugar" on labels, "dextrose," "fructose," "lactose," "sorbitol," "mannitol," "xylitol," and "honey" indicate a product contains sugar.
9. Over-the-counter cold medications containing epinephrine-like compounds (including ephedrine, pseudoephedrine, phenylpropanolamine, phenylephrine, and epinephrine) can raise blood glucose levels and should only be used with a physician's approval.
10. *Planning ahead:* Keep the following items on hand in case of colds, flu, or other kinds of illnesses:
    - Thermometer
    - Urine test strips for ketones (check expiration date periodically)
    - Approved over-the-counter cold and flu medicines
    - Syringes or prescription for them (if insulin is not usually taken but is part of a sick day plan)
    - Short-acting insulin (keep refrigerated)
    - Extra prescriptions for all medications usually taken (or have on file at pharmacy)
    - Nonperishable foods such as noncaffeinated soft drinks (regular and diet), regular gelatin, popsicles, sport drinks, saltines, and canned fruit juices

11. Call the physician if any of the following occurs:
    - Vomiting over several hours
    - Diarrhea recurring within 6 hours
    - Difficulty breathing
    - Blood glucose levels greater than 240 mg/dl for 24 hours if using oral medications; blood glucose levels greater than 240 mg/dl for two consecutive tests (4 hours apart) after taking supplemental insulin
    - Blood glucose levels less than 60 mg/dl
    - Moderate to large amounts of ketones in urine and no improvement after at least 12 hours
    - Signs of dehydration such as dry skin or mouth, sunken eyes, or weight loss
    - Sickness that continues from 12 to 48 hours without improvement
    - Increased fatigue
    - Stomach or chest pain
    - Temperature that stays at higher than 101° F
    - Acute loss of vision
12. When calling the physician, he or she will want to know blood glucose levels and urine ketone levels, how long the illness has lasted, what medicines have been taken, temperature, how much has been eaten or drunk, and other symptoms that have been experienced.
13. If necessary to go to the emergency department, staff should be informed of the diabetes.

In summary, in all cases the client must be advised to (1) maintain a steady intake of food every day, (2) replace the carbohydrate value of solid foods with that of liquid or soft foods as needed, (3) monitor blood and urine frequently for sugar and ketone levels, and (4) contact the physician if the illness lasts more than a day or so.

References

American Diabetes Association: *Traveling with diabetes supplies*, Alexandria, Va, 2004 (updated), Author. Retrieved February 9, 2006, from *www.diabetes.org/advocacy-and-legalresources/discrimination/public_accommodation/travel.jsp*.

Diabetes Mall: FAA regulations for diabetes supplies, *Diabetes News*, Oct 7, 2001. Retrieved January 17, 2006, from *www.diabetesnet.com/news/news100701.php*.

Diabetes Mall: *Air travel with diabetes*, San Diego, Author. Retrieved January 17, 2006, from *www.diabetesnet.com/diabetes_information/diabetes_travel.php*.

FAA Office of Public Affairs Press Releases: *FAA Advises air travelers on airport, airline security measures*, Washington, DC, 2001 (October 8), U.S. Department of Transportation. Retrieved January 17, 2006, from *www.faa.gov/apa/pr/pr.cfm?id=1435*.

Hernandez CL: Traveling with diabetes, *Diabetes Self-Manage*, Nov/Dec 2003. Retrieved June 28, 2006, from *www.diabetesselfmanagement.com*.

Irons MJ: Fighting colds and flu, *Diabetes Self-Manage*, Jan/Feb 1998. Retrieved June 28, 2006, from *www.diabetesselfmanagement.com*.

National Diabetes Information Clearinghouse: *What I need to know about eating and diabetes*, NIH Publication No. 02-5043, Bethesda, Md, 2002 (May), National Institute of Diabetes and Digestive and Kidney Diseases, National Institutes of Health.

DIABETES EDUCATION PROGRAM

Goal: Person-Centered Self-Care

In past years the traditional medical model has guided diabetes education in its methods, language, and respective roles assumed. Professionals have viewed themselves as having major authoritative roles and have assigned to the person with diabetes the more passive role of "patient." With notable exceptions in certain places, this model has been followed in most cases. However, with the increasing movement toward changing roles of practitioners and consumers in the healthcare system, persons with diabetes are assuming a more active voice in planning and conducting their own care. Several barriers in our traditional system stem from three sources: (1) our culture, (2) our healthcare delivery system, and (3) our professional training habits. Essentially, much of the core problem focuses on communication. For example, a list of words we use too commonly that may be objectionable to persons with diabetes, along with the preferred language, include the following:

- *"Diabetic" used as a noun:* The word *diabetic* is an adjective and should not be used alone as a noun. Use instead the phrase *person with diabetes.*
- *Compliance:* The word *compliance* raises red flags in minds of persons with diabetes. It is a purely medical term and connotes an authoritative physician position. Instead, the word *adherence* should be used, which has been adopted by national committees and associations working in the field of diabetes. The word *adherence* indicates placement of more decision-making responsibility on the person with diabetes to determine courses of action in varying situations, which is, of course, the necessity.
- *Patient:* Instead of *patient,* the phrase *person with diabetes* should be used. Persons with diabetes, like any other person, are patients only when they are in the hospital or seeing a physician for an illness.
- *Cheating:* A particularly abusive word in the minds of many persons with diabetes, especially parents of children and young people with diabetes, is the word *cheating.* This flagrant language abuse suggests dishonesty or failure to live up to an external code. By and large, persons with diabetes do not "cheat." They may kid themselves, or they may be inaccurate in their reporting, but they do not cheat. Instead phrases such as *having difficulty* or *having a problem with* should be used.

Contents: Tools for Self-Care

A plan for diabetes education must recognize the need for building self-sufficiency and responsibility within persons with diabetes and their families. It should provide practical guidelines that build on necessary skills that a person with diabetes must have for the best possible control, as well as additional surrounding factors related to life situations and psychosocial needs. Content areas include needs in relation to the nature of diabetes, nutrition and basic meal planning, insulin (or oral medication) effects and how to regulate them, monitoring of blood glucose, how to deal with illness, and, if relevant, urine ketones (see the *Case Study* box, "The Woman With Type 2 Diabetes Mellitus").

Educational Materials: Person-Centered Standards

A broad, confusing array of diabetes education materials are available. Some are excellent, and some should be discarded. Whatever is used should measure up to several basic person-centered requirements by doing the following:

- Give the intended receiver credit for having some intelligence and wanting new information
- Inform persons fully and completely, giving both sides when experts disagree—as they surely do on occasion
- Appeal to various levels of audience, ranging from basic to sophisticated
- Never be patronizing, dehumanizing, or childish

CASE STUDY

The Woman With Type 2 Diabetes Mellitus

Angela is a 35-year-old woman diagnosed 2 years ago with type 2 diabetes mellitus (T2DM). She has three children whose birth weights were in the range of 4.5 to 5 kg (10 to 11 lb). The children, now teenagers, show no signs of diabetes, and their weights are reported to be within normal limits despite their mother's fondness for cooking. Her husband, an underpaid construction worker, is slightly overweight.

Approximately 6 months ago, Angela was seen with a complaint of a series of infections that lasted longer than usual during the past 2 months. At that time she was measured as 165 cm (5 ft 5 in) and 71 kg (156 lb). Her glucose tolerance test was positive. She was seen for follow-up twice during the following month, each time showing hyperglycemia and glycosuria. At the second follow-up, an oral antidiabetic medication was prescribed, and she was referred for medical nutrition therapy (MNT).

Angela did not keep this appointment or her subsequent medical appointment. She was not seen again until 1 month ago, when she was seen in the emergency department with ketoacidosis. She responded well to treatment and was placed on a 1200-kcal diet and a mixture of intermediate- and rapid-acting insulin given in two injections a day. Her discharge plan included a referral for MNT consultation session and diabetes education classes.

Questions for Analysis

1. What factors do you think contributed to the ketoacidosis? Why?
2. What relation do these factors have to diabetes control?
3. Why did Angela first appear to have T2DM?
4. Assume that Angela administers insulin before breakfast and before the evening meal. What additional information is necessary to develop an individualized meal plan?
5. Identify any personal factors that may affect Angela's follow-through with her treatment plan. Do you anticipate any problems?
6. If so, how would you attempt to help her solve them?
7. Outline a diabetes education plan for Angela.

Health Promotion

Nutrition Questions From Persons With Diabetes

Persons with diabetes have many questions about their diets especially when they are newly diagnosed and anxieties are high. They do not want just a "yes" or "no" answer. For any item of concern, they want to know if it can be used at all and if use is limited, why, and by how much. Questions about alcohol and various sweeteners are common.

Alcohol and Diabetes: Do They Mix?

People with diabetes should follow the same sensible drinking guidelines as people without diabetes, as follows[62-66]:

* Use alcohol only in moderation (1 drink/day for women, 2 drinks/day for men).
  1 drink = 12 oz regular beer, 5 oz wine, or 1.5 oz of 80-proof distilled spirits (whiskey, scotch, rye, vodka, brandy, cognac, rum).
* Never drink alcohol on an empty stomach.
* Some medications may not mix with alcohol; check with physician or pharmacist.
* Never drink and drive.
* Never drink if pregnant or trying to become pregnant.
* Above all, use common sense.

Having diabetes should not prevent consumption of alcohol; however, some considerations must be made. Alcohol can cause hyperglycemia and hypoglycemia. Alcohol moves very quickly from the stomach into the bloodstream; it does not require digestion or metabolism. Approximately 30 to 90 minutes after an alcoholic drink is consumed, alcohol in the bloodstream is at its highest concentration. Because the liver plays the biggest role in removing alcohol from the blood, it stops making glucose while cleansing alcohol from the body. If blood glucose levels are falling during the same time, hypoglycemia can occur very quickly. For those taking insulin or oral hypoglycemic agents, they too are lowering blood glucose levels. This is why two shots of whiskey on an empty stomach lowers blood sugar dramatically.

Alcohol is high in kcalories (and low in food value) and can raise blood glucose, especially if mixed with sweet mixers, fruit juices, or ice cream. Two ounces of 90-proof alcohol contain almost 200 kcal. Wine coolers, liqueurs, and port wines are also high in sugar and kcalories. This can interfere with weight loss goals and practicing tight control. Alcohol also increases serum cholesterol levels, although this effect is transient. And it can lead to hyperlipoproteinemia with high triglyceride levels in susceptible persons, including persons with diabetes, when it is excessive. Alcohol can also make neuropathy and retinopathy worse.

For clients who choose to use alcohol, they should ask themselves the following three basic questions:

1. Is my diabetes under control?
2. Does my healthcare provider agree that I am free from health problems that alcohol can make worse (e.g., high blood pressure, neuropathy)?
3. Do I know how alcohol can affect me and my diabetes?

If "yes" is the answer to all three questions, then it is okay for him or her to have an occasional drink. In addition to the sensible drinking guidelines listed earlier, the following recommendations should also be considered:

* Discuss the use of alcohol with your physician or dietitian.
* Drink with caution, and carry identification.
* Choose drinking buddies wisely. (Make sure at least one friend or trusted companion knows that you have diabetes and is aware of what should be done in case of hypoglycemia.)
* Have a snack before going to bed to prevent hypoglycemia during sleep.
* Do not drink if you are practicing tight control (because alcohol impairs judgment); have neuropathy, hypertriglyceridemia, or hypertension; or are taking Diabinese (which causes nausea, flushing, headache, or dizziness when mixed with alcohol); or Glucophage (which can cause lactic acidosis).
* Always sip alcoholic drinks slowly.
* If you are a male client and taking insulin, you can include two alcoholic beverages in addition to your regular meal plan. If you are a female client, you can include one alcoholic beverage. Do not omit food in exchange for an alcoholic drink.
* If you are not taking insulin (and watching your weight), you should substitute alcohol for fat choices and in some cases extra starch choices (sweet wines, sweet vermouth, and wine coolers).

Can I Use Fructose in My Diabetic Diet?

How would you answer this question from your diabetic client? Fructose has been touted as a sweetener for persons with diabetes because it is a naturally occurring sugar that is as much as 1 to 1½ times as sweet as sucrose. But can the person with diabetes use it safely?

Although fructose as a sweetener is not for all persons with diabetes, generally you can reply, "Yes, but with qualifications." The following should be considered:

* Advertising claims promoting fructose are sometimes so misleading that many consumers mistakenly believe that it can be used as a "free" food. However, fructose has the same nutritive value as other sugars—4 kcal/g. Persons with T1DM should especially be instructed to use fructose as carefully as they use any other food with a caloric and carbohydrate value.

- The quantity must be limited. If used, the maximum amount is 75 g/day.
- Consumption of fructose in large amounts may have adverse effects on plasma lipids.
- The sweetness of fructose varies with temperature, acidity, and dilution. It has been used satisfactorily in some cooked desserts. However, with high temperatures, a rise in pH, and increased concentration of solution, its sweetness is reduced.

TO SUM UP

Whatever methods or materials we use, one central fact remains: the person who has diabetes is the most important and a fully equal member of the diabetes care team. Interdisciplinary approaches and strategies that involve this recognition can be developed.

Diabetes mellitus is a syndrome composed of many metabolic disorders collectively characterized by hyperglycemia and other symptoms. Treatment relies heavily on a basic type of therapy—a carefully controlled diet. Diabetes is classified in four categories: T1DM, T2DM, GDM, and prediabetes.

Blood glucose levels are controlled primarily by hormones of pancreatic islet cells: insulin, which facilitates passage of glucose through cell membranes via special membrane receptors; glucagon, which ensures adequate levels of glucose to prevent hypoglycemia; and somatostatin, which controls the actions of insulin and glucagon to maintain normal blood glucose levels. Diabetes results from inadequate insulin secretion or insulin resistance from too few receptor sites. Symptoms range from polydipsia, polyuria, polyphagia, and signs of abnormal energy metabolism to fluid and electrolyte imbalances, acidosis, and coma in seriously uncontrolled conditions.

T1DM affects about 5% to 10% of all persons with diabetes. It often develops during childhood or adolescence. Treatment involves blood glucose self-monitoring, insulin administration, and regular meals and exercise to balance insulin activity. T2DM occurs mostly in adults, particularly those who are overweight. Acidosis is rare. Treatment consists of weight management and exercise. The food plan for both types of diabetes should be low in saturated fats and cholesterol to reduce cardiovascular risk. Moderate regular exercise increases efficiency of insulin and aids in weight management. GDM occurs in 2% to 5% of all pregnancies.

QUESTIONS FOR REVIEW

1. Describe the major characteristics of T1DM and T2DM. Explain how these characteristics influence differences in nutrition therapy. List and describe medications used to control these conditions.
2. Identify and explain symptoms of uncontrolled diabetes mellitus.
3. Describe three major complications of uncontrolled diabetes and therapy used in the DCCT designed to achieve and maintain normal blood glucose levels and help avoid these complications.
4. Glenn just found out that he has diabetes mellitus. He is a sedentary, 45-year-old man who is 170 cm (5 ft 8 in) tall and weighs 94 kg (210 lb). No medications were prescribed for him. What is his BMI? If he decides to drink, how much alcohol could be allowed and how should he fit it into his diet? Defend your answer. Glenn wants to help his children reduce their chances of developing diabetes. What advice would you offer?

REFERENCES

1. American Diabetes Association: *National diabetes fact sheet,* Alexandria, Va, 2005, Author. Retrieved February 9, 2006, from *www.diabetes.org/uedocuments/NationalDiabetesFactSheetRev.pdf.*
2. American Diabetes Association: Position statement: diagnosis and classification of diabetes mellitus, *Diabetes Care* 28(suppl):S37, 2005.
3. American Diabetes Association: Direct and indirect costs of diabetes in the United States, Alexandria, Va, 2002, Author. Retrieved January 17, 2006, from *www.diabetes.org/diabetes-statistics/cost-of-diabetes-in-us.jsp.*
4. Whitehouse FW: Classification and pathogenesis of the diabetes syndrome: a historical perspective, *J Am Diet Assoc* 81(3):243, 1982.
5. Nestle et al: A case of diabetes mellitus, *N Engl J Med* 81:127, 1982.
6. Bliss M: *The discovery of insulin,* Chicago, 1982, University of Chicago Press.
7. Atkinson MA, Maclaren NK: The pathogenesis of insulin dependent diabetes, *N Engl J Med* 331:1428, 1994.
8. McKeigue PM et al: Relation of central obesity and insulin resistance with high diabetes prevalence and cardiovascular risk in South Asians, *Lancet* 337:382, 1991.
9. Dowse GK et al: Abdominal obesity and physical inactivity as risk factors for NIDDM and impaired glucose tolerance in Indian, Creole, and Chinese Mauritians, *Diabetes Care* 14(4):271, 1991.
10. Connell JE, Thomas-Doberson D: Nutritional management of children with insulin-dependent diabetes mellitus: a review by the Diabetes Care and Education Dietetic Practice Group, *J Am Diet Assoc* 91(12):1556, 1991.
11. Kissebah AH et al: Relation of body fat distribution to metabolic complications of obesity, *J Clin Endocrinol Metab* 54:254, 1982.
12. American Diabetes Association: Position statement: standards of medical care for patients with diabetes mellitus, *Diabetes Care* 28(suppl): S4, 2005.
13. American Diabetes Association: Type 2 diabetes in children and adolescents, *Pediatrics* 105:671, 2000.
14. American Diabetes Association: Type 2 diabetes in children and adolescents, *Diabetes Care* 23:381, 2000.
15. Pinhas-Hamiel O: Type 2 diabetes: not just for grownups anymore, *Contemp Pediatr* 1:102, 2001.
16. Sinha R et al: Prevalence of impaired glucose tolerance among children and adolescents with marked obesity, *N Engl J Med* 346:802, 2002.

17. Levetan C: Into the mouths of babes: the diabetes epidemic in children, *Clin Diabetes* 19:102, 2001.

18. Rosenbloom AL et al: Emerging epidemic of type 2 diabetes in youth, *Diabetes Care* 22:345, 1999.

19. Dabelea D, Snell-Bergeon JK, Heartsfield CL et al: Increasing prevalence of gestational diabetes mellitus (GDM) over time and by birth cohort. *Diabetes Care* 28:579, 2005.

20. Tuomilehto J et al: Prevention of type 2 diabetes mellitus by changes in lifestyle among subjects with impaired glucose tolerance, *N Engl J Med* 344:13453, 2001.

21. Pan XR et al: Effects of diet and exercise in preventing NIDDM in people with impaired glucose tolerance: the DaQing IGT and Diabetes Study, *Diabetes Care* 20:537, 1997.

22. National Institutes of Diabetes and Digestive and Kidney Diseases: *Diet and exercise dramatically delay type 2 diabetes: diabetes medication metformin also effective,* Bethesda, Md, 2001 (August 8), National Institutes of Health. Retrieved January 17, 2006, from *www.niddk.nih.gov/welcome/releases/8_8_01.htm.*

23. Polonsky KS et al: Non–insulin-dependent diabetes mellitus—a genetically programmed failure of the beta cell to compensate for insulin resistance, *N Engl J Med* 334(12):777, 1996.

24. Walston J et al: Time of onset of non–insulin-dependent diabetes mellitus and genetic variation in the β3-adrenergic receptor gene, *N Engl J Med* 333(6):343, 1995.

25. Wendorf M, Goldfine ID: Archeology of NIDDM—excavation of the thrifty genotype, *Diabetes* 40:161, 1991.

26. Bell GI: Molecular defects in diabetes mellitus, *Diabetes* 40:413, 1991.

27. Porte D Jr, Schwartz MW: Diabetes complications: why is glucose potentially toxic? *Science* 272(5262):699, 1996.

28. Clarke CM Jr, Lee DA: Prevention and treatment of the complications of diabetes mellitus, *N Engl J Med* 332(18):1210, 1995.

29. Diabetes Control and Complications Trial Research Group: The effect of intensive treatment of diabetes on the development and progression of long-term complications in insulin-dependent diabetes mellitus, *N Engl J Med* 329:977, 1993.

30. Barner CW et al: WAVE: a pocket guide for a brief nutrition dialogue in primary care, *Diabetes Educ* 27:352, 2001.

31. Franz MJ et al: Evidence-based nutrition principles and recommendations for the treatment and prevention of diabetes and related complications, *Diabetes Care* 25:148, 2002.

32. American Diabetes Association: Translation of the diabetes nutrition recommendations for health care institutions, *Diabetes Care* 25(suppl):61S, 2002.

33. American Dietetic Association: Nutrition recommendations and principles for people with diabetes mellitus, *J Am Diet Assoc* 94(5):504, 1994.

34. Schlundt DG et al: Situational obstacles to dietary adherence for adults with diabetes, *J Am Diet Assoc* 94(8):874, 1994.

35. American Diabetes Association: Implications of the Diabetes Control and Complications Trial (position statement), *Diabetes Care* 25:S25, 2002.

36. Delahanty LM, Halford BN: The role of diet behaviors in achieving improved glycemic control in intensively treated patients in the Diabetes Control and Complications Trial, *Diabetes Care* 16:1453, 1993.

37. Harris MI, Eastman RC: Is there a glycemic threshold for mortality risk? *Diabetes Care* 21:331, 1998.

38. Delahanty L et al: Expanded role of the dietitian in the Diabetes Control and Complications Trial: implications for clinical practice, *J Am Diet Assoc* 93(7):758, 1993.

39. Lyon RB, Vinci DM: Nutrition management of insulin-dependent diabetes mellitus in adults: review by the Diabetes Care and Education Dietetic Practice Group, *J Am Diet Assoc* 93(3):309, 1993.

40. The Oxford Center for Diabetes, Endocrinology and Metabolism Diabetes Trials Unit: *UK prospective diabetes study,* Oxford, England, 1998, Author. Retrieved January 17, 2006, from *http://www.dtu.ox.ac.uk/ukpds/results.html.*

41. Robertson KE: What the UKPDS really says about cardiovascular disease and glycemic control, *Clin Diabetes* 17:109, 1999.

42. Ousman Y, Sharma M: The irrefutable importance of glycemic control, *Clin Diabetes* 19:71, 2001.

43. American Diabetes Association: Implications of the United Kingdom Prospective Diabetes Study (position statement), *Diabetes Care* 25:S28, 2002.

44. Thomas AM, Gutierrez YM: *American Dietetic Association guide to gestational diabetes mellitus,* Chicago, 2005, American Dietetic Association.

45. American Diabetes Association: Gestational diabetes mellitus (position statement), *Diabetes Care* 25(suppl):94S, 2002.

46. Reader D, Sipe M: Key components of care for women with gestational diabetes, *Diabetes Spectrum* 14:188, 2001.

47. American Diabetes Association: Gestational diabetes mellitus (position statement), *Diabetes Care* 24:77S, 2001.

48. Anderson EJ et al: The DCCT Research Group: nutrition interventions for the intensive therapy in the Diabetes Control and Complications Trial, *J Am Diet Assoc* 93(7):768, 1993.

49. Thom S: Humalog (insulin lispro): nutritional implications and educational considerations, *On Cutting Edge* 17(4):8, 1996.

50. Trautmann ME et al: Intensive insulin therapy with insulin lispro in patients with type I diabetes reduces the frequency of hypoglycemia episodes, *Endocrinol Diabetes* 104:25, 1996.

51. Setter SM: New drug therapies for the treatment of diabetes, *On Cutting Edge* 19(2):3, 1998.

52. Hayes C: Pattern management: a tool for improving blood glucose control with exercise, *On Cutting Edge* 17(4):4, 1996.

53. Joyce M, King J: Consideration in selecting appropriate blood glucose monitoring devices, *On Cutting Edge* 17(4):16, 1996.

54. Gregory RP et al: Nutrition management of a collegiate football player with insulin-dependent diabetes: guidelines and a case study, *J Am Diet Assoc* 94(4):775, 1994.

55. Beebe C: Implementation of the 1994 Nutrition Recommendations in Clinical Practice: NIDDM, *On Cutting Edge* 16(2):11, 1995.

56. Metzger BE, Coustan DR, eds: Proceedings of the fourth international workshop conference on gestational diabetes mellitus, *Diabetes Care* 21(suppl):1B, 1998.

57. Rizzo T et al: Correlations between antepartum maternal metabolism and intelligence of offspring, *N Engl J Med* 325:911, 1991.

58. Diabetes Prevention Program Research Group: The diabetes prevention program: recruitment methods and results, *Control Clin Trials* 23:157, 2002.

59. Ross TA, Boucher JL, O'Connell BS: *American Dietetic Association guide to diabetes medical nutrition therapy and education,* Chicago, 2005, American Dietetic Association.

60. American Diabetes Association: Position statement: nutrition principles and recommendations in diabetes, *Diabetes Care* 27(suppl):S36, 2004.

61. Chapman KM et al: Applying behavioral models to dietary education of elderly diabetic patients, *J Nutr Educ* 27(2):75, 1995.

62. American Diabetes Association: *Alcohol, alcohol, everywhere: but is it safe to drink?* Alexandria, Va, Author. Retrieved February 9, 2006, from *www.diabetes.org/type-1-diabetes/alcohol.jsp.*

63. Detroit Medical Center, Wayne State University: *Nutrition for diabetics: use of alcohol,* Detroit, 1999, iMcKesson LLC. Retrieved January 17, 2006, from *www.sinaigrace.org/health_info/topics/nutr3311.html.*

64. Franz MJ et al: Evidence-based nutrition principles and recommendations for the treatment and prevention of diabetes and related complications, *Diabetes Care* 25:148, 2002.

65. Joslin Diabetes Center: *Managing diabetes: fitting alcohol into your meal plan,* Boston, 2006, Author. Retrieved January 17, 2006, from *www.joslin.org/education/library/index.shtml.*

66. Stockwell P: *Alcohol and diabetes,* 1993-2003, Edward Reid. Retrieved January 17, 2006, from *www.faqs.org/faqs/diabetes/faq/part3/section-20.html.*

FURTHER READINGS AND RESOURCES

Readings

Gregory RP et al: Nutrition management of a collegiate football player with insulin-dependent diabetes: guidelines and a case study, *J Am Diet Assoc* 94(7):775, 1994.

This interesting account of balancing insulin, high level of physical activity, and a daily training diet of 6200 kcal relates a sample game day schedule of meals and interval blood tests with related amounts of a sports drink before the game, at half-time, and after the game. This college athlete had no problem finishing the 11-game season (his senior year) with excellent game performances.

Warshaw H: *Guide to healthy restaurant eating,* ed 2, Chicago, 2002, American Diabetes Association.

This useful book reviews more than 3500 menu items from over 55 major restaurant chains. Nutrition information is included for kcalories, fat, percent kcalories from fat, saturated fat, cholesterol, sodium, carbohydrate, fiber, and protein with serving sizes and/or exchanges for each item. Restaurant pitfalls and strategies for "defensive" restaurant dining are included.

Websites of Interest

- National Diabetes Education Program (NDEP); the NDEP is a federally sponsored initiative that involves public and private partnerships to improve the treatment and outcomes for people with diabetes through a variety of activities; the NDEP publications include a newsletter, materials for people with diabetes (in several languages), materials for healthcare providers, materials for organizations, and media kits; single copies of most materials are available free of charge or can be downloaded from the NDEP website: *http://ndep.nih.gov;* (1-800-860-8747).

- American Diabetes Association (ADA); the ADA publishes many health professional and client materials in addition to its scientific journals; in an annual supplement to *Diabetes Care,* the ADA reissues its practice guidelines that address a wide array of clinical issues, including nutrition; these guidelines can be downloaded from the ADA website free of charge; local information about ADA activities can be obtained from either the website or the 800 number; diabetes self-management educational programs that are reviewed and receive ADA "recognition" are covered by Medicare and other third-party payers: *www.diabetes.org;* (1-800-DIABETES).

- Diabetes Care and Education (DCE) Practice Group of the American Dietetic Association; the DCE publishes *On the Cutting Edge,* a theme-centered newsletter on timely topics related to nutrition and diabetes; educational materials developed by the DCE are available for purchase from the ADA; the DCE website provides information about the Medicare MNT benefits for persons with diabetes, Health Care Financing Administration (HFCA) rules for ADA Education Recognition Programs reimbursement, and Current Procedural Terminology (CPT) codes for MNT; the website also provides information about the DCE publications and email listserv: *www.dce.org; www.eatright.org.*

- Centers for Disease Control and Prevention, National Center for Chronic Disease Prevention and Health Promotion, Diabetes Public Health Resource; the website has information about the Diabetes Control Program in each state and diabetes-related statistics such as the rise in the prevalence and incidence of diabetes; the National Diabetes Fact Sheet *CDC Information* is available as a downloadable file: *www.cdc.gov/diabetes;* (1-877-CDC-DIAB).

- National Institutes of Diabetes and Digestive and Kidney Diseases (NIDDK), National Diabetes Information Clearinghouse (NDIC); the NIDDK website provides information about its diabetes-related clinical trials and other research programs, a directory of diabetes organizations, health education programs, and diabetes-related topics; downloadable files include *Diabetes Dateline,* an NIDDK newsletter; client education materials; and information for health professionals; the NIDDK website also includes the National Diabetes Information Clearinghouse, which disseminates information about online and print materials and provides access to database searches for diabetes-related references: *www.niddk.nih.gov/health/diabetes/diabetes.htm.*

- American Association of Diabetes Educators (AADE); as a multidisciplinary organization of health professionals who teach about diabetes, the AADE and its website provide information about the scope of practice and standards related to diabetes education; the website also has information and AADE publications: *http://aadenet.org.*

CHAPTER 22

Renal Disease

Sara Long

This chapter reviews basic kidney function and pathophysiology of kidney diseases. Nutrition assessment methodology and nutritional recommendations for chronic kidney disease (CKD), maintenance dialysis therapy, postrenal transplantation, acute renal failure (ARF), renal stones, and urinary tract infection (UTI) are discussed.

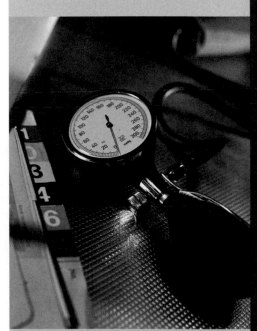

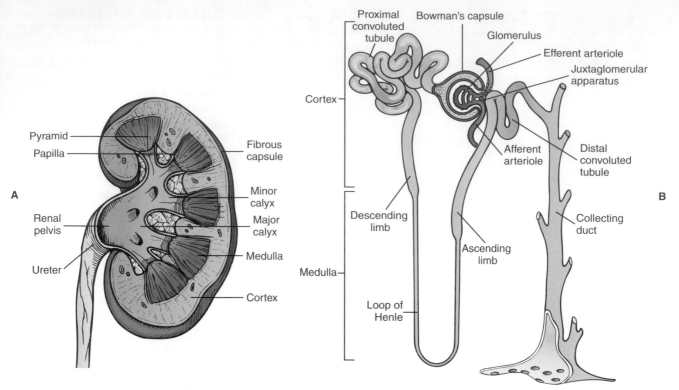

FIGURE 22-1   A, Longitudinal section of the kidney. **B,** Nephron of the kidney. *(From Lewis SM, Collier IC, Heitkemper MM: Medical-surgical nursing: assessment and management of clinical problems, ed 4, St. Louis, 1996, Mosby.)*

BASIC KIDNEY FUNCTION

Main functions of the kidney are excretory, regulatory, and endocrine. The excretory function serves to remove potentially toxic metabolic waste products such as urea, major end product of protein metabolism, from the blood. The regulatory function controls electrolyte, acid-base, and fluid balance. The result is maintenance of proper serum concentrations of sodium, potassium, calcium, phosphorus, chloride, bicarbonate, and hydrogen ions. The endocrine functions include conversion of the biologically inactive form of vitamin D (25-hydroxycholecalciferol) to the biologically active vitamin D (1,25-dihydroxycholecalciferol), synthesis of erythropoietin (needed for red blood cell production in the bone marrow), and synthesis and release of renin, which regulates systemic blood pressure.[1,2]

These functions are accomplished by the unique architecture of the nephron, the basic functioning unit of the kidney. Each human adult kidney consists of approximately 1 million nephrons (Figure 22-1). The key structures of the nephron are the glomerulus and the tubules.[2]

Glomerulus

At the head of each nephron, blood enters in a single capillary and then branches into a group of collateral capillaries.

This tuft of collateral capillaries is held closely together in a cup-shaped membrane. This cup-shaped capsule is named *Bowman's capsule* for the young English physician Sir William Bowman. In 1843 Bowman established the basis of plasma filtration and consequent urine secretion from the interrelationship of blood-filled glomeruli and enveloping membrane. The filtrate formed here is cell free and virtually protein free.

Tubules

Continuous with the base of Bowman's capsule, nephron tubules wind in a series of convolutions toward their terminal in the renal pelvis. The following list details specific reabsorption functions performed by the four sections of the tubule:

1. *Proximal tubule:* In the first section nearest the glomerulus, major nutrient reabsorption occurs. Essentially 100% of the glucose and amino acids and 80% to 85% of the water, sodium, potassium, chloride, and most other substances are reabsorbed. Only 15% to 30% of the filtrate remains to enter the next section.
2. *Loop of Henle:* This narrowed midsection of the renal tubule is named for the German anatomist Friedrich Henle, who in 1845 first demonstrated its unique structure and function in creating the necessary fluid

pressures for ultimately forming concentrated urine. At this narrowed midsection, the thin loop of the tubule dips into the central renal medulla. Here, through a balanced system of water and sodium exchange through sodium pumps in the limbs of the loop (the countercurrent system), important fluid density is created surrounding the loop. This area of increased density in the central part of the kidney is important to concentrate urine through osmotic pressure as the lower collecting tubule later passes through this same area of the kidney.

3. *Distal tubule:* This latter portion of tubule functions primarily in providing acid-base balance through secretion of ionized hydrogen. It also conserves sodium by reabsorbing it under the influence of the hormones aldosterone and vasopressin (also called antidiuretic hormone [ADH]).

4. *Collecting tubule:* In this final widened section of the tubule, filtrate is concentrated to save water and form urine for excretion. Water is absorbed under the influence of pituitary hormone vasopressin (ADH) and osmotic pressure of the more dense surrounding fluid in this central part of the kidney. Resulting volume of urine, now concentrated and excreted, is only 0.5% to 1% of the original water and solutes filtered at the beginning in Bowman's capsule.

It is through these specialized anatomic components that the kidney serves to maintain homeostasis of the body's internal environment.[1,2]

CHRONIC KIDNEY DISEASE

Chronic renal failure is a disease syndrome in which progressive, irreversible losses of excretory, endocrine, and metabolic capacities of the kidney occur as a result of kidney damage. Determination of renal function requires evaluation of glomerular filtration rate (GFR), which is accomplished through clearance tests. Clearance tests measure the rate at which substances are cleared from the plasma by the glomerulus.[3] In clinical practice, GFR is best approximated by using prediction equations and factoring in serum creatinine concentration, age, gender, race, and body size. Recommended prediction equations for adults are the Modification of Diet in Renal Disease (MDRD) study and Cockroft-Gault equations.[4] A normal GFR is 125 ml/min/1.73 m^2.[3] As kidney disease progresses, GFR falls. Chronic renal failure progresses slowly over time and may include periods during which kidney function remains stable. However, once the disease progresses to end stage (GFR <15 ml/min/1.73 m^2), continuance of life requires the initiation of maintenance dialysis therapy or subsequent kidney transplantation[5] (see also the *Case Study* box, "The Patient With Chronic Renal Failure").

CKD is a public health problem. Incidence and prevalence of end-stage renal disease (ESRD) have doubled in the United States during the past decade.[6] In 1998 the prevalence rate was 1160 per million. In 1999 the rate increased to 1217 per million.[7] Point prevalence on December 31, 1998, was more than 1160 per million population, of which 835 per million population were receiving dialysis replacement therapy. Of the group being treated by dialysis, 97 per million were over 70 years of age compared with 2.1 per million being children[4] (see also the *Focus on Culture* box, "Kidney Failure: Another Equal Opportunity Disease?"). The total cost for the ESRD program continues to increase. In 1997 the cost was $15.64 billion; in 1998, $16.7 billion; and in 1999, $17.9 billion.[6,7]

Life expectancy for a person with ESRD is significantly below that of the general U.S. population. For example, a 40- to 44-year-old person on dialysis has a projected 6.6 to 10.9 years of additional life compared with the expected 37.4 years for a person of the same age without disease.[7] CKD is accompanied by significant comorbidities, including cardiovascular disease (CVD), malnutrition, and anemia. Lost working days and income, frequent intercurrent illness, and psychosocial adjustments all lend to a difficult life quality.

The most common causes of ESRD are diabetic nephropathy and hypertension. In 1999 43% of new cases of CKD were the result of diabetes and 26% were the result of hypertension.[7] Other common causes of

---

nephron Microscopic anatomic and functional unit of the kidney that selectively filters and resorbs essential blood factors, secretes hydrogen ions as needed for maintaining acid-base balance, and then resorbs water to protect body fluids and forms and excretes a concentrated urine for elimination of wastes. The nephron includes the renal corpuscle (glomerulus), the proximal convoluted tubule, the loop of Henle, the distal convoluted tubule, and the collecting tubule, which empties the urine into the renal medulla. The urine passes into the papilla and then to the pelvis of the kidney. Urine is formed by filtration of blood in the glomerulus and by the selective reabsorption and secretion of solutes by cells that constitute the walls of the renal tubes. There are approximately 1 million nephrons in each kidney.

medulla Inner tissue substance of the kidney.

dialysis Process of separating crystalloids and colloids in solution by the difference in their rates of diffusion through a semipermeable membrane; crystalloids pass through readily, and colloids pass through only very slowly or not all.

CASE STUDY

The Patient With Chronic Renal Failure

Mr. Steinberg is 45 years old, married, and works as a city planner for a large municipal government. He cited a recent history of nausea, anorexia, hematuria, and swollen ankles during a physical examination. His wife reported he had been tiring more easily than usual during the past year. A history of prior illnesses proved negative, except for a severe case of influenza with sore throat 10 years before during an epidemic when he was stationed with the Army overseas. Tests were ordered, and the patient was advised to return in a week for review of the test results and sooner if there were any changes in his symptoms.

Mr. Steinberg did return, with additional symptoms of headaches and occasionally blurred vision. At that time his blood pressure was 160/98 mm Hg, his temperature was 37.5° C (99.6° F), and he had lost 4 kg (8¾ lb). Laboratory tests showed albumin and red and white blood cells in the urine, with an elevated blood urea nitrogen (BUN); a phenolsulfonphthalein (PSP) test indicated a reduced filtration rate. The diagnosis was chronic renal failure.

The physician discussed the diagnosis and its serious prognosis with Mr. and Mrs. Steinberg, giving them benefits and disadvantages of both hemodialysis and kidney transplantation. Antihypertensive medication was prescribed along with other drugs to minimize discomfort.

During the following weeks Mr. Steinberg continued to lose weight, had increasing joint pain, and became anemic. He found it increasingly difficult to maintain his hectic schedule of frequent meetings, conferences, and public speeches because of gastrointestinal bleeding, increasing nausea, and occasional muscle spasms. Small mouth sores made eating very difficult.

Finally the Steinbergs informed the physician of their decision to accept the kidney transplant as a means of controlling the disease process. They were referred to the clinical dietitian (RD) for renal diet counseling to control protein, sodium, potassium, phosphate, and fluids, as well as to ensure adequate kcalories. After discussing these needs for nutritional maintenance before surgery, the RD helped them develop a meal plan based on Mr. Steinberg's food preferences. Food selection and preparation were discussed in detail, with many ideas for building in as much variety and taste appeal as possible.

The Steinbergs' follow-up with the food plan was excellent. One month later the laboratory values were almost normal, blood pressures averaged 140/88 mm Hg, the headaches and blurred vision had virtually disappeared, and Mr. Steinberg had gained 3.2 kg (7 lb) of his lost weight. The nutrient supplements, including the amino acid analogues, were taken each day as instructed.

Fortunately a kidney donor was soon found, and with the aid of drug control of immune responses the transplant surgery was apparently a success. Mr. Steinberg convalesced well at home, kept all follow-up visits with the healthcare team, and has continued to be asymptomatic 1 year following surgery.

Questions for Analysis

1. Identify a metabolic imbalance caused by renal failure that may account for each symptom presented by Mr. Steinberg.
2. What would be the objectives in care of renal failure such as Mr. Steinberg was experiencing?
3. What factors affect the amount of protein needed by persons with chronic renal failure? What amounts are usually used? Why? What are the amino acid analogues used with the low-protein diet, and why are they used?
4. What factors affect the amount of sodium needed by persons with chronic renal failure? How much is usually recommended?
5. Why is it important to control potassium levels? How much is recommended? What clinical signs presented by Mr. Steinberg may indicate that he had not been getting enough potassium?
6. Why is control of phosphate important in the diet for chronic renal failure? What additional means may be used to control it?
7. What factors affect fluid balance in chronic renal failure? How much is usually allowed?
8. What is the basic principle of the low-protein dietary regimen? List and explain each factor in the diet and potential problems in its management.
9. Outline a general teaching plan you would use to instruct the Steinbergs about the presurgical and postsurgical dietary needs.

 FOCUS ON CULTURE

Kidney Failure: Another Equal Opportunity Disease?

Of the 20 million Americans currently living with kidney disease, a disproportionate number are blacks. This reflects an incidence rate that is fourfold higher than that of their European American counterparts and is most commonly attributed to the increased prevalence of high blood pressure, diabetes, and a familial history of the disease. But not only are blacks at a higher risk for developing kidney disease, they also seem to acquire it earlier in life with almost half not knowing they have the condition until dialysis is required.

This is a startling realization, considering early interventions can limit the damage done to the kidneys. Later diagnosis of kidney disease can result in higher rates of chronic problems, dialysis dependency, and the need for transplantation. The difficulty is that relatively few blacks receive screening or intervention. Adding to the problem, with diabetes being the number one risk factor for kidney disease, one third of the cases of diabetes among blacks go undiagnosed, demonstrating the need for further screening.

According to the National Kidney Foundation, blacks represent 13% of the American population but make up 35% of those on kidney transplant waiting lists. Consequently, there is an increased transplant demand for blacks but a moderately low donor ship rate, compounding the problem.

The following five primary reasons influence low African-American donorship:

1. Lack of transplant awareness
2. Religious myths and misconceptions
3. Distrust of the medical community

4. Fear of premature declaration of death after signing a donor card
5. Fear of potential preference for races other than blacks

Whether this problem stems from lack of education, lack of healthcare, or genetic factors, the fact remains that blacks possess many risk factors affecting renal health. Screenings and education about blood glucose and blood pressure control at a younger age along with lifestyle and medication interventions have been shown to have dramatic results in kidney health; unfortunately, only a small percentage actually receive these screenings or treatment. This problem is a major one that is made all the more disheartening by the unnecessary suffering involved. Hopefully with increased visibility brought to kidney disease the incidence rate in the black population will decline.

References

Freedman B et al: The familial risk of end-stage renal disease in African Americans, *Am J Kidney Dis.* 21(4):387, 1993.

National Kidney and Urologic Diseases Information Clearinghouse, National Institute of Diabetes and Digestive and Kidney Diseases, National Institutes of Health, Bethesda, Md. Available at *http://kidney.niddk.nih.gov/index.htm.*

National Kidney Foundation, New York. Available at *www.kidney.org/.*

Reif M, Hall P: *Kidney failure among African Americans,* Cincinnati, Ohio, 2001, Net Wellness. Retrieved January 18, 2006, from *www.netwellness.org/healthtopics/kidney/faq2.cfm*

Tarver-Carr M et al: Excess risk of chronic kidney disease among African-American versus white subjects in the United States: a population-based study of potential explanatory factors, *J Am Soc Nephrol* 13:2363, 2002.

TABLE 22-1	Simplified Classification of Chronic Kidney Disease by Diagnosis

Disease	Major Types (Examples)
Diabetic kidney disease	Type 1 and type 2 diabetes
Nondiabetic kidney disease	Glomerular diseases (autoimmune diseases, systemic infections, drugs, neoplasia)
	Vascular diseases (large vessel disease, hypertension, microangiopathy)
	Tubulointerstitial diseases (urinary tract infection, stones, obstruction, drug toxicity)
	Cystic diseases (polycystic kidney disease)
Diseases in the transplant	Chronic rejection
	Drug toxicity (cyclosporine or tacrolimus)
	Recurrent diseases (glomerular diseases)
	Transplant glomerulopathy

From National Kidney Foundation: K/DOQI clinical practice guidelines for chronic kidney disease: evaluation, classification and stratification, *Am J Kidney Dis* 39(suppl 1):S1, 2002.

kidney failure include glomerulonephritis, cystic kidney disease, and urologic disease.[7] Table 22-1 outlines the classification of kidney disease.

Pathophysiology of Glomerular Disease

The majority of nondiabetic glomerular diseases are the result of immune-mediated mechanisms. Although renal injury induced by antibody alone is known to occur, mechanisms involved in renal injury resulting from antigen-antibody complex formation are better understood. Antigen-antibody complex formation occurs as a result of antibody reacting either to circulating antigens or to native kidney antigens expressed on renal cell membranes. Immune complex deposition may occur within the glomerular basement membrane (GBM), between the GBM and epithelial cell (subepithelial), between the GBM and endothelial cell (subendothelial), or within the mesangial matrix. The pattern of immune complex deposition within the glomerulus is helpful diagnostically because different diseases have characteristic patterns.[4,8] For example, membranous nephropathy is characterized in part by subepithelial immune complex deposition (Figures 22-2 and 22-3).

Deposition of immune complexes leads to activation of the complement system, which mediates injury through inflammatory or noninflammatory mechanisms. Chemotactic complement components formed as products of the activated complement cascade result in the migration of inflammatory cells into glomeruli. These cells, which

include platelets, macrophages, and polymorphonuclear neutrophils (leukocytes), all produce products that are either directly cytotoxic or serve as mediators for further cell or matrix injury (e.g., proteases, reactive oxygen species, lipid mediators, and cytokines). When subepithelial immune complexes activate complement, a noninflammatory mechanism is responsible for glomerular injury.[8,9]

Treatment of Kidney Disease

The approach to treatment of kidney disease has shifted focus from diagnosis and treatment of established kidney diseases to detection and treatment at much earlier stages.[4] Studies in patients with diabetic nephropathy have demonstrated the clinical course of this disease can be significantly improved if specific interventions are instituted early in development of the disease. These include annual screening for microalbuminuria (≥ 30 mg/day or 20 μg/min of albumin in the urine); improving glycemic control; aggressive antihypertensive therapy with angiotensin-converting enzymes or angiotensin receptor blockers; and lifestyle modifications that include weight loss, reduction in salt and alcohol intake, and exercise.[10]

Less traditional interventions that have been explored for their beneficial effects on renal disease include nutrients such as amino acids and carbohydrates. A class of nutrients that continues to be investigated for potential benefits on progression of renal disease is omega-3 fatty acids (see the discussion under the heading "Health Promotion" later in this chapter).

Through their initiative entitled "K/DOQI: Kidney Disease Outcomes Quality Initiative," The National Kidney Foundation recently published clinical practice guidelines for evaluation, classification, and stratification of CKD.[4] A main rationale for development of these clinical guidelines was accumulation of evidence that adverse effects of CKD including kidney failure, CVD, and premature death can be prevented or delayed by earlier testing and treatment of CKD.[4]

K/DOQI guidelines for CKD recommend all individuals during health evaluations be evaluated as to whether

glomerulonephritis A form of nephritis affecting the capillary loops in an acute short-term infection. It may progress to a more serious chronic condition leading to irreversible renal failure.

complement A complex series of enzymatic proteins occurring in normal serum that interact to combine with and augment (fill out, complete) the antigen-antibody complex of the body's immune system, producing lysis when the antigen is an intact cell; composed of 11 discrete proteins or functioning components, activated by the immunoglobulin factors IgG and IgM.

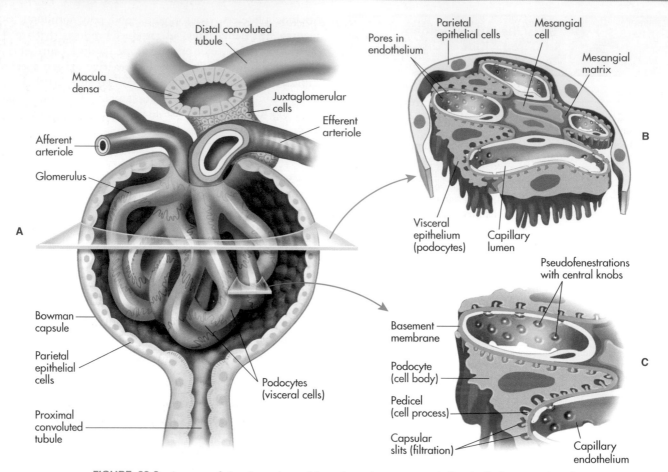

FIGURE 22-2   Anatomy of the glomerulus and juxtaglomerular apparatus. **A,** Longitudinal cross-section of glomerulus and juxtaglomerular apparatus. **B,** Horizontal cross-section of glomerulus. **C,** Enlargemt of glomerular capillary filtration membrane. *(From McCance K, Huether S:* Pathophysiology: the biologic basis for disease in adults and children, *ed 5, St. Louis, 2006, Mosby/Elsevier..)*

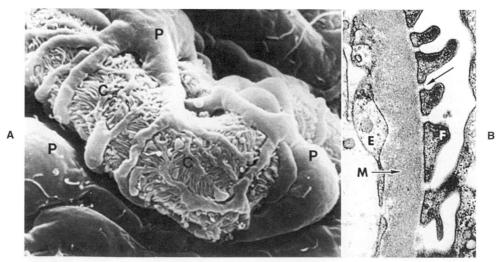

FIGURE 22-3   Glomerular capillary. **A,** Scanning electron micrograph of normal glomerular capillary *(C)* enclosed by podocytes *(P)* with primary processes and interdigitating foot processes. **B,** Glomerular capillary wall showing foot processes of endothelial podocytes *(F),* filtration slit membrane *(arrow),* basement membrane *(M),* and fenestrated endothelium *(E)* (magnification, ×40,000). *(From Kissane JM, ed:* Anderson's pathology, *ed 9, St. Louis, 1990, Mosby.)*

TABLE 22-2	Stages of Chronic Kidney Disease Clinical Presentations		
Stage	**Description**	**GFR Range (ml/min/1.73 m^2)**	**Clinical Presentations***
	At increased risk	≥90 (without markers of damage)	CKD risk factors
1	Kidney damage with normal or ↑ GFR	≥90	Markers of damage (nephrotic syndrome, nephritic syndrome, tubular syndromes, urinary tract symptoms, asymptomatic urinalysis abnormalities, asymptomatic radiologic abnormalities, hypertension due to kidney disease)
2	Kidney damage with mild ↓ GRF	60-89	Mild complications
3	Moderate ↓ GFR	30-59	Moderate complications
4	Severe ↓ GFR	15-29	Severe complications
5	Kidney failure	<15 (or dialysis)	Uremia, cardiovascular disease

From National Kidney Foundation: K/DOQI clinical practice guidelines for chronic kidney disease: evaluation, classification and stratification, *Am J Kidney Dis* 39(suppl 1):S1, 2002.

GFR, Glomerular filtration rate; *CKD,* chronic kidney disease.

*Includes presentations from preceding stages. Chronic kidney disease is defined as either kidney damage or GFR <60 ml/min/1.73 m^2 for ≥3 months. Kidney damage is defined as pathologic abnormalities or markers of damage, including abnormalities in blood or urine tests or imaging studies.

they are at increased risk of having or developing renal disease. Patients are to be considered at risk if they have diabetes, hypertension, autoimmune diseases, systemic infections, exposure to drugs or procedures associated with acute decline in kidney function, recovery from acute kidney failure, age greater than 60 years, family history of kidney disease, or reduced kidney mass.[4] Table 22-2 identifies stages of disease and associates each stage with a level of GFR and clinical manifestations. As the GFR falls below 60 ml/min/1.73 m^2, nutrition intervention becomes an important component of medical care.

Malnutrition, Morbidity, and Inflammation

Malnutrition is a significant comorbidity of chronic renal failure, including patients on hemodialysis or peritoneal dialysis therapy.[11,12] Prevalence of malnutrition and characterization of nutritional status of the predialysis patient with chronic, progressive disease have not been definitively described. The largest set of data concerning nutritional status of the patient with chronic kidney disease is available from the MDRD study.[13] This study reported correlations between GFRs, diet intake, and indexes of nutritional status, including serum albumin, transferrin, and body weight. The earliest relationship reported was for GFRs equivalent to serum creatinine levels in the ranges of approximately 2.3 and 2.5 mg/dl for females and males, respectively (GFR = 35 ml/min/1.73 m^2). As kidney failure progressed as evidenced by worsening GFR, there was a deterioration in nutritional status. Because the MDRD study excluded patients who presented with malnutrition, overall prevalence of malnutrition in this patient group could not be calculated.

Nutritional status of the patient on maintenance dialysis therapy has been widely documented. Surveys report 23% to 76% of patients on hemodialysis and 18% to 50% of patients on peritoneal dialysis therapy are malnourished.[11] Life-threatening malnutrition is present in 5% to 10% of patients, and moderate malnutrition is present in an additional 20% to 40%.[14] Factors contributing to malnutrition in patients with renal failure are listed in Box 22-1.

It is now recognized that malnutrition is an important risk factor for death.[15,16] In a study of more than 14,000 hemodialysis patients, Lowrie and Lew[15] found those with a serum albumin concentration of less than 2.5 g/dl had a risk of death 20 times higher than patients with albumin levels of greater than 4.0 g/dl. Patients with albumin levels of 3.5 to 4.0 g/dl had a risk of death 2 times higher than patients with albumin levels greater than 4.0 g/dl. Other indexes of nutritional status have since been identified to be important predictors of mortality; these include levels of serum cholesterol, creatinine, and prealbumin. As a result, it has been hypothesized that malnutrition is a main cause of death in the dialysis patient population.

hemodialysis Removal of certain elements from the blood according to their rates of diffusion through a semipermeable membrane—e.g., by a hemodialysis machine.

peritoneal dialysis Dialysis through the peritoneum into and out of the peritoneal cavity.

BOX 22-1 | **Factors Contributing to the Presence of Malnutrition in Patients With Chronic Renal Failure**

1. Anorexia due to the following:
   - Nausea, emesis, medications
   - Uremia/uremic state of metabolism
   - Underdialysis
   - Accumulation of uremic toxins not completely removed by dialysis
2. Metabolic acidosis
3. Endocrine disorders (insulin resistance, hyperparathyroidism, impaired response to insulin-like growth factor I)
4. Comorbidity (infections, intercurrent illnesses)
5. Reduced nutrient intake
6. Dialysis related to the following:
   - Inadequate dose
   - Catabolism (bioincompatible membrane)
   - Loss of amino acids and protein to the dialysate
   - Reuse with bleach
7. Psychosocial
   - Depression
   - Inability to purchase or prepare food adequately
   - Loss of or poorly fitting dentures

From Wolfson M: Causes, manifestations, and assessment of malnutrition in chronic renal failure. In Kopple J, Massry S, eds: *Nutritional management of renal disease*, Philadelphia, 1997, Williams & Wilkins.

TABLE 22-3 | **Proposed Features of Type 1 and Type 2 Malnutrition**

	Type 1	Type 2
Serum albumin	Normal/low	Low
Comorbidity	Uncommon	Common
Presence of inflammation	No	Yes
Food intake	Low	Low/normal
Resting energy expenditure	Normal	Elevated
Oxidative stress	Increased	Markedly increased
Protein catabolism	Decreased	Increased
Reversed by dialysis and nutritional support	Yes	No

From Stenvinkel P et al: Are there two types of malnutrition in chronic renal failure? Evidence for relationships between malnutrition, inflammation and atherosclerosis (MIA syndrome), *Nephrol Dial Transplant* 15(7):953, 2000, by permission of Oxford University Press.

Interventions to improve serum albumin and other markers of nutritional status have had mixed results. It has been recently hypothesized that the parameters reflecting malnutrition are influenced not only by nutritional status but also by an inflammatory process that may or may not be related to the presence of active CKD.[17-19] The inflammatory response is mediated by cytokines including interleukin-1, interleukin-6, and tumor necrosis factor-alpha. Cytokines induce anorexia, decreases in fat mass, loss of lean muscle mass, augmented catabolism, and decreases in serum levels of albumin, prealbumin, and transferrin. Similar changes are induced by malnutrition. Studies have demonstrated increased levels of these cytokines in surveys of hemodialysis and peritoneal dialysis patients.[20]

Several parameters used for nutrition assessment and nutrition monitoring are negative acute-phase reactant proteins (ARPs), including albumin, prealbumin, and transferrin. In response to inflammation, hepatic synthesis and serum levels of the above negative ARPs diminish. At the same time, synthesis and serum levels of positive ARPs increase; these include C-reactive protein (CRP), serum amyloid A, and ferritin. In dialysis patients, serum albumin concentration is negatively associated with positive ARPs.[21] Therefore indicators traditionally viewed to be signs of malnutrition, such as decreased serum concentrations of albumin and prealbumin, loss of muscle mass, and weight loss, may not be the result of malnutrition but may instead be the result of an inflammatory response or some combination of inflammation and malnutrition. Clinical or biologic stimuli/stimulus activating a proinflammatory response with symptoms of malnutrition is currently unknown. Hypotheses include unrecognized clinical infection, bioincompatible membranes, oxidative stress, increased production of glycosylated end products, endothelial dysfunction, or vascular disease.[17-21]

The main cause of death in patients with ESRD is CVD.[22] In dialysis patients the death rate from CVD is 10 to 20 times higher than that in the general population.[23] Atherosclerosis is an inflammatory disease characterized by increased adhesiveness of the endothelium for platelets, leukocytes, increased vascular permeability, formation of vasoactive cytokines, and growth factors. CRP is a powerful predictor of cardiovascular events. Elevated levels are commonly observed in patients with chronic renal disease.

Elevated CRP levels in renal patients suggest a chronic state of inflammation. Stenvinkel and colleagues[17] have hypothesized interactions exist between malnutrition, inflammation, and CVD, referred to as the malnutrition, inflammation, atherosclerosis (MIA) syndrome. It is possible some patients are malnourished as a result of (1) anorexia and hypercatabolism related specifically to renal disease, (2) inflammation and CVD, and (3) a mixed type of malnutrition (Table 22-3 and Figure 22-4). These newer hypotheses are the beginning of a different approach to treatment of malnutrition in renal disease. As understanding of the causes of malnutrition and discrimination of nutrition parameters become possible, more successful interventions can be developed.

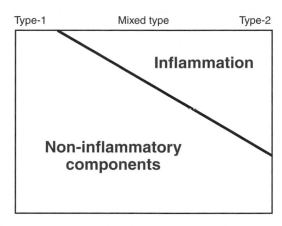

FIGURE 22-4 Proposed relative contribution of noninflammatory components (e.g., low intake of protein and energy because of uremic anorexia, underdialysis, physical activity) and the inflammatory components of malnutrition in patients with type 1 and type 2 malnutrition, respectively. *(From Stenvinkel P et al: Are there two types of malnutrition in chronic renal failure? Evidence for relationships between malnutrition, inflammation and atherosclerosis {MIA syndrome},* Nephrol Dial Transplant 15{7}:953, 2000, *by permission of Oxford University Press.)*

NUTRITION ASSESSMENT OF PATIENTS WITH KIDNEY DISEASE

Evaluating and monitoring nutritional status are vital components of nutrition care of the patient with kidney disease. High prevalence of malnutrition, large number of aberrations in normal metabolism, and complications including anorexia and catabolism all indicate need for consistent monitoring. Nutrition assessment is best completed by a registered dietitian who has received special training in renal nutrition care.

When completing a nutrition assessment, an array of indexes, each representing a specific data category, are measured independently and then evaluated collectively to ascertain nutritional status of the renal patient. Table 22-4 lists the data categories that encompass the nutrition assessment of the renal patient. Specific indexes used to evaluate biochemical values are listed in Table 22-5. Following is a review of indexes most commonly measured from each data category.[24-26]

Subjective global assessment (SGA) is an approach to completing a nutrition assessment that has been validated in the ESRD population. However, current efforts for identifying methods for nutrition assessment are focusing on developing objective methodologies.

Clinical

Medical History

The medical history should include any information about the patient's appetite, food intake, and ability to metabolize food. This requires past medical and surgical history, current medical diagnosis and problems, prescribed medications, drug use including alcohol, bowel habits, and weight history. Record of any major organ or gastrointestinal diseases, surgeries, or previous symptoms of malabsorption or other digestive problems, including nausea, vomiting, and diarrhea, should be noted. Impairment in fluid and electrolyte balance, hypertension/hypotension, proteinuria, and any previous symptoms of uremia that affect appetite, food intake, digestion, or nutritional status should also be noted.

Psychosocial History

This evaluates the patient's mental status, as well as factors regarding economics, education level, physical home environment, food shopping and preparation capabilities, and available support systems. The goal is to create an individualized intervention the patient or patient's support system can understand and apply. Factors that might compromise nutritional status include depression or improper food preparation and storage equipment. This component of the assessment process helps identify patients requiring social services to assist with economic needs or special services to provide regular access to food and medications.

Demographics

Information on age, marital status, gender, and ethnicity is needed to assess nutritional status. Many reference standards used to classify clinical indexes adjust for gender and age. Knowledge of ethnicity affects ability to individualize nutrition therapy; marital status helps identify support systems.

Physical Activity

Assessment of the patient's physical capabilities is needed to maintain activities of daily living and proper level of physical exercise for psychologic and physical therapeutics. The following questionnaires have been validated for the purpose of measuring physical activity and physical functioning in the ESRD patient population: the Stanford 7-Day Physical Activity Recall, Physical Activity Scale for the Elderly, Human Activity Profile, and Medical Outcomes Study Short-Form 36-item questionnaire.

Current Medical and Surgical Issues

Identification of nutritional implications of medical and surgical problems is imperative for the nutrition assessment procedure. For the patient with chronic, progressive disease, this requires acknowledgment of any newly diagnosed medical/surgical illnesses.

---

proteinuria The presence of an excess of serum proteins, such as albumin, in the urine.

| TABLE 22-4 | **Nutrition Assessment Parameters in Chronic Kidney Disease** |
</br>

Parameter	What It Measures	Components

History and physical examination	Past and present nutritional status; areas that should be addressed when developing a plan of care	Review of medical record
		Patient, family, and/or caregiver interview
		Psychosocial history
		Ability to obtain, prepare, ingest, and enjoy food
		Mental status
		Educational level
		Functional status
		Person responsible for shopping/preparing food
		Patient's functional status (activities of daily living)
		Diet histories
		  • Usual food intake
		  • Food intake patterns
		  • Factors affecting intake
		Religious/cultural beliefs
		Use of supplements and alternative or complementary therapies
		Past diet restrictions (and education)
		Patient's ability to chew, swallow, taste, and smell foods
		Changes in appetite and eating pattern
		Food preferences, allergies, and intolerances
		Use of alcohol
		Practice of pica

Anthropometric assessment	Weight status; nutritional status; distribution of body fat, lean muscle mass, and bone	Body weight (can be difficult to determine due to fluid retention) Estimated dry weight or edema-free body weight (BW_{ef}) Hemodialysis: weight postdialysis Peritoneal dialysis: weight after drainage of dialysate with peritoneum empty Interdialytic weight gains Fluid gains between hemodialysis treatments Height Initial measurement essential Recumbent bed height, arm span, or knee height may be used if patient cannot stand Estimation of frame size Body mass index Estimated of body composition Skinfold thicknesses
Energy and nutrient requirements	Must be individually assessed based on type of dialysis, cause of kidney disease, and other comorbidities	kcal per kg formulas
Subjective global assessment	Useful measure of protein-energy nutritional status in maintenance dialysis patients	4-item, 7-point scale Medical history Weight change during previous 6 months Dietary intake GI symptoms Physical examination Visual assessment of subcutaneous tissue and muscle mass
Biochemical parameters	Monitored on ongoing basis to assess nutritional status	See Table 22-5

Data from Barbá PD, Goode JL: Nutrition assessment in chronic kidney disease. In Byham-Gray L, Wiesen K, eds: *A clinical guide to nutrition care in kidney disease,* Chicago, 2004, American Dietetic Association.

TABLE 22-5 | Biochemical Parameters for Assessing Nutritional Status

Parameter	Substance	Normal Range	CKD Range
Visceral protein stores	Albumin	3.5-5.0 g/dL	WNL for laboratory or ≥4.0 g/dL
	Prealbumin (transthyretin)	15-36 mg/dL	>30 mg/dL
	Transferrin	Females: 15%-50% Males: 20%-50%	WNL
	C Reactive protein (CRP)	0.8 mg/dL	2-15 mg/dL
Static (Somatic) protein reserves	Serum creatinine	Females: 0.5-1.1 mg/dL Males: 0.6-1.2 mg/dL	2-15 mg/dL
Other estimates of protein reserves	Nitrogen balance		
Fluid, electrolyte, and acid-base status	Sodium	135-145 mEq/L	WNL
	Potassium	3.5-5.0 mEq/L	3.5-6.0 mEq/L
	Chloride		
	Calcium	WNL for laboratory	Normal: 8.4-10.2 mg/dL; preferably at low end of normal (8.4-9.5 mg/dL)
	Phosphorus	3.0-4.5 mg/dL	3.5-5.5 mg/dL
	CO_2		22-25 mEq/L
	Glucose	70-105 mg/dL	WNL <200 nonfasting before dialysis; intake has influence
Indirect indices of renal function and dialysis adequacy	Serum creatinine	Females: 0.5-1.1 mg/dL Males: 0.6-1.2 mg/dL	2-15 mg/dL
	Blood urea nitrogen (BUN)	10-20 mg/dL	60-80 mg/dL in anuric; well dialyzed and eating adequate protein
	URR (urea reduction ratio)	N/A	>65%
	eKT/V (equilibrated clearance of urea during dialysis)	N/A	>1.2
	Kt/V (hemodialysis)	N/A	1.2
	Kt/V (peritoneal dialysis)	N/A	2.0-2.2
Anemia	Hemoglobin	Females: 12-16 g/dL Males: 14-18 g/dL	Variable 11-12 g/dL
	Ferritin	Females: 10-150 mg/mL Males: 12-300 mg/mL	≥100 ng/mL, but no know benefit >800
	Serum iron	Females: 50-170 µg/dL Males: 60-175 µg/dL	WNL
Hyperlipidemia	Serum cholesterol	<200 mg	WNL <150 mg, evaluate for nutrient deficit
	Triglycerides	Females: 35-135 mg/dL Males: 40-160 mg/dL	WNL <200 mg/dL
Renal osteodystrophy	Calcium	WNL for laboratory	Normal: 8.4-10.2 mg/dL; preferably at low end of normal (8.4-9.5 mg/dL)
	Alkaline phosphatase	30-85 ImU/mL	WNL for laboratory
	Parathyroid hormone (PHT) (i) intact	10-65 pg/mL	150-300 pg/mL
	Biointact (3rd generation)	60-140 pg/mL	80-160 pg/mL

Data from Barbá PD, Goode JL: Nutrition assessment in chronic kidney disease. In Byham-Gray L, Wiesen K, eds: *A clinical guide to nutrition care in kidney disease*, Chicago, 2004, American Dietetic Association; and Wilkens KG: Medical nutrition therapy for renal disorders. In Mahan K, Escott-Stump S, eds: *Krause's food, nutrition, & diet therapy*, ed 11, Philadelphia, 2004, Saunders.

WNL, Within normal limits.

Diet and Food Intake

This category relies on subjective patient reporting to evaluate qualitative and quantitative aspects of food intake. One of the most useful outputs from this category is calculation of nutrient intake. Other outputs include information related to past and current food intake (qualitative and quantitative), eating patterns, and specific food preferences. This information allows an approximation of the diet's adequacy. It also helps to identify nutrient factors that may be contributing to medical problems. Qualitative data are essential for formulation of individual diet therapy, including meal plans and menus.

Diet History

Nutrition history is usually obtained at the initial meeting. It is an all-inclusive collection of some objective but primarily subjective information concerning the patient's food, such as aversions, allergies, preferences, and intake. Information on previous and current diet intake assists in devising interventions to improve diet or devising an acceptable therapeutic meal plan. The most commonly used tools to obtain food intake information differ in approach to data collection, retrospective versus prospective, and whether the information is a qualitative description of intake versus a quantitative one.

Food Record.

A food record provides qualitative and approximate quantitative food intake information that is best collected prospectively. The minimal time recommended for data collection is 3 days; a reasonable maximum is 5 days. The patient should provide intake information for both weekends and weekdays so that variability can be determined. For the dialysis patient, it is strongly recommended the food record include intake for dialysis as well as nondialysis days, in addition to weekend versus weekday pattern. A difference in food intake between dialysis and nondialysis days has been noted in both type and amount of food selected.

The patient should be provided with instructions on how to approximate food portion sizes and servings of fluid to ensure accurate reporting. Use of food models is very helpful. The food record should include time of day of any intake (both meals and snacks), names of foods eaten, approximate amount of food ingested, method of preparation, and special recipes or steps taken in the food preparation. The same instructions apply to fluid intake. Brand names are requested when available.

Some patients find it is more convenient to record food intake at the end of the day. This is an inferior method because the data collection becomes retrospective and more subject to error. Calculation of intake of total protein, protein quality, carbohydrate, fat, fatty acid classes, and other selected nutrients is best completed by a computerized nutrient analysis program.

24-Hour Food Recall.

The 24-hour food recall is an interactive tool in which the clinician assists the patient in remembering qualitative and quantitative food intake via prompting. The clinician can sit with a patient during dialysis and slowly help the patient recall the previous day's intake of both food and fluid. Food models or drawings can be used to help the patient identify portion size. One 24-hour recall, however, does not provide sufficient information to ascertain total food intake.

A variation of the 24-hour recall for a dialysis patient is to meet with the patient during three consecutive treatments, or at least four sessions within a 2-week period, and obtain one 24-hour recall at each visit. Effort should be made to obtain a recall for a weekend day, a dialysis day, and a nondialysis day. To obtain a total food intake on a dialysis day, the practitioner can ask the patient what he or she had to eat so far that day and record it. The patient or family member can finish recording for the rest of the day, or the clinician can meet with the patient at the next session to help him or her recall what was eaten for the rest of that day. Calling the patient's home on a daily basis to obtain the needed information is an option but is not practical.

Food Frequency Questionnaires.

Food frequency questionnaires (FFQs) approximate nutrient intake by identifying periodicity of intake of specific foods within food groups that are significant sources of a particular nutrient or nutrients (e.g., dairy products are a good source of calcium, vitamin D, and protein). A food frequency consists of listing foods according to group, such as vegetables, fruits, dairy, protein, and so forth. The patient is questioned as to how often he or she eats this food per day, per week, and per month. An approximation of adequacy of intake of specific nutrients can be calculated from the results. Although FFQs have not been widely used to assess the intake of renal patients, a recent study in hemodialysis patients provides preliminary data indicating the Block (version 98) FFQ can be a useful tool for this purpose.[27]

Biochemical Values

Serum biochemical values are used to assess and monitor nutritional status over time. Selected serum values pertain to visceral protein stores, static protein reserves, overall protein nutriture, immune competence, iron stores, and vitamin, mineral, and trace element status. In addition to these components, nutrition assessment involves evaluating fluid, electrolyte, and acid-base status; renal function; dialysis adequacy for the patient receiving replacement therapy; serum lipid levels; and bone health.

Visceral Protein Stores

Serum levels of albumin, transferrin, prealbumin, and retinol-binding protein (RBP) are biochemical markers most often used to assess visceral protein stores, monitor response to nutrition intervention, and identify which patients are at risk for development of complications or are responding poorly to medical/surgical treatment. The assumption—not yet proved—is that serum concentration represents hepatic protein synthetic mass and indirectly the functional protein mass of the internal viscera (i.e., heart, lung, kidneys, intestines).[24]

Serum Albumin. Albumin, the most abundant plasma protein, functions to maintain plasma oncotic pressure and serves as a major carrier protein for drugs, hormones, enzymes, and trace elements. Clinically significant hypoalbuminemia occurs with different types of malnutrition besides kidney disease (e.g., protein-energy kwashiorkor, uncomplicated), in both children and adults. In these conditions, hypoalbuminemia usually indicates other metabolic derangements, as well as a poor prognosis. From these observations, serum albumin became a part of routine nutrition assessment of the hospitalized patient and subsequently the renal patient.

Causes of significant hypoalbuminemia associated with malnutrition are not known. (See the previous discussion of the MIA syndrome under the heading "Malnutrition, Morbidity, and Inflammation.") Although serum albumin levels have been used extensively in clinical practice, research studies, and nutritional surveys to assess nutritional status of the chronic and end-stage renal patient population, reliability and sensitivity of this parameter have been questioned. Concerns are independent of conditions that change serum albumin as a marker of visceral protein stores. Use of albumin for assessment purposes has been criticized because of its long half-life, averaging 14 to 20 days, and large body pool, 4 to 5 mg/kg, making albumin slow to respond to changes in visceral protein stores. It is therefore a late marker of malnutrition.[12,21]

Prealbumin (Thyroxine-Binding Prealbumin, Transthyretin). Prealbumin is a carrier protein for RBP and thus has a major role in transport of thyroxine. Its short half-life of 2 to 3 days and its small body pool make it more sensitive than albumin to changes in protein status. This was the first visceral protein found to be low in healthy children who were eating marginal amounts of protein. In primates, prealbumin reflects overall nitrogen balance during starvation and refeeding. Decreases in serum levels occur independently of nutritional status when there is acute metabolic stress, including trauma, minor stress, and inflammation. Serum concentration has also been observed to decrease in liver disease and with iron supplementation. Prealbumin can be useful as a nutritional marker after acute metabolic stress.

Low molecular weight of prealbumin (approximately 54,980 daltons) precludes its use as a marker of nutritional status in patients with chronic renal disease who

have a decreased GFR. Prealbumin levels have been reported to be elevated in the euvolemic patient with chronic renal failure. In hemodialysis patients, high levels have been observed and are attributed to decreased renal catabolism. A decline in the proportion of circulating free prealbumin versus that complexed with RBP may explain the diminished catabolism and therefore elevated levels. A concentration of less than 30 mg/dl (normal range, 10 to 40 mg/dl) may indicate malnutrition in the hemodialysis patient and has recently been associated with an increased risk of death. These studies indicate prealbumin level may serve as a better nutrition assessment tool and predictor of patient outcome than the traditionally used serum albumin in the dialysis population.[14,16]

Retinol-Binding Protein. This protein circulates in a 1:1 molar ratio with prealbumin and transports the alcohol fraction of vitamin A. Its short half-life of 10 to 12 hours and small body pool enable it to respond quickly and specifically to changes in protein status. RBP is not an appropriate marker of nutritional status for the patient with chronic renal disease or ESRD because it is catabolized in renal proximal tubular cells. With renal disease, half-life is reported to be prolonged, and serum levels increase. Other limitations of RBP for nutrition assessment are that serum levels become low in hyperthyroidism, vitamin A deficiency, and acute catabolic states (i.e., levels change inversely with acute-phase proteins).

Transferrin (Siderophilin). The main function of transferrin is to bind ferrous iron and to transport iron to the bone marrow. Its half-life of 8 to 10 days and small body pool enable it to respond more rapidly to short-term changes in protein status, compared with albumin. Studies in malnourished children, as well in hospitalized patients, have demonstrated a correlation between transferrin and the severity and prognosis of disease, as well as an improvement in serum levels with nutrition intervention.[24]

Before it was practical to measure transferrin levels, total iron-binding capacity (TIBC) was thought to be equivalent to the amount of iron required to saturate plasma transferrin. This assumption turned out to be true only in normal and iron-deficient subjects. The most common

hyperthyroidism Abnormally increased activity of the parathyroid gland, resulting in excessive secretion of parathyroid hormone, which usually helps regulate serum calcium levels in balance with vitamin D hormone; excess secretion occurs when the serum calcium level falls below normal, as in chronic renal disease or in vitamin D deficiency.

estimate is obtained from TIBC using this formula: transferrin = $(0.8 \times$ TIBC$) - 43$. However, this formula has not been validated as an estimate of serum transferrin in the renal patient, and a direct measure is recommended. Use of this protein in nutrition assessment of the renal patient is confounded by many factors that influence serum levels. Iron deficiency increases hepatic synthesis and plasma levels. Reduced transferrin concentrations are observed in association with uremia, protein-losing enteropathy, nephropathy, acute catabolic states, chronic infections, and iron loading. In chronic renal failure, transferrin is reliable for the evaluation of iron status. Most patients on renal replacement receive erythropoietin therapy and iron supplementation. Use of transferrin should be reserved for those patients who have a stable erythropoietin regimen with adequate iron replacement.

Insulin-Like Growth Factor I (Somatomedin C).
Insulin-like growth factor I (IGF-I) is a serum protein with mitogen properties and insulin-like activities; it may be a sensitive biochemical indicator of nitrogen balance. With a half-life of 2 to 6 hours, IGF-I represents an acute-phase response. Studies of hospitalized, hypercatabolic patients indicate that IGF-I is a better marker of nitrogen balance than other serum proteins. In humans, IGF-I levels fall during fasting and increase with refeeding, and IGF-I has been reported to be a reliable marker of malnutrition in children. A serum concentration below 300 ng/ml indicates a poor nutritional status in hemodialysis patients.

Static Protein Reserves (Somatic Protein, Muscle Stores)
Measures of muscle mass are thought to be good indicators of static protein reserves because approximately 60% of total body protein is contained in muscle. Skeletal muscle is the predominant source of amino acid mobilization during periods of nutritional deficiency. Both anthropometric and biochemical markers are used to assess muscle mass. Anthropometric techniques are discussed later in this chapter under the heading "Body Composition."

Urinary and Serum Creatinine.
Creatinine is formed at a relatively constant rate from creatine, a compound found predominantly in muscle; therefore urinary creatinine is proportional to muscle creatine content and hence to total body muscle mass. Urinary excretion of creatinine correlates with lean body mass measured by isotope dilution and 40 K total body counting techniques.

For the patient with renal insufficiency or deteriorating renal function, urinary creatinine cannot be used for nutrition assessment purposes. There is no role for urinary creatinine excretion in nutrition assessment for the end-stage patient who has zero or insignificant residual renal function and accumulates creatinine.

For a chronic renal patient with a stable GFR and for the dialysis patient, changes in serum creatinine over time (about 3 months) may indicate a change in muscle mass. Verification of a change in muscle mass based on the serum creatinine must be confirmed by assessing other parameters of somatic protein stores, as well as by evaluating the patient's weight, overall food intake, and biochemical markers of visceral stores.

Immune Competence.
A comprehensive nutrition assessment includes tests of immune function. Total lymphocyte count and delayed cutaneous hypersensitivity responses are tests of humoral immunity and have limited use in nutrition assessment because of altered host defenses. Use of serum complement system components and serum immunoglobulins to test humoral immunity is complex because of discrepancies concerning which proteins are altered in renal failure or improve with adequate nutrition.

Body Weight

Initial assessment of body weight and monitoring of weight change over time represent critical components of the nutrition assessment process. Weight loss in excess of 5% to 10%, depending on the patient's overall nutritional status, or substandard weight for height should be considered a risk factor for malnutrition. Interrelationships between weight loss over time and outcome in the renal patient population have not yet been reported.

Body mass index (weight [kg]/height [m^2]), current weight, usual weight, ideal body weight, percent usual weight, percent ideal body weight, and particularly percent weight change over a defined time period are important parameters of body weight. A database or sheet in the patient's chart committed to record body weight is recommended for every patient.

Body Composition

Measures of body composition to ascertain fat stores and lean body mass are included. Other than the initial investment for skinfold calipers and an accurate tape measure, anthropometry is an inexpensive technique. Measurements obtained are compared with standards that classify the patient as normal, "at risk" for malnutrition, or having a type and degree of malnutrition. In general, measurements below the 35th to 40th percentile suggest mild depletion; below the 25th to 35th percentile, moderate depletion; and below the 25th percentile, severe depletion.

Anthropometry
Fat Stores.
Approximately half of human fat is found in the subcutaneous layer. Therefore measurement of subcutaneous fat provides a reasonably accurate index of total body fat. Triceps skinfold thickness and subscapular skinfold are commonly used to quantify adipose tissue thickness on the limbs and trunk. Other body points that can be measured to ascertain adipose stores using

skinfold thickness are biceps, abdomen, suprailiac, medial calf, and anterior thigh. Loss of fat from subcutaneous stores occurs proportionally; therefore repeat measures from a selected group of sites in an individual patient can provide reliable information on trends of adipose stores. In dialysis patients, it is recommended arm measures be completed using the nonaccess arm. Otherwise, the right arm is recommended for use in measurements.

Skeletal Muscle (Somatic Protein Mass, Static Protein Reserves). Anthropometric measures of muscle mass can serve as an indirect assessment of muscle stores because approximately 60% of total body protein is located in skeletal muscle. In response to poor nutrition, skeletal muscle is the primary source of amino acids. The most commonly used anthropometric measures to assess skeletal muscle are midarm muscle circumference (MAMC) and midarm circumference (MAC). There are several limitations to these anthropometric measures: a 10% error occurs between measurements even when performed by the same clinician, and there is a poor correlation reported between visceral stores and upper arm measurements. Therefore anthropometric measures alone cannot be relied on to evaluate muscle and fat stores. Anthropometric measures are best used in conjunction with data from the other categories (see Table 22-4).

Advanced Methods of Body Composition Analysis

Methods available to determine fat-free mass are measures of body water, potassium, nitrogen, and calcium and two electrical approaches, bioelectrical impedance (BIA) and electromagnetic scanning, referred to as TOBEC and EMSCAN, respectively. Techniques to estimate total body fat other than anthropometry are inert gas absorption, infrared interactance, total body carbon using neutron activation, computed tomography, magnetic resonance imaging, and dual-energy x-ray absorptiometry (DEXA). Although several of these techniques have been used for body composition analysis in renal patients, they have not been adopted for routine use.

ALTERED NUTRIENT REQUIREMENTS WITH CHRONIC KIDNEY DISEASE

Nutrition intervention for patients with CKD includes modifications for sodium, fluid, potassium, phosphorus, calcium, vitamin D, iron, calories, and protein. Although global recommendations are available, nutrition care must be individualized based on serum chemistry levels, fluid balance, and nutritional status. These concerns are addressed in the following discussion (see also the *Diet-Medications Interactions* box, "Common Drugs Used for Renal Disorders and Potential Food-Drug Interactions").

Sodium and Potassium

As kidney function declines, ability of the nephrons to maintain sodium balance through sodium excretion diminishes. However, an adaptive mechanism results in undamaged nephrons' being able to excrete a higher percentage of filtered sodium, with the effect being a decrease in the fractional reabsorption and an increase in fractional excretion of sodium by renal tubules. As GFR falls to 10 ml/min, a 2.0- to 3.0-g sodium restriction may be required to maintain both sodium and fluid balance. Clinical symptoms of excessive sodium intake include shortness of breath, hypertension, congestive heart failure, and edema. Alternatively, a patient who continues to have a urine output of at least 1000 ml/day may be able to maintain sodium balance on an unrestricted intake.[28]

Kidney regulation of potassium balance is obtained by renal excretion of potassium in an amount equal to that absorbed by the gastrointestinal tract. Potassium balance is dependent on the ability of the tubules to continue to secrete potassium into the ultrafiltrate. This ability will decrease as kidney failure progresses. Once the patient becomes oliguric or GFR drops to about 10 ml/min, dietary potassium restriction to approximately 2.5 g/day is required to maintain the serum levels within the normal range of 3.5 to 5.5 mEq/L.[28]

Phosphorus, Calcium, and Vitamin D

The consequence of abnormalities of calcium, phosphorus, and vitamin D metabolism seen in chronic kidney disease is development of bone diseases, which are referred to as renal osteodystrophy. Diagnoses include osteoporosis, osteosclerosis, osteomalacia, and osteitis fibrosa. The healthy kidney filters about 7 g of phosphorus per day, of which 80% to 90% is reabsorbed by the renal tubules and the remaining 10% is excreted into urine. Phosphorus balance can be maintained until the GFR falls under 20 ml/min. At that point, phosphorus accumulation occurs in the serum. In addition, conversion of vitamin D to the active form 1,25-dihydrocholecalciferol is diminished, resulting in low serum calcium levels and elevated parathyroid hormone levels. Dietary intervention for bone disease management is dietary phosphorus restriction to 5 to 10 mg of phosphorus per kilogram of body weight per day. In addition to dietary phosphate restriction, most patients require oral calcium and/or oral or intravenous vitamin D or vitamin D analogues. Serum parathyroid hormone, calcium, and phosphorus levels must be monitored closely to avoid excesses and deficiencies that can exacerbate the bone disease.[28,29]

---

osteodystrophy Defective bone formation.

DIET-MEDICATIONS INTERACTIONS

Common Drugs Used for Renal Disorders and Potential Food-Drug Interactions

Drug	Potential Food Drug Interaction
Pyelonephritis and Urinary Tract Infections	
Ceftriaxone and gentamicin	• Sufficient water and fluids should be consumed.
	• Monitor glucose changes in persons with DM.
	• Avoid use with alcohol
Sulfisoxazole (Gantrisin)	• Can deplete folacin and vitamin K.
Trimethoprim (Trimpex), trimethoprim/sulfamethoxazole (Bactrim, Septra, Cotrim)	• May cause diarrhea, GI distress, and stomatitis.
	• Sufficient fluid intake necessary.
Nitrofurantoin (Furadantin, Macrodantin)	• Should be taken with food or milk.
	• Adequate dietary protein necessary.
	• Nausea, vomiting, anorexia common.
Quinolones: Ofloxacin (Floxin), norfloxacin (Noroxin), ciprofloxacin (Cipro), trovafloxacin (Trovan)	• Milk, yogurt, and calcium supplements should be avoided when taking Cipro. Caffeine intake should be limited.
	• Floxin or Maxaquin should be taken separately from vitamin supplements. Nausea is one side effect.
Urolithiasis/Nephrolithiasis (Kidney Stones)	
Allopurinol (Zyloprim) and probenecid (usually used instead of or in conjunction with purine-restricted diet)	• Drink 10-12 glasses of fluid daily.
	• Avoid concomitant intake of vitamin C supplements.
	• Maintain alkaline urine.
	• Side effects include nausea, vomiting, diarrhea, and abdominal pain.
Thiazide diuretics	• Increase intake of high-potassium foods.
	• Control sodium intake.
	• Increase magnesium intake.
	• Dry mouth or GI distress may occur.
D-Penicillamine	• Requires B_6 and zinc supplementation.
	• Increase fluid intake with cystinuria.
	• Take 1-2 hours before/after meals.
	• Stomatitis, diarrhea, nausea, vomiting, abdominal pain may occur.
Demerol, etc.	• Dry mouth, constipation, nausea, vomiting can occur.
Acute Renal Failure	
Exchange resins (Kayexalate)	• Take separately from calcium and antacids by several hours.
Sorbitol	• Bloating, flatulence, or diarrhea may occur.
Chronic and End-Stage Renal Disease	
Phosphate binders: calcium acetate or calcium carbonate	• Nausea and vomiting.
Ergocalciferol (vitamin D analogue)	• Additional water necessary to prevent constipation.
	• Monitor fluids carefully if urine output is decreased.
	• Avoid long-term use.
Recombinant human erythropoietin (r-HuEPO)	• Iron supplements necessary.
	• Do not take iron supplement at same time as calcium.
Hemodialysis	
Kayexalate	• Take separately from calcium supplements or antacids.
Transplantation (patients are usually on three to four of the five drugs listed below)	
Corticosteroids (Prednisone, Solu-Cortef)	• Increased catabolism or proteins.
	• Negative nitrogen balance.
	• Hyperphagia.
	• Ulcers.
	• Decreased glucose tolerance.
	• Sodium and fluid retention.
	• Impaired calcium absorption and osteoporosis.
	• Cushing's syndrome.
	• Obesity.
	• Muscle wasting.
	• Increased gastric secretion.

Data from Escott-Stump S: *Nutrition and diagnosis-related care,* ed 5, Philadelphia, 2002, Lippincott Williams & Wilkins.
DM, Diabetes mellitus; *GI,* gastrointestinal.

🔵 DIET-MEDICATIONS INTERACTIONS—cont'd

Common Drugs Used for Renal Disorders and Potential Food-Drug Interactions

Drug	Potential Food Drug Interaction
Transplantation—cont'd	
Cyclosporine	• Nausea, vomiting, and diarrhea.
	• Hyperlipidemia and hyperkalemia may occur.
	• Elevated glucose and lipids.
Immunosuppressants (Muromonab, Orthoclone [OKT3], antithymocyte globulin [ATG]}	• Nausea, anorexia, diarrhea, and vomiting.
	• Fever.
	• Stomatitis.
Azathioprine (Imuran)	• Leucopenia, thrombocytopenia.
	• Oral and esophageal sores.
	• Macrocytic anemia.
	• Pancreatitis.
	• Vomiting, diarrhea.
	• Folate supplementation may be needed.
	• Dietary modifications (liquid or soft diet, use of oral supplements) may be needed.
Tacrolimus (Prograf, FK506)	• GI distress, nausea, vomiting, diarrhea.
	• Hyperglycemia.

Iron

Because of the diminished ability of the failing kidney to synthesize adequate amounts of erythropoietin, most patients with chronic renal failure develop anemia if left untreated. Recommended levels for hematocrit are 33% to 36%; for hemoglobin, 11 to 12 g/dl. These target levels are accomplished through administration of recombinant human erythropoietin (r-HuEPO) and 10 to 18 mg oral iron. Doses are individualized. If left untreated, adverse clinical events can occur, including increased mortality rates, malnutrition, angina, cardiac enlargement, and impaired immunologic response.[30,31]

Calories and Protein

Historically, dietary protein was restricted in patients with chronic renal disease to levels as low as 0.3 g of protein per kilogram of body weight per day when supplemented with essential amino acids or nitrogen-free analogues called *keto-acids*. A more common protein restriction was 0.6 g/kg/day. Rationale for the restriction was based on observations in animals and human studies that, in general, high-protein diets resulted in proteinuria, mortality, and renal damage, whereas restriction of dietary protein resulted in improvements.[25] There are a large number of human studies that have demonstrated low-protein diets initiated early in chronic renal failure improve uremic symptoms by decreasing formation of nitrogenous compounds. These diets were to be calorically dense, in the range of 35 kcalories (kcalories or kcal)/kg to promote protein sparing and minimize formation of protein metabolic byproducts. However, beneficial effects of these diets on preventing progression of kidney disease were never demonstrated. Patients often became malnourished. Whether this was because of inability to adhere to the diet or from some other catabolic event was not discriminated in the majority of studies.[25]

In 1990, the MDRD study was implemented to test, in a large multicenter trial, use of low-protein diets in delaying progression of renal disease.[13] Two groups of patients were studied. Group A patients had GFRs in the range of 25 to 55 ml/min/1.73 m^2 and were randomized to a diet of 1 or more g of protein per kilogram per day or 0.6 g/kg/day. Mean blood pressures were maintained at 105 or 92 mm Hg. Group B patients had GFRs in the range of 13 to 24 ml/min/1.73 m^2 and were assigned diets containing 0.6 or 0.3 g of protein per kilogram per day plus a keto-acid supplement. Blood pressure goals were the same. Renal function was monitored for 2.2 years by measuring ^{125}I-iothalamate renal clearance. The MDRD study results demonstrated that neither the low-protein diet nor the blood pressure control decreased the loss of GFR.

The K/DOQI guidelines for CKD include recommendations for protein and calories based on a comprehensive review of the literature.[4] These guidelines recommend 0.6 g protein per kilogram of body weight per day when GFR is less than 25 ml/min and the patient is not on dialysis. For individuals who do not want to follow this diet or are unable to maintain adequate caloric intake, a diet providing protein in the amount of 0.75 g/kg/day is recommended to be considered. At this same level of GFR, caloric intake for patients younger than 60 years of age is recommended to be 35 kcal/kg/day; for those 60 years of age or older, 30 to 35 kcal/kg/day. Other diet recommendations that integrate current data concerning protein, calories, fatty acids, vitamins, and minerals until additional data are available are listed in Table 22-6.

TABLE 22-6	Recommended Dietary Nutrient Intake for Patients With Chronic Renal Failure Not Undergoing Dialysis[a,b,c]

Nutrient	Recommendation
Protein: low-protein diet (g/kg/day)	GFR <25 ml/min: 0.6 g protein/kg/day; if patient unable to maintain adequate intake of calories or will not accept this diet, 0.75 g protein/kg/day
Energy (kcal/kg/day)	GFR <25 ml/min: 35 kcal/kg/day if <60 years of age; 30-35 kcal/kg/day if ≥60 years of age
Fat (percentage of total energy intake)[d,e]	30
Polyunsaturated/saturated fatty acid ratio[e]	1.0:1.0
Carbohydrate[e,f]	Remainder of nonprotein calories
Total fiber intake (g/day)[e]	20-25
Minerals (range of intake)	
Sodium (mg/day)	1000-3000[g]
Potassium (mEq/day)	40-70
Phosphorus (mg/kg/day)	5-10[h]
Calcium (mg/day)	1400-1600[i]
Magnesium (mg/day)	200-300
Iron (mg/day)	≥10-18[j]
Zinc (mg/day)	15
Water (ml/day)	Up to 3000 as tolerated[g]
Vitamins	Diet may be supplemented with these quantities
Thiamin (mg/day)	1.5
Riboflavin (mg/day)	1.8
Pantothenic acid (mg/day)	5
Niacin (mg/day)	20
Pyridoxine HCl (mg/day)	5
Vitamin B_{12} (μg/day)	3
Vitamin C (mg/day)	60
Folic acid (mg/day)	1
Vitamin A	Refer to chapter text for additional information
Vitamin D	Refer to chapter text for additional information
Vitamin E (IU/day)	15
Vitamin K	None[k]

Modified from Kopple J: Nutrition management of nondialyzed patients with chronic renal failure. In Kopple JD, Massey SG, eds: *Nutritional management of renal diseases,* Philadelphia, 1997, Williams & Wilkins; with data from National Kidney Foundation: K/DOQI clinical practice guidelines for chronic kidney disease: evaluation, classification and stratification, *Am J Kidney Dis* 39(suppl 1):S1, 2002.

   GFR, Glomerular filtration rate.

   [a]GFR >4-5 ml/min/1.73 m^2 and <25 ml/min/1.73 m^2.

   [b]The protein intake is increased by 1.0 g/day of high-biologic-value protein for each g/day of urinary protein loss.

   [c]When recommended intake is expressed per kilogram of body weight, this refers to the patient's normal weight, as determined from the NHANES data, or adjusted body weight.

   [d]Refers to percentage of total energy intake (diet plus dialysate); if triglyceride levels are very high, the percentage of fat in the diet may be increased to about 40% of total calories; otherwise, 30% of total calories is preferable.

   [e]These dietary recommendations are considered less crucial than the others. They are emphasized only if the patient has a specific disorder that may benefit from this modification or has expressed interest in his dietary prescription and is complying well with more important aspects of the dietary treatment.

   [f]Should be primarily complex carbohydrates.

   [g]Can be higher in patients who have greater urinary losses.

   [h]Phosphate binders (aluminum carbonate or hydroxide, or calcium carbonate, acetate, or citrate) often are needed to maintain normal serum phosphorus levels.

   [i]Dietary intake usually must be supplemented to provide these levels. Higher daily calcium intakes are commonly ingested because of the use of calcium binders of phosphate.

   [j]At least 10 mg/day for males and nonmenstruating females; ≥18 mg/day for menstruating females.

   [k]Vitamin K supplements may be needed for patients who are not eating and who receive antibiotics.

MEDICAL NUTRITION THERAPY

As of January 2002, Medicare began to provide payment for medical nutrition therapy for patients with chronic renal insufficiency. The Institute of Medicine (IOM) defines chronic renal insufficiency as the stage of renal disease associated with a reduction in renal function not severe enough to require dialysis or transplantation (GFR = 13 to 50 ml/min/1.73 m^2).[4,32] The Renal Practice Group of the American Dietetic Association (ADA) recently published guidelines for care for the patient with kidney disease that includes expected outcomes of medical nutrition therapy.[33] These guidelines identify outcome assessment parameters, expected outcome of therapy, and ideal/goal value of indexes being monitored (Table 22-7).

TABLE 22-7	Expected Outcomes of Medical Nutrition Therapy for Adults With Chronic Kidney Disease Not Requiring Dialysis Replacement Therapy

Expected Outcomes of Medical Nutrition Therapy

Outcome Assessment Factors	Expected Outcome of Therapy	Ideal/Goal Value
Clinical Outcomes	**Measure <30 Days Before Nutrition Session**	
Biochemical Parameters		
Blood urea nitrogen, creatinine	Levels stabilized	Levels stabilized
Albumin	Level maintained within goal range (stabilized in nephrotic syndrome)	3.5-5.0 g/dl (may be lower in nephrotic syndrome)
Potassium	Level maintained within goal range	3.5-5.5 mEq/L
Phosphorus	Level progressing toward goal range	2.5-5.0 mg/dl
Calcium	Level progressing toward goal range	8.5-10.5 mg/dl
Serum glucose (premeal)	Maintained within goal range	80-120 mg/dl
HbA1c (diabetes)	Maintained within goal range	<7%
Cholesterol	Level progressing toward goal range	120-240 mg/dl
Triglycerides (fasting)	Level progressing toward goal range	<200 mg/dl
Creatinine clearance/GFR	Decline minimized	Stabilized
Hematologic Parameters		
Hematocrit/hemoglobin	Adequate erythropoiesis maintained	Hematocrit 33%-36%; hemoglobin 11.0-12.0 g/dl
Ferritin	Adequate iron stores maintained for erythropoiesis	Ferritin 100-800 ng/ml
Transferrin saturation		Transferrin saturation 20%-50%
Anthropometrics		
Weight	Reasonable weight achieved/ maintained	Within reasonable body weight (body mass index, 20-25 kg/m^2)
	Adequate body mass maintained	Adequate muscle/fat stores
Clinical Signs and Symptoms		
	Level of functional ability maintained	Optimum functional ability
		Minimum gastrointestinal symptoms
	Good appetite maintained	Food intake >80% recommended intake
	Appropriate blood pressure control maintained	Blood pressure within appropriate limits
Patient/Caregiver Behavioral Outcomes		**MNT Goals**
Food selection/meal planning	Exhibits positive changes in food selection and amounts	1. Makes appropriate food choices and takes medications as prescribed
	If diabetic, times meals and snacks appropriately	2. Maintains appropriate protein intake
		3. Maintains lab values within acceptable limits
		4. If diabetic, maintains stable glucose levels through appropriate dietary practices
		5. If no medical limitations, maintains an exercise program
Nutrient needs	Identifies foods with a significant protein content	
Potential food/drug interactions	Verbalizes potential food/drug interactions	
Exercise	If no medical limitations, gradually increases or continues physical activity level	

Modified from American Dietetic Association: *Guidelines for nutrition care of renal patients*, ed 3, Chicago, 2002, Author.

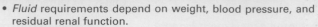

PERSPECTIVES IN PRACTICE
Peritoneal Dialysis

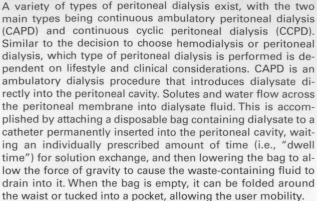

A variety of types of peritoneal dialysis exist, with the two main types being continuous ambulatory peritoneal dialysis (CAPD) and continuous cyclic peritoneal dialysis (CCPD). Similar to the decision to choose hemodialysis or peritoneal dialysis, which type of peritoneal dialysis is performed is dependent on lifestyle and clinical considerations. CAPD is an ambulatory dialysis procedure that introduces dialysate directly into the peritoneal cavity. Solutes and water flow across the peritoneal membrane into dialysate fluid. This is accomplished by attaching a disposable bag containing dialysate to a catheter permanently inserted into the peritoneal cavity, waiting an individually prescribed amount of time (i.e., "dwell time") for solution exchange, and then lowering the bag to allow the force of gravity to cause the waste-containing fluid to drain into it. When the bag is empty, it can be folded around the waist or tucked into a pocket, allowing the user mobility.

The exchange takes place via osmosis and diffusion, with the rate being determined in part by the amount of dextrose in the solution. The most common dialysate solutions are 1.5%, 2.5%, or 4.25% dextrose in 1.5 to 2 L of solution. Actual rate of solute transport, type of number of peritoneal dialysis exchanges, and solution dwell times vary among patients. Each patient is prescribed an individualized dialysis prescription that includes the number and type of dialysate solutions to use each day and the length of dwell times. A method to determine membrane function and the optimal peritoneal dialysis method for each patient is the peritoneal equilibration test. Peritoneal solute and solvent movement rates vary among patients and over time can vary even within the same patient. Therefore clinical monitoring of dialysis adequacy is important. Patients using CAPD as a renal replacement therapy have greater mobility than those on hemodialysis and typically have a more liberal diet in regard to dietary potassium, phosphorus, and total fluid intake due in large part to the more continuous nature of the therapy. Protein requirement is higher and can be a challenge for some patients. Table 22-6 lists the nutritional recommendations for patients on peritoneal dialysis. Special nutrient considerations are as follows:

- *Protein and amino acid* losses average 5 to 15 g/24 hr; amino acid losses average 3 g/day (see Table 22-8 for protein requirements).
- *Potassium* requirements depend on the number of solution exchanges, whether the patient has any residual renal function, and the individual clearance characteristics of the patient's peritoneal membrane. On average, potassium recommendation is 3 to 4 g/day. Some patients will require potassium supplementation.
- *Phosphorus-binding antacids* are not as needed because of improved control of phosphorus blood levels with CAPD use.
- *Dietary sodium* is usually restricted to 2 to 4 g/day. The recommendation must be individualized in accordance to the patient's fluid status, blood pressure, and thirst.

- *Fluid* requirements depend on weight, blood pressure, and residual renal function.

CAPD poses nutrition-related problems related to weight gain from the dialysate and, on the other end of the spectrum, anorexia because of glucose absorption from the dialysate.

One method available to calculate glucose absorption in an individualized manner is the D/D_0 formula: grams of glucose absorbed.

$$\text{Glucose (g)} = (1\ D/D_0) \times G_i$$

where D_0 is initial dextrose in the dialysate at zero hours (g); D is remaining dextrose in the dialysate after an appropriate dwell time (g); D/D_0 is fraction of glucose remaining in the dialysate; and G_i is initial glucose instilled:

13 g/L for 1.5% dextrose
22 g/L for 2.5% dextrose
38 g/L for 4.25% dextrose

In addition to posing possible weight management problems, extra dextrose can lead to elevated triglycerides and low-density lipoprotein (LDL) levels and depressed levels of protective high-density lipoproteins (HDLs), thus increasing risk of coronary heart disease in long-term users.

Nutritionists and nurses who counsel patients being transferred from hemodialysis to CAPD regimen may find that patients need guidance in adjusting to their new diet. The following guidelines may be helpful:
- Increase potassium intake by eating a wide variety of fruits and vegetables each day.
- Encourage liberal fluid intake to prevent dehydration.
- Encourage complex carbohydrates while avoiding overindulging in concentrated sweets to help control triglyceride and HDL levels.
- Maintain lean body weight by incorporating the kcalories provided by the dialysate into the total meal plan (to be calculated and explained to the patient by the renal dietitian).

References

National Kidney Foundation: K/DOQI clinical practice guidelines for nutrition in chronic renal failure, *Am J Kidney Dis* 35(suppl 2):S9, 2000.

National Kidney Foundation: Kidney disease outcomes quality initiative (K/DOQI): practice guidelines for peritoneal dialysis adequacy, *Am J Kidney Dis* 37(suppl 1):S55, 2001.

Passadakis T, Vagemezis V, Oreopoulos D: Peritoneal dialysis: better than, equal to, or worse than hemodialysis? Data worth knowing before choosing a dialysis modality, *Perit Dial Int* 21:25, 2001.

Valderrabano F, Lopez-Gomez J: Quality of life in end-stage renal disease patients, *Am J Kidney Dis* 38(3):443, 2001.

Wiggins K: *Guidelines for nutrition care of renal patients*, ed 3, Chicago, 2002, American Dietetic Association.

Maintenance Hemodialysis

Since the advent of the artificial kidney machine, a number of kidney dialysis centers have been established for treatment of progressive chronic renal insufficiency. Home units are also available, although considerable skill and expense are required to operate them. Much of the cost is paid under a provision of Medicare. A patient requiring maintenance hemodialysis usually requires two or three treatments per week, with each treatment lasting $2\frac{1}{2}$ to 5 hours.

During treatment the patient's blood circulates through the dialysis solution in an artificial kidney (the dialyzer), maintaining normal blood levels of life-sustaining substances the patient's own kidneys can no longer accomplish. An alternative form of peritoneal dialysis is practical for long-term ambulatory therapy at home (see the *Perspectives in Practice* box, "Peritoneal Dialysis").

TABLE 22-8	Nutritional Recommendations for Patients on Hemodialysis and Peritoneal Dialysis Therapy	
Nutrient	**Hemodialysis**	**Peritoneal Dialysis**
Protein (g/kg)*	1.2 IBW	1.2-1.3 IBW
Energy (kcal/kg or kJ/kg)* If patient <90% or >115% of median standard weight, use aBW_{ef}	30-35 (125-145) if ≥60 years of age and 35 (145) if <60 years of age	30-35 (125-145) if ≥60 years of age and 35 (145) if <60 years of age
Phosphorus	800-1200 mg/day or <17 mg/kg*	1200 mg/day or <17 mg/kg*
Sodium	2000-3000 mg/day (88-130 mmol/day)	Individualized based on blood pressure and weight; CAPD and APD: 3000-4000 mg/day (130-175 mmol/day)
Potassium	40 mg/kg* or approximately 2000-3000 mg/day (50-80 mmol/day)	Generally unrestricted with CAPD and APD (approximately 3000-4000 mg/day [80-105 mmol/day]) unless serum level is increased or decreased
Fluid	500-1000 ml/day + daily urine output	CAPD and APD approximately 2000-3000 ml/day based on daily weight fluctuations, urine output, ultrafiltration, and blood pressure; unrestricted if weight and blood pressure are controlled and residual renal function = 2-3 L/day
Calcium	Approximately 1000-1800 mg/day; supplement as needed to maintain normal serum level	Approximately 1000-1800 mg/day; supplement as needed to maintain normal serum level

From Goldstein DJ, McQuiston B: Nutrition and renal disease. In Coulston A, Rock C, Monson E, eds: *Nutrition in the prevention and treatment of disease,* San Diego, 2001, Academic Press.
*For continuous ambulatory peritoneal dialysis (CAPD) and automated, or "cycler," peritoneal dialysis (APD) include dialysate calories.

Diet of a patient on kidney dialysis is a vital aspect of maintaining biochemical control. Several basic objectives govern each individually tailored diet, designed to (1) maintain adequate protein and calorie intake, (2) prevent dehydration or fluid overload, (3) maintain normal serum potassium and sodium blood levels, and (4) maintain acceptable phosphate and calcium levels.

Protein and Calories

The K/DOQI initiative completed a comprehensive evaluation regarding protein and energy intake for patients receiving maintenance hemodialysis and peritoneal dialysis therapy.[33] The recommendation is patients on hemodialysis therapy maintain a protein intake of 1.2 g per kilogram of body weight per day. Patients receiving peritoneal dialysis are recommended to receive 1.2 to 1.3 g /kg /day. Calorie intake is advised to be 35 kcal/kg/day for those who are younger than 60 years and 30 to 35 kcal/kg /day for individuals 60 years or older.[33]

Fluid

Fluid intake is recommended to be equal to approximately 500 ml/day, plus an amount equal to urinary output, if any. Total intake must account for additional fluids in foods consumed. Even with this restriction, there is an expected daily weight gain between dialysis treatments. Interdialytic weight gain is ideally no greater than 2% to 5% body weight or no greater than an average of 2.5 kg.[32]

Sodium, Potassium, and Phosphorus

To control body fluid retention and hypertension, sodium should be limited to 2000 to 3000 mg/day. This restriction helps to prevent pulmonary edema or congestive heart failure from fluid overload.

Potassium restriction is imperative to prevent hyperkalemia. Potassium accumulation can induce cardiac arrhythmias or cardiac arrest. Thus, a dietary allowance of 2000 to 3000 mg/day is usually followed.

To prevent serum phosphorus levels from exceeding 4.0 to 6.0 mg/dl and to prevent bone disease, dietary phosphorus is recommended to be 800 to 1200 mg/day or less than 17 mg/kg.

Vitamins

During dialysis treatments, water-soluble vitamins from the blood are lost in dialysate filtered out of circulating blood. A daily supplement providing water-soluble vitamins is recommended. Table 22-8 summarizes dietary recommendations for patients receiving hemodialysis and peritoneal dialysis.

Peritoneal Dialysis

An alternative form of dialysis, peritoneal dialysis, allows dialysate solutions to flow directly through a catheter port established through the abdominal wall into the abdominal cavity. The solution is typically a dextrose-salt

TO PROBE FURTHER

KIDNEY TRANSPLANTATION

Approximately 273,000 Americans receive maintenance dialysis as their kidney replacement. Some patients await transplantation.[1,2] Others cannot consider a transplant because of medical and/or psychosocial issues. Overall, kidney transplantation remains the treatment of choice for the majority of patients with end-stage renal disease (ESRD). Advances in solid organ transplantation and immunosuppressive therapy have resulted in improved patient survival and improved viability of transplanted kidneys.[1-4]

Nearly 50% of all kidney transplant recipients will be alive with a successful functioning transplant 10 years after transplantation.[2] One-year cadaver kidney success rates are 89%, and 5-year success rates are 65%. In comparison, success rates for recipients of living-donor kidneys are 97% at 1 year and 78% at 5 years. A patient who is trouble free for the first 3 months after the transplantation has an excellent prognosis. Most common causes of death after the first year are cardiovascular disease (CVD), infection, and cancer.[2]

The patient who receives a kidney transplant has a challenging first year. Visits to the transplant team occur an average of 2 or 3 times per week during the first month and once per week for up to 3 months after the surgery. Visits then drop to once monthly during the first year if there are no problems. After the first year it is recommended patients have their laboratory parameters monitored every 1 to 2 months.[2-4]

Medication regimens are challenging for the transplant recipient. Immunosuppressive agents, lipid-lowering drugs, antihypertensives, and hypoglycemic agents are needed for quite some time. There can be significant side effects to these medicines, and adherence to the rigid medication schedule is critical for successful allograft survival. Medical problems that can develop during the first year include infections such as cytomegalovirus, hyperlipidemia, bone disease, diabetes, CVD, hypertension, and dental problems. Weight gain as a side effect of medications can also become a problem (see text for nutritional recommendations for the kidney transplant recipient).[1-4]

Morbidity and mortality rates for kidney transplantation are clinically significant. These statistics should improve as advances in the technology of the surgery and pharmacologic management occur over time. Not every patient will medically qualify for transplantation, and every candidate must be assessed for his or her ability to meet the demands of the posttransplantation period. In the future, perhaps availability of organs for transplantation will be increased by improvements in living related surgeries, development of artificial organs, and/or, most optimistically, finding a cure for progressive kidney disease.[1-4]

References

1. Baiardi F et al: Effects of clinical and individual variables on quality of life in chronic renal failure patients, *J Nephrol* 15(1):61, 2002.
2. Braun WE: Update on kidney transplantation: increasing clinical success, expanding waiting lists, *Cleve Clin J Med* 69(6):501, 2002.
3. Matas A et al: Life satisfaction and adverse effects in renal transplant recipients: a longitudinal analysis, *Clin Transplant* 16(2):113, 2002.
4. Centers for Medicare and Medicaid Services: 2001 Annual report: End Stage Renal Disease Clinical Performance Measures Project, *Am J Kidney Dis* 39(suppl 2):S1, 2002.

solution. High osmolality of the solution causes waste materials to diffuse across the saclike peritoneum lining the abdominal cavity (see the *Perspectives in Practice* box, "Peritoneal Dialysis"). Then this dialysate collection of waste materials flows back into the dialysate bag for disposal. The peritoneal membrane serves as the filtering mechanism.[25]

There are two main types of peritoneal dialysis, as follows:

1. Continuous ambulatory peritoneal dialysis (CAPD), in which a dialysis solution in a plastic pouch is infused and drained via gravity each day (24 hours), 5 times at 4-hour intervals
2. Continuous cyclic peritoneal dialysis (CCPD), in which three or four machine-delivered exchanges are given at night, about 3 hours each, leaving about 2 L of dialysate solution in the peritoneal cavity for 12 to 15 hours during the day

Nutritional concerns specific to peritoneal dialysis involve calories contributed by the dialysate, which are usually 1.5%, 2.5%, or 4.25% dextrose in 1.5 to 2 L of solution, and fluid and potassium intake can be liberalized compared with hemodialysis because of the enhanced clearance of potassium.

Kidney Transplantation

Incident rates for kidney transplantation have increased 6.3% annually from 1995 to 1999.[7] There are currently 101,000 individuals living with a functioning kidney transplant (see the *To Probe Further* box, "Kidney Transplantation"). Patients with kidney transplants often face nutritional challenges related to posttransplantation medications. Hyperlipidemia, weight gain, and abnormal blood glucose levels can result, often because of side effects of the antirejection medications such as corticosteroids and cyclosporin A.[34] In addition, transplant recipients are at increased risk for CVD. The death rate from CVD is 40% in this patient population, and 60% of patients develop hypercholesterolemia.[34-36] Therefore nutrition therapy for the kidney transplant recipient is designed to control blood lipids, blood glucose, and blood pressure within normal ranges; to maintain normalized electrolyte imbalances; to prevent weight gain; and to promote good nutritional health.[35,36] A low-fat diet and exercise plan are generally

TABLE 22-9	Nutritional Guidelines for Adult Kidney Transplant Recipients

Nutrient	Prescription	Purpose
First 6-8 Weeks After Transplantation and During Treatment for Acute Rejection		
Protein	1,3-1,5 g/kg	Counteract protein catabolism; promote wound healing
Calories	30-35 kcal (125-145 kJ)/kg	Meet postsurgery energy demands and allow protein to be used for anabolism
After 6-8 Weeks		
Protein	1.0 g/kg	Minimize muscle protein wasting
Calories	Sufficient to achieve optimal weight for height	Achieve/maintain optimal weight
At All Times		
Carbohydrates	Consistent carbohydrate intake; increase fiber content	Meet energy demands; promote bowel regularity
Fats	No more than 30% of calories; cholesterol <300 mg/day	Reduce posttransplant hyperlipidemia; help prevent progression of atherosclerosis
Potassium	Variable; restrict or supplement as necessary based on serum level	Maintain acceptable potassium level
Sodium	2-4 g (87-175 mmol) may be necessary	Maintain blood pressure control in salt-sensitive individuals; minimize edema
Calcium	1000-1500 mg	Minimize further bone demineralization; correct calcium/phosphorus imbalance
Phosphorus	1200-1500 mg; some patients may require supplements	Minimize further bone demineralization; correct calcium/phosphorus imbalance
Fluids	Ad libitum	Maintain adequate hydration

Modified from American Dietetic Association: *Manual of clinical dietetics*, ed 6, Chicago, 2000, Author.

recommended.[7,34,35] A summation of nutritional guidelines for this patient group is provided in Table 22-9.

Acute Renal Failure

The catabolic ARF patient, most frequently encountered in the intensive care setting, presents a management challenge to the entire team of physicians, nurses, dietitians, respiratory therapists, dialysis staff, pharmacy, and other technicians. These patients are in negative nitrogen balance and generate much urea resulting from the catabolic process. Infection is a major threat, and it aggravates the existing malnutrition.

Disease Process

Renal failure may occur as an acute phase with sudden shutdown of renal function following some metabolic insult or traumatic injury to normal kidneys. The situation is often life threatening, and mortality rate associated with renal failure is high. Survival is less than 50%, especially after surgery.[37,38] In this medical emergency, the nutritionist and nurse play important supportive roles. Immediate and continuing nutrition support is essential.

ARF may have various causes, as follows: (1) severe injury such as extensive burns or crushing injuries that cause widespread tissue destruction; (2) infectious diseases such as peritonitis; (3) traumatic shock after surgery on the abdominal aorta; (4) toxic agents in the environment such as carbon tetrachloride or poisonous mushrooms; or (5) immunologic drug reactions in allergic or sensitive persons, such as penicillin reaction.[37-39]

Clinical Symptoms

The major sign of ARF is oliguria, diminished urine output, often accompanied by proteinuria or hematuria. This diminished urine output is brought on by underlying tissue problems that characterize ARF. Usually there is blockage of tubules caused by cellular debris from tissue trauma or urinary failure with backup retention of filtrate materials.[39]

Oliguria. Diminished urinary output is a cardinal symptom, often with proteinuria or hematuria accompanying the

peritoneum A strong smooth surface—a serous membrane—lining the abdominal/pelvic walls and the undersurface of the diaphragm, forming a sac enclosing the body's vital visceral organs within the peritoneal cavity.

oliguria Secretion of a very small amount of urine in relation to fluid intake.

hematuria The abnormal presence of blood in the urine.

small output. Water balance becomes a crucial factor. The course of the disease is usually divided into an oliguric phase followed by a diuretic phase. The urinary output during the oliguric phase varies from as little as 20 to 200 ml/day.

Anorexia, Nausea, and Lethargy.
During this initial phase of ARF the patient may be lethargic and anorectic and experience nausea and vomiting. Blood pressure elevation and signs of uremia may be present. Oral intake is usually difficult in this catabolic period.[40]

Increasing Serum Urea Nitrogen and Creatinine Levels.
During the initial catabolic period after injury, surgery, or some other metabolic dysfunction, the serum urea nitrogen level increases along with the creatinine level. These increases result from tissue breakdown of muscle mass. Blood potassium, phosphate, and sulfate levels also increase, and sodium, calcium, and bicarbonate levels decrease.[40]

General Medical Management
Usually after initial conservative medical therapy, recovery occurs in a few days to 6 weeks. However, in more complicated cases in which the oliguria continues for 4 to 5 days, more aggressive therapy, including hemodialysis and total parenteral nutrition (TPN), is instituted.

Basic Treatment Goals.
Treatment must be individualized, adjusted according to progression of the illness, type of treatment being used, and the patient's response. In general, however, basic therapy objectives are as follows[40]:

- Reduce and minimize protein breakdown.
- Prevent protein catabolism, and minimize uremic toxicity.
- Prevent dehydration or overhydration.
- Correct acidosis carefully.
- Correct electrolyte depletions, and avoid excesses.
- Control fluid and electrolyte losses from vomiting and diarrhea.
- Maintain optimal nutritional status.
- Maintain appetite, general morale, and sense of well-being.
- Control complications—hypertension, bone pain, nervous system problems.

Nutritional Requirements for Patients With Acute Renal Failure
The ARF patient's nutrition requirements are directly influenced by type of renal replacement therapy (if any), nutritional and metabolic status, and degree of hypercatabolism. Current recommendations for protein and calories for this patient population are defined in the following discussion.[37-42]

Protein is expressed as grams per kilogram of ideal body weight per day. Protein sources containing both essential and nonessential amino acids should be provided.

For patients whose ARF is expected to resolve in a few days and who will not need dialysis, 0.55 to 1 g of protein is recommended.[37,38] The patient's nutritional and metabolic status and renal diagnosis determine exact dose. For patients receiving acute hemodialysis the recommendation is 1.2 to 1.3 g of protein; for those on acute intermittent or CAPD, 1.2 to 1.5 g; and for those on chronic renal replacement therapies, 1.5 to 2.0 g.[37,38]

When energy requirements cannot be measured directly, calorie requirements can usually be met by providing 35 to 50 kcal/kg ideal body weight, reserving the upper limit of the range for patients who are severely catabolic and whose nitrogen balance does not improve at lower intakes. In general, 60% of calories should be provided as carbohydrate and 20% to 35% as fat. Any patient receiving TPN for more than 5 to 7 days should receive 50 to 100 g of lipids as an emulsion, to avoid essential fatty acid (EFA) deficiency.[37-41]

Total fluid intake for any patient depends on amount of residual renal function (i.e., is the patient oliguric? anuric?) and fluid and sodium status. In general, fluid intake can be calculated by adding to the 24-hour urine output 500 ml for insensible losses.

Supplementation of minerals, electrolytes, and trace elements is determined by monitoring serum and urine levels, when appropriate, to prevent excess or deficiency states from arising. Although specific vitamin requirements of ARF patients are not known, the following guidelines are available[37-41]:

- Supplementation of vitamin A is not recommended for at least 2 weeks because levels are elevated with chronic renal failure.
- Vitamin K supplements should be given particularly to patients who are taking antibiotics that suppress intestinal growth of bacteria that usually synthesize it.
- To avoid vitamin B_6 deficiency, 10 mg of pyridoxine hydrochloride per day (8.2 mg of pyridoxine per day) is recommended.
- Limiting ascorbic acid to 60 to 100 mg/day prevents increased oxalate production and serum oxalate levels.

Route of Nutrition Support.
Criteria for deciding which route of nutrition support to use, enteral or parenteral, for critically ill patients have become increasingly complex. In addition to increased costs associated with the parenteral route, some studies report an increased incidence of infectious complications with parenteral, compared with enteral, nutrition.[43] Parenteral nutrition has also been associated with atrophy of gut mucosa, reduced levels of secretory immunoglobulin A, enhanced bacterial and endotoxin translocation, and exaggerated hormonal and metabolic responses to septic challenge.[40] Therefore patients with catabolic ARF should be evaluated for route of nutrient delivery; enteral nutrition should be used if the gut is functional.[43]

Because uremia is a potent catabolic signal, metabolic studies in patients with ARF and CRF have traditionally limited the intake of nonessential amino acids in an attempt to reduce urea production. Proteins of high biologic value, but in quantities much smaller than are usually given (less than 0.5 g/kg/day), were administered along with adequate calories, usually in the form of glucose. The same approach was used with TPN. A central venous infusion of an essential amino acid solution and a hypertonic dextrose solution was frequently administered to provide calories and a small quantity of essential nitrogen. It was thought this approach would prevent malnutrition and at the same time reduce protein catabolism and minimize the rise in blood urea nitrogen (BUN) level.[38]

This clinical approach to nutrition therapy has not reduced mortality rates.[37,42] In the mid-1990s aggressive use of dialysis (early intervention and large doses) and use of parenteral solutions (for those not candidates for enteral) containing mixed amino acids, dextrose, and lipids were becoming standard practice. Dialysis therapy can be adjusted to the patient in terms of clearing catabolic products and allowing for increased administration of protein and calories. Continuous renal replacement therapy (CRRT) has made possible aggressive nutrition support for hypercatabolic patients who have failing kidney function.[37-40]

Debate continues about optimal amino acid composition of TPN solutions.[43] Despite some question about the relative nephrotoxicity of certain amino acids, current recommendations call for formulations containing mixed amino acids, essential and nonessential. There is currently no conclusive evidence specialized formulations such as those additionally enriched with branched-chain amino acids have a beneficial effect on outcome.

Because available data on nutrition therapy for ARF are both limited and conflicting, no treatment plan can be enthusiastically advocated for such patients. Depending on whether dialysis is initiated or not, general recommendations for protein are 0.6 to 1.4 g/kg/day. Adequate kcalories should also be provided (30 to 35 kcal/kg/day). Percentage of increases in protein and calorie needs in catabolic ARF patients is generally related to the precipitating event. Not only must protein and calorie requirements be estimated, but also altering intake of vitamins and electrolytes should be considered in view of the degree of renal dysfunction. Strategies for fluid and electrolyte management include continuous renal replacement therapies such as continuous arteriovenous hemodialysis (CAVHD). These treatment modalities can allow for sufficient nutrition while avoiding fluid and electrolyte complications. Dialysis interventions require close monitoring and assessment to allow ongoing adjustment of the total treatment regimen.[37-42]

Noncatabolic patients may not require dialysis therapy if normal fluid and electrolyte balance can be maintained and blood urea nitrogen (BUN) does not exceed 80 mg/dl. This group of ARF generally results from ingestion of nephrotoxic drugs or exposure to contrast dyes used for diagnostic imaging. These patients are not normally nutritionally depleted and have lower urea generation rates. Oral and enteral feedings are preferred as long as the gastrointestinal tract is functioning normally. However, catabolic ARF patients are most frequently encountered in the intensive care setting. Despite improvements in dialysis technology and intensive care medicine, mortality rate of critically ill patients with ARF remains over 50%.[37,38] Work is being conducted with this patient population to improve the approaches of study design so better intervention studies can be conducted in the future.[42]

KIDNEY STONE DISEASE

Disease Process

Kidney stone disease is an ancient medical problem. Since the days of Hippocrates, records of its incidence have appeared in medical documents. It continues to be a prevalent health problem. Multiple stone attacks affect 12% to 20% of American men and 5% to 10% of women during their lifetimes, with most of the stones today composed of calcium oxalate mixed with varying proportions of calcium phosphate.[44] Kidney stone disease appears to be chronic and recurrent. Basic cause is unknown, but many predisposing risk factors have been found to be involved with calcium, protein, and sodium, with sodium—mostly in the form of dietary salt (NaCl)—receiving the most attention.[44] Although basic cause of kidney stones remains unknown, many factors contribute directly or indirectly to their formation. These factors relate to the nature of the urine itself or to conditions of urinary tract environment. According to the concentration of urinary constituents, major stones formed are calcium stones, struvite stones, uric acid stones, and cystine stones (Figure 22-5).

Major Types of Stones
Calcium Stones.   Most kidney stones are composed of calcium compounds, usually calcium oxalate or calcium oxalate mixed with calcium phosphate. In persons who form stones, which is a familial tendency, the urine produced is supersaturated with these crystalloid elements, and there is a lack of normal urine substances that prevent

---

blood urea nitrogen (BUN) The nitrogen component of urea in the blood; a measure of kidney function; elevated levels of BUN indicate a disorder of kidney function.

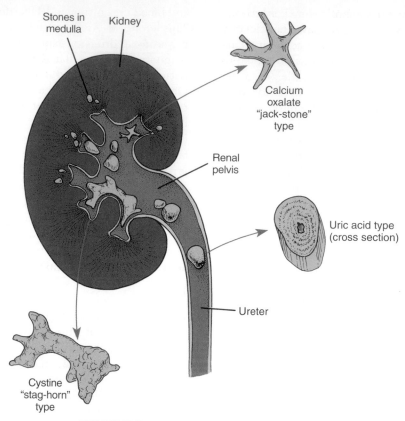

FIGURE 22-5   Renal stones in kidney, pelvis, and ureter.

the crystals from forming stones.[45] Theories as to how excessive urinary calcium may result include the following:

- *Excess calcium intake:* This results from prolonged use of large amounts of milk, alkali therapy for peptic ulcer, use of a hard water supply, or supplemental calcium.[46,47]
- *Excess salt (NaCl) intake:* Recent research, both salt-loading studies and reports of free-living populations, confirms earlier observations that high intakes of NaCl result in hypercalciuria.[44]
- *Excess vitamin D:* Hypervitaminosis D may cause increased calcium absorption from the intestine as well as increased withdrawal from bone.
- *Prolonged immobilization:* Body casting or immobilization from illness or disability may lead to withdrawal of bone calcium and increased urinary concentration.
- *Hyperparathyroidism:* Primary hyperparathyroidism causes excess calcium excretion. About two thirds of the persons with this endocrine disorder have kidney stones, but this disorder accounts for only about 5% of total calcium stones.
- *Renal tubular acidosis:* Excess excretion of calcium is caused by defective ammonia formation.
- *Idiopathic calciuria:* Some persons, even those on a low-calcium diet, for unknown reasons may excrete as much as 500 mg of calcium per day.

- *Oxalate:* Because of a metabolic error in handling oxalates, about half of the calcium stones are compounds with this material. Oxalates occur naturally only in a few food sources (see Appendix H) and individual absorption/excretion rates influence availability. Studies in normal volunteers consuming oxalate-rich foods have indicated that the increased urinary oxalate values were not proportional to the oxalate values of food.[45] Only eight foods caused a significant increase in urinary oxalate excretion: spinach, rhubarb, beets, nuts, chocolate, tea, wheat bran, and strawberries. Nutrition therapy for stone-forming individuals may be limited to restriction of these eight foods, with results monitored by laboratory analysis of urine composition.
- *Animal protein:* A diet high in animal protein, such as the typical American diet, has been linked to increased excretions of calcium, oxalate, and urate. A vegetarian type of diet has been recommended by some investigators as a wise choice for stone-forming persons.
- *Dietary fiber:* Added dietary fiber has been found to reduce risk factors for stone formation, especially calcium stones.

Struvite Stones.   Next to calcium stones in frequency are struvite stones, composed of a single compound—magnesium ammonium phosphate ($MgNH_4PO_4$). These are often called "infection stones" because they are associated with UTIs. The offending organism in the infection is *Proteus mirabilis*. This is a urea-splitting bacterium that contains urease, an enzyme that hydrolyzes urea to ammonia. Thus urinary pH becomes alkaline. In the ammonia-rich environment struvite precipitates and forms large, "stag-horn" stones. Surgical removal is usually indicated.

Uric Acid Stones.   Excess uric acid excretion may be caused by an impairment in intermediary metabolism of purine, as occurs in gout. It may also result from a rapid tissue breakdown in wasting disease.

Cystine Stones.   A heredity metabolic defect in renal tubular reabsorption of the amino acid cystine causes this substance to accumulate in urine. This condition is called *cystinuria*. Because this is a genetic disorder, it is characterized by early onset and a positive family history. This is one of the most common metabolic disorders associated with kidney stones in children before puberty.

Urinary Tract Conditions

Physical changes in urine and organic stone matrix provide urinary tract conditions that lead to formation of kidney stones.

Physical Changes in the Urine.   Susceptible persons form stones when physical changes in the urine predispose to such formation. Such physical conditions include the following:

- *Urine concentration:* Concentration of urine may result from a lower water intake or from excess water loss, as in prolonged sweating, fever, vomiting, or diarrhea.
- *Urinary pH:* Changes in urinary pH from its mean 5.85 to 6 may be influenced by diet or altered by ingestion of acid or alkali medications.

Organic Stone Matrix.   Formation of an organic stone matrix provides the necessary core or nucleus (nidus) around which crystals may precipitate and form a mucoprotein-carbohydrate complex. In this complex, galactose and hexosamine are the principal carbohydrates. Some possible sources of these organic materials include (1) bacteria masses from recurrent UTIs; (2) renal epithelial tissue of the urinary tract that has sloughed off, possibly because of vitamin A deficiency; and (3) calcified plaques (Randall's plaques) formed beneath the renal epithelium in hypercalciuria. Irritation and ulceration of overlying tissue cause the plaques to slough off into the collecting tubules.

Clinical Symptoms

Severe pain and numerous urinary symptoms may result, with general weakness and sometimes fever. Laboratory examination of urine and chemical analysis of any stone passed help determine treatment.

General Treatment

Fluid Intake.   Large fluid intake produces a more dilute urine and is a foundation of therapy. Dilute urine helps to prevent concentration of stone constituents.

Urinary pH.   An attempt to control solubility factor is made by changing urinary pH to an increased acidity or alkalinity, depending on the chemical composition of the stone formed. An exception is calcium oxalate stones because solubility of calcium oxalate in urine is not pH dependent. Conversely, however, calcium phosphate is soluble in an acid urine.

Stone Composition.   When possible, dietary constituents of the stone are controlled to reduce the amount of the substance available for precipitation.

Binding Agents.   Materials that bind stone elements and prevent their absorption in the intestine cause fecal excretion. For example, sodium phytate is used to bind calcium, and aluminum gels are used to bind phosphate. Glycine and calcium have a similar effect on oxalates.

Alternative Remedies.   A number of herbs are also used to help prevent the development of kidney stones (see the *Complementary and Alternative Medicine {CAM}* box, "Common Herbal Treatments for Kidney Stones").

Nutrition Therapy

Nutrition therapy is directly related to the stone chemistry.

Calcium Stones.   Traditional dietary approach for calcium stones has been to limit dietary calcium intake to about 400 mg/day. This has raised concerns regarding effects on bone density when used long term.[47,48] In addition, because calcium stones have an alkaline chemistry, an acid ash diet has been thought to help create a urinary environment less conducive to the precipitation of the basic stone elements. Classification of food groups is based on the pH of the metabolic ash produced (see Appendix I). An acid ash diet increases the amount of meat, grains, eggs, and cheese. It limits the amounts of vegetables, milk, and fruits. An alkaline ash diet outlines the opposite use of these foods. Use of cranberry juice has been promoted to assist in acidification of urine. However, commercially prepared cranberry juices on the consumer market are too dilute to be effective because they contain only about 26% cranberry juice. Thus an inordinate volume would be required to achieve any consistent effectiveness as a urinary acidifying agent. Instead, to effect a sustained acidifying of urinary pH most physicians rely on drugs.

A recent study by Borghi and colleagues[48] indicates a calcium-rich diet low in salt and animal protein significantly reduces recurrence of kidney stones in men. In this study 120 men with recurrent calcium oxalate stones and

COMPLEMENTARY AND ALTERNATIVE MEDICINE (CAM)
Common Herbal Treatments for Kidney Stones

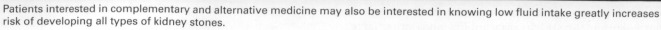

Patients interested in complementary and alternative medicine may also be interested in knowing low fluid intake greatly increases risk of developing all types of kidney stones.

Herb	Efficacy	Side Effects and/or Risks	Drug Interaction
Citrate	May help prevent oxalate and acid stones by binding with calcium in urine, reducing the amount of calcium available to form calcium oxalate stones. It also alkalizes urine, inhibiting development of calcium oxalate and uric acid stones.		• Increases serum levels of ephedra, flecainide, mecamylamine, methamphetamine. • Decreases serum levels of lithium, methotrexate, salicylates, sulfonylureas, tetracyclines. • Hyperkalemia when taking ACE inhibitors, potassium-sparing diuretics.
Calcium	Calcium supplements might slightly increase kidney stone risk, whereas dietary calcium reduces risk of kidney stones.	Higher intakes are associated with increased risk of prostate cancer.	• Concurrent use of calcium with pheasant's eye (Adonis vernalis) increases risk of cardiac toxicity. • Calcium channel blockers may be affected by combinations of calcium supplements and high doses of vitamin D. • May decrease blood level of atenolol (beta blocker) and possibly other beta-blockers. • Interferes with absorption of tetracyclines, levothyroxine. • Excess intake can interfere with absorption of iron, zinc, magnesium, iodine, manganese, and copper.
Magnesium (magnesium oxide or magnesium hydroxide)	No strong evidence that magnesium prevents calcium oxalate stones.	Should not be taken by those with severe heart or kidney disease without consultation with a healthcare provider.	• May decrease absorption of psyllium.
Vitamin B_6 (pyridoxamine)	Weak evidence that vitamin B_6 might help prevent calcium oxalate stones.	Vitamin B_6 deficiency increases amount of oxalate in urine. Large doses may cause nausea, vomiting, and potential risk of neurotoxicity.	• None found.
GLA (gamma-linolenic acid) (omega-6 oils, omega-6 fatty acids, evening primrose oil, black currant oil, borage oil)	No evidence available.	No adverse effects have been noted.	• Increases bleeding time when used with anticoagulant therapy. • GLA is synergistic with paclitaxel.

References

Bratman S, Girman AM: *Mosby's handbook of herbs and supplements and their therapeutic uses,* St. Louis, 2003, Mosby/Elsevier Science.

Herr SM: *Herb-drug interaction handbook,* ed 2, Nassau, NY, 2002, Church Street Books.

ACE, Angiotensin-converting enzyme.

hypercalciuria were randomized to receive a normal calcium diet (30 mmol/day, n = 60) with a dietary protein restriction of 52 g/day and salt restriction of 50 mmol/day. The other 60 men in the study were randomized to receive the traditional low-calcium diet, 10 mmol/day. At the end of 5 years 20% of the patients on the normal-calcium, low-protein and low-sodium diet and 38% of the men on the low-calcium diet had relapses. Relative risk for the normal-calcium diet compared with the low-calcium diet was 0.49. Urinary calcium levels dropped in both group, but urinary oxalate excretion fell in the normal-calcium group and increased in the men on the low-calcium diet. Although exact mechanisms are still being debated, the study does indicate a low–animal protein diet and low-sodium diet with normal calcium intake protects against recurrence of kidney stones compared with the traditional low-calcium diet.

Uric Acid Stones. Approximately 4% of the total incidence of renal calculi are uric acid stones. Because uric acid is a metabolic product of purines, dietary control of this precursor is indicated. Purines are found in active tissue such as glandular meat, other lean meat, meat extractives, and, in lesser amounts, plant sources such as whole grains and legumes. An effort to produce an alkaline ash to help increase the urinary pH is indicated.

Cystine Stones. Approximately 1% of total stones produced are cystine; this condition is a relatively rare genetic disease. Cystine is a nonessential amino acid produced from the essential amino acid methionine; thus a diet low in methionine is used. This diet is used with high fluid intake and alkaline diet therapy.

URINARY TRACT INFECTION

Disease Process

The term *urinary tract infection* refers to a wide variety of clinical infections in which a significant number of microorganisms are present in any portion of the urinary tract.[49,51] A common form is cystitis, an inflammation of the bladder that is very prevalent in young women. At least 20% of women experience a UTI during their lifetime, of which the vast majority are cases of uncomplicated cystitis.[49,50] The condition is called recurrent UTI if three or more bouts are experienced in 1 year.

The majority of cases are caused by aerobic members of the fecal flora, especially *Escherichia coli.*[51] Presence of these organisms in urine is termed *bacteriuria.* Urine produced by the normal kidney is sterile and remains so as it travels to the bladder. In UTI, however, the normal urethra has microbial flora; therefore any voided urine generally contains many bacteria. Bacteriuria is present when the quantity of organisms is more than 100,000/ml of urine. The female anatomy is more conducive to entry of these bacteria into the urinary tract. Recurrent cystitis occurs mostly in young and otherwise healthy women who have infections that usually correspond with sexual activity and continued diaphragm use. In most cases simply changing to another birth control method will solve the problem. Cystitis is characterized by frequent voiding and burning on urination.

Treatment

Currently antibiotic treatment of UTI has been cut back a great deal. General nutritional measures include acidifying urine by taking vitamin C (because cranberry juice is not effective) and drinking plenty of fluids to produce a dilute urine. Control of UTI is an important measure because it is a risk factor in stone formation. Current medical research shows promise for the development of new vaccines to prevent UTIs.[51]

RESOURCES

The renal diet is complex and presents a challenge to practitioners and even more so to patients. A basic resource, the National Renal Diet educational series, provides valuable guides. These standardized guidelines for nutrition intervention and patient education in renal disease have been developed by the collaborative work of renal dietitians from the American Dietetic Association Renal Dietitians Dietetic Practice Group and the National Kidney Foundation Council on Renal Nutrition. The Professional Guide can be used in conjunction with ADA's other guides for the care of renal disease patients. Because dietary management must be tailored to the stage of the disease and method of treatment, the series of materials contains a professional guide and six client booklets, each designed with special food lists to meet specific needs of the various renal disease requirements. These ADA resources give the practitioner a comprehensive basis for individualizing dietary instructions and provide the patient and family with a practical guide for everyday decisions and plans for food choices.

The Council on Renal Nutrition of the National Kidney Foundation is an expert resource for information. Membership includes a subscription to the *Journal of Renal Nutrition,* a quarterly publication geared toward nutritionists, scientists, and physicians interested and working in the fields of nephrology and renal nutrition. For contact information, see the *Websites of Interest* section at the end of this chapter.

Importance of nutritional status and care has been documented to have a role in patient outcomes; therefore interest in renal nutrition and the number of online resources have substantially increased. (See the *Websites of Interest* section at the end of this chapter for a listing of websites that provide excellent information and links to other sites pertaining to renal nutrition and nephrology.)

Health Promotion

Omega-3 Fatty Acids and Renal Disease

Recent statistics available report there are currently 300,000 Americans living with the diagnosis of ESRD.[52] Despite countless research efforts, mechanisms responsible for the progressive nature of renal disease remain elusive. Historically, nutrition science has been an inherent component of research directed toward identifying nutrient manipulations that ameliorate kidney disease, metabolic abnormalities associated with chronic renal insufficiency, and mechanisms by which nutrients modulate factors involved in promoting exacerbation of existing disease. In all of these research areas, dietary protein, phosphorus, and caloric deprivation have been more widely studied than other nutrients. However, more recently there has been a shift of research interest directed toward dietary EFAs. This shift is in response to a growing body of evidence indicating that fatty acid substitution of cell membrane phospholipids modulates biochemical pathways implicated in both the pathophysiology of progressive kidney disease and CVD so prominent in the renal patient population.

It has been demonstrated that altering availability of EFAs can influence the natural course of several important diseases in the mammalian organism. For example, epidemiologic studies of the Dutch, Japanese, and native Greenland Eskimo populations attribute their low incidence of heart disease to a fish diet high in omega-3 fatty acids. Several investigations exploring the effects of polyunsaturated fatty acid–supplemented diets in experimental immune and nonimmune models of renal disease have been reported.[52-58] Beneficial observations have included an improved lipid profile, prolonged survival, and improved renal function.

Dietary EFAs are direct precursors to the biologically diverse and potent class of compounds called eicosanoids. EFAs can also modulate cellular production of interleukins. Several chronic inflammatory and renal diseases are characterized in part by an overproduction of eicosanoids and interleukins. These facts, which have been demonstrated in animal and some human studies, suggest that manipulation of dietary fatty acids might contribute a therapeutic influence by altering proinflammatory and other activated pathways in disease processes. In vitro, manipulation of fatty acids has been found to modify macrophage function, production of vasoactive substances, and membrane signal transduction.[57] Alteration of phospholipid fatty acid composition in cell membranes achieved through manipulation of cell medium fatty acid content has been observed to affect many cellular properties; examples include cell membrane fluidity, receptor binding, cell-mediated transport, ion channels, eicosanoid formation, and intracellular calcium concentration.[52-58]

Although studies in humans have been few in number, recent reports are encouraging. Kutner et al[53] explored the effect of fish consumption in 216 incident dialysis patients. Patient survival was followed for 3 years. This study found fish intake was associated with patient survival. Patients who ate fish were 50% less likely to die during the study interval. Donadio[54] demonstrated in human trials that omega-3 fatty acids have a beneficial effect on immunoglobulin A nephropathy (IgAN). IgAN is the most prominent cause of glomerulosclerosis in the world. It affects young adults of whom 20% to 40% will develop progressive renal disease and ultimately kidney failure. Rationale for interest in omega-3 fatty acids in IgAN was based on the effect of these fatty acids on altering production of eicosanoids and inflammatory mediators. In clinical trials Donadio and colleagues observed that patients with IgAN treated with 1.8 g of eicosapentaenoic acid (EPA) and 1.2 g of docosahexaenoic acid (DHA) had a slower loss of renal function. In a different trial, patients treated with placebo had a higher rate of developing renal failure than those treated with EPA and DHA.

Additional research is needed to elucidate beneficial effects of omega-3 fatty acid intake in patients with chronic renal disease. However, the current body of research indicating inflammatory mechanisms responsible for the high prevalence of CVD in this patient population and the interrelationships between markers of malnutrition and inflammation certainly encourage continued research in the role of omega-3 fatty acids in modulating these common biochemical pathways.

TO SUM UP

Through its unique functional units, the nephrons, the kidneys act as a filtration system, reabsorbing substances the body needs, secreting additional hydrogen ions to maintain a proper pH balance in the blood, and excreting unnecessary materials in a concentrated urine.

Renal function may be impaired by a variety of conditions. These include inflammatory and degenerative diseases, infection and obstruction, chronic diseases such as hypertension and diabetes, environmental agents such as insecticides and solvents and other toxic substances, and some medications and trauma. Some clinical conditions affecting structure and function include glomerulonephritis, acute and chronic renal failure, renal calculi, and UTI.

CKD and its result, ESRD, are treated by dialysis—hemodialysis or peritoneal dialysis—and kidney transplantation. The diet for CKD needs to include ample calories and protein with restrictions for GFR of less than 25 ml/min/1.73 m^2 only if the patient is able to maintain adequate caloric intake. Dialysis patients must be monitored closely for calories, protein, fluid, and electrolyte balance. All of the diets need to be individualized to ensure overall nutritional adequacy and adherence. Monitoring of nutritional status is important for all patients.

QUESTIONS FOR REVIEW

1. For each of the following conditions, outline nutritional components of therapy, explaining impact of each on kidney function: glomerulonephritis, ARF (renal insufficiency), and chronic renal failure.

2. Identify four clinical conditions that impair renal function. Give an example of each, describing its effect on various structures in the kidney.

3. List nutritional factors that must be monitored in individuals undergoing renal dialysis.

4. Summarize the rationale and nutrient recommendations for patients who have received a renal transplant.

5. Outline nutrition therapy used for patients with various types of kidney stones. Describe each type of stone and explain the rationale for each aspect of therapy.

6. For what condition is a UTI a predisposing factor? What general nutrition principles are recommended in the treatment of such infections?

REFERENCES

1. Gonyea JP, McCarthy M: Overview: pathophysiology of the kidney. In Byham-Gray L, Wiesen K, eds: *A clinical nutrition guide to nutrition care in kidney disease,* Chicago, 2004, American Dietetic Association.

2. Banasik JL: Renal function. In Copstead LC, Banasik JL, eds: *Pathophysiology,* ed 3, St. Louis, 2005, Elsevier/Saunders.

3. Gregory MC: Renal function tests. In Jones S, ed: *Clinical laboratory pearls,* New York, 2001, Lippincott Williams & Wilkins.

4. National Kidney Foundation: K/DOQI clinical practice guidelines for chronic kidney disease: evaluation, classification and stratification, *Am J Kidney Dis* 39(suppl 1):S1, 2002.

5. Zawada E: Initiation of dialysis. In Daugirdas J, Plake P, Ing T, eds: *Handbook of dialysis,* ed 2, Philadelphia, 2001, Lippincott Williams & Wilkins.

6. U.S. Renal Data System: Annual data report II: incidence and prevalence of ESRD, *Am J Kidney Dis* 34:S40, 1999.

7. U.S. Renal Data System: Excerpts from the USRDS 2001 annual data report: atlas of end-stage renal disease in the United States, *Am J Kidney Dis* 38(suppl 3):S1, 2001.

8. Couser W: Mediation of immune glomerular injury, *J Am Soc Nephrol* 1:13, 1990.

9. Lu CY, Salant DJ: Renal immunology and pathology, *Curr Opin Nephrol Hypertens* 7(3):27, 1998.

10. American Diabetes Association: Diabetic nephropathy, *Diabetes Care* 25(suppl 1):S85, 2002.

11. Qureshi AR et al: Factors influencing malnutrition in hemodialysis patients: a cross-sectional study, *Kidney Int* 53:773, 1998.

12. Goldstein DJ, Callahan C: Strategies for nutritional intervention in patients with renal failure, *Miner Electrolyte Metab* 24(1):82, 1997.

13. Klahr S et al: The effects of dietary protein restriction and blood pressure control on the progression of chronic renal failure: modification of diet in renal disease study group, *N Engl J Med* 330:878, 1994.

14. Chertow G, Lazarus M: Malnutrition as a risk factor for morbidity and mortality in maintenance patients. In Kopple J, Massry S, eds: *Nutritional management of renal disease,* Philadelphia, 1997, Williams & Wilkins.

15. Lowrie EG, Lew NL: Death risk in hemodialysis patients: the predictive value of commonly measured variables and an evaluation of death rate between facilities, *Am J Kidney Dis* 15:458, 1990.

16. Owen WF: Nutritional status and survival in end-stage renal disease patients, *Miner Electrolyte Metab* 2:(1):72, 1997.

17. Stenvinkel P et al: Are there two types of malnutrition in chronic renal failure? Evidence for relationships between malnutrition, inflammation and atherosclerosis (MIA syndrome), *Nephrol Dial Transplant* 15(7):953, 2000.

18. Kaysen G: Role of inflammation and its treatment in ESRD patients, *Blood Purif* 20:70, 2002.

19. Bistrian BR: Interaction between nutrition and inflammation in end-stage renal disease, *Blood Purif* 18(4):333, 2000.

20. Don BR, Kaysen G: Assessment of inflammation and nutrition in patients with end-stage renal disease, *J Nephrol* 13(4):249, 2000.

21. Kaysen G: Malnutrition and the acute-phase reaction in dialysis patients—how to measure and how to distinguish, *Nephrol Dial Transplant* 15(10):1521, 2000.

22. Hasselwander O: Oxidative stress in chronic renal failure, *Free Radic Res* 29(1):1-11, 1998.

23. Eikelboom J, Hankey G: Associations of homocysteine, C-reactive protein and cardiovascular disease in patients with renal disease, *Curr Opin Nephrol Hypertens* 10:377, 2001.

24. Goldstein DJ: Assessment of nutritional status in renal disease. In Mitch WE, Klahr S, eds: *Nutrition and the kidney,* ed 4, Philadelphia, 2002, Lippincott Williams & Wilkins.

25. Goldstein DJ, McQuiston B: Nutrition and renal disease. In Coulston A, Rock C, Monson E, eds: *Nutrition in the prevention and treatment of disease,* San Diego, 2001, Academic Press.

26. Wolfson M: Causes, manifestations, and assessment of malnutrition in chronic renal failure. In Kopple J, Massry S, eds: *Nutritional management of renal disease,* Philadelphia, 1997, Williams & Wilkins.

27. Kalantar-Zadeh K et al: Food intake characteristics of hemodialysis patients as obtained by food frequency questionnaire, *J Ren Nutr* 12:17, 2002.

28. Biesecker R, Stuart N: Nutrition management of the adult hemodialysis patient. In Byham-Gray L, Wiesen K, eds: *A clinical nutrition guide to nutrition care in kidney disease,* Chicago, 2004, American Dietetic Association.

29. Bro S, Olgaard K: Effects of excess parathyroid hormone on nonclassical target organs, *Am J Kidney Dis* 30:606, 1997.

30. Frankenfield D et al: Anemia management of adult hemodialysis patients in the U.S.: results from the 1997 Core Indicators project, *Kidney Int* 57:578, 2000.

31. Tarng D et al: Erythropoietin hyporesponsiveness: from iron deficiency to iron overload, *Kidney Int* 55:S107, 1999.

32. Renal Dietitians Dietetic Practice Group, Wiggins K, ed: *Guidelines for nutrition care of renal patients,* ed 3, Chicago, 2002, American Dietetic Association.

33. National Kidney Foundation: K/DOQI clinical practice guidelines for nutrition in chronic renal failure, *Am J Kidney Dis* 35(suppl 2):S9, 2000.

34. Weil SE: Nutrition in the kidney transplant recipient. In Danovitch GM, ed: *Handbook of kidney transplantation,* ed 2, Boston, 1996, Little, Brown.

35. Jaggers H, Allman M, Chan M: Changes in clinical profile and dietary considerations after renal transplantation, *J Renal Nutr* 6:12, 1996.

36. Blue L: Adult kidney transplantation. In Hasse J, Blue L, eds: *Comprehensive guide to transplant nutrition,* Chicago, 2002, American Dietetic Association.

37. Weiner Feldman R: Nutrition in acute renal failure, *J Renal Nutr* 4(2):97, 1994.

38. Matarese L: Assessment and nutrition management of the patient with renal disease. In Winkler M, Lysen L, eds: *Suggested guidelines for nutrition and metabolic management of adult patients receiving nutrition support,* ed 2, Chicago, 1993, American Dietetic Association.

39. Bickford A, Schatz SR: Nutrition management in acute renal failure. In Byham-Gray L, Wiesen K, eds: *A clinical nutrition guide to nutrition care in kidney disease,* Chicago, 2004, American Dietetic Association.

40. Monson P, Mehta R: Nutrition in acute renal failure: a reappraisal for the 1990s, *J Renal Nutr* 4(2):58, 1994.

41. Druml W: Nutritional management of acute renal failure. In Jacobson H, Striker G, Skaher S, eds: *The principles and practices of nephrology,* St. Louis, 1995, Mosby.

42. Mehta R et al: Refining predictive models in critically ill patients with acute renal failure, *J Am Soc Nephrol* 13(5):1350, 2002.

43. Burtis WJ et al: Dietary hypercalciuria in patients with calcium oxalate kidney stones, *Am J Clin Nutr* 60(3): 1995.

44. Massy LK, Whiting SJ: Dietary salt, urinary calcium, and kidney stone risk, *Nutr Rev* 53(5):131, 1995.

45. Massy LK et al: Effect of dietary oxalate and calcium on urinary oxalate and risk of formation of calcium oxalate kidney stones, *J Am Diet Assoc* 93(8):901, 1993.

46. Curhan GC et al: Comparison of dietary calcium with supplemental calcium and other nutrients as factors affecting the risk for kidney stones, *Ann Intern Med* 126(7):497, 1997.

47. Coe FL et al: Diet and calcium: the end of an era? *Ann Intern Med* 126(7):553, 1997.

48. Borghi L et al: Comparison of two diets for the prevention of recurrent stones in idiopathic hypercalciuria, *N Eng J Med* 346(2):77, 2002.

49. Service RE: New vaccines may ward off urinary tract infections, *Science* 276(5312):533, 1997.

50. Dranov P: Urinary tract infection, *Am Health* 14(4):66, 1995.

51. Langermann S et al: Prevention of mucosal *Escherichia coli* infection by FimH-adhesin-based system vaccination, *Science* 276(5312):607, 1997.

52. U.S. Renal Data System: Annual data report: executive summary, *Am J Kidney Dis* 34:S9, 1999.

53. Kutner N et al: Association of fish intake and survival in a cohort of incident dialysis patients, *Am J Kidney Dis* 39(5):1018, 2002.

54. Donadio J: The emerging role of omega-3 polyunsaturated fatty acids in the management of patients with IgA nephropathy, *J Ren Nutr* 11(3):122, 2001.

55. Donadio J et al: A controlled trial of fish oil in IgA nephropathy, *N Engl J Med* 331:1194, 1994.

56. Goldstein DJ et al: Fish oil ameliorates renal injury and hyperlipidemia in the Milan normotensive rat model of focal glomerulosclerosis, *J Am Soc Nephrol* 6:1468, 1995.

57. Goldstein DJ, Wheeler DC, Salant DJ: The effects of omega-3 fatty acids on complement-mediated glomerular epithelial cell injury, *Kidney Int* 50:1863, 1996.

58. Weise W et al: Fish oil has protective and therapeutic effects on proteinuria in passive Heymann nephritis, *Kidney Int* 43:359, 1993.

FURTHER READINGS AND RESOURCES

Readings

National Kidney Foundation: Kidney disease outcomes quality initiative (K/DOQI): practice guidelines for peritoneal dialysis adequacy, *Am J Kidney Dis* 37(suppl 1):S55, 2001.
One of the publications from the K/DOQI series, this supplement addresses the main aspects of peritoneal dialysis care and offers to the clinician relevant applicable guidelines based on an extensive review and analysis of the medical literature that can be used to guide clinical management.

Ikizler T et al: Association of morbidity with markers of nutrition and inflammation in chronic hemodialysis patients: a prospective study, *Kidney Int* 55:1945, 1999.
This article provides an analysis of clinical parameters reflective of malnutrition and inflammation that are associated with clinical outcomes.

National Kidney Foundation: Kidney disease outcomes quality initiative: clinical practice guidelines for the treatment of anemia of chronic renal failure, *Am J Kidney Dis* 37(suppl 1):S182, 2001.
One of the publications from the K/DOQI series, this supplement provides applicable guidelines that the clinician can use to manage the anemia associated with CKD.

Daugirdas J, Van Stone J, Boag J: Hemodialysis apparatus. In Daugirdas J, Blake P, Ing T, eds: *Handbook of dialysis,* ed 3, Philadelphia, 2001, Lippincott Williams & Wilkins.
An excellent overview of what equipment is needed for hemodialysis therapy and how it all works.

Albright RC: Acute renal failure: a practical update, *Mayo Clin Proc* 76:67, 2001.
An excellent update on the management of patients with ARF.

Herselman M et al: Protein-energy malnutrition as a risk factor for increased morbidity in long term hemodialysis patients, *J Ren Nutr* 10:7, 2000.
Interesting data demonstrating that malnutrition is associated with morbidity in dialysis patients.

Websites of Interest

- *Journal of Renal Nutrition;* this site also provides links to the homepage of the National Kidney Foundation and the Council on Renal Nutrition: *www.jrnjournal.org.*
- National Kidney Foundation: *www.kidney.org.*
- American Dietetic Association: *www.eatright.org.*
- Hypertension, Dialysis and Clinical Nephrology (HDCN): *www.hdcn.com.*
- Nephrology News and Issues Online (NephrOnline): *www.nephronline.com.*
- International Society on Renal Nutrition and Metabolism: *www.renalnutrition.com.*
- *Journal of the American Society of Nephrology: www.jasn.org.*
- *American Journal of Kidney Diseases: www.ajkd.org.*

CHAPTER 23

Metabolic Stress

Sara Long

In this chapter various surgical procedures are discussed with a focus on surgical procedures and situations that could bear a large nutritional consequence, particularly thermal injuries (or burns). Understanding the surgical procedure performed, with knowledge of nutritional and absorptive function and capacity of the alimentary tract, is imperative to providing optimal nutrition care of surgery patients (see also the **Focus on Culture** *box, "Physiologic Changes Related to the Aging Process That Can Affect Surgery"). An understanding of the body's response to metabolic stress is also important when determining optimal timing and type of nutrition intervention for the patient.*

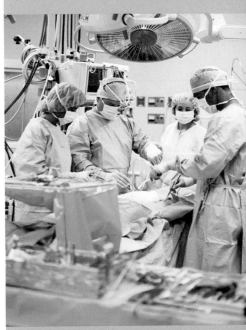

◆ FOCUS ON CULTURE

Physiologic Changes Related to the Aging Process That Can Affect Surgery

Physiologic Change	Effects	Potential Postoperative Complications
Cardiovascular		
↓ Elasticity of blood vessels	↓ Circulation to vital organs	Shock (hypotension), thrombosis with pulmonary embolism
↓ Cardiac output	Slower blood flow	boli, delayed wound healing, postoperative confu-
↓ Peripheral circulation		sion, hypervolemia, decreased response to stress
Respiratory		
↓ Elasticity of lungs and chest wall	↓ Vital capacity	Atelectasis, pneumonia, postoperative confusion
↓ Residual lung volume	↓ Alveolar volume	
↓ Forced expiratory volume	↓ Gas exchange	
↓ Ciliary action	↓ Cough reflex	
Fewer alveolar capillaries		
Urinary		
↓ Glomerular filtration rate	↓ Kidney function	Prolonged response to anesthesia and drugs, overhy-
↓ Bladder muscle tone	Stasis of urine in bladder	dration with intravenous fluids, hyperkalemia, uri-
Weakened perineal muscles	Loss of urinary control	nary tract infection, urinary retention
Musculoskeletal		
↓ Muscle strength	↓ Activity	Atelectasis, pneumonia, thrombophlebitis, constipa-
Limitation of motion		tion or fecal impaction
Gastrointestinal		
↓ Intestinal motility	Retention of feces	Constipation or fecal impaction
Metabolic		
↓ γ-Globulin level	↓ Inflammatory response	Delayed wound healing, wound dehiscence or evis-
↓ Plasma proteins		ceration
Immune System		
Fewer killer T-cells	↓ Ability to protect against invasion	Wound infection, wound dehiscence, pneumonia, uri-
↓ Response to foreign antigens	by pathogenic microorganisms	nary tract infection

From Keeling AW, Muro A, Long BC: Preoperative nursing. In Phipps WJ et al, eds: *Medical-surgical nursing: concepts and clinical practice,* ed 5, St. Louis 1995, Mosby.

Extent of Body Reserves of Nutrients

Nutrient	Time Required to Deplete Reserves in Well-Nourished Individuals
Amino acids	Several hours
Carbohydrate	13 hours
Sodium	2-3 days
Water	4 days
Zinc	5 days
Fat	20-40 days
Thiamin	30-60 days
Vitamin C	60-120 days
Niacin	60-180 days
Riboflavin	60-180 days
Vitamin A	90-365 days
Iron	125 days (women), 750 days (men)
Iodine	1000 days
Calcium	2500 days

From Guthrie HA: *Introductory nutrition,* ed 7, St. Louis, 1989, Times Mirror/Mosby College Publishers.

NUTRITIONAL NEEDS OF GENERAL SURGERY PATIENTS

Preoperative Nutrition

Nutritional needs of surgery patients vary based on several factors, including the patient's disease process, other comorbidities, and baseline nutritional status. Many general surgery patients are adequately nourished preoperatively and therefore do not have any special nutrient requirements (see the *Perspectives in Practice* box, "Energy and Protein Requirements in General Surgery Patients"). The disease itself often lends to poor nutrient intake and a hypermetabolic state that places the patient at nutritional risk. Malnutrition is associated with altered immune function, poor wound healing, and increased morbidity and mortality rates.[1] It is estimated that more than 50% of hospitalized patients are malnourished on both hospital admission and hospital discharge.[2-5] Ideally, for optimal outcomes a malnourished patient should be nutritionally repleted for 7 to 10 days before surgery if time permits.[6]

PERSPECTIVES IN PRACTICE
Energy and Protein Requirements in General Surgery Patients

Nutritional needs of general surgery patients vary based on several factors, including the patient's disease process, other comorbidities, surgery to be performed, and baseline nutritional status. For example, compare the following patient situations.

Adequately Nourished Preoperative Patient
For the patient with normal energy and nitrogen balance, approximately 25 kcal/kg/day and 0.8 to 1.0 g/kg/day of protein should maintain these balances.

Adequately Nourished Postoperative Patient
After surgery, if no complications occurred, energy requirements remain about the same—25 kcal/kg/day. Protein requirements increase slightly due to increased metabolism and need for wound healing in the postoperative period to 1.0 to 1.1 g/kg/day.

Adequately Nourished Stressed Patient
This patient is assumed to have adequate nutrient stores; therefore replenishment is not the goal. Metabolic stress increases metabolic and catabolic rates, making energy and protein needs elevated. Energy needs are estimated at 25 to 30 kcal/kg/day; protein needs, 1.2 to 1.5 g/kg/day. Postoperatively the patient should be reassessed, and protein needs may increase up to 2 g/kg/day.

Nutritionally Depleted Nonstressed Patient
Upcoming Surgery: Gastrointestinal Tract Resection Resulting From Obstruction
Because of reduced dietary intake, this patient's nutrient stores (mostly glycogen and fat) may be depleted. In the nonstressed state, protein stores are spared for the most part. Energy needs are similar to those of the nourished preoperative patient at 25 kcal/kg/day. However, protein needs are slightly elevated to 1.0 to 1.2 g/kg/day. Postoperatively this patient's energy needs will remain near the same at 25 kcal/kg/day, but protein needs are increased to 1.2 to 1.5 g/kg/day.

Nutritionally Depleted Stressed Patient
This patient has elevated requirements for both energy and protein because of cytokine and hormonal shifts causing a hypermetabolic and hypercatabolic state. Energy needs are 25 to 30 kcal/kg/day with caution to avoid overfeeding. Overfeeding in a hypermetabolic state can result in hyperglycemia, hypercarbia, hepatic steatosis, and overall immune suppression. Protein needs are elevated to 1.5 to 2.0 g/kg/day. Postoperatively the nutrient needs remain about the same. At this point the goal is to minimize loss of lean body mass, not to replenish it. Once the patient is stable and anabolic, calories can be increased to 35 kcal/kg/day as needed for rehabilitation.

References

A.S.P.E.N. Board of Directors: Guidelines for the use of parenteral and enteral nutrition in adult and pediatric patients, *J Parent Enteral Nutr* 26:1SA, 2002.

Frankenfield D: Energy and macrosubstrate requirements. In American Society for Enteral and Parenteral Nutrition: *The science and practice of nutrition support: a case-based core,* ed 3, Dubuque, Iowa, 2001, Kendall/Hunt.

Unless the gastrointestinal (GI) tract is nonfunctional, nutrient provision should be provided enterally rather than parenterally.[7] Following are some guidelines:

- *Energy:* Adequate calories should be consumed to prevent loss of endogenous stores of carbohydrate, fat, and protein. Carbohydrates should constitute the majority of calories (50% to 60%). A minimum of approximately 150 g of carbohydrates per day is needed for central nervous system function.

- *Protein:* Most patients do not have excessive preoperative protein requirements, but body stores should be assessed. Adequate protein status is imperative to facilitate optimal wound healing.

- *Vitamins and minerals:* Any deficiency state such as anemia should be corrected. Electrolytes and fluids should be normalized and in balance with correction of dehydration, acidosis, or alkalosis.

One often-overlooked factor is the use of medicinal herbs. Many patients do not think to disclose the ingestion of herbal supplements when they are asked about medications during the preoperative interview, but some of these substances can complicate surgery. The *Diet-Medications Interactions* box, "Medicine or Poison?," lists some common herbal supplements that can create complications during surgery.

Immediate Preoperative Period

Typical dietary preparation for surgery involves giving nothing by mouth 8 to 12 hours before surgery. The rationale is to ensure the stomach is empty of food and liquids to prevent vomiting or aspiration during surgery or anesthesia recovery. In an emergency situation, gastric suction is used to remove stomach contents. With surgery involving the GI tract, food and fecal matter may interfere with the procedure itself and cause contamination. Therefore before lower GI surgery, a low-residue diet may be prescribed to reduce fecal residue. Although restricting dietary intake may prevent risks of anesthesia, it can also impair the patient's ability to respond to the metabolic stress of surgery.

Postoperative Nutrition

Nutrient provision in the postoperative period depends on several factors, including surgical procedure performed and anticipated time to resumption of oral intake, complications of surgery and postoperative clinical

DIET-MEDICATIONS INTERACTIONS

Medicine or Poison?

"Poisons and medicines are oftentimes the same substances given with different intents."

Peter Mere Latham (1789-1875)

Medicinal herbs and pharmaceutical drugs: Both can be therapeutic at one dose and toxic at another. Patients may not think to include herbal supplements when reporting medications used during the preoperative interview. Possible surgical complications vary depending on the herbal supplement used. Following are some common herbal supplements that may cause surgical complications.

Herb	Common Uses	Possible Surgical Complication
Dan Shen (*Salvia miltiorrhiza*)	Antibacterial, antihepatotoxin, mild sedative, antiinflammatory	May cause bleeding
Dong quai (*Angelica sinensis*)	Menstrual disorders, menopause	May cause bleeding (interferes with warfarin)
Echinacea (*Echinacea purpurea*)	Prevent and treat common cold, treat infections, enhance wound healing	May interfere with effectiveness of immunosuppressant drugs given to prevent transplant rejection; may interfere with body's immune functioning after surgery, could impair wound healing
Ephedra* (*Ma huang*, Herbal Exstasy, Chinese ephedra)	Sinus congestion, weight loss (ephedrine/caffeine)	May cause cardiovascular problems (increased heart rate, arrhythmias, heart attack or stroke); interaction with anesthesia can lead to abnormal heartbeat; for patients taking maintenance doses of MAOIs, interaction with anesthesia and MAOIs may result in life-threatening hypertension and coma
Feverfew (*Tanacetum parthenium*)	Migraine headaches (prophylaxis), rheumatoid arthritis	May cause bleeding
Garlic (*Allium* spp.)	Atherosclerosis, hyperlipidemia, hypertension, antithrombotic effects, chemoprevention, insect repellant, antimicrobial	May cause bleeding or interfere with normal clotting
Ginkgo (*Ginkgo biloba*)	Alzheimer's disease and non-Alzheimer's dementia, ordinary age-related memory loss, improving memory and mental function in the young, intermittent claudication, premenstrual syndrome, altitude sickness, tinnitus	May cause bleeding
Ginseng (*Panax ginseng*)	Enhancing immunity, improving mental activity, diabetes, athletic performance	May cause bleeding (interferes with warfarin)
Goldenseal (*Hydrastis Canadensis*)	Antimicrobial, expectorant	May cause or worsen hypertension
Kava (*Piper methysticum*)	Anxiety	May enhance sedative effects of anesthesia
Licorice† (*Glycyrrhiza glabra*)	Peptic ulcer disease, expectorant/antitussive	May increase blood pressure
St. John's wort (*Hypericum perforatum*)	Major depression of mild to moderate severity, polyneuropathy	Can increase or decrease effect of some drugs used during and after surgery
Valerian (*Valeriana officinalis*)	Insomnia, anxiety	May interfere with effects of anesthesia

NOTE: Different herbs stay in the body for different lengths of time. An individual taking herbs may need to stop taking them 1 or 2 weeks before surgery.

References

Bratman S, Girman AM: *Mosby's handbook of herbs and supplements and their therapeutic uses,* St. Louis, 2003, Mosby.

Escott-Stump S: *Nutrition and diagnosis-related care,* ed 5, Philadelphia, 2002, Lippincott Williams & Wilkins.

Fugh-Berman A: Herb-drug interactions, *Lancet* 355:134, 2000.

Kuhn MA, Winston D: *Herbal therapy and supplements: a scientific and traditional approach,* Philadelphia, 2001, Lippincott.

Mayo Clinic Staff: *Herbal supplements and surgery: what you need to know,* Rochester, Minn, 2003, Mayo Foundation for Medical Education and Research. Available at *www.mayoclinic.com.* Accessed August 14, 2005.

MAOI, Monoamine oxidase inhibitor.

*Ephedra was banned by the U.S. Food and Drug Administration in December 2003.

†Most licorice candy contains little or no herbal licorice. Consumers should consult the product ingredients. "Licorice flavoring" is safer than "licorice extract" or "natural licorice" for these purposes.

TABLE 23-1	Influences on Resting Energy Expenditure

Clinical Condition	REE (%)*
Elective uncomplicated surgery	Normal
Major abdominal, thoracic, and vascular surgery	
ICU + mechanical ventilation	105-109 ± 20-28
Cardiac surgery	
ICU + mechanical ventilation	119 ± 21
Multiple injury	
ICU + mechanical ventilation	138 ± 23
Spontaneous ventilation	119 ± 7
Head and multiple injury,	
ICU + mechanical ventilation	150 ± 23
Head injury	
ICU + spontaneous ventilation	126 ± 14
ICU + mechanical ventilation	104 ± 5
Infection	
Sepsis + spontaneous ventilation	121 ± 27
ICU + septic shock + mechanical ventilation	135 ± 28
Sepsis + mechanical ventilation	155 ± 14
Septic shock + mechanical ventilation	102 ± 14
Multiple injury + sepsis + mechanical ventilation + TPN	191 ± 38

Modified from Chiolero R, Revelly JP, Tappy L: Energy metabolism in sepsis and injury, *Nutrition* 13(suppl):45S, 1997, with permission from Elsevier.

*Values are percentage of reference value (±SD).

REE, Resting energy expenditure; *ICU,* intensive care unit; *TPN,* total parenteral nutrition.

BOX 23-1	Selected Methods for Estimating Energy Requirements

Harris-Benedict Basal Energy Expenditure (BEE) Equation

$$\text{Male: } 66.5 + 13.8(W) + 5.0(H) - 6.8(A)$$
$$\text{Female: } 655.1 + 9.6(W) + 1.9(H) - 4.7(A)$$

where W is weight (in kilograms); H, height (in centimeters); and A, age (in years).

NOTE: To predict total energy expenditure (TEE), add an injury/activity factor of 1.2 to 1.8 depending on the severity and nature of illness.

Ireton-Jones Energy Expenditure Equations (EEEs)

Spontaneously Breathing Patients

$$\text{EEE (s)} = 629 - 11(A) + 25(W) - 609(O)$$

Ventilator-Dependent Patients

$$\text{EEE (v)} = 1784 - 11(A) + 5(W) + 244(G) + 239(T) + 804(B)$$

where *EEE* is given in kcal/day; *v*, ventilator-dependent; *s*, spontaneously breathing; *A*, age (in years); *W*, body weight (in kilograms); *G*, Gender (female = 0, male = 1); *V*, ventilator support (present = 1, absent = 0); *T*, diagnosis of trauma (present = 1, absent = 0); *B*, diagnosis of burn (present = 1, absent = 0); and *O*, obesity >30% above ideal body weight (IBW) (from 1959 Metropolitan Life Insurance tables; present = 1, absent = 0).

status, and preoperative nutritional status. The well-nourished patient undergoing elective surgery will typically resume oral feeding by postoperative day 3 to 7, depending on return of bowel function. In this situation, supplemental nutrition in the form of enteral and parenteral nutrition is not indicated. The malnourished patient who is undergoing elective or emergency surgery and not anticipated to be able to meet his or her nutritional needs orally for a period of 7 to 10 days should receive specialized nutrition support.[6] This nutrition support should be provided enterally rather than parenterally to minimize incidence of complications.[6] Duration of this therapy will then depend on the patient's clinical status and transition to an adequate oral dietary consumption.

Energy Requirements

In the immediate postoperative period, especially in the critically ill, the goal of nutrition support is maintenance of current lean body mass, not repletion, and should serve as an adjunct to other critical therapies. Numerous factors are present that limit effectiveness of exogenously administered nutritional substrates in preventing catabo-

lism regardless of the level of support. It should not be expected to convert a catabolic, septic patient into an anabolic state at this time. Many undesirable metabolic complications can occur in attempting to do so, such as hypercapnia, hyperglycemia, hypertriglyceridemia, hepatic steatosis, and azotemia.[7-11] Once the hypermetabolic process is corrected, anabolism is favored and repletion can occur.

There are multiple methods for determining energy requirements. Indirect calorimetry involves actual measurement of energy expenditure and remains the "gold standard."[12] However, there are many disadvantages to this method, including increased cost, trained personnel, and inaccurate readings in patients with an FiO_2 of 50% or greater, malfunctioning chest tubes, endotracheal tubes, or bronchopleurofistulas. Because of these flaws, many institutions do not have the technology available and rely on predictive equations. Predicting energy needs can be difficult because of uncertainties regarding multiple factors of energy expenditure (Table 23-1).[13] Predictive equations (Box 23-1) may overestimate energy needs for those mechanically ventilated and sedated, and neuromuscular paralysis can decrease energy requirements by as much as 30%.[14-16] Calculated results are only as accurate as the variables used in the equation. Obesity and resuscitative water weight complicate use of these equations and lead to a tendency for overfeeding.[17] It is unclear as to whether ideal body weight (IBW) or actual body weight should be used in predictive energy equations. It has been reported that obese patients should receive 20 to 30 kilocalories (kcalories or kcal)/kg IBW per day,[18] as well as use of adjusted body weight, particularly in those greater than 130% IBW.[17] Predictive equations have been developed to account for obesity, using actual body weight, as well as trauma, burns, and ventilatory status.[19] Patino and colleagues[20] reported a hypocaloric-hyperproteinic nutrition regimen provided during the first days of the flow phase of the adaptive response to injury, sepsis, and critical illness. The regimen consists of a daily supply of 100 to 200 g of glucose and 1.5 to 2.0 g of protein per kilogram IBW. Overall, energy requirements for surgery patients range from 20 to 35 kcal/kg usual body weight per day.[21]

Protein Requirements

Dietary protein is required to build new and maintain existing body tissue and has many functions in the body. Protein can also be oxidized directly for adenosine triphosphate (ATP) and is critical to the body's ability to perform gluconeogenesis. Therefore protein is an important energy substrate in addition to its role in tissue building and repair.

Protein requirements in the surgical patient are typically elevated, particularly in the critically ill. Increased requirements are the result of need for tissue synthesis and wound healing, maintenance of oncotic pressure, adequate blood volume, maintenance of immune function, and energy substrate. Stressed critically ill patients require protein in the range of 1.5 to 2.0 g/kg/day.[20] Achieving positive nitrogen balance is nearly impossible immediately after metabolic insult, but after the primary insult is controlled or resolved, positive nitrogen balance is feasible. Protein requirements do not decrease with increasing age. Reduction in lean body mass and obligatory loss of protein during physiologic stress increase protein requirements for the critically ill older patient to those similar to those for a younger patient.[22] Protein tolerance as opposed to protein requirement often determines amount of protein delivered. Onset of azotemia, impaired renal or hepatic function, signals the need to reduce protein delivery. Most studies that examined graded protein intakes in septic, injured, or burned patients have found no protein-sparing benefit to giving protein in excess of the above recommendations.[23]

Fluid Requirements

Water is the medium within which all systems and subsystems function. It is necessary in digestion, absorption, transport, and utilization of nutrients, as well as elimination of toxins and waste products. Water also provides structure to cells and is a vital component of thermoregulation. Water is the most abundant substance in the human body, accounting for approximately 60% of body weight of adult males and 50% of body weight of adult females. The majority of water intake comes from ingested fluid and food; a small amount is produced as a

TABLE 23-2	Normal Daily Fluid Gains and Losses in Adults		
Fluid Gains		**Fluid Losses**	
Sensible		**Sensible**	
Food	1000 ml	Urine	1500 ml
Fluid	1200 ml	Feces	100 ml
		Sweat	50 ml
Insensible		**Insensible**	
Oxidative metabolism	350 ml	Skin	500 ml
		Lungs	400 ml
TOTAL	2550 ml	TOTAL	2550 ml

From Whitmire SJ: Fluid and electrolytes. In Gottschlich MM, ed: *The science and practice of nutrition support: a case-based core curriculum,* Dubuque, Iowa, 2001, Kendall/Hunt, with permission from the American Society for Enteral and Parenteral Nutrition (A.S.P.E.N.). A.S.P.E.N. does not endorse the use of this material in any form other than its entirety.

byproduct of metabolic processes, primarily carbohydrate metabolism. The main source of water loss is in the form of urine. However, sizeable amounts are also lost insensibly through skin and respiratory tract. Smaller amounts of water are lost in sweat and feces (Table 23-2).

Normal body water requirements can be estimated using a variety of methods. The National Research Council recommends 1 ml/kcal energy expenditure for adults with average energy expenditure living under average environmental conditions. Fluid requirements increase with several conditions, including fever, high altitude, low humidity, profuse sweating, watery diarrhea, vomiting, hemorrhage, diuresis, surgical drains, and loss of skin integrity (e.g., burns, open wounds).

Therefore fluid balance is of vital concern after surgery. Patients often receive large volumes of fluid intraoperatively. These volumes are normally diuresed postoperatively, but occasionally the patient may require diuretics to facilitate this. Typically surgical patients are provided with intravenous fluids until oral intake is resumed and tolerated to maintain fluid balance. Daily weight measurement of the patient provides a guideline for fluid balance.

Vitamins and Minerals

Adequate levels of vitamins and minerals are very important for optimal postoperative recovery. Vitamin C serves many functions in the body. In addition to being an antioxidant, it is required for synthesis of collagen, carnitine, and neurotransmitters and for immune-mediated and antibacterial functions of white blood cells. Iron is an essential component of hemoglobin, which is necessary for oxygen transport; of myoglobin, which is necessary for muscle iron storage; and in cytochromes, which are necessary for the oxidative production of cellular energy. Vitamin K is essential in the blood-clotting mechanism.

Surgical patients with elevated enteric losses (e.g., ostomy, stool, fistula) are at risk for several trace element deficiencies (e.g., zinc, copper). If losses exceed 800 ml/day, extra supplementation of micronutrients should be considered. Various GI operations may also place a surgical patient at risk for several micronutrient deficiencies, depending on the location of bowel resected.

Diets

Oral Diet

The preferred route of nutrient delivery is for the patient to be able to consume adequate nutrients through an oral diet. Fortunately the majority of surgical patients can accomplish this by postoperative day 7 at the latest. Routine intravenous fluids are intended to provide hydration and electrolytes, not energy and protein requirements. For example, 1 L of routine intravenous fluids of a 5% dextrose solution provides 50 g of dextrose, with an energy value of only 170 kcal; no protein is provided. If adequate calories and protein are not consumed, the patient's diet may be supplemented. Often the addition of between-meal feedings consisting of soft, high-protein foods is adequate. However, sometimes commercially available oral supplements may be provided because they are a concentrated source of energy, protein, and vitamins/minerals.[24] Not all patients tolerate these supplements because they tend to be very sweet and patients develop taste fatigue. Every effort should be made to maximize the patient's diet for his or her diet preferences to improve inadequate dietary consumption.

Routine Postoperative Diets

A diet order is typically prescribed postoperatively once the patient exhibits adequate bowel function (e.g., flatus, bowel sounds present). Historically the first diet order is a clear liquid diet (Box 23-2). This diet contains hyperosmolar fluids, calories from primarily simple sugars, very little protein, and a fair amount of sodium and chloride. Because this diet is incomplete and very unpalatable, patients should be advanced to either a full liquid or soft/regular diet as soon as the clear liquid diet is tolerated. These diets are complete diets in that calorie, protein, and vitamin/mineral requirements can be met if adequate amounts are consumed. Recently this historical diet progression after GI surgery was challenged.[25] Patients randomized to a regular diet as their first postoperative diet after abdominal surgery had equal tolerance and improved nutrient intake compared with those receiving a clear liquid diet.

Specialized Nutrition Support

If an oral diet is not tolerated or feasible, then enteral or parenteral nutrition may be provided. Enteral nutrition is indicated for patients with an adequately functional GI tract and oral nutrient intake that is insufficient to meet estimated needs.[6] Enteral nutrition maintains nutri-

---

BOX 23-2 | Typical Foods in Postoperative Diets

Clear Liquid
Broth
Clear juice (apple, grape, cranberry)
Jello
Sodas (Sprite, ginger ale)
Tea
Coffee

Full Liquid
Juice (any)
Milk
Milkshakes
Ice cream
Cream soups
Thinned oatmeal, corn grits
Scrambled eggs (in some institutions)
Oral liquid nutritional supplements (e.g., Ensure, Boost)

Soft/Regular
Juice
Canned fruits
Cooked vegetables
Soft meats (baked chicken, stews, roasts)
Scrambled eggs
Pancakes, biscuits, muffins
Soups
Soft sandwiches (egg, tuna, chicken salad, turkey, ham and cheese)
Soft starches (mashed potatoes, pasta, rice)
Milk, tea, coffee
Ice cream
Puddings, yogurt
Soft desserts (cake, pies, soft cookies)

---

tional, metabolic, immunologic, and barrier functions of the intestines; it is less expensive and safer than parenteral nutrition.[26] Although enteral nutrition is the preferred route of nutrient delivery, it is not innocuous and there are some situations where enteral feeding is not feasible (Box 23-3) and parenteral nutrition should be used. Expected length of therapy, clinical condition, risk of aspiration, and medical expertise usually determine route of administration and type of access for tube feedings. There are multiple methods for obtaining enteral access (Box 23-4), all of which carry various degrees of expertise, risk, and expense. Nasoenteric or oroenteric tubes are generally used when therapy is anticipated to be of short duration (e.g., less than 4 weeks) or for interim access before placement of a long-term device. Long-term access requires a percutaneous or surgically placed feeding tube. It is not always clear when enteral nutrition will be tolerated. If the individual's needs are not met enterally, then

---

sepsis Presence in the blood or other tissues of pathogenic microorganisms or their toxins; conditions associated with such pathogens.

parenteral nutrition may be implemented for either full nutrient provision or concurrently with enteral delivery to provide the balance of nutrients not tolerated.

The majority of postoperative surgical patients can tolerate a standard enteral formulation that provides their energy and protein requirements. Recently research studies have evaluated use of "immune-enhancing" enteral formulas in postoperative GI cancer patients, trauma patients, and patients with critical illness. These formulas are supplemented with various "immune-enhancing" nutrients, including L-arginine, L-glutamine, omega-3 fatty acids, nucleic acids, and various vitamins and minerals.

BOX 23-3 | Indications for Parenteral Nutrition

Indications
- Bowel obstruction
- Persistent intolerance of enteral feeding (e.g., emesis, diarrhea)
- Hemodynamic instability
- Major upper gastrointestinal bleed
- Ileus
- Unable to safely access intestinal tract

Relative Indications
- Significant bowel wall edema
- Nutrient infusion proximal to recent gastrointestinal anastomosis
- High-output fistula (>800 ml/day)

BOX 23-4 | Methods of Enteral Access

Short Term (<4 weeks)
Nasoenteric Feeding Tube
Spontaneous passage
Bedside-prokinetic agent

Active Passage
Bedside-assisted
Endoscopic
Fluoroscopic
Operative

Long Term (>4 weeks)
Percutaneous Feeding Tube
Percutaneous endoscopic
  Gastric (PEG)
  Gastric/jejunal (PEG/J)
  Direct jejunal (DPEJ)

Laparoscopic
Gastrostomy
Jejunostomy

Surgical
Gastrostomy
Jejunostomy

When these diets were used in these surgical populations, decreases in infectious complications and hospital length of stay were noted.[6,27]

NUTRITIONAL CONCERNS FOR PATIENTS UNDERGOING ALIMENTARY CANAL SURGERY

The digestive tract is a metabolically active organ involved in digestion, absorption, and metabolism of many nutrients; therefore various surgical interventions involving the GI tract can result in malabsorption and maldigestion and nutritional deficiencies (Table 23-3).

Head and Neck Surgery

These patients often present for surgery malnourished due to their disease state. Many times surgical intervention is required because of a tumor that may be inhibiting the patient's ability to chew and swallow normally. Typically, loss of this ability is what makes the patient seek medical attention. Patients with head and neck cancer usually have a long history of alcohol and tobacco use, which may also affect optimal nutritional status.

Depending on the patient's treatment, optimization of nutrition preoperatively is ideal. This also depends on the individual's disease progression and ability to swallow. Many times preoperative treatment involves radiation and/or chemotherapy to reduce the tumor size. In these situations ability to swallow may worsen due to negative side effects of these therapies. Ideally, placement of a percutaneous endoscopic gastrostomy (PEG) feeding tube can be performed to allow for nutrition, hydration, and medication administration to maintain and/or improve nutritional status preoperatively. The patient may also still be able to swallow soft foods or liquids, which should be maximized for caloric and protein density. If a PEG tube is not placed preoperatively, it can be placed intraoperatively or a nasoenteric tube may be placed. These feeding tubes are then used postoperatively until the patient is able to resume an oral diet.

Esophageal Surgery

There are several medical conditions affecting the esophagus that can prevent swallowing and thus nutrient intake. Common conditions include corrosive injuries and perforation, achalasia, gastroesophageal reflux disease (GERD), and partial or full obstruction caused by cancer, congenital abnormalities, or strictures. These conditions usually require surgical intervention involving removal of a segment or the entire esophagus (see the *Case Study* box, "The Patient With Esophageal Cancer"). The esophageal tract is then replaced with either the stomach (gastric pull-up) or the intestine (colonic/jejunal interposition). A gastric pull-up procedure involves drawing the stomach up to the esophageal stump, causing displacement of the stomach into the thoracic cavity. This procedure results in a reduction of stomach volume

capacity, with potential delayed gastric emptying and dumping syndrome (Figure 23-1). The colonic/jejunal interposition procedure involves forming a new conduit by anastomosing the selected portion of bowel between the esophagus and stomach. Complications following

TABLE 23-3	Common Gastrointestinal Operations and Nutritional Consequences
Location	**Potential Consequences**
Esophagus	
Resection/replacement	Weight loss due to inadequate intake
Gastric pull-up	↑ Protein loss due to catabolism
Colonic interposition	May require enteral/parenteral nutrition until oral intake appropriate
	Antidumping diet; may malabsorb fat/fat-soluble vitamins, simple sugars, and various vitamins/minerals
	Early satiety due to reduced storage capacity (gastric pull-up)
Stomach	
Partial gastrectomy/ vagotomy	Early satiety due to reduced storage capacity
	Delayed gastric emptying of solids due to stasis
	Rapid emptying of hypertonic fluids
Total gastrectomy	Weight loss due to dumping/malabsorption, early satiety, anorexia, inadequate intake, unavailability of bile acids and pancreatic enzymes due to anastomotic changes
	Malabsorption may lead to anemia, metabolic bone disease, protein-calorie malnutrition
	Bezoar formation
	Vitamin B_{12} deficiency due to lack of intrinsic factor
Intestine*	
Proximal	Malabsorption of vitamins/minerals (Ca^{2+}, Mg^{2+}, iron, vitamins A and D)
Gastric bypass	Protein-calorie malnutrition from malabsorption due to dumping, unavailability of bile acids and pancreatic enzymes due to anastomotic changes
	Bezoar formation
Distal	Malabsorption of vitamins/mineral (water soluble—folate, vitamins B_{12}, C, B_1, B_2, pyridoxine)
	Protein-calorie malnutrition due to dumping
	Fat malabsorption
	Bacterial overgrowth if ileocecal valve resected
Colon	Fluid and electrolyte (K^+, Na^+, Cl^-) malabsorption

*Note that consequences may occur only with extensive disease process and resection.

malabsorption and maldigestion Malabsorption is a syndrome in which normal products of digestion do not traverse the intestinal mucosa and enter the lymphatic or portal venous branches. Maldigestion, which may be clinically similar to malabsorption, describes defects in the intraluminal phase of the digestive process caused by inadequate exposure of chyme to bile salts and pancreatic enzymes. Clinical symptoms of malabsorption include diarrhea, steatorrhea, and weight loss. Laboratory signs include depressed serum fat-soluble vitamin levels, accelerated prothrombin time, hypomagnesemia, and hypocholesterolemia. Patients with symptoms of malabsorption should have a laboratory work-up to determine the presence and degree of nutrient loss.

gastroesophageal reflux disease (GERD) Describes symptoms that result from reflux of gastric juices, and sometimes duodenal juices, into the esophagus. Symptoms include substernal burning (heartburn), epigastric pressure sensation, and severe epigastric pain. Prolonged and severe GERD can lead to esophageal bleeding, perforation, strictures, Barrett's epithelium, adenocarcinoma, and pulmonary fibrosis (from aspiration). Conservative dietary therapy involves weight reduction; restriction of carbonated beverages, caffeine, fatty foods, peppermint, chocolate, and ethanol; small frequent meals; and wearing of loose clothing to promote symptomatic relief.

dumping syndrome Constellation of postprandial symptoms that result from rapid emptying of hyperosmolar gastric contents into the duodenum. The hypertonic load in the small intestine promotes reflux of vascular fluid into the bowel lumen, causing a rapid decrease in the circulating blood volume. Rapid symptoms of abdominal cramping, nausea, vomiting, palpitations, sweating, weakness, reduced blood pressure, tremors, and osmotic diarrhea occur. Symptoms of early dumping begin 10 to 30 minutes after eating; late dumping syndrome occurs 1 to 4 hours after a meal. Late dumping is a result of insulin hypersecretion in response to the carbohydrate load dumped into the small intestine. Once the carbohydrate is absorbed, the hyperinsulinemia causes hypoglycemia, which results in vasomotor symptoms such as diaphoresis, weakness, flushing, and palpitations. Individuals who have undergone gastrointestinal surgery resulting in a reduced or absent gastric pouch are more prone to dumping syndrome.

CASE STUDY

The Patient With Esophageal Cancer

Kevin is a 54-year-old accountant seen by his family physician for pain with swallowing and difficulty swallowing solid foods for the past 6 weeks. This has resulted in continued weight loss and fatigue. Kevin was referred to the gastrointestinal medicine service for further evaluation. After a series of tests that included endoscopy and biopsy, Kevin was found to have esophageal cancer with the tumor lying in the midesophagus. He was then referred to the gastrointestinal surgery service for surgical evaluation.

A medical history revealed that Kevin smoked two packs of cigarettes per day, drank three martinis per day, and was cachectic. A referral was sent to the dietitian for nutritional evaluation and recommendations for optimizing his nutritional status for surgery. A nutrition history revealed that during the past 6 weeks, his diet had progressively decreased in consistency to the point where he could tolerate only liquids and some soft solid foods such as mashed potatoes, oatmeal, and applesauce. At a height of 178 cm (5 ft 10 in), Kevin's weight had dropped from 80 kg (176 lb) to 63 kg (139 lb), leaving him at 79% of his usual body weight. His blood work revealed a serum albumin level of 3.0 g/dl and prealbumin of 13.2 mg/dl. He no longer could stand long enough to make himself a meal and had to take a bath rather than shower because he became too tired. He was not currently taking any medications because he could not swallow them. His current diet order was a full liquid diet.

Assessment of calorie and protein requirements estimated that Kevin required approximately 1800 kcal (basal energy expenditure + 25%) and 75 to 95 g of protein (1.2 to 1.5 g/kg) daily. Because he could eat some solid foods, the dietitian changed him to a soft diet. He modified Kevin's diet so that it contained soft, high protein–containing solids and liquids that he stated he could eat and ordered a 48-hour calorie count. A liquid multivitamin was also provided. Kevin was now able to eat enough calories and protein for 14 days preoperatively that he gained 3 kg (7 lb); his albumin increased to 3.1 g/dl, and prealbumin increased to 17 mg/dl.

He underwent an esophagectomy with a gastric pull-up. A feeding jejunostomy tube was placed intraoperatively. Kevin was started on low-rate enteral feedings on postoperative day 2, which were gradually advanced to his goal requirements over the next 2 days. He was not allowed to eat until postoperative day 7 after a swallowing study for anastomotic evaluation. Once his diet was initiated and tolerated, his tube feedings were provided nocturnally because he was not able to consume 100% of his nutritional needs orally. He was discharged home with an oral postgastrectomy diet and nocturnal tube feedings to provide about 50% of his nutritional needs for 10 days, at which time his nutrition would be reevaluated.

Questions for Analysis

1. Evaluate the preoperative nutrition assessment data. Why were the particular energy and protein assessment factors chosen?
2. What dietary modifications accompany a postgastrectomy diet?
3. Why was Kevin placed on a postgastrectomy diet when his stomach was not resected?
4. At what point should his enteral tube feedings be discontinued?

---

this procedure include swallowing difficulties, strictures, and leakage at the anastomotic site.

Preoperative nutrition for these patients may be a tolerated oral diet, often liquids because of dysphasia and obstruction. If a patient is unable to consume his or her full nutrient needs orally, then a feeding tube may be placed if the esophagus is not obstructed. A PEG tube is not indicated if a gastric pull-up procedure is to be performed because the stomach is used to make the esophageal conduit and a hole resulting from a gastrostomy tube would be contraindicated. These patients may require preoperative parenteral nutrition if the esophagus is obstructed. Intraoperatively, a jejunal feeding tube may be placed to allow for postoperative enteral nutrition until the anastomosis heals and oral intake is resumed. If enteral access is not obtained intraoperatively, then parenteral nutrition is indicated because these patients may not resume oral intake for 7 to 10 days.

For patients with chronic GERD, a Nissen fundoplication procedure may be performed. This is the most commonly performed antireflux procedure operation for patients with gastroesophageal reflux refractory to medical management. This procedure involves wrapping the stomach around the base of the esophagus, near the lower esophageal sphincter; this places pressure and narrows the lower esophageal opening to prevent reflux (Figure 23-2). Patients are typically placed on a pureed diet for 2 weeks after this procedure with small frequent meals, no gulping of liquids, and crushed or liquid medications. After this time solid foods are gradually added to the diet

with future avoidance of bread products, nuts, and seeds because these can become lodged in the lower esophagus and cause an obstruction.

Gastric Surgery

A number of nutrition problems may develop after gastric surgery, depending on the type of surgical procedure and the patient's response. There are several indications for gastric surgery, including tumor removal, ulcer disease, perforation, hemorrhage, Zollinger-Ellison syndrome, gastric polyposis, and Ménétrier's disease. A vagotomy is often performed to eliminate gastric acid secretion. Vagotomy at certain levels can alter the normal physiologic function of the stomach, small intestine, pancreas, and biliary system. Total gastric and truncal vagotomy procedures impair proximal and distal motor function of the stomach. Digestion and emptying of solids are retarded while emptying of liquids is accelerated.[28] These vagotomy procedures are commonly accompanied by a drainage procedure (antrectomy or pyloroplasty) that helps the stomach to empty. Nutrition complications associated with vagotomy and pyloroplasty include dumping syndrome, steatorrhea, and bacterial overgrowth.

A total gastrectomy involves removal of the entire stomach. A storage reservoir may be created using a section of jejunum. A subtotal or partial gastrectomy involves removal of a portion of the stomach accompanied by a reconstructive procedure. A Billroth I (gastroduodenostomy)

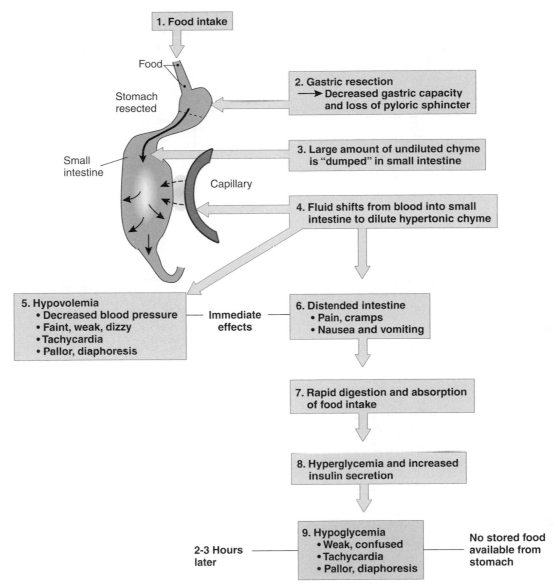

FIGURE 23-1 Dumping syndrome (postgastrectomy). *(From Gould BE: Pathophysiology for health professions, ed 2, Philadelphia, 2002, Saunders.)*

anastomosis A surgical joining of two ducts to allow flow from one to the other.

sphincter A circular band of muscle fibers that constricts a passage or closes a natural opening in the body (e.g., lower esophageal sphincter, pyloric sphincter).

Zollinger-Ellison syndrome A condition characterized by severe peptic ulceration, gastric hypersecretion, elevated serum gastrin, and gastrinoma of the pancreas or the duodenum. Total gastrectomy may be necessary.

gastric polyposis An abnormal condition characterized by the presence of numerous polyps in the stomach.

Ménétrier's disease (giant hypertrophic gastritis) Rare disease characterized by large folds of nodular gastric rugae that may cover the wall of the stomach, causing anorexia, nausea, vomiting, and abdominal distress.

vagotomy Cutting of certain branches of the vagus nerve, performed with gastric surgery, to reduce the amount of gastric acid secreted and lessen the chance of recurrence of a gastric ulcer.

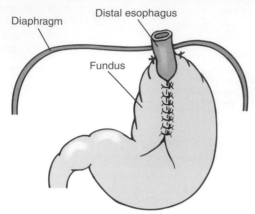

FIGURE 23-2   Nissen fundoplication. *(From Lewis SM, Heitkemper MM, Dirksen SR: Medical-surgical nursing: assessment and management of clinical problems, ed 5, St. Louis, 2000, Mosby.)*

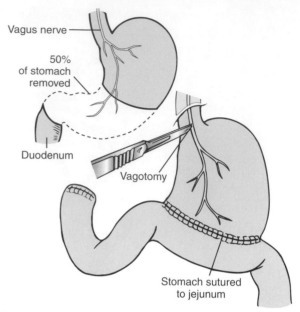

FIGURE 23-4   Billroth II (gastrojejunostomy). *(From Lewis SM, Heitkemper MM, Dirksen SR: Medical-surgical nursing: assessment and management of clinical problems, ed 5, St. Louis, 2000, Mosby.)*

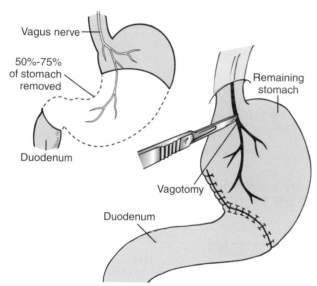

FIGURE 23-3   Billroth I (gastroduodenostomy). *(From Lewis SM, Heitkemper MM, Dirksen SR: Medical-surgical nursing: assessment and management of clinical problems, ed 5, St. Louis, 2000, Mosby.)*

involves an anastomosis of the proximal end of the intestine (duodenum) to the distal end of the stomach (Figure 23-3). A Billroth II (gastrojejunostomy) involves an anastomosis of the stomach to the side of the jejunum, which creates a blind loop (Figure 23-4). Any gastric surgery carries some potential for development of malnutrition. Common consequences include weight loss, dumping syndrome, malabsorption, anemia, and metabolic bone disease. Dumping syndrome, epigastric fullness, nausea, and vomiting often occur in the early postoperative period. These symptoms are managed with dietary modifications and antiemetic medications.[28]

Generally after gastric surgery, small frequent oral feedings are resumed according to the patient's tolerance (Box 23-5). For the first 2 weeks after surgery, soft, bland foods with a low fiber content should be consumed in small portions. Simple sugars, lactose, and fried foods

should be avoided; beverages should be consumed at least 30 minutes before and after meals; and foods high in complex carbohydrates and protein should be emphasized. Generally these diet modifications are necessary for only the short term because most patients can resume a regular diet. However, some individuals may need an antidumping diet indefinitely. For individuals who were malnourished preoperatively, a small-bowel feeding tube may be placed intraoperatively. Low-rate enteral feedings using a standard formulation may be initiated on postoperative day 1. Tube feedings are adjusted according to the patient's clinical progress and tolerance of an oral diet. Patients may be discharged home with nocturnal tube feedings until their oral diet consumption is optimal. Oral supplements may be provided to increase nutrient intake; however, they need to be isotonic, containing no simple sugars, to avoid dumping. Unfortunately, most oral liquid supplements are hyperosmolar, containing simple sugars, and therefore are not well tolerated after gastric surgery. Parenteral nutrition is indicated only if enteral access is not available and the patient is malnourished and not able to tolerate adequate nutrients orally.

Anemia is a common consequence of gastric surgery. Anemia can be attributed to a deficiency or malabsorption of one or more nutrients, including iron, vitamin B_{12}, and folate. Assimilation of vitamin B_{12} requires liberation of the vitamin from protein and binding of the vitamin to intrinsic factor, both of which occur in the stomach. Failure of either of these reactions to occur results in vitamin B_{12} malabsorption, which with time produces anemia.[28] Total gastrectomy patients require periodic intramuscular vitamin B_{12} injections. Metabolic

BOX 23-5 | Postgastrectomy Antidumping Diet

Principles of the Diet

After surgery some discomfort or diarrhea may occur. Therefore to reduce the likelihood of those symptoms a healthy, nutritionally complete diet should be followed. Each person may react to food differently. Foods should be reintroduced into the diet slowly.

Steps of the Diet

1. Intake of complex carbohydrates is unlimited (e.g., bread, vegetables, rice, potatoes).
2. Intake of simple sugars (e.g., sugar, candy, cake, pies, jelly, honey) should be kept to a minimum. Artificial sweeteners may be used.
3. Fat intake should be moderate (≤30% total calories).
4. Protein should be unlimited because it helps with wound healing (e.g., meats, legumes).
5. Milk contains lactose, which may be hard to digest. Introduce milk and milk products slowly several weeks after surgery.
6. Eat small, frequent meals, approximately six meals per day, to avoid loading the stomach.
7. Limit fluids to 4 oz (½ cup) during mealtimes. This prevents the rapid movement of food through the upper gastrointestinal tract.
8. Drink fluids 30 to 45 minutes before and after eating to prevent diarrhea.
9. Relatively low-roughage foods and raw foods are allowed as tolerated after postoperative day 14.
10. Eat and chew slowly.
11. Avoid extreme temperatures of foods.

Sample Menu

Breakfast

Scrambled egg, 1
Toast, 1 slice
Margarine, 1 tsp
Low-sugar jelly, 1 tsp
Banana, 1 small

Midmorning Snack

Canned fruit, water packed, ½ cup
Graham crackers, 2 squares

Lunch

Bread, 2 slices
Ham, 2 oz
Cheese, 1 oz
Mustard, 2 tsp
Canned fruit, water packed
Yogurt, sugar-free, 4 oz

Midafternoon Snack

Saltine crackers, 3 squares
Peanut butter, 1 tbsp

Dinner

Chicken breast, 3 oz
Mashed potatoes, ½ cup
Green beans, ½ cup
Margarine, 2 tsp
Yogurt, sugar-free, 4 oz

Evening Snack

Sugar-free pudding, ½ cup
Vanilla wafers, 3 pieces

---

bone disease can be a late complication of gastric surgery. The cause of metabolic bone disease varies with the surgical procedure. The Billroth II procedure is associated with more complications than is the Billroth I because it bypasses the duodenum and upper jejunum (the site of calcium absorption). Procedures that destroy the pylorus can result in rapid gastric emptying, which may contribute to development of metabolic bone disease. Rapid gastric emptying not only reduces absorption time but also, when fats are malabsorbed, can lead to formation of insoluble calcium soaps.[28] Fat malabsorption can also lead to vitamin D malabsorption, which leads to impaired metabolism of calcium and phosphorus.

Intestinal Surgery

Surgical resections of the small and large intestine are usually well tolerated. If excessive amounts of bowel are removed, nutritional consequences can arise depending on the location resected. If more than 50% of the small intestine is removed, short-bowel syndrome may occur. This syndrome is characterized by severe diarrhea or steatorrhea, malabsorption, and malnutrition. Often the patient may require long-term parenteral nutrition to maintain his or her nutritional status and fluid and electrolyte balance (see Chapter 18).

Pancreaticoduodenectomy (Whipple Procedure)

In cases of ampullary, duodenal, and pancreatic malignancies, a pancreaticoduodenectomy may be performed. This procedure, one of the most difficult and technically demanding in GI surgery, involves resecting the distal stomach, distal common duct, pancreatic head, and duodenum. Three anastomoses—pancreaticojejunostomy, choledochojejunostomy, and gastrojejunostomy (Billroth II)—must be performed. In the past few years a pyloric-sparing Whipple procedure has become more prominent, resulting in a Billroth I anastomosis. This procedure carries fewer postoperative nutritional concerns than the other, which results in a Billroth II anastomosis (Figure 23-5).

Ileostomy and Colostomy

In cases of intestinal lesions, obstruction, or inflammatory bowel disease of the entire colon or when diversion

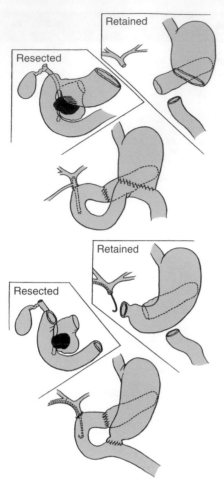

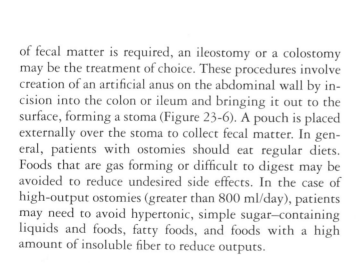

FIGURE 23-5   Whipple procedure. *(From Hardy JD, ed:* Hardy's textbook of surgery, *ed 2, Philadelphia, 1988, JB Lippincott.)*

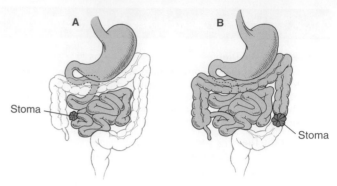

FIGURE 23-6   **A,** Ileostomy. **B,** Colostomy.

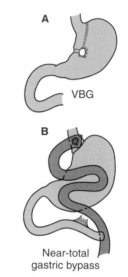

FIGURE 23-7   **A,** Vertical banded gastroplasty (VBG). **B,** Roux-en-Y gastric bypass.

of fecal matter is required, an ileostomy or a colostomy may be the treatment of choice. These procedures involve creation of an artificial anus on the abdominal wall by incision into the colon or ileum and bringing it out to the surface, forming a stoma (Figure 23-6). A pouch is placed externally over the stoma to collect fecal matter. In general, patients with ostomies should eat regular diets. Foods that are gas forming or difficult to digest may be avoided to reduce undesired side effects. In the case of high-output ostomies (greater than 800 ml/day), patients may need to avoid hypertonic, simple sugar–containing liquids and foods, fatty foods, and foods with a high amount of insoluble fiber to reduce outputs.

Bariatric Surgery

In the past several years, surgery for treatment of obesity has become more prevalent. Probably the most common procedure for weight loss in the world is the vertical banded gastroplasty (VBG), or gastric stapling (Figure 23-7, *A*). This technique is performed under general anesthesia and requires about 4 to 5 days in the hospital postoperatively. The VBG procedure limits food intake by creating a small pouch (½ oz) in the upper stomach with a narrow outlet (½ inch) reinforced by a mesh band to prevent stretching. The pouch fills quickly and empties slowly with solid food, producing a feeling of fullness. Overeating results in pain or vomiting, thus restricting food intake. This procedure is preferred for those people who engage in "bulk" or "binge" eating. The disadvantage of this procedure is that weight loss is not as great as that with other procedures. It does not restrict the intake of high-caloric liquids, and the pouch can stretch with overeating. As a result, 20% of people do not lose weight, and only half of people lose at least 50% of their excess weight with a VBG.

The Roux-en-Y gastric bypass (see Figure 23-7, *B*) is a combination of gastric stapling and intestinal bypass. It promotes weight loss by (1) restricting the amount of food a person can ingest by reducing the holding capacity of the stomach and (2) interfering with complete absorption of nutrients by shortening the length of small

BOX 23-6 | Postoperative Diet for Gastric Bypass Procedure for Morbid Obesity

Stage I: Clear liquids   Begin once liquids allowed; continue for two to three meals
Stage II: Gastric bypass liquids   Begin after clear liquids tolerated; continue for 3 to 4 weeks
Stage III: Pureed   Begin after postoperative week 4; continue for 1 to 2 weeks
Stage IV: Soft, solids   Begin after postoperative week 6; continue indefinitely

Gastric Bypass Liquids

Nonfat milk
Blenderized soups
100% Fruit juice (diluted ½ water, ½ juice)
Vegetable juice (e.g., V8, tomato)
Sugar-Free Carnation Instant Breakfast powder mixed with nonfat milk
Grits, oatmeal, cream of wheat, mashed potatoes (thinned down enough that it could go through a straw)
Nonfat, sugar-free milkshakes
Thinned baby food
Sugar-free drinks (e.g., sodas, tea)

Eating Guidelines

Small meals: each "feeding" should be ≤4 oz total (½ cup)
Six to eight "feedings" per day to consume adequate nutrients
60 minutes between meals and drinking fluids
Eat slowly and chew food well; each "feeding" should last at least 30 minutes
Avoid sugars (sucrose, honey, corn syrup, fructose) and sugar-containing beverages and foods/candy
Low-fat foods only (avoid fried foods, gravies, excessive margarine, butter, high-fat meats, and breads)
Eat high-protein foods (milk, yogurt, soft meats, eggs)
Avoid soft, calorie-dense foods (e.g., ice cream, chocolate, cheese, cookies)
Avoid obstructive foods (e.g., tough, fibrous red meat, bread made from refined flour, celery, popcorn, nuts, seeds, membranes of citrus fruits)

Take a daily complete multivitamin (liquid or chewable)
Calcium supplements (1500 mg/day)

Sample Menu (After 8 Weeks)

Breakfast

Banana, ¼ medium
Scrambled egg, 1 egg
Toast, white, ½ slice
Margarine, ½ tsp

Morning Snack

Graham crackers, 2
Pudding, sugar-free made with nonfat milk, ½ cup

Lunch

Broiled chicken breast, 2 oz
Carrots, boiled, ¼ cup
Margarine, 1 tsp
Pasta salad, ¼ cup

Afternoon Snack

Canned fruit, water packed, ½ cup

Dinner

Baked or broiled fish, 2 oz
Green beans, ¼ cup
Potato, baked, ½ small
Margarine, ½ tsp

Evening Snack

Cheese, American, 1 oz
Saltine crackers, 2 squares

NOTE: Consume nonfat milk or yogurt between meals, throughout the day. Drink/eat no more than 2 to 3 oz at a time for a daily total of 2 cups.

---

intestine through which the food travels. Unlike the VBG, this procedure discourages intake of high-calorie sweets by producing nausea, diarrhea, and other unpleasant symptoms. With this procedure a small gastric pouch (15 ml) is made near where stomach and esophagus meet. The small pouch and remainder of the stomach are divided from each other with staples. An opening is made in the pouch where a portion of the small intestine is connected. This new connection between the pouch and the small intestine is called a Roux-en-Y limb. Food then travels down the esophagus and bypasses nearly all of the stomach and first 2 feet of small intestine. Complications related to gallstones, which tend to form during rapid weight loss, can be prevented by removal of the gallbladder. This procedure is intended for people who "graze" during the day on high-calorie and sugar-containing foods, as well as eating large amounts. Box 23-6 lists a sample meal plan after gastric bypass surgery.

Like any major abdominal operation, these bariatric surgical procedures carry risks such as bleeding, infection, bowel blockage due to scar tissue formation, hernia through the incision, and anesthesia risks. The most serious risk is leakage of fluid from the stomach or intestines resulting in abdominal infection and reoperation. There are additional risks directly related to being obese; these include blood clots in legs or lungs, pneumonia, and cardiac complications. Less-immediate risks are ulcers in the stomach or intestine, dumping syndrome, bezoar formation, obstruction

bariatrics The field of medicine that focuses on the treatment and the control of obesity and diseases associated with obesity.

bezoar A hard ball of hair or vegetable fiber that may develop within the stomach and intestines; can cause an obstruction, requiring removal. Formed because of reduced gastric motility, decreased gastric mixing and churning, and reduced gastric secretions.

of stoma, and malnutrition from too rapid weight loss and loss of vitamins and minerals. From 10 to 15 per 100 people experience some complications from the gastric bypass; death may occur from complications in 1 or 2 per 100 patients. Because this procedure is not risk free, strict criteria for eligibility should be made. Generally those who have at least 100 lb excess body weight (or a body mass index of ≥ 40 kg/m^2) and have significant obesity-related medical problems and for whom all other serious attempts at weight reduction have failed may be candidates. A thorough medical and nutritional/behavioral evaluation is necessary to determine eligibility.

Other Related Problems

Enteric Fistulas

Enteric fistulas are abnormal communications between a portion of the intestinal tract and another organ (internal) or between the intestinal tract and the surface of the body (external or enterocutaneous).[28] The most common sites of origin are the pancreas and the large and small intestines. The majority of enteric fistulas result from surgical wound dehiscence or necrosis from bowel ischemia. Inflammatory bowel disease, cancer, trauma, and radiation to the abdomen can also lead to fistula development.

Several metabolic complications can arise as a result of an enteric fistula, including fluid and electrolyte losses, malnutrition, and sepsis. The route of nutrition intervention depends on the location of the fistula. Proximal fistulas may require that a patient be placed on parenteral nutrition if enteral access distal to the fistula cannot be achieved. This is because eating, and thus nutrients in the proximal bowel, stimulates GI secretions, thereby complicating fistula management and the likelihood of spontaneous fistula closure. Fistulas located in the distal bowel, particularly the colon, may have low output (less than 500 ml/day) and thus allow for oral intake of low residue or even elemental feedings. High-output fistulas (greater than 500 ml/day) most likely will not close spontaneously and require surgical correction.

Chylous Ascites and Chylothorax

Chylous leaks into the peritoneal and thoracic cavities can follow surgical injury or trauma to the lymphatic ducts and obstruction due to cancer or congenital anomalies. Leakage of chyle into the abdominal or thoracic cavity can cause ascites, pleural effusions, abdominal pain, anorexia, hypoalbuminemia, hyponatremia, hypocalcemia, hypocholesterolemia, and elevated alkaline phosphatase.[28] Chylous leaks may resolve with conservative management alone, although surgical repair can be required to ligate the duct. Conservative management involves reducing the chyle flow, which is normally 1500 to 5500 ml/day. Dietary intake (fat and fluid), blood pressure, and portal blood flow contribute to the production of chyle. Dietary manipulation is the main means of reducing chyle flow. Because

dietary long-chain triglycerides (LCTs) are incorporated into chylomicrons, restriction of these fats in the diet is imperative. Depending on severity of the chyle leak and patient's response, the patient may be allowed oral dietary intake with no LCT, enteral feeding with no LCT, or parenteral nutrition. Medium-chain triglycerides (MCTs) are allowed enterally because these are absorbed directly via the portal vein, not the lymphatic system. A diet without or limited to less than 4% of calories as LCTs is not advised for more than 10 to 14 days because it lacks essential fatty acids (linoleic and linolenic acid) and the patient can develop a deficiency. Resolution of lymphatic leaks conservatively can take up to 6 weeks; therefore adequate nutrition during this period is important to maintain nutritional status.

NUTRITIONAL NEEDS IN THERMAL INJURIES

Trauma and burn patients exhibit similar metabolic alterations as previously described except metabolic alterations often occur to a much greater extent. Few traumatic injuries result in a hypermetabolic state comparable to that of a major burn. An understanding of the etiology of metabolic response and implications for nutritional requirements is necessary with traumatic and burn injuries for a nutrition care plan to be designed to minimize the effects of hypermetabolism and hypercatabolism and for support immunocompetence to be developed.

Metabolic Response to Injury

Stressed patients undergo several metabolic phases as a series of "ebb and flow" states reflecting a patient's response to the severity of the stress. The initial ebb phase occurs immediately after injury and is associated with shock. If the injured patient survives, ebb phase evolves into the flow phase. Table 23-4 lists hormonal, metabolic, and clinical outcome comparisons between the two phases.

Clinical efforts in the ebb phase are focused on maintaining heart action and blood circulation. The flow state is a hyperdynamic phase in which substrates are mobilized for energy production while increased cellular activity and hormonal stimulation are noted. There is an energy expenditure distinction for each phase, making the goals of nutrition therapy variable depending on the stage in question. During ebb phase there is a decrease in metabolic needs. Typically due to hemodynamic instability and need for resuscitation, nutrition intervention is not pursued during this phase. Flow phase brings hypermetabolism, yielding increased proteolysis and nitrogen loss, accelerated gluconeogenesis, hyperglycemia and increased glucose utilization, and retention of salt and water. Mobilization of protein, fat, and glycogen is believed

TABLE 23-4	Ebb and Flow Phases	
	Ebb Phase	**Flow Phase**
Hormonal and non-hormonal	↑Glucagon ↑Adrenocorticotropic hormone (ACTH)	↑Counterregulatory hormones (epinephrine, norepinephrine, glucagon, cortisol) ↑Insulin ↑Catecholamines ↑Cytokines (tumor necrosis factor alpha, interleukins-1, -2, and -6)
Metabolic	Circulatory insufficiency ↑ heart rate (vascular constriction) ↓Digestive enzyme production ↓Urine production	Hyperglycemia ↓Protein synthesis/↑amino acid efflux ↑Gluconeogenesis ↑Glycogenolysis ↑↑Urea nitrogen excretion/net (−) nitrogen balance
Clinical outcomes	Hemodynamic instability	Fluid and electrolyte imbalances Mild metabolic acidosis ↑Resting energy expenditure

Data from Cresci G, Martindale R: Nutrition in critical illness. In Berdanier C et al, eds: *Handbook of nutrition and food,* Boca Raton, Fla, 2002, CRC Press; and Cresci G: Metabolic stress. In Matarese L, Gottschlich M, eds: *Contemporary nutrition support practice,* ed 2, Philadelphia, 2003, WB Saunders.

to be mediated through release of cytokines such as tumor necrosis factor alpha, interleukins-1, -2, and -6, and counterregulatory hormones such as epinephrine, norepinephrine, glucagon, and cortisol. Circulating levels of insulin are also elevated in most metabolically stressed patients, but responsiveness of tissues to insulin, especially skeletal muscle, is severely blunted. This relative insulin resistance is believed to be due to the effects of the counterregulatory hormones. The hormonal milieu normalizes only after the injury or metabolic stress has resolved. As long as the patient is in a hyperdynamic catabolic state, optimal nutrition support is needed but can only at best approach zero nitrogen balance in attempts to minimize further protein wasting.

Burn Wounds

Size and depth of the burn wound affect its healing process and overall prognosis (Figure 23-8). Burns are usually classified by degree using the **rule of nines,** as follows:

1. *First-degree burns:* erythema involving cell necrosis above the basal layer of the epidermis
2. *Second-degree burns:* erythema and blistering, and necrosis within the dermis
3. *Third-degree burns:* full-thickness skin loss, including fat layer
4. *Fourth-degree burns:* exposed bone and tendon

Burns of first- and second-degree depths generally reepithelialize without surgical intervention. Third-degree burns will not heal independent of excision and grafting. Fourth-degree burns typically involve the use of muscle

flaps because skin grafting onto bone is not a viable therapy option.

Extent of the burn directly affects fluid resuscitation, surgical needs, immunocompetence, metabolic sequelae, and nutrition intervention. Second- and third-degree burns covering 15% to 20% or more of the total body surface area (TBSA), or 10% in children and older adults, usually cause extensive fluid loss and require intravenous fluid and electrolyte replacement therapy. Burns of severe depth covering more than 50% of the TBSA are often fatal, especially in infants and older adults. Thermal injury permits the loss of heat, water, nitrogen, whole proteins, and micronutrients through the open wound. Loss of the protective skin barrier allows microorganisms to access subcutaneous tissue and potentiates systemic infectious processes, which contribute to postburn hypermetabolic state. Loss of plasma volume and electrolytes through the open wound predispose the burned patient to acid-base

chyle The fat-containing, creamy white fluid that is formed in the lacteals of the intestine during digestion, is transported through the lymphatics, and enters the venous circulation via the thoracic duct.

rule of nines Describes the percentage of the body surface represented by various anatomic areas. For example: each upper limb, 9%; each lower limb, 18%; anterior and posterior trunk, each 18%; head and neck, 9%; and perineum and genitalia, 1%.

erythema Redness of the skin produced by coagulation of the capillaries.

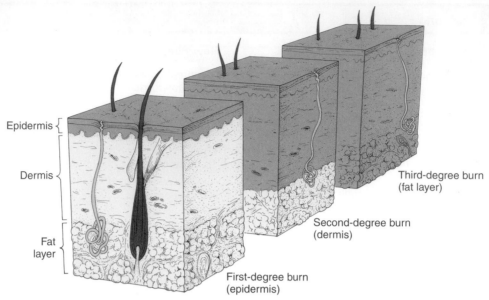

Epidermis

Dermis

Fat layer

Third-degree burn (fat layer)

Second-degree burn (dermis)

First-degree burn (epidermis)

FIGURE 23-8   Depth of skin area involved in burns.

imbalance and cardiovascular, pulmonary, and renal instability. Adequate fluid and electrolyte resuscitation during the first 24 to 48 hours of postburn hypovolemia is essential for hemodynamic stability. Extensive fluid shifts, unique to burn injury, drive the characteristic edema process of resuscitation by increasing intracellular and interstitial fluid volumes. Fluids given during the resuscitative period should be titrated in accordance with urine output to prevent both overresuscitation and underresuscitation. The replacement of extracellular sodium chloride, most commonly in the form of lactated Ringer's solution, is obligatory for successful resuscitation.[29]

In addition, certain herbs and botanicals have been suggested for use in patients with thermal injuries. The *Complementary and Alternative Medicine (CAM)* box, "Feel the Burn?," outlines these herbs and provides additional information on their efficacy, safety, and potential drug interactions.

Nutrition Therapy After Burn Injury

Thermal injury induces hypermetabolism of varying intensity and duration depending on extent and depth of the body surface affected, presence of infection, and efficacy of early treatment. Energy requirements peak at approximately postburn day 12 and typically slowly normalize as the percentage of open wound decreases with reepithelialization or skin grafting.

Energy.   Burn patients require individualized nutrition plans to provide optimal energy and protein to accelerate muscle and protein synthesis and minimize proteolysis. There are numerous predictive equations to estimate energy needs. Several studies have reviewed the accuracy of predictive equations in determining energy requirements

in burn patients. Consensus appears that predictive equations tend to overestimate energy expenditure, and the preferred method of determining energy requirements is by using indirect calorimetry. If indirect calorimetry is not available in the clinical situation, it is suggested resting energy expenditure can be estimated at 50% to 60% above the Harris-Benedict equation for burns of more than 20% of TBSA.[30]

Carbohydrate.   During the flow phase of metabolic stress, hyperglycemia is present due to the increased glucagon-to-insulin ratio that activates gluconeogenesis. Tissue insulin resistance further exacerbates glucose intolerance. Despite these metabolic aberrations, carbohydrate should be the primary energy source provided for the burned patient. For burns exceeding 25% TBSA, carbohydrate should compose 60% to 65% of the calories.[29] Patients should be monitored closely for hyperglycemia and glucosuria with exogenous insulin provided to maintain blood glucose levels at less than 180 mg/dl.[6] Complications of hyperglycemia include osmotic diuresis with resulting dehydration and hypovolemia, lipogenesis, fatty liver, and carbon dioxide retention inhibiting ventilatory weaning.

Protein.   Trauma, burns, and sepsis initiate a cascade of events that leads to accelerated protein degradation, decreased rates of synthesis of selected proteins, and increased amino acid catabolism and nitrogen loss. Clinical consequences of these metabolic alterations may increase morbidity and mortality rates of patients, causing serious organ dysfunction and impaired host defenses. Therefore trauma and burn patients require increased amounts of protein in attempts to minimize endogenous proteolysis as

COMPLEMENTARY AND ALTERNATIVE MEDICINE (CAM)
Feel the Burn?

The following herbs and botanical supplements have been suggested for use with thermal injury.

Herb/Botanical and Use in Burns	Efficacy	Safety Issues	Drug Interactions
Aloe (Aloe vera) Topical gel used to heal burns and reduce burn pain.	There is no evidence aloe promotes burn healing; research indicates aloe significantly delays healing of second-degree burns.	Occasional allergic reaction. Considered safe, but comprehensive safety studies are lacking.	None are known. Aloe gel may be a useful adjuvant therapy when combined with hydrocortisone acetate cream. If gel is taken internally, it can reduce absorption of many medications.
Echinacea (E. purpurea, E. pallida, E. angustifolia) Used topically to enhance wound healing.	Several research studies have provided evidence that various Echinacea species can significantly reduce duration and severity of illness, but there is little to demonstrate efficacy in wound healing.	Oral echinacea causes few side effects; most common reports include bad taste and minor GI symptoms.	E. angustifolia (the most popular species in North America) root might inhibit CYP3A4.
Garlic (Allium spp.) Used orally and topically to fight infections.	Little research, if any, is available to substantiate this claim.	Garlic is on the FDA's GRAS list. Raw garlic taken in excessive doses can cause numerous symptoms such as stomach upset, heartburn, nausea, vomiting, diarrhea, flatulence, facial flushing, rapid pulse, and insomnia. Topical garlic can cause skin irritation, blistering, even third-degree burns.	When taken with anticoagulants, NSAIDs, antiplatelet agents, or other herbs that exert anticoagulation effects (feverfew, ginkgo), garlic may increase bleeding time. Blood glucose level may be decreased with hypoglycemic agents.
Gotu kola (Centella asiatica) Used in Europe as treatment for scarring	No substantial evidence to support this claim.	Rare allergic reactions to topical gotu kola.	None known.
Plantain (Plantago ovata, P. psyllium, P. lanceolata, P. major) Used topically for skin inflammation.	Efficacy has not been validated scientifically.	Safe. Long-term use shows no toxicity.	None known.
St. John's wort (Hypericum perforatum) Hypericum tincture or oil is used topically for inflammation and burns.	Speeds healing of burns.	Noted side effects are related to ingested herb.	Interactions related to ingested herb.

References

Bascom A et al: Professional guide to complementary and alternative therapies, Springhouse, Pa, 2001, Springhouse.
Bratman S, Girman AM: Mosby's handbook of herbs and supplements and their therapeutic uses, St. Louis, 2003, Mosby.

Escott-Stump S: Nutrition and diagnosis-related care, ed 5, Philadelphia, 2002, Lippincott Williams & Wilkins.
Kuhn MA, Winston D: Herbal therapy and supplements: a scientific and traditional approach, Philadelphia, 2001, Lippincott.

GI, Gastrointestinal; FDA, Food and Drug Administration; GRAS, generally recognized as safe; NSAID, nonsteroidal antiinflammatory drug.

well as to support the large losses from wound exudate. Providing 20% to 25% of calories as protein to those with burns of greater than 25% TBSA promotes improved nutrition laboratory values, immunity, nitrogen balance, and survival.[31] Overall recommendations are to provide protein in the amount of 1.5 to 2.0, rarely up to 3.0 g/kg body

lactated Ringer's solution Sterile solution of calcium chloride, potassium chloride, sodium chloride, and sodium lactate in water administered to replenish fluid and electrolytes.

weight per day in attempts to minimize protein losses. Providing these higher levels of protein requires continuous monitoring of fluid status, blood urea nitrogen, and serum creatinine due to high renal solute load. In addition to quantity of protein provided, protein quality is also significant. Use of high-biologic protein is preferred for burn patients. Whey protein has been further endorsed over casein due to its beneficial effects on burned children, improvement in tube feeding tolerance, enhanced solubility at low gastric pH, greater digestibility, and improved nitrogen retention. Pharmacologic doses of the single amino acids arginine and glutamine have also been explored as to their benefit in critical illness and burns.

Fat. Lipid is an important component of a trauma or burn patient's diet for many reasons, one being an isosmotic concentrated energy source at 9 kcal/g. Dietary lipid is also a carrier for fat-soluble vitamins, as well as a provider of the essential fatty acids linoleic and linolenic acid. Even though lipids are required in critical illness, excess lipid can be detrimental. Excessive lipid administration has been associated with hyperlipidemia, fatty liver immune suppression, and impaired clotting ability. For burn and multiple trauma patients, the recommended amount of total fat delivery is 12% to 15% of total calories. A minimum of 4% of calories in the diet should consist of essential fatty acids to prevent deficiencies, which often equates to about 10% of total calories as fat because most sources do not solely contain essential fatty acid. Formulations supplemented with fish oil, a rich source of n-3 fatty acids (eicosapentaenoic acid [EPA] and docosahexaenoic acid [DHA]) and canola oil (a-linolenic acid) are of particular interest for their potential antiinflammatory and immune-enhancing benefits.[30]

Vitamins and Minerals. Micronutrients function as coenzymes and cofactors in metabolic pathways at the cellular level. With increased energy and protein demands associated with traumatic and burn injury, one would expect there to also be increased need for vitamins and minerals. In addition, increased nutrient losses from open wounds and altered metabolism, absorption, and excretion would also be suspect for requirements beyond that of the Recommended Dietary Allowances. Various vitamins and minerals have also been found to aid with wound healing, immune function, and other biologic functions. Unfortunately, little concrete data are available to support exact requirements during these hypermetabolic states. However, in addition to a daily multivitamin burn patients may benefit from additional vitamin A (5000 IU/1000 kcal of enteral nutrition), vitamin C (500 mg twice daily), and zinc (45 mg elemental zinc per day).

Nutrient Delivery

Oral intake is generally adequate in children and adults with burns of less than 25% TBSA and in young children and infants with less than 15% TBSA. Adequate oral intake can be achieved by providing patient food preferences, high-calorie, high-protein supplements, and modular calorie and protein enhancement of foods.[29] However, patients with burns of greater than 25% TBSA often require enteral tube feeding. Gastric feedings are frequently interrupted in burn patients for multiple reasons such as the presence of gastric ileus, dressing changes, physical therapy, prone positioning, respiratory treatments, and surgery. Enteral feeding is well tolerated in burn patients when delivered in the small intestine because the small bowel maintains its absorptive capacity. Therefore a nasoenteric feeding tube is preferred. Small-bowel feeding may also reduce incidence of aspiration. Enteral nutrient delivery should be initiated as soon as postinjury allows during the resuscitative period. Early enteral feedings, within the first 6 hours after the burn, have been shown to decrease the level of catabolic hormones, improve nitrogen balance, maintain gut mucosal integrity, lower the incidence of diarrhea, and decrease hospital stay.[32] A full-strength, intact protein formula at low rate (20 to 30 ml/hr) advanced by 5 to 20 ml/hr to the desired volume is typically tolerated.[29] Parenteral nutrition is indicated only if enteral nutrition is not tolerated or grossly inadequate because it has been associated with metabolic and immunologic complications.[32] Whenever possible, low-rate enteral feedings should accompany parenteral nutrition to prevent villous atrophy.

Health Promotion

Immunonutrition

It is known that malnutrition leads to suppressed immune responses. Providing nutrition support using standard enteral formulations has shown improvements in various clinical indexes of nutritional status when adequate calories and protein are given; however, there is a lack of demonstrated effect on morbidity and mortality. During the past two decades the field of immunology has exploded and expanded into nearly every area of medicine, including nutrition. Certain dietary components have been classified as "immune-enhancing nutrients." Compared with standard nutrients, an immune-enhancing nutrient is a substance that provides positive effects on the immune system when provided in certain quantities. Of the many immune-enhancing nutrients identified in human clinical trials, the ones that appear to be most beneficial are L-arginine, L-glutamine, nucleotides, omega-3 fatty acids (EPA and DHA), and various vitamins and minerals (zinc and vitamins A, E, and C). Several special enteral nutrient formulations have been categorized as immune-enhancing formulations (IEFs). Each of these formulas contains various combinations and/or levels of these immune-enhancing nutrients.[33]

Glutamine is known to be a major fuel source for rapidly dividing cells such as enterocytes, reticulocytes, and lymphocytes. In normal metabolic states, glutamine is a nonessential amino acid. However, during times of metabolic stress, glutamine is implicated as being conditionally essential because it is needed for maintenance of gut metabolism, structure, and function. Despite the accelerated skeletal muscle release of amino acids, blood glutamine levels are not increased after burns. In fact, decreased plasma glutamine levels have been reported after severe burn, multiple trauma, or multiple organ failure.[34]

A number of studies have shown beneficial effects with supplemental glutamine, its precursors (ornithine α-ketoglutarate and α-ketoglutarate), or glutamine dipeptides (alanine-glutamine, glycine-glutamine). These studies deliver glutamine in pharmacologic doses of 25% to 35% of the dietary protein. Supplemental glutamine has been shown to have multiple benefits that include increased nitrogen retention and muscle mass, maintenance of the GI mucosa and its permeability, preserved immune function and reduced infections, and preserved organ glutathione levels. These protective effects of glutamine supplementation could have significant effects on morbidity and mortality rates in trauma and burn patients. Safety and cost-effectiveness of glutamine supplementation in trauma and burns continue to be researched.

Arginine, like glutamine, is considered a conditionally essential amino acid. Arginine is the specific precursor for nitric oxide production, as well as a potent secretagogue for anabolic hormones such as insulin, prolactin, and growth hormone. Under normal circumstances, arginine is considered a nonessential amino acid because it is adequately synthesized endogenously via the urea cycle. However, research suggests that during times of metabolic stress, optimal amounts of arginine are not synthesized to promote tissue regeneration or positive nitrogen balance.

Studies in animal and humans have investigated the effects of supplemental arginine in various injury models. Positive outcomes from supplementation include improved nitrogen balance, wound healing, and immune function and increased anabolic hormones, insulin and growth hormone. The outcomes are of special interest in the posttrauma and postburn patient during the flow phase when enhancement of these processes would yield the greatest advantage. However, despite these positive effects, caution with excessive arginine supplementation is warranted in burn patients because of its potential adverse effects on nitric oxide production.

Even though *lipids* are required, excess lipid can be detrimental. Excessive lipid administration has been associated with hyperlipidemia, fatty liver immunosuppression, and impaired clotting ability. All long-chain fatty acids share the same enzyme systems because they are elongated and desaturated with each pathway competitive in nature based on substrate availability. Dietary fatty acids modulate the phospholipid cell membrane composition and the type and quantities of eicosanoids produced. Prostaglandins of the 3 series (PGE_3) and series 5 leukotrienes have proved to be antiinflammatory and immune-enhancing agents. Also, PGE_3 is a potent vasodilator. These concepts have received considerable attention for the potential of n-3 fatty acids to enhance immune function and reduce acute and chronic inflammation.

In most standard enteral formulations, the fat source is predominantly n-6 fatty acids with a portion coming from MCTs. Formulations supplemented with fish oil, a rich source of n-3 fatty acids (EPA and DHA) and canola oil (a-linolenic acid), are available. Clinical trials utilizing these formulations have shown positive benefits in patients with psoriasis, rheumatoid arthritis, burns, sepsis, and trauma. These benefits are thought to be due to alterations in eicosanoid and leukotriene production, with decreased arachidonic acid metabolites (e.g., PGE_2), as well as increased production of the less biologically active trienoic prostaglandins and pentaenoic leukotrienes.

Clinical Outcomes With Immune-Enhancing Formulas

Trauma Outcomes. Immune-enhancing formulas (IEFs) have been used in trauma patients and are associated with decreased incidence of intraabdominal abscess, multiple organ failure, infections, and systemic inflammatory response syndrome (SIRS), as well as decreased hospital length of stay and days of therapeutic antibiotic use.

Intensive Care Unit/Sepsis Outcomes. The intensive care unit population involves a very heterogeneous group, making data interpretation difficult. This population involves differing severity and pathologic processes of various disease states. Studies conducted with this population have differences in study design and methods of reporting data, adding to the complexity of comparing results between investigations. A few studies have been conducted with various diagnoses, such as cardiac failure, pulmonary failure, transplantation, trauma, and GI surgery. Positive outcomes in the form of decreased incidence of infections, requirement for mechanical ventilation, incidence of bacteremia, and length of stay were reported when using IEFs.

Surgery Outcomes. Research in surgical populations using IEFs has been performed with preoperative, postoperative, or combined nutrition therapies. The majority of procedures performed in these studies involved upper GI cancer or head and neck cancer surgery. Significantly improved outcomes in the IEF groups include fewer infections and wound complications, decreased severity of complications, and shorter postoperative and hospital length of stay.[35]

Other Populations (Burns, Head Injury, Human Immunodeficiency Virus/Acquired Immunodeficiency Syndrome). Study of the use of IEFs in these patient populations is limited. Currently only two studies investigating the effect of IEFs on immune function and nutritional status of acquired immunodeficiency syndrome (AIDS) patients have been published. Improved weight gain was found in one of the studies when IEF was provided but not in the other study.[36] Burn patients appear to benefit when provided with IEFs, exhibiting decreased infections and length of hospital stay. Head injury patients theoretically should benefit from IEFs because of severe hypermetabolism and the likelihood of infectious complications. However, there are no clinical data available to support this theory. More research using IEFs in these populations is needed.

TO SUM UP

Nutritional status of the patient should be addressed before the patient is even considered for surgery. If the patient has any nutrient deficiencies, these should be corrected before surgery if time allows. Postoperatively the patient should be provided with nutrition as soon as feasible to improve surgical outcomes.

Postoperative nutrition may be provided in a number of ways. The oral route is preferred; however, often it is not feasible or adequate to support metabolic needs. Enteral or parenteral nutrition may be provided for those unable to achieve adequate nutrient intake and absorption orally. Enteral feeding is preferred over parenteral. Because alimentary tract surgery often alters the flow of nutrients, resulting in several potential metabolic and nutrition complications, postoperative diets are described to help minimize these effects.

QUESTIONS FOR REVIEW

1. Discuss requirements for energy, protein, vitamins, and minerals and means of providing them during the various stages of surgery (preoperative, immediately preoperative, postoperative).
2. Describe potential nutritional consequences that may result after surgery of the head and neck, esophagus, stomach, and intestine.
3. Develop a menu plan for a patient undergoing gastric bypass surgery for morbid obesity; include all phases of the diet progression.
4. Describe metabolic alterations that occur during metabolic stress.
5. Develop a nutrition care plan for a patient sustaining third-degree burns covering 40% TBSA.

REFERENCES

1. Klein S et al: Nutrition support in clinical practice: review of published data and recommendations for future research directions, *J Parenter Enteral Nutr* 21:133, 1997.
2. Vitello J: Prevalence of malnutrition in hospitalized patients remains high, *J Am Coll Nutr* 12:589, 1993.
3. Naber T et al: Prevalence of malnutrition in nonsurgical hospitalized patients and its association with disease complication, *Am J Clin Nutr* 66:1232, 1997.
4. Coats K et al: Hospital-associated malnutrition: a reevaluation 12 years later, *J Am Diet Assoc* 93:27, 1993.
5. Kelly I et al: Still hungry in hospital: identifying malnutrition in acute hospital admissions, *Q J Med* 93:93, 2000.
6. A.S.P.E.N. Board of Directors: Guidelines for the use of parenteral and enteral nutrition in adult and pediatric patients, *J Parenter Enteral Nutr* 26:1SA, 2002.
7. VA TPN Cooperative Study: Perioperative total parenteral nutrition in surgical patients, *N Engl J Med* 325:525, 1991.
8. Cerra B et al: Applied nutrition in ICU patients: a consensus statement of the American College of Chest Physicians, *Chest* 111:769, 1997.
9. Klein C, Stanek G, Willes C: Overfeeding macronutrients to critically ill adults: metabolic complications, *J Am Diet Assoc* 98:795, 1998.
10. Pomposelli JJ et al: Early postoperative glucose control predicts nosocomial infection rate in diabetic patients, *J Parenter Enteral Nutr* 22:77, 1998.
11. Pomposelli JJ, Bistrian BR: Is total parenteral nutrition immunosuppressive? *New Horiz* 2:224, 1994.
12. Flancbaum L et al: Comparison of indirect calorimetry, the Fick method, and prediction equations in estimating the energy requirements of critically ill patients, *Am J Clin Nutr* 69:461, 1999.
13. Chiolero R, Revelly JP, Tappy L: Energy metabolism in sepsis and injury, *Nutrition* 13(suppl):45S, 1997.
14. Frankenfield DC et al: Validation of several established equations for resting metabolic rate in obese and nonobese people, *J Am Diet Assoc* 103:1152, 2003.
15. Frankenfield DC, Roth-Yousey L, Compher C: Comparison of predictive equations for resting metabolic rate in healthy nonobese and obese adults: a systematic review, *J Am Diet Assoc* 105:775, 2005.
16. Barton RG: Nutrition support in critical illness, *Nutr Clin Pract* 10:129, 1994.
17. Cutts M et al: Predicting energy needs in ventilator-dependent critically ill patients: effect of adjusting weight for edema or adiposity, *Am J Clin Nutr* 66:1250, 1997.
18. Marik P, Varon J: The obese patient in the ICU, *Chest* 113:492, 1998.
19. Ireton-Jones CS et al: Equations for estimation of energy expenditures in patients with burns with special reference to ventilatory status, *J Burn Care Rehab* 13:330, 1992.
20. Patino J et al: Hypocaloric support in the critically ill, *World J Surg* 23:553, 1999.
21. Cresci GA, Martindale RG: Nutrition support in trauma. In American Society for Enteral and Parenteral Nutrition: *The science and practice of nutrition support: a case-based core,* ed 3, Dubuque, Iowa, 2001, Kendall/Hunt.
22. Campbell W et al: Increased protein requirements in elderly people: new data and retrospective reassessments, *Am J Clin Nutr* 60:501, 1994.
23. Dabrowski G, Rombeau J: Practical nutritional management in the trauma intensive care unit, *Surg Clin North Am* 80:92, 2000.
24. Keele AM et al: Two-phase randomized controlled clinical trial of prospective oral dietary supplements in surgical patients, *Gut* 40:343, 1997.
25. Jeffery KM et al: The clear liquid diet is no longer a necessity in the routine postoperative management of surgical patients, *Am Surg* 62:167, 1996.

26. Lipman T: Grains or veins: is enteral nutrition really better than parenteral nutrition? A look at the evidence, *J Parenter Enteral Nutr* 22:167, 1998.

27. Heyland DK et al: Should immunonutrition become routine in critically ill patients? A systematic review of the evidence, *JAMA* 286:944, 2001.

28. Sullivan M, Alonso E: Gastrointestinal and pancreatic disease. In Matarese L, Gottschlich M, eds: *Contemporary nutrition support practice,* Philadelphia, 1998, WB Saunders.

29. Mayes T, Gottschlich M: Burns and wound healing. In American Society for Enteral and Parenteral Nutrition: *The science and practice of nutrition support: a case-based core,* ed 3, Dubuque, Iowa, 2001, Kendall/Hunt.

30. Khorram-Sefat R et al: Long-term measurements of energy expenditure in severe burn injury, *West J Surg* 23:115, 1999.

31. Alexander JW et al: Beneficial effects of aggressive protein feeding in severely burned children, *Ann Surg* 192:505, 1980.

32. Rose J et al: Advances in burn care. In Cameron J et al, eds: *Advances in surgery,* vol 30, Chicago, 1996, Mosby-Year Book.

33. Hillhouse J: Immune-enhancing enteral formulas: effect on patient outcome, *Support Line* 23:16, 2001.

34. Martindale R, Cresci G: The use of immune enhancing diets in burns, *J Parenter Enteral Nutr* 25(suppl):S24, 2001.

35. Sax H: Effect of immune enhancing formulas in general surgery patients, *J Parenter Enteral Nutr* 25(suppl):S19, 2001.

36. Schloerb P: Immune-enhancing diets: products, components, and their rationales, *J Parenter Enteral Nutr* 25(suppl):S3, 2001.

FURTHER READINGS AND RESOURCES

Readings

Cerra FB: How nutrition intervention changes what getting sick means, *J Parenter Enteral Nutr* 14(suppl 5):164, 1990.

This article provides a good review of three basic factors that influence what is observed at an ill patient's bedside when considering the effects of nutrition intervention: (1) the disease process inherent in the metabolic response to injury, (2) the presence of starvation, and (3) the presence of the nutrition intervention.

Hustler DA: Nutritional monitoring of a pediatric burn patient, *Nutr Clin Pract* 6:11, 1991.

This experienced dietitian-specialist on a burn-center team provides a case report of a young boy who sustained mostly full-thickness burns over 56% of his total body surface area. She describes in detail the challenge of initial evaluation and therapy, constant close monitoring, and appropriate responses to changing needs.

Tynes JJ et al: Diet tolerance and stool frequency in patients with ileoanal reservoirs, *J Am Diet Assoc* 92(7):861, 1992.

This brief report of a survey of patients with ileoanal reservoirs provides much helpful background information about this recently developed alternative surgical procedure to the ileostomy, with practical guidance for nutritional management and patient counseling.

Websites of Interest

- U.S. Surgical: *www.ussurg.com/uss/index.html.*
- American Academy of Physical Medicine and Rehabilitation: *www.aapmr.org.*
- American Botanical Council: *www.herbalgram.com.*

C H A P T E R 24

Acquired Immunodeficiency Syndrome (AIDS)

Sara Long

In this chapter of our clinical series, we focus on acquired immunodeficiency syndrome (AIDS). This modern-day plague has eluded medical science's search for a cure and left countless numbers of infected and dying young adults and children in its wake.

Here we examine the background of the AIDS epidemic and nature of the human immunodeficiency virus-1 (HIV-1). We review the current state of medical management and its relation to nutritional status in the course of the disease. As knowledge of the disease process has grown during the past two decades, it has become increasingly evident that nutrition support plays a vital role in the care of HIV-infected and AIDS patients.

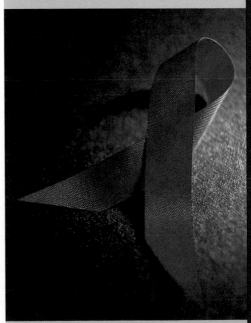

EVOLUTION OF HIV AND THE AIDS EPIDEMIC

In the late 1970s, physicians on the east and west coasts of the United States, centered in New York City and San Francisco, became puzzled about an uncommon medical problem appearing among their patients.[1] No known cause of immune suppression could be found. Nonetheless, they were suffering and dying from complications of common infections, largely pneumonia, ordinarily handled easily by the human immune system and usual antibiotics or other antibacterial drugs. Its virus source and pandemic effects were soon to become alarmingly evident worldwide.

Evolution of HIV

Social Change

Where did this new deadly virus come from, and how did it gain such strength? Apparently, HIV represents not a new virus but an old one that in recent years has grown deadly in humans as it gained strength during the social upheavals of the 1960s and 1970s. The uprooting effect of this rapid social change and urbanization allowed the virus to spread rapidly through world populations and to reproduce aggressively in its human host.

Parasitic Nature of Virus

No virus can have a life of its own; by their structure and nature, all viruses are parasites. They are mere shreds of genetic material, a small packet of genetic information encased in a protein coat. They contain only a small chromosome of nucleic acids (ribonucleic acid [RNA] or deoxyribonucleic acid [DNA]), usually with fewer than five genes. They can live only through a host, whom they invade and infect. There they hijack the host's cell machinery to run off a multitude of copies of themselves. Their purpose is to make as many self-copies as they can. Today's viruses are those that succeeded in that task over time and are, like all plants and animals, simply descendants of earlier forms. Scientists agree that the human immunodeficiency viruses HIV-1 and HIV-2 are genetically similar to viruses found in African primates such as monkeys and apes (simian immunodeficiency virus [SIV]) and were probably transmitted to humans in an earlier age.

The earliest known case of AIDS was recently identified in an African blood sample collected in 1959 from a Bantu man who lived in the Democratic Republic of Congo, an area from which the current epidemic is believed to have spread.[2] This sample is the oldest HIV infection discovered so far, indicating that it predates the time at which the virus divided into several of the current varieties that now infect different parts of the world. Over the years HIV has mutated into many different subtypes. Africa is home to 70% of the adults and 80% of the children living with HIV infection in the world.[3]

Although the course of the present worldwide epidemic is difficult to predict, there is a growing sense of guarded optimism among the leading scientists based on the current research agenda, especially among the increasing number of young, newly trained scientists with new ideas, and a changing U.S. culture of AIDS research that embraces more cooperative team attitudes.[4-7]

Disease Progression

The individual clinical course of HIV infection varies substantially. Four distinct stages mark the progression of the disease and are usually referred to as (1) asymptomatic stage, (2) early symptomatic stage, (3) late symptomatic stage, and (4) advanced HIV disease stage.

Primary HIV Infection

HIV infects cells that express the $CD4^+$ receptor on their surface, including T-helper cells, monocytes, macrophages, and dendritic cells. After initial attachment to the $CD4^+$ molecule, HIV fuses with and then enters the cell's cytoplasm, sheds its envelope coat, and releases its contents. Reverse transcription takes place creating viral DNA, which is integrated into the host DNA.[8] The virus may then remain dormant or become activated, at which time new virions are reassembled and shed from the cell into the circulation to infect another host cell. Lymphoid tissue (lymph nodes, adenoids, tonsil, spleen) contain the highest concentration of HIV-infected cells during the latent period, which can last up to 10 years before clinical manifestation of the disease occurs.

Approximately 5 to 30 days (median, 14 days) after initial exposure and infection, a mild flulike syndrome (fever, adenopathy, sore throat, rash, myalgia, arthralgia, diarrhea, nausea, and vomiting) may occur, lasting about 1 week. Antibody tests for HIV do not usually test positive at this time. This brief response corresponds to the process of *seroconversion,* the development of antibodies to the viral infection. Subsequent HIV testing will be positive. Signs of enlarged lymph nodes, or persistent generalized lymphadenopathy (PGL), persist in about 30% of cases. An extended asymptomatic period usually continues for the next 10 to 12 years. However, this seemingly inactive period of relative wellness can be deceiving.

Asymptomatic Stage

During the asymptomatic stage of infection, viral replication continues and cellular destruction takes place in many tissues and organs of the body.[8] There also is a steady decline in the $CD4^+$ T-cell levels, a drop of 40 to $80/\mu l$ for every year of infection. With use of viral load measurement, it has been established HIV load correlates with $CD4^+$ cell counts and with disease progression. Healthy, uninfected individuals have a $CD4^+$ cell count of 500 to $1500/\mu l$ of blood. Early detection and treatment may prevent local propagation of HIV.

Early Symptomatic Stage

After the extended asymptomatic HIV-positive stage, which may last as long as 12 years, a period of associated infectious illnesses begins. This stage develops when CD4$^+$ cell counts drop to about 500/μl and HIV viral load increases to greater than 10,000/ml.[9] At this point even the most common infections, known as *opportunistic infections (OIs)*, have an open opportunity to take effect, spread, and cause systemic disease. Common symptoms observed during this pre-AIDS period include candidiasis, herpes zoster, cervical dysplasia, pelvic inflammatory disease, listeriosis, and peripheral neuropathy.

Late Symptomatic Stage

The late symptomatic stage begins when the CD4$^+$ T-cell count in blood falls to less than 200/μl and viral load counts increase to greater than 100,000/ml.[10] Diseases such as tuberculosis or Kaposi's sarcoma (the most common AIDS-associated malignancy) occur; at counts below 200/mm^3, *Pneumocystis carinii* pneumonia and *Toxoplasma gondii* (protozoan parasites able to infect a number of body organs) appear; and at counts under 50/mm^3, cytomegalovirus (CMV) or lymphoma can flourish[11] (see the *Case Study* box, "AIDS in a Young Man"). When the virus finally destroys sufficient white cells and the CD4$^+$ count decreases to less than 50/μl, the immune system is severely impaired, resulting in multiple OIs and malignancies. Death usually occurs in less than 1 year.

U.S. Public Health Service Responsibilities

In any major epidemic the U.S. Public Health Service and its related agencies have the major task of monitoring and stopping the spread of a disease. Thus they carry responsibilities in two major areas: (1) surveillance, including testing and counseling, and (2) community education and prevention through interrupting the spread of the epidemic, vaccine research, and treatment.

Surveillance

Throughout the AIDS epidemic, as knowledge of this new disease and its nature has grown, the U.S. Centers for Disease Control and Prevention (CDC) in Atlanta has worked with state and territorial health departments and has been involved in constant worldwide knowledge exchange to conduct accurate and comprehensive AIDS surveillance in the United States.[11] Since the mid-1980s such seroprevalence studies have provided a massive amount of information about HIV spread in various population groups and have helped the CDC develop early classification guidelines for medical teams caring for HIV-infected patients. Periodic CDC revisions of surveillance criteria reflect advances in the care and understanding of disease caused by HIV infection. In accord with current knowledge and the evolution of the

HIV epidemic among demographic groups, the CDC has expanded the AIDS surveillance definition to include any HIV-seropositive person with a CD4$^+$ (specific T-lymphocyte subset analysis) cell count of less than 200/μl of blood.[11]

Because of the tremendous life-changing impact of a positive HIV-1 test result to the individual and his or her family and loved ones, public health testing programs have developed a coordinated pretest and posttest counseling component, especially in clinics serving high-risk areas.[12] First, a brief pretest interview assesses personal knowledge of HIV infection, provides risk-reduction education, and offers the HIV test. Then those who accept the HIV testing are given a 2-week return appointment for a longer follow-up review of test results and counseling concerning healthcare and personal needs.

Education and Prevention

The U.S. Department of Health and Human Services (USDHHS), through its Public Health Service and Food and Drug Administration (FDA) divisions, has provided national health promotion and disease prevention objectives for the year 2010 that call for the expansion of HIV education and prevention efforts.[13] Wide community involvement in the community-based process of developing any health promotion or disease prevention program is essential for its successful outcome. This need has been shown, for example, in the mobilizing of community leadership and resources to plan and implement interventions in other health problems such as heart disease or changing lifestyle habits (e.g., smoking) that contribute to lung disease.

Community-support need is particularly true with HIV infection. Despite its burdening social stigma, it is

---

virus Minute infectious agent, characterized by lack of independent metabolism and by the ability to reproduce with genetic continuity only with living host cells. They range in decreasing size from about 200 nanometers (nm) down to only 15 nm. (A nanometer is a linear measure equal to one billionth of a meter; it is also called a millimicron.) Each particle (virion) consists basically of nucleic acids (genetic material) and a protein shell, which protects and contains the genetic material and any enzymes present.

pandemic A widespread epidemic, distributed through a region, a continent, or the world.

parasite An organism that lives on or in an organism of another species, known as the host, from whom all life cycle nourishment is obtained.

lymphoma General term applied to any neoplastic disorder (cancer) of the lymphoid tissue.

CASE STUDY

AIDS in a Young Man

David is a 32-year-old man who was recently admitted to the hospital with a history of weight loss, painful difficulty swallowing, and watery diarrhea. He has been in a long-term, monogamous relationship with his partner for 6 years. David works as an accountant at a large firm. Six months ago, David started to notice he was losing weight involuntarily and he began having large-volume, loose stools. He developed thrush in his mouth about 3 months before admission, which caused the odynophagia. About 1 week before admission a high temperature developed in David that did not respond to analgesics. He also complained of shortness of breath, chest tightness, and a dry cough. Physical examination revealed a weight loss of 11.3 kg (25 lb) and oral candidiasis; the chest radiographic examination was positive for *Pneumocystis carinii* pneumonia (PCP). David was admitted to receive intravenous antibiotics (trimethoprim-sulfamethoxazole [TMP-SMX]) and intravenous fluconazole, an antifungal. A stool culture revealed cytomegalovirus (CMV), and therefore intravenous ganciclovir, an antiviral agent, was initiated. David's oral intake was noted to be extremely poor; he also developed severe nausea and vomiting as a result of the medications and the infectious processes. His average daily volume of diarrhea also increased to 1800 ml/day. Results of the nutrition assessment were as follows:

Height (cm)	177.8 cm
Weight (kg)	61.4
Usual weight (kg)	72.7
Percent weight loss	15.5
Body weight (percent of usual)	84
Triceps skinfold	25th percentile
Midarm muscle circumference	25th percentile
CD4^{++}	118
Serum potassium (mEq/dl)	3.1
Blood glucose (mg/dl)	70
Blood urea nitrogen (mg/dl)	32
Creatinine (mg/dl)	0.4
Serum albumin (mg/dl)	2.8
Serum osmolality	325
Calculated basal energy expenditure (BEE)	2450 kcal/day

Questions for Analysis

1. Name and describe nutritional complications of oral candidiasis, gastrointestinal CMV infection, and PCP. How does treatment affect nutritional status?
2. Based on laboratory and anthropometric data, does David appear to be malnourished? What is your specific, objective evidence? What type of malnutrition does he exhibit?
3. Assess David's hydration status. What data could help you determine this?
4. What are the acute or immediate nutrition goals? What about long-term goals?
5. What type of nutrition support (enteral or parenteral) would you administer to David to prevent further nutritional depletion?

reaching into all communities in some form, cutting short the lives of children, adolescents, and young adults in ever-increasing numbers. Such a deadly pandemic warrants mobilization and coordination of the most realistic and effective preventive strategies possible for all ethnic and socioeconomic community groups to change sexual risk-taking behavior at all levels—local, national, and international.[14] New drugs are continually being developed, but prevention of the spread of the disease is key.[14]

NATURE OF THE DISEASE PROCESS

Action of HIV on the Immune System

HIV-1 and HIV-2 are members of a class of viruses called retrovirus because their unique life cycle involves a reverse transcription of RNA into DNA in the cell nucleus, which is then integrated into the host cell DNA.[2] The virus consists of an outer envelope with attached surface proteins covering the outer protective shell and an inner shell that contains the small strands of RNA genetic material and enzymes, including the reverse transcriptase. Of the virus's nine genes, four apparently less essential ones are poorly understood. After entering the body, the virus attaches to host cells, mostly the actively replicating T-helper (CD4$^+$) white blood cells, major lymphocytes of the body's immune system. There it integrates itself into the host cell's DNA copying system, infecting and eventually killing the host cell. Rapidly increasing masses of virus particles erupt from the dying cells in small buds to immediately infect new cells.

Methods of Transmission and Groups at Risk

Throughout the world, sexual behavior is central to the epidemic spread of HIV infection and AIDS. An estimated 71% of HIV infections worldwide are a result of heterosexual behavior, and 15% are a result of homosexual behavior; only a relatively small proportion of cases are a result of intravenous drug use with contaminated needles.[2] In 1997 it was estimated there were between 650,000 and 900,000 cases of AIDS in the United States. Approximately 40,000 individuals are infected and die of the disease yearly. The CDC and the Public Health Service indicated that AIDS cases by type of transmission reported in 1999 were as follows[15]:

- 46% Male homosexual/bisexual behavior
- 30% Heterosexuals
- 18% Injecting drug users
- 1% Perinatal transmission
- Less than 1% blood transfusions
- Less than 1% hemophiliacs

The remaining cases were listed as "no risk reported." Women and young people, particularly nonwhites, are increasingly at risk. Persons in the South and Northeast accounted for higher percentages of reported cases than the previous year.[14]

Mother-to-child HIV transmission has been drastically reduced in the United States in recent years—from a high of 2500 in 1992 to fewer than 400 perinatal HIV infections annually (see also the *Focus on Culture* box, "Special Considerations for Children With AIDS"). HIV can be transmitted through breast milk, and therefore HIV-infected women are advised to avoid breast-feeding their infants.[14]

FOCUS ON CULTURE

Special Considerations for Children With AIDS

Malnutrition, particularly inadequate calories and protein, and dehydration are serious issues in children with AIDS. In adults, the disease affects nutritional status. In children, not only is nutritional status affected, but also growth and development can be significantly impaired, resulting in growth failure. There is a strong relationship between early nutritional status—poor growth, cachexia, poor oral intake, decreased absorption of nutrients and increased energy expenditure—and mortality risk.

Nutrition assessments should be performed routinely in all children with AIDS so that any problems can be identified and treated as they occur and nutritional deficits can be minimized. Assessments should include evaluation of anthropometrics, visceral protein stores, red blood cell indexes, and electrolytes. Appetite, intake, and feeding ability should also be assessed. Developmental delays can also increase the risk for developing failure to thrive.

Providing adequate calories to maintain linear growth and support weight gain can be difficult as a result of chronic infections, fever, and medications. In 1994 the Centers for Disease Prevention and Control (CDC) revised the criteria for wasting in HIV-infected children under 13 years of age, and they are as follows:

- Persistent weight loss of more than 10% of baseline
- Decrease of at least two percentiles on the weight-for-age chart in children younger than 1 year of age *or*
- Two consecutive measurements more than 30 days apart of less than the 5th percentile on the weight-for-height chart and chronic diarrhea (>2 loose stools daily for >30 days) or documented or constant fever for more than 30 days

Diarrhea and malabsorption can result in dehydration, which can be very serious in infants and young children, and the onset may occur suddenly. To prevent dehydration, offer Popsicles, Jell-O, juices, and other beverages often. Oral rehydration fluids, such as Pedialyte, will also help to replace electrolytes lost with acute or chronic diarrhea.

The following lists contains suggestions to provide supplemental calories and nutrient intake:

- Use a calorie-dense formula (24 to 27 kcal/oz) for infants. Add glucose polymers or medium-chain triglycerides to formulas, or reduce the amount of water added to powdered formulas to boost calories.
- Try liquid medical nutritional supplements, such as PediaSure, to provide supplemental calories.
- Add fats such as butter, margarine, or mayonnaise to foods to boost calories.
- Encourage nutrient-dense snacks such as raisins and peanuts or peanut butter.
- For the older, lactose-tolerant child, add skim milk powder to whole milk to boost calories and proteins.

- Make adjustments in diet consistency and temperatures to overcome eating difficulties associated with disease complications and any other eating problems.
- For lactose-intolerant children with AIDS, use soy-based infant formulas instead of milk.
- Add Lactaid (the enzyme lactase) to milk for better tolerance and digestion.
- Use low-lactose dairy foods such as yogurt and mild cheddar cheese, if tolerated.

Vitamin and mineral supplements in amounts one or two times the Recommended Dietary Allowance (RDA) may ensure adequate intake of these nutrients and contribute to meeting increased requirements that occur during hypermetabolic states. Attention should also be given to drug-nutrient interactions and other effects of these drugs on nutritional status.

Caregivers need to be particularly careful about food safety and sanitation. Safe food preparation is as important for children as it is for adults with HIV/AIDS, and the same food safety guidelines also apply.

Proper procedures and sanitary formula preparation must be followed for infants being bottle-fed. Infants should not be put to bed with a bottle of milk or juice, because they are easily contaminated. Unpasteurized milk and milk products should never be given, because they may be a source of *Salmonella* and other microorganisms that can cause intestinal infections.

Children should never be fed any food directly from a jar to avoid possible bacterial contamination of the remaining food from the child's mouth. Fruits and vegetables should be peeled or cooked, and meat, chicken and fish should be well cooked. All utensils and dishes should be washed in a dishwasher or in hot sudsy water.

References

Ball CS: Global issues in pediatric nutrition: AIDS, *Nutrition* 14(10):767, 1998.

Beisel WR: Nutrition in pediatric HIV infection, *J Nutr* 126(10 suppl): 2611S, 1996.

Fields-Gardner C: HIV and children: the nutrition story. II. Nutrition in pediatric HIV disease, *BETA* July:37, 1998. Retrieved February 22, 2006, from *www.sfaf.org/treatment/beta/b37/b37kids2.html*.

Grossman M: Special problems in the child with AIDS. In Sande MA, Volberding PA, eds: *The medical management of AIDS*, ed 2, Philadelphia, 1990, WB Saunders.

Nutrition intervention in the care of persons with HIV—position of the American Dietetic Association and Dietitians of Canada, *J Am Diet Assoc* 100:708, 2000.

Raiten DJ: Nutrition and HIV infection: a review and evaluation of the extant knowledge of the relationship between nutrition and HIV infection, *Nutr Clin Pract* 6(3):S1, 1991.

Groups at Risk

Persons at greatest risk of HIV infection are those who, if sexually active, are not consistently practicing responsible and safer sexual behavior, which consists of (1) consistent and correct condom use for protection (the regular latex male sheath, female polyurethane condom, or cervical cap approved for use by the FDA) and (2) reduction in high-risk sexual practices, such as avoidance of sex with multiple partners and persons at risk for HIV.[14] Others at

> **retrovirus** Any of a family of single-strand RNA viruses having an envelope and containing a reverse coding enzyme that allows for a reversal of genetic transcription from RNA to DNA rather than the usual DNA to RNA, the newly transcribed viral DNA then being incorporated into the host cell's DNA strand for the production of new RNA retroviruses.

risk are injection drug users who share needles. Because the public-donated blood supply for transfusions has been thoroughly cleared of HIV infection through a rigorous double-testing program, this route of infection risk by blood units for medical purposes has virtually been eliminated.

Diagnosis of HIV Infection

Testing Procedures

HIV infection is diagnosed by detection of the virus or serologic response to the virus. HIV infection can be identified by the detection of specific antibodies, as is done in the routine screening of blood and blood products for transfusion and in most epidemiologic studies. The recommended procedure for virus detection is a two-step process. The first step is enzyme-linked immunosorbent assay (ELISA) screening. Second, suspected positive samples from the ELISA screening are followed with Western blot testing for confirmation. Both of these tests are highly sensitive and specific, and both are used to confirm the results before informing the individual. Because a positive test is such a personal and life-changing event, most experienced physicians caring for HIV-infected patients repeat all positive tests again, even when they have been confirmed by Western blotting, before informing the individual. Requirements for the testing procedure include pretest and posttest counseling to cover such issues as the following:

- Medical significance of the test, whether positive or negative
- Limitations of the test
- Information about HIV-1 and AIDS, how they are spread, and how to prevent their spread
- Medical, nutrition, and psychosocial care availability
- Confidentiality concept involved with documentation in the medical record; possible social and legal results of testing, personal needs, and support system

Viral load assays are used to assess prognosis, determine the need for antiretroviral therapy and type of antiretroviral therapy to use, and monitor the progression of the disease. Viral load is inversely correlated with the $CD4^+$ cell count.

Clinical Symptoms and Illnesses

Early clinical symptoms that may follow initial exposure to the virus add further confirmation to the HIV-seropositive testing procedures. These initial symptoms, as well as possible associated illnesses and diseases that characterize later HIV stages, have been generally described earlier in discussion of basic disease progression. Some examples of these common OIs that manifest depending on $CD4^+$ cell count range are listed in Table 24-1.

TABLE 24-1	Common Infectious Complications of AIDS

Microorganism	Nutritional Implications
Parasites	
Pneumocystis carinii	Dyspnea, fever, weight loss
Toxoplasma gondii	Fever
Cryptosporidium	Malabsorption, diarrhea
Isospora belli	Diarrhea
Microspora	Malabsorption, diarrhea
Entamoeba histolytica	Diarrhea
Giardia lamblia	Diarrhea
Acanthamoeba	Meningoencephalitis
Bacteria	
Campylobacter	Abdominal pain, cramping, bloody diarrhea, fever
Legionella	Fever
Listeria monocytogenes	Fever
Mycobacterium avium-intracellulare	Fever, weight loss, diarrhea, malabsorption
Salmonella	Diarrhea, bacteremia
Shigella	Abdominal pain, bloody diarrhea, fever
Fungi	
Aspergillus	Fungemia, fevers, weight loss
Candida albicans	Thrush, stomatitis, esophagitis, nausea
Cryptococcus neoformans	Fever, nausea, vomiting
Histoplasma capsulatum	Fever, weight loss, dysphagia
Viruses	
Cytomegalovirus	Esophagitis, colitis, diarrhea
Herpes simplex virus	Ulcerative mucocutaneous lesions, stomatitis, esophagitis, pneumonia
Epstein-Barr virus	Oral hairy leukoplakia
Hepatitis B	Nausea, vomiting, fever
Herpes zoster	Mucocutaneous lesions

Data from American Dietetic Association: *Manual of clinical dietetics,* ed 6, Chicago, 2000, Author; Gold JWM: HIV-1 infection: diagnosis and management, *Med Clin North Am* 76(1):1, 1992; Bernard EM et al: Pneumocystosis, *Med Clin North Am* 76(1):107, 1992; and Ralten DJ: Nutrition and HIV infection: a review and evaluation of the extent of knowledge of the relationship between nutrition and HIV infection, *Nutr Clin Pract* 6(3):1S, 1991.

Basic Role of Nutrition in HIV Disease Process

Nutrition support plays a vital role throughout the HIV disease process in three basic areas. First, it is a vital component of care for the involuntary weight loss and body tissue wasting caused by disease effects on metabolism, reflected in the severe state of protein-energy malnutrition. Second, and fundamental in all conditions associated with the body's basic immune system, nutrition is an intimate and integral component of care through specific roles of key nutrients in maintaining the body's immunocompetence. Furthermore, for many of the associated diseases, individual nutritional status influences the impact of morbidity and mortality regardless of disease process. Third, many of the new drug therapies, especially the protease inhibitors, cause lipodystrophy, reduced levels of high-density lipoprotein cholesterol, hypertriglyceridemia, hyperglycemia, and insulin resistance. Long-term consequences include an elevated risk of cardiovascular disease in this population.

MEDICAL MANAGEMENT

Current Basic Goals

Medical management of HIV-1 infection in all of its stages is constantly evolving as medical research seeks to eliminate, or at least suppress, the virus. Intensive current research is aimed at preventing progressive immunodeficiency, stopping HIV-1 transmission to uninfected persons, and restoring depressed immune function to normal to prevent AIDS-associated complications. Thus present basic medical management objectives are threefold, as follows:

1. To delay progression of the infection and improve the patient's immune system
2. To prevent opportunistic illnesses
3. To recognize the infection early and provide rapid treatment for any complications of immune deficiency, including infections and cancers

Initial Evaluation: AIDS Team

Initial medical evaluation of a newly diagnosed HIV-infected patient is critical. It requires ongoing comprehensive care by the AIDS team of professional medical, nutrition, nursing, and psychosocial healthcare specialists. Box 24-1 outlines an initial evaluation guide for beginning the care of a person with newly identified HIV-1 infection. These guidelines emphasize the special coordinated care by all members of the AIDS team and importance of personal nutrition and psychosocial support.

BOX 24-1 Initial Evaluation of Newly Diagnosed HIV-Infected Patients

Routine History and Physical Examination

History of exposure to infectious complications of AIDS
Assessment of baseline mental status
Baseline laboratory studies
- Complete blood count (CBC), differential, platelets
- Biochemistry screening profile
- Urinalysis
- Chest radiographic examination
- Tuberculin test with anergy panel
- Serologic test for syphilis
- Serologic test for *Toxoplasma*
- T-lymphocyte subsets
- Serologic test for hepatitis B (optional)

Nutrition assessment, counseling, support, and follow-up
Psychosocial and financial status assessment

Referral to and Involvement in Psychosocial Support

Social worker, nurse, psychologist or psychiatrist, patient support group, community support group, and agencies
Rehabilitation program for substance abusers
Planning for family members and children, including issues of testing and providing for their care

Modified from Gold JWM: HIV-1 infection: diagnosis and management, *Med Clin North Am* 76(1):1, 1992.

Antiretroviral Drug Therapy

As of the end of 2000 there were 15 FDA-approved antiretroviral drugs available in the United States. Antiretroviral therapy consists of three classifications of agents: (1) nucleoside reverse transcriptase inhibitors (NRTIs) such as zidovudine (AZT) and didanosine (ddI), (2) nonnucleoside reverse transcriptase inhibitors (NNRTIs) such as nevirapine (NVP), and (3) protease inhibitors (PIs) such as saquinavir, indinavir, and ritonavir. Antiretroviral agents are commonly given as part of a two- or three-drug regimen, or "cocktail," known as highly active antiretroviral therapy, or HAART. Guidelines set by the International AIDS Society-USA (IAS-USA) recommend treatment of patients with viral loads greater than 30,000 copies/ml regardless of $CD4^+$ cell count, of patients with viral loads between 5000 and 30,000 copies/ml who have $CD4^+$ cell counts below 500/μl, and of patients with $CD4^+$ cell counts below 350/μl regardless of viral load.[16] A summary of drugs used to treat various aspects of HIV/AIDS is found in Table 24-2.

Nucleoside Reverse Transcriptase Inhibitors

These agents are nucleoside analogues that become phosphorylated by host enzymes, after which they are incorporated into newly formed DNA. Transcription ceases, thus halting replication of the virus before incorporating into the host genome.[17]

Nonnucleoside Reverse Transcriptase Inhibitors

These agents work by binding directly to reverse transcriptase, which causes a conformational change in the enzyme, rendering it nonfunctional.[18]

Protease Inhibitors

These antiretrovirals work by preventing cleavage of protein precursors by inhibiting the protease enzyme. Resultant proteins that are formed cannot be packaged into mature virus and therefore are not virulent.[19] Studies have shown that PIs can reduce the amount of virus in the blood.

TABLE 24-2	Approved and Investigational Drugs Used to Treat HIV/AIDS

Generic	Trade Name
Nucleoside Reverse Transcriptase Inhibitors (NRTIs)[a]	
Abacavir	Ziagen, ABC
Abacavir/lamivudine	Epzicom
Abacavir/lamivudine/ zidovudine	Trizivir
Didanosine	Videx, ddI
Emtricitabine	Emtriva, FTC
Emtricitabine/tenofovir disoproxil fumarate	Truvada
Lamivudine	Epivir, 3TC
Lamivudine and zidovudine	Combivir
Stavudine	Zerit, d4T
Tenofovir disoproxil fumarate	Viread, M\PMPA, Prodrug, TDF
Zalcitabine	Hivid, ddC
Zidovudine	Retrovir, AZT, ZDV

NRTIs under investigation: Alovudine, Amdoxivir, DPC 817, Elvucitabine, Racivir

Generic	Trade Name
Nonnucleoside Reverse Transcriptase Inhibitors (NNRTIs)[a]	
Delavirdine	Rescriptor, DLV
Efavirenz	Sustiva, EFV
Nevirapine	Viramune, NVP

NNRTIs under investigation: Calanolide A, Capravirine, TMC125

Generic	Trade Name
Protease Inhibitors (PIs)[b]	
Amprenavir	Agenerase, APV
Atazanavir	Reyatiz, ATV, ATZ
Fosamprenavir	Lexiva, 908, 1-APV, GW433908
Lopinavil/Ritonavir	Kaletra, LPV/RTV
Nelfinavir	Viracept, NFV
Ritonavir	Norvir, RTV
Saquinavir	Fortovase, Invirase, SQV
Tipranavir	Aptivus

PIs under investigation: TMC114

Generic	Trade Name
Entry and Fusion Inhibitors[c]	
Enfuvirtide	Fuzeon, T-20

Fusion inhibitors under investigation: AMD070, BMS-488043, GSK-873,140 (aplaviroc), Peptide T, PRO 542, SCH-C, SCH-D (vicriviroc), TNX-355, UK-427,857 (maraviroc)

Generic	Trade Name
Opportunistic Infections (OIs) and Other Drugs[d]	
Acyclovir	Zovirax, ACV
Adefovir dipivoxil	Hepsera
Aldesleukin	Proleukin, IL-2, Interfeukin-2, recombinant human, rIL-2
Amphotericin B	Abelecet, AmBisome, Amphocin, Amphotec, Fungizone

Generic	Trade Name
Azithromycin	Zithromax
Clarithromycin	Biaxin
Doxorubicin	Liposomal (Doxil, Adriamycin)
Dronabinol	Marinol, THC
Entecavir	Baraclude
Epoetin alfa	Epogen, Procrit, r-HuEPO
Etoposide	Etopophos (phosphate salt), Toposar, VePesid
Fluconazole	Diflucan
Ganciclovir	Cytovene, Vitrasert
Globulin, Immune	Gamma-P I.V., Polygram S/D, IGIV, Immune Globulin Intravenous (Human)
Interferon alfa-2	Intron A (2b), Roferon-A (2a)
Isoniazid	Nydrazid, INH
Itraconazole	Sporanox
Megestrol	Megace
Paclitaxel	Onxol, Taxol, Paxene
Peginterferon alfa-2	PEG-Intron (2b), Pegasys (2a)
Pentamidine	NebuPent
Poly-L-lactic acid	New-Fill, Sculptra
Ribavirin	Copegus, Rebetol, Virazole
Rifabutin	Mycobutin
Rifampin	Rifadin, Rimactane
Somatropin	Serostim, Growth hormone (human), Human growth hormone
Sulfamethoxazole/ Trimethoprim	Bactrim, Septra, Cotrimoxazole
Testosterone	Androderm, Androgel, Depo-Testosterone, Sustanon
Trimetrexate	Neutrexin
Valganciclovir	Valcyte

Drugs under investigation: Poly(I)-Poly(C12U)

Integrase Inhibitors[e]

None listed

Integrase inhibitors under investigation: L-000870810

Microbicides Drugs[f]

None

Vaginal and rectal microbicides that hinder transmission of sexually transmitted diseases, including HIV, are being investigated: C31G, Carbopol 974P, Carrageenan, Cellulose sulfate, Cyanovirin-N, Dextran sulfate, Hydroxyethyl cellulose, PRO 2000, UC-781.

Data from U.S. Department of Health and Human Services: *AIDSinfo: drugs,* Rockville, Md, Author. Available at *http://aidsinfo.nih.gov.* Accessed September 23, 2005; and U.S. Food and Drug Administration: Drugs used in the treatment of HIV infection, Rockville, Md, 2005 (October), Author. Retrieved February 21, 2006, from *www.fda.gov/oashi/aids/virals.html.*

[a]NRTIs and NNRTIs prevent reverse transcriptase from making more copies of the HIV genome.

[b]PIs prevent protease from breaking apart long strands of viral proteins to make the smaller, active proteins HIV needs to reproduce.

[c]Fusion inhibitors are specific types of entry inhibitors that prevent fusion between HIV's outer envelope and the cell's outer membrane.

[d]OIs are illnesses caused by organisms that do not usually cause disease in persons with healthy immune systems. Common OIs in people living with AIDS include *Pneumocystis carinii* pneumonia; cryptosporidiosis; histoplasmosis; other parasitic, viral, and fungal infections; and some types of cancers such as Kaposi's sarcoma.

[e]Integrase inhibitors prevent integrase from inserting HIV's genetic material into an infected cell's genetic material.

[f]Microbicides destroy microbes such as viruses and bacteria.

DIET-MEDICATIONS INTERACTIONS

Protease Inhibitor Drug-Nutrient Side Effects and Interactions

Protease Inhibitor Drugs	Drug Side Effects	Comments
Saquinavir (Invirase)	Diarrhea, nausea, abdominal cramps	Take after a high-kcalorie, high-fat meal for best absorption; grapefruit juice decreases absorption
Indinavir (Crixivan)	Taste changes, nausea, vomiting, diarrhea, elevated blood cholesterol, hypertriglyceridemia, and hyperglycemia	Best absorbed on an empty stomach or a non-fat light snack Increase fluids to about 24 oz/day (consider weight and age) High-calorie diet
Ritonavir (Norvir)	Diarrhea, nausea, vomiting; elevated liver function tests, anorexia, abnormal feelings in mouth (burning, prickling); hypercholesterolemia, hypertriglyceridemia	Take with high-kcalorie, high-fat foods
Nelfinavir (Viracept)	Nausea, diarrhea, loose stools	Take with food
Amprenavir (Agenerase)	Nausea, vomiting, diarrhea, flatulence	Do not take with a high-fat meal
Nevirapine* (Viramune)	Skin rash, mouth sores, general fatigue; elevated liver function tests	May take with food or an empty stomach

Data from Heller LS, Shattuck L: Nutrition support with children with HIV/AIDS, *J Am Diet Assoc* 97(5):473, 1997. Some data from AIDS Project Los Angeles: *Nutritional considerations for protease inhibitors*, Los Angeles, Author. Available at *www.apla.org*. Accessed September 23, 2005.

*Nevirapine is in the drug category of nonnucleoside reverse transcriptase inhibitors.

NOTE: All protease inhibitors have the potential for causing hypercholesterolemia, hypertriglyceridemia, and hyperglycemia, along with body composition changes (lipodystrophy).

NOTE: A high-fat/high-calorie meal is defined as 1006 kcal, 48 g protein, 57 g fat, 60 g carbohydrate (the nutritional breakdown for this meal for the best absorption rates).

Rigid adherence to drug regimens is crucial to therapeutic efficacy of the drugs. Noncompliance, because of either the side effects, which can be severe, or around-the-clock administration that is required, increases risk of drug resistance. There are many side effects from these drugs, which may contribute to noncompliance with drug regimens as listed in the *Diet-Medications Interactions* box, "Protease Inhibitor Drug-Nutrient Side Effects and Interactions." Side effects such as nausea and diarrhea may require diet modifications (see Chapter 19). Efficacy of NNRTIs and NRTIs has been found to diminish over time because the virus has the ability to mutate and thus becomes resistant to drugs currently available. Use of combination therapy, or "cocktails," with two or three of the drugs that have complementary actions, achieves more effective results over longer periods of time, especially in reducing reservoirs of infection hidden in lymph tissues.[20,21] To keep HIV levels as low as possible, it is recommended PIs be taken with at least two other anti-HIV drugs, the combination known as *HAART.* However, this multidrug therapy, requiring dozens of pills daily along with a long list of sometimes unbearable side effects, and their often complicated medication-meal schedules, is very expensive, often costing more than $15,000 per year.[22]

Self-Testing Monitoring Kits

The growing AIDS-related market has led to the development of self-testing kits used by patients and their physicians to help make treatment decisions. Most of these monitors measure levels of white blood cells with a $CD4^+$ receptor, the receiving point used by surface protein of the HIV to infect cells. These measures indicate how much damage has been done to the immune system.

Continuing Vaccine and Research and Developments

A safe and effective vaccine against HIV is essential for global control of the AIDS pandemic. Vaccine development is an extremely lengthy and costly process. There are many political and social hurdles and obstacles that must be overcome, including the question as to who will pay for such an enormous venture. In addition, a vaccine must be safe, effective, stable at a wide range of temperatures, and effective against more than one strain of HIV/AIDS. Although funding for HIV vaccine research has increased more than 100% from fiscal year 1997 to fiscal year 2000, an effective vaccine has yet to be developed.[23]

Global Perspective

Worldwide more than 50 million people have been infected with HIV/AIDS, and 16 million have died, surpassing tuberculosis and malaria as the leading infectious cause of death worldwide, according to data released by the Joint United Nations Programme on HIV/AIDS (UNAIDS) and the World Heath Organization (WHO).[24] In 1999 a record 2.8 million people died—more than any prior year—and an estimated 5.4 million people contracted HIV. Of people living with HIV infection, 95% live in developing countries, with more than two thirds of the total living in sub-Saharan Africa. Four of five HIV-positive women and 87% of HIV-positive children in the world live in Africa.[24] HIV is spreading rapidly in South Africa, Zimbabwe, Botswana, and India. China, Cambodia, Myanmar, Thailand, Vietnam, and Latin America are showing increasing levels of HIV infection.[24] Social ramifications are significant; millions of children are becoming orphans each year.

Undoubtedly epidemiology and treatment of HIV-1 infection will change rapidly over the next few years. Patients will live longer and have improved quality of life. Nonetheless, with longer life and treatment for known complications, new complications will probably appear, such as uncommon infections, neurologic disease, or wasting syndromes. The medical management of AIDS will continue to require highly involved healthcare professionals and patients, as well as community support.

Basic Approach: Individual Status and Needs

Although answers will eventually come to many of our puzzling questions, HIV infection is still an elusive, epidemic, terminal disease, and its treatment varies according to individual status and needs—medical, nutritional, and psychosocial. Research breakthroughs will help light the course, but in every case, healthcare professionals and patients must remain highly involved, seeking the best possible individual care each step of the way.

There are many causes of malnutrition in HIV infection. Thus at any point nutritional recommendations and support must be individualized and integrated with other therapies. Nutrition care plans must provide a comprehensive view of disease process through each stage, specific drug use, and the patient's wishes. All patients diagnosed as HIV infected should be considered to be at nutritional risk. Although the patient may be in an earlier, asymptomatic period, the disease process, its complications, or treatments will eventually take their toll on the person's nutritional status. Nutritional status of any HIV-infected person may be compromised in numerous ways. At all times each patient must be viewed within the context of his or her own disease and individual lifestyle.

HIV Wasting

Severe Malnutrition and Weight Loss

Before development of antiretroviral agents, weight loss and cachexia were a predominant and eventual outcome of HIV disease. Multiple pathologic processes contribute to weight loss commonly seen in patients with AIDS, including the drug regimens, malignancies, fevers, enteropathy, OIs, increased resting energy metabolism, lack of finances for food, and depression. Weight loss tends to be episodic; acute episodes of weight loss were found to be associated with acute OIs, whereas chronic weight loss

was found to be associated with gastrointestinal disease and malabsorption.[25] Malnutrition itself suppresses cellular immune function. So striking is this chronic, relentless body wasting of AIDS that early in the AIDS epidemic outbreak in Uganda, Africa, it was given the name "slim disease."[26] Body wasting in AIDS is characterized by loss of body cell mass, primarily muscle protein. Death occurs when body weight reaches two thirds of normal weight and body cell mass reaches half of normal values. This designation implies that death may be more often a result of malnutrition, specifically negative nitrogen balance, than the direct effects of infection or malignancy.[27] Also, attendant diseases of the wasting process play a major role in the decreased quality of life, debilitating weakness, and fatigue seen in patients with AIDS.

Factors Contributing to Wasting

Wasting seen in persons with HIV infection or AIDS may be a result of any of the following processes, alone or in any combination:

- *Inadequate food intake:* Both clinicians and persons with HIV infection and AIDS indicate, from their combined clinical observations and personal experience, that an important factor in the profound weight loss is severe anorexia. This state is probably related to both the patient's personal life-changing situation and the body's physiologic changes from the disease. Anorexia and its resulting decreased food intake, insufficient to meet body needs, clearly contribute to the body wasting.[28]
- *Anorexia:* Pharmacologic appetite stimulants, such as megestrol acetate (Megace) and dronabinol (Marinol), have shown promising results. Megestrol acetate is a derivative of progesterone that was found to increase appetite in women who were given the medication as an adjunct to their oncologic therapy for breast cancer. Studies have shown megestrol acetate to enhance appetite, improve weight gain, and enhance sense of well-being in both cancer and HIV/AIDS patients.[29] An increase in fat mass rather than lean body mass may occur because megestrol acetate lowers the level of serum testosterone in patients with AIDS,[30] an effect that is not reversed by testosterone supplementation. Overall, megestrol acetate is generally well tolerated, especially in the liquid form; however, its costs can be prohibitive. Megestrol acetate may cause an exacerbation of hyperglycemia and therefore should not be prescribed to diabetics or those experiencing hyperglycemia secondary to medications. Dronabinol is another pharmacologic agent useful for anorexia, as well as helpful in treating nausea and vomiting. Side effects include altered mental status, anxiety, confusion, emotional lability, and hallucinations, which may be undesirable in older patients and patients whose job requires mental acuity. Dronabinol has not been

shown to be more effective than megestrol acetate in the treatment of anorexia.

- *Malabsorption of nutrients:* From early reports, as well as continuing clinical experience, diarrhea and malabsorption have been common in persons with HIV infection and AIDS. Diarrhea and malabsorption have been related to food (especially lactose) intolerances, antiretroviral therapy, other medications used to treat OIs, villous atrophy resulting from malnutrition or repeated bowel infections, low serum albumin levels, zinc deficiency or excess, and inadequate or absent digestive enzymes or bile salts.[31]
- *Altered metabolism:* Many persons with HIV infection and AIDS have a tendency to have an increased resting energy metabolism and become hypermetabolic, especially during an acute infectious episode. Other metabolic abnormalities include depletion of body cell mass, depletion of total body nitrogen, and body composition changes that occur with HAART.

Treatment of HIV Wasting

Nutrition Assessment

The initial nutrition assessment must be comprehensive to provide the baseline information necessary for beginning and continuing nutrition care, including nutritional supplementation, early in the course of the disease.[32,33] Table 24-3 provides guidelines the team clinical dietitian uses to calculate daily calorie and protein needs, and assess weight changes. Calculations and evaluations are required especially for selected patients—children and adults—on special nutrition support therapies, either enteral or parenteral.[34]

A nutrition assessment should be conducted for all patients at all stages of HIV-related diseases to monitor status routinely and identify potential problems early. Initially nutrition assessment and intervention will help in devising practical medication-meal schedules, providing medical nutrition therapy to preserve lean body mass and prevent weight loss, identifying potential symptoms that may interfere with adequate food intake, and monitoring anthropometric and biochemical indexes as indicated in Table 24-4.

TABLE 24-3	Estimated Energy and Protein Requirements

Adults: minimum 35-40 kcal/kg and 1-2 g protein/kg

Children: Recommended Dietary Allowances

Age	Energy (kcal/kg)	Protein (g/kg)
0-6 mo	108	2.2
6-12 mo	98	1.6
1-3 yr	102	1.2
4-6 yr	90	1.1
7-10 yr	70	1.0

Formula for catch-up growth:

$$\text{Kcal/kg and protein g/kg} = \frac{\text{RDA for weight/age} \times \text{Median weight/height}}{\text{Actual weight}}$$

Modified from Henderson R: Nutrition support of persons living with human immunodeficiency virus infection. In Matarese LE, Gottschlich MM, eds: *Contemporary nutrition support practice: a clinical guide,* Philadelphia, 1998, WB Saunders.

TABLE 24-4	Nutrition Assessment Parameters

Extent of Malnutrition (Adults)			
	Mild	**Moderate***	**Severe***
Albumin (g/dl)	3.0-3.5	2.4-2.9	<2.4
Transferrin (mg/dl)	150-200	100-150	<100
Thyroxine binding prealbumin (g/L)	1.0-1.5	0.5-1.0	<0.5
Ideal body weight (%)	80-90	70-79	<69
Usual body weight (%)	85-95	75-84	<74
Weight loss/unit time	<5%/mo	<2%/wk	<2%/wk
	<7.5%/3 mo	>5%/mo	
	<10%/6 mo	<7.5%/3 mo	
		<10%/6 mo	

Anthropometry	Normal Male	Normal Female
Triceps skinfold (mm)	12.5	16.5
Midarm circumference (cm)	29.3	28.5

Modified from Nutrition assessment parameters. In American Dietetic Association: *Manual of clinical dietetics,* ed 6, Chicago, 2000, Author; and Hickey MS: Nutritional support of patients with AIDS, *Surg Clin North Am* 71(3):645, 1991, with permission from Elsevier.

*Nutrition therapy indicated.

Further, person-centered nutrition care required for all HIV-infected patients is evident in ongoing nutrition assessment (see the *Health Promotion* section near the end of this chapter). Special attention is given to any taste and smell losses, which reduce appetite and food intake. These losses in appetite may be aided by increased flavor enhancement in food preparation.[35] This type of detailed initial nutrition interview includes investigation of the patient's medical history, physical and anthropometric data, biochemical indexes, full medication review, living situation, dietary intake, general socioeconomic status, and assistance needs. All patients, at first contact with a health professional, should be referred to the HIV/AIDS team clinical dietitian for screening to evaluate the degree of any nutrition problems.[36] Together with the patient, the dietitian can then initiate a plan for personal ongoing nutrition care and support.

Micronutrients and Antioxidant Therapy

The role of micronutrients, that is, vitamins and minerals, in therapeutic amounts as part of the treatment of AIDS is the focus of much current research. Ongoing studies have focused on the antioxidant capacities of six basic micronutrients—vitamins A, C, and E and beta carotene and the trace minerals iron and zinc[37] (Table 24-5). Studies have shown an increase in oxidative stress resulting from metabolic overproduction of reactive oxygen intermediates and a weakened antioxidant defense system in HIV-positive individuals.[38] Supplementation with megadoses of vitamins and minerals is increasingly common, and although persons with HIV/AIDS do have increased needs, a megadose of certain micronutrients (selenium, zinc) may be detrimental to the immune system. More research is needed in this area to obtain a more accurate assessment of the need for vitamins, minerals, and antioxidants.

Alternative Therapies

Persons with HIV infection and AIDS are particularly vulnerable to alternative therapies and supplements. In 1990 it was estimated that in the United States approximately 425 million visits were made to alternative practitioners, representing $13.7 billion in expenditures, including $10.3 billion in out-of-pocket expenses.[39] Alternative treatments used by persons with HIV infection and AIDS include, but are not limited to, Ayurvedic medicine, homeopathic medicine, traditional Chinese medicine, acupuncture, chiropractic, massage therapy, reflexology, therapeutic touch, and qi gong. A full description of these therapies is beyond the scope of this chapter; however, it may be found in other resources. Herbal therapies are also commonly used among this population. Hundreds and maybe thousands of herbal preparations are consumed by millions of people in the United States. Herbals targeted toward persons with HIV/AIDS include bitter melon, compound Q, curcumin, astragalus, echinacea, milk thistle, Siberian ginseng, SPV-30, aloe vera, alpha lipoic acid, Iscador, *N*-acetylcysteine (NAC), and shark cartilage. A significant interaction has been described between the herbal therapy St. John's wort (*Hypericum perforatum*), which is commonly taken for depression, and the PI indinavir (Crixivan). St. John's wort decreases blood levels of indinavir by 49% to 99%.[40] The FDA warns that St. John's wort may also significantly reduce blood concentrations of all HIV PIs and possibly other drugs, including those antiretrovirals in the NNRTI class. A description of these and other commonly used herbals,

---

TABLE 24-5	**Micronutrients Immune Response Deficiency and Supplement Effects**

Micronutrient	Immune Response Deficiency	Supplement Effects
Vitamins		
Vitamin A	Impaired response; increased infections and subsequent mortality	Improves immunity; excess is toxic
Beta carotene	Impaired immunity, increased cancer risk	Enhances response, CD4 T cells
B vitamins	Reduced lymphoid tissue	Vitamin B_{12} enhances skin test, mitogen response; vitamin B_6 does not enhance above reactions
Vitamin C	Impaired phagocytosis	May enhance immune function
Vitamin E	T-, B-cell dysfunction	Enhances immunity, skin test response, and function
Minerals		
Copper	Impaired function of macrophages	Good repletion, but excess can be toxic
Iron	Reduced immune response	Excess can harm
Selenium	Low intake, cancer risk	Repletion contributes to survival; excess can impair immunity
Zinc	Loss of T-cell immunity	Improves with moderate supplementation; excess can harm

Modified from Cunningham-Rundles S et al: Micronutrient and cytokine interaction in congenital pediatric HIV infection, *J Nutr* 126(10S):2674S, 1996, with permission from the American Society for Nutritional Sciences.

along with their mechanisms of actions and side effects, can be found in a variety of pharmacology and pharmaceutical textbooks, Office of Dietary Supplements within the National Institutes of Health, and FDA publications.

Nutrition Intervention

Major goals of medical nutrition therapy during HIV infection, as recommended by the HIV/AIDS Practice Group of the American Dietetic Association,[41] are as follows:

- To optimize nutritional status, immunity, and overall well-being
- To prevent the development of specific nutrient deficiencies
- To prevent loss of weight and lean body mass
- To maximize the effectiveness of medical and pharmacologic treatments
- To minimize healthcare costs

It is the position of The American Dietetic Association and Canadian Dietetic Association that nutrition intervention, medical nutrition therapy, and education should be components of the total healthcare provided to persons infected with HIV.[41] Suggested guidelines for developing such patient-centered care plans are outlined in Box 24-2. For those persons receiving nutrition support in special enteral or parenteral forms, the dietitian should work with the HIV/AIDS team physician and other members of the nutrition support team to develop an appropriate feeding mode, using enteral means or parenteral feeding via peripheral or central veins (see Chapter 18).

Treatment of HIV-Associated Wasting

For some patients, control of viral load with antiretroviral agents is accompanied by weight gain. However, weight gain may be accompanied by adipose tissue gain versus lean body mass. The primary goal should be repletion of lean body cell mass. The first step is to improve nutritional intake—adequate calories and protein, vitamins and minerals, and medical nutritional supplements as necessary.

HAART-Associated Metabolic and Body Composition Changes.   Although HAART has revolutionized medical treatment of HIV and AIDS and reduced incidence of malnutrition and infections, adverse effects of HAART continue to be a major obstacle to patient compliance and

---

BOX 24-2 | Guidelines for Developing Patient-Centered Care Plans

Symptom Management

Loss of Appetite

Eat a snack or small meal every 2 to 3 hours because large portions may fill you up too much.

Eat more food in the morning when your appetite is best.

Eat favorite foods whenever you feel like it.

Eat foods that contain a lot of protein and calories (peanut butter and jelly sandwiches, milkshakes, pizza).

Avoid low-calorie foods or low-fat/fat-free foods.

Take medicines with juice, chocolate milk, or an instant breakfast drink instead of water, unless your physician or nurse tells you not to.

Try 10 to 15 minutes of mild exercise before eating to stimulate your appetite.

If fatigue is a problem, keep easy-to-prepare foods on hand, such as frozen meals, canned soups, and eggs; have family members or friends prepare foods or arrange for home delivery of foods.

Nausea and Vomiting

Avoid fried, greasy, spicy, and very sweet foods.

Eat bland, well-cooked, easy-to-digest foods such as rice, noodles, potatoes, chicken, turkey, custard, yogurt, and oatmeal.

Try eating dry, salty foods such as crackers and toast first thing in the morning and sipping on flat sodas and weak ginger or mint tea throughout the day to calm your stomach.

If food odors are a problem, eat cold or lukewarm food, and stay out of the kitchen while foods are being cooked.

Avoid eating your favorite foods while nauseated.

Do not lie down for 2 hours after eating meals.

Sore Mouth or Throat

Eat foods that are soft and smooth in texture such as mashed potatoes, yogurt, pudding, custards, oatmeal, and scrambled eggs.

Avoid spicy, acidic, hard, and hot foods—they can irritate your mouth.

Cold foods such as ice cream and Popsicles can be soothing to your mouth.

Add gravies or cream sauces to meats and vegetables before eating to make them easier to swallow.

Soak dry foods such as bread and cookies in milk or other beverage before eating.

Use a straw to drink beverages and soup to help ease discomfort.

Diarrhea

Avoid foods that may make diarrhea worse such as milk and milk products; greasy and fatty foods; high-fiber foods and foods that cause gas; and carbonated, caffeinated, and alcoholic beverages.

Eat foods that may help control diarrhea such as bananas, applesauce, rice, and gummy bears.

Eat well-cooked, easy-to-digest foods like canned peaches, cooked carrots, baked chicken and fish, potatoes, and noodles.

Drink eight or more glasses of fluids such as sports drinks, apple juice, and broth each day.

Eat foods that are high in minerals such as potatoes, bananas, fish, and meat.

Try a BRAT diet—bananas, rice, applesauce, and toast—for a couple of days.

Modified from Keithley JK, Swanson B: Minimizing HIV/AIDS malnutrition, *Medsurg Nurs* 7(5):261, 1998, with permission from Janetti Publications, Inc.

a limiting factor that drives the cost-benefit ratio for pharmacologic therapy. Lipodystrophy and its related fat distribution complications have become the major nutrition issues in patients being treated with PIs. Lipodystrophy syndrome consists of changes in body shape that are caused by abnormal redistribution of fat. Fat accumulates in the abdominal area (truncal and visceral obesity), in the axillary pads, and in the dorsocervical pads ("buffalo hump") but decreases in the legs, arms, and nasolabial and cheek pads.[42] Lipodystrophy, although not life threatening, can cause varying degrees of depression, anxiety, social withdrawal, and low self-esteem, which can ultimately lead to poor medication compliance. Many patients discontinue therapy, risking progression of HIV infection. HAART can also cause hyperlipidemia (especially hypertriglyceridemia and hypercholesterolemia) and insulin resistance, which can significantly increase the risk of developing cardiovascular disease. This is a major concern and potentially a major deterrent to early or continuous therapy. Overall, the risk of myocardial infarction in HIV-infected patients taking PIs appears to be twofold to threefold higher than in the general population.[43] Persons on HAART are also at increased risk of developing diabetes, hypertension, and osteoporosis.

Obtaining baseline anthropometrics (waist-hip ratio, bioelectric impedance analysis, skinfold measurements) and serial measurements (i.e., at each clinic visit) is important for monitoring changes in body composition. Baseline measurements of triglycerides, total cholesterol and lipoproteins (high-density lipoprotein [HDL], low-density lipoprotein [LDL], very low-density lipoprotein [VLDL]), blood glucose, and blood pressure should be obtained. They should also be obtained at each clinic visit to monitor for changes. Diet, exercise, and pharmacologic agents are useful in the treatment of lipodystrophy syndrome. Patients with abnormal LDL, HDL, and total cholesterol levels may benefit from following the therapeutic lifestyle changes (TLC) diet (see Chapter 20 for details), which emphasize grains, cereals, legumes, fruits, vegetables, lean meats, poultry, fish, and low-fat dairy products. Diet-resistant hyperlipidemia may need to be controlled with lipid-lowering agents. Currently researchers are trying to determine which drugs can be used safely and effectively in persons on anti-HIV drugs. Individuals with insulin resistance and hyperglycemia will need counseling for carbohydrate counting (see Chapter 21). An individual with hypertriglyceridemia will need to limit intake of simple carbohydrates and alcohol. Exercise, especially weight training, may help prevent muscle wasting in the arms, legs, and buttocks, whereas aerobic exercise may help control abdominal visceral fat accumulation. Clinical trials are ongoing to determine actual benefits.

Use of Anabolic Agents in HIV and AIDS.

Use of anabolic agents has been recommended as an effective way of improving gains in lean body mass. Anabolic agents such as oxandrolone and nandrolone decanoate are known to promote protein anabolism and are generally safe when taken as prescribed.[44] Recombinant human growth hormone (rhGH), whose trade name is Serostim, is the most extensively studied anabolic agent; it has also been shown to significantly improve lean body mass and nitrogen balance in treatment of HIV/AIDS wasting.[45] Human growth hormone therapy may help control some of the body composition changes seen in some individuals with lipodystrophy. There are many potential side effects of anabolic agents, including gynecomastia, testicular atrophy and decreased fertility, salt retention, lipid and carbohydrate abnormalities, and acne. In addition, anabolic agents are frequently very expensive (approximately $18,000 per year); however, Medicaid has approved reimbursement for this treatment.[46] Resistance or weight training is strongly recommended as a safe and effective method for maintaining and improving lean body mass in all individuals who are physically able to exercise.

Nutrition Counseling, Education, and Supportive Strategies

Counseling Principles

An adolescent client once aptly defined a counselor as "someone to talk to while I make up my mind." Client-centered counseling in the care of persons with HIV infection and AIDS must be just that. Professionals and patients must remain involved throughout the progressive course of the disease because the patient's wishes and needs are ultimately paramount in various treatments and decisions about care. The basic goal of nutrition counseling is to make the fewest possible changes in the person's lifestyle and food patterns necessary to promote optimal nutritional status while providing maximum comfort and quality of life. In this person-centered care process, several counseling principles are particularly pertinent, as follows:

- *Motivation:* Changed behavior in any area requires motivation, desire, and ability to achieve one's goals. Until the patient perceives food patterns and behaviors as appropriate goals, it is best to wait for a better time and begin with establishing a general supportive climate in which to continue working together. Any specific obstacle raised by the patient, such as time, physical limitations, money, or increased anxiety, can be met with related suggestions to think about. Priorities among needs should be recognized in the care plan, and items should be introduced according to order of importance and immediacy of the patient's nutrition problems.
- *Rationale:* Any diet or food behavior change, with possible benefits and risks, must be clearly explained to the patient. The question "Why?" is always important to everybody.
- *Provider-patient agreement:* In the best interests of all concerned, the patient and healthcare provider must

COMPLEMENTARY AND ALTERNATIVE MEDICINE (CAM)
Are Persons With HIV/AIDS Vulnerable to Nutritional Quackery?

People with chronic diseases, such as AIDS, that lack curative therapy and have poor prognoses are susceptible to claims of unproved therapies and nutrition quackery. The following questionable practices are some of the nutritional quackery being touted as treatments for HIV infection.

Megadoses of Nutrients

Large doses of vitamins A and C, selenium, and zinc have been recommended to restore cell-mediated immunity by increasing T-cell number and activity. The value of such large doses has not been established in controlled clinical studies. In fact, the opposite is true; megadoses of these nutrients can be dangerous. Chronic intakes of vitamin A in excess of 25,000 IU/day can be toxic, especially to the liver. Doses of vitamin C above 2000 mg can cause diarrhea, nausea, and gastrointestinal upset; increase the risk of kidney stones; and cause a urine test to test falsely positive for diabetes. Chronic intakes of excess zinc, as little as 25 mg/day, can cause gastrointestinal distress, nausea, and impaired immune function. Selenium is also toxic in high chronic doses. It is recommended that persons with HIV/AIDS take two multivitamin-mineral supplements per day to ensure intake of 200% of the Recommended Dietary Allowance (RDA) for vitamins and minerals.

Dr. Berger's Immune Power Diet

In his 1985 book, Stuart M. Berger[1] states that poor health is caused by "immune hypersensitivity" to many foods such as milk, wheat, corn, yeast, soy, sugar, and eggs. He suggests a 21-day elimination diet for foods believed to cause allergies, followed by a reintroduction phase and then a maintenance diet, to prevent food sensitivities and "revitalize" the immune system. The usefulness of this diet has not been tested or proved by scientific studies. The diet promoted in Berger's book (high in fruits and vegetables and low in fat and calcium) may cause malnutrition, and the suggestion that moldy food be consumed to test for allergy to molds is dangerous to persons who are immunocompromised. His claims are unsubstantiated.

Antiviral AL 721

This compound, developed in Israel and approved by the Food and Drug Administration (FDA) for clinical trials, is composed of "active lipids" (AL) mixed in a ratio of 70% neutral lipid, 20% lecithin, and 10% phosphatidylethanolamine—hence the 721 designation. It has been hypothesized that AL 721 can reduce or inhibit HIV infection. Clinical trials found little toxicity but no consistent trends in T-cell quantification or HIV cultures. AL 721 made at home from soy or egg yolk lecithin or obtained already mixed may be impure and can spoil easily if stored improperly.

Yeast-Free Diet (Anticandidiasis Diet)

Candida infection, which causes oral and esophageal thrush, is common in individuals who are immunocompromised.

Authors of this diet suggest that certain persons have "candidiasis hypersensitivity" and that by following the diet (restricted in carbohydrates, yeast, sugar, processed foods, fruits [initially], and milk), this disorder can be successfully treated. The American Academy of Allergy, Asthma, and Immunology has been strongly critical of these concepts. Because the diet is limited in carbohydrates, an individual may develop ketosis, which can cause nausea and headache. This diet may also be too low in calories for individuals with HIV infection/AIDS.

Colonic Therapy

Colonic irrigation is touted to detoxify the large intestine to reduce poisons and wastes in the body. Not only is the procedure expensive, but also it is not FDA approved for "cleansing" the body of wastes. Colon cleansing is only approved and medically indicated before a colonoscopy/sigmoidoscopy. There is also great potential for harm because colonic irrigation can cause severe cramps, pain, perforation of the large intestine resulting in serious infection, and electrolyte losses, especially potassium. There is no medically substantiated reason for a person with HIV infection/AIDS (or anyone, for that matter) to have a colonic irrigation.

Macrobiotic Diet

A macrobiotic diet is based on an Oriental philosophy that it will restore balance and harmony between yin and yang forces and thereby improve health. However, it is very low in fat and high in fiber: 50% (by volume) whole grain cereals, 20% to 30% vegetables, 10% to 15% cooked beans or seaweed; and 5% miso (fermented soy paste) or tamari broth soup. This regimen can produce protein-calorie malnutrition and provides inadequate intake of riboflavin, niacin, and calcium in adults, as well as pyridoxine and vitamins B_{12} and D in children (in addition to those nutrients mentioned for adults).

These diets and other alternative therapies require further study in controlled clinical trials.

Reference

1. Berger SM: *Dr. Berger's immune power diet*, New York, 1985, New American Library Trade.

Bibliography

Anderson JA: Position statement on candidiasis hypersensitivity, *J Allerg Immunol* 78:271, 1986.

Jarvis WT: *Colonic irrigation*, Peabody, Mass, 1995, National Council Against Health Fraud.

Raiten DJ: Nutrition and HIV infection: a review and evaluation of the extant knowledge of the relationship between nutrition and HIV infection, *Nutr Clin Pract* 6(3):S1, 1991.

agree to the change. Any change should be structured around daily routines and include any caregivers as needed. The nutrition counselor should provide any needed information and encouragement throughout the process.

- *Manageable steps:* All information given and actions agreed on should proceed in manageable steps, as small as necessary, in order of complexity and difficulty. Information overload can discourage anyone. But here the particular stress load at any point can be intolerable for the patient. At such points of stress, patients are also more vulnerable to the lure of unproved HIV/AIDS therapies (see the *Complementary and Alternative Medicine {CAM}* box, "Are Persons With HIV/AIDS Vulnerable to Nutritional Quackery?").

Personal Food Management Skills

The patient's living situation and general practical skills in planning, purchasing, and preparing food must be considered. Any need for information and guidance in developing skills in any aspect of procuring food, or in sources of needed help, should be provided.

Community Programs

Information may be needed about any available community food programs, such as Meals-on-Wheels, for delivery of prepared meals at times when the patient is too ill to get out for food. A number of these programs in various hard-hit inner cities on the east and west coasts of the United States, for example, as well as in central cities, have developed to meet these needs, and in some cases they also provide home health and nutrition care services.[47-50] Also, information may need to be provided about food assistance programs such as food stamps or food commodities (see Chapter 10), for which the lower-income person may qualify.

Psychosocial Support

Every aspect of care provided should be given within a form and context that also provides genuine psychosocial support. All healthcare providers working with HIV-infected patients must be particularly sensitive to the special psychologic and social issues that confront persons with AIDS. Major stress areas may include issues relating to autonomy and dependency, a sense of uncertainty and fear of the unknown, grief, change and loss, fear of symptoms, fears of abandonment, and spiritual questions that arise when someone confronts a life-threatening illness. Common emotions are hostility, denial, withdrawal, depression, anxiety, guilt, and confusion. All of these at one time or another may significantly influence treatment. Healthcare providers must always be aware and assess how the patient and caregivers are relating to the disease, using assistance of social workers, clinical psychologists, or psychiatrists as needed.[51,52] Stress reduction groups, including exercise training, are helpful, as they have proved to be in other life-threatening situations such as patients with cancer or coronary heart disease.[53]

Most important, however, healthcare workers must examine their own values and fears regarding sexual orientation, sexual behavior, intravenous drug use, and fears of AIDS transmission. Preconceived judgments are easily picked up by patients and threaten the provider-patient relationship. Before they can be effective with patients, all healthcare workers must first confront their own fears and prejudices and learn to let go of such judgmental behavior.

Health Promotion

The ABCDs of Nutrition Assessment in AIDS

The initial nutrition assessment visit with an HIV-infected patient is an important beginning point for continuing nutrition care that is to follow. This encounter serves both informational and relational functions. It provides necessary baseline information for planning practical individual nutrition support. More important, it establishes the essential provider-patient relationship, the human context within which this continuing nutrition care and support will be provided as needed. The basic ABCDs of nutrition assessment will provide a practical guide with special assessment (the letters *E* and *F*) added for HIV-infected patients, as outlined in the following sections.[54,55]

Anthropometry

- Age, sex, height
- Weight: current, usual, percent of usual, ideal, percent of ideal, weight loss over defined time period
- Midarm measures: circumference, triceps skinfold thickness; calculated midarm muscle circumference

Biochemical Indexes

- Serum proteins: albumin, prealbumin, transferrin
- Liver function tests (evaluate liver function)
- Blood urea nitrogen, serum electrolytes (evaluate renal function)
- Urinary urea nitrogen excretion over 24 hours (nitrogen balance)
- Creatinine height index
- Complete blood cell count (evaluate for anemia)
- Fasting glucose (evaluate for hyperglycemia or hypoglycemia)

Clinical Observations

- General signs of nutritional status
- Drug effects

Diet Evaluation

- Usual intake, current intake, restrictions, modifications (use both 24-hour recall and food diaries)
- Nutritional supplements, vitamin-mineral supplements
- Food allergies, intolerances
- Activity level (general kilocalories [kcalories or kcal] expended per day)
- Support system (caregivers to help with nutrition care plan)

Environmental, Behavioral, and Psychologic Assessment

- Living situation, personal support
- Food environment, types of meals, eating assistance needed

Financial Assessment

- Medical insurance
- Income, financial support through caregivers
- Current medical and other expenses
- Ability to afford food, enteral supplements, added vitamins and minerals

TO SUM UP

The viral evolution and current worldwide spread of HIV infection have reached epidemic proportions and are still growing. Disease progression follows three distinct stages: HIV infection, AIDS-related complex (ARC) with associated opportunistic illnesses, and full-blown AIDS with complicating diseases leading to death. This overall disease progression from initial infection to death lasts about 10 to 12 years. The Public Health Service and the CDC of the USDHHS have responsibilities for monitoring the disease and providing leadership in research and treatment development, based on collaborative information exchange with scientists worldwide.

During the initial decade of the epidemic in the 1980s, scientists learned the nature and life cycle of the new mutation of HIV and its transmission modes and population groups at risk. Development of diagnostic testing procedures has enabled population surveillance and individual detection of disease and personal care to proceed. A fundamental role of nutrition support in this personal care of HIV-infected individuals has become evident.

Medical management of HIV infection, which is without a vaccine or cure, involves supportive treatment of associated illnesses and complicating diseases. In the terminal HIV stage the virus eventually gains sufficient strength to destroy white blood cells of the host's immune system, and death follows.

Current ongoing research involves study of the role of micronutrients in oxidation processes in the cell. Nutritional management focuses on providing personal individual nutrition support to counteract the severe body wasting and malnutrition characteristic of the disease. The process of nutrition care involves comprehensive nutrition assessment and evaluation of personal needs, planning care with each patient and caregivers, and meeting practical food needs. Throughout the care process, nutrition counseling, education, and strategic services also help provide psychosocial support to each patient.

QUESTIONS FOR REVIEW

1. Describe the evolutionary history of HIV-1 and its current worldwide epidemic spread. How is it transmitted, and why do you think it has spread so rapidly? Identify major population groups at risk.
2. Describe the nature of the AIDS virus and its action in the human body. What is a retrovirus?
3. Describe the progression of HIV infection in terms of its stages of development from initial infection to death.
4. Identify the drugs currently used in the medical management of HIV/AIDS, and describe any associated actions, side effects, or toxicities that may relate to dietary management.
5. Discuss the causes of HIV wasting and its medical and nutrition therapies.

6. Outline the basic parts of a comprehensive initial nutrition assessment of a patient with HIV infection/AIDS.
7. Describe the general process of planning nutrition care on the basis of the patient assessment information and the main types of nutrition problems in HIV infection/AIDS. Devise a related plan of action for each type of problem. Can you give an example of how you might follow up to see what worked or did not work and make adjustments accordingly?

REFERENCES

1. Piot P: AIDS: a global response (editorial), *Science* 272(5270):1855, 1996.
2. Tuofu Z et al: An African HIV-1 sequence from 1959 and implications for the origin of the epidemic, *Nature* 391(6667):594, 1998.
3. Joint United Nations Programme of HIV/AIDS (UNAIDS): *AIDS epidemic update,* Geneva, Switzerland, Dec 2000, Author.
4. Cohen J: The changing of the guard, *Science* 272(5270):1876, 1996.
5. Holmberg SD: The estimated prevalence and incidence of HIV in 96 large U.S. metropolitan areas, *Am J Public Health* 86(5):642, 1996.
6. Stein Z, Susser M: AIDS—an update on global dynamics (editorial), *Am J Public Health* 97(6):901, 1997.
7. Cohen J: AIDS therapy: failure isn't what it used to be . . . but neither is success, *Science* 279(5354):1133, 1998.
8. Flaskerud JH, Ungvarski PJ: Overview and update of HIV disease. In Ungvarski PJ, Flaskerud JH, eds: *HIV/AIDS: a guide to primary care management,* ed 4, Philadelphia, 1999, WB Saunders.
9. Sax P: Viral load testing, *AIDS Clin Care* 8(4):31, 1996.
10. Ryan F: *Virus X: tracking the new killer plaques,* Boston, 1997, Little, Brown.
11. Gold JWM: HIV-1 infection: diagnosis and management, *Med Clin North Am* 76(1):1992.
12. Otten MW et al: Changes in sexually transmitted disease rates after HIV testing and posttest counseling, Miami, 1988 to 1989, *Am J Public Health* 83(4):529, 1993.
13. U.S. Department of Health and Human Services: *Healthy People 2010,* ed 2, 2 vols, Washington, DC, 2000, U.S. Government Printing Office. Available at *www.healthypeople.gov.* Accessed February 16, 2006.
14. Centers for Disease Control and Prevention, Public Health Service: *HIV prevention strategic plan through 2005,* Atlanta, 2001, Author.
15. Centers for Disease Control and Prevention, Public Health Service: Guidelines for national human immunodeficiency virus case surveillance, including monitoring for immunodeficiency virus infection and acquired immunodeficiency syndrome, *MMWR* 48(RR13):1, 1999.
16. Carpenter CCJ: Antiretroviral therapy in adults: updated recommendations of the International AIDS Society-USA Panel, *JAMA* 283(3):381, 2000.
17. Samuel R, Suh B: Antiretroviral therapy 2000, *Arch Pharmacol Res* 23(5):425, 2000.
18. Miller V et al: Clinical experience with non-nucleoside reverse transcriptase inhibitors, *AIDS* 11(suppl A):S157, 1997.
19. Flexner C: HIV-protease inhibitors, *N Engl J Med* 338(18):1281, 1998.
20. Cohen J: Stubborn HIV reservoirs vulnerable to new treatments, *Science* 276(5314):898, 1997.

21. Cavert W et al: Kinetics of response in lymphoid tissues to anti-retroviral therapy of HIV-1 infection, *Science* 276(5314):960, 1997.

22. Office of AIDS Research, NIH: *Research overview, 2000,* Bethesda, Md, 2000, National Institutes of Health.

23. *HIV/AIDS: Confronting the global pandemic—Canada's contribution,* Toronto, June 1-2, 2000 (conference).

24. Temesgen Z: Overview of HIV infection, *Ann Allergy Asthma Immunol* 83:1, 1999.

25. Macallan DC: Wasting in HIV infection and AIDS, *J Nutr* 129(1):S238, 1999.

26. Serwadda D et al: Slim disease: a new disease in Uganda and its association with HTLV-III infection, *Lancet* 2:849, 1985.

27. Macallan DC et al: Energy expenditure and wasting in human immunodeficiency virus infection, *N Engl J Med* 333(2):83, 1995.

28. American Gastroenterological Association Medical Position Statement: Guidelines for the management of malnutrition and cachexia, chronic diarrhea, and hepatobiliary disease in patients with HIV infection, *Gastroenterology* 111:1722, 1996.

29. Oster MH et al: Megestrol acetate in patients with AIDS and cachexia, *Ann Intern Med* 121(6):400, 1994.

30. Engelson ES et al: Effects of megestrol acetate therapy upon body composition and serum testosterone in patients with AIDS (abstract), *Clin Res* 42:281A, 1994.

31. Adinolfi AJ: Symptom management in HIV/AIDS. In Durham JD, Lashley FR, eds: *The person with HIV/AIDS: a nursing perspective,* ed 3, New York, 2000, Springer.

32. Stack JA et al: High-energy, high-protein, oral, liquid, nutrition supplementation in patients with HIV infection: effect on weight status in relation to incidence of secondary infection, *J Am Diet Assoc* 96(4):337, 1996.

33. Chlebowski RT et al: Dietary intake and counseling, weight maintenance, and the course of HIV infection, *J Am Diet Assoc* 95(4):428, 1995.

34. Heller LS, Shattuck D: Nutrition support for children with HIV/AIDS, *J Am Diet Assoc* 97(5):473, 1997.

35. Graham CS et al: Taste and smell losses in HIV infected patients, *Physiol Behav* 58(2):287, 1995.

36. Fields-Gardner C et al: *A clinician's guide to nutrition and HIV and AIDS,* Chicago, 1997, American Dietetic Association.

37. Kotler DP: Antioxidant therapy and HIV infection: 1998, *Am J Clin Nutr* 67:7, 1998.

38. Los Angeles County Commission on HIV Health Services: *Guidelines for implementing HIV/AIDS medical nutrition therapy protocols,* Los Angeles, Oct 1997, Author.

39. Anastasi JK: Alternative and complementary therapies. In Ungvarski PJ, Flaskerud JH, eds: *HIV/AIDS: a guide to primary care management,* ed 4, Philadelphia, 1999, WB Saunders.

40. Piscitelli SC et al: Indinavir concentrations and St. John's wort, *Lancet* 355(9203):547, 2000.

41. Young JS: HIV and medical nutrition therapy, *J Am Diet Assoc* 97(10):S161, 1997.

42. Kotler DP: *Lipodystrophy—it just gets more complicated,* Eighth Annual Conference on Retroviruses and Opportunistic Infections, Chicago, Feb 6, 2001.

43. Scerola D et al: Reversal of cachexia in patient treated with potent antiviral therapy, *AIDS Read* 10(6):365, 2000.

44. Loss JC: The use of anabolic agents in HIV disease, *Support Line* 21(3):23, 1999.

45. Schambelan M, Mulligan K, Grunfeld C: Recombinant growth hormone in patients with HIV-associated wasting: a randomized, placebo-controlled trial, *Ann Intern Med* 125:873, 1996.

46. FDC Reports: *Serono Serostim required on state Medicaid formularies, HCFA says,* vol 66, Chevy Chase, Md, 1999, FDC Reports.

47. Luder E et al: Assessment of nutritional, clinical, and immunologic status of HIV-infected, inner-city patients with multiple risk factors, *J Am Diet Assoc* 95(6):655, 1995.

48. Topping CM et al: A community-based, interagency approach by dietitians to provide meals, medical nutrition therapy, and education to clients with HIV/AIDS, *J Am Diet Assoc* 95(6):683, 1995.

49. Kraak VI: Home-delivered meal programs for homebound people with HIV/AIDS, *J Am Diet Assoc* 95(4):476, 1995.

50. Udine LM, Rorthkopf MM: Utilization of home health care services in HIV infection: a pilot study in Ohio, *J Am Diet Assoc* 94(1):83, 1994.

51. Antoni MH et al: Cognitive-behavior stress management intervention buffers distress responses and immunologic change following notification of HIV-1 seropositivity, *J Consult Clin Psychol* 59(6):906, 1991.

52. Jacobsberg LB, Perry S: Psychiatric disturbances, *Med Clin North Am* 76(1):99, 1992.

53. LaPerriere A et al: Aerobic exercise training in an AIDS risk group, *Int J Sports Med* 12(suppl 1):S53, 1991.

54. Fields-Gardner C: Position of the American Dietetic Association and the Canadian Dietetic Association: Nutrition intervention in the care of persons with human immunodeficiency virus infection, *J Am Diet Assoc* 94(9):1042, 1994.

55. Trujillo EB et al: Assessment of nutritional status, nutrient intake, and nutrition support in AIDS patients, *J Am Diet Assoc* 92(4):477, 1992.

FURTHER READINGS AND RESOURCES

Readings

Nowak MA, McMichael AJ: How HIV defeats the immune system, *Sci Am* 273(2):58, 1995.

> *This article provides interesting background in a case study, and its accompanying editorial, of perinatal transmission of AIDS at birth with apparent clearance afterward, in a boy now 5 years old and in kindergarten, and a discussion of the controversial question of breast-feeding by HIV-positive mothers.*

Websites of Interest

- National Association of People With AIDS: *www.napwa.org.*
- The Foundation for AIDS Research (amFAR): *www.amfar.org.*
- Medscape: *http://hiv.medscape.com.*
- Centers for Disease Control and Prevention, Division of HIV/AIDS Prevention (DHAP): *www.cdc.gov/hiv/dhap.htm.*
- National Institute of Allergy and Infectious Diseases (NIAID), Division of Acquired Immunodeficiency Syndrome: *www.niaid.nih.gov/daids/default.htm.*
- National Institutes of Health Office of AIDS Research: *www.nih.gov/od/oar.*
- Association of Nutrition Services Agencies (ANSA): *www.aidsnutrition.org.*
- Direct AIDS Alternative Information Resources (DAAIR): *www.daair.org.*
- AIDS.org News: *www.aids.org/news.html.*
- National AIDS Treatment Advocacy Project: *www.natap.org.*
- American Dietetic Association: *www.eatright.org.*

CHAPTER 25

Cancer

Sara Long

This chapter focuses on cancer, one of the major diseases in the Western world. We examine the nature of the cancer process and its treatments and seek to relate these processes to nutritional factors involved.

Here we look at nutrition and cancer in two basic areas: the role of nutrition in cancer development and prevention and its role in cancer therapy and rehabilitation. Cancer development and its prevention are discussed in relation to the interplay of environment, the body's defense system, and nutritional factors that govern each. During medical therapy for the disease process, nutrition support plays a large role in the effectiveness of therapy and quality of life. To understand these nutritional relationships we must understand the nature of cancer as a growth process, the physiologic basis of cancer and structure and function of cells, and the body's defense systems in immunity and in the healing process.

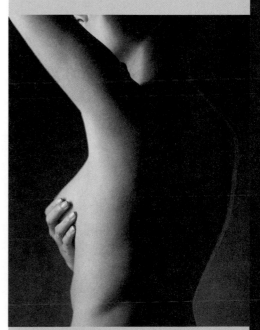

FOCUS ON CULTURE

Americancer?

America has long been known as a destination for those hoping to start a new life. Since the days when immigrants poured through Ellis Island, the dream of becoming an American citizen has been idealized as a way of life with immense opportunity and freedom. But along with this American dream, could immigrants be putting themselves and their children at risk for cancer?

Over the last couple of decades several researchers have investigated the risk of developing cancer with immigrants' assimilation to the American way of life. First-generation immigrants gave researchers a unique view on the effects American customs, dietary patterns, and environments have on the development of various forms of cancer. Unpredictably, these immigrants showed little discrepancy from their native counterparts in cancer rates; it was only in subsequent generations that variances were of consequence. It seemed first-generation immigrants were more likely to adhere to traditions from their homeland and accordingly remained in sync with their native health history.

This phenomenon is important because it shows external factors play a considerable role in increasing cancer risk. Although genetic predisposition is also a factor, diet and other lifestyle choices of the common American diet can be examined for their shortcomings through these migrant studies. Moreover, preventative characteristics of immigrants' culture can be examined and implemented for a possible constructive effect on cancer risk.

Although assimilation of immigrants into the culture and "negative" practices of America is an inevitable consequence, this trend has been able to show effects that domestic habits, including diet, can have on development of cancer. Although much research has yet to be concluded, this information is incredibly valuable and could potentially help examine particular environments, lifestyles, and dietary practices that could be modified to help reduce risk and fight the national cancer crises in America.

References

Herrinton J et al: Ovarian cancer: incidence among Asian migrants to the United States and their descendants, *J Natl Cancer Inst* 86:1336, 1994.

Karagas TM: *Migrant studies: cancer epidemiology and prevention,* New York, 1996, Oxford University Press.

King S, Schottenfeld D: The "epidemic" of breast cancer in the U.S.—determining the factors, *Oncology* 10:4, 1996.

Li F, Pawlish K: *Cancers in Asian-Americans and Pacific Islanders: migrant studies,* New York, 1999-2006, Chinese American Medical Society. Retrieved February 23, 2006, from *www.camsociety.org/issues/fredli.htm.*

McCredie M, What have we learned from studies of migrants? *Cancer Causes Control* 9:1, 1998.

THE PROCESS OF CANCER DEVELOPMENT

Multiple Forms of Cancer

The health toll of cancer continues to extract its price in human disease and death, despite ongoing efforts by the scientific and healthcare communities. In 1971 the United States first initiated a nationwide moratorium to fight the disease with the National Cancer Act. In 1995 the Assistant Secretary for Health and the Surgeon General chaired an initiative called Healthy People 2000. This program, cocoordinated by the U.S. Department of Health and Human Services and the National Cancer Institute of the National Institutes of Health (NIH), began a national initiative on health goals and objectives. It sought to focus the attacks on cancer into several priority areas. Building on these initiatives, *Healthy People 2010* was launched in 1999. It is a set of health objectives for the nation to achieve during the first decade of the new century.[1]

In its latest report the NIH statistical cancer review program Surveillance, Epidemiology, and End Results (SEER) has indicated an overall decline in the incidence of cancer by 0.8% per year between 1990 and 1997.[2] However, when reported in aggregate, due in large part to an older and expanding population, the incidence expressed in numbers of cases of overall cancer deaths continues to increase.[3] The World Health Organization estimates 35% of human cancers in the Western world are diet related.[4]

The American Cancer Society estimates that in the year 2006 approximately 564,830 Americans will die from cancer. In its multiple forms, cancer has become one of our major health problems, second only to heart disease, and accounts for approximately 23% of the total deaths in the United States each year (see the *Focus on Culture* box, "Americancer?").[3]

Breast cancer is the most common form of cancer among women in the United States. The incidence of breast cancer has continued to rise for the past two decades.[5] Prostate cancer is the leading cancer diagnosed among men in the United States.[5] Cancer of the lung is the second most common cancer and leading cause of cancer death among both men and women.[5]

Difficulties in the study of cancer have arisen from its varying nature and multiple forms. The word cancer is a general term used to designate any one of many malignant tumors, or neoplasms (new growths), forming in various body tissue sites. There are many different forms of cancer, varying worldwide and changing with population migrations. There are multiple causes and often conflicting research results because of the large number of variables involved. We would be more correct, then, to use the plural term *cancers* in discussing this great variety of neoplasms.

To better understand cancer development we should view it as a growth process that has its physiologic basis in the structure and function of cells. Because nutrition is fundamental to all tissue growth, we need to look briefly at

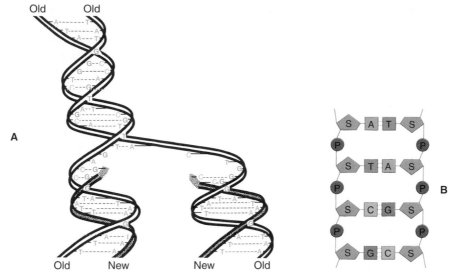

FIGURE 25-1   DNA structure. **A,** The "unzipping" of DNA to form new RNA strands. Note the cross-links connecting the strands: *A,* adenine; *T,* thymine; *C,* cytosine; *G,* guanine. **B,** Diagram of a portion of DNA structure. An enlargement of a four-bar twist of the DNA molecule.

the cancer cell to understand the relationship of nutritional factors to cancer. This "misguided cell" and its tumor tissue represent normal cell growth that has gone wild.

The Cancer Cell

Molecular mechanisms that influence conversion of a normal cell into a cancerous cell have been extensively studied and continually evolve on the basis of new scientific theories. It was originally thought that the scientific basis of all cancers was a single metabolic disturbance in cell replication caused by some sort of mutation. However, in the latter half of the twentieth century it was determined that because the normal cell cycle of division and replication is governed by multiple signals, loss of the controlled state as it occurs during neoplastic development must proceed through multiple steps.[6] In fact, it is now generally understood that cancer develops through a series of four distinct steps: initiation, promotion, development, and progression.[7]

In adult humans about 3 to 4 million cells complete the normal life-sustaining process of cell division every second, in large part without mistake, guided by a genetic code unique to each living being. How are the process and rate of cell reproduction maintained so precisely in normal cells? And, more important, why is this normal, precise regulation of cell reproduction and function lost in cancer cells, and why do cancer cells then remain mutant and malformed, functionally imperfect, incapable of normal cell life?

The first part of the answer lies in the nature of the cell's genetic material and its regulating components. Specific genetic material in the cell's nucleus is arranged as chromosomes, containing deoxyribonucleic acid (DNA). Specific sites along chromosome threads are called *genes.* Each gene carries specific information that controls synthesis of specific proteins and transmits genetic heritage. A single chromosome thread is made up of hundreds of genes arranged end to end, and each gene of DNA is made up of about 600 to several thousand smaller subunits called *nucleotides.* The nucleic acids, DNA and its companion ribonucleic acid (RNA), compose the controlling system by which both the cell and thus the organism sustain life. The structure of DNA is that of a very large polynucleotide made up of many individual mononucleotides, each one of which has three parts: (1) a sugar (deoxyribose), (2) a phosphate, and (3) a specific nitrogenous base—adenine, cytosine, guanine, or thymine. It is the ladderlike pairing of these nitrogenous bases (as shown in Figure 25-1) that incorporates the "genetic code" and enables the DNA to transmit messages to guide protein structure. DNA appears as a twisted ladder or spiral staircase in structure and thus is called a *helix,* the Greek word that means "coil."

Gene Control of Cell Reproduction and Function
The Normal Cell

New cells are created by division of preexisting cells, a process in which the preexisting cell's genetic pattern is

---

cancer A malignant cellular tumor with properties of tissue invasion and spreading to other parts of the body.

neoplasm Any new tissue growth that is abnormal, uncontrolled, and progressive.

exactly replicated in the new cell. Normally each particular cell's structure and function operate in an orderly manner under gene control, directing the cell's specific processes of protein synthesis. Gene action, however, may be switched on and off, depending on the position of a cell in the body, the stage of body development, and the external environment. Specific regulator genes control such function by producing a repressor substance as needed to regulate operator genes and structural genes. This orderly regulation of induction and repression in cell activity, however, may be lost with mutation of these regulatory genes. Control is also lost when a specific gene for some reason moves from its position to another location on the chromosome. There are four types of such mutated genes presently thought to contribute to tumor development: oncogenes, tumor suppressor genes, DNA repair genes, and genes that influence programmed cell death.[6]

The Cancer Cell

A cell may become malignant when one of these potentially cancer-causing genes is translocated and reinserted into a highly active part of the DNA. This has been shown to occur, for example, in patients with Burkitt's lymphoma and the blood cancer acute nonlymphocytic leukemia (i.e., the cancer cell appears to be derived from a normal cell that has mutated and lost control over cell reproduction).

Cancer Tumor Types

On this basis of cell nature and differentiation, it is possible to classify cancer tumor types according to the type of originating tissue; for example, those arising from connective tissues are called sarcomas and those arising from epithelial tissues are called carcinomas. We can also classify tumor types by extent or degree of cell tissue change. Tumor stages are defined in relation to rate of growth, degree of autonomy, and invasiveness.

Relation to the Aging Process

Because the incidence of cancer increases with age, a relationship exists between cancer development and the aging process in cells, tissues, and organ systems.

Causes of Cancer Cell Development

It is thus evident the basic cause of cancers is a mutation of genes that govern normal cell reproduction.

Chemical and Environmental Carcinogens

One of the first indications chemical carcinogens exist in the environment came from a British investigator, Percival Pott, when he discovered chimney sweeps had an increased incidence of scrotal cancer; it was determined the common denominator among cancer victims was exposure to soot.[8] Chemical carcinogens interfere with structure or function of regulatory genes by binding to DNA bases in such a way that the likelihood it will undergo a mutation during DNA repair or replication is increased. This mutation can thus lead to neoplastic transformation.[8] Exposure to such agents may be by individual choice, as in cigarette smoking, which accounts for nearly 90% of all lung cancers,[5] making tobacco smoke the single most lethal carcinogen in the United States. Smoking also causes cancer in other primary sites such as the larynx, oral cavity, and oropharynx. Smoking contributes to cancer of the upper respiratory tract, esophagus, bladder, and pancreas, with the degree of malignancy depending on the frequency of smoking and duration of the habit, especially when started at a young age. Although the prevalence of cigarette smoking among people 18 years of age and over has decreased since 1987, prevalence of smoking among the vulnerable age-group of children and teenagers continues to rise with inevitable long-term mortality risks.

Other exposure comes via general environmental substances, such as pesticide residues, water and air pollutants, food additives and contaminants, and occupational hazards. However, many of our natural environmental agents can carry more hazard potential, depending on the dose. The principle that "the dose makes the poison" applies to all substances, including carcinogens, natural or synthetic. These potentially carcinogenic substances may cause cancer either by mutation, altering the regulation of gene function, or by activating a dormant virus.

Radiation

Radiation sufficient to damage DNA causes breakage and incorrect rejoining of chromosomes. Such radiation damage may be ionizing, such as from x-rays, radioactive materials, and atomic exhausts or wastes, or it may be nonionizing, such as from sunlight. Ultraviolet radiation in sunlight is one of the most prominent sources of environmental carcinogens. It is highly genotoxic but does not penetrate the skin. Our longtime pursuit of the bronzed-god look has taken a large toll: sun-related skin cancer rates have risen rapidly in the United States and Europe, afflicting younger and younger persons. The common forms on the head and neck—basal cell carcinoma and squamous cell carcinoma—are easily cured by surgical removal. However, a far more lethal form, malignant melanoma, occurs in skin cells that produce the pigment melanin and accounted for approximately 7800 deaths in 2001 alone.[3] In the United States the incidence varies with latitude, with the greater number occurring in the southern states. It is thought exposure to high levels of sunlight in childhood is a strong determinant of risk for development of melanoma; however, sun exposure in adulthood also plays a role.[9] The rising incidence probably results from increased recreational exposure to sunlight, as well as the potential "greenhouse effect" of decreased protective ozone layers.[10]

Oncogenic Viruses

Although oncogenes were first found in viruses, their evolutionary history indicates they are also present and functioning in normal vertebrate cells in the form of proto-oncogenes. It is their abnormal expression, or activation by mutation, that can lead to cancerous growth. Viruses may be thought of as a major risk factor for cancer development, exceeded only by tobacco use.

A virus is little more than a packet of genetic information encased in a protein coat (see Chapter 24). It contains a small chromosome, DNA or RNA, with a relatively small number of genes, usually fewer than five and never more than several hundred. In contrast, cells of complex organisms have tens of thousands of genes. Generally, when viruses produce disease, they act as parasites, taking over the cell machinery to replicate themselves. Numerous oncogenic, or tumor-producing, viruses have been identified. A tumor virus is a type of transforming virus capable of producing tumors only in hosts in which the virus can replicate. They transform cells by integrating a DNA copy of the virus (termed a *provirus*) into the host cell genome. If a proto-oncogene is contained in the region, the provirus integration then alters the structure or function of the proto-oncogene and thereby promotes tumor development.[8] Human papilloma virus (HPV) is now recognized as the main cause of cervical cancer.[11] Retroviruses are implicated in a number of mammary tumors and skin cancer.[12] Other viruses implicated in the causes of cancer include the Epstein-Barr virus (lymphomas), hepatitis B and C (hepatocellular carcinoma), and human immunodeficiency virus (Kaposi's sarcoma).

Epidemiologic Factors

Studies of cancer distribution and occurrence in relation to such factors as race, diet, region, sex, age, heredity, and occupation show variable and conflicting results. It is becoming increasingly clear, for example, that racial differences in cancer incidence between blacks and whites in the United States are great, with more cancer cases among blacks than among whites. However, it is also clear these differences have nothing to do with race but have much to do with poverty, which has implications for nutritional status, healthcare, education, and resources. World incidence of cancer does vary a great deal from country to country, and that of specific cancer types varies from 6- to 300-fold, with incidence rates in the United States being appreciably greater than those in many other countries.

Also, racial incidence of cancer seems to change as population groups migrate and acquire the different cancer characteristics of the new population. Although specific dietary factors have been hard to pinpoint in the cause of cancer, worldwide epidemiologic studies show significant correlation of death from breast cancer, for example, with the consumption of fat in the diet and of liver cancer with the consumption of alcohol.

Stress Factors

The idea that emotions may play a part in malignancy is not new. Galen, a second-century Greek physician, wrote of such relationships, as have many different kinds of "healers" since that time. However, these relationships are difficult to measure. Even with great technologic and scientific advances, Western medicine holds fast to its basic tenet that a thing must be measurable under controlled conditions to be said to exist.

Nonetheless, increasing observations are being made of relationships between cancer and less-measurable factors of stress. Clinicians and researchers have reported psychic trauma, especially the loss of a central relationship, seems to carry with it a strong cancer correlation. Cause of a possible relationship between such trauma and cancer may lie in two physiologic areas: (1) damage to the thymus gland and immune system and (2) neuroendocrine effects mediated through the hypothalamus, pituitary, and adrenal cortex. This automatic "cascade of physiologic events" triggered by stress may well provide the neurologic currency that converts anxiety to malignancy. Such a stressful state may also make a person more vulnerable to other factors that are present, influencing integrity of the immune system, food behaviors, and nutritional status. Once cancer occurs, however, patients with cancer have many options for easing their distress and improving the quality of their lives through supportive relations and current positive medical approaches to pain management.[13,14]

---

oncogene Any of various genes that, when activated as by radiation or a virus, may cause a normal cell to become cancerous; viral genetic material carrying the potential of cancer and passed from parent to offspring.

sarcoma A tumor, usually malignant, arising from connective tissue.

carcinoma A malignant new growth made up of epithelial cells, infiltrating the surrounding tissue and spreading to other parts of the body.

radiation A highly controlled treatment for cancer, using radioactive substances in limited, controlled exposure to kill cancerous cells.

malignant melanoma A tumor tending to become progressively worse, composed of melanin (the dark pigment of the skin and other body tissues), usually arising from the skin and aggravated by excessive sun exposure.

THE BODY'S DEFENSE SYSTEM

Components of the Immune System

The human body's defense system is remarkably efficient and complex. Several components of special type cells protect not only against external invaders such as bacteria and viruses but also against internal "aliens" such as malignant tumor cells. These malignant cells from developing tumors in the body can spread invading cells into other body tissues and form secondary tumors, or metastases, that become life threatening.

Two major populations of cells provide the immune system's primary line of defense for detecting and destroying malignant cells that arise daily in the body. These cells mediate specific cellular immunity and humoral immunity, as well as providing supportive backup biologic systems. These two populations of lymphoid cells, or lymphocytes, a type of white blood cell, develop early in life from a common stem cell in fetal liver and bone marrow (Figure 25-2). They then differentiate and populate peripheral lymphoid organs during latter stages of gestation. One type is called T cells, traced from thymus-derived cells. The other type, B cells, is preprocessed by the liver and bone marrow.

T Cells

After precursor cells migrate to the thymus, the T-cell population is differentiated in this small gland, which lies posterior to the sternum and anterior to the great vessels partially covering the trachea. The majority of the circulating small lymphocytes in blood, lymph, and certain areas of the lymph nodes and spleen are T cells. These cells recognize invading antigens by means of specific specialized receptors on their surfaces. When T cells meet an antigen—a foreign intruder, a "nonself," or an alien substance such as abnormal cancer cells—they proliferate and initiate specific cellular immune responses, as follows:

- They activate phagocytes, special cells that have intracellular killing and degrading mechanisms for destroying invaders.
- They cause an inflammatory response through chemical mediators released by the antigen- stimulated T cells.

In the early 1970s, Burnet[15] proposed the theory of immune surveillance of cancer wherein most cancer tumors are rejected by the immune system and occasional failure to do so leads to cancer development. It was subsequently discovered most tumors express tumor antigens that can then be targets for rejection responses. Furthermore, T cells recognize these antigens in a different way than antibodies recognize them.[16] Harnessing this ability in the patient with cancer, scientists developed gene therapy, which has been used to create these cytotoxic T-lymphocytes specific for specific tumor types. Many strategies are being developed to deploy this immune-mediated destruction of tumors. For example, bone marrow transplantation has developed to infuse T cells from healthy donors against well-defined tumor antigens into the blood of patients with cancer with that specific tumor type.

B Cells

The B-cell population matures first in bone marrow and then, after migration, in the solid peripheral lymphoid tissues of the body—lymph nodes, spleen, and gut. These cells are responsible for synthesis and secretion of

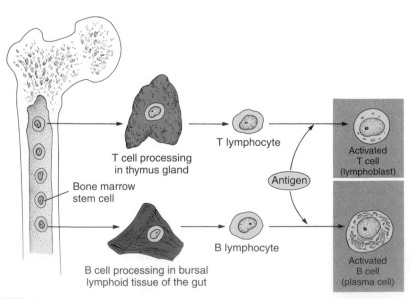

FIGURE 25-2 Development of the T and B cells, lymphocyte components of the body's immune system.

specialized protein known as antibodies. When the B cells contact an antigen, they increase and initiate specific humoral immune responses, as follows:

- They produce specific antibodies or immunoglobulins in the blood.
- They produce a particular antibody secretion, immunoglobulin A, in the bowel and upper respiratory mucosa.

This combination of antigen and antibody then activates the complement system, which attracts phagocytes and initiates the inflammatory response for healing.

Relation to Nutrition

Immune System

Integrity of the body's immune system components requires nutrition support. Acute starvation causes thymic atrophy and has immunosuppressive effects.[17,18] Severely malnourished persons show changes in structure and function of the immune system with atrophy of the liver, bowel wall, bone marrow, spleen, lymphoid tissue, and diaphragm muscles.[19] Sound nutrition can help to maintain normal immunity and combats sustained attacks in malignancy. Early use of vigorous nutrition support for patients with cancer may help to provide recovery of normal nutritional status, including immunocompetence, thereby improving their response to therapy and prognosis.[20]

The Healing Process

Tissue integrity, essential for the healing process, is maintained through protein synthesis. Such strength of tissue is a front line of the body's defense system. This process of healing requires optimal nutritional intake to support (1) cell function and structure of all its parts involving DNA, RNA, amino acids, and proteins and (2) integrity of all of the immune system components.

IMPACT OF CANCER THERAPY ON NUTRITION

Current cancer therapy takes four major forms: surgery, radiation, chemotherapy, and bone marrow transplantation. Medical treatments for cancer entail physiologic stress. These results include toxic tissue effects, often with damage to cell DNA structure and changes in normal body function. Thus the benefit achieved is not without attendant problems. Nutrition support seeks to alleviate these problems and to enhance the potential success for cancer therapy.

Surgery

Operable Tumors

Early diagnosis of operable tumors has led to successful surgical treatment of a large number of patients with cancer. Success of any surgery depends in large measure on sound nutritional status of the patient (see Chapter 23); this is especially true of patients with cancer because their general condition may be weakened. Prevention of problems through early detection and surgical treatment has significantly increased cancer cure rates. Surgical treatment may also be used with other forms of therapy for removal of single metastases or for prevention and alleviation of symptoms. Optimal nutritional status preoperatively and maximal nutrition support postoperatively are fundamental to the healing process.

Medical Nutrition Therapy of the Oncology Surgery Patient

Nutrition therapy of the patient with cancer undergoing surgery takes on the following two goals:

1. To support the general healing process and overall body metabolism
2. To modify the diet or feeding regimen in appropriate ways to compensate for the surgical site involved

Beyond regular nutritional needs surrounding any surgical procedure and its healing process, gastrointestinal surgery poses special problems for normal eating and digesting and absorbing of food nutrients (Table 25-1). Clinical examples include esophageal and stomach resections, as follows:

- *Head and neck surgery,* or resections in the oropharyngeal area, is sometimes necessitated by presence of cancer. In such cases, food intake is greatly affected. A creative variety of food forms and semiliquid textures, as well as modes of feeding, must be devised. Often mechanical problems of food ingestion make long-term tube feeding necessary (see Chapter 18).
- *Gastrectomy* may cause numerous postgastrectomy "dumping" problems requiring frequent, small, low-carbohydrate feedings (see Chapter 23). Vagotomy contributes to gastric stasis. Various intestinal resections or tumor excisions may cause steatorrhea because of general malabsorption, fistulas, or stenosis.
- *Pancreatectomy* causes loss of digestive enzymes with ensuing malabsorption and weight loss; it also induces insulin-dependent diabetes mellitus.

Radiation

After discovery of radiation in the nineteenth century, scientists soon found it could damage body tissue. Continued study of its use and control revealed normal tissue could largely withstand an amount of radiation that would damage and destroy cancer tissue. The subsequent role of radiation in cancer treatment has developed around controlled use with two types of tumors: (1) those responsive to radiation therapy, or radiotherapy, within a dose level tolerable to health of normal tissue and (2) those that

TABLE 25-1	Nutrition-Related Side Effects of Cancer Treatment

Treatment Modality	Nutrition-Related Side Effects
Upper Gastrointestinal Surgery	
Radical resection of oropharyngeal area	Chewing and swallowing difficulties
Esophagectomy	Gastric stasis, hypochlorhydria, steatorrhea, and diarrhea secondary to vagotomy, early satiety, regurgitation
Gastrectomy	Dumping syndrome, malabsorption, achlorhydria, lack of intrinsic factor and R protein, hypoglycemia, and early satiety
Intestinal Resection	
Jejunum	Decreased efficiency of absorption and many nutrients
Ileum	Vitamin B_{12} deficiency, bile salt losses with diarrhea or steatorrhea, hyperoxaluria and renal stones, calcium and magnesium depletion, and fat-soluble vitamin deficiencies
Massive bowel resection	Life-threatening malabsorption, malnutrition, metabolic acidosis, and dehydration
Ileostomy and colostomy	Complication of salt and water balance
Blind-loop syndrome	Vitamin B_{12} malabsorption
Pancreatectomy	Malabsorption and diabetes mellitus
Radiation Therapy	
Oropharyngeal area	Destruction of sense of taste and smell, xerostomia and odynophagia, oral mucositis and ulceration, loss of teeth, and osteonecrosis
Thorax and mediastinum	Esophagitis with dysphagia; fibrosis with esophageal stricture
Abdomen and pelvis	Bowel damage, acute and chronic, with diarrhea, malabsorption, stenosis and obstruction, ulceration and fistula formation

Modified from Shils ME, editor: *Modern nutrition in health and disease,* ed 10, Philadelphia, 2006, Lippincott Williams & Wilkins.

can be targeted without damage to overlying vital organ tissue.

Forms of Radiation Therapy

Radiation therapy damages the DNA of cells; therefore cells cannot continue to divide and grow. Radiation used in cancer therapy is produced from the following three main sources:

1. In external beam irradiation (or x-ray), radiation is directed at the patient externally from a linear accelerator. This type of radiation frequently causes nutrition-related side effects.
2. In brachytherapy, highly radioactive isotopes, such as cobalt 60, are placed directly into or next to the tumor to deliver a highly localized dose. Nutritional side effects do not generally occur from this type of radiotherapy.
3. In stereotaxis, radiation is delivered in a narrow beam to difficult-to-reach places such as brain tumors.

Medical Nutrition Therapy of the Radiation Oncology Patient

Radiotherapy may be used alone or in conjunction with other therapies both for curative and palliative care for approximately 50% of all patients with cancer at some time during the course of their disease. Radiation

enteritis will influence nutritional status and therapy a great deal, depending on the site and intensity of treatment. Clinical examples include irradiation to head, neck, and abdominal cavity, as follows:

- *Head and neck* irradiation will affect oral mucosa and salivary secretions, as well as the esophagus, influencing taste sensations and sensitivity to food temperature and texture. Common side effects include mucositis, xerostomia, loss of taste, and alteration in or loss of smell. Other means of tempting appetite through food appearance and aroma, as well as texture, must be developed. Nutritional management may be further compounded by the curtailment of food intake caused by anorexia and nausea. Esophagitis from head and neck radiation may be so severe as to cause esophageal fibrosis or stricture. In this scenario, dilation of the esophagus is sometimes attempted, to create a passageway large enough to swallow a bolus of food, but if unsuccessful, a feeding tube often becomes necessary for nutrition support.
- *Abdomen* irradiation may produce denuded bowel mucosa, loss of villi, and absorbing surface area with tissue edema and congestion; vascular changes occur as a result of intimal thickening, thrombosis, ulcer formation, or inflammation. In the intestinal wall there may be fibrosis, stenosis, necrosis, or ulceration. General

malabsorption or fistulas may develop, as well as hemorrhage, obstruction, and diarrhea, all contributing to nutrition problems.

Chemotherapy

Drug Development

Chemotherapy refers to use of chemical agents to treat cancer in a systemic manner; these agents are delivered intravenously and therefore elicit their effects throughout the body. Many of the most effective chemotherapy agents currently in use have been developed only within the past few years. Therapeutic use of a chemotherapy agent is based on two general principles related to rate and mode of action.

Rate of Action

The so-called cell or log (logarithm)-kill hypothesis of the action of chemotherapeutic agents on tumors indicates a single dose can be only as much as 99.9% effective in killing the tumor cells. Thus if as large a tumor as is compatible with life can be treated with a drug tolerable at a toxicity level that is 99.9% effective, the tumor is gradually reduced with successive doses that cause "fractional killing" with each dose. This process finally brings the tumor within the capability of the body's own immune system to take over and make the final kill and cure. The smaller the tumor, either because of early detection or initial treatment by surgery or radiation, the greater the possible effectiveness of the chemotherapeutic agents. Also, the following two other principles of dosage rate for greater effectiveness are important:

- Aggressive use of maximal tolerable dosages in repeated series
- Use of several drugs combined for a synergistic effect

Many malignancies such as leukemias, lymphomas, and testicular cancer are now successfully treated by such combination therapy.[21] However, most common cancers, such as breast, lung, colorectal, and prostate, require an overall program that involves surgery and radiation for a maximal cure rate.

Mode of Action

Chemotherapeutic agents are effective because they disrupt normal processes in the cell responsible for cell growth and reproduction. Some agents interfere with DNA synthesis. Others disrupt DNA structure and RNA replication. Others prevent cell division through mitosis, cause hormonal imbalances, or make unavailable specific amino acids necessary for protein synthesis. It is this diversity in mode of action that provides a basis for grouping drugs into certain classes of chemotherapeutic agents, as follows:

- Alkaloids
- Alkylating agents
- Antibiotics
- Antimetabolites
- Enzymes
- Hormones

They are usually used in combined therapy or as adjuvant therapy in conjunction with surgery or radiation.

Toxic Effects

Chemotherapeutic agents have the same effects on rapidly reproducing normal cells as they do on the rapidly reproducing cancer cells. Interference with normal function is most apparent in normal cells of the bone marrow, gastrointestinal tract, and hair follicles, accounting for a number of the toxic side effects and problems in nutritional management, as follows:

- *Bone marrow effects* include interference with production of red blood cells (anemia), white blood cells (infections), and platelets (bleeding). Many healthcare practitioners subscribe to the use of a neutropenic diet during these instances, in which potentially microbially contaminated food ingredients, such as raw, unwashed vegetables and other foods, are eliminated.
- *Gastrointestinal effects* include nausea and vomiting, stomatitis, anorexia, ulcers, and diarrhea.
- *Hair follicle effects* include alopecia (baldness) and general hair loss.

Modes of Drug Use

Chemotherapy may be used alone or in conjunction with other treatments such as surgery or radiotherapy to increase the cure rate.

Chemotherapy Research

Researchers are working to find substances, in either food or drugs that can prevent or halt cancer development. Their goal is to develop drugs or modify foods as a preventive strategy for people at high risk for cancer.[22] There is considerable evidence to suggest many plant-derived extracts contain compounds that can inhibit the process of carcinogenesis effectively.[23] These chemical compounds produced by plants or in persons eating the plants are now termed *phytochemicals* (see discussion in Chapter 6). For example, members of this group of compounds include alpha- and beta-carotene found in carrots; beta-cryptoxanthin found in oranges, peaches,

---

palliative Care affording relief but not cure; useful for comfort when cure is still unknown or obscure.
stomatitis Inflammation of the oral mucosa, especially the buccal tissue lining the inside of the cheeks, but it also may involve the tongue, palate, floor of mouth, and the gums.

and tangerines; and lutein found in vegetables such as tomatoes, green beans, spinach, and other green vegetables. There are many of these phytochemicals, found in a wide variety of vegetables and fruits, that provide specific health benefits. Another group, called disease-preventive agents, is being studied. This group—the dithiolthiones found in cruciferous vegetables such as broccoli, cauliflower, and cabbage—are potential preventive agents.[23] Phytochemicals can inhibit carcinogenesis by inhibiting phase I and II enzymes, scavenging DNA reactive agents, suppressing the abnormal proliferation of preneoplastic lesions, and inhibiting certain properties of the cancer cell.[24,25] Moreover, ingestion of specific beneficial bacteria, known as probiotics, may have anticarcinogenic effects in colon cancer.[26]

Major nutritional concerns during chemotherapy relate to (1) gastrointestinal symptoms caused by the effect of toxic drugs on rapidly developing mucosal cells, (2) anemia associated with bone marrow effects, and (3) general systemic toxicity effect on appetite (see the *Diet-Medications Interactions* box, "Nutritional Side Effects of Chemotherapeutic Agents"). Stomatitis, nausea, diarrhea, and malabsorption contribute to many food intolerances. Antiemetic drugs such as prochlorperazine (Compazine) may be used (Table 25-2); such drugs act on the vomiting center in the brain to prevent the nausea response. Prolonged vomiting seriously affects fluid and electrolyte balance, especially in older adult patients, and needs to be controlled. In patients with breast cancer, relief from nausea has been achieved with use of the

---

💊 DIET-MEDICATIONS INTERACTIONS

Nutritional Side Effects of Chemotherapeutic Agents

Side Effects	Chemotherapy Agents	Side Effects	Chemotherapy Agents
Nausea and vomiting	Bleomycin	Diarrhea	Fludarabine
	Busalfan		Methotrexate
	Cisplatin		5-Fluorouracil
	Cyclophosphamide		Flutamide
	Doxorubicin		Vincristine
	Ifosfamide		Vinorelbine
	Interferon alfa		Paclitaxel
	Interleukin		Docetaxel
	Fludarabine		Doxorubicin
	Flutamide	Oral ulceration	Fludarabine
	Leuprolide		Methotrexate
	Methotrexate		Mitomycin
	Mitomycin		Bleomycin
	5-Fluorouracil		Doxorubicin
	Vincristine		Dactinomycin
	Vinorelbine		5-Fluorouracil
	Paclitaxel		Vincristine
	Rituximab		Vinorelbine
	Tamoxifen citrate		Paclitaxel
	Trastuzumab		Docetaxel
	Docetaxel	Gastrointestinal ulceration	Methotrexate
Anorexia	Bleomycin		Ara-C
	Busalfan		Procarbazine hydrochloride
	Cisplatin	Abdominal or epigastric pain	Methotrexate
	Cyclophosphamide		Cyclophosphamide
	Doxorubicin		Dactinomycin
	Ifosfamide		Prednisone
	Interferon alfa		Dexamethasone
	Interleukin	Constipation	Vincristine
	Fludarabine		
	Mitomycin		
	Methotrexate		
	5-Fluorouracil		
	Vincristine		
	Vinorelbine		
	Paclitaxel		
	Docetaxel		

Data from McCallum PD, Polisena CG, eds: *The clinical guide to oncology nutrition*, Chicago, 2000, American Dietetic Association; Coulston AM, Rock CL, Monsen ER, eds: *Nutrition in the prevention and treatment of disease*, San Diego, 2001, Academic Press; and Shils ME: Nutrition and diet in cancer. In Shils ME, Young VR, eds: *Modern nutrition in health and disease*, Philadelphia, 1988, Lea & Febiger.

TABLE 25-2 | Medications Used to Control Nausea and Vomiting in Patients Receiving Chemotherapy

Antiemetics

Class	Drug	Route – Oral	Route – Rectal	Route – Injectable	Mechanism of Action	Site of Action	Side Effects	Comments
Phenothiazines	Perphenazine (Trilafon)	X		X	DA	CTZ	EPS, sedation, hypotension	Prochlorperazine is the most effective agent in this class; perphenazine may be effective with high IV doses; prochlorperazine is available in sustained released capsule which should not be crushed
	Prochlorperazine (Compazine)	X	X	X				
	Promethazine (Phenergan)	X	X	X				
	Thiethylperazine (Torecan)	X	X	X				
Butyrophenones	Droperidol (Inapsine)	X		X	DA	CTZ	EPS, sedation	
	Haloperidol (Haldol)	X	X	X				
Substituted benzamide	Metoclopramide (Reglan)	X	X	X	DA or 5-HT3 in high doses	CTZ	EPS, sedation, fatigue, diarrhea, nausea	Also used in early satiety and anorexia
Serotonin antagonists	Dolasetron (Anzemet)	X		X	5-HT3	CTZ, PGSEC	Headache, diarrhea, constipation, ECG changes, somnolence	Increased effect with corticosteroids
	Granisetron (Kytril)	X		X			Headache, diarrhea, constipation, somnolence	
	Ondansetron (Zofran)	X		X				
Benzodiazepines	Lorazepam (Ativan)	X		X	BDZ	Unknown	Sedation, confusion, amnesia, slurred speech	Effective for anticipatory nausea/anxiety; lorazepam may be placed under the tongue
	Diazepam (Valium)	X		X				
Corticosteroids	Dexamethasone (Decadron)	X		X	Unknown	Unknown	Increased appetite, mood change, anxiety, euphoria, headache, metallic taste, hyperglycemia	Most effective when used with 5-HT3
Anticholinergics	Scopolamine (TransDerm)		Patch		ACH	Emetic center	Urinary retention, dry eyes, constipation	Effective for nausea related to motion
Cannabinoids	Dronabinol (Marinol)	X			Unknown	CNS	Mood changes, increased appetite, hypotension, tachycardia	Well tolerated in younger patients; may crush

From Kennedy LD: Common supportive drug therapies used with oncology patients. In MacCallum PD, Polisena CG, eds: *The clinical guide to oncology nutrition*, Chicago, 2000 American Dietetic Association.

DA, Dopamine antagonist; *CTZ,* chemoreceptor trigger zone; *EPS,* extrapyramidal side effects; *IV,* intravenous; *5-HT3,* serotonin3 (5-hydroxytryptamine₃) antagonist; *PGSEC,* peripheral gastrointestinal stimulation to emetic center; *ECG,* electrocardiographic; *BDZ,* benzodiazepine; *ACH,* anticholinergic; *CNS,* central nervous system.

antiemetic drug megestrol acetate (Megace), a synthetic female sex hormone similar to the natural hormone progesterone. However, results have shown that although megestrol acetate can increase appetite and weight gain in patients with cancer, it has no effect on lean body mass; rather weight gain appears to be related solely to increases in fat mass.[27,28] Two drugs that act as serotonin blockers, granisetron hydrochloride (Kytril) and ondansetron hydrochloride (Zofran), administered in combination therapy with dexamethasone, an adrenal cortical steroid, have been shown to control episodic nausea and vomiting.[29]

In some cases of chronic long-term drug therapy, special nutritional management restricting conditioned, or learned, food aversions to odors and colors has been effective. For example, patients receiving periodic treatments of the drug cisplatin (Platinol), who had a special diet of three meals a day of plain colorless, odorless foods, including items such as cottage cheese, applesauce, vanilla ice cream, and other predetermined foods, experienced little nausea and increased food intake.[30] Potential for development of conditioned food aversions while on long-term chemotherapy is diminished by use of food having little or no odor or color because drug-related dysgeusia (perverted sense of taste) and dysosmia (impaired sense of smell) are correlated with visual olfactory stimulation factors.[30,31]

Certain chemotherapeutic drugs also have special effects. For example, monoamine oxidase (MAO) inhibitors may be used for pretreatment relief of mental and emotional depression or for palliative therapy. These antidepressant drugs cause well-known pressor effects when used with tyramine-rich foods (see Appendix J). Thus these foods should be avoided when using such drugs.

NUTRITION THERAPY

Therapeutic Goals

In general, nutrition therapy deals with the following two types of cancer-related issues:

1. Those alterations in nutritional status related to the disease process itself
2. Those related to medical treatment of the disease

Basic objectives of nutrition therapy in cancer are to (1) meet increased metabolic demands of the disease and prevent catabolism as much as possible and (2) alleviate symptoms resulting from the disease and its treatment through adaptations of food and the feeding process.

Alterations in Nutritional Status Related to the Disease Process

Basic feeding challenges governing nutrition therapy are caused by general systemic effects of the neoplastic disease process and by specific responses related to type of cancer.

General Systemic Effects of the Neoplastic Disease Process Affecting Nutrition Therapy

Malnutrition is the most common secondary diagnosis in patients with cancer and is a prognostic indicator for poor response to cancer therapy and shortened survival time.[32] The disease process causes three basic systemic effects—(1) anorexia, (2) altered metabolic state, and (3) negative nitrogen balance—which are often accompanied by a continuing weight loss. These effects may vary widely with individual patients, according to type and stage of the disease, from mild, scarcely discernible responses to the extreme forms of debilitating cachexia seen in advanced disease, and they are estimated to cause more than 50% of the cancer deaths.[33,34]

Cachexia is not a local effect but rather arises from distant metabolic effects (i.e., it is a type of paraneoplastic syndrome). Although some have suggested tumor and host compete for nutrients, this is unlikely, given that some patients with cancer with very large tumors show no signs of cachexia.[34] This extreme weight loss and weakness are caused by abnormalities in fat, muscle, and glucose metabolism, mediated in part by natural body defense substances such as tumor necrosis factor and cytokines. First, there is evidence the cancer's catabolic effects may result in an increase in fat breakdown, brought about by tumor necrosis factor.[34] Second, a reduced rate of somatic protein synthesis and an increased rate of protein degradation have been noted, also brought about by tumor necrosis factor. Third, there is evidence the wasting in patients with cancer is caused in part by abnormalities in metabolism of glucose.[34] The drug hydrazine sulfate seems to correct this metabolic error, allowing patients to conserve more energy and show modest improvements in survival, but no remissions have been documented.[35]

Anorexia is frequently accompanied by depression or discomfort during normal eating. This contributes further to a limited nutrient intake at the very time the disease process causes an increased metabolic rate and nutrient demand. Often this imbalance of decreased intake and increased demand creates a negative nitrogen balance, an indication of body-tissue wasting. Sometimes a true tissue loss of protein is masked by outward nitrogen equilibrium as the growing tumor retains nitrogen at the expense of the host, further compounding the problem.

Nutritional Effects Related to the Type of Cancer

In addition to the generalized wasting syndrome known as *cachexia* discussed here, specific nutrition problems individually present themselves depending on the site or organ involved. Of foremost significance are tumors that cause obstruction or lesions in the gastrointestinal tract or adjacent tissue. In fact the cancer may reduce intake or absorption of nutrients via (1) altered oral intake, (2) malabsorption of nutrients and subsequent diarrhea,

(3) functional and motility problems arising from surgical procedures or tumor growth, (4) fluid and electrolyte imbalances, (5) hormonal imbalances (e.g., diabetes that has been caused by pancreatectomy for pancreatic cancer), and (6) anemia.

Abdominal radiation may cause intestinal damage, with tissue edema and congestion, decreased peristalsis, or endarteritis in small blood vessels.[36] The liver is somewhat more resistant to damage from radiation in adults, but children are more vulnerable than adults.

Individualizing Nutrition Therapy for Cancer

Two important principles of nutrition therapy, vital in any sound nutrition practice but especially essential in care of patients with cancer, provide the basis for planning the nutrition care of each patient, as follows (see also the *Case Study* box, "Patient With Cancer"):

1. Personal nutrition assessment
2. Vigorous nutrition therapy to maintain good nutritional status and support medical treatment

Nutrition Screening and Assessment

It is far more difficult to replenish a nutritionally depleted patient than to maintain a good nutritional status from the outset of the disease process. Therefore a primary goal in nutrition therapy is to prevent a depleted state. Initial assessment for baseline data and regular monitoring thereafter during treatment are necessary. A detailed personal history is essential to determining individual needs, desires, and tolerances. To be valid the interview should be conducted as a conversation, using verbal and nonverbal probes and pauses rather than a cross-fire of separate questions and answers (see Chapter 16).

Nutrition Therapy and Plan of Care

Based on careful individual nutrition diagnosis, the clinical dietitian conducts a thorough nutrition assessment and prepares a nutrition diagnosis for optimal nutrition therapy to meet needs. This nutrition therapy outline is then incorporated into the nutrition care plan as the clinical dietitian works with other members of the healthcare staff to carry it out. Primary care provided by a dietitian and nurse on a regular basis is a necessary part of oncology team practice. This early, vigorous care often makes the difference in the success rate of medical therapy. Thus working closely with the oncology nurse and physician, the clinical dietitian assesses personal needs, determines nutritional requirements, plans and manages nutrition care, monitors progress and responses to therapy, and makes adjustments in care according to status and tolerances.

Determining Nutritional Needs

Each nutrient factor related to tissue protein synthesis and energy metabolism requires careful attention. Increased needs for energy, protein, vitamins and minerals, and fluid are based on demands made by the disease and its treatment. Individual needs and food tolerances vary, but general guidelines are the same.

Energy. Great energy demands may be placed on the patient with cancer. These demands result from a hypermetabolic state that exists in some patients with cancer and from tissue-healing requirements. Of this total dietary kcalories value, sufficient carbohydrate (at least 45% to 50% of total calories) to spare protein for vital tissue synthesis is essential. For the adult patient with good nutritional status, approximately 25 to 30 kilocalories (kcalories or kcal)/kg body weight/day will provide for maintenance needs. A more malnourished patient may require more calories, depending on the degree of malnutrition and body trauma. Carbohydrate should supply the majority of energy intake, with fat making up about 30% of total calories.

Providing a malnourished patient with cancer with nutrition support must be done with caution. Overfeeding must be avoided to minimize the risk of "refeeding syndrome," in which severe intracellular electrolyte and fluid shifts may occur.

Dietary Fat. Some studies have related excessive dietary fat to cancer metastasis and effectiveness of cancer

---

CASE STUDY

Patient With Cancer

Catherine is a 35-year-old mother of three young children. She was admitted to the hospital with multiple enterocutaneous fistulas 3 weeks ago at which time she weighed 52 kg (116 lb). She is 165 cm (5 ft 5 in) tall. Catherine has a history of recurrent cervical cancer for which she had a hysterectomy 4 months before admission. During chemotherapy that followed, she had regular bouts with nausea and anorexia. Surgery was performed again. Her fistulas continued to drain for 2 weeks postoperatively, during which she tolerated clear liquids only. An intravenous drip of 10% glucose and 45% normal saline was ordered to supplement fluids and kcalories. This week she developed peritonitis and has had a fever with a maximum temperature of 39° C (102° F) over the past 24 hours. Her weight has dropped to 41 kg (90 lb); drainage from the fistulas has become odorous. The patient was placed in isolation today and was advised by her physician that he intended to start her on total parenteral nutrition (TPN) and conduct some more tests to determine her progress.

Questions for Analysis

1. What types of nutrition assessment procedures would be used by the TPN team for planning Catherine's nutrition therapy? Explain the purpose of each.
2. Calculate Catherine's energy and protein needs, and account for increased needs.
3. Why did Catherine develop nausea and anorexia during chemotherapy? What are the implications of this for recovery? Outline a plan for evaluating and controlling nausea and vomiting in patients undergoing chemotherapy.
4. What personal concerns would you expect Catherine to have? What resources would you use to help her obtain the personal and physical support she probably needs?

therapy.[37,38] However, in deciding whether to alter components of the diet of the patient with cancer, it is important to note the patient's usual intake and recent intake and relative efficacy of this diet change at the particular stage of disease of the patient. Certainly in early stages of cancer a reduction in fat may be beneficial; however, in later states of disease, a primary goal of therapy is to increase the caloric density of the diet, and limiting fat will be counterproductive to that end.

Protein.   Tissue protein synthesis, a necessary component of healing and rehabilitation, requires essential amino acids and nitrogen. Efficient protein use, which depends on an optimum protein/calorie ratio, promotes tissue building, prevents tissue wastage (catabolism), and helps make up tissue deficits. An adult patient with good nutritional status will need about 0.8 to 1.2 g/kg/day of protein to meet maintenance needs and ensure anabolism. A malnourished patient may need up to two times more protein to replenish tissue and restore positive nitrogen balance.

Vitamins and Minerals.   Adequate intakes of vitamins and trace elements are important for normal tissue function and healing and for maintenance of immune function. However, care must be given to avoiding megavitamin and trace mineral alternative therapy in cancer treatment. Excessive dosages for vitamins can have deleterious health effects, may interfere with immune function, and may accelerate rate of growth of some cancers.[39] Key vitamins and minerals control protein and energy metabolism through their roles in cell enzyme systems. They also play a necessary part in structural development and tissue integrity. B-complex vitamins in general serve as necessary coenzyme agents in energy and protein metabolism. Vitamins A and C are necessary for development and integrity of body tissues. Vitamin A also has a significant role in protective immunity and cell differentiation; vitamin C has significant antioxidant, enzymatic, and immune biologic functions related to cancer.[40,41] Increased dietary consumption of vegetables and fruits is the best way to obtain these vitamins. Vitamins A, E, and D may alter expression of certain oncogenes.[42] Vitamin D hormone ensures proper calcium and phosphorus metabolism in bone and blood serum. Vitamin E protects the integrity of cell wall materials and hence tissue integrity. Many minerals function in structural and enzymatic roles in vital metabolic and tissue-building processes. Thus an optimal intake of vitamins and minerals, at least to the Recommended Dietary Allowance (RDA) levels but frequently augmented with supplements according to individual patient nutritional status, is indicated.

Fluids.   Most adults require water in the amount of approximately 35 ml/kg/day, or between 1500 and 2000 ml/day. Adequate fluid intake is important for the following two reasons:

1.   To replace gastrointestinal losses or losses caused by infection and fever
2.   To help the kidneys dispose of metabolic breakdown products from destroyed cancer cells as well as from toxic drugs used in treatment

For example, some toxic drugs such as cyclophosphamide (Cytoxan) require as much as 2 to 3 L of forced fluids daily to prevent hemorrhagic cystitis.

Alternative Therapy With Herbal Products.   In recent years many cancer patients have turned toward herbal therapy as an alternative to chemotherapy, radiation, or surgery. Many herbal therapies have not been adequately tested and have been found to have toxic effects (see the *Complementary and Alternative Medicine {CAM}* box, "Alternative Therapy: Commonly Recommended Herbal Products").

The healthcare practitioner must have some basic understanding of therapeutic claims and dangers of some of these herbal products. Although many cancer patients should not have all hopes for a cure dashed, it behooves the healthcare team to caution patients about the use of these products and to point out those products that are unproven and could be unsafe.

NUTRITIONAL MANAGEMENT OF SELECTED CANCER-RELATED SYMPTOMS

The specific feeding method used depends on the individual patient's condition. However, the classic dictum of nutritional management should prevail: "If the gut works, use it." Details of available enteral and parenteral modes of nutrition support are provided in Chapter 18. If at all possible, an oral diet with supplementation is the most desired form of feeding, of course. A carefully designed personal plan of care based on nutrition assessment data and including adjustments in texture, temperature, food choices, and tolerances, as well as family food patterns, can often meet needs (see the *Perspectives in Practice* box, "Promoting Oral Intake in Patients With Cancer"). Often the hospitalized patient's diet can be supplemented with familiar foods from home as the clinical nutritionist plans with the family. Personal food tolerances will vary according to the current treatment and nature of the disease. A number of adjustments in food texture, temperature, amount, timing, taste, appearance, and form can be made to help alleviate symptoms stemming from common problems in successive parts of the gastrointestinal tract.

Difficulties in eating may be caused by loss of appetite, problems in the mouth, or swallowing problems.

COMPLEMENTARY AND ALTERNATIVE MEDICINE (CAM)
Alternative Therapy: Commonly Recommended Herbal Products

Patients diagnosed with cancer often develop a sense of desperation resulting from feelings of helplessness. Lack of knowledge regarding what is happening in their bodies can lead them to seek out CAM to combat their cancer. When patients take an active role in their treatment, it has been shown to have a positive therapeutic effect. But as for the treatments themselves, results are less optimistic. The fact is that for the most part, alternative cancer treatments are unproven, unscientific, and ineffective methods that in some cases interfere with lifesaving proven treatments.

It is easy to see why CAM would be an attractive alternative to traditional chemotherapy or radiation treatments because those traditional methods are taxing on the body and not 100% effective. But it is important for patients to understand the severity and results of the CAM they use. Although some treatments are as harmless (and possibly helpful) as prayer and touch therapy, others involve invasive risky procedures. Each therapy should be judged on a case-by-case basis as it relates to the condition of the patient. The following list contains a few examples and information about some more well-known CAM treatments.

Herb	Claim	Efficacy	Safety	Current Recommendations
Chaparral	Analgesic Expectorant Diuretic Emetic Antiinflammatory	Studies have shown no anticancer effect.	Long-term use in rats led to lesions in mesentery, lymph nodes, and kidneys. One documented case of liver disease in humans. Removed from the generally recognized as safe (GRAS) list.	Not recommended.
Echinacea	Immune stimulant, wound healer	Widely used in Germany to treat the common cold and respiratory and urinary tract infections. Needs more research	Significant side effects have not been observed. Allergies are always possible.	May be used with caution. Not recommended for longer than 8 consecutive weeks. Not recommended during pregnancy or lactation.
Essiac	Developed by Canadian nurse Rene Cassie to treat cancer.	No anticancer effects.	Not safe for consumption and is illegal to distribute in the United States.	Not recommended.
Ginger	Digestive aid Stimulant Diuretic Antiemetic	Found to be useful in treating motion sickness. Antiemetic properties are due to the local action on the stomach, not on the central nervous system.	No toxicities have been reported. Very large overdoses may cause central nervous system depression and cardiac arrhythmias. Thrombocytopenia has been reported in people taking large doses.	May be used for temporary relief of nausea.
Hoxey herbs	Anticancer agent	No benefit has ever been documented. Note that the originator Harry Hoxey died of prostate cancer while treating himself with his formula.	Not recommended.	Not recommended.

Data from American Cancer Society: *Complementary and alternative therapies*, Atlanta, 2006, Author. Available at *www.cancer.org/docroot/ETO/ETO_5.asp*. Accessed February 23, 2006; Molseed L: Alternative therapies in oncology. In MacCallum PD, Polisena CG, eds: *The clinical guide to oncology nutrition*, Chicago, 2000, American Dietetic Association; and Edzard E, Casselith B: The prevalence of complementary/alternative medicine in cancer, *Cancer* 83 (4):777, 1998.

AIDS, Acquired immunodeficiency disease.

Continued

Herb	Claim	Efficacy	Safety	Current Recommendations
Kombucha tea (Manchurian tea or Kargasok tea)	Immune system stimulator	Unsubstantiated claims of antitumor activity.	Home-brewed "mushroom" usually passed to friends and family members. Susceptible to microbial contamination. Acidosis, aspergillosis, nausea, vomiting, and jaundice have been reported.	Not recommended.
Milk thistle	Liver protector (active ingredient is silymarin)	Appears to protect undamaged liver cells from toxins. May be helpful in cirrhosis and hepatitis.	No adverse effects have been noted.	Safe for use. May have beneficial effects.
Mistletoe (American and European)	American—stimulates smooth muscle, increases blood pressure, increases uterine and intestinal contractions European—decreases blood pressure, antispasmodic, calmative agent	Extracts of the European form have been used as a palliative cancer treatment. There is little evidence supporting effectiveness.	Berries are poisonous, and some evidence suggests that the leaves may also be poisonous.	Not recommended.
Pau D'arco	Powerful tonic Blood builder Anticancer agent Also used to treat diabetes, rheumatism, and ulcers	Has been shown to have activity against cancer in animals but causes severe side effects in humans.	Toxic—induces nausea, vomiting, anemia, and bleeding in humans.	Not recommended.
Peppermint	Digestive aid Antispasmodic	Stimulates bile flow. Stimulates tonus of the lower esophageal sphincter. Appetite stimulant.	Safe for adults. Not recommended for children due to increased choking reflex with menthol.	Safe for adults. Not recommended for children.
Pokeroot	Cathartic Emetic Narcotic Anticancer Dyspepsia Glandular swelling	No efficacy has been demonstrated for any claim except that it is a strong emetic and cathartic.	Extremely toxic. Causes gastroenteritis, hypotension, and hyporespiration. Fatal in children.	Not recommended.

The despair that cancer triggers can lead many to look for additional treatment regimens, some safe and some potentially dangerous. The act of finding and using these alternative or complementary treatments has been proven a therapeutic practice and can give the patient a sense of control in an otherwise chaotic process. Even so, the bottom line remains that patients should be urged to provide total disclosure of all alternative treatments so any adverse side effects can be discussed and avoided.

Name	What It Is	Claims and Risks
Cancell (Protocel, Crocinic Acid, Cantron)	A dark liquid initially produced by a chemist who received its formulation in a dream; this treatment is sometimes used in place of traditional cancer medications.	Although promoted as a cure to all cancers and even AIDS, there have been no studies to support this claim. Formulation of *Cancell* is not totally known, partially due to the fact different manufacturers use different names and ingredients. Although banned, this therapy is still sold and used as a dietary supplement under various names. Possible interactions, flulike symptoms, fatigue, and lack of other treatments could pose considerable risks to the patient using this method.

COMPLEMENTARY AND ALTERNATIVE MEDICINE (CAM)—cont'd
Alternative Therapy: Commonly Recommended Herbal Products

Name	What It Is	Claims and Risks
Colon therapy (colonic, enema irrigation)	Cleansing the large intestine through water or some other liquid formulation.	Touted as a prevention method, colon therapy is literally the removal of waste and "toxins" from the large intestine. There is no scientific evidence supporting any claims of colon therapy or even that toxins accumulate in the large intestine. Procedures are rather invasive and can result in electrolyte imbalance, fluid overload, allergic reactions, intestinal tears, and even death.
Spirituality, religion, and prayer	This is generally a belief in something greater than oneself that exhibits control over lives and events.	Although there is no doubt prayer and other religious methods are therapeutic to many, clinical trials of effectiveness are sketchy at best. However, there is virtually no risk of side effects unless patient refuses traditional treatments in lieu of religious practices.
Heat therapy	Exposing parts or all of the body to high temperatures to increase effectiveness of other treatments	There has been some evidence supporting the claims of this therapy; however, more research is needed. The high death rate relating to whole body heat therapy has been cause for some concern, as well as burns and blisters stemming from the localized heat treatments.

PERSPECTIVES IN PRACTICE
Promoting Oral Intake in Patients With Cancer

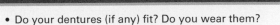

Encouraging and maintaining adequate oral intake for patients with cancer represents one of the most difficult aspects of cancer treatment. It is time consuming and often frustrating but may be one of the most rewarding experiences in patient care. By identifying feeding problems, initiating appropriate interventions, and providing individual education, adequate oral nutrition is promoted. The dietitian is the key figure for coordinating the nutrition program, but its success requires the full support and cooperation of the entire healthcare team, especially the nurse.

The patient interview is one of the most important parts of nutrition assessment. Information that helps identify adequacy of current nutritional intake and potential nutrition problems is obtained during the interview. The following list of questions may assist in gathering accurate information about the patient's ability to obtain oral nutrition:

- How would you describe your appetite?
- Has it changed recently?
- Are you eating differently than you have most of your life?
- Do you usually eat three meals each day? Has this changed recently?
- Are you nauseated or experiencing vomiting? Is this food or medication related? How long have you been experiencing this? How often do you vomit or feel nauseated?
- Do you have a bowel movement every day? Has this changed?
- Do you have diarrhea? If so, do you think this may be food related?
- Do food smells or cooking odors bother you?
- Do you have difficulty chewing?

- Do your dentures (if any) fit? Do you wear them?
- Do you have difficulty swallowing?
- Is your mouth dry? Does your saliva seem to be different? Is it thicker or decreased in amounts?
- Do you find it easier to drink liquids than to eat solid foods?
- What were you able to eat yesterday? (Obtain a brief 24-hour dietary recall.)
- Are you unable to eat certain foods right now?
- Do some foods taste different to you? Can you give an example?
- Have you ever taken any high-kcalorie, high-protein supplements? When? What kind? How often? Were you able to tolerate them?
- Do you take a multivitamin supplement?
- Do you have any food allergies or intolerances? Are these new, or have you always experienced these intolerances?
- Do you prepare your own meals? If so, do you ever feel too tired to prepare something to eat?

The success of the interview depends on the dietitian's professional competence, interviewing skills, and bedside manner. If the dietitian establishes a feeling of comfort and trust with the patient, the opportunity to accomplish successful dietary interventions is great.

References

Bloch AS: Nutrition and cancer: the paradox, *Diet Curr* 23(2):1, 1996.
Marian M: Cancer cachexia: prevalence, mechanisms, and interventions, *Support Line* 20(2):3, 1998.
Nahikian-Nelms ML: Encouraging oral intake. In Bloch AS, ed: *Nutrition management of the cancer patient*, Rockville, Md, 1990, Aspen.

Loss of Appetite

Anorexia is a major problem and curtails food intake when it is needed most. It is a general systemic effect of the cancer disease process itself, often further induced by cancer treatment and progressively enhanced by personal anxiety, depression, and stress of the illness. Such a vicious cycle, if not countered by much effort, can lead to more malnutrition and the well-recognized starvation "cancer cachexia," a syndrome of emaciation, debilitation, and malnutrition (Table 25-3).[34]

A vigorous program of eating, not dependent on appetite for stimulus, must be planned and maintained with patient and family. It is helpful sometimes to develop protein and caloric goals, discussing the role of nutrients and key foods in combating the disease and

TABLE 25-3	Dietary Modifications for Nutrition-Related Side Effects of Cancer
Side Effect	**Suggested Dietary Modifications**
Anorexia	Provide small, frequent meals.
	Offer high-calorie, high-protein, nutrient-dense foods.
	Encourage consumption of the highest calorie, highest protein foods first.
	Suggest commercially available nutritional supplements, as tolerated.
	Avoid foods with offensive odors.
	Encourage favorite foods.
Altered perception of taste and odor	Maximize use of herbs and seasonings to enhance flavor of foods.
	If the flavor and aroma of red meats are offensive, avoid these foods and use alternative protein-rich foods such as chicken, fish, cheese, eggs, and milk.
	Serve cold foods and beverages more often than hot foods and beverages.
	Vary appearance (i.e., color and texture) of foods.
	Prepare and serve food in glass or porcelain rather than metal pans or dishes.
Stomatitis and mucositis	Provide foods in liquid, semisolid, or pureed form.
	Avoid tart, citric, or acidic foods and beverages.
	Avoid extremes in temperature.
	Avoid excessively seasoned and spicy foods.
	Avoid dry, coarse foods; serve foods with sauces or gravies.
	Encourage foods that melt or are liquid or soft textured at room temperature.
	Avoid carbonated beverages.
Xerostomia	Moisten foods with sauces, gravies, liquid, melted butter, mayonnaise, or yogurt.
	Encourage naturally soft, moist foods.
	Encourage sipping of liquids throughout the day.
	Avoid alcohol.
Dysphagia	Provide foods in liquid, semisolid, or pureed form.
	Maximize calorie and protein density of food as possible.
	Use commercially available liquid nutritional supplements.
Nausea and vomiting	Give small, frequent meals.
	Give dry foods without added fats or sauces, such as dry toast.
	Give liquids only between meals.
	Avoid greasy, fried, high-fat foods.
	Avoid foods with strong odors.
Diarrhea	Provide small, frequent meals.
	Encourage plenty of liquids to prevent dehydration.
	Avoid greasy, fried, high-fat foods.
	Consider limiting dietary lactose if these foods exacerbate symptoms.
	Avoid high-fiber foods.
	Avoid gassy, cruciferous vegetables, such as broccoli and cauliflower.
	Avoid caffeine.

Modified from Dobbin M, Harmuller VW: Suggested management of nutrition-related symptoms. In MacCallum PD, Polisena CG, eds: *The clinical guide to oncology nutrition,* Chicago, 2000, American Dietetic Association.

providing support for therapy. With such support both patient and family are better able to build a positive mental attitude toward the diet as an integral part of treatment and are thus more able to accept responsibility for this aspect of therapy. Often this positive attitude of the vital role patients play in their own treatment is a means of gaining some sense of control of their own lives, a sense frequently lost in the bewildering world of cancer and its therapy.

The overall goal is to provide food with as much nutrient density as possible so every bite will count. If appetite is better in the morning, a good breakfast should be emphasized. Food texture may be varied as tolerated, with appeal to sensory perceptions of color, aroma, and taste. A series of small meals with a wide variety of foods is better tolerated than regular larger meals. Getting some exercise before meals and maintaining surroundings that reduce stress may also help in the eating process.

Mouth Problems

Eating difficulties may stem from sore mouth, stomatitis, or taste changes. Sore mouth often results from chemotherapy or from radiation to the head and neck area. It is increased by any state of malnutrition or from infections such as candidiasis (thrush), with numerous ulcerations of the oral and throat mucosa. Frequent small meals and snacks—soft in texture, bland in nature, and cool or cold in temperature—are often better tolerated. There may also be alterations in the tongue's taste buds, causing taste distortion ("taste blindness") and inability to distinguish the basic tastes of salt, sweet, sour, or bitter, with consequent food aversions. Because the aversion is often toward basic protein foods, a high-protein, high-energy liquid drink supplement may be needed. Dental problems may also contribute to mouth difficulties and should be corrected. Salivary secretions are also affected by cancer treatment; therefore foods with a high liquid content should be used. Solid foods may be swallowed more easily with the use of sauces, gravies, broth, yogurt, or salad dressings. A food processor or blender can render foods in semisolid or liquid forms and make them easier to swallow. If the swallowing problem is especially severe because of tumor growth or therapy, guides for a special swallowing training program, including progressive food textures, exercises, and positions, can be followed.

Gastrointestinal Problems

Eating difficulties may include nausea and vomiting, general indigestion, bloating, or specific surgery responses such as the postgastrectomy "dumping" syndrome (see Chapter 23). Nausea is often enhanced by foods that are hot, sweet, fatty, or spicy; these can be avoided according to individual tolerance. Other lower gastrointestinal problems may include general diarrhea, constipation, flatulence, or specific lactose intolerance or surgery responses, such as occur with intestinal resections and various ostomies. Helpful guidance for patients with colostomies, ileostomies, or ileoanal reservoirs is necessary (see Chapter 23). Effect of chemotherapy or radiation treatment on mucosal cells secreting lactase contributes to lactose intolerance. In such cases a nutrient supplement formula that is lactose free or a soy-milk formula should be used.

A number of commercial nutrient supplement products are available. A comparative review of these products will provide the basis for developing a formulary in the hospital setting for a limited number of such products (see Chapter 18). A food processor or blender can be used at home to produce creative solid and liquid food combinations from regular foods for interval liquid supplementation.

Patients with cancer need plenty of encouragement and a feeling of autonomy or personal control for the optimal success of a dietary plan. Sometimes it becomes necessary to make small attainable goals of specific foods and amounts to be consumed. If the patient can be made to view food as important as medication in their daily routine, better success will be likely.

Feeding in Terminal Illness

Although many advances have been made in detection and treatment of cancer, mortality rates for some cancers have not declined and have actually increased for some cancers.[3] In working with patients with cancer, one can automatically see that the progressive weight loss and malnutrition that occur, caused by the primary tumor and its spread, and lead to profound nutritional depletion cause a great deal of personal turmoil, increased morbidity, and overall reduced quality of life. For some patients a time comes when spread of the disease overcomes the body's capacity to combat it. When the patient is no longer able to eat, enteral tube feeding or parenteral feeding may be considered. Ultimately, however, ethical questions about continued feeding efforts are faced in many cases (see the *To Probe Further* box, "When Does Feeding Become an Ethical Issue?"). Answers lie with the patient, as long as possible, and with the family. But sensitive and supportive counseling is needed from the cancer team members, especially the clinical dietitian and nurse responsible for administering the continued feeding and for personal care.

candidiasis Infection with the fungus of the genus *Candida,* generally caused by *C. albicans,* so named for the whitish appearance of its small lesions; usually a superficial infection in moist areas of the skin or inner mucous membranes.

TO PROBE FURTHER

WHEN DOES FEEDING BECOME AN ETHICAL ISSUE?

Plato believed the moral person and the physician both should abide by the Hippocratic principle of medicine: "Above all, do no harm." In recent times others have returned to Plato's use of this medical model of ethics. Current writers assert that an ethic of care rests on the "premise of nonviolence—that no one should be hurt."

Technology such as enteral and parenteral nutrition may sometimes support a caring intent and compassionate spirit, whereas at other times such modern technology becomes a value in and of itself with its own standard of efficiency. Enteral and parenteral feeding techniques may be used to maintain indefinitely patients who are unable to take food orally.

Concerned ethical thinkers use the following moral principles for decisions in regard to life-sustaining treatment that encompasses enteral or parenteral nutrition: benefit to patient, respect for patient autonomy or self-determination, maintenance of moral integrity of health professionals, and justice in distributing scarce medical resources among eligible patients. They offer helpful views to guide clinicians in coming to a reasoned and defensible resolution of moral conflict.

Alternatives to Artificial Nutrition

All options of nutrition support should be explored, not simply the consideration of "Give food or fluids" versus "Do not give food or fluids." Dietitians are particularly useful in identifying alternative feeding strategies. The full range of therapeutic options should be carefully explored instead of assuming that the choices are "Let the patient die" or "Keep the patient alive."

Patient Prognosis for Recovery of Functions

A widely held ethically defensible view is that aggressive means of life prolongation becomes less morally desirable in proportion to the inability of the patient to regain what he or she considers to be useful function. Persistent vegetative state and permanent loss of consciousness are examples of extreme cases where recovery of function is not possible. Accurately determining the prognosis for recovery is essential.

Total Management Plans and Goals of Therapy

The patient's prognosis and nature of the illness might determine whether the goal of medical care is to attempt cure, to manage a chronic illness that cannot be cured so as to maintain maximal patient function, or to allow a terminally ill patient to die with maximal comfort and symptom control.

Nutrition treatment may make sense within one plan of care but no sense at all in another.

Wishes of the Patient or Patient Surrogate

It is legally and ethically acceptable that in almost all cases the voluntary choice of an informed patient should override all other concerns. When the patient cannot choose, a surrogate or other substitute decision maker who is familiar with the patient's values and wishes may be consulted.

Ability of the Patient to Choose

It is important to assess the patient's ability to make the particular medical care choice relevant to the matter at hand. In some circumstances, expert psychiatric or psychologic evaluation is needed to determine this.

Benefits and Burdens of Artificial Treatment

The medical team often tends to overestimate benefits and underestimate burdens of treatments they use routinely. When the means of administering nutrition become invasive and painful, then burdens may become substantial. Restraining the patient or repeated blood draws to monitor effects of total parenteral nutrition may be deemed burdens unacceptable to the patient. Patients may feel being kept alive by artificial means is an indignity itself and life is no longer useful or meaningful to them. Spiritual and emotional burdens should be assessed equally with physical burdens in making accurate assessments of moral obligations to patients.

Modern medical technology has produced circumstances that caregivers and patients alike have never faced before. Decisions regarding nutrition and hydration in terminally ill patients are becoming more frequent. Ethical and moral questions do not always have black or white solutions; there are gray areas to consider. The ethical task for dietitians may be to achieve balance between what works and who cares.

References

Brody H, Noel MB: Dietitians' role in decisions to withhold nutrition and hydration, *J Am Diet Assoc* 91(5):580, 1991.

Dalton S: What are the sources and standards of ethical judgment in dietetics? *J Am Diet Assoc* 91(5):545, 1991.

Edelstein S, Anderson S: Bioethics and dietetics: education and attitudes, *J Am Diet Assoc* 91(5):546, 1991.

Wall MG et al: Feeding the terminally ill: dietitians' attitudes and beliefs, *J Am Diet Assoc* 91(5):549, 1991.

NUTRITION AND CANCER: THE FINAL ANALYSIS

What, then, are our overall final conclusions? As Bloch, an experienced oncology nutrition specialist, has well reminded us, we see nutrition has a dual role in relation to cancer—both prevention and therapy.[29]

Preventive Role

Nutrition and health professionals have a major wellness role in maintaining health and preventing illness, especially in relation to cancer. This role is embodied in the American Cancer Society's dietary guidelines, as follows[43]:

1. Choose most of the foods you eat from plant sources.
    - Eat five or more servings of fruits and vegetables each day.
    - Eat other foods from plant sources, such as breads, cereals, grain products, rice, pasta, or beans, several times each day.
2. Limit your intake of high-fat foods, particularly from animal sources. Choose foods low in fat. Limit consumption of meats, especially high-fat meats.
3. Be physically active; achieve and maintain a healthy weight. Be at least moderately active for 30 minutes

or more on most days of the week. Stay within your healthy weight range.

4. Limit consumption of alcoholic beverages, if you drink at all.

These guidelines are similar to the overall *Dietary Guidelines for Americans 2005* (see Chapter 1). They are displayed in the 2005 *MyPyramid Food Guidance System* and emphasized in national and state health initiatives, including encouraging Americans to eat more servings of fruits and vegetables every day.[44] This emphasis stems from certain compounds found in plants, thus called phytochemicals ("plant chemicals"), which ongoing research indicates have promising effects in chemoprevention of cancer.[23] As indicated, these compounds include food nutrients—vitamins A (and its analogues), C, and E—as well as nonnutritive substances such as indoles, isothiocyanates, dithiolthiones, and organosulfur.[24,25]

Therapeutic Role

For the patient with cancer, the clinical dietitian must shift into a therapeutic role, in which the patient is central in diet planning during disease stages and therapy effects. Nutrition therapy must now focus constantly on proactive assessment with early and continuing preventive measures to intervene wisely before malnutrition occurs. For example, anticipate possible gastrointestinal needs or psychosocial situations that relate to appetite, eating various foods, or drug effects. Provide information concerning mouth care, symptoms experienced, or drug actions and effects. The cancer diagnosis need not be a ticket to starvation. With appropriate pain control and treatment for chemotherapy and radiation-induced side effects, patients with cancer can continue to eat well through the latter stages of their disease. The clinical dietitian and healthcare team should work closely together with the patient to plan meals and snacks based on food preferences and dislikes, subjective intolerance of certain foods, and difficulties in chewing and swallowing.

Health Promotion

Toward the Prevention of Cancer

Studies of geographic, socioeconomic, chronologic, and immigration patterns of cancer distribution indicate the vast majority of cases of cancer are primarily caused by environmental factors. The logical conclusion is that reduction of these causative factors may reduce or eliminate most forms of cancer.[45-51]

The American Cancer Society suggests that two thirds of all cases of cancer in the United States are caused by only two factors: inhaled smoke and ingested food. Tobacco, alone or in combination with alcohol, remains the most important cause of cancer, accounting for about one of every three cancer deaths in the United States. Cigarettes are the most important cause of tobacco-related cancer, but other forms of tobacco (chewing tobacco and snuff) are also established carcinogens. Cancer risk of ex-smokers remains elevated compared with lifetime nonsmokers. However, quitting smoking, even late in life after heavy long-term abuse, greatly reduces cancer risk when compared with the risk of continued smoking. Despite the rhetoric of tobacco companies, even regular smokers of low-tar cigarettes have a much higher cancer risk than nonsmokers.[45-51]

Alcohol, in addition to its synergistic effects with tobacco, increases risk of cancers of the oral cavity, pharynx, liver, and esophagus. Alcohol use has also been consistently linked to colorectal cancer and female breast cancer. Liquor, wine, and beer seem to be equal in effect on cancer risk.

Major incriminating dietary factors that appear now to be carcinogenic are the food changes that contrast current Western diets with those of our Paleolithic hunter-gatherer ancestors. We have reduced the amount of energy we obtain from starchy foods by one half to two thirds. We have decreased our intake of dietary fiber by 75%. We have more than doubled the proportion of energy we derive from fat and changed from mostly unsaturated fats to saturated fats. We have increased our salt intake fivefold, and sugar now accounts for one fifth of our total energy intake. The diet of our ancestors was energy dilute, whereas our modern diet is energy dense.[45-51]

Many studies link what we eat and do not eat to development of cancer. Direct relationships between preserved or salty foods and nasopharynx and stomach cancer have been consistently observed in case control and correlational studies. Generous ingestion of fresh fruits and vegetables has consistently been found to decrease the risk of stomach cancer. Epidemiologic studies suggest a relation between high-animal-fat, low-fiber intakes and colorectal cancer. The basis for this relationship lies in decreased transit time through the colon associated with high-fiber diets and increased water content in the intestinal lumen that dilutes other nutrients such as animal fat.

Considerable, although not yet conclusive, evidence exists that ascorbic acid has a protective effect against cancer of the esophagus, larynx, and oral cavity. Nutrients such as vitamin A, beta-carotene, vitamin E, and ascorbic acid are thought to lower cancer risk in patients with elevated risk for cancers of the lung, esophagus, colon, and skin. Clinical and laboratory studies support findings that adequate intakes of vitamin D and calcium are associated with reduced incidence of colorectal cancer. These studies did not necessarily use supplemental amounts of these nutrients in addition to the RDAs but were based more on low levels of intake of these nutrients, which would parallel the low levels of fresh fruit and vegetable intakes that are prevalent in our society.

The majority of the causes of cancer—such as tobacco, alcohol, animal fat, obesity, and ultraviolet light—are associated with lifestyle, that is, personal choices and not environmental causes. This fact reinforces the basic truth that the best cure is prevention. Lifestyle changes, including regular exercise, are the best prevention.[45-51]

TO SUM UP

Cancer is a term applied to abnormal, malignant growths in various body tissue sites. The cancerous cell is derived from a normal cell that loses control over cell reproduction. Cancer cell development occurs via mutation, carcinogens, radiation, and oncogenic viruses. It is also influenced by many epidemiologic factors such as diet, alcohol, and smoking, as well as physical and psychologic stress factors. Cell development is mediated by the body's immune system, primarily its T cells, a type of white blood cell found in blood, lymph, and certain parts of the lymph nodes and spleen, and B cells, which manufacture and secrete antibodies.

Cancer therapy consists primarily of surgery, radiation, and chemotherapy. Supportive nutrition therapy for the patient with cancer should be highly individualized and depends on the response of each body system to the disease and to the treatment itself. It is based on a thorough nutrition assessment and provided by a number of routes—oral, tube feeding, peripheral vein, and total parenteral nutrition. The oral route is preferred if at all possible. Nutrient requirements and feeding mode must be designed for the specific physical and psychologic needs of individual patients.

QUESTIONS FOR REVIEW

1. What is cancer? Identify and describe several major causes of cancer cell formation.
2. How does your body attempt to defend itself against cancer? What nutritional factors may diminish this ability?
3. List and describe the rationale and mode of action of the types of therapies used to treat cancer.
4. Differentiate those factors challenging cancer recovery that are associated with the disease versus the type of therapy used.
5. Outline the general procedure for the nutritional management of a patient with cancer.

REFERENCES

1. U.S. Department of Health and Human Services: *Healthy people 2010: with understanding and improving health and objectives for improving health,* ed 2, 2 vols, Washington, DC, 2000, U.S. Government Printing Office.
2. Ries LAG et al: The annual report to the nation on the status of cancer, with a special section on colorectal cancer, 1970-1997, *Cancer* 88:2398, 2000.
3. Greenlee RT et al: Cancer statistics 2001, *CA Cancer J Clin* 51:15, 2001.
4. Miller AB: *Diet in cancer prevention,* Online WHO Database, 2001, World Health Organization. Available at *www.who.int/library/database/index.en.shtml.*
5. Miller AB et al: *Racial/ethnic patterns of cancer in the United States, 1988-1992,* Publication No. 956-4104, Bethesda, Md, 1996, National Cancer Institute.
6. Klein G: Fould's dangerous ideas revisited: the multistep development of tumors 40 years later, *Adv Cancer Res* 72:1, 1998.
7. Reif AE, Hearen T: Consensus on synergism between cigarette smoke and other environmental carcinogens in the causation of lung cancer, *Adv Cancer Res* 76:161, 1999.
8. Ross J: Structure and function of the gene. In Abeloff MD et al, eds: *Clinical oncology,* ed 2, New York, 2000, Churchill Livingstone.
9. Whiteman DC, Whiteman CA, Green AC: Childhood sun exposure as a risk factor for melanoma: a systematic review of epidemiologic studies, *Cancer Causes Control* 12:69, 2001.
10. deGruijl FR: Skin cancer and solar UV radiation, *Eur J Cancer* 35:2003, 1999.
11. Franco EL, Duarte-Franco E, Ferenczy A: Cervical cancer: epidemiology, prevention and the role of human papillomavirus infection, *CMAJ* 164:1017, 2001.
12. Sourvinos G, Tsatsanis C, Spandidos DA: Mechanisms of retrovirus-induced oncogenesis, *Folia Biol (Praha)* 46:226, 2000.
13. Holland JC: Cancer's psychological challenges, *Sci Am* 275(3):158, 1996.
14. Foley KM: Controlling the pain of cancer, *Sci Am* 275(3):164, 1996.
15. Burnet FM: Immunologic surveillance in neoplasia, *Transplant Rev* 7:3, 1971.
16. Boon T et al: T-lymphocyte response. In Abeloff MD et al, eds: *Clinical oncology,* ed 2, New York, 2000, Churchill Livingstone.
17. Matarese G: Leptin and the immune system: how nutritional status influences immune response, *Eur Cytokine Netw* 11:7, 2000.
18. Carlson GL: The influence of nutrition and sepsis upon wound healing, *J Wound Care* 8(9):471, 1999.
19. Dureil B, Matuszczak Y: Alteration in nutritional status and diaphragm muscle function, *Reprod Nutr Dev* 38:175, 1998.
20. Bozzetti F et al: Perioperative total parenteral nutrition in malnourished gastrointestinal cancer patients: a randomized clinical trial, *J Am Soc Parenter Enteral Nutr* 24:7, 2000.
21. Hellman S, Vokes EE: Advancing current treatments for cancer, *Sci Am* 275(3):118, 1996.
22. Watzl B, Watson RR: Role of alcohol abuse in nutrition immunosuppression, *J Nutr* 122:733, 1992.
23. Greenwald P: Chemoprevention of cancer, *Sci Am* 275(3):96, 1996.
24. Kelloff GJ et al: Progress in cancer chemoprevention: development of diet-derived chemopreventive agents, *J Nutr* 130:467S, 2000.
25. Walaadkhan AR, Clemens MR: Effect of dietary phytochemicals on cancer development, *Int J Mol Med* 1(4):742, 1998.
26. Vanderhoof JA: Probiotics: future directions, *Am J Clin Nutr* 73(suppl):1152S, 2001.
27. Aulas JJ: Alternative cancer treatments, *Sci Am* 275(3):162, 1996.
28. Loprinzi CL et al: Body composition changes in patients who gain weight while receiving megestrol acetate, *J Clin Oncol* 11:152, 1993.
29. Bloch AS: Nutrition and cancer: the paradox, *Diet Curr* 23(2):1, 1996.

30. Menashiam L et al: Improved food intake and reduced nausea and vomiting in patients given a restricted diet while receiving cisplatin chemotherapy, *J Am Diet Assoc* 92(2):58, 1992.

31. Darbinian J, Coulston A: Impact of chemotherapy on the nutritional status of the cancer patient. In Bloch AS, ed: *Nutrition management of the cancer patient*, Rockville, Md, 1990, Aspen.

32. Wilson RL: Optimizing nutrition for patients with cancer, *Clin J Oncol Nurs* 4(1):23, 2000.

33. Tayek JA, Chlebowski RT: Metabolic response to chemotherapy in colon cancer patients, *J Parenter Enter Nutr* 16(suppl 6):65, 1992.

34. Shaw JHF et al: Leukine kinetics in patients with benign disease, non-weight losing cancer and cancer cachexia: studies at the whole body level and the response to nutritional support, *Surgery* 109:37, 1991.

35. Tisdale MJ: Wasting in cancer, *J Nutr* 129(1):243S, 1999.

36. Polisena GG: Nutrition concerns in the radiation therapy patient. In McCallum PD, Polisena CG, eds: *The clinical guide to oncology*, Chicago, 2000, American Dietetic Association.

37. Djuric Z et al: Effects of a low-fat diet on levels of oxidative damage to DNA in human peripheral nucleated blood cells, *J Natl Cancer Inst* 83(11):766, 1991.

38. Burns CP, Spector AA: Effects of lipids on cancer therapy, *Nutr Rev* 48(6):233, 1990.

39. Molseed L: Alternative therapies in oncology. In McCallum PD, Polisena CG, eds: *The clinical guide to oncology nutrition*, Chicago, 2000, American Dietetic Association.

40. Ross C: Vitamin A and protective immunity, *Nutr Today* 27(4):18, 1992.

41. Henson DE et al: Ascorbic acid: biologic functions and relation to cancer, *J Natl Cancer Inst* 83(8):547, 1991.

42. Prasad KN, Edwards-Prasad J: Expressions of some molecular cancer risk factors and their modification by vitamins, *J Am Coll Nutr* 9(1):28, 1990.

43. American Cancer Society: *Guidelines for nutrition in cancer prevention*, Atlanta, 1999, American Cancer Society.

44. Foerster SB et al: California's "5-a-Day-For Better Health" campaign: an innovative population-based effort to effect large-scale dietary change, *Am J Prev Med* 11:124, 1995.

45. Garland CF et al: Can colon cancer incidence and death rates be reduced with calcium and vitamin D? *Am J Clin Nutr* 54:193S, 1991.

46. Henderson BE et al: Toward the primary prevention of cancer, *Science* 254:1131, 1991.

47. Kalman DS, Villani LJ: Exercise and the cancer patient, *On-Line* 6(1):1 [American Dietetic Association].

48. Leffell DJ, Brash DE: Sunlight and skin cancer, *Sci Am* 275(1):52, 1996.

49. Trichopoulos D et al: What causes cancer? *Sci Am* 275(3):80, 1996.

50. Willett WC et al: Strategies for minimizing cancer risk, *Sci Am* 275(3):88, 1996.

51. Wynder EL: Primary prevention of cancer: planning and policy considerations, *J Natl Cancer Inst* 83(7):475, 1991.

FURTHER READINGS AND RESOURCES

Readings

Bloch AS, ed: *Nutrition management of the cancer patient*, Rockville, Md, 1990, Aspen.
This helpful reference by an experienced oncology dietitian and her contributors provides a comprehensive background for a better understanding of the complexities of caring for cancer patients.

Bloch AS, Thomson CA: Position of the American Dietetic Association: phytochemicals and functional foods, *J Am Diet Assoc* 95(4):493, 1995.

Steinmetz KA, Potter JD: Vegetables, fruit, and cancer prevention: a review, *J Am Diet Assoc* 96(10):1027, 1996.
These two statements, one an American Dietetic Association position paper and the other a review of the role of certain foods in cancer prevention, provide important information for counseling.

Kalman D, Villani LJ: Nutritional aspects of cancer-related fatigue, *J Am Diet Assoc* 97(6):650, 1997.
This article describes the fatigue associated with cancer and its treatment and ways in which all cancer team members may contribute to using nutritional management to minimize these side effects and broaden the patient's nutritional limits and food choices.

Websites of Interest

- American Cancer Society: *www.cancer.org/docroot/home/index.asp*
- National Cancer Institute: *www.cancer.gov/*
- OncoLink (University of Pennsylvania): *www.oncolink.com/*
- Breastcancer.org: *www.breastcancer.org/*
- WebMD: *www.webmd.com/diseases_and_conditions/cancer.htm*
- American Association for Cancer Research: *www.aacr.org/*
- M.D. Anderson Cancer Center (University of Texas): *www.mdanderson.org/*

CHAPTER 26

Chronic Disabling Conditions and Rehabilitation

Ethan Bergman and Nancy Buergel

This chapter completes our clinical nutrition series. In addition to the primary care clinical problems we reviewed in preceding chapters of this section, we conclude with a focus on chronic disabling diseases that require rehabilitative care.

Persons who have sustained severe injury or illness often require extended specialized care. These long-term needs result from the stress of disabling injury or illness, which carries added physical, mental, and social burdens. Such situations often involve profound trauma and devastating effects that call for tremendous coping resources.

In this final chapter we examine the supportive role of nutrition therapy in the rehabilitative process. We look at musculoskeletal disease, neuromuscular disease, and progressive neurologic disorders. In each case we see personalized nutrition care plays a vital role in the healing and restoring process. Such care demands special knowledge and skills.

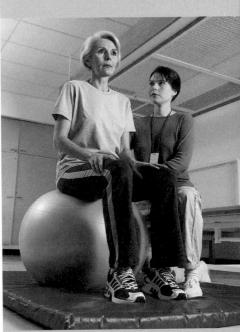

Copyright 2006 JupiterImages Corporation.

◆ FOCUS ON CULTURE

Cultural Aspects of Dietary Adherence

Compliance with nutrition education during rehabilitation is achieved by only 50% of patients, with fewer than 20% maintaining long-term changes. This can be an intimidating and discouraging fact for many dietitians and nutrition educators to deal with. Yet, it is the job of the nutrition professional to identify obstacles that may affect compliance and try to work through them with their patients. One obstacle in dietary compliance that merits particular consideration is cultural food practices and traditions. Cultural practices can often be overlooked, but if these practices are used in association with a healthy eating plan, they can potentially increase short- and long-term adherence and overall health.

Culture itself can have a huge effect on the way patients perceive the rehabilitation process. Their views of the human body's physical, mental, and spiritual states can modify the effectiveness of any form of rehabilitation, including the nutritional aspect. In most cases the health professional is able to grasp only a superficial level of understanding about a particular culture and as such must strive for an openness of mind that will allow him or her to appreciate obstacles the particular client might encounter.

Culturally specific dietary interventions, both professional and peer led, have been shown to improve eating habits in a variety of different ethnic and racial minority populations. This almost certainly relates to the fact that most cultures think of food as more than simply a source of nutritional value; food is part of celebration, tradition, and comfort. If a dietary change instituted a total overhaul of their traditional diet, it is unlikely that there will be any significant success. On the other hand, by using dietary customs and foodstuffs are already imbedded in their routine, the odds of compliance rise considerably.

When working with a diverse population, healthcare professionals can often think of cultural differences as a stumbling block. Lack of personal knowledge pertaining to the culture of a patient can lead to total avoidance of the topic. Conversely, by altering this mindset, learning about cultural aspects, and using them as a tool, dietary adherence after rehabilitation can be easier for the client and result in higher success rates.

Cultural Dietary Assessment Tools
- Identify cultural beliefs and how the patient practices these.
- Identify individual beliefs about health as they apply to culture and beliefs.
- Identify patients' support system: community, family, spiritual/religious.
- Recognize possible cultural barriers that could interfere with therapy.
- Focus on cultural foods that DO fit into a specific diet plan, not on ones that do not.

Implementation of Cultural Dietary Plans
- Customize a diet plan that adheres to cultural dietary practices.
- Produce education materials that are written at a suitable level and are linguistically and culturally appropriate.
- Use translators and peers to facilitate.
- Employ culturally suitable approaches to therapy (talking circles, prayers, use of elders as leaders).
- Understand and incorporate holidays, values, and traditions into the diet plan.

References

Chyun D et al: Coronary heart disease prevention and lifestyle interventions: cultural influences, *J Cardiovasc Nurs* 18(4):302, 2003.

Hartvell D, Henry J: Dietary advice for patients undergoing coronary artery bypass surgery: falling on deaf ears? *Int J Food Sci Nutr* 54:37, 2003.

Kiokkalainen M et al: Difficulties in changing the diet in relation to dietary fat intake among patients with coronary heart disease, *Eur J Clin Nutr* 53:120, 1999.

NUTRITION THERAPY AND REHABILITATION

Goals of Supportive Care and the Role of the Dietitian

Care for those with chronic disabling disease or injury is guided by positive goals. Successful support is rooted in a positive philosophy based on the optimal potential of each person affected. This approach requires a specialized team working with the patient and family to meet individualized needs. Within each situation, two goals are fundamental in planning care: (1) prevention of further disability and (2) restoration of potential function. Healthcare workers and their clients have developed many creative care techniques to meet these twin goals. Together with other specialized therapists on an individual's rehabilitation team, the registered dietitian functions as the nutrition specialist and carries out the following responsibilities[1]:

- *Nutrition screening:* An initial screening to identify clients with nutrition problems potentially leading to malnutrition.

- *Nutrition assessment:* A comprehensive process to evaluate nutritional status of the client by using medical, dietary, and medication histories; laboratory data; and anthropometric measurements such as weight and height.

- *Nutrition care plan:* A plan developed to care for the client's short-term and long-term needs in a culturally appropriate manner. Part of the care plan may include nutrition education and counseling, involving work with the individual client, family, and other caregivers to best understand and achieve the nutrition goals[2] (see also the *Focus on Culture* box, "Cultural Aspects of Dietary Adherence").

- *Nutrition monitoring:* Periodic evaluation to determine if the care plan is effective and if clinical changes have occurred that may alter the continuing therapy.

In addition to clinical nutrition therapy responsibilities, the dietitian has other related responsibilities, including coordination of community services. These may include referrals and communication with centers and agencies involved in home healthcare, rehabilitation, public health, vocation, financial assistance, or other services.

TO PROBE FURTHER

WHAT ARE THE ETHICAL CONCERNS?

As with all areas of medicine, there is considerable debate over the ethical considerations of disability and rehabilitation. Issues such as life-sustaining treatment, withholding nutrition and hydration, and assisted death all fall under the main heading of quality of life. Since the time of Hippocrates there have been many controversial definitions in the evolution of clinical ethics; however, it mainly means to search for the good and right option when one faces a choice about a potential action. Religious, cultural, and legal factors may all play a part in ethics but do not singly affect the outcome.

The 1976 New Jersey Supreme Court decision that recognized the right of Karen Ann Quinlan's family to withdraw medical treatment they believed she would not have wanted was a landmark in the advent of modern clinical ethics. One of the recommendations handed down by the justice system relating to this case was that alternative means of resolving ethical dilemmas should be developed by healthcare institutions, specifically mentioning an *ethics committee*. Also developed at this point was the *Quinlan formula* that aided professionals in resolving dilemmas of this nature.

Rehabilitation for catastrophic illness or injury is complex and labor intensive. It requires interaction between patient, caregivers, and staff to achieve the best possible outcome. Strong emotions and psychologic barriers are inevitable at the onset of hospitalization, as well as throughout rehabilitation, often shaping the course of treatment. At the crux of ethical decision making is compassion for the individual and commitment to creating a healing environment.

It is helpful to have advance directives in place for each patient upon admission so these decisions are clear, but this is not always the case. Other useful tools are clinical pathways that act as a roadmap, indicating how to proceed based on a particular clinical situation. The ultimate goal is to care for a patient "holistically," considering all aspects and caring for him or her as an individual with decision-making capabilities either now or at a previous point in life.

In March 2005, for the first time in the history of the United States, the U.S. Congress met in a special session to pass a piece of legislation for one person, Terri Schiavo. Ms. Schiavo was a Florida woman who was in a persistent vegetative state. She became a public figure when her husband, Michael Schiavo, and her parents became embroiled over the continued use of a feeding tube to provide nutrition for her. Mr. Schiavo wanted the tube removed, and Ms. Schiavo's parents wanted it maintained.

In 1990, when Ms. Schiavo was 27 years old, she suffered from cardiac arrest, possibly because of a potassium imbalance. As a result, she lived in a persistent vegetative state. In 1998 Michael Schiavo petitioned the court to remove the feeding tube against the wishes of Ms. Schiavo's parents. The judge determined that there was convincing evidence Ms. Schiavo would choose to remove the tube if she were able to make that decision. An appeals court upheld the first judge's decision, and the Florida Supreme Court declined to review it. The parents continued and presented new evidence and had the case reviewed once more. The original court decision was upheld.

The court battle and the publicity surrounding the Schiavo case centered around the wishes of the client, Terri Schiavo. Because Ms. Schiavo had not signed an advance directive determining her end-of-life wishes, the court battle ensued. If Ms. Schiavo had signed an advance directive with regard to surviving on a feeding tube, there would not have been an issue to resolve.

References

Annas GJ: "Culture of life" politics at the bedside—the case of Terri Schiavo, *N Engl J Med* 352(16):1710, 2005.

In re Quinlan, 355 A.2d 647 (NJ 1976), *cert denied*, 429 US 1992.

Quill T: Terri Schiavo—a tragedy compounded, *N Engl J Med* 352(16):1630, 2005.

Sakakihara Y: Ethical attitudes of Japanese physicians regarding life-sustaining treatment for children with severe neurological disabilities, *Brain Dev* 22(2):113, 2000.

Shevell M: Ethical issues in neurodevelopmental disabilities, *Curr Opin Pediatr* 11(6):508, 1999.

Stanley AL: Withholding artificially provided nutrition and hydration from disabled children: assessing their quality of life, *Clin Pediatr* 39(10):575, 2000.

Team Approach Method

In some devastating cases, obstacles may seem almost insurmountable. Chronic incurable disease or a poor prognosis can be overwhelming to clients and their caregivers; the client's initial reaction is often one of defeat, resignation, or withdrawal. However, the healthcare team can draw on its tremendous resources to set positive goals and meet the various needs of clients. Rehabilitation team specialists include the physician (physiatrist), clinical dietitian, nurse, occupational therapist, physical therapist, psychologist, speech pathologist, and social worker. These sensitive and skilled specialists lend their particular expertise, insights, and resources to identify and meet specific personal needs.

At all times, however, these healthcare specialists remember the most important member of the team is the client; they always work with, not for, the client and family to help develop solutions. Goal setting is always personal. These three partners—professional specialists, client, and family—form a greater healthcare team. Rehabilitation is always a shared, supportive undertaking, whatever the individual client's limitations or outcome (see the *To Probe Further* box, "What Are the Ethical Concerns?").

> disability A mental or physical impairment that prevents an individual from performing one or more gainful activities; not synonymous with handicap, which implies serious disadvantage.
>
> advance directives Instructions for medical treatment given by a patient while he or she has decisional capacity to do so.
>
> clinical pathways Clear standards or protocols for patient care that are designed to promote cost efficiency, better outcomes, and faster recovery.

Socioeconomic and Psychologic Factors

Social Attitudes

General attitudes of society toward disabled persons vary between extremes of overprotection and avoidance. These social attitudes are not easily changed. Deformities or severe illness may make some people uncomfortable, perhaps because they are reminded of their own vulnerability and mortality. Others may be unsure how to work with ill or disabled individuals or choose to completely ignore them. However, disabled persons do have varying special needs, and social avoidance of these needs manifests itself as obstacles to basic mobility: there are doorways not made for wheelchairs, unmanageable stairs and curbing, lack of access to public transportation, and many more daily barriers. At the opposite extreme, overprotection robs a person of his or her dignity and smothers the will to fight against surrounding odds and develop self-acceptance. Balance is needed. Social attitudes toward people of disability will be more helpful if they exist between the two extremes of overprotection and avoidance.

Economic Problems

Care for a person with a disabling injury or severe illness can be a long and costly process: a major area of exploration for the healthcare team is one of financial resources. A skilled financial expert can work with insurance companies and the patient's personal finances to get the best care with the least possible monetary burden. Continuing long-term economic problems may revolve around the client's employment capabilities or earning capacities and the cost of providing care.

Living Situation

Disabled persons face many practical problems in everyday living. Whether a person needs long-term hospital care or can maintain independent living, perhaps with an attendant, depends on a number of physical and situational factors. If the person can maintain a home, then necessary special equipment for maximal self-care enables the person to do more things for himself or herself and helps preserve his or her sense of agency and self-worth.[3] Depending on the disability, chewing, swallowing, and manipulating eating utensils may be problems. These issues often result in problems maintaining food quality, desirable food temperatures, and adequacy of intake that can ultimately lead to malnutrition.

Psychologic Barriers

Positive resolution of many practical and emotional problems requires tremendous psychologic adjustment. Every person with physical body trauma struggles with self-image and, understandably, may withdraw in defeat and exhaustion. Changes that occur during rehabilitation processes test both inner strength and physical stamina: depending on personal resources and strengths, an individual may or may not be able to function. Much of the healthcare team's keen insight and concern are directed toward supporting each person's efforts to meet individual needs. That many disabled persons do reach self-care goals in some measure is evident in the remarkable achievements some of them attain, despite or perhaps because of their difficulties.

Psychosocial Implications of the Inability to Self-Feed

Sometimes a person is unable to make the transition to self-feeding due to an inability to physically move the food to the mouth or the inability to swallow. When alternate means of nutrient intake are necessary, another psychologic adjustment is needed. Many individuals in this circumstance feel anger, frustration, fear, sadness, and a sense of grief because of their inability to complete this basic, fundamental task.

Disabled persons who are unable to self-feed may feel a sense of hopelessness that disrupts their ability to function in other ways, such as interacting socially with family and friends. They may become clinically depressed and require psychologic counseling and antidepressant medication. Clinical signs of depression include lethargy, social withdrawal, irritability, fatigue, self-loathing, and suicidal thoughts.[4]

Special Needs of Older Disabled Persons

America is aging because Americans are living longer. The Federal Interagency Forum on Aging Related Statistics states that by 2050 there will be almost 87 million people 65 years old or older living in the United States.[5] During the next decade the most rapid population increase will be among those older than 85 years. From 2000 to 2010 the number of individuals in the United States 85 years and over is projected to increase from 4.2 million to 6.1 million. This increase is expected to continue, and by 2050 the projected number over 85 years is 20.9 million.

With older age comes an increased number of disabled older adults. The age-adjusted proportion of older Americans with a chronic disability declined from 25% in 1984 to 20% in 1999. However, because there are more older Americans, the total number with chronic disabilities increased from 6.2 million to 6.8 million in the same time frame. According to the National Institute on Aging (NIA), about 79% of people age 70 years or older have at least one of seven potentially disabling conditions (arthritis, hypertension, heart disease, diabetes, respiratory diseases, stroke, and cancer).[5,6] Increased services, including rehabilitation services, are needed, but rehabilitation needs of older persons differ from those of younger people.

National Long-Term Care Survey Results

Fortunately, during the past decade there has been a sharp decline in the observed rate of disability for people 65 years old or older. In a landmark study, researchers used the 1982 disability rates from the National Long-Term Care Survey (NLTCS) for people 65 years old or older to estimate the numbers of disabled persons in each future year using data from the Census Bureau projections. They then used subsequent waves of the NLTCS to determine the actual numbers of disabled persons and compared that with their estimates. Using this method, they observed 1.6 million fewer disabled older people in the United States in 1998 than there would have been if the disability rate had not changed since 1982. These decreases in disability have been confirmed using multiple databases and have been shown to benefit both men and women and both minority and nonminority populations. The latest preliminary findings from the 1999 NLTCS suggest the rate of decline in chronic disability is continuing and may be accelerating in a downward trend.[7]

Life-Changing Events of Aging

Although chronic disability is declining, the aging American population will still require special care because of their changing needs. Three life-changing events of aging determine needs: retirement, chronic illnesses, and general physical decline.

Vocational Rehabilitation

Without adequate planning, many older persons experience stressful disorientation with retirement. After a lifetime of active involvement in a familiar working environment, retirees suddenly lack a sense of stability and identity. Supportive activities focus on vocational planning and the effective use of leisure time. At this point, many persons have not been accustomed to viewing leisure activities in a positive manner and need help in making this adjustment. In addition, vocational programs can help persons find gainful employment after they retire from work and can also help retired healthy Americans find ways of contributing their wisdom and skills to younger workers in their field of specialty. In turn, such activity can enhance the health and social assets of the older person.

Residual Disabilities From Illnesses

In the age period of 60 to 75 years (the young-old), rehabilitation is focused on problems of chronic diseases of aging—heart disease, hypertension, stroke, and cancer. Chronic illnesses may also be related to damaging health behaviors such as alcoholism, smoking, excessive calorie intake from foods high in fat and salt, and a sedentary lifestyle. Survival after a heart attack or stroke occurs more often with modern medical care. Early efforts at rehabilitation help prevent disability, avoid complications, and restore reasonable function.

Physical Decline in Aging

In persons from 75 to 85 years of age and older (the old-old), disability increases sharply. Much of this increase comes from falls and resulting fractures, chronic brain failure, disorders in locomotion, impaired senses of perception, and increased problems with drug reactions and interactions. Older persons may have several different diseases and take a number of different drugs or receive a variety of medical treatments. In this age-group, minor disabilities often result in major handicaps. Mental and physical dependency may require supportive care in the home or long-term care facility. The Global Burden of Disease Project reported the leading causes of worldwide disability are different than the leading causes of death and includes 6 neuropsychiatric disorders among the top 20 causes of disability.[8]

Common health problems in both young-old and old-old groups involve nutrition care as well. These problems include arthritis, cardiorespiratory and cardiovascular insufficiency, depression, sensory deprivation, infections, skin and foot disorders, and nutritional deficiencies from poor dental health and fad diets.

Disease and disability do not affect only older adults. Many disabled groups include young people, and many older adults continue to be fit and healthy. However, the increasing age of the general population inevitably brings with it an increasing number of older adults with chronic disease and various disabilities of aging. Even minor disabilities may cause major handicaps in everyday living, and minor injuries may bring major debilitating results. In any case, goals of rehabilitation care are to prevent further disability and to restore the maximal function available.

PRINCIPLES OF NUTRITION THERAPY

Prevention of Malnutrition

Calories

Part of the responsibility of the registered dietitian in rehabilitation is to assess calorie and nutrient needs of the client and periodically monitor the client's intake to ensure current nutritional needs are being met. The rehabilitative process of physical therapy involves hard work. The patient tires easily, and energy intake must be sufficient to meet the energy output demands. Excess calories must be avoided to prevent obesity, but sufficient energy for physical activity and tissue metabolism is essential.

---

handicap A mental or physical defect that may or may not be congenital, which prevents the individual from participating in normal life activities; implies disadvantage.

Protein

Protein is needed to maintain general strength of tissue structure and function. Tissue and organ integrity protects against catabolism, infections, negative nitrogen balance, and pressure sores. Dietary protein in optimal quantity (15% to 20% of total kcalories) and quality ensures the necessary supply of all essential amino acids required for tissue synthesis. In addition to these general needs, severe trauma such as that involved in spinal cord injury (SCI) brings special needs to meet the catabolic response.

Carbohydrate

For persons with physical trauma, general energy needs are great. These needs are met by dietary carbohydrate as the body's major fuel source (approximately 50% to 60% of kcalories). Severe trauma requires maximal carbohydrate, especially in the early stages after injury. Protein helps to provide needed energy but is primarily used for other purposes such as tissue rebuilding and integrity. Thus sufficient carbohydrate-rich foods are important to provide the needed energy, as well as to prevent protein catabolism and negative nitrogen balance.

Fat

Fat is a calorically dense form of energy that supplies essential fatty acids and adds palatability to the diet. The general dietary recommendation that fat supply about 25% to 30% of the total kcalories is usually sufficient. There are certain circumstances, however, such as the disabled client with diabetes or chronic obstructive pulmonary disease, where percentage of calories from fat may be adjusted above 30% of total calories from fat.

Vitamins and Minerals

Optimal intake of vitamins and minerals is needed for metabolic activity and maintenance of tissue reserves. Normal Dietary Reference Intake (DRI, including Recommended Daily Allowance [RDA] and Adequate Intake [AI]) standards for age and sex are adequate in most cases. However, a deficiency state such as anemia indicates need for supplementation. In some rehabilitation centers, multivitamin preparations are given routinely to ensure adequate amounts.

Restoration of Eating Ability

Normal Development of the Eating Process

In normal growth and development of a child, the feeding and eating process develops through an overlapping and interdependent series of physical and psychologic stages. Usual activities of eating—swallowing, chewing, hand and utensil use—gradually develop with motor ability. Learning comes with much practice and patience.

In a sense, the injured person must "start over" and gradually relearn these basic skills.

With an understanding of these normal patterns, the disabled person works with the professional team of occupational and physical therapists, dietitians, and nurses to find adaptive procedures to restore basic eating ability. For each client the eating process will require individual attention to the following aspects:

- Nature and degree of motor control
- Eating position
- Use of adaptive utensils (see Figures 26-1 and 26-2)
- Support of individual needs

For example, blind persons will need a description of the food served, its placement on the plate (named usually in a clockwise direction), and a follow-up training course in preparing food with a number of assistive tools and techniques.

The personal food plan must fulfill basic nutrition needs, and amounts must be increased according to additional metabolic demands. Furthermore, appetite and motivation must be supported to accomplish the task. Sensory stimuli such as variety in food texture, temperature, color, and flavor can enhance appetite and help motivate the learning of new adapted modes of eating. Also, "comfort foods" or familiar ethnic dishes and well-liked foods can encourage the client with the sometimes frustrating and difficult process of relearning how to eat.

Independence in Daily Living

With each disabled person the goal is to achieve as much independence in daily living as possible. Maximal use is made of individual neuromotor resources and emotional reserves, and self-help devices are used as needed to aid these personal resources. A large number of creative devices are available. The U.S. Department of Health and Human Services, Bureau of Primary Care provides a list of assistive devices for those who have limited use of their hands, including eating and dressing devices.[9] Healthcare products specially designed to help with eating are sold by a number of companies. These include the universal cuff that provides a secure grasp on a variety of handle shapes and sizes, an ideal product for persons who have limited use of their hands. Figures 26-1 and 26-2 illustrate examples of specialized eating devices.

Chronic Medical Conditions

A number of chronic conditions can illustrate various areas of need for nutrition therapy. Briefly reviewed here are examples of such conditions in three types of problems, as follows:

1. Musculoskeletal disease
2. Neuromuscular injury and disease
3. Progressive neurologic disorders

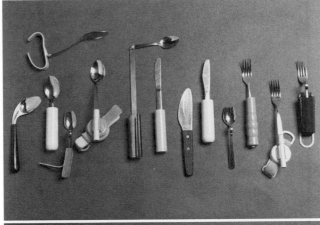

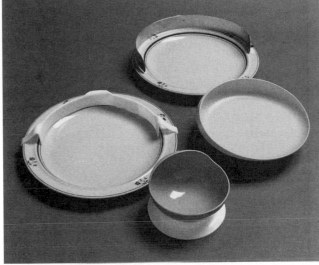

FIGURE 26-1 A number of small and relatively inexpensive feeding aids are available to meet the needs of individuals with disabilities. **A,** Utensil adaptations help with length, grasping, and range of motion. **B,** Plate guards and scoop bowls provide an edge to help place food on the utensil. *(From Olson DA, DeRuyter F: Clinician's guide to assistive technology, St. Louis, 2002, Mosby.)*

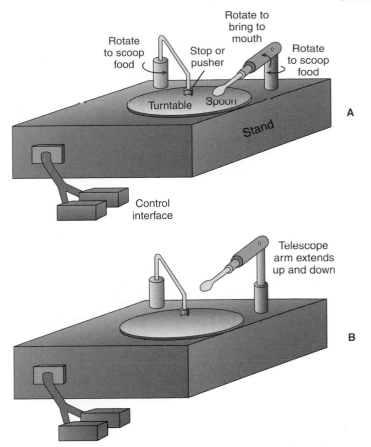

FIGURE 26-2 Two types of electromagnetic feeders for more advanced assisted feeding. **A,** The spoon is attached to a lever arm that is moved to mouth level. **B,** The spoon is attached to a telescoping arm that moves it to mouth level. *(Redrawn from Cook AM, Hussey SM: Assistive technologies: principles and practice, ed 2, St. Louis, 2002, Mosby.)*

MUSCULOSKELETAL DISEASE

Rheumatoid Arthritis

Clinical Characteristics

The general term *arthritis* comes from the Greek word *arthron,* meaning "joint." Rheumatoid Arthritis (RA) affects 5% to 11% of the U.S. population. The incidence rises with age, and peak age for onset of disease is between 25 and 55.[10]

Its underlying chronic, systemic, inflammatory disease process usually begins in the young adult years and affects women twice as often as men. The cause of RA is unknown, though infectious, genetic, and hormonal factors can all play a role in its development. It is a severe type of autoimmune disorder in which the body's immune system acts against its own tissue. It mainly attacks joints of the hands, arms, and feet, causing them to become extremely painful, stiff, and even deformed. Severe disease is associated with larger joints such as the hips, and a life-threatening joint complication can occur when the cervical spine is affected. The precise triggering antigen is still unknown.

Joint damage occurs because of tissue change in the synosheaths. The synovium becomes inflamed and secretes more fluid, leaving the joint swollen and fatigued. Later the cartilage becomes rough and pitted, eventually

pressure sores Long-term bed-bound or immobile patients risk the development of pressure sores at points of bony protuberances, where prolonged pressure of body weight in one position cuts off adequate blood circulation to that area, causing tissue death and ulceration.

synosheath Protective pliable connective tissue surrounding the bony collagen mesh and fluid that come together in the synovial area between major bone heads in joints, which allows normal padded and lubricated joint movement and motion.

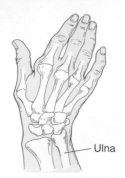

FIGURE 26-3 Arthritic hand showing ulnar drift.

affecting the underlying bone. Progressive joint deformity usually advances rapidly, with joint destruction taking place 1 to 2 years after appearance of the disease (Figure 26-3).

This disability dramatically affects activities of daily living, especially the fundamental necessity of obtaining and eating food. Results of RA include destruction of wrist ligaments and tendons, with weakened finger and handgrip strength, and limited finger movement (see Figure 26-3). All of these changes limit the ability to self-feed, shop for food, or prepare food. Also, elbow and shoulder involvement hinders bringing food to the mouth. Tissue damage at the temporomandibular joint (TMJ) of the jaw limits normal opening and closing of the mouth and may alter chewing ability.

Other nonjoint effects of RA—anemia due to chronic disease, decrease in salivary secretions, dysphagia, and bone disease—further complicate nutrition problems, leading to overall malnutrition. In children and adolescents the malnutrition resulting from the juvenile form of RA can cause serious growth retardation.

Medical Management

Medical treatment of RA, as defined by the American College of Rheumatology (ACR),[11] involves four approaches to therapy and control of the inflammatory process. First, an emphasis is put on early diagnosis and treatment. A second approach is the use of combinations of disease-modifying antirheumatic drugs (DMARDs). A third emphasis is the use of agents that target cytokines, such as drugs that target tumor necrosis factor (TNF) alpha and interleukin-1. The fourth emphasis is recognition that assessment of treatment outcomes should include an analysis of important coexisting illnesses, particularly cardiovascular disease and osteoporosis.[12]

Medications used to treat RA are divided into three categories: nonsteroidal antiinflammatory drugs (NSAIDs), corticosteroids, and DMARDs. Aspirin and other NSAIDs remain mainstays of medical therapy, especially in combination with other medications. NSAIDs are used in the first few weeks when the client is suffering from pain and stiffness before a diagnosis of RA has been made and are commonly given in enteric-coated preparations to avoid gastric irritation. Efforts are underway to determine the best combination of NSAIDs and other medications to reduce the gastrointestinal complications, but to date the quality of the investigations are low.[13] In addition to NSAIDs, cyclooxygenase-2 (COX-2) inhibitors are also commonly used. COX-2 inhibitors are favorable because the risk of gastrointestinal bleeding with long-term use is significantly reduced. Currently there is one available COX-2 inhibitor on the market, celecoxib (Celebrex).

Corticosteroids suppress the inflammatory response in RA. Because corticosteroids are effective at slowing the progression of RA, they are used in 30% to 60% of RA patients. They are controversial, however, due to their side effects, including thinning skin, cataracts, osteoporosis, hypertension, and hyperlipidemia. When given, they are accompanied by supplemental calcium (1 to 1.5 g/day), and vitamin D (800 IU/day).[14]

If rest, exercise, and use of NSAIDs are ineffective after several months, aggressive therapy with DMARDs may be in order, especially when used in combination.[15] Included in this group are gold compound (injectable varieties like gold sodium thiomalate [Myochrysine] and aurothioglucose [Solganal], or oral medications such as auranofin [Ridaura]); antibiotics such as D-penicillamine; antimalarial medications such as hydroxychloroquine sulfate (Plaquenil); and antineoplastic/anticancer drugs such as methotrexate.

In the past few years, a promising medication called etanercept (Enbrel) has become a first-line agent for the treatment of RA. Etanercept acts by inhibiting the inflammatory protein TNF. Other new medications include infliximab (Remicade),[16] which also blocks TNF, and leflunomide (Arava), which works to block growth of new cells. Remicade is available as an intravenous injection taken on a regular basis, whereas Arava is taken as a daily oral medication.[17]

Agents for pain relief and function improvement, such as glucosamine sulfate, hyaluronic acid, or chondroitin, have been found to be mildly effective treatment for patients with mild to moderate pain due to RA. A statistical analysis, called meta-analysis, was conducted for all randomized, placebo-controlled trials of either glucosamine sulfate or chondroitin for hip or knee arthritis. Of the 500 initially identified studies, 15 met the randomized, placebo-controlled criteria. These 15 studies included 1775 patients. One in five patients showed improvements in joint mobility and also had reduced narrowing of joint spaces. Effective onset of improvements was several weeks in these cases.[18] It is also found that glucosamine does not contribute to risk of gastrointestinal bleeding.[19,20] Another meta-analysis showed that hyaluronic acid was also mildly effective.[21] When irreversible destruction of cartilage occurs in advanced stages of the disease, reconstructive joint surgery along with physical therapy and occupational therapy may be employed.

Nutritional Management

In all settings, planning of nutrition therapy must begin with early assessment of individual patient status and needs, especially to detect any degree of malnutrition. Initial history must then assess potential food-drug interactions. The history should include any "nonconventional" treatments for RA as well, such as dietary supplements and practices that may not be scientifically proved.

Special functional assessment of eating ability is also necessary. Such assessments should include attention to any swallowing problem from lack of salivary secretions and dysphagia. Standard nutrition assessment is also essential. Nutritional needs can be determined and monitored based on the following data:

- *Energy:* Energy needs vary widely and must be determined on an individual basis. In general, needs will involve basal energy expenditure plus added calories for increased metabolic activity factors (MAFs), such as stress of disease activity, sepsis, fever, skeletal injury, or surgery. If the client is receiving physical therapy, an additional physical activity factor is used. Total calories are increased as needed to achieve desirable weight gain during growth or decreased if indicated for obese adults. Follow-up monitoring determines any needed adjustments in energy estimates.

- *Protein:* Protein needs vary with protein status, surgical therapy, proteinuria, and nitrogen balance. A well-nourished adult patient needs about 0.5 to 1 g of protein/kg/day during quiet disease periods. An increase to 1.5 to 2 g/kg/day is needed during active inflammatory disease periods. DRI standards for age and sex can guide protein needs for children to meet basic growth needs. States of malnutrition will require more.

- *Vitamins and minerals:* Standard recommendations for vitamins and minerals are used. Specific supplementation may be used if needed, such as supplying calcium and vitamin D if bone disease is involved or if the patient is undergoing steroid therapy.

- *Special enteral and parenteral feeding:* Tube feeding may be used either to supplement oral intake or to supply total nutrition support. Parenteral nutrition support is reserved for preoperative and postoperative needs or when bowel rest is indicated (see the *Case Study* box, "Managing Nutritional Status for a Patient on a Tube-Feeding Formula").

Some researchers have investigated the potential for a vegetarian diet—more specifically a vegan diet using uncooked foods to relieve symptoms of RA. This is often referred to as the "living foods" diet. It consists of uncooked berries, fruits, vegetables, roots, nuts, germinated seeds, and sprouts, that is, rich sources of antioxidants, carotenoids, vitamins C and E, and flavonoids, and polyphenolic compounds such as quercetin, myricetin, and kaempherol. The diet is also high in fiber.[22]

Some reports have concluded a large number of people subjectively benefited from a vegan diet.[23,24] However, much more study is needed regarding this mode of therapeutic treatment for RA. It is difficult for young, healthy individuals to meet protein and vital nutrient requirements (B_{12} and iron) following a vegan diet. Older adults and disabled individuals, already managing an array of obstacles, would face an even greater challenge to incorporate this laborious diet into their therapeutic plan.

In addition, attention may be given to other dietary modifications under study that have shown therapeutic promise. Results indicate supplementation with fish oils containing omega-3 fatty acids suppresses synthesis of cytokines and eicosanoids, lessening their potent inflammatory activities. However, it is unlikely fish oil supplementation will have a major impact on the treatment of RA, although it might be used as an adjunct therapy without major side effects.[25]

The course of RA is unpredictable. The disease is usually progressive, and some degree of permanent disability usually results. After years of disease, many persons are capable of self-care with rehabilitation training and are fully employable.[26] Continuing optimal nutrition therapy is important to maintenance care and to help ensure that clients optimize their potential quality of life.

Osteoarthritis

This milder form of arthritis commonly called osteoarthritis (OA) in older adults is more appropriately called *degenerative joint disease (DJD)* because there is minimal inflammation involved. It is estimated DJD encompasses between 60% and 70% of joint diseases overall and affects approximately 44% of persons over the age of 40 years in the United States. As an age-related disease, DJD is on the rise in the United States because the segment of the population over 65 is growing. It is chronic and may progress, limiting movement of affected joints: mainly the hands, knees, and hips. Marked disability is uncommon, but DJD may become a chronic disabling disease in older adults.[27] There is no cure for the disease process, which ultimately destroys cartilage between the rubbing heads of bones in involved joints. However, damaged joints can be replaced by **arthroplasty**, surgical removal of the degenerated joint, and replacement with a

---

cytokines Substances, produced in tissues, that can cause inflammatory changes in tissue cells (e.g., tumor necrosis factor and interleukin-1).

arthroplasty Plastic surgery of nonfunctioning body joints to form movable joints with replacement metal or plastic materials.

CASE STUDY

Managing Nutritional Status for a Patient on a Tube-Feeding Formula

Charles, a 30-year-old white man with Baltic myoclonic epilepsy for 15 years, was ordered by the home care agency to have a nutrition consultation. He was unable to communicate and had a percutaneous endoscopic gastrostomy (PEG) tube for feeding and 24-hour nursing care at home. Charles had a stage III pressure ulcer and was on a therapeutic bed at a 45-degree angle. He was repositioned every 2 hours to aid in wound healing and prevent further decline. His medical history was significant for hemolytic anemia due to anti-seizure medications, fevers, and electrolyte imbalances from fluid overload.

Charles was well supported by family and healthcare professionals.

He received an enteral formula, which was estimated to provide 2300 kcal and 75 g of protein. He also received approximately 200 ml of water every 4 hours, and the tube was flushed with 50 ml of water after all formula and medications were administered. His fluid was restricted to no greater than 3000 ml/day, and the nurses indicated that it was sometimes difficult to achieve less than this amount due to his number of medications. Nursing provided range-of-motion exercises daily, but he received no other physical rehabilitative therapy.

His medications included phenobarbital every 8 hours, 60 mg every day and 90 mg twice a day; valproic acid 120 mg every 6 hours; Pepcid 20 mg twice a day; Klonopin 4 mg 3 times a day; Dilantin 100 mg every 8 hours; Colace 15 ml every day; Proventil inhaler via trach every 8 hours; folic acid 2 mg; potassium chloride (KCl) 30 mEq; ferric phosphate every day; and a bowel regimen with milk of magnesia and Dulcolax as needed.

His laboratory study results at the initial assessment included calcium (Ca) 8.1 mg/dl ↓, phosphorus (P) 2.8 mg/dl, albumin (Alb) 2.7 g/dl ↓, hemoglobin (Hb)/hematocrit (Hct) 10.5 g/dl ↓/30.2% ↓, cholesterol 115 mg/dl ↓, sodium (Na) 128 mEq/l ↓, potassium (K) 4.2 mEq/l, glucose 59 mg/dl ↓, Dilantin 6.7 μg/ml ↓, zinc (Zn) 22 μg/dl ↓, iron (Fe) 48 μg/dl.

Charles was 183 cm (6 ft) tall and weighed approximately 70 kg (155 lb). It was suspected that he had lost weight in the last year, but the amount was unknown because he had no bed scale. His ideal weight was 78 kg (172 lb). Estimated requirements for anabolism were 3017 kcal 126 g of protein, and approximately 3000 ml of fluid per day. In light of his pressure ulcer, moderately depleted visceral protein stores (partly dilutional), low cholesterol, and recent weight loss, the following steps were suggested:

1. Increase the formula administration to meet estimated requirements for anabolism.
2. If formula administered is tolerated but does not result in weight gain, consider changing formulas to one that is more calorically dense to provide more calories but not additional volume from free water to prevent hyponatremia and fluid overload.
3. Add a multivitamin infusion (MVI) without Fe to ensure adequate nutrient intake.
4. Change the FePhos to FeSO$_4$.
5. Add 220 mg ZnSO$_4$ bid and an additional 500 mg vitamin C to facilitate wound healing.
6. Increase Dilantin: be sure to give it 1 hour after and 2 hours before feeding.
7. Keep accurate intake and output (I&O) reports.

Family and agency were instructed to call the registered dietitian with questions or concerns.

At a 6-month follow up, the dietitian found all of the recommendations were instituted as suggested. Laboratory study results were as follows: Alb 3.0 g/dl ↓, Na 139 mEq/l, K 4.9 mEq/l, Cl 100 mEq/l, CO$_2$ 31 mEq/l, blood urea nitrogen (BUN) 12 mg/dl, Cr 0.3 mg/dl ↓, glucose 96 mg/dl, cholesterol 130 mg/dl ↓, Hb/Hct 11.6 g/dl ↓/33.0% ↓, Dilantin 11.5 μg/ml.

At this stage, Charles had a debridement of his stage III pressure ulcer and was granulating tissue well. He appeared to be gaining weight according to a subjective nursing assessment. His estimated weight at this juncture was 180 lb, and the nurses reported difficulty in turning him due to the weight gain. The tube feeding was unchanged except for the increased calories administered. There was an increase in constipation and a recent urinary tract infection reported. He appeared nonedematous and comfortable. His abdomen was soft, but the family was complaining that he looked "pudgy." His estimated needs decreased to approximately 2300 kcal and 95 g of protein per day with the 25-lb weight gain.

Lactulose was added to his bowel regimen as an as-needed medication; however, nurses reported using it almost daily because other medications were not treating his high impactions. There was also a question of consistent care in turning him and giving bowel medications as prescribed. He continued to tolerate his tube feeding without other apparent problems.

The dietitian recommended the following steps:

1. Continue medications and supplements as ordered.
2. Give 120 ml of warm prune juice via G-tube, and flush with 50 ml of water.
3. Warm tube feeding rather than administering cold from refrigerator to aid in bowel stimulation.
4. Change to original lower caloric density tube feeding.
5. Maintain adequate flushing to prevent dehydration and constipation, but keep careful I&O reports to prevent edema.
6. Ensure all staff maintain a consistent turning schedule and range-of-motion activities.

Questions for Analysis

1. What can the registered dietitian do if a question of inconsistent care becomes an issue in the home? With whom should she speak first?
2. How would you calculate the required volume and administration schedule of an enteral tube feeding? How would you monitor the patient tolerance of the tube feeding?
3. How accurate are estimated requirements if height and weight cannot be adequately obtained? Are there other methods the registered dietitian could have used to track his progress?
4. What other ways could the constipation have been managed? What do you believe was the greatest cause of the constipation?
5. Why did his serum albumin level remain low given the amount of protein he received from his tube feeding? Should the registered dietitian have ordered other laboratory studies to assess protein status?

joint made of metal or plastic components. Hip replacements have been performed since the early 1960s, and the technique is now being refined and applied to other joints. In general, appropriate pain-controlling medication and therapeutic nutrition for general health promotion help relieve symptoms of DJD. Glucosamine sulfate has some effectiveness in treating the pain associated with DJD. It has gained some recognition and favor in the medical field because it is relatively inexpensive and

has little to no side effects, yet it has been shown to mildly stimulate proteoglycan synthesis by chondrocytes and has mild antiinflammatory properties.

The American Pain Society has published guidelines for treating osteoarthritis pain. Pain treatment includes combining pharmacologic therapies such as NSAIDs and COX-2 with nonpharmacologic therapies such as cold, heat, assistive and adaptive aids, and weight loss for those who are obese.[28]

Osteoporosis

The metabolic bone disorder osteoporosis is the most common skeletal disorder in the United States. According to the National Osteoporosis Foundation (NOF), 10 million Americans have osteoporosis and an additional 18 million have low bone mass, putting them at a high risk for developing osteoporosis. The American College of Obstetricians and Gynecologists (ACOG) indicates 13% to 18% of women over 50 years of age have osteoporosis and another 37% to 50% have low bone mass, referred to as osteopenia. Osteoporosis is referred to as the "silent disease" because bone loss occurs without symptoms. The first sign of the problem might not be until a person experiences a fracture. At this point the disease is in its advanced stages, when damage can already be profound. Hip fracture results in significant morbidity and mortality (15% and 20%, respectively). Thoracic spinal fracture due to osteoporosis can also result in pain; deformity; loss of independence; and reduced function of the cardiovascular, respiratory, and digestive systems.[29,30]

Osteoporosis is the result of the body not forming sufficient new bone or of the body reabsorbing too much bone, or both. The latter is typically a situation that occurs in old age. Calcium and phosphate are the two minerals responsible for normal bone formation. If calcium intake is not sufficient throughout the early years in life or if the body does not absorb sufficient calcium from the diet, bone tissue may suffer. Other causes of osteoporosis include hyperparathyroidism, hyperthyroidism, Cushing's syndrome, immobilization, bone malignancies, certain genetic disorders, and excessive corticosteroid use.

Approximately 80% of postmenopausal women in the United States have osteoporosis. Overall, one in two women and one in eight men over age 50 will experience osteoporosis-related fractures. This is primarily because of the decline in estrogen production in women and androgen production in men. After age 70, osteoporosis affects men and women equally as a slow, steady rate of bone loss. Increasing risk of fracture develops over many decades, and these fractures in older adults are a major cause of disabling illness and death. Bones of the vertebrae and hip are equally vulnerable, but hip fractures are more serious.[31] In 2001, direct medical expenditures relating to osteoporotic fractures was estimated at $17 billion.[32]

The best line of defense against osteoporosis is prevention: much of the research today is in the development of medications for prevention. In postmenopausal women, medical treatment of postmenopausal osteoporosis in women is often managed with estrogen replacement therapy (ERT).[33]

ERT, however, is not without controversy. In 2003 the Women's Health Initiative (WHI) published results of a randomized controlled trial on estrogen and progesterone on fractures in women and concluded that there was no evidence of net benefit. Accordingly, the WHI

BOX 26-1	Risk Factors for Osteoporotic Fracture in Postmenopausal Women

History of prior fracture
Family history of osteoporosis
White
Dementia
Smoking
Low body weight and body mass index
Estrogen deficiency*
    Early menopause (age <45 years or bilateral oophorectomy)
    Prolonged premenopausal amenorrhea (>1 year)
Long-term low calcium intake
Alcoholism
Impaired eyesight despite adequate correction
History of falls
Inadequate physical activity

Data from National Institutes of Health: Osteoporosis prevention, diagnosis, and therapy, *NIH Consensus Statement* 17(1):1, 2000.
   *A patient's current use of hormone therapy does not preclude estrogen deficiency.

recommends that estrogen and progesterone not be used for prevention or treatment of osteoporosis.[34] The ACOG, on the other hand, supports use of estrogen and progesterone for bone protection when it is appropriate based on benefit versus risk.[35]

Medical Management

In medical management it is very important to identify individuals who have osteoporosis or are at risk because of low bone mineral density (BMD). The U.S. Preventive Services Task Force recommends that all women over 65 years of age be screened for bone density using dual energy x-ray absorptiometry (DEXA) at the femoral neck. Those women who are 60 to 64 years should also be screened if they have additional risk factors for osteoporosis.[36] Box 26-1 lists risk factors for osteoporosis fractures.

A number of new medications for prevention and treatment of osteoporosis are currently available and approved by the Food and Drug Administration (FDA). Teriparatide, a synthetic parathyroid hormone available by daily injection, stimulates new bone formation and can reduce fracture rates by about 70% in postmenopausal women, but it also is associated with negative side effects including dizziness, cramping, nausea, headache, and hypercalcemia.[37] Alendronate, a bisphosphonate, is a potent inhibitor of bone resorption and has been effective towards increasing bone mineral density when taken daily for 10 years.[38] Use of bisphosphonates have resulted in reduced fracture incidence by 40% to 60% in postmenopausal women. However, they are also associated with stomach pain and other gastrointestinal tract problems such as nausea, vomiting, and diarrhea. Other preventive medications include risedronate, raloxifene, and calcitonin.. These are all classified as antiresorptive medications; they affect the

TABLE 26-1	Medications Used to Manage Osteoporosis

Medication	Comments
Estrogen replacement therapy (ERT)/hormone replacement therapy (HRT)	Available as pill, skin patch; low dose; increased risk of uterine cancer when taken alone—recommended to be taken with the hormone progestin for women who have an intact uterus to prevent cancer, although the issue of a relationship between breast cancer and estrogen is still to be determined
Alendronate sodium (Fosamax)	Classified as a bisphosphonate; best if taken on an empty stomach with a full glass of water; normally prescribed to be taken once a week
Risedronate (Actonel)	Classified as a bisphosphonate; taken daily on an empty stomach with a large glass of water
Raloxifene (Evista)	Classified as a selective estrogen receptor modulator (SERM); taken daily in pill form with or without meals; unlike estrogens, SERMs do not appear to stimulate uterine or breast tissue, thereby minimizing the risk for these types of cancer
Calcitonin (Miacalcin)	Naturally occurring hormone involved in calcium regulation and bone metabolism; protein available as injection or nasal spray
Parathyroid hormone (PTH)	Stimulates bone formation unlike the other antiresorptive drugs mentioned above; treatment with PTH is still experimental; most effective when given 1-2 yr and followed by antiresorptive medications to maintain the benefits

TABLE 26-2	Dietary Reference Intakes for Calcium and Vitamin D

Age	Calcium (mg)	Vitamin D (μg)
Birth-6 mo	210*	5*
6 mo-1 yr	270	5
1-3 yr	500	5
4-8 yr	800	5
9-13 yr	1300	5
14-18 yr	1300	5
19-30 yr	1000	5
31-50 yr	1000	5
51-70 yr	1200	10
>70 yr	1200	15
Pregnant		
<18 yr	1300	5
19-30 yr	1000	5
31-50 yr	1000	5

From Food and Nutrition Board, Institute of Medicine: *Dietary reference intakes for calcium, phosphorus, magnesium, vitamin D, and fluoride,* Washington, DC, 1997, National Academies Press. Retrieved March 6, 2006 from *www.nal.usda.gov/fnic/etext/000105.html.*
  *These are all daily values.
  mg, Milligrams; *μg,* micrograms.

bone remodeling cycle by slowing or stopping bone resorption or breakdown. As a result, new formation continues at a greater rate than bone resorption, and bone density may increase. Table 26-1 summarizes medications currently used to prevent and treat osteoporosis.

Isoflavones, a class of phytoestrogens that are found in soy products and red clover, may have beneficial effects on bone density. However, there have been few randomized controlled trials with humans using isoflavones. Therefore it is difficult to support the use of isoflavones to prevent or treat osteoporosis.[30]

Nutritional Management

Peak bone mass occurs around age 30 and needs to be sustained through a healthy diet and physical activity.[39] Development of osteoporosis in men and women responds to nutrition therapy. Successful prevention and

treatment includes a well-balanced diet with a calcium intake of at least 1000 mg/day and 5 μg /day of vitamin D for adults 19 to 50 years old. These recommended amounts increase for adults over 50 years old to 1200 mg/day of calcium and 10 μg/day of vitamin D. The amount of daily intake of calcium and vitamin D varies according to age, sex, and circumstances such as pregnancy and lactation (Table 26-2). These amounts are based on the 1997 recommendations of the National Academy of Sciences (NAS). It is also important to note the NAS suggests a Tolerable Upper Intake Level (UL) for calcium of 2500 mg/day and for vitamin D of no greater than 50 μg daily for anyone over the age of 1. An appropriate UL for those under age 1 has not been established yet for calcium but is set at 25 μg for vitamin D. These ULs include the use of supplements, as well as food, for obtaining calcium and vitamin D. The body can properly handle about 500 mg of calcium at one time, whether from food or supplements. Vitamin D is potentially the most toxic of all vitamins, so care should be taken in recommendations made to clients concerning vitamin D supplementation. Other nutrient-related considerations are discussed in Box 26-2.

Depending on the degree of hand joint involvement, self-feeding devices may assist eating.

Individuals of all ages are encouraged to participate in regular physical activity. Weight-bearing activity such as running tends to cause the most trauma to the bones,

| BOX 26-2 | Nutrition-Related Considerations and Osteoporosis |

Phosphorus Nutrition

Bone mineral, hydroxyapatite, is made of calcium phosphate. Not much attention has been paid to phosphorus intake because most people have an abundance of phosphorus in their diets. However, it is estimated that 10% to 15% of older women have intakes of less than 70% of the recommended intake for phosphorus. In cases where the individual under consideration has limited phosphorus in his or her diet, a calcium phosphate supplement may be warranted.

The DASH Diet and Bone Health

The Dietary Approaches to Stop Hypertension (DASH) diet is advocated to reduce blood pressure by increasing fruit, vegetable, and whole grain intake while reducing sodium intake. However, recent studies indicate the DASH diet may also be helpful in reducing bone loss and potentially reducing the risk of fracture. The DASH diet has been shown to reduce bone markers that indicate increased bone turnover, indicating the DASH Diet may be helpful in reducing bone loss. Both serum osteocalcin, a marker of bone formation, and C-terminal telopeptide of type I collagen (CTX), a marker of bone resorption, were reduced, indicating a reduced rate of bone turnover. Although still preliminary, these results provide fodder for more research on the beneficial effects of including a wide variety of fruits, vegetables, and whole grains on bone health.

Soft Drinks in Schools

Contracts between soft drink producers and school districts for exclusive pouring rights encourages students directly and indirectly to consume soft drinks. Schools benefit from this arrangement by receiving compensation from the soft drink producer, but the students are encouraged to consume soft drinks, potentially at the displacement of milk and calcium in the diet. Coupled with the obesity epidemic and potential for dental cavities from high-sugar-content soft drinks, the American Academy of Pediatrics includes in its policy statement on Organizational Principles (to guide and define the child healthcare system and/or improve the health of all children) that a clearly defined, districtwide policy that restricts the sale of soft drinks will safeguard against health problems such as obesity, osteoporosis, and dental decay.

References

American Academy of Pediatrics Committee on School Health: Soft drinks in schools. *Pediatrics* 113(1):152, 2004.
Doyle L, Cashman KD: The DASH diet may have beneficial effects on bone health, *Nutr Rev* 62(5):215, 2004.
Heaney RP: Phosphorus nutrition and the treatment of osteoporosis. *Mayo Clin Proc* 79(1):91, 2004.

stimulating osteoblast activity and boosting bone density and mass.

NEUROMUSCULAR INJURY AND DISEASE

The Growing Problem of Neurologic Injuries

According to the American Heart Association, traumatic injury from accidents is the leading cause of death in the first four decades of life and the fourth leading cause of death for all ages.[40] Each year 11,000 spinal cord injuries occur; 52% of these injuries result in paraplegia and 47% in quadriplegia. There are an estimated 50 million Americans affected by diseases or disorders of the spinal cord and brain, including 250,000 cases of SCI.[41] The lengthy list of disorders includes SCI, memory loss, addiction, schizophrenia, learning disability, depression, stroke, brain injury, dementia, and increased tendency toward suicide violence.

With current advances in emergency medicine, the number of persons surviving traumatic brain and SCI has increased dramatically. Proper nutrition therapy after these injuries in the acute care and rehabilitative setting is essential.

Traumatic or Acquired Brain Injury

Approximately 1.5 million people sustain traumatic brain injury every year.[42] An estimated 5.3 million Americans, a little more than 2% of the population, now live with disabilities resulting from a brain injury. Each year 80,000 Americans experience the onset of long-term disability after a traumatic brain injury.[43] Vehicular crashes are the leading cause of brain injury (50%), followed by violence, mostly with firearms, and falls in older adults. The cost of brain injury in the United States is estimated to be $56.3 billion annually.[44]

Brain injuries fall into one of the following two groups:

1. *Traumatic brain injury (TBI):* A traumatic brain injury occurs when an outside force impacts the head hard enough to cause the brain to move within the skull or if the force causes the skull to break and directly hurts the brain. This injury is an assault to the brain, not of a degenerative or congenital nature, caused by an external physical force that may produce a diminished or altered state of consciousness, resulting in impaired cognitive abilities or physical functioning. It can also result in disturbance of behavioral or emotional functioning.

2. *Acquired brain injury (ABI):* An acquired brain injury is an injury that is not hereditary, congenital, degenerative, or induced by birth trauma. An acquired brain injury is an injury to the brain that has occurred after birth. Examples of ABI include anoxia due to airway obstruction.

Postinjury Metabolic Alterations

When brain injury occurs, there is a primary injury and a resultant set of secondary injuries. Primary injury to the brain occurs from the force of direct contact with the source of the trauma plus inertial forces following initial impact. The type of impact received will contribute to the type and extent of the initial assault to the brain. A secondary set of injuries will follow, which are probably caused by a series of mechanisms. These may include membrane damage resulting from either oxidative stress free-radical cascade; inflammation; or from neurotoxicity due to the release of neurotransmitters, disrupting the cells' ionic equilibrium.[42]

The brain is the control center of body functions and activities. Because of this, a brain injury brings an immediate cascade of systemic metabolic and protective responses that affect the entire body and its resources. When the systemic inflammatory response is activated, a sustained state of hypermetabolism develops. Ultimately, if the process continues unchecked, a sequence of organ failures may follow. Any complication prolongs the hypermetabolic phase, and the increasing protein catabolism causes depletion of lean body mass.[45] Increased energy expenditure and urinary nitrogen excretion mark this increased metabolic demand in response to trauma.

Initial Nutrition Management

Immediate goals of the care team are control of the injury, maintenance of oxygen transport, and metabolic support. Immediate nutrition support is vital to meet the hypermetabolic drain on the body tissue resources for increased energy, protein, and fluid demands. Regular monitoring of energy needs is essential, often more than once a day. Most trauma centers now use indirect calorimetry at the bedside with a mobile calorimeter unit.

Early nutrition support may be delivered via the enteral or parenteral route. Delayed gastric emptying after TBI has led some to advocate early percutaneous endoscopic gastrostomy or jejunal (PEG/PEJ) feeding.[46,47] Success has been reported using enteral feedings as early as 2 to 3 days after injury, primarily to keep bowel function intact. Total parenteral nutrition (TPN) is a practical option because it can be started within the first 24 hours after injury and may be immediately adjusted to the nutritional requirements of each patient according to daily metabolic profile and urinary nitrogen analysis.[48] Providing TPN and enteral nutrition in combination therapy is commonly used to preserve gut integrity while achieving nutrient requirements. TPN is gradually tapered when the enteral formula is well tolerated and considered adequate.[49]

Rehabilitative Nutrition

Nutritional rehabilitation for the person with TBI or ABI presents a complex of individual problems that require skilled and sensitive nutritional management. Individualized care plans are designed to focus on immediate- and long-range plans for the patient. To develop individual nutrition care plans, the rehabilitation dietitian works closely with other team members, such as the nurse, occupational therapist, speech pathologist, cognitive rehabilitation therapist, and physical therapist. Together they assess the degree of dysphagia, difficulty with chewing and swallowing, level of language deficit and communication, and ability to perform basic activities of daily living skills, including food preparation and eating. Short- and long-range goals, as well as strategies to reach these goals, are developed along with many practical suggestions for adapting food forms and textures to meet eating problems.

Spinal Cord Injury

Postinjury Management

The cervical region of the spine at the neck is the most mobile portion of the spine and hence the most vulnerable site for spinal cord injuries. Spinal cord damage disrupts transmission of impulses from the brain to peripheral nerves and muscles, so muscle function below the level of injury is lost, resulting in paralysis, immobilization, and complicated illnesses. According to the Christopher Reeve Paralysis Foundation, there are an estimated 250,000 to 400,000 spinal cord–injured individuals living in the United States. Each year catastrophic SCI in the United States produces some 11,000 new survivors.[50,51] Because of advanced medical care, the number of survivors, and consequent costs, is increasing each year.

Many of these SCIs are a result of automobile accidents (37%); other factors include violence (28%), falls (21%), and sports injuries (6%). Forty-seven percent of the injuries result in quadriplegia (loss of movement and sensation in both the arms and legs), and 52% result in paraplegia (loss of movement and sensation in the lower body). SCIs cost the nation at least $9.7 billion per year for medical care, equipment, and disability support. Initial hospitalization (an average of 15 days of acute care and then 44 days in rehabilitation), adaptive equipment, and home modification costs after injury average $140,000 per patient. Trauma and rehabilitation costs alone are almost $250,000 for each SCI individual.[50,51]

There are no known repairs for spinal cord injuries, but there is some promising research being conducted. The following four strategies exist for repairing the injured spinal cord[52]:

1. Promoting regrowth of the injured nerves by using nerve growth stimulants or substances that suppress inhibitors of neuronal extensions
2. Bridging spinal cord lesions with scaffolds that are saturated with nerve growth factors to promote axon growth
3. Repairing damaged myelin in order to restore nerve impulse conductivity in the damaged area
4. Enhancing central nervous system plasticity by enhancing the growth of spared, intact nerve fibers above and below the site of injury

Nutrition Management

Protein-energy malnutrition is common in individuals with SCI. About half of hospitalized patients and two thirds of the patients admitted to a rehabilitation unit exhibit clinical signs of malnutrition.[53,54] Malnutrition increases the risk for development of pressure sores, and fat mass excess due to immobility increases cardiovascular and respiratory risks for SCI patients. They are predisposed to development of diabetes mellitus and bony fractures as well.[55]

SCI patients are usually well nourished at the time of sudden injury. Thus the goal of starting the feeding process as early as possible helps to counteract the initial acute phase of spinal shock and prevents onset of a nutritional decline and secondary illness. Enteral feeding tubes placed beyond the pylorus usually make it possible to start nutrition support within 3 to 5 days. There is a wide variation in metabolic rate and energy needs, but they tend to be lower than those of other trauma patients as a result of decreased metabolic activity of denervated muscle.[56] The higher the injury on the spinal column, the greater the denervated muscle mass and the lower the measure of energy expenditure. Daily guidelines for energy needs are approximately 23 kilocalories (kcalories or kcal)/kg for quadriplegics and 28 kcal/kg for paraplegics.[56]

Rehabilitation Nutrition

When the acute phase passes and the patient is stabilized, usually 2 to 3 months after injury, the extended rehabilitation training phase begins. This complex process is designed to restore the client to the best functional capacity possible and to promote independent living.[57] The goal of rehabilitation is to prevent and treat any complications associated with SCI. Combined therapies are used from the team of rehabilitation specialists: physiatrist, registered dietitian, registered nurse, physical therapist, occupational therapist, speech therapist, psychologist, social worker, and vocational counselor. Nutrition Nutritional management involves individual assessment and care of (1) basic energy-nutrient needs and feeding capacities and (2) complications associated with SCI.

Basic Nutritional Needs

Energy needs are based on sufficient calories to maintain an ideal body weight somewhat below that given for a comparable person in standard weight-height tables for healthy populations. For example, general weight goals for paraplegics have been recommended at 10 to 15 lb below standard body weight, and for quadriplegics, 15 to 20 lb below standard weight.[56] Excess weight gain is common in clients with SCI as a result of decreased metabolic rate that persists from the preceding acute postinjury phase and continued relative immobilization.[58] Obesity contributes to a patient's medical problems and

adds difficulty for caregivers in the frequent turning necessary in bed to prevent pressure sores and in transfers between bed and wheelchair. Adequate protein intake is essential for maintaining muscle mass and tissue integrity in order to prevent negative nitrogen balance, ulcer formation, or infection. Palatable high-protein supplements between meals may be needed to maintain an adequate intake. The client may be at risk for vitamin or mineral deficiencies if appetite and food intake are poor as a result of depression or fatigue. A standard multiple vitamin-mineral preparation is often recommended to ensure nutritional adequacy.

Associated Complications

Several nutrition-related complications in rehabilitation for patients with SCI require special attention, as follows:

- *Pressure sores:* Caused by immobilization, pressure sores are loss of pressure sensation around bony prominences, involving decreased blood circulation, skin breakdown, and ulcer formations that are open to infection and difficult to heal. Pressure sores occur in 60% of quadriplegic patients and 52% of paraplegics. Nutritional factors involved include anemia, which reduces oxygen supply to tissues; excessive weight loss, which reduces padding of bony prominences; and low levels of plasma proteins such as albumin, which lead to edema and loss of skin elasticity. Protein deficiency requires an increased protein intake. More severe ulcers require more intense nutrition intervention, with protein needs of 1.5 to 2 g/kg of body mass. Although not a panacea, vitamin C and zinc supplementation can aid in the healing process when combined with proper diet.[54]

- *Hypercalciuria:* Immobility leads to an imbalance in calcium metabolism with a loss of bone calcium and its increased excretion in the urine. Over the long term this loss of bone calcium leads to osteoporosis, which has been found to be present and progressive in 88% of the patients with SCI, affecting denervated musculoskeletal tissue below the level of injury. Bone fractures occur in about 7% of these patients. A balance of calcium–vitamin D therapy and a prudent control of excessive protein and sodium intakes, which cause increased calcium withdrawal, is indicated.

- *Kidney stones:* Hypercalciuria also contributes to formation of kidney stones. Neurogenic effects after SCI cause loss of normal bladder control, resulting in problems of urinary reflux, retention, incontinence, infection, and stone formation.[59] Regular catheterization is necessary to prevent accumulation of bacteria and solutes such as calcium and other particles that can easily form stones. A high fluid intake of 2 to 3 L/day must be a part of the overall nutrition care plan to dilute the urine and reduce the solute concentration.

- *Neurogenic bowel:* Gastrointestinal complications from loss of normal neuromuscular controls include decreased peristalsis and loss of bowel control. A regularly scheduled program for emptying the bowel is necessary. Remedies vary but could include prune juice with lemon, glycerin suppositories, a high-fiber diet with ample fluid to prevent fecal impaction, and regular toileting. A daily schedule and accurate recording of results are recommended to promote regularity and limit the need for enemas or manual evacuation of stool.

- *Depression:* During the initial days of shock and survival, the full impact of the disability is not comprehended by the client. When transfer to the rehabilitation unit occurs and the full extent of the disability is realized, a period of depression, even anger, is a normal part of the personal grieving and healing process. Its severity and duration depend in large measure on the patient's personal strengths and resources, but it also requires sensitive yet realistic support of the family and the rehabilitation team for the serious and demanding work of rehabilitation to be successful. The dietitian must help ensure that adequate energy, protein, and fluid intake is maintained. Optimum nutritional status is achieved with appetizing foods, especially when the client's spirit is low. Even subtle improvements in muscle mass and function from nutrition therapy can be a source of strength for the client's mind and body.

Cerebrovascular Accident (Stroke)

Brain injury resulting from a stroke causes varying degrees of nerve damage and body paralysis. According to the American Heart Association, cerebrovascular disease (CVD) from underlying atherosclerosis ranks first as a cause of death among Americans. CVD resulted in over 930,000 deaths in 2001. Stroke alone ranks third as a cause of death and is a major cause of disability in the United States. Every year about 700,000 people experience a new or recurrent stroke in the United States. In recent years the incidence of strokes has declined, largely as a result of improvement in control of hypertension and increased public education concerning hypertension. The length of time to recover from a stroke depends on its severity. From 50% to 70% of survivors regain functional independence, but 15% to 30% are permanently disabled. Institutional care is required by 20% of stroke victims at 3 months after onset. In 1999, $4.8 billion ($14,752 per patient discharge) was paid to Medicare beneficiaries discharged from short-stay hospitals for stroke. An additional $1.5 billion was paid for those who experienced transient ischemic attacks or precerebral occlusions.[60] Dysphagia occurs in up to half of patients after a stroke; in most it is transient with only about 1 in 10 patients having any swallowing problems at 6 months. Persistent dysphagia may be due to a lack of bilateral cerebral hemisphere representation of the oral and pharyngeal musculature involved in swallowing.[61] Safe feeding methods may require a swallowing evaluation using a videofluoroscopic modified barium swallow to determine if the client is at risk for aspiration. Clients are fed with a nasoenteric or enterostomy tube if swallowing is deemed unsafe.[62] Further rehabilitative care follows the same general goals and methods discussed in this chapter.

Developmental Disabilities

During the developmental period of childhood, neuromuscular conditions such as cerebral palsy (CP), epilepsy, spina bifida, and Down syndrome cause eating problems that can contribute to poor growth and delayed development (see also the *To Probe Further* box, "Special Education for Special Kids").

Cerebral Palsy

CP is a general term for nonprogressive disorders of muscle control of movements and posture. It affects some 500,000 children and adults in the United States at the rate of 2 to 4 children per 1000. Approximately 5000 infants are diagnosed with the condition each year.[63] It is not a disease, and it has no "cure" per se, although training and therapy can help to improve function. CP has many causes and usually results from brain damage that occurs during fetal development or shortly after birth, probably as a result of *hypoxia,* poor oxygen supply to the brain. Other causes include premature birth, low birth weight, Rh or A-B-O blood type incompatibility between mother and infant, infection of the mother with German measles or other viral diseases in early pregnancy, and bacteria that directly or indirectly attack the infant's central nervous system.

Most affected children fall into the following three principal types:

1. Spastic—muscles of one or more limbs permanently contracted, making normal movements very difficult or impossible
2. Athetoid—involuntary writhing movements
3. Ataxic—disturbed sense of balance and depth perception

An individual may possess more than one type. These continuous involuntary movements increase energy needs; research reports indicate increased resting metabolic rates that are approximately 15% higher than those of non-CP control subjects.[64] Because the immune system is often compromised in persons with developmental disabilities, they are at high risk for problems related to food safety. Thus all caregivers involved should have food safety training.[65,66]

TO PROBE FURTHER

SPECIAL EDUCATION FOR SPECIAL KIDS

Advances in technology, science, and medicine have made it possible for more children with disabilities to function in the public education system: more children are able to complete an education now than ever before. By law, all eligible school-age children and youth with disabilities are entitled to receive a free appropriate public education (FAPE). The federal law that supports special education and related service programming for children and youth with disabilities is called the Individuals With Disabilities Education Act (IDEA). IDEA was formerly known as EHA or Education for the Handicapped Act, which was enacted in 1975. EHA has a long history of amendments to improve the services that it covers, including special funding incentives for states to make FAPE available for all school-age children with disabilities ages 3 through 5. Provisions were also included to help states develop early intervention programs for infants and toddlers with disabilities.

In 1990 among the amendments to the EHA was a name change to IDEA. One primary purpose of the IDEA is to ensure that all children with disabilities have available to them a "free appropriate public education" that emphasizes special education and related services designed to meet unique needs and prepare students for employment and independent living. This means services are provided at public expense, under public supervision and direction, and without charge. Disabilities include mental retardation, hearing impairment or deafness, speech or language impairment, visual impairment or blindness, serious emotional disturbance, orthopedic impairment, autism, traumatic brain injury, or specific learning disability.

Special education is defined as instruction that is specially designed, at no cost to caregivers, to meet a child's unique needs. Specially designed includes adapting the content, methodology, or delivery of instruction to make it possible for the child to meet certain standards of education that apply to all children within the jurisdiction of the public agency. Special education can be conducted in the classroom, the home, the hospital, institutions, and other settings. Special education must be provided to students in what is known as the least restrictive environment. Some related services also covered under this law include speech-language pathology and audiology; psychologic, physical, and occupational therapy; therapeutic recreation; early identification and assessment of childhood disabilities, counseling services for students, as well as parents or caregivers; orientation and mobility services; and social work in schools.

Final regulations currently guiding the school systems' design and implementation of their special education and related services were published in the 1997 IDEA Amendments document located in the *Federal Register*. Because state policies can vary widely, caregivers are encouraged to obtain a copy of their state's policy either through the school district or the state director of special education. The National Information Center for Children and Youth With Disabilities (NICHCY), located in Washington, DC, is another resource for caregivers and students. The IDEA, its amendments, and regulations can be obtained by contacting the Office of Special Education Programs (OSEP) at the U.S. Department of Education.

References

Committee on Labor and Human Resources: *Report to accompany S. 717,* Washington, DC, 1997, U.S. Government Printing Office.

Family Educational Rights and Privacy Act (P.L. 93-380), CFR Title 34, Part 99, 1988.

Flippo KF, Inge KJ, Barcus JM: *Assistive technology: a resource for school, work, and community,* Baltimore, 1995, Paul H. Brookes.

Individuals With Disabilities Education Act Amendments of 1997 (PL 105-17), 20 USC Chapter 33, Sections 1400-1485, 1997.

U.S. Department of Education: Assistance to states for the education of children with disabilities and the early intervention program for infants and toddlers with disabilities: final regulations, *Federal Register* 64(48):12406, 1999.

Mental retardation, with an intelligence quotient (IQ) below 70, occurs in about 75% of persons with CP, mostly in the spastic group. Important exceptions occur, mostly among those with the athetoid type; some of these individuals are highly intelligent. With patient and skillful care, features of the condition can improve throughout childhood. Improvements in methods used in obstetrics and neonatal care have led to reduced incidence of injury and death of mothers and infants. With interventions such as folate supplementation to pregnant women, immunizations, and avoidance of potentially toxic substances, it is expected that the cerebral palsy rate should diminish. But to date this has not occurred. This is partly because rates of preterm births (less than 37 weeks of gestation) and very preterm births (less than 32 weeks of gestation) have remained the same over the last 15 years.[67]

Early nutrition therapy for CP patients focuses mainly on feeding problems. When the infant or young child cannot obtain sufficient nourishment as a result of oral motor dysfunction, there is a problem with body growth. Nutritional status, health, and body growth are most af-fected in children with the greatest motor dysfunction.[68,69] When satisfactory oral feeding is not possible or when oral feeding is interrupted for a prolonged period because of illness or surgery, enteral nutrition support via nasoenteric or gastrostomy tube feeding may be necessary. For patients with severe CP, tube feeding improves quality of life for both the child and the family, despite minor complications.[70,71]

Oral feeding can pose numerous problems, both functional and behavioral. Feeding problems resulting from oral motor dysfunction (e.g., difficulties in sucking, swallowing, or chewing), gross motor/self-feeding impairment, lack of appetite, and food aversions can significantly reduce energy and nutrient intake, as can prolonged

> spina bifida A congenital defect in the fetal closing of the neural tube to form a portion of the lower spine, leaving the spine unclosed and the spinal cord open in various degrees of exposure and damage.

assisted feeding and use of pureed foods. In persons with severe physical and developmental difficulties, malnutrition and growth failure are common.

Early and ongoing nutrition assessment, intervention, and counseling are essential components of rehabilitation team care. In cases where accurate height measures to assess growth are difficult because of joint contractures, spasticity, or inability to stand, reasonably accurate stature can be calculated from knee height measures, using the standard equations given in Table 26-3.[72] In children with CP, growth retardation persists with age. Studies have shown that at age 2 years they are 2% shorter than their peers, and at 8 years of age they are 10% shorter.[73] As adults, persons with spastic CP need about 500 extra kcal/day to cover added energy need for *athetosis,* the continuous involuntary writhing motions of the disease.[74] Many still have feeding problems, but exercise helps promote better nutrition.[75] Other nutritional concerns are food intolerance, food allergies, drug-nutrient interactions, constipation, and reflux.[76]

Epilepsy

Epilepsy, literally "seizures," is a neuromuscular disorder in which abnormal electrical activity in the brain causes recurring transient seizures. Normally the brain regulates all human activities, thoughts, perceptions, and emotions through the regular, orderly, electrical excitation of its nerve cells. During an epileptic seizure, however, an unregulated, chaotic electrical discharge occurs. Seizures often appear spontaneously, or in some cases they may be set off by some stimulus such as a flashing light. This brain dysfunction may develop for no obvious reason, or there may be an inherited predisposition. In other cases it may result from a wide variety of diseases or injuries such as birth trauma, a metabolic imbalance in the body, head injury, brain infection (meningitis, encephalitis), stroke, brain tumor, drug intoxication, or alcohol or drug withdrawal states.

According to the American Epilepsy Society, epilepsy and seizures affect about 2.3 million Americans and result in an estimated $12.5 billion in medical costs and lost or reduced earnings and production. Approximately 10% of all Americans will experience a seizure sometime in their lives, and 3% will have had a diagnosis of epilepsy by age 80.[77]

Usually the disorder starts in childhood or adolescence. It plateaus from ages 15 to 65 years and then rises again among older adults.[77] About a third of these persons will outgrow the condition and will not need medication. Another third find their seizures well controlled by drug treatment and require less medication over time. The remaining third find that their condition remains the same or becomes increasingly resistant to drug therapy.

Physicians now have more drug options than ever before to treat epilepsy. Before 1990 six antiepileptic drugs (AEDs) were available for treatment of all forms of epilepsy. These are carbamazepine, phenobarbital, phenytoin, primidone, valproic acid, and ethosuximide. Since then, eight new AEDs have been approved by the U.S. Food and Drug Administration for clients with epilepsy whose care is not sufficient using only the existing drugs. The new drugs are felbamate, gabapentin (Neurontin), lamotrigine (Lamictal), topiramate (Topamax), tiagabine (Gabitril), oxcarbazepine (Trileptal), levetiracetam (Keppra), and zonisamide (Zonegran). Vigabatrin, though not currently approved in the United States, is also a possibility for future use with adults who experience partial seizures. Partial seizures begin with an electrical discharge in one limited area of the brain and may be related to head injury, brain infection, stroke, or tumor, but in most cases the cause is unknown.

These new drugs have shown some advantages in effectiveness compared with existing drugs. For example, gabapentin has been shown to be effective in treatment of newly diagnosed clients with partial epilepsy.[78,79] Anticonvulsant drugs like valproic acid are often the first line of treatment for epilepsy and in most cases do lessen seizure frequency. In cases of Lennox-Gastaut syndrome, a severe form of epilepsy that usually begins in early childhood and is difficult to treat, newer AEDs such as lamotrigine and topiramate have proved to be effective and well-tolerated treatments for associated seizures.[80] Each client needs to be evaluated for the most effective and appropriate means of controlling his or her seizures,

---

TABLE 26-3	Recommended Equations for Estimating Stature From Knee Height*

Age/Sex Group	Equation
Black Males	
6-18 yr	Stature = (Knee height × 2.18) + 39.60
18-60 yr	Stature = (Knee height × 1.79) + 73.42
White Males	
6-18 yr	Stature = (Knee height × 2.22) + 40.54
18-60 yr	Stature = (Knee height × 1.88) + 71.85
Black Females	
6-18 yr	Stature = (Knee height × 2.02) + 46.59
18-60 yr	Stature = (Knee height × 1.86) – (age × 0.06) + 68.10
White Females	
6-18 yr	Stature = (Knee height × 2.15) + 43.21
18-60 yr	Stature = (Knee height × 1.87) – (age × 0.06) + 70.25

From Chumlea WMC, Guo SS, Steinbaugh ML: Prediction of stature from knee height for black and white adults and children with application to mobility-impaired or handicapped persons, *J Am Diet Assoc* 94(12):1385, 1994, with permission from the American Dietetic Association.

*Equations are based on normal, healthy individuals. Stature and knee height are measured in centimeters.

and factors such as drug side effects must be considered. For example, phenobarbital, phenytoin, and carbamazepine have been associated with decreased bone mineral density.[81] These drugs may not be good long-term solutions for someone who has a significant risk of osteoporosis.

When medications fail to control seizure activity, other treatments are available such as vagal nerve stimulation (VNS) and a ketogenic diet. VNS was approved for use by the Food and Drug Administration in 1997 as an adjunctive therapy in adult and adolescent clients over the age of 12 years. A flat, round battery about the size of a silver dollar is surgically implanted in the chest wall. Electrodes are threaded under the skin and wound around the vagus nerve in the neck. The therapy works by sending small regular pulses of electrical energy to the brain via the vagus nerve. The healthcare team initially programs electrical impulses, and the patient has the option to activate the impulses if he or she feels a seizure is about to occur. Although seizures are rarely eliminated completely, the majority of people who undergo VNS implantation experience fewer seizures and have a better sense of control.[82] VNS has also been shown to be effective in pediatric populations younger than 12 years.[83] Even with the effectiveness of VNS, clients still may require antiepileptic medication.

Nutrition management of epilepsy functions in several areas of care. First, it helps to ensure an appropriate diet for normal growth during childhood and adolescence and for health maintenance in adulthood. Second, it seeks to ameliorate side effects of the anticonvulsant drugs used (see the *Diet-Medications Interactions* box, "Anticonvulsant Drugs Used to Control Basic Types of Epilepsy and Their Nutrition-Related Side Effects"). Some commonly used drugs and their relation to food and nutrients are shown in the *Diet-Medications Interactions* box. Third, if a ketogenic diet is used, the clinical dietitian is responsible for its calculations and education of staff, patient, and family in its use. This special high-fat, low-carbohydrate diet was developed to control epilepsy before current anticonvulsant drugs became widely available in the 1940s. It is still successfully used with some children possessing intractable myoclonic epilepsy that resists drug therapy.[84] In addition to the effectiveness of the ketogenic diet for seizure control, the diet may also help reduce costs for healthcare in this population.[85] The ketogenic mechanism of seizure control is not clearly understood, although the mechanism may involve having a threshold level of ketones present, which may help control seizures by disrupting nerve transmission at the synapse.[86] Details of the strict calculations required to achieve the necessary ratio of high fat to low carbohydrate are outlined

DIET-MEDICATIONS INTERACTIONS

Anticonvulsant Drugs Used to Control Basic Types of Epilepsy and Their Nutrition-Related Side Effects

Most Commonly Used Drug	Drug Trade Name	Nutrition-Based Side Effects
Grand Mal (Tonic/Clonic) Seizures		
Phenytoin (adults)	Dilantin	Nausea, vomiting, and constipation; reduced taste sensation; vitamins D and K catabolism; reduced serum calcium, vitamins B_6 and B_{12}, folate, and serum magnesium levels; overgrowth of gums
Phenobarbital	Luminal	Increased appetite or anorexia, nausea, vomiting, vitamins D and K catabolism, reduced bone density
Primidone	Mysoline	Gastrointestinal upset, weight loss
Carbamazepine	Tegretol	Nausea, vomiting, diarrhea, abdominal pain, xerostomia (dry mouth), glossitis (sore tongue), stomatitis (sore mouth), increased blood urea nitrogen
Petit Mal (Absence of Seizures)		
Ethosuximide	Zarontin	Gastrointestinal upset, nausea, vomiting, anorexia, weight loss
Valproic acid	Depakene, Depakote	Nausea, vomiting, indigestion, diarrhea, abdominal pain, constipation, anorexia and weight loss, or increased appetite and weight gain
Clonazepam	Klonopin	Hyperactivity, short attention span, impulsive behavior, weight gain
Partial Seizures		
Phenytoin (adults)	Dilantin	Nausea, vomiting, and constipation; reduced taste sensation; vitamins D and K catabolism; reduced levels of serum calcium, vitamins B_6 and B_{12}, folate, and serum magnesium; overgrowth of gums
Phenobarbital	Luminal	Increased appetite or anorexia, nausea, vomiting, vitamins D and K catabolism, reduced bone density
Carbamazepine	Tegretol	Nausea, vomiting, diarrhea, abdominal pain, xerostomia (dry mouth), glossitis (sore tongue), stomatitis (sore mouth), increased blood urea nitrogen

in the American Dietetic Association's *Pediatric Manual of Clinical Dietetics.*[87]

There are concerns about using a ketogenic diet with children because it may result in poor growth. Liu and colleagues[88] recommend that adequate amounts of energy and protein be included with a higher proportion of polyunsaturated to saturated fats. Supplementation of vitamins and minerals should also be considered.

The ketogenic diet is normally initiated in a hospital setting with a starvation period with fluid restriction. There is concern this fasting period with fluid restriction may have negative effects, especially in a pediatric population. Kim and colleagues[89] have provided evidence that the initial fasting period may not be necessary to provide the same beneficial effects on seizure control as long as the client reaches the ketogenic state.

Other dietary interventions are also possible and have shown some potential for effectiveness. The Atkins diet raises the levels of ketones, similarly to the ketogenic diet, but offers more protein, which would potentially be beneficial for a growing child. A calorie-restricted diet has been shown to reduce seizure activity in animal models without the presence of ketones. Use of omega-3 and omega-6 polyunsaturated fatty acids has had some success in reducing seizures.[86]

Spina Bifida

In the United States, spina bifida is the most commonly occurring type of neural tube defect (NTD), a congenital malformation of the spine that contributes to serious developmental disabilities.[90] It develops during early embryonic life when the neural tube, which forms the spinal cord, does not close completely, leaving part of one or more vertebrae of the spinal cord exposed at birth. Because the vertebral canal usually closes within 4 weeks of conception, this congenital defect can often be diagnosed early in the pregnancy by ultrasound scanning or by high levels of alpha fetoprotein in the amniotic fluid or maternal blood. Therefore appropriate genetic counseling can be provided for the parents. Recent discovery of the cell enzyme error involved indicates that folic acid (folate) and vitamin B_{12} supplementation at time of conception through the first few months of pregnancy reduces a woman's risk that the baby will develop this devastating neural tube defect.[91,92] Mandatory fortification of cereal grain products with folate went into effect in January 1998. Between October 1998 and December 1999 the reported prevalence of spina bifida declined 31%, and the presence of anencephaly, absence of the cerebral hemispheres, was reduced by 16%. There was an estimated reduction in the number of NTD-affected pregnancies from 4000 in 1995 to 1996 to 3000 in 1999 to 2000.[93]

The defect can occur anywhere along the spine but is more common in the lower back. One group study of children with myelomeningocele indicates the neuro-logic damage that occurs depends on the severity and level of the lesion on the spine.[94] The incidence is about 1 per 1000 babies born, but it increases with either very young or old maternal age. A mother who has had one affected child is 10 times more likely to have another affected child.

There are three main forms of spina bifida, as follows:

1. *Spina bifida occulta:* This is the least serious and most common form. The name indicates an "unseen cleft in the spine." It often goes unnoticed in otherwise healthy children except for a small dimple over the area of the underlying abnormality.
2. *Myelomeningocele:* Also known as *myelocele,* this is the most severe form, and the child is usually severely disabled. Here the spinal cord *(myelo)* and its enveloping membranes *(meninges)* protrude from the spine in a sac *(cele).*
3. *Meningocele:* This form is less severe than myelomeningocele, because the nerve tissue of the spinal cord usually remains intact. Outer skin covers the bulging sac, and therefore there usually are no functional problems. Ideally, necessary surgical repairs are performed in the first few days of life.

Nutritional management of children with spina bifida focuses on growth pattern and individual degree of problems of growth retardation and short stature, low muscle mass and weakness, deformities or paralysis of lower extremities, and reduced ability to control bladder and bowels. Normal growth charts have been revised for use with nutrition assessment of these children.[95] Nutrition care plans give attention to the main problems of short stature and poor growth, increased weight, and constipation. Obesity is a particular problem because of several factors: (1) low basal metabolic rate related to lowered amount of lean body mass, (2) little physical activity related to the disabled condition and dependency on a wheelchair, and (3) use of food and overfeeding by parents or other caregivers to reward or show love or to counteract what is seen as frailty or weakness caused by the disability. All of these factors become part of ongoing nutrition counseling. Most children born with spina bifida live well into adulthood as a result of caring professionals and the sophisticated medical techniques available today.

A growing concern is development of a latex allergy, which is a common secondary condition associated with spina bifida. A latex allergy produces symptoms of watery eyes, wheezing, hives, rash, swelling, and, in severe cases, anaphylaxis. Research has shown people with spina bifida are more susceptible because they are repeatedly exposed to latex products early in life and repeatedly due to medical procedures. Some common products that contain latex are catheters, elastic bandages, baby bottle nipples, pacifiers, medical gloves, and balloons.

Down Syndrome

A chromosomal abnormality accounts for the mental retardation and characteristic appearance of children with Down syndrome, a condition first described in the nineteenth century by the English physician John L.H. Down (1828-1896). Its cause remained a mystery until 1959, when modern researchers discovered persons with Down syndrome had one too many chromosomes in each of their cells: 47 instead of the normal 46. Because the extra chromosome is usually number 21, Down syndrome is also called trisomy 21. The two parent chromosomes numbered 21 fail to separate into daughter cells during the first stage of sperm or egg cell formation, and some eggs or sperm are thus formed with an extra number 21 chromosome. If one of these takes part in fertilization, the resulting baby will have the extra chromosome and Down syndrome. This event is more likely if the mother is over 35 years of age, indicating that defective egg formation, rather than sperm formation, is usually the cause.[96] Expression of the genes in a trisomy 21 condition is altered and results in modified protein production, neurobiologic development, and finally abnormal physiologic function when compared with the nontrisomy individual. However, exact dysfunction remains poorly understood.[97]

Down syndrome occurs in about 1 in 1000 infants born. This rate has decreased from about 1 in 700 births with the number of terminated pregnancies resulting from early detection.[96] The rate rises steeply with increased maternal age to about 1 in 40 among mothers over 40 years. Currently there are more than 350,000 people living in the United States with this syndrome. Degree of mental retardation varies, with an IQ anywhere between 30 and 80, but all are capable of limited learning. Up to 50% of these individuals have congenital heart defects, which can be surgically corrected. More than 25% develop Alzheimer's disease after the age of 35, and 15% to 20% have a greater chance of developing a curable form of leukemia as a newborn and up to age 3.[98] Despite complications associated with Down syndrome, these children are usually affectionate, cheerful, and friendly and get along well with family and friends. They thrive to their full potential in a loving family.

Early intervention in Down syndrome is important to ensure longevity and highest possible quality of life. Congenital heart defects are common in individuals with Down syndrome. Rate of congenital defects does not differ between ethnic groups. An analysis of median age of death indicates there has been a striking improvement in longevity among white Down syndrome individuals. However, there has not been the same increase in longevity in other ethnic groups. This difference may be caused by differential availability of access to early intervention.[99] Prenatal diagnosis of Down syndrome is made by chromosome analysis, and screening can be conducted to help identify those who may need chromosome analysis. Currently in the United States a blood screening test for chromosome anomalies is given to all women in the first trimester of pregnancy. This is followed by prenatal cytogenic diagnosis if indicated. The screening method has a 69% detection rate at present and a 5% false-positive rate. There is much effort being made to increase sensitivity of the blood test to reduce or eliminate invasive testing such as amniocentesis.[96]

Nutrition therapy for individuals with Down syndrome focuses on delayed feeding skills; inappropriate, excessive, or inadequate intakes of food energy and nutrients; and poor eating habits. Diets need to be individualized because these children tend to gain excess weight if they are given the intakes recommended for children who do not have Down syndrome.[98]

Early intervention often occurs in Down patients because they are commonly diagnosed before or at birth. Common problems found in Down patients include congenital heart disease, hearing loss, and ophthalmologic problems. Thyroid disease and celiac disease are common, and development of diabetes may also occur with Down patients.[100] An awareness of these potential problems is important for the healthcare provider and for the family to allow prevention and early detection as the Down syndrome infant gets older. Encouraging physical activity is also important to helping reduce the risk of obesity and diabetes.

PROGRESSIVE NEUROLOGIC DISORDERS

Progressive neurologic disorders, especially through the middle and older years of adulthood, have disabling effects on the personal lives of many individuals. Examples reviewed here illustrate some of these effects and nutrition approaches to providing support.

Parkinson's Disease

Parkinson's disease is a long-known neurologic disease, first described by the English physician James Parkinson (1755-1824) nearly two centuries ago, when in 1817 he described its characteristic symptoms in "An Essay on the Shaking Palsy."[101] According to the World Parkinson's Disease Association, more than 4 million people worldwide have Parkinson's disease. It is a common disorder reported in every race, region of the world, and age-group, although the average age of onset is 55 years.

---

alpha fetoprotein A fetal antigen in amniotic fluid that provides an early pregnancy test for fetal malformations such as neural tube defect.

Ten percent of total cases affect those under age 40, and about 1% of all people over 60 years of age are affected. The onset of motor symptom dysfunction usually occurs after the age of 40 years, rising in incidence with advancing age.

Complete underlying origins of Parkinson's disease remain unknown. There appears to be a genetic influence in some cases, as well as an environmental influence. Most people with Parkinson's disease do not have a family history of the disorder: only about 15% of patients have a close relative with the disease.[102] Several different genetic factors influencing the onset of Parkinson's disease have been identified. For example, a parkin gene has been identified on chromosome 6 in several families that have early-onset, autosomal recessive parkinsonism. In these families at least one family member had been diagnosed with Parkinson's disease at 45 years of age or younger. Other Parkinson's risk factor genes have been identified, and similar discoveries are on the rise. At this time, however, routine genetic testing is not recommended for Parkinson's disease.[103]

There is some evidence that environmental factors may be related to incidence of Parkinson's disease. In 1983 a group of patients were by accident exposed to a toxic by-product of illegal pethidine production. Pethidine (meperidine) is a fast-acting opioid analgesic drug, sold under the name of Demerol. These individuals developed levodopa-responsive parkinsonism. Some researchers speculate that a trigger such as the toxic by-product above may in many cases be related to onset of the disease.[102]

Another theory concerning the development of Parkinson's disease involves iron status. Iron deficiency in early stages of life, despite correction with iron supplementation, may play a role in neurologic degeneration. It is not possible, however, to ascertain this information until an autopsy is performed.[104] Iron is known to accumulate at sites of brain pathologic processes in patients with Parkinson's disease, though postmortem examination cannot distinguish whether iron accumulation caused the damage or resulted from damage.[105] Parkinson's disease affects the basal ganglia, a cluster of nerve cells at the central base of the brain. Signals from the brain's motor cortex pass, via the brainstem reticular formation and the spinal cord, to the muscles, which contract. Other signals pass through the basal ganglia, which provides a damping effect to help smooth and control signal flow to reticular formation and spinal cord, thus preventing uncoordinated muscle contraction responses. This damping effect is produced by the balancing action of two neurotransmitters: (1) dopamine, which is made in the basal ganglia and is necessary for the damping effect, and (2) acetylcholine, a widespread neurotransmitter in the body. Dopamine stimulates signal flow, whereas acetylcholine inhibits it. In Parkinson's disease, degeneration of key parts of the basal ganglia causes a lack of dopamine within this part of the brain, thus preventing the basal ganglia from modifying nerve pathways that control muscle function. Muscles become overly tense, causing joint rigidity and a general body stiffness, a fine constant tremor even at rest, and slow movements.[102]

Medical Management

Although there is no cure for Parkinson's disease, there are an array of treatments that may help with symptomatic treatment of tremors and with preventing disease progression. Three forms of treatment are used: drugs, surgical interventions, and physical treatments.

Drug management has helped to minimize the symptoms for many patients. Medications include those that promote dopamine synthesis, such as levadopa and dopa-decarboxylase inhibitor. Other medications include those that activate specific receptors such as dopamine agonists and those that prolong dopamine availability such as monoamine oxidase type B (MAO-B) inhibitors. Other drugs prolong levadopa availability such as catechol-O-methyltransferase (COMT) inhibitors. COMT inhibitors are taken with levodopa. They prolong the duration of symptom relief by blocking the action of the enzyme, which breaks down levodopa before it reaches the brain. COMT inhibitors are usually started when a patient begins to experience a natural "wearing off" of the levodopa as the disease progresses. A more consistent exposure of levodopa to the brain aids in more independent function on the part of the patient. It improves the patient's ability to perform activities of daily living. Box 26-3 provides a list of medications commonly prescribed.

Neurosurgery for people with Parkinson's disease is done to restore functional balance in affected nervous tissue. There are three target areas for the surgeries: thalamus, globus pallidus, and subthalamic nucleus. Surgery may involve central nervous system lesions at one or more of these sites. Also, chronic stimulating electrodes may be implanted at these sites. In addition, reconstructive surgery may be used to implant fetal mesencephalic cells or other cells that produce dopamine.[106]

Nutrition Management

There is not a specific diet all Parkinson's patients should follow. The main emphasis should be on meeting nutrition needs of the individual, though general concerns include providing enough energy and protein to prevent weight loss and muscle atrophy. Also, the Parkinson's patient should emphasize sufficient fiber and fluid to reduce the risk of constipation. Calcium intake is a concern to help maintain the bone mass and strength of the affected individual. Energy requirements vary according to the severity of the symptoms. A Parkinson's patient who has dyskinesias (impaired ability for voluntary muscle movement), with much muscle involvement, may be using as much energy as a non-Parkinson's patient who has moderate activity. Increased Parkinson's movement may relate to weight loss in the advanced stages of the disease.

<table>
<tr><td>

BOX 26-3 | **Medications Used to Treat Parkinson's Disease**

Promote Dopamine Synthesis

Levadopa
Dopa-decarboxylase inhibitor

Activate Specific Receptors

Dopamine agonists
  Apomorphine
  Bromocriptine
  Cabergoline
  Dihydroergocryptine
  Lisuride
  Pergolide
  Piribedil
  Pramipexole
  Ropinirole

Prolong Dopamine Activity

MAO-B inhibitor: selegiline

Prolong Levadopa Bioavailability

COMT inhibitors
  Entacapone
  Tolcapone

Other Medications

Levodopa
Sinemet (levodopa/carbidopa)
Symmetrel (amantadine hydrochloride)
Anticholinergics (trihexyphenidyl, benztropine mesylate, procyclidine)
Eldepryl (selegiline or deprenyl)
Dopamine agonists: Parlodel (bromocriptine), Permax (pergolide), Mirapex (pramipexole), Requip (ropinirole)
COMT inhibitors: Tasmar (tolcapone), Comtan (entacapone)

From Rascol O et al: Treatment interventions for Parkinson's disease: an evidence based assessment, *Lancet* 359(9317):1589, 2002, with permission from Elsevier.

MAO-B, Monoamine oxidase type B; *COMT,* catechol-*O*-methyltransferase.
</td></tr>
</table>

Amino acids compete with levodopa to get across the blood-brain barrier. Because of this, treatment in the 1980s restricted protein intake to enhance uptake of levodopa into the brain. This may be beneficial for a small number of patients, but a protein-restricted diet is potentially harmful especially for those who are prone to malnutrition. With other improvements in treatment, such as controlled-release levodopa and surgical interventions, use of protein-restricted diets has declined. Rather than restricting protein, patients who may have problems with medication absorption should redistribute their protein throughout the day and avoid taking their levadopa with foods high in protein.

Other points of emphasis of nutrition therapy are bowel dysfunction; dysphagia; nausea, vomiting, and anorexia; delayed gastric emptying; hypotension when standing; bradykinesia; depression; and impaired cognitive function. Bowel dysfunction resulting in constipation, impaction, and obstruction are serious problems often found in the Parkinson's patient. Several factors contribute to this state, including a reduction in gastric motility associated with Parkinson's disease itself, as well as medication side effects, lack of exercise, and low fiber and fluid intake. Management of bowel dysfunction includes increasing fiber and fluid in the diet as well as increasing physical activity within the individual's abilities. Pharmacotherapy, use of medications that enhance bowel motility, may also be used to enhance bowel function.

More than 50% of Parkinson's patients experience dysphagia, especially in later stages of the disease. Aspiration contributes to death in many Parkinson's patients. A swallowing examination should be performed by a trained speech therapist. The assessment may result in changes to food texture, fluid viscosity, and temperature. In general, cold foods stimulate swallowing, and sour foods tend to provide stimuli for the oral and pharyngeal coordination of swallowing to occur.

Common side effects of levodopa include severe nausea that affects food intake. This problem is most often associated with initiation of the drug and tends to improve as the patient develops a tolerance to the drug. Taking the medications with a small snack such as crackers may be helpful in reducing nausea in patients who experience gastrointestinal distress or discomfort. Strategies for improving gastric emptying include eating small meals and taking medications 15 to 30 minutes before meals. Medications enhancing gastric motility, such as domperidone, may also be helpful.

Hand tremors make obtaining and preparing food, as well as eating movements of carrying food from the bowl or plate to the mouth, difficult. Thus, for example, soups should be avoided and more textured foods used. As the disease progresses, there may be problems with chewing, swallowing, or aspiration of small food items such as peas or nuts, as well as discomfort from constipation, flatulence, or delayed gastric emptying. The following changes may be helpful: small frequent meals of increased carbohydrate and decreased fat, chewing thoroughly and eating slowly with special utensils as needed, with appropriate energy intake to maintain optimal weight and adequate fiber and fluid to prevent constipation. Swallowing difficulties may necessitate changes in food texture appropriate for individuals with dysphagia (see Chapter 19).

Individuals with Parkinson's disease who suffer from bradykinesia (abnormal slowness of movement) have problems with slowness and stiffness. These individuals may benefit from small portions of food that are not over-

---

dyskinesia Impairment of the power of voluntary movement.
bradykinesia Very slow movement.

whelming. Also, changes in texture and size of pieces that are more appropriate for the patient should be made before presenting the meal to the patient to avoid embarrassment.

Hypotension with standing, also known as orthostatic hypotension, may result in falling or fainting when a Parkinson's patient stands. This seems to be related to advanced stages of the disease plus medication and dehydration resulting from less-than-adequate fluid intake. Patients with orthostatic hypotension may benefit from increased fluid intake and, if appropriate, increased sodium intake. This may be accomplished by encouraging adding salt at the table or consuming salty foods.

Depression and impaired cognitive function are common in Parkinson's patients. As many as 40% of patients may be depressed, and as many as 30% may suffer from dementia. These patients are at high risk for malnutrition because their emotional or mental status may result in an inability to prepare or consume adequate calories.[107]

Unintentional weight loss and body composition changes are common in Parkinson's patients. They are at greater nutritional risk than a matched population and should have continuing nutrition assessment and guidance to prevent this complication.[108]

Factors reported in epidemiologic studies relate to incidence of Parkinson's disease with high levels of iron intake in both sexes and high milk product intake in men. Factors reported in epidemiologic studies show inverse correlations of incidence of Parkinson's disease with low circulating levels of homocysteine, as well as with high caffeine intake. Those who were folate deficient and hyperhomocysteinemic had a greater chance of suffering from Parkinson's disease, though more research is needed in these areas to establish cause and effect. Administration of coenzyme Q has been shown to slow rate of deterioration in patients with early-stage Parkinson's disease according to one study. But again, more investigation is needed to establish efficacy of this treatment modality.[109]

Huntington's Chorea

First described in a landmark 1872 paper by American physician George Huntington (1850-1916), Huntington's chorea is an uncommon genetic disease in which degeneration of basal ganglia of the brain results in chorea (rapid, jerky, involuntary movements) and dementia (progressive mental impairment). In 1993 a large group of scientists from six institutions discovered the defective gene that causes the disease, opening the way to future therapeutic interventions and possibly a cure.[110] Cases of symptomatic effects beginning in childhood are rare. This genetic disease is inherited in an autosomal dominant pattern. The highest concentration of persons worldwide with Huntington's chorea is one family in the little town of San Luis on the shores of Lake Maracaibo high in the Andes mountains of Venezuela.[111] In the United States the disease develops in about 5 of 100,000

persons. Generally symptoms do not appear until middle adulthood (ages 35 to 50), so affected persons may have children before knowing they have the disease. Continuing study has identified the gene mutation that causes an abnormal protein product the researchers have called *huntingtin*.[112] Formation of this protein occurs when an abnormal expansion of the DNA sequence results in insertion of the amino acid glutamine into the primary sequence of proteins, resulting in insoluble protein aggregates. These insoluble proteins invade nuclei of nerve cells, which eventually shut down function of the cell and may cause cell death.[113]

Medical Management

As a result of recent advances in genetics, a test is now available for young adults whose parents have Huntington's chorea to learn, with 95% accuracy, if they carry the gene and thus have the disorder. This test can then help them decide whether to have children themselves. There is no known cure; therefore medical management helps to lessen the characteristic chorea, which affects face, arms, and trunk with random grimaces, twitches, and general clumsiness. The drug chlorpromazine (Thorazine), the most widely used antipsychotic drug for its tranquilizing effect (it suppresses brain centers that control abnormal emotions and behaviors), has been found to be useful in lessening mental impairment due to Huntington's. Thorazine has resulted in fewer behavior changes, as well as improvements in decisions, apathy, irritability, and memory loss.

Nutritional Management

Excessive muscular activity involved with Huntington's requires adequate energy and nutrient intake to prevent malnutrition and excess weight loss. As the disease progresses, patients become cachectic (a profound state of ill health and malnutrition resulting in emaciation and lean body loss) and, despite adequate food intake, demonstrate a progressive catabolic state. Nutrition counseling involves planning energy-nutrient-dense diets to combat malnutrition, usually 1.2 to 1.5 g of protein per kilogram of body weight. Also helpful is assistance with dysphagia or feeding problems and the provision of adequate fiber to combat the drug side effect of constipation.[114] Persons with advanced disease accompanied by dysphagia, marasmus, and depression may best be supported with an enteral formula. Bolus feedings via a PEG tube or other long-term enteral method is recommended due to the constant movement and risk of displacing the tube.

There is some evidence caloric restriction, while maintaining good nutrition and fewer meals, delayed onset of Huntington's Disease in mice and also caused mice with Huntington's Disease to live longer. This suggests the same might be true of humans who inherit the Huntington's gene.[115] More investigation needs to be done to substantiate these benefits.

Guillain-Barré Syndrome

Two twentieth-century French neurologists, Georges Guillain (1876-1961) and Jean Alexander Barré (1880-1965), first described this acute postinfectious polyneuritis. It is less commonly referred to as Landry's ascending paralysis. Guillain-Barré is a rare form of damage to peripheral nerves in which the myelin sheaths covering nerve axons, and sometimes the axons themselves, deteriorate, causing loss of nerve conduction and partial or complete paralysis. Nerve inflammation occurs particularly where their roots leave the spine, impairing both movement and sensation. Muscular weakness in the legs, often accompanied by numbness and tingling, progresses upward to trunk and arms, as well as face and head. A low-grade fever persists, and there may be urinary tract infection, respiratory failure requiring a ventilator, and personality changes. This acute syndrome is an autoimmune reaction, often following a viral infection or sometimes an immunization, such as the swine flu vaccine given readily in 1976. Two thirds of Guillain-Barré patients have reported they had an infection in the weeks preceding onset of the syndrome. Evidence indicates there is an association with *Campylobacter jejuni, Mycoplasma pneumoniae,* cytomegalovirus, and Epstein-Barr virus, and infection with one of these microorganisms often precedes Guillain-Barré syndrome. The infection and resultant syndrome is associated with axonal degeneration, slow recovery, and sometimes severe residual disability.[116] Incidence worldwide is about 1 to 3 per 100,000 annually and occurs in all age-groups, although rarely in infants. The incidence varies by age-group and tends to have peaks in late adolescence and early adulthood, as well as in older adults. Increased incidence in older adults may be due to a weakened immune system with age. Adolescents and young adults have a higher risk of cytomegalovirus and *Campylobacter* infection, which correlates with the onset of Guillain-Barré syndrome.[117]

Medical Management

Assessing effectiveness of treatments is difficult because individual effects are highly variable and improvement may be spontaneous and occur without any intervention. However, acute care is often necessary for close monitoring of the acute condition, especially if a breathing difficulty occurs. In severe cases, plasma exchange (PE) or plasmapheresis, in which blood plasma is withdrawn from the patient, treated to remove antibodies, and replaced, may be done. PE is potentially more dangerous with patients who have unstable blood pressure or who may be susceptible to coagulation. Most people completely recover from Guillain-Barré without specific treatment other than general supportive care, but many take several months to regain their ability to walk and function normally. However, some are left with permanent weakness in affected areas. One year after contraction, 5% of Guillain-Barré syndrome patients will die

and 15% are still unable to walk without assistance. Disabilities in ambulation due to leg weakness and possibly feeding disabilities due to arm and trunk damage may need attention from professional staff.[118]

Nutritional Management

During early acute phases, enteral or parenteral nutrition support may be necessary, with attention to increased energy and protein needs in the formula solutions. Respiratory distress requiring ventilator assistance can be problematic. In this case it is crucial not to overfeed the patient. Popular high-fat formulations that claim to decrease CO_2 production can cause delayed gastric emptying and further gastrointestinal complications and therefore should be avoided.[119] Food consistency and texture may need to be adjusted in early oral feedings to accommodate any chewing and swallowing problems from weak facial and throat muscles. Continuing attention to energy and nutrient needs during convalescence is required to restore lost body weight and muscle mass.

Amyotrophic Lateral Sclerosis

Medical Management

Amyotrophic lateral sclerosis (ALS) also is called *Lou Gehrig disease* for the famous U.S. baseball player who developed ALS at the height of his successful Major League career. ALS is the most common of the motor neuron diseases, affecting approximately 1 person in 10,000.[120] In these rare neuron disorders, nerves that control muscular activity degenerate within the brain and spinal cord. Researchers report discovery of the gene causing a hereditary form of the disease.[121,122] The gene, superoxide dismutase-1 *(SOD1),* controls synthesis of an enzyme that helps cells get rid of highly toxic and destructive superoxide free radicals, which are produced by a variety of oxidative cell reactions.[123] If the enzyme was abnormal because of the defective ALS gene, free cell radicals might build up, causing the death of the motor neurons affected in ALS. As it is now, the relentless nerve degeneration of ALS progresses to involve muscles of respiration and swallowing, usually killing its victims in about 3 years.[123]

---

chorea A wide variety of ceaseless involuntary movements that are rapid, complex, and jerky, yet appear to be well coordinated; characteristic movements of Huntington's disease.

amyotrophic lateral sclerosis (ALS) A progressive neuromuscular disease characterized by the degeneration of the neurons of the spinal cord and the motor cells of the brainstem, causing a deficit of upper and lower motor neurons; death usually occurs in 2 to 3 years.

Identifying the responsible defective gene has led to more knowledge of how the progressive destructive course of ALS may be slowed, controlled, or prevented. Riluzole remains the only drug to slow disease progression, although interventions such as noninvasive ventilation and gastrostomy also extend survival.[124] Research on ALS indicates a virus in the spinal cord may be partially responsible for escalation of the disease state.[125] Scientists are optimistic about the theory of a virus, because any virus has potential for a vaccine (as with polio) or treatment with antiretroviral medications (as with human immunodeficiency virus [HIV]). There is also some evidence that a toxin derived from a person's diet may play a role in ALS development.[126]

Other environmental influences, such as neurotrauma related to athletic competition, have been suggested and investigated.[127] Veterans of the 1991 Persian Gulf War are contracting ALS at twice the rate of the general population, although cause and effect has not been established because of the small sample size.[128] Results do suggest, however, environment may affect incidence of ALS in the population.

Nutritional Management

Nutrition therapy and counseling focus on increased energy intake and adjusting nutrient needs as the disease progresses. Weakness of hands and arms, as well as problems with chewing, swallowing, delayed or absent response of the gag reflex, and risk of aspiration, will require eating assistance and modification of food textures. Frequent small meals are better tolerated than a few large meals. In advanced stages, enteral and parenteral nutrition support can supply needed energy and nutrients in a variety of individualized formulas.[129,130]

Multiple Sclerosis

Multiple sclerosis (MS) is a progressive disease of the central nervous system that destroys scattered patches of insulating myelin, the fatty covering of nerve fibers in the brain and spinal cord that protects the neurons and facilitates the passage of neuromuscular impulses. The precise cause of MS is unknown, but it is an autoimmune disease in which the body's defense system begins to treat myelin tissue in the central nervous system as a foreign substance and gradually sets out to destroy it, with subsequent scarring left in its wake.

In these denuded patches, nonfunctional plaques of scar tissue replace myelin whereby nerve fiber can no longer conduct normal electrical impulses. The severity of the condition varies markedly from person to person. An as-yet-unknown genetic factor is probably involved in development of MS because relatives of affected persons are eight times more likely than others to develop the disease. Environment seems to play a role. MS is five times more common in temperate zones, such as the United States and Europe, than in the tropics. Perhaps it is induced by a virus picked up in the first 15 years of life in these temperate climates. Approximately two thirds of persons affected experience beginning symptoms between ages 20 and 40 years, twice as many women than men are affected, and it is most commonly found in white populations. In the relatively high-risk temperate areas incidence of MS is about 1 in 1000 people. Depending on how extensive tissue involvement is and which parts of the brain and spinal cord are affected, effects of MS vary widely from mild periodic feelings of tingling, numbness, constriction, or stiffness in any part of the body to more severe disabling disease. Symptoms may also include urinary bladder urgency, dizziness, loss of balance, fatigue, and depression.

Diagnosis of the disease should be made by a physician with MS experience, based on objective evidence of two or more neurologic signs using magnetic resonance imaging (MRI) with gadolinium contrast. The MRI should show evidence of brain lesions. A second MRI at least 3 months later will help identify new lesions and track progression of existing lesions. It is important to rule out other potential contributors to the symptoms such as vascular disease, spinal cord compression, vitamin B_{12} deficiency, central nervous cord infection such as Lyme disease or syphilis, and other inflammatory conditions such as systemic lupus erythematosus.

Medical Management

Although there is no cure for MS, there are five disease-modifying drugs approved by the Food and Drug Administration to treat MS patients. Four of the treatments are used in initial management of the disease to help slow progression and reduce symptoms. The fifth is used for worsening forms when the individual with MS is in relapse. Three of the four initial treatments are beta interferons, intramuscular interferon beta-1a (Avonex), subcutaneous interferon beta-1a (Rebif), and interferon beta-1b (Betaseron). Beta interferons are cytokines, which have their therapeutic effects by modulating immune function and have antiviral activities. They have been shown to reduce relapses by about one third. In double-blind placebo-controlled trials, beta interferon treatments were shown to reduce lesions on MRIs by 50% to 80% and to improve the patient's quality of life.[131,132] There may be side effects associated with beta interferon use such as flulike symptoms, injection site reactions, worsening of preexisting spasticity, depression, and anemia. The fourth drug used for initial treatment of MS works through a different mechanism: glatiramer is a polypeptide mixture designed to mimic and compete with myelin sheath protein. It has been shown to reduce relapses by about one third and is generally well tolerated. A fifth drug, mitoxantrone, is recommended for use with patients experiencing worsening forms of MS. Mitoxantrone has been shown to reduce relapses by 67%.

Side effects include nausea and alopecia. Mitoxantrone is used only with severe cases and only for 2 to 3 years because of its cumulative toxic effects on the heart.

The best time to start treatment is early after diagnosis to reduce lesion progression and irreversible damage, because treatment modalities are most effective at reducing new lesions rather than repairing old lesions.[131]

Nutritional Management

Individuals with MS respond to basic nutrition therapy that supplies adequate energy and nutrients to achieve optimal nutrition status. Similar to other neuromuscular diseases, assistance with symptomatic gastrointestinal problems, elimination, and dysphagia is instituted as needed.[133] If steroid therapy is initiated, dietary sodium maybe reduced. Nasoenteric or gastrostomy tube feeding may be needed in advanced stages of the disease to provide enteral nutrition support and is generally well tolerated.[134]

There are no well-supported data that diet has a profound effect on treatment of MS; however, a low-fat, low-calorie, low-saturated fat diet may help to manage some symptoms associated with the disease.[135] Prevention of MS has been the debate for many years. One study indicates a diet rich in fruits, vegetables and whole grains may be preventative and an increased risk of MS may be related to high energy and animal food intake, but evidence is not conclusive.[136] Often "diets" touted to prevent MS are confused by the general public as treatment regimens. For example, it has been suggested that high consumption of animal fat, high-energy foods, and low intake of fish products and plant components may play a role in the "etiology" of MS,[136] but there is no evidence that eating high amounts of plant foods and fish products has any great effect on the prevention, prognosis, or progression of the disease.

Myasthenia Gravis

Cause for the neuromuscular disease myasthenia gravis (MG) is unknown. MG occurs in about 14 of every 100,000 persons, eventually causing the affected person to become paralyzed as a result of inability of neuromuscular junctions to transmit nerve fiber signals to the voluntary muscles. The most common form of MG is a chronic autoimmune disorder in which antibodies from the body's immune system attack acetylcholine receptors and gradually destroy the receptors in voluntary muscles that are responsible for picking up nerve impulses. As a result, affected muscles respond to nerve impulses only weakly or not at all.[137]

According to the Myasthenia Gravis Foundation of America, only about 2 to 5 new cases of this rare disease per 100,000 people are diagnosed annually. It affects more women than men in a ratio of 3:2. Although it can occur at any age, it usually occurs from ages 20 to 30 in women and from ages 50 to 70 in men.[138] Facial muscles are usually affected first, causing drooped eyelids, double vision, and sometimes a lack of facial animation with an absent stare appearance. Weak muscles of the face, throat, larynx, and neck cause difficulties in speaking and eating. As muscles in the arms and legs become affected, problems with other daily living activities such as food procurement and preparation, as well as dressing, personal hygiene, and climbing stairs, also develop. In severe cases, respiratory muscles in the chest weaken and cause breathing difficulty.

Medical Management

Treatment involves administration of corticosteroids and immunosuppressive drugs. Further temporary relief for the severely compromised patient may be obtained through immune system modulation by plasmapheresis or by intravenous immunoglobulin (IVIG) administration. Because the disease is caused by circulating autoantibodies, exchanges of the patient's antibody-containing blood for antibody-free blood may be helpful in warding off a crisis.[137]

Antibodies produced by the disease attack receptors on muscle cells that bind acetylcholine neurotransmitter necessary for muscle contraction, thus effectively reducing stimulation of muscle cells and weakening muscle action. Anticholinesterase agents used to treat MG, such as neostigmine (Prostigmin) or pyridostigmine (Mestinon), increase the amount of the neurotransmitter acetylcholine at the nerve ending by blocking the action of the enzyme that normally breaks it down.[139] Blocking action of these drugs increases levels of the acetylcholine transmitter by allowing more of it to accumulate in the synaptic cleft between nerve and muscle fiber endings, thus permitting the remaining receptors to function more efficiently. Corticosteroids (prednisone) and immunosuppressants like azathioprine (Imuran) may be used to suppress the abnormal action of the immune system that occurs in MG.

Nutritional Management

Nutrition therapy has three main goals, as follows:

1. To maintain optimal energy-nutrient intake for muscle strength and good nutritional status
2. To solve any associated eating problems
3. To help counteract drug side effects of nausea and vomiting

---

myasthenia gravis (MG) A progressive neuromuscular disease caused by faulty nerve conduction resulting from the presence of antibodies to acetylcholine receptors at the neuromuscular junction.

The previously mentioned drugs should be taken with liquid or food to lessen stomach irritation. Other suggestions are to adjust meal patterns to accommodate the individual. Provide the largest meal at breakfast, when the patient is more rested, and then frequent small meals throughout the day; take medications 1 hour before eating when strength is best; modify food texture to decrease excessive chewing; and supplement with enteral feedings as needed.

Alzheimer's Disease

Alzheimer's disease was named for the German neurologist Alois Alzheimer (1864-1915), who in 1907 first described the characteristic neurofibrillary tangles found in the postmortem brain of a 51-year-old demented woman named Auguste who died in 1906.[140,141] Also referred to as senile dementia Alzheimer's type (SDAT), the disease is a form of progressive dementia in which nerve cells degenerate in the brain and the brain substance shrinks. The hallmark of the disease is the development of abnormal intracellular filaments in tangles of neurofibrils and extracellular deposits of amyloid-forming protein in senile plaques (amyloid plaques) and cerebral blood vessels, as first reported by Alzheimer. Density of these plaques has become the basis for the postmortem diagnosis of Alzheimer's disease; there is no absolute diagnostic test for the disease during life, although there is an assessment instrument, the Mini-Mental State Examination (MMSE), which is commonly used to assess cognitive changes with dementia patients. Coupled with clinical examination, MMSE assessments may result in accurate diagnosis 90% of the time. The MMSE assesses six areas of function: orientation, registration, attention and calculation, recall, language, and ability to copy a figure. A score of 23 or less on the 30-question scale suggests that the person suffers from dementia. The MMSE has limitations in that is does not specify the cause of the dementia. It also may fail to detect mild dementia.

Alzheimer's disease accounts for 60% to 80% of dementia cases over the age of 65 years. It afflicts between 2.7% and 11.7% of the population over the age of 65 years and about half of the population over the age of 85 years.[142]

In addition to its human cost to patient and family, Alzheimer's disease levies a tremendous social and financial burden. Currently more than 4.5 million Americans have been diagnosed. Care for these patients costs about $100 billion dollars annually. The Alzheimer's Association estimates there may be 16 million cases in the United States by the year 2050. With the rapidly increasing population of persons over 85 years, the healthcare problem of Alzheimer's disease is assuming enormous proportions. By 2010, Medicare costs for beneficiaries with Alzheimer's are expected to increase 54.5%, from $31.9 billion in 2000 to $49.3 billion.

There is no known single cause for Alzheimer's disease, though researchers have learned a great deal about factors that play a role in its onset. Rare, familial types of Alzheimer's have been discovered in a few hundred families worldwide. Individuals who inherit the specific gene carried in affected families are almost guaranteed to develop Alzheimer's by the time they reach 65 years of age. Some may develop the disease as early as 30 years of age. Other factors related to the onset of Alzheimer's disease that offer preliminary hope are aspects of maintaining general health as a person ages: controlling blood pressure, weight, and blood cholesterol while exercising the body and mind and remaining socially active.

One theory behind the development of SDAT is oxidative stress. Many researchers have investigated this area, reviewing flavonoids, antioxidants, and dietary restriction as methods to both prevent the onset of Alzheimer's and treat it.[143,144]

Other dietary factors being investigated concerning onset of Alzheimer's disease include dietary folate and fish and omega-3 fatty acid intake. Elevated plasma homocysteine is a strong risk factor for Alzheimer's disease. Adequate dietary folate is known to reduce plasma homocysteine and may therefore reduce the risk of Alzheimer's. However, additional research is needed to substantiate this potential role of dietary folate.[145] Fish oils and fish consumption, at least on a weekly basis, may reduce the risk of Alzheimer's disease according to a study of 8500 individuals who were 65 years old and older based on a self-administered food frequency questionnaire. However, better-controlled studies need to be done to substantiate this.[146]

Progression of Alzheimer's disease has been divided into three broad stages, as follows[147]:

1. *Stage one:* the early period of increasing forgetfulness and anxious depression
2. *Stage two:* a middle period of severe memory loss of recent events, disorientation, and personality changes
3. *Stage three:* the final period of severe confusion, psychosis, memory loss, personal neglect, inability to leave the bed, feeding problems, full-time nursing care, and finally death from an infection such as pneumonia

Medical Management

Once a person has been diagnosed with Alzheimer's disease, an individual treatment plan must be formed. This plan should include methods for slowing the decline in cognitive function such as the use of cholinesterase inhibitor therapy. The treatment plan should also include management of other conditions that are present such as Parkinson's disease or heart disease, because the patient will lose the ability to care for these problems. Treatment of behavior and mood symptoms related to Alzheimer's disease is also important. Methods and resources supporting both the

Alzheimer's patient and caregivers will be helpful in making the multiple transitions that may occur over the course of the disease, because the patient's symptoms and needs will continue to change.

In stage one, the physician should provide information about expectations regarding drug therapy. The physician should also discuss patient and caregiver preferences regarding choices that will inevitably be made in the future concerning care and end-of-life decisions. In stage two, with changes in the patient's behavior, the caregiver may need assistance in dealing emotionally with the changes, as well as support to physically manage the patient. In the third stage of Alzheimer's, the caregiver may require additional support to help with daily living activities, as well as guidance concerning placement and terminal care.[148,149]

There is no treatment for the disease itself, except for suitable day-to-day nursing and social care for both the patient and the family. Keeping the patient well nourished, occupied, and physically active helps to lessen anxiety and personal distress, especially in the early stages when the person is sufficiently aware of his or her condition.[150] A regular exercise program, combined with education for caregivers concerning techniques for behavior management, has been shown to improve the physical health of the affected individual and to reduce depression. Physical activity may also reduce the frailty that often accompanies Alzheimer's patients as they progress through the disease.[151] Some use of antianxiety medication often helps improve difficult behavior and enables the patient to sleep more restfully. Family counseling and respite care are essential.

Research into drug therapy continues, though at present, cholinesterase inhibitors (ChEIs) are regarded as the standard treatment of Alzheimer's disease. Four ChEIs have been approved by the Food and Drug Administration for the treatment of mild to moderate Alzheimer's disease. These are tacrine (Cognex), donepezil (Aricept), rivastigmine (Exelon), and galantamine (Reminyl). These compounds are effective because they increase the concentration of acetylcholine at nerve cell synapses by inhibiting breakdown of acetylcholine. These drugs may relieve behavioral and psychologic symptoms of Alzheimer's disease, but the effects may be extremely variable, with no improvement in some patients, whereas others make dramatic improvements.[148]

A host of alternative treatments for Alzheimer's is also emerging with the millennial trend moving toward alternative medicine. In most cases there is insufficient scientific evidence backing the majority of products available on the market. The latest news available on some of the more popular products is presented in the *Complementary and Alternative Medicine (CAM)* box, "Alternative Treatments for Alzheimer's Disease."

Nutritional Management

Nutrition therapy in each stage of Alzheimer's disease becomes increasingly difficult and challenging. Cognitive losses may have profound effects on nutritional intake for several reasons. The Alzheimer's patient may lack the attention needed to eat or may not be able to concentrate long enough to eat enough food to provide sufficient calories and nutrients to sustain daily needs. The patient may also have memory problems related to the use of utensils or the act of swallowing. The patient may be combative or refuse to go into the dining room where the food is available. Appropriate caregiver education about interventions may be helpful in minimizing the negative effects of dementia-related eating problems.

Adequate nutrition throughout the course of the disease is essential to improve physical well-being, help maximize the patient's functioning, and improve the quality of life. Nutrition-related changes occur at each progressive stage of the illness, as shown in Table 26-4, and illustrate the major goals of maintaining adequate nutrition and preventing malnutrition and devising practical ways of dealing with feeding problems.[152] Because these patients may be more active, they tend to have lower body weight and may require higher energy intakes than normal older adults. They often require high-caloric supplements to help supply added nourishment. In general, they have more risk factors and major indicators of poor nutritional status than the overall older adult population.[153] The following four major factors help promote optimal intake in long-term care:

1. Using skillful individual feeding techniques
2. Selecting appropriate food consistency
3. Providing adequate time in which to feed
4. Focusing on the midday meal when peak cognitive abilities occur

Health Promotion

Outcomes Measurement

In the United States the number of persons reporting disabling conditions from 1994 to 1995 was 54 million.[153] During 1996, direct medical costs for persons with disability were $260 billion. Rising healthcare costs are just one of the reasons behind developing outcome standards. A second rationale for developing outcome standards is for the practitioner to have a reliable tool to compare data

---

amyloid A glycoprotein substance having a relation to starchlike structure but more a protein compound; an abnormal complex material forming characteristic brain deposits of fibrillary tangles always found in postmortem examinations of patients with Alzheimer's disease, the only means of definitive diagnosis; found in various body tissues that, when advanced, form lesions that destroy functional cells and injure the organ.

COMPLEMENTARY AND ALTERNATIVE MEDICINE (CAM)
Alternative Treatments for Alzheimer's Disease

Product	Description
Metrifonate	Metrifonate is a cholinesterase inhibitor that has been investigated for use with mild to moderate AD cases. It has been found effective in areas of cognition and global functioning compared to placebo in four randomized, double-blind controlled trials. However, development of this agent has been stopped based on side effects including muscle weakness and respiratory paralysis.[a]
Memantine	Memantine has been approved for use in the treatment of dementia in Germany for over 10 years and has recently been approved for use in the European Union. It has been useful in moderate to severe cases of AD. The FDA is currently reviewing this drug.[a]
Antioxidants vitamin E and selegiline	Vitamin E is a lipid-soluble vitamin obtained naturally from foods or supplemented. Because of its antioxidative effect, it may aid in the breakdown of free radicals that may be the cause of damage to brain cells. Selegiline is a drug used in the therapy of Parkinson's disease. It is defined as a selective MAO-B inhibitor. Selegiline was originally developed as an antidepressant. Selegiline has been medically approved for use only in treatment of Parkinson's disease. In a double-blind randomized placebo-controlled study, fewer patients in the vitamin E group (2000 IU/day) and the selegiline (5 mg bid) reached one of the four endpoints (death, institutionalization, loss of two of three basic daily functions, or severe dementia) compared to the control group. Because of potential side effects of gastrointestinal tract distress and prolonged bleeding, a lower dose of 400 IU/day is recommended if vitamin E is chosen as a therapeutic regimen. If vitamin E is tolerated, there is no need to use selegiline. The U.S. RDA for vitamin E is 30 IU/day.[a-d]
Estrogen	Oral conjugated equine estrogen has not been shown to be an effective treatment modality for AD in postmenopausal women. Therefore estrogen is not recommended to treat AD patients. However, there is increasing evidence that estrogen may have positive effects on the risk and may delay the time of onset of AD in postmenopausal women.[a]
Ginkgo biloba	Ginkgo biloba is a plant extract that has both antioxidant and antiinflammatory properties to protect cell membranes and to regulate neurotransmitter function. Researchers have linked Ginkgo biloba (120 to 240 mg/day for 3 to 6 months) with small but significant improvement in cognition function in four randomized, placebo-controlled trials. However, research is needed to determine if there are improvements in activities of daily living and social behavior. There are no data concerning the safety of using ChEIs in conjunction with Ginkgo biloba. One known risk associated with gingko is hemorrhaging if taken with other anticoagulants, because it is known to reduce the ability of the blood to clot.[e,f]
Huperzine A	Huperzine A is a moss extract that traditionally has been used in Chinese medicine for centuries. It acts as an acetylcholinesterase inhibitor. It has been shown to be just as effective as the leading FDA-approved medications, but it is unregulated and manufactured under no uniform standards. Therefore it is not recommended and is considered dangerous.
Coenzyme Q10	Also known as ubiquinone, coenzyme Q10 is an antioxidant that occurs naturally in the body and is necessary for normal cell reactions. Little is known about coenzyme Q10 and its consideration to treat Alzheimer's disease.

AD, Alzheimer's disease; *FDA,* Food and Drug Administration; *MAO-B,* monoamine oxidase type B; *RDA,* Recommended Dietary Allowance; *ChEI,* cholinesterase inhibitor.

[a]Grossberg GT, Desai AK: Management of Alzheimer's disease, *J Gerontol A Biol Sci Med Sci* 58A(4):331, 2003.

[b] Miller JW: Vitamin E and memory: is it vascular protection? *Nutr Rev* 58(4):109, 2000.

[c]Huntington's disease. In Escott-Stump S, ed: *Nutrition and diagnosis-related care,* ed 4, Philadelphia, 1997, Lippincott Williams & Wilkins.

[d] Duan W et al: Dietary restriction normalizes glucose metabolism and BDNF levels, slows disease progression, and increases survival in huntingtin mutant mice, *Proc Nat Acad Sci* 100(5):2911, 2003.

[e] Pritchard J, Hughes RAC: Guillain-Barré syndrome, *Lancet* 363(9427):2186, 2004.

[f] LeBars PL et al: A placebo-controlled, double-blind, randomized trial of an extract of Ginkgo biloba for dementia: North American EGb study group, *JAMA* 278(16):1327, 1997.

to make an accurate assessment of a patient. Practically every specialty has a set of standards. In disability and rehabilitation, a commonly reported standard is the Functional Independence Measure (FIM). FIM is an objective method of obtaining functional performance information from a patient. From this seven-point test, the observer can make a determination as far as the patient's length of stay or discharge plan. This information is essential in this age of cost containment.[154-158]

A traditional assessment method is determining the patient's activities of daily living (ADLs). ADLs include mobility around the home, getting to and from the toilet, transfer from chair, transfer from bed, feeding, dressing, and bathing. With either of these methods, a point system is used to determine a specific outcome, leaving less room for subjective interpretations that would otherwise be obtained strictly from an interview process with patient and caregivers. That is not to presume subjective

TABLE 26-4	Progression of Alzheimer's Disease

Stage	General Symptoms	Nutrition-Related Effects
1 (Early)	Loss of memory	Difficulty in shopping, cooking
	Decrease in social and vocational skills	Forgetting to eat
	Careless work, housekeeping, finances	Changes in taste and smell
	Easily lost	Unusual food choices
	Personality changes	Degeneration of appetite regulation
	Recognition of faces	
	Well-oriented to time	
2 (Middle)	Inability to recall names	Increased energy requirement from agitation
	Disorientation to time	Holding food in mouth
	Delusions	Forgetting to swallow
	Depression	Losing ability to use utensils
	Agitation	Using spoon only
	Language problems	Eating with hands
3 (Final)	Complete disorientation	No recognition of food
	Forgetting own name	Refusal to eat or open mouth for feeding
	Not recognizing family	Need for nasogastric feeding
	Loss of verbal skills	
	Loss of basic self-care skills	
	Urinary and fecal incontinence	
	Bed-bound	

Data from Gray GE: Nutrition and dementia, *J Am Diet Assoc* 89(12):1795, 1989.

assessment does not have a place in patient care, but rather to point out the importance of objective methods in making logical conclusions about patient outcomes.[154-158]

Other assessment methods that have been developed and are routinely used throughout hospitals and rehabilitation settings are the Glasgow Coma Scale score, the Revised Trauma Score, the Fugl-Meyer Assessment (FMA) and the Neurobehavioral Cognitive Status Examination (NCSE) for motor and cognitive abilities; Spinal Pain Independence Measure (SPIM) for patients with chronic low back pain disability; the Spinal Cord Independence Measure (SCIM), recently revised by Catz-Itzkovich, to more sensitively measure the functional performance of patients with spinal cord lesions; the Office of Population Censuses and Surveys Scale (OPCS) and the Amputee Activity Score (AAS), to measure specifically the function for an amputee; and the Test of Playfulness (ToP), used primarily with children with disabilities to measure interactions between the child and his or her environment and activity.[154-158]

As with any assessment tool, reliability and validity between users is of primary significance. By choosing a method described above, the observer can easily assess a patient's disability and make a logical determination based on factual information.

TO SUM UP

Individuals facing chronic disabling illness and injury confront a myriad of complex challenges, including social, financial, physical, and psychologic barriers. The team approach, involving family and friends in addition to health professionals, becomes an essential basis of care.

Basic principles of nutrition care involve the prevention of malnutrition and restoration of eating ability. The role of the nutritionist is to assess individual nutrition requirements to meet basal energy expenditure (BEE) needs, adjust for metabolic activity factors (MAFs) resulting from any underlying disease process, and consider requirements to meet the energy needs of physical therapy and other activities. There must be sufficient intake to meet basic energy and macronutrient requirements. Vitamin and mineral supplements may be needed to guard against deficiencies.

To restore eating ability the occupational therapist and nurse play significant roles in promoting adequate swallowing, chewing, and hand and utensil use skills. To meet individual nutrient needs the nutritionist must assess eating skills, estimate eating desire (sensory stimuli, "comfort foods"), and help the client develop new ways of eating with various self-help devices.

Chronic disabling conditions that require special nutrition attention and modification to treat underlying disease effects include (1) musculoskeletal disease, such as various forms of arthritis; (2) neuromuscular injury and disease, caused by a sudden brain or spinal cord injury or a stroke or by developmental disabilities resulting from cerebral palsy, epilepsy, or spina bifida; and (3) progressive neurologic disorders, such as Parkinson's and Huntington's diseases, ALS, multiple sclerosis, or dementia as seen in Alzheimer's disease.

QUESTIONS FOR REVIEW

1. What are two major goals of rehabilitative therapy for chronic disabling conditions? How do the basic principles of nutrition therapy help meet these goals?

2. Describe functions of major nutrients in preventing or retarding the catabolic process that often occurs in long-term disabling illness or injury.

3. Select six different disease processes or injuries discussed that result in eating disabilities. Describe the nature of the disease or injury, and relate it to the disability involved. Outline the medical and nutrition therapy used in each case, giving the rationale for the nutritional management.

REFERENCES

1. Moore C: The dietitian in clinical practice. In Winterfeldt EA, Bogle ML, Ebro LL: *Dietetics, practice and future trends,* Gaithersburg, Md, 1998, Aspen.

2. Lacey K, Pritchett E: Nutrition care process and model: ADA adopts road map to quality care and outcomes management, *J Am Diet Assoc* 103(8):1061, 2003.

3. Verbrugge LM et al: The great efficacy of personal and equipment assistance in reducing disability, *Am J Public Health* 87(3):384, 1997.

4. National Institute of Neurological Disorders and Stroke: *Poststroke rehabilitation fact sheet,* Bethesda, Md, 2006, National Institutes of Health. Retrieved March 3, 2006, from *www.ninds.nih.gov/disorders/stroke/poststrokerehab.htm.*

5. National Center for Health Statistics: *National vital statistics report, United States life tables, 2002,* Washington, DC, 2004 (November 10), Author.

6. Federal Interagency Forum on Aging-Related Statistics: *Older Americans 2004: key indicators of well-being—highlights,* Washington, DC, 2004 (modified 2005), Administration on Aging, U.S. Department of Health and Human Services. Retrieved March 3, 2006, from *www.agingstats.gov/chartbook2004/highlights.html.*

7. Manton KG, Stallard E, Corder LS: The dynamics of dimensions of age-related disability 1982 to 1994 in the U.S. elderly population, *J Gerontol A Biol Sci Med Sci* 53(1):B59, 1998.

8. The leading causes of disability worldwide, 1990, in years of life lived with disability, *BMJ* 325:947, 2002.

9. Bureau of Primary Health Care, Health Resources and Services Administration: *Assistive devices,* Rockville, Md, U.S. Department of Health and Human Services. Retrieved March 3, 2006, from *http://bphc.hrsa.gov/nhdp/ASSISTIVE_DEVICES_OT.htm.*

10. Pisetsky DS, St. Clair EW: Progress in the treatment of rheumatoid arthritis, *JAMA* 286(22):2787, 2001.

11. American College of Rheumatology Subcommittee on Rheumatoid Arthritis Guidelines: Guidelines for the management of rheumatoid arthritis: 2002 update, *Arthritis Rheum* 46:328, 2002.

12. O'Dell JR: Therapeutic strategies for rheumatoid arthritis, *N Engl J Med* 350(25):2591, 2004.

13. Hooper L et al: The effectiveness of five strategies for the prevention of gastrointestinal toxicity induced by non-steroidal antiinflammatory drugs: systematic review, *BMJ* 329(7472):948, 2004.

14. O'Dell JR. Therapeutic strategies for rheumatoid arthritis, *N Engl J Med* 350(25):2591, 2004.

15. Schnabel A: Disease-modifying antirheumatic drugs: enhancing efficacy by combination, *Lancet* 363(9410):670, 2004.

16. Preboth M: Infliximab for the treatment of rheumatoid arthritis, *Am Fam Physician* 65(11):2384, 2002.

17. Olsen NJ, Stein M: New drugs for rheumatoid arthritis, *N Engl J Med* 350(21):2167, 2004.

18. Glucosamine improves joint mobility for 1 in 5 patients with osteoarthritis, *BMJ* 327(7427):1296, 2003.

19. Hochberg MC: What a difference a year makes: reflections on the ACR recommendations for the medical management of osteoarthritis, *Curr Rheumatol Rep* 3:473, 2001.

20. Hochberg MC: Pharmacological therapy of osteoarthritis, *Best Pract Res Clin Rheumatol* 15:583, 2001.

21. Lo GH et al: Intra-articular hyaluronic acid in treatment of knee osteoarthritis: a meta-analysis, *JAMA* 290(23):3115, 2003.

22. Agren JJ et al: Divergent changes in serum sterols during a strict uncooked vegan diet in patients with rheumatoid arthritis, *Br J Nutr* 85(2):137, 2001.

23. Muller H, de Toledo FW, Resch KL: Fasting followed by vegetarian diet in patients with rheumatoid arthritis: a systematic review, *Scand J Rheumatol* 30(1):1, 2001.

24. Hanninen O et al: Antioxidants in vegan diet and rheumatic disorders, *Toxicology* 155(1-3):45, 2000.

25. Tidow-Kebritchi S, Mobarhan S. Effects of diets containing fish oil and vitamin E on rheumatoid arthritis, *Nutr Rev* 59(10):335, 2001.

26. Westhoff G, Listing J, Zink A: Loss of physical independence in rheumatoid arthritis: interview data from a representative sample of patients in rheumatologic care, *Arthritis Care Res* 13(1):11, 2000.

27. Gorevic PD: Osteoarthritis: a review of musculoskeletal aging and treatment issues in geriatric patients, *Geriatrics* 59(8):28, 2004.

28. Vallerand AH: Treating arthritis pain, *Nurse Pract* 28(4):7, 2003.

29. Kanis JA et al: Risk of hip fracture according to the World Health Organization criteria for osteopenia and osteoporosis, *Bone* 27(5):585, 2000.

30. Clinical management guidelines for obstetricians and gynecologists: osteoporosis, *Obstet Gynecol* 103(1):203, 2004.

31. Wolf RL et al: Update on the epidemiology of osteoporosis, *Curr Rheumatol Rep* 2(1):74, 2000.

32. National Osteoporosis Foundation: *Fast facts on osteoporosis,* Washington, DC, Author. Retrieved March 3, 2006, from *www.nof.org/osteoporosis/diseasefacts.htm.*

33. Snelling AM et al: Modifiable and nonmodifiable factors associated with osteoporosis in postmenopausal women: results from the Third National Health and Nutrition Examination Survey, 1988-1994, *J Womens Health Gend Based Med* 10(1):57, 2001.

34. Cauley JA et al: Effects of estrogen plus progesterone on risk of fracture and bone mineral density: the Women's Health Initiative Randomized Trial, *JAMA* 290:1729, 2003.

35. American College of Obstetricians and Gynecologists: *Statement of the American College of Obstetricians and Gynecologists on hormone therapy for the prevention and treatment of postmenopausal osteoporosis,* Washington, DC, 2003, Author. Retrieved March 3, 2006, from *www.acog.org/from_home/publications/press_releases/nr10-07-03.cfm.*

36. U.S. Preventive Services Task Force: Screening for osteoporosis in postmenopausal women: recommendations and rationale, *Ann Intern Med* 137(6):526, 2002.

37. Wilson JF: New treatments for growing scourge of brittle bones, *Ann Intern Med* 140(2):153, 2004.

38. Bone HG et al: Ten years' experience with alendronate for osteoporosis in postmenopausal women, *N Engl J Med* 350(12):1189, 2004.

39. Prince RL, Kerr DA: What strategies can women use to optimize bone health at this stage of life? *Med J Aust* 173(suppl):S106, 2000.

40. American Heart Association: *Leading causes of death: 1998, biostatistical fact sheet,* Dallas, 2001, Author.

41. Christopher Reeve Foundation: *SCI facts,* Short Hills, NJ, 1999, Author. Retrieved March 3, 2006, from *www.christopherreeve.org/site/c.geIMLPOpGjF/b.1402847/k.EE60/SCI_Facts.htm.* (Statistics published by the University of Alabama National Spinal Cord Injury Statistical Center, Centers for Disease Control and Prevention.)

42. Lovaski D, Kerr ME, Alexander S: Traumatic brain injury research: a review of clinical studies, *Crit Care Nurs Q* 23(4):24, 2001.

43. Anonymous: TBI state demonstration grants, *J Head Trauma Rehabil* 15(1):750, 2000.

44. Thurman D: The epidemiology and economics of head trauma. In Miller L, Hayes R, eds: *Head trauma: basic, preclinical, and clinical directions,* New York, 2001, Wiley and Sons.

45. Pepe JL, Barba CA: The metabolic response to acute traumatic brain injury and implications for nutritional support, *J Head Trauma Rehabil* 14(5):462, 1999.

46. Klodell CT et al: Routine intragastric feeding following traumatic brain injury is safe and well tolerated, *Am J Surg* 179(3):168, 2000.

47. Yanagawa T et al: Nutritional support for head injured patients, *Cochrane Database Syst Rev* (2):CDC001530, 2000.

48. Kirby DF et al: Early enteral nutrition after brain injury by percutaneous endoscopic gastrojejunostomy, *J Parenter Enteral Nutr* 15(3):298, 1991

49. Silkroski M: Transitional feeding. In, *Tube feeding: practical guidelines and nursing protocols,* Gaithersburg, Md, 2001, Aspen.

50. Rice DR, Max W: Annotation: the high cost of injuries in the United States, *Am J Public Health* 86(1):14, 1996.

51. Berkowitz et al: *Spinal cord injury: an analysis of medical and social costs,* The University of Alabama at Birmingham National Spinal Cord Injury Statistical Center, The National Spinal Cord Injury Association, New York, 1998, Demos Medical Publishing.

52. Schwab ME: Repairing the injured spinal cord, *Science* 295(5557):1029, 2002.

53. Cruse JM et al: Review of immune function, healing of pressure ulcers, and nutritional status in patients with spinal cord injury, *J Spinal Cord Med* 23(2):129, 2000.

54. Cruse JM et al: Facilitation of immune function, healing of pressure ulcers, and nutritional status in spinal cord injury patients, *Exp Mol Pathol* 68(1):384, 2000.

55. Desport JC et al: Total body water and percentage fat mass measurements using bioelectrical impedance analysis and anthropometry in spinal cord-injured patients, *Clin Nutr* 19(3):185, 2000.

56. Monroe MB et al: Lower daily energy expenditure as measured by a respiratory chamber in subjects with spinal cord injury compared with control subjects, *Am J Clin Nutr* 68(6):1223, 1998.

57. Rouch W: Are pushy axons a key to spinal cord repair? *Science* 276(5321):1917, 1997.

58. Yankelson S: Traumatic brain injury. In Gines DJ, ed: *Nutrition management in rehabilitation,* Gaithersburg, Md, 1990, Aspen.

59. Audran M, Legrand E: Hypercalciuria, *Joint Bone Spine* 67(6):509, 2000.

60. Health Care Financing Administration: *Health care financing review: statistical supplement,* Tables 29 and 30, Washington, DC, 2001, Author. Available at *www.cms.hss.gov/reviews/supp.* Accessed December 29, 2004.

61. O'Neill PA: Swallowing and prevention of complications, *Br Med Bull* 56(2):457, 2000.

62. Finestone HM: Safe feeding methods in stroke patients, *Lancet* 355(9216):1662, 2000.

63. Koman LA, Smith BP, Shilt JS: Cerebral palsy, *Lancet* 363(9421):1619, 2004.

64. Johnson RK et al: Total energy expenditure in adults with cerebral palsy as assessed by doubly labeled water, *J Am Diet Assoc* 97(9):966, 1997.

65. Walter A et al: Food safety training needs exist for staff and consumers in a variety of community-based homes for people with developmental disabilities, *J Am Diet Assoc* 97(6):611, 1997.

66. Hogan SE, Evers SE: A multinational rehabilitation program for persons with severe physical and developmental disabilities, *J Am Diet Assoc* 97(2):162, 1997.

67. Nelson KB: Can we prevent cerebral palsy? *N Engl J Med* 349(18):1765, 2003.

68. Sullivan PB et al: Impact of feeding problems on nutritional intake and growth: Oxford Feeding Study II, *Develop Med Child Neurol* 44(7):461, 2002.

69. Fung EB et al: Feeding dysfunction is associated with poor growth and health status in children with cerebral palsy, *J Am Diet Assoc* 102(3):361, 2002.

70. Smith SW, Camfield C, Camfield P: Living with cerebral palsy and tube feeding: a population-based follow up study, *J Pediatr* 135(3):307, 2000.

71. Harrington M, Lyman B: Special considerations for the pediatric patient. In Silkroski M, Guenter P, eds: *Tube feeding: practical guidelines and nursing protocols,* Gaithersburg, Md, 2001, Aspen.

72. Hogan SE: Knee height as a predictor of recumbent length for individuals with mobility-impaired cerebral palsy, *J Am Coll Nutr* 18(2):201, 1999.

73. Johnson RK, Ferrara MS: Estimating stature from knee height for persons with cerebral palsy: an evaluation of estimating equations, *J Am Diet Assoc* 91(10):1283, 1991.

74. Stallings VA et al: Body composition in children with spastic quadriplegic cerebral palsy, *J Pediatr* 126:1883, 1995.

75. Ferrang TM et al: Dietary and anthropomorphic assessment of adults with cerebral palsy, *J Am Diet Assoc* 92(9):1083, 1992.

76. Gonzalez L, Nazario CM, Gonzalez MJ: Nutrition related problems of pediatric patients with neuromuscular disorders, *P R Health Sci J* 19(1):35, 2000.

77. Brodie MJ, Dichter MA: Antiepileptic drugs, *N Engl J Med* 334(2):168, 1996.

78. Morantz CA: Recommendations for prescribing new antiepileptic drugs, *Am Fam Physician* 70(6):1167, 2004.

79. Jarrar RG, Buchhalter JR: Therapeutics in pediatric epilepsy. I. The new antiepileptic drugs and the ketogenic diet, *Mayo Clinic Proc* 78(3):359, 2003.

80. Schmidt D, Bourgeois B: A risk-benefit assessment of therapies for Lennox-Gastaut syndrome, *Drug Saf* 22(6):467, 2000.

81. LaRoche SM, Helmers SL: The new antiepileptic drugs: clinical applications, *JAMA* 291(5):615, 2004.

82. Chadwick D: Vagal-nerve stimulation for epilepsy, *Lancet* 357(9270):1726, 2001.

83. Murphy JV et al: Vagal nerve stimulation in refractory epilepsy: the first 100 patients receiving vagal nerve stimulation at a pediatric epilepsy center, *Arch Ped Adolesc Med* 157(6):560, 2003.

84. Edelstein SF, Chisholm M: Management of intractable childhood seizures using the non-MCT oil ketogenic diet in 20 patients, *J Am Diet Assoc* 96(11):1181, 1996.

85. Mandel A et al: Medical costs are reduced when children with intractable epilepsy are successfully treated with the ketogenic diet, *J Am Diet Assoc* 102(3):396, 2002.

86. Stafstrom CE: Dietary approaches to epilepsy treatment: old and new options on the menu, *Epilepsy Curr* 4(6):215, 2004.

87. Nevin-Folino NL, ed: *Pediatric manual of clinical dietetics,* ed 2, Chicago, 2003, American Dietetic Association.

88. Liu YMC et al: A prospective study: growth and nutritional status of children treated with the ketogenic diet, *J Am Diet Assoc* 103(6):707, 2003.

89. Kim DW et al: Benefits of the nonfasting ketogenic diet compared with the initial fasting ketogenic diet, *Pediatrics* 114(6):1627, 2004.

90. Mitchell LE et al: Spina bifida, *Lancet* 364(9448):1885, 2004.

91. Gross SM et al: Inadequate folic acid intakes are prevalent among young women with neural tube defects, *J Am Diet Assoc* 101(3):342, 2001.

92. Lucock M: Folic acid: nutritional biochemistry, molecular biology, and role in disease processes, *Mol Genet Metab* 71(1-2):121, 2000.

93. Mersereau P et al: Spina bifida and anencephaly before and after folic acid mandate—United States, 1995-1996 and 1999 and 2000, *JAMA* 292(3):325, 2004.

94. Atencio PL et al: Effect of level of lesion and quality of ambulation on growth chart measurements in children with myelomeningocele, *J Am Diet Assoc* 92(7):858, 1992.

95. Dustrude A, Prince A: Provision of optimal nutrition care in myelomeningocele, *Top Clin Nutr* 5(2):34, 1990.

96. Roizen NJ, Patterson D: Down's syndrome, *Lancet* 361(9365):1281, 2003.

97. Capone GT: Down syndrome: genetic insights and thoughts on early intervention, *Infants Young Child* 17(1):45, 2004.

98. Luke A et al: Nutrient intake and obesity in prepubescent children with Down syndrome, *J Am Diet Assoc* 96(12):1262, 1996.

99. Quenhe Y, Rasmussen SA, Friedman JM: Mortality with Down's syndrome in the USA from 1983 to 1997: a population based study, *Lancet* 359(9311):1019, 2002.

100. Roizen NJ: The early interventionist and the medical problems of the child with Down syndrome, *Infants Young Child* 16(1):88, 2003.

101. Youdim MBH, Riederer P: Understanding Parkinson's disease, *Sci Am* 276(1):52, 1997.

102. Samii A, Nutt JG, Ranson BR: Parkinson's disease, *Lancet* 363(9423):1783, 2004.

103. Siderowf A, Stern M: Update of Parkinson disease, *Ann Int Med* 138(8):641, 2003.

104. Pinero D, Jones B, Beard J: Variations in dietary iron alter behavior in developing rats, *J Nutr* 131(2):311, 2001.

105. Shoham S, Youdim MB: Iron involvement in neural damage and microgliosis in models of neurodegenerative diseases, *Cell Mol Biol* 46(4):743, 2000.

106. Rascol O et al: Treatment interventions for Parkinson's disease: an evidence based assessment, *Lancet* 359(9317):1589, 2002.

107. Cushing ML, Traviss KA, Calne SM: Parkinson's disease: implication for nutritional care, *Can J Diet Pract Res* 63(2):81, 2002.

108. Beyer PI et al: Weight change and body composition in patients with Parkinson's disease, *JAMA* 95(9):979, 1995.

109. Frankish H: Coenzyme Q10 could slow functional decline in Parkinson's disease, *Lancet* 360(9341):1227, 2002.

110. Revkin A: Hunting down Huntington's, *Discover* 14(12):98, 1993.

111. Wexler NS et al: Huntington's disease in Venezuela and gene linkage, *Cytogenet Cell Genet* 37:605, 1984.

112. Barinaga M: An intriguing new lead on Huntington's disease, *Science* 271(5253):1233, 1996.

113. Josefson D: Molecular basis underlying Huntington's chorea found, *BMJ* 315(7106):446, 1997.

114. Huntington's disease. In Escott-Stump S, ed: *Nutrition and diagnosis-related care,* ed 4, Philadelphia, 1997, Lippincott Williams & Wilkins.

115. Duan W et al: Dietary restriction normalizes glucose metabolism and BDNF levels, slows disease progression, and increases survival in huntingtin mutant mice, *Proc Nat Acad Sci* 100(5):2911, 2003.

116. Pritchard J, Hughes RAC: Guillain-Barré syndrome, *Lancet* 363(9427):2186, 2004.

117. Newswanger DL, Warren CR: Guillain-Barré syndrome, *Am Fam Physician* 69(10):2405, 2004.

118. Hadden RDM, Hughes RAC: Management of inflammatory neuropathies, *J Neurol Neurosurg Psychiatry* 74(2 suppl):ii9, 2003.

119. A.S.P.E.N. Board of Directors: Guidelines for the use of parenteral and enteral nutrition in adult and pediatric patients, *J Parenter Enteral Nutr* 17(suppl 4):1SA, 1993.

120. McNamara JO, Fridovich I: Did radicals strike Lou Gehrig? *Nature* 362(6415):20, 1993.

121. Rosen DR et al: Mutations in Cu/Zn superoxide dismutase gene are associated with familial amyotrophic lateral sclerosis, *Nature* 362(6415):59, 1993.

122. Marx J: Gene linked to Lou Gehrig's disease, *Science* 259(5100):1393, 1993.

123. Wiedau-Pazas M et al: Altered reactivity of superoxide dismutase in familial amyotrophic lateral sclerosis, *Science* 271(5247):515, 1996.

124. Al-Chalabi A, Leigh PN: Recent advances in amyotrophic lateral sclerosis, *Curr Opin Neurol* 13(4):397, 2000.

125. Berger MM et al: Detection and cellular localization of enterovirus RNA sequences in spinal cord of patients with ALS, *Neurology* 54(1):20, 2000.

126. Hampton T: Food chain of evidence points to a brain toxin, *JAMA* 290(21):2788, 2003.

127. Piazza O, Siren AL, Ehrenreich H: Soccer, neurotrauma and amyotrophic lateral sclerosis: is there a connection? *Curr Med Res Opin* 20(4):505, 2004.

128. Dyer O: Veterans of the first Gulf War are developing amyotrophic lateral sclerosis, *BMJ* 327(7418):766, 2003.

129. Hardiman O: Symptomatic treatment of respiratory and nutritional failure in amyotrophic lateral sclerosis, *J Neurol* 247(4):245, 2000.

130. Strong MJ, Rowe A, Rankin RN: Percutaneous gastrojejunostomy in amyotrophic lateral sclerosis, *J Neurol Sci* 169(1-2):128, 1999.

131. Calabresi PA: Diagnosis and management of multiple sclerosis, *Am Fam Physician* 70(10):1935, 2004.

132. Denis L et al: Long-term treatment optimization in individuals with multiple sclerosis using disease-modifying therapies: a nursing approach, *J Neurosci Nurs* 36(1):10, 2004.

133. Thomas FJ, Wiles CM: Dysphagia and nutritional status in multiple sclerosis, *J Neurol* 246(8):677, 1999.

134. Annoni JM et al: Percutaneous endoscopic gastrostomy in neurological rehabilitation: a report of six cases, *Disabil Rehabil* 20(8):308, 1998.

135. Timmerman GM, Stuifbergin AK: Eating patterns of women with multiple sclerosis, *J Neurosci Nurs* 31(3):152, 1999.

136. Ghadirian P et al: Nutritional factors in the aetiology of multiple sclerosis: a case-control study in Montreal, Canada, *Int J Epidemiol* 27(5):845, 1998.

137. Antozzi C: Myasthenia gravis and myasthenic syndrome, *Neurol Sci* 24:s260, 2003.

138. Howard J: Myasthenia gravis—a summary, Myasthenia Gravis Foundation of America. Retrieved April 27, 2006 from www.myasthenia.org/information/summary.htm

139. Guyton AC, Hall JE: *Textbook of medical physiology,* ed 9, Philadelphia, 1996, WB Saunders.

140. Alzheimer A: Uber eine eigenartige Erkrankung der Hirnrinde, *Allgemeine Zeitschrift fur Psychiatrie* 64:146, 1907. (English translation, *Arch Neurol* 21:109, 1969.)

141. O'Brien C: Auguste D and Alzheimer's disease, *Science* 273(5271):28, 1996.

142. Cummings JL et al: Guidelines for managing Alzheimer's disease. I. Assessment, *Am Fam Physician* 65(11):2263, 2002.

143. Commenges D et al: Intake of flavonoids and risk of dementia, *Eur J Epidemiol* 16(4):357, 2000.

144. Mattson MP: Emerging neuroprotective strategies for Alzheimer's disease: dietary restriction, telomerase activation, and stem cell therapy, *Exp Gerontol* 35(4):489, 2000.

145. LeBoeuf R: Homocysteine and Alzheimer's disease, *J Am Diet Assoc* 103(3):304, 2003.

146. Morris MC et al: Consumption of fish and n-3 fatty acids and risk of incident of Alzheimer disease, *Arch Neurol* 60(7):940, 2003.

147. Grossberg GT, Desai AK: Management of Alzheimer's disease, *J Gerontol A Biol Sci Med Sci* 58A(4):331, 2003.

148. Cummings JL et al: Guidelines for managing Alzheimer's disease. II. Treatment, *Am Fam Physician* 65(12):2525, 2002.

149. Rolland Y et al: Feasibility of regular physical exercise for patients with moderate to severe Alzheimer's disease, *J Nutr Health Aging* 4(2):109, 2000.

150. Teri L et al: Exercise plus behavioral management in patients with Alzheimer disease, *JAMA* 290(15):2015, 2003.

151. Poehlman ET, Dvorak RV: Energy expenditure in Alzheimer's disease, *J Nutr Health Aging* 2(2):155, 1998.

152. Renvall NJ et al: Nutritional care of ambulatory residents in special care units for Alzheimer's patients, *J Nutr Elder* 12(4):5, 1993.

153. Prevalence of disabilities and associated health conditions among adults—United States, 1999, *MMWR Morb Mortal Wkly Rep* 50(7):120, 2001.

154. Cameron D et al: The clinical utility of the test of playfulness, *Can J Occup Ther* 68(2):104, 2001.

155. Fong KN, Chan CC, Au DK: Relationship of motor and cognitive abilities to functional performance in stroke rehabilitation, *Brain Inj* 15(5):443, 2001.

156. Itzkovich M et al: Spinal Pain Independence Measure: a new scale for assessment of primary ADL dysfunction related to LBP, *Disabil Rehabil* 23(5):186, 2001.

157. Jagger C et al: Patterns of onset of disability in activities of daily living with age, *J Am Geriatr Soc* 49(4):404, 2001.

158. Panesar BS, Morrison P, Hunter J: A comparison of three measure of progress in early lower limb amputee rehabilitation, *Clin Rehabil* 15(2):157, 2001.

FURTHER READINGS AND RESOURCES

Readings

In addition to the websites and references listed at the end of the text, following is a summary of some additional resources that may prove helpful.

Thornton H, Jackson D, Turner-Stokes L: Accuracy of prediction of walking for young stroke patients by use of the FIM, *Physiother Res Int* 6(1):14, 2001.

This article scientifically evaluates the commonly used FIM, or Functional Independence Measure, for its precision and identifies factors influencing accuracy.

Halstead LS: The John Stanley Coulter lecture: the power of compassion and caring in rehabilitation healing, *Arch Phys Med Rehabil* 82(2):149, 2001.

This article is an excellent and timely review of the complementary and alternative side of medicine as it relates to rehabilitation. The authors review seven articles from the literature and provide examples of research-based interventions with potential for enhancing outcomes in traditional rehabilitation populations.

Ahronheim JC, Moreno JD, Zuckerman C: *Ethics in clinical practice,* ed 2, Gaithersburg, Md, 2000, Aspen Publishers.

This text is a must-have for any practicing clinician interested in the ethical questions facing our society today. It covers an array of topics and contains 31 case studies with detailed question and answer format following each case.

Shoham S, Youdim MB: Iron involvement in neural damage and microgliosis in models of neurodegenerative diseases, *Cell Mol Biol* 46(4):743, 2000.

This is an excellent article that explains the study of iron accumulation at sites of the brain. Among the diseases mentioned are Parkinson's disease, Huntington's chorea, and multiple sclerosis.

Yanagawa T et al: Nutritional support for head-injured patients, *Cochrane Database Syst Rev* (2):CD001530, 2000.

This review from Japan suggests that early enteral feeding may be associated with better outcomes in terms of survival and disability. Because enteral nutrition support is commonly required for patients sustaining injury or with chronic illness, it is crucial that the caregiver have some understanding of its relevance.

Cummings JL et al: Guidelines for managing Alzheimer's disease. I. Assessment, *Am Fam Physician* 65(11):2263, 2002.

Cummings JL et al: Guidelines for managing Alzheimer's disease. II. Treatment, *Am Fam Physician* 65(12):2525, 2002.

These two articles are good resources concerning the assessment and treatment of Alzheimer's patients from a family physician perspective, including clinical diagnostic tools and pharmacologic treatment.

Websites of Interest

- Alzheimer's Association: *www.alz.org.*
- American Epilepsy Society: *www.aesnet.org.*
- American Heart Association (and Stroke 2000 Statistical Update): *www.americanheart.org.*
- Brain Injury Association of America: *www.biausa.org.*
- Christopher Reeve Foundation: *www.apacure.org.*
- Epilepsy Foundation: *www.efa.org.*
- Huntington's Disease Society of America: *www.hdsa.org.*
- Myasthenia Gravis Foundation of America, Inc.: *www.myasthenia.org.*
- National Dissemination Center for Children with Disabilities: *www.nichcy.org.*
- National Institute on Aging, National Institutes of Health: *www.nih.gov/nia.*
- National Multiple Sclerosis Society: *www.nationalmssociety.org.*
- National Osteoporosis Foundation: *www.nof.org.*
- National Spinal Cord Injury Association: *www.spinalcord.org.*
- Office of Special Education and Rehabilitative Services (OSERS), U.S. Department of Education, Individuals With Disabilities Education Improvement Act (IDEA) of 2004: *www.ed.gov/offices/OSERS/IDEA/index.html.*
- Parkinson's Disease Foundation: *www.pdf.org.*
- Spina Bifida Association: *www.sbaa.org.*
- United Cerebral Palsy: *www.ucp.org.*
- World Federation of Neurology Amyotrophic Lateral Sclerosis: *www.wfnals.org.*
- World Parkinson Disease Association: *www.wpda.org.*

APPENDIXES

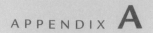

Caffeine Content of Foods

Caffeine Content	Serving (mg)
Coffee, 6-oz Cup	
Brewed, drip method	103
Brewed, percolator method	75
Instant, 1 rounded tsp	57
Decaffeinated	2
Flavored, regular and sugar-free	25-75
Espresso, 1 oz	40
Tea	
3-minute brew, 6-oz cup	36
Instant, 1 rounded tsp in 8 oz of water	25-35
Decaffeinated, 5-minute brew, 6-oz cup	1
Cola Beverages, 12 oz	
Regular or diet	35-50
Decaffeinated	Trace

Caffeine Content	Serving (mg)
Cherry Colas, Dr. Pepper, Mr. Pibb, 12 oz	
Regular or diet	35-50
Decaffeinated	Trace
Mellow Yellow, 12 oz	
Regular or diet	52
Mountain Dew, 12 oz	
Regular or diet	54
Cocoa and Chocolate	
Cocoa beverage, 6-oz cup	4
Chocolate milk, 8 oz	8
Chocolate, sweet, semisweet, dark, milk, 1 oz	8-20
Chocolate, baking, unsweetened, 1 oz	58
Chocolate-flavored, syrup, 1 oz	5
Chocolate pudding, ½ cup	4-8

Data from Pennington JA: *Bowes and Church's food values of portions commonly used,* ed 17, Baltimore, 1998, Lippincott-Williams & Wilkins.

Soluble, Insoluble, and Total Fiber Content in Selected Plant Foods

Food	Serving Size	Total* Fiber (g)	Soluble Fiber (g)	Insoluble Fiber (g)
Cereals				
All-Bran	⅓ cup	8.6	1.4	7.2
Cheerios	1¼ cup	2.5	1.2	1.3
Corn flakes	1 cup	0.5	0.1	0.4
Oatmeal, cooked	½ cup	2.0	0.9	1.1
Shredded wheat	⅔ cup	3.5	0.5	3.0
Special K	1 cup	0.9	0.2	0.7
Grains				
Macaroni, white, cooked	½ cup	0.7	0.4	0.3
Macaroni, whole wheat, cooked	½ cup	2.1	0.4	1.7
Popcorn, popped	3 cups	2.0	0.1	1.9
Rice, white, cooked	⅓ cup	0.5	Trace	0.5
Rice, brown, cooked	⅓ cup	0.4	0.1	0.3
Wheat bran	½ cup	12.3	1.0	11.3
Wheat germ	3 tbsp	3.9	0.7	3.2
Breads				
Bagel, plain	½	0.7	0.3	0.4
Corn bread	½-inch cube	1.4	0.3	1.1
Oatmeal bread	1 slice	2.4	0.6	1.8
Pumpernickel bread	1 slice	2.7	1.2	1.5

Food	Serving Size	Total* Fiber (g)	Soluble Fiber (g)	Insoluble Fiber (g)
Rye bread	1 slice	1.8	0.8	1.0
White bread	1 slice	0.6	0.3	0.3
Whole wheat bread	1 slice	1.5	0.3	1.2
Hamburger bun	½	0.7	0.2	0.5
Pretzels, hard	¾ oz	0.8	0.2	0.6
Fruit				
Apple	1 small	2.8	1.0	1.8
Applesauce, canned	½ cup	2.0	0.7	1.3
Apricots, raw, with skin	2	1.7	0.9	0.8
Apricots, canned	4 halves	1.2	0.5	0.7
Banana	½ small	1.1	0.3	0.8
Blueberries	¾ cup	1.4	0.3	1.1
White grapes, with skin	15 small	0.6	0.3	0.3
Cantaloupe, cubed	1 cup	1.1	0.3	0.8
Orange	1 small	2.9	1.8	1.1
Orange juice	¾ cup	0.4	0.2	0.2
Pear, fresh, with skin	1 medium	4.0	2.2	1.8
Raisins, dried	2 tbsp	0.4	0.2	0.2
Strawberries	1¼ cup	2.8	1.1	1.7

Data from American Dietetic Association: *Manual of clinical dietetics,* ed 5, Chicago, 1996; and Duyff RL: *American Dietetic Association complete food and nutrition guide,* ed 2, Hoboken, NJ, 2002, John Wiley & Sons.

*The total dietary fiber may not equal the sum of the soluble and insoluble fiber due to rounding.

Food	Serving Size	Total* Fiber (g)	Soluble Fiber (g)	Insoluble Fiber (g)
Vegetables				
Asparagus, cooked	½ cup	1.8	0.7	1.1
Broccoli, cooked	½ cup	2.4	1.2	1.2
Brussels sprouts, cooked	½ cup	3.8	2.0	1.8
Carrots, raw	1 (7½ inches)	2.3	1.1	1.2
Carrots, cooked	½ cup	2.0	1.1	0.9
Cauliflower, cooked	½ cup	1.0	0.4	0.6
Corn, canned	½ cup	1.6	0.2	1.4
Iceberg lettuce	1 cup	0.5	0.1	0.4
Peas, frozen, cooked	½ cup	4.3	1.3	3.0
Sweet potato, cooked	⅓ cup	2.7	1.2	1.5
Spinach, cooked	½ cup	1.6	0.5	1.1
Tomato, raw	1 medium	1.0	0.1	0.9
Tomato sauce	⅓ cup	1.1	0.5	0.6
V8 juice	½ cup	0.7	0.2	0.5

Food	Serving Size	Total* Fiber (g)	Soluble Fiber (g)	Insoluble Fiber (g)
Legumes				
Black-eyed peas, canned	½ cup	4.7	0.5	4.2
Chick peas, dried, cooked	½ cup	4.3	1.3	3.0
Kidney beans, red, canned	½ cup	7.9	2.0	5.9
Lentils, dried, cooked	½ cup	5.2	0.6	4.6
Lima beans, canned	½ cup	4.3	1.1	3.2
Vegetarian baked beans	½ cup	6.3	2.1	4.2
Soybeans	½ cup	5.4	2.4	3.0
Nuts and Seeds				
Peanut butter, creamy	1 tbsp	1.0	0.3	0.7
Peanuts, roasted	10 large	0.6	0.2	0.4
Walnuts	2 whole	0.3	0.1	0.2
Sunflower seeds	1 tbsp	0.5	0.2	0.3
Added Ingredients				
Oat bran	1 tbsp	0.9	0.4	0.5
Flaxseed	1 tbsp	1.6	0.8	0.7
Psyllium	1 tbsp	6.0	4.8	1.2

Centers for Disease Control and Prevention (CDC) Growth Charts

2 to 20 years: Boys
Body mass index-for-age percentiles

NAME _____

RECORD # _____

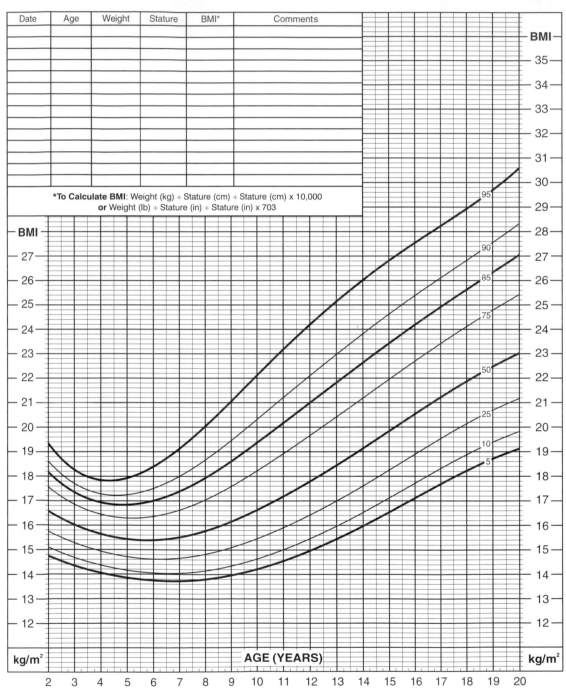

Date	Age	Weight	Stature	BMI*	Comments

*To Calculate BMI: Weight (kg) ÷ Stature (cm) ÷ Stature (cm) x 10,000
or Weight (lb) ÷ Stature (in) ÷ Stature (in) x 703

AGE (YEARS)

Published May 30, 2000 (modified 10/16/00).
SOURCE: Developed by the National Center for Health Statistics in collaboration with
   the National Center for Chronic Disease Prevention and Health Promotion (2000).
   http://www.cdc.gov/growthcharts

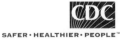
SAFER · HEALTHIER · PEOPLE™

2 to 20 years: Girls
Body mass index-for-age percentiles

NAME _____

RECORD # _____

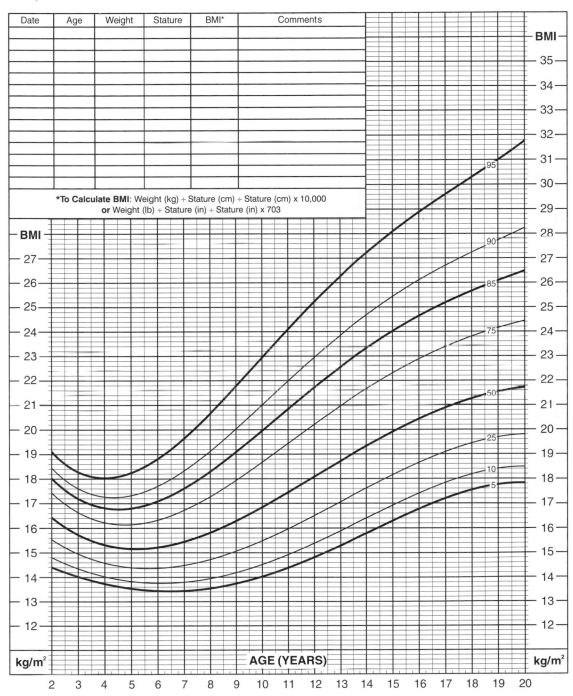

Date	Age	Weight	Stature	BMI*	Comments

*To Calculate BMI: Weight (kg) ÷ Stature (cm) ÷ Stature (cm) x 10,000
or Weight (lb) ÷ Stature (in) ÷ Stature (in) x 703

AGE (YEARS)

kg/m²

Published May 30, 2000 (modified 10/16/00).
SOURCE: Developed by the National Center for Health Statistics in collaboration with
the National Center for Chronic Disease Prevention and Health Promotion (2000).
http://www.cdc.gov/growthcharts

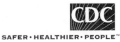

SAFER · HEALTHIER · PEOPLE™

Birth to 36 months: Boys
Head circumference-for-age and
Weight-for-length percentiles

NAME _____

RECORD# _____

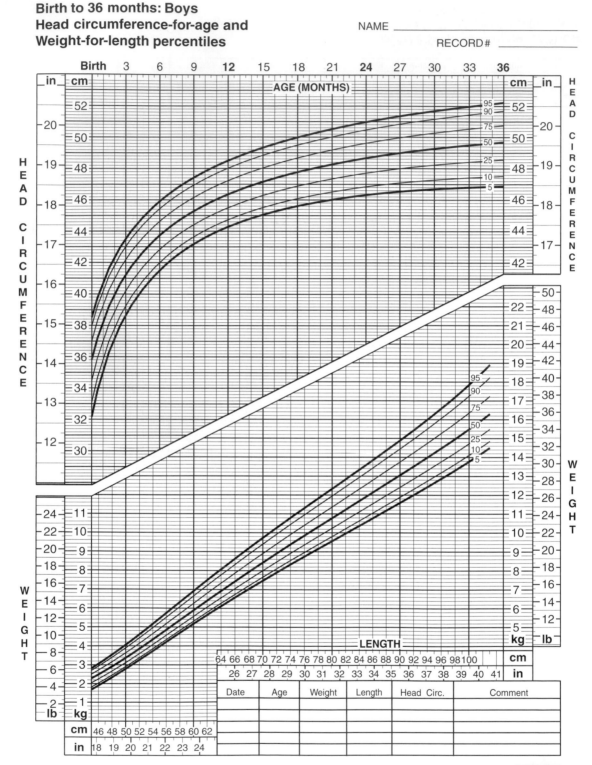

Published May 30, 2000 (modified 10/16/00).
SOURCE: Developed by the National Center for Health Statistics in collaboration with
the National Center for Chronic Disease Prevention and Health Promotion (2000).
http://www.cdc.gov/growthcharts

SAFER · HEALTHIER · PEOPLE™

Birth to 36 months: Girls
Head circumference-for-age and
Weight-for-length percentiles

NAME _____

RECORD # _____

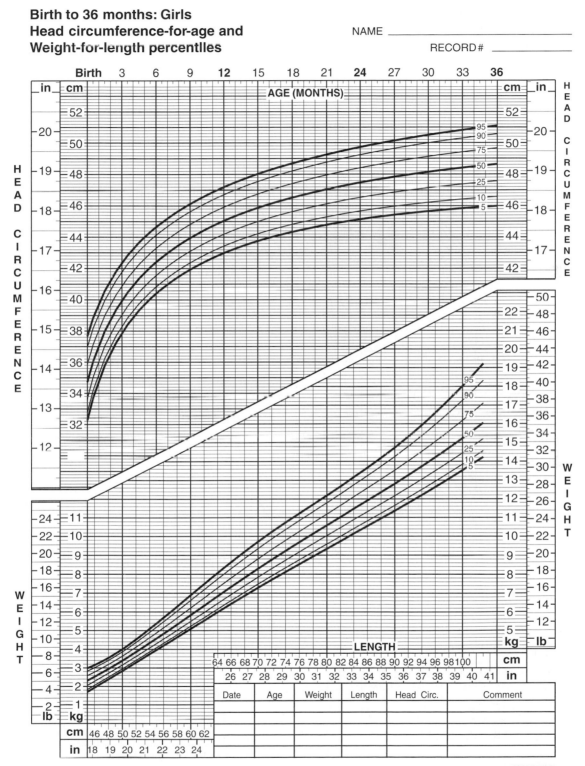

Published May 30, 2000 (modified 10/16/00).
SOURCE: Developed by the National Center for Health Statistics in collaboration with
the National Center for Chronic Disease Prevention and Health Promotion (2000).
http://www.cdc.gov/growthcharts

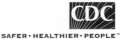

SAFER·HEALTHIER·PEOPLE™

2 to 20 years: Boys
Stature-for-age and Weight-for-age percentiles

NAME _____

RECORD# _____

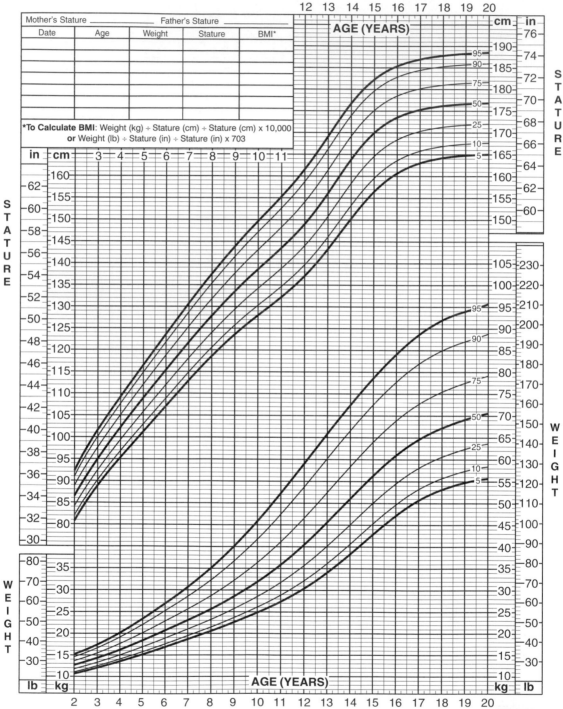

Mother's Stature _____ Father's Stature _____

Date	Age	Weight	Stature	BMI*

*To Calculate BMI: Weight (kg) ÷ Stature (cm) ÷ Stature (cm) x 10,000
or Weight (lb) ÷ Stature (in) ÷ Stature (in) x 703

AGE (YEARS)

Published May 30, 2000 (modified 11/21/00).
SOURCE: Developed by the National Center for Health Statistics in collaboration with
the National Center for Chronic Disease Prevention and Health Promotion (2000).
http://www.cdc.gov/growthcharts

SAFER · HEALTHIER · PEOPLE™

2 to 20 years: Girls
Stature-for-age and Weight-for-age percentiles

NAME _____

RECORD# _____

Mother's Stature		Father's Stature		
Date	Age	Weight	Stature	BMI*

*To Calculate BMI: Weight (kg) ÷ Stature (cm) ÷ Stature (cm) x 10,000
or Weight (lb) ÷ Stature (in) ÷ Stature (in) x 703

AGE (YEARS)

12 13 14 15 16 17 18 19 20

STATURE

95
90
75
50
25
10
5

in cm   3   4   5   6   7   8   9   10   11

AGE (YEARS)

2   3   4   5   6   7   8   9   10   11   12   13   14   15   16   17   18   19   20

WEIGHT

Published May 30, 2000 (modified 11/21/00).
SOURCE: Developed by the National Center for Health Statistics in collaboration with
the National Center for Chronic Disease Prevention and Health Promotion (2000).
http://www.cdc.gov/growthcharts

SAFER · HEALTHIER · PEOPLE™

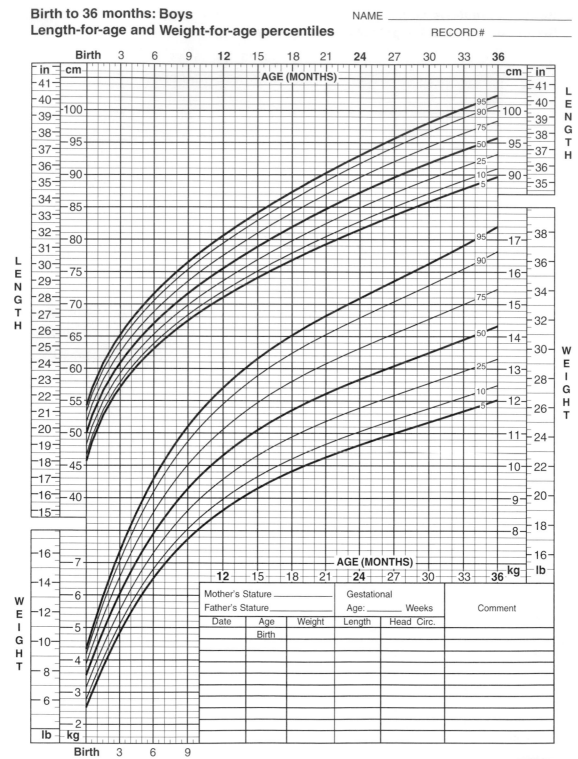

Birth to 36 months: Boys
Length-for-age and Weight-for-age percentiles

NAME _____

RECORD# _____

Published May 30, 2000 (modified 4/20/01).
SOURCE: Developed by the National Center for Health Statistics in collaboration with
the National Center for Chronic Disease Prevention and Health Promotion (2000).
http://www.cdc.gov/growthcharts

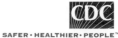

Birth to 36 months: Girls
Length-for-age and Weight-for-age percentiles

NAME _____

RECORD# _____

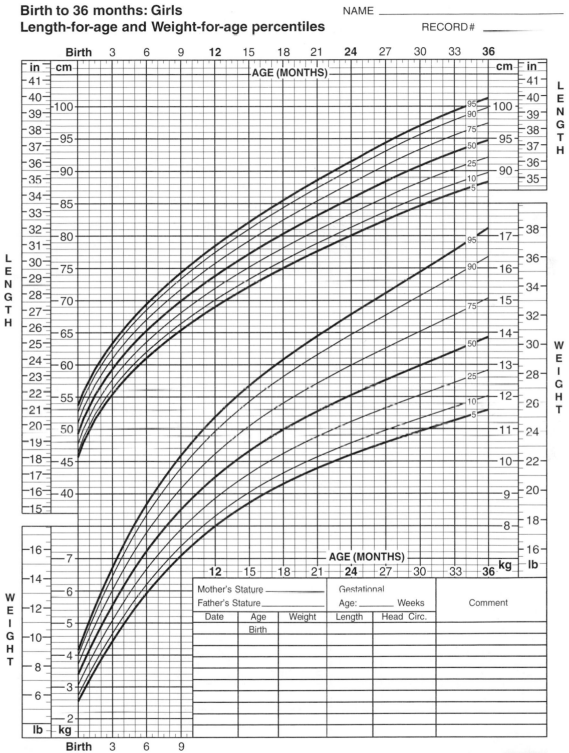

Published May 30, 2000 (modified 4/20/01).
SOURCE: Developed by the National Center for Health Statistics in collaboration with
the National Center for Chronic Disease Prevention and Health Promotion (2000).
http://www.cdc.gov/growthcharts

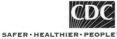

SAFER · HEALTHIER · PEOPLE™

Weight-for-stature percentiles: Boys

NAME _____

RECORD# _____

Date	Age	Weight	Stature	Comments

Percentile curves labeled: 95, 90, 85, 75, 50, 25, 10, 5

STATURE

cm: 80 85 90 95 100 105 110 115 120

in: 31 32 33 34 35 36 37 38 39 40 41 42 43 44 45 46 47

Published May 30, 2000 (modified 10/16/00).
SOURCE: Developed by the National Center for Health Statistics in collaboration with
the National Center for Chronic Disease Prevention and Health Promotion (2000).
http://www.cdc.gov/growthcharts

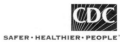

SAFER · HEALTHIER · PEOPLE™

Weight-for-stature percentiles: Girls

NAME _____

RECORD # _____

Date	Age	Weight	Stature	Comments

STATURE

cm 80 85 90 95 100 105 110 115 120

in 31 32 33 34 35 36 37 38 39 40 41 42 43 44 45 46 47

95
90
85
75
50
25
10
5

Published May 30, 2000 (modified 10/16/00).
SOURCE: Developed by the National Center for Health Statistics in collaboration with
the National Center for Chronic Disease Prevention and Health Promotion (2000).
http://www.cdc.gov/growthcharts

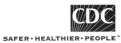

SAFER · HEALTHIER · PEOPLE™

Body Mass Index: Obesity Values (Second of Two BMI Tables)

	36	37	38	39	40	41	42	43	44	45	46	47	48	49	50	51	52	53	54
Height (inches)							**Body Weight (pounds)**												
58	172	177	183	186	191	196	201	205	210	215	220	224	229	234	239	244	248	253	258
59	178	183	188	193	198	203	208	212	217	222	227	232	237	242	247	252	257	262	267
60	184	189	194	199	204	209	215	220	225	230	235	240	245	250	255	261	266	271	276
61	190	195	201	206	211	217	222	227	232	238	243	248	254	259	264	269	275	280	285
62	196	202	207	213	218	224	229	235	240	246	251	256	262	267	273	278	284	289	295
63	203	208	214	220	225	231	237	242	248	254	259	265	270	278	282	287	293	299	304
64	209	215	221	227	232	238	244	250	256	262	267	273	279	285	291	296	302	308	314
65	216	222	228	234	240	246	252	258	264	270	276	282	288	294	300	306	312	318	324
66	223	229	235	241	247	253	260	266	272	278	284	291	297	303	309	315	322	328	334
67	230	236	242	249	255	261	268	274	280	287	293	299	306	312	319	325	331	338	344
68	236	243	249	256	262	269	276	282	289	295	302	308	315	322	328	335	341	348	354
69	243	250	257	263	270	277	284	291	297	304	311	318	324	331	338	345	351	358	365
70	250	257	264	271	278	285	292	299	306	313	320	327	334	341	348	355	362	369	376
71	257	265	272	279	286	293	301	308	315	322	329	338	343	351	358	365	372	379	386
72	265	272	279	287	294	302	309	316	324	331	338	346	353	361	368	375	383	390	397
73	272	280	288	295	302	310	318	325	333	340	348	355	363	371	378	386	393	401	408
74	280	287	295	303	311	319	326	334	342	350	358	365	373	381	389	396	404	412	420
75	287	295	303	311	319	327	335	343	351	359	367	375	383	391	399	407	415	423	431
76	295	304	312	320	328	336	344	353	361	369	377	385	394	402	410	418	426	435	443

From NIH/National Heart, Lung, and Blood Institute: *Appendix V: Body mass index chart (chart 2), Clinical guidelines on the identification, evaluation, and treatment of overweight and obesity in adults,* Bethesda, Md, June 1998, National Institutes of Health.

To use the table, find the appropriate height in the left-hand column. Move across to a given weight. The number at the top of the column is the BMI of that height and weight. Pounds have been rounded off.

NOTE: For lower body mass index values, see Table 5-4 on p. 96.

Means, Standard Deviations, and Percentiles of Triceps Skinfold Thickness (mm) by Age for Males and Females of 1 to 50 Years

| Age (yr) | N | Mean | SD | Percentiles | | | | | | | | |
				5	10	15	25	50	75	85	90	95
Males												
1.0-1.9	681	10.4	2.9	6.5	7.0	7.5	8.0	10.0	12.0	13.0	14.0	15.5
2.0-2.9	677	10.0	2.9	6.0	6.5	7.0	8.0	10.0	12.0	13.0	14.0	15.0
3.0-3.9	717	9.9	2.7	6.0	7.0	7.0	8.0	9.5	11.5	12.5	13.5	15.0
4.0-4.9	708	9.2	2.7	5.5	6.5	7.0	7.5	9.0	11.0	12.0	12.5	14.0
5.0-5.9	677	8.9	3.1	5.0	6.0	6.0	7.0	8.0	10.0	11.5	13.0	14.5
6.0-6.9	298	8.9	3.8	5.0	5.5	6.0	6.5	8.0	10.0	12.0	13.0	16.0
7.0-7.9	312	9.0	4.0	4.5	5.0	6.0	6.0	8.0	10.5	12.5	14.0	16.0
8.0-8.9	296	9.6	4.4	5.0	5.5	6.0	7.0	8.5	11.0	13.0	16.0	19.0
9.0-9.9	322	10.2	5.1	5.0	5.5	6.0	6.5	9.0	12.5	15.5	17.0	20.0
10.0-10.9	334	11.5	5.7	5.0	6.0	6.0	7.5	10.0	14.0	17.0	20.0	24.0
11.0-11.9	324	12.5	7.0	5.0	6.0	6.5	7.5	10.0	16.0	19.5	23.0	27.0
12.0-12.9	348	12.2	6.8	4.5	6.0	6.0	7.5	10.5	14.5	18.0	22.5	27.5
13.0-13.9	350	11.0	6.7	4.5	5.0	5.5	7.0	9.0	13.0	17.0	20.5	25.0
14.0-14.9	358	10.4	6.5	4.0	5.0	5.0	6.0	8.5	12.5	15.0	18.0	23.5
15.0-15.9	356	9.8	6.5	5.0	5.0	5.0	6.0	7.5	11.0	15.0	18.0	23.5
16.0-16.9	350	10.0	5.9	4.0	5.0	5.1	6.0	8.0	12.0	14.0	17.0	23.0
17.0-17.9	337	9.1	5.3	4.0	5.0	5.0	6.0	7.0	11.0	13.5	16.0	19.5
18.0-24.9	1752	11.3	6.4	4.0	5.0	5.5	6.5	10.0	14.5	17.5	20.0	23.5
25.0-29.9	1251	12.2	6.7	4.0	5.0	6.0	7.0	11.0	15.5	19.0	21.5	25.0
30.0-34.9	941	13.1	6.7	4.5	6.0	6.5	8.0	12.0	16.5	20.0	22.0	25.0
35.0-39.9	832	12.9	6.2	4.5	6.0	7.0	8.5	12.0	16.0	18.5	20.5	24.5
40.0-44.9	828	13.0	6.6	5.0	6.0	6.9	8.0	12.0	16.0	19.0	21.5	26.0
45.0-49.9	867	12.9	6.4	5.0	6.0	7.0	8.0	12.0	16.0	19.0	21.0	25.0

From Frisancho AR: *Anthropometric standards for the assessment of growth and nutritional status*, Ann Arbor, 1990, The University of Michigan Press.

Age (yr)	N	Mean	SD	Percentiles								
				5	10	15	25	50	75	85	90	95
Females												
1.0-1.9	622	10.4	3.1	6.0	7.0	7.0	8.0	10.0	12.0	13.0	14.0	16.0
2.0-2.9	614	10.5	2.9	6.0	7.0	7.5	8.5	10.0	12.0	13.5	14.5	16.0
3.0-3.9	652	10.4	2.9	6.0	7.0	7.5	8.5	10.0	12.0	13.0	14.0	16.0
4.0-4.9	681	10.3	3.0	6.0	7.0	7.5	8.0	10.0	12.0	13.0	14.0	15.5
5.0-5.9	673	10.4	3.5	5.5	7.0	7.0	8.0	10.0	12.0	13.5	15.0	17.0
6.0-6.9	296	10.4	3.7	6.0	6.5	7.0	8.0	10.0	12.0	13.0	15.0	17.0
7.0-7.9	330	11.1	4.2	6.0	7.0	7.0	8.0	10.5	12.5	15.0	16.0	19.0
8.0-8.9	276	12.1	5.4	6.0	7.0	7.5	8.5	11.0	14.5	17.0	18.0	22.5
9.0-9.9	322	13.4	5.9	6.5	7.0	8.0	9.0	12.0	16.0	19.0	21.0	25.0
10.0-10.9	329	13.9	6.1	7.0	8.0	8.0	9.0	12.5	17.5	20.0	22.5	27.0
11.0-11.9	302	15.0	6.8	7.0	8.0	8.5	10.0	13.0	18.0	21.5	24.0	29.0
12.0-12.9	323	15.1	6.3	7.0	8.0	9.0	11.0	14.0	18.5	21.5	24.0	27.5
13.0-13.9	360	16.4	7.4	7.0	8.0	9.0	11.0	15.0	20.0	24.0	25.0	30.0
14.0-14.9	370	17.1	7.3	8.0	9.0	10.0	11.5	16.0	21.0	23.5	26.5	32.0
15.0-15.9	309	17.3	7.4	8.0	9.5	10.5	12.0	16.5	20.5	23.0	26.0	32.5
16.0-16.9	343	19.2	7.0	10.5	11.5	12.0	14.0	18.0	23.0	26.0	29.0	32.5
17.0-17.9	291	19.1	8.0	9.0	10.0	12.0	13.0	18.0	24.0	26.5	29.0	34.5
18.0-24.9	2588	20.0	8.2	9.0	11.0	12.0	14.0	18.5	24.5	28.5	31.0	36.0
25.0-29.9	1921	21.7	8.8	10.0	12.0	13.0	15.0	20.0	26.5	31.0	34.0	38.0
30.0-34.9	1619	23.7	9.2	10.5	13.0	15.0	17.0	22.5	29.5	33.0	35.5	41.5
35.0-39.9	1453	24.7	9.3	11.0	13.0	15.5	17.0	23.5	30.0	35.0	37.0	41.0
40.0-44.9	1391	25.1	9.0	12.0	14.0	16.0	19.0	24.5	30.5	35.0	37.0	41.0
45.0-49.9	962	26.1	9.3	12.0	14.5	16.5	19.5	25.5	32.0	35.5	38.0	42.5

Means, Standard Deviations, and Percentiles of Upper Arm Muscle Area (cm^2) by Height (cm) for Boys and Girls of 2 to 17 Years

| Height (cm) | N | Mean | SD | Percentiles | | | | | | | | |
				5	10	15	25	50	75	85	90	95
Boys: 2 to 11 Years												
87-092	94	12.9	2.2	9.3	10.4	10.6	11.2	12.9	14.2	15.0	15.8	16.5
93-098	373	13.7	2.4	10.2	10.9	11.2	12.1	13.5	15.3	15.9	16.5	17.0
99-104	587	14.6	3.1	10.9	11.7	12.2	13.0	14.5	15.9	16.5	17.1	18.4
105-110	587	15.7	3.1	12.0	12.8	13.3	14.1	15.4	17.0	17.8	18.6	19.8
111-116	588	16.7	2.9	12.6	13.6	14.3	15.0	16.6	18.1	18.9	19.6	20.7
117-122	496	18.1	3.5	14.1	14.5	15.0	16.1	17.7	19.7	20.7	21.6	23.4
123-128	376	19.5	3.6	15.0	15.9	16.3	17.4	19.2	21.2	22.3	23.2	24.2
129-134	359	21.6	4.3	16.1	17.3	18.4	19.3	21.1	23.2	24.7	25.3	27.9
135-140	354	22.9	4.2	17.2	18.1	18.9	20.4	22.6	24.9	26.1	27.2	30.2
141-146	325	25.1	5.2	19.3	20.1	20.8	21.9	24.0	27.2	29.0	30.5	34.0
147-152	266	27.5	4.8	21.2	22.4	23.2	24.8	27.0	29.8	31.8	32.9	34.4
153-158	150	29.8	7.2	22.3	23.2	24.3	25.4	28.4	32.2	34.8	36.9	40.1
159-164	65	32.5	6.5	23.7	24.5	25.3	27.5	31.9	35.6	39.7	41.4	44.5
Boys: 12 to 17 Years												
141-146	31	26.8	4.7	20.7	21.4	22.7	24.1	25.6	30.3	32.8	33.9	36.3
147-152	90	28.2	4.1	22.4	23.4	24.1	25.6	27.5	30.2	33.1	34.2	36.1
153-158	181	31.4	6.4	22.7	24.9	26.1	27.5	30.4	34.1	36.4	39.1	41.5
159-164	218	35.0	7.7	23.7	26.7	27.8	30.2	34.1	38.6	41.5	44.3	48.4
165-170	323	40.8	9.3	28.1	29.7	31.5	34.2	40.0	45.6	49.0	52.9	58.9
171-176	431	46.6	9.9	32.8	35.2	36.6	39.5	45.8	52.6	56.0	59.1	66.0
177-182	431	50.3	9.3	36.1	38.7	40.8	43.4	49.5	56.4	59.4	62.6	65.9
183-188	269	53.4	11.2	38.3	41.3	42.8	46.1	52.6	57.8	63.0	67.5	74.3
189-194	99	55.4	9.9	41.4	44.2	45.7	48.9	53.9	60.3	65.0	68.5	74.0

From Frisancho AR: *Anthropometric standards for the assessment of growth and nutritional status,* Ann Arbor, 1990, The University of Michigan Press.

Height (cm)	N	Mean	SD	Percentiles								
				5	10	15	25	50	75	85	90	95
Girls: 2 to 10 Years												
87-092	154	12.6	2.1	9.5	10.1	10.5	11.0	12.6	14.2	14.8	15.5	16.2
93-098	384	13.2	2.1	10.1	10.7	11.0	11.8	13.2	14.4	15.3	15.8	16.9
99-104	533	14.1	2.3	10.6	11.2	11.7	12.5	14.0	15.5	16.4	16.9	18.0
105-110	550	14.8	2.4	11.3	11.9	12.4	13.2	14.6	16.3	17.3	17.9	18.9
111-116	543	15.9	2.8	12.3	13.0	13.5	14.2	15.7	17.4	18.4	19.1	20.3
117-122	465	17.0	2.8	13.0	13.9	14.4	15.2	16.7	18.5	19.6	20.3	21.4
123-128	372	18.2	2.8	14.2	15.0	15.5	16.2	17.9	19.6	20.8	21.6	22.9
129-134	333	20.1	4.6	15.3	16.1	16.8	17.6	19.7	21.7	22.9	23.8	25.4
135-140	303	21.6	4.2	16.1	17.4	18.1	19.2	21.1	23.8	24.8	26.3	27.9
141-146	258	23.3	4.0	17.6	18.5	19.5	20.5	23.0	25.8	27.9	28.8	30.6
147-152	161	25.2	5.2	18.5	20.0	20.7	21.7	24.4	27.8	30.0	31.2	32.9
153-158	66	26.7	6.7	19.4	20.1	22.4	23.0	25.4	29.2	31.8	34.0	38.2
Girls: 11 to 17 Years												
141-146	53	23.8	4.4	17.1	19.3	19.5	21.0	23.4	25.5	27.9	28.6	33.4
147-152	119	25.2	4.6	18.5	19.7	20.9	22.0	24.3	28.0	29.8	30.3	34.4
153-158	305	29.1	6.4	20.8	22.0	23.0	24.7	28.3	32.9	35.0	37.5	39.2
159-164	587	32.2	7.1	23.3	24.8	26.0	27.7	31.2	35.7	38.0	40.1	43.5
165-170	715	34.2	7.4	25.0	26.6	27.8	29.5	33.2	37.6	40.2	42.8	46.9
171-176	367	34.9	8.0	25.9	27.1	28.0	29.9	33.7	38.0	41.2	43.5	47.6
177-182	113	37.8	8.4	28.6	29.5	30.5	31.7	35.9	41.1	45.9	47.8	58.2

Means, Standard Deviations, and Percentiles of Upper Arm Muscle Area (cm^2) by Age for Adult Males of Small, Medium, and Large Frames

| Age (yr) | N | Mean | SD | Percentiles | | | | | | | | |
				5	10	15	25	50	75	85	90	95
Males With Small Frames												
18.0-24.9	443	45.6	10.6	30.8	33.8	35.8	38.7	44.6	51.3	55.2	58.1	63.2
25.0-29.9	318	48.2	9.8	33.5	36.8	39.2	41.8	47.6	53.5	57.7	61.2	63.7
30.0-34.9	237	49.6	10.2	35.0	37.5	38.9	42.0	58.8	56.4	60.0	62.7	66.9
35.0-39.9	212	51.2	10.4	34.7	38.7	40.9	44.1	50.7	57.5	61.7	63.8	70.0
40.0-44.9	210	51.5	10.1	34.9	38.1	40.6	44.2	51.6	58.2	61.6	64.5	66.9
45.0-49.9	220	49.7	10.8	32.8	36.5	38.9	42.9	49.1	55.7	59.5	63.3	68.8
50.0-54.9	225	49.1	11.2	33.8	36.0	38.2	41.5	47.6	55.5	60.7	63.8	69.3
55.0-59.9	204	47.9	10.1	31.2	35.4	37.8	41.7	47.8	54.3	58.8	61.4	64.2
60.0-64.9	318	48.7	11.2	32.5	36.3	38.7	41.4	48.0	54.6	59.6	62.2	68.0
65.0-69.9	446	45.1	10.7	26.7	31.5	34.7	37.6	44.7	52.5	56.1	58.5	62.7
70.0-74.9	314	43.5	10.3	27.7	30.8	32.9	36.1	43.4	49.6	53.4	56.6	59.9
Males With Medium Frames												
18.0-24.9	875	50.5	10.5	35.5	38.2	40.8	43.6	49.5	56.5	60.8	63.2	69.3
25.0-29.9	626	54.0	11.3	37.0	40.1	42.9	46.8	53.2	60.9	65.6	67.7	73.0
30.0-34.9	472	55.0	10.4	38.5	42.2	44.8	48.0	54.3	61.8	65.7	68.6	72.7
35.0-39.9	416	56.7	11.7	39.9	43.1	45.2	48.8	55.9	64.0	69.0	71.6	75.6
40.0-44.9	413	56.7	11.0	39.2	42.6	45.8	49.2	56.3	64.0	68.0	71.1	74.4
45.0-49.9	433	56.6	11.2	39.0	42.6	45.6	49.4	55.9	63.7	69.6	72.8	76.2
50.0-54.9	440	55.3	11.7	37.6	41.8	44.5	47.7	54.2	62.5	65.9	69.6	74.1
55.0-59.9	403	55.4	10.8	39.2	42.5	44.4	48.5	54.8	62.2	66.7	69.5	75.0
60.0-64.9	627	52.3	10.8	34.5	38.3	41.6	45.0	52.1	59.2	63.3	66.3	70.4
65.0-69.9	886	49.8	10.5	33.4	37.2	39.6	43.0	49.2	56.7	60.1	62.4	68.1
70.0-74.9	626	47.8	10.8	30.8	34.6	36.9	40.6	47.5	54.4	59.1	62.0	66.8

From Frisancho AR: *Anthropometric standards for the assessment of growth and nutritional status,* Ann Arbor, 1990, The University of Michigan Press.

NOTE: Values for males age 18 years and older have been adjusted for bone area by subtracting 10.0 cm^2 from the calculated mid–upper arm muscle area.

Age (yr)	N	Mean	SD	Percentiles								
				5	10	15	25	50	75	85	90	95
Males With Large Frames												
18.0-24.9	431	55.7	12.2	37.6	40.8	43.0	47.3	54.6	63.5	67.0	71.6	76.7
25.0-29.9	305	60.3	12.0	42.6	45.7	48.4	52.6	60.4	67.3	72.8	75.8	81.2
30.0-34.9	230	62.8	13.4	44.2	46.9	49.2	53.3	62.6	70.6	75.3	78.8	84.0
35.0-39.9	203	61.6	13.3	43.2	46.0	48.9	51.8	59.9	70.3	76.6	79.4	82.8
40.0-44.9	204	61.8	12.3	44.9	47.4	49.6	53.2	60.0	69.8	74.4	79.4	83.7
45.0-49.9	214	61.1	13.0	42.9	46.3	48.1	52.4	59.6	67.5	71.1	74.9	86.4
50.0-54.9	214	60.5	12.8	41.8	46.0	47.8	51.6	59.4	67.6	72.5	77.6	85.4
55.0-59.9	198	60.2	12.0	42.3	45.0	47.9	52.9	59.8	66.9	71.8	75.3	83.8
60.0-64.9	311	57.9	12.1	38.9	43.9	46.8	50.1	57.5	65.8	69.0	71.8	77.4
65.0-69.9	439	54.5	12.7	35.6	39.4	41.7	46.0	53.7	62.7	66.9	70.7	75.6
70.0-74.9	310	52.0	12.4	33.2	38.3	40.3	43.6	51.6	59.0	63.8	67.2	72.2

Means, Standard Deviations, and Percentiles of Upper Arm Muscle Area (cm^2) by Age for Adult Females of Small, Medium, and Large Frames

Age (yr)	N	Mean	SD	Percentiles								
				5	10	15	25	50	75	85	90	95
Females With Small Frames												
18.0-24.9	651	26.2	6.0	18.2	19.6	20.7	22.5	25.5	29.2	31.2	32.8	36.2
25.0-29.9	486	27.8	7.4	19.5	20.6	21.6	23.2	26.9	30.8	33.3	35.2	38.1
30.0 34.9	413	28.6	7.8	19.1	21.6	22.4	24.5	27.8	31.4	33.7	36.2	38.8
35.0-39.9	368	29.8	10.1	19.7	21.4	22.9	24.4	28.8	32.5	35.4	37.5	42.2
40.0-44.9	350	29.8	6.6	20.9	22.1	23.4	25.7	28.9	33.2	36.0	37.9	41.8
45.0-49.9	241	29.2	7.4	19.1	21.5	22.6	24.3	28.3	33.3	36.1	38.7	41.2
50.0-54.9	256	30.3	7.3	20.8	22.1	23.9	25.5	29.1	33.4	36.7	38.5	41.3
55.0-59.9	223	30.9	7.6	20.4	22.3	23.6	25.8	30.2	34.8	37.6	41.3	45.1
60.0-64.9	351	31.9	8.7	20.9	22.4	23.6	25.8	31.2	36.4	39.1	41 1	46.2
65.0-69.9	491	31.3	8.1	19.4	22.1	23.7	25.7	30.6	35.4	39.8	41.8	45.7
70.0-74.9	367	32.0	9.9	20.3	22.5	24.1	25.9	30.3	36.1	39.8	42.6	47.3
Females With Medium Frames												
18.0-24.9	1296	29.3	7.0	19.8	21.9	23.2	24.9	28.4	32.8	35.2	37.2	40.7
25.0-29.9	964	30.0	7.2	20.7	22.1	23.3	25.0	29.0	33.9	36.8	39.0	43.3
30.0-34.9	814	32.0	9.1	21.4	23.1	24.2	26.3	30.8	36.1	39.4	41.8	46.4
35.0-39.9	728	32.7	8.4	21.4	23.6	24.9	27.3	31.4	37.3	40.8	43.0	47.0
40.0-44.9	696	33.7	12.1	21.2	23.2	25.1	27.2	31.6	37.7	43.1	47.1	52.3
45.0-49.9	484	33.8	8.8	22.2	23.6	25.5	27.9	32.2	37.9	42.5	45.4	49.6
50.0-54.9	502	35.0	9.7	22.8	25.2	26.2	28.5	33.7	40.0	43.5	46.7	51.4
55.0-59.9	442	36.3	11.5	23.7	25.3	26.6	28.7	34.5	41.5	44.9	49.2	53.4
60.0-64.9	695	35.1	9.1	23.0	25.3	26.5	29.2	33.9	39.9	43.7	46.1	49.4
65.0-69.9	971	35.7	10.0	22.4	24.8	26.4	29.1	34.6	40.7	44.5	48.1	51.9
70.0-74.9	731	35.3	9.7	22.2	24.3	26.1	28.9	34.0	40.0	44.4	46.7	51.3

From Frisancho AR: *Anthropometric standards for the assessment of growth and nutritional status,* Ann Arbor, 1990, The University of Michigan Press.
NOTE: Values for females age 18 years and older have been adjusted for bone area by subtracting 6.5 cm^2 from the calculated mid–upper arm muscle area.

Age (yr)	N	Mean	SD	Percentiles								
				5	10	15	25	50	75	85	90	95
Females With Large Frames												
18.0-24.9	641	34.4	10.7	21.9	23.8	25.3	27.3	31.9	38.7	43.9	47.5	55.8
25.0-29.9	471	36.7	11.5	22.2	25.4	26.8	29.3	34.5	42.0	46.8	50.3	60.1
30.0-34.9	392	38.8	12.3	24.0	25.8	27.3	30.1	36.3	45.1	50.7	55.1	61.2
35.0-39.9	357	41.6	14.4	23.9	27.4	29.1	32.2	39.1	47.2	53.7	61.0	72.1
40.0-44.9	344	43.5	16.6	26.2	28.8	30.5	32.9	40.3	49.5	54.4	58.7	71.6
45.0-49.9	236	43.0	15.8	25.0	28.0	29.4	32.5	39.7	49.0	58.3	62.8	69.9
50.0-54.9	246	42.4	13.1	25.1	28.4	30.1	33.4	39.6	49.5	54.8	59.7	68.4
55.0-59.9	213	45.2	16.9	27.0	30.0	32.4	35.8	42.0	51.0	58.5	62.2	65.7
60.0-64.9	341	43.1	14.2	26.6	29.1	31.2	33.9	40.7	49.8	54.8	57.5	67.6
65.0-69.9	482	42.5	13.4	26.4	28.4	30.6	33.5	40.0	48.7	55.3	58.7	66.5
70.0-74.9	363	41.5	11.6	25.7	28.8	30.2	32.8	40.1	48.7	51.4	54.8	60.3

Means, Standard Deviations, and Percentiles of Upper Arm Fat Area (cm^2) by Age for Males and Females of 1 to 74 Years

| Age (yr) | N | Mean | SD | Percentiles | | | | | | | | |
				5	10	15	25	50	75	85	90	95
Males												
1.0-1.9	681	7.5	2.2	4.5	4.9	5.3	5.9	7.4	8.9	9.6	10.3	11.7
2.0-2.9	672	7.4	2.3	4.2	4.8	5.1	5.8	7.3	8.6	9.7	10.6	11.6
3.0-3.9	715	7.6	2.4	4.5	5.0	5.4	5.9	7.2	8.8	9.8	10.6	11.8
4.0-4.9	707	7.3	2.5	4.1	4.7	5.2	5.7	6.9	8.5	9.3	10.0	11.4
5.0-5.9	676	7.4	3.1	4.0	4.5	4.9	5.5	6.7	8.3	9.8	10.9	12.7
6.0-6.9	298	7.7	4.1	3.7	4.3	4.6	5.2	6.7	8.6	10.3	11.2	15.2
7.0-7.9	312	8.1	4.2	3.8	4.3	4.7	5.4	7.1	9.6	11.6	12.8	15.5
8.0-8.9	296	8.9	5.0	4.1	4.8	5.1	5.8	7.6	10.4	12.4	15.6	18.6
9.0-9.9	322	10.1	6.2	4.2	4.8	5.4	6.1	8.3	11.8	15.8	18.2	21.7
10.0 10.9	333	12.0	7.3	4.7	5.3	5.7	6.9	9.8	14.7	18.3	21.5	27.0
11.0-11.9	324	13.6	9.4	4.9	5.5	6.2	7.3	10.4	16.9	22.3	26.0	32.5
12.0-12.9	348	13.9	9.6	4.7	5.6	6.3	7.6	11.3	15.8	21.1	27.3	35.0
13.0-13.9	350	13.0	9.2	4.7	5.7	6.3	7.6	10.1	14.9	21.2	25.4	32.1
14.0-14.9	358	13.3	10.2	4.6	5.6	6.3	7.4	10.1	15.9	19.5	25.5	31.8
15.0-15.9	356	12.8	9.0	5.6	6.1	6.5	7.3	9.6	14.6	20.2	24.5	31.3
16.0-16.9	350	13.9	9.5	5.6	6.1	6.9	8.3	10.5	16.6	20.6	24.8	33.5
17.0-17.9	337	12.9	8.9	5.4	6.1	6.7	7.4	9.9	15.6	19.7	23.7	28.9
18.0-24.9	1752	16.9	10.8	5.5	6.9	7.7	9.2	13.9	21.5	26.8	30.7	37.2
25.0-29.9	1250	18.8	11.6	6.0	7.3	8.4	10.2	16.3	23.9	29.7	33.3	40.4
30.0-34.9	940	20.4	11.4	6.2	8.4	9.7	11.9	18.4	25.6	31.6	34.8	41.9
35.0-39.9	832	20.1	10.5	6.5	8.1	9.6	12.8	18.8	25.2	29.6	33.4	39.4
40.0-44.9	828	20.4	11.2	7.1	8.7	9.9	12.4	18.0	25.3	30.1	35.3	42.1
45.0-49.9	867	20.1	11.0	7.4	9.0	10.2	12.3	18.1	24.9	29.7	33.7	40.4
50.0-54.9	879	19.4	10.3	7.0	8.6	10.1	12.3	17.3	23.9	29.0	32.4	40.0
55.0-59.9	807	19.2	10.2	6.4	8.2	9.7	12.3	17.4	23.8	28.4	33.3	39.1
60.0-64.9	1259	19.1	10.2	6.9	8.7	9.9	12.1	17.0	23.5	28.3	31.8	38.7
65.0-69.9	1773	18.0	9.8	5.8	7.4	8.5	10.9	16.5	22.8	27.2	30.7	36.3
70.0-74.9	1250	17.5	9.4	6.0	7.5	8.9	11.0	15.9	22.0	25.7	29.1	34.9

From Frisancho AR: *Anthropometric standards for the assessment of growth and nutritional status,* Ann Arbor, 1990, The University of Michigan Press.

Age (yr)	N	Mean	SD	Percentiles								
				5	10	15	25	50	75	85	90	95
Females												
1.0-1.9	622	7.3	2.3	4.1	4.6	5.0	5.6	7.1	8.6	9.5	10.4	11.7
2.0-2.9	614	7.7	2.3	4.4	5.0	5.4	6.1	7.5	9.0	10.0	10.8	12.0
3.0-3.9	651	7.8	2.5	4.3	5.0	5.4	6.1	7.6	9.2	10.2	10.8	12.2
4.0-4.9	680	8.0	2.6	4.3	4.9	5.4	6.2	7.7	9.3	10.4	11.3	12.8
5.0-5.9	672	8.5	3.4	4.4	5.0	5.4	6.3	7.8	9.8	11.3	12.5	14.5
6.0-6.9	296	8.7	3.9	4.5	5.0	5.6	6.2	8.1	10.0	11.2	13.3	16.5
7.0-7.9	329	9.8	4.5	4.8	5.5	6.0	7.0	8.8	11.0	13.2	14.7	19.0
8.0-8.9	275	11.3	6.5	5.2	5.7	6.4	7.2	9.8	13.3	15.8	18.0	23.7
9.0-9.9	321	13.1	7.3	5.4	6.2	6.8	8.1	11.5	15.6	18.8	22.0	27.5
10.0-10.9	329	14.1	7.7	6.1	6.9	7.2	8.4	11.9	18.0	21.5	25.3	29.9
11.0-11.9	302	16.3	9.7	6.6	7.5	8.2	9.8	13.1	19.9	24.4	28.2	36.8
12.0-12.9	323	16.9	8.9	6.7	8.0	8.8	10.8	14.8	20.8	24.8	29.4	34.0
13.0-13.9	360	19.1	11.0	6.7	7.7	9.4	11.6	16.5	23.7	28.7	32.7	40.8
14.0-14.9	370	20.4	11.0	8.3	9.6	10.9	12.4	17.7	25.1	29.5	34.6	41.2
15.0-15.9	309	20.7	11.4	8.6	10.0	11.4	12.8	18.2	24.4	29.2	32.9	44.3
16.0-16.9	343	23.5	10.9	11.3	12.8	13.7	15.9	20.5	28.0	32.7	37.0	46.0
17.0-17.9	291	23.9	13.0	9.5	11.7	13.0	14.6	21.0	29.5	33.5	38.0	51.6
18.0-24.9	2588	25.2	13.4	10.0	12.0	13.5	16.1	21.9	30.6	37.2	42.0	51.6
25.0-29.9	1921	28.1	14.7	11.0	13.3	15.1	17.7	24.5	34.8	42.1	47.1	57.5
30.0-34.9	1619	31.6	16.1	12.2	14.8	17.2	20.4	28.2	39.0	46.8	52.3	64.5
35.0-39.9	1453	33.6	16.8	13.0	15.8	18.0	21.8	29.7	41.7	49.2	55.5	64.9
40.0-44.9	1390	34.3	16.2	13.8	16.7	19.2	23.0	31.3	42.6	51.0	56.3	64.5
45.0-49.9	961	36.0	17.2	13.6	17.1	19.8	24.3	33.0	44.4	52.3	58.4	68.8
50.0-54.9	1004	36.7	15.9	14.3	18.3	21.4	25.7	34.1	45.6	53.9	57.7	65.7
55.0-59.9	879	37.6	17.7	13.7	18.2	20.7	26.0	34.5	46.4	53.9	59.1	69.7
60.0-64.9	1389	37.1	16.0	15.3	19.1	21.9	26.0	34.8	45.7	51.7	58.3	68.3
65.0-69.9	1946	34.7	15.1	13.9	17.6	20.0	24.1	32.7	42.7	49.2	53.6	62.4
70.0-74.9	1463	32.9	14.6	13.0	16.2	18.8	22.7	31.2	41.0	46.4	51.4	57.7

Normal Constituents of Blood and Urine in Adults

Normal Constituents of Blood in the Adult

Physical Measurements

Viscosity (serum—water as unity)		1.00-1.24
Bleeding time (Simplate method)	Minutes	3.0-9.5
Prothrombin time (plasma)	Seconds	10-14
Sedimentation rate (Westergren method)		
Men	mm/hr	Less than 20
Women	mm/hr	Less than 30

Hematologic Studies

Red blood cells		
Men	10^{12} per L	4.5-6.0
Women	10^{12} per L	4.0-5.0
White blood cells	10^9 per L	4-11
Lymphocytes	%	20-40
Neutrophils	%	50-70
Monocytes	%	4-8
Eosinophils	%	0-4
Basophils	%	0-2
Platelets	10^9 per L	150-400

Proteins

Total protein (serum)	g/dl	6.0-8.0
Albumin (serum)	g/dl	3.5-5.0
Globulin (serum)	g/dl	2.0-3.5
Albumin:globulin ratio		1.5:1-2.5:1
Fibrinogen	mg/dl	200-400
Hemoglobin		
Men	g/dl	13.5-18.0
Women	g/dl	12.0-16.0

Nitrogen Constituents

Urea N (Blood urea nitrogen) (serum)	mg/dl	6-20
Creatinine (whole blood)	mg/dl	0.5-1.5
Uric acid (whole blood)		
Men	mg/dl	4.5-6.5
Women	mg/dl	2.5-5.5

Abbreviations and conversion factors:

dl = deciliter
ml = milliliter
μg = microgram

$$mEq/L = \frac{mg\backslash L}{Equivalent\ weight}$$

$$Equivalent\ weight = \frac{Atomic\ weight}{Valence\ of\ element}$$

g = gram
mEq = milliequivalent

$$mmol\ (millimole)/L = \frac{mg\backslash L}{Molecular\ weight}$$

vol % (volume percent) = mmol/L $\times$ 2.24

Carbohydrates and Lipids

Glucose (whole blood)	mg/dl	70-90
Ketones—as acetone	mg/dl	0.3-2.0
Fats (total lipids) (serum)	mg/dl	570-820
Cholesterol (total) (serum)	mg/dl	140-200
Bilirubin (total—adults) (serum)	mg/dl	0.2-1.3

Blood Gases

CO_2 content (serum)	mmol/L	22-28
CO_2 content (arterial blood)		
Men	mm Hg	35-48
Women	mm Hg	32-45
Oxygen capacity (whole blood) (varies with hemoglobin level)	vol %	16-24
Oxygen saturation		
Arterial blood	%	95-98
Venous blood	%	60-85

Acid-Base Constituents

Sodium	mEq/L	135-145
Potassium (serum)	mEq/L	3.5-5.5
Calcium	mg/dl	9.0-11.0
	mEq/L	4.5-5.5
Magnesium (serum)	mEq/L	1.5-2.5
Phosphorus, inorganic	mg/dl	2.8-4.5
Chlorides, expressed as Cl (serum)	mEq/L	95-105
Lactic acid	μg/dl	5-20
Base bicarbonate HCO_3 (serum)	mEq/L	20-30
pH (blood or plasma at 38° C)		7.35-7.45

Miscellaneous

Alkaline phosphatase (serum)	U/L	38-126
Iron	μg/dl	50-150
Ascorbic acid	mg/dl	0.4-1.5
Carotene (serum)	μg/dl	10-85

Normal Constituents of Urine in the Adult

Urine Constituents

Creatine	<100 mg/24 hr
Creatinine	0.8-2.0 g/24 hr
Protein	None
Urea	20-35 g/24 hr
Uric acid	250-750 mg/24 hr
Acetone bodies	None
Bile	None
Calcium	100-250 mg/24 hr
Chloride	110-250 mEq/24 hr
Glucose	None
Sodium	40-250 mEq/24 hr

Physical Measurements

Specific gravity	1.003-1.030
Reaction (pH) (depends on diet)	4.0-8.0
Volume	800-1600 ml/24 hr

Exchange Lists for Meal Planning

Foods are listed with their serving sizes, which are usually measured after cooking. When you begin, measuring the size of each serving will help you learn to "eyeball" correct serving sizes. The following chart shows the amount of nutrients in one serving from each list:

Groups/Lists	Carbohydrate (g)	Protein (g)	Fat (g)	Calories
Carbohydrate Group				
Starch	15	3	0-1	80
Fruit	15	—	—	60
Milk				
Fat-free, low-fat	12	8	0-3	90
Reduced-fat	12	8	5	120
Whole	12	8	8	150
Other carbohydrates	15	Varies	Varies	Varies
Nonstarchy vegetables	5	2	—	25
Meat and Meat Substitutes Group				
Very lean	—	7	0-1	35
Lean	—	7	3	55
Medium-fat	—	7	5	75
High-fat	—	7	8	100
Fat Group	—	—	5	45

The Exchange Lists are the basis of a meal-planning system designed by a committee of the American Diabetes Association and The American Dietetic Association. Although designed primarily for people with diabetes and others who must follow special diets, the Exchange Lists are based on principles of good nutrition that apply to everyone. Copyright 2003 American Diabetes Association, Inc., The American Dietetic Association. Used with permission.

STARCH LIST

Cereals, grains, pasta, breads, crackers, snacks, starchy vegetables, and cooked beans, peas, and lentils are starches. In general, one starch is as follows:

- ½ cup of cooked cereal, grain, or starchy vegetable
- ⅓ cup of cooked rice or pasta
- 1 oz of a bread product, such as 1 slice of bread
- ¾ to 1 oz of most snack foods (Some snacks may also have added fat.)

Nutrition Tips

1. Most starch choices are good sources of B vitamins.
2. Foods made from whole grains are good sources of fiber.
   - A serving from the Bread list, on average, has 1 g of fiber.
   - A serving from the Cereals and Grains list or the Crackers and Snacks list, on average, has 2 g of fiber.
   - A serving from the Starchy Vegetables list, on average, has 3 g of fiber.
3. Beans, peas, and lentils are good sources of protein and fiber.
   - A serving from this group, on average, has 6 g of fiber.

Selection Tips

1. Choose starches made with little fat as often as you can.
2. Starchy vegetables prepared with fat count as one starch and one fat.
3. For many starchy foods (e.g., bagels, muffins, dinner rolls, buns), a general rule of thumb is 1 oz equals 1 carbohydrate serving. However, bagels or muffins range widely in size. Check the size you eat. Also, use the Nutrition Facts on food labels when available.
4. Beans, peas, and lentils are also found on the Meat and Meat Substitutes list.
5. A waffle or pancake is about the size of a compact disc (CD) and about ¼ inch thick.
6. Because starches often swell in cooking, a small amount of uncooked starch becomes a much larger amount of cooked food.
7. Most of the serving sizes are measured or weighed after cooking.
8. Always check Nutrition Facts on the food label.

One starch exchange equals 15 g of carbohydrate, 3 g of protein, 0–1 g of fat, and 80 calories.

Bread	
Bagel, 4 oz	¼ (1 oz)
Bread, reduced-calorie	2 slices (1½ oz)
Bread, white, whole wheat, pumpernickel, rye	1 slice (1 oz)
Bread sticks, crisp, 4 inches × ½ inch	4 (⅔ oz)
English muffin	½
Hot dog or hamburger bun	½ (1 oz)
Naan, 8 × 2 inch	¼
Pancake, 4 inches across, ¼ inch thick	1
Pita, 6 inches across	½
Roll, plain, small	1 (1 oz)
Raisin bread, unfrosted	1 slice (1 oz)
Tortilla, corn, 6 inches across	1
Tortilla, flour, 6 inches across	1
Tortilla, flour, 10 inches across	⅓
Waffle, 4½ inches square or across, reduced-fat	1
Cereals and Grains	
Bran cereals	½ cup
Bulgur	½ cup
Cereals, cooked	½ cup
Cereals, unsweetened, ready-to-eat	¾ cup
Cornmeal (dry)	3 tbsp
Couscous	⅓ cup
Flour (dry)	3 tbsp
Granola, low-fat	¼ cup
Grape-Nuts	¼ cup
Grits	½ cup
Kasha	½ cup
Millet	⅓ cup
Muesli	¼ cup

Oats	½ cup
Pasta	⅓ cup
Puffed cereal	1½ cups
Rice, white or brown	⅓ cup
Shredded wheat	½ cup
Sugar-frosted cereal	½ cup
Wheat germ	3 tbsp

Starchy Vegetables

Baked beans	⅓ cup
Corn	½ cup
Corn on the cob, large	½ cob (5 oz)
Mixed vegetables with corn, peas, or pasta	1 cup
Peas, green	½ cup
Plantain	½ cup
Potato, baked with skin	¼ large (3 oz)
Potato, boiled	½ cup or ½ medium (3 oz)
Potato, mashed	½ cup
Squash, winter (acorn, butternut, pumpkin)	1 cup
Yam, sweet potato, plain	½ cup

Crackers and Snacks

Animal crackers	8
Graham crackers, 2½ -inch square	3
Matzoh	¾ oz
Melba toast	4 slices
Oyster crackers	24
Popcorn (popped, no fat added, or low-fat microwave)	3 cups
Pretzels	¾ oz
Rice cakes, 4 inches across	2
Saltine-type crackers	6

Snack chips, fat-free or baked (tortilla, potato)	15-20 (¾ oz)
Whole-wheat crackers, no fat added	2-5 (¾ oz)

Beans, Peas, and Lentils

(count as 1 starch exchange, plus 1 very lean meat exchange)

Beans and peas (garbanzo, pinto, kidney, white, split, black-eyed)	½ cup
Lima beans	⅔ cup
Lentils	½ cup
Miso 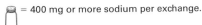	3 tbsp

Starchy Foods Prepared With Fat

(count as 1 starch exchange, plus 1 fat exchange)

Biscuit, 2½ inches across	1
Chow mein noodles	½ cup
Corn bread, 2-inch cube	1 (2 oz)
Crackers, round butter-type	6
Croutons	1 cup
French-fried potatoes, oven-baked (see also the Fast Foods list)	1 cup (2 oz)
Granola	¼ cup
Hummus	⅓ cup
Muffin, 5 oz	⅕ (1 oz)
Popcorn, microwaved	3 cups
Sandwich crackers, cheese or peanut butter filling	3
Snack chips (potato, tortilla)	9-13 (¾ oz)
Stuffing, bread (prepared)	⅓ cup
Taco shell, 6 inches across	2
Waffle, 4½ inches square or across	1
Whole wheat crackers, fat added	4-6 (1 oz)

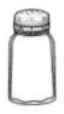

= 400 mg or more sodium per exchange.

Common Measurements

3 tsp = 1 tbsp
4 tbsp = ¼ cup
5⅓ tbsp = ⅓ cup
4 oz = ½ cup
8 oz = 1 cup
1 cup = ½ pint

FRUIT LIST

Fresh, frozen, canned, and dried fruits and fruit juices are on this list. In general, one fruit exchange is:

- 1 small fresh fruit (4 oz)
- ½ cup of canned or fresh fruit or unsweetened fruit juice
- ¼ cup of dried fruit

Nutrition Tips

1. Fresh, frozen, and dried fruits have about 2 g of fiber per choice. Fruit juices contain very little fiber.
2. Citrus fruits, berries, and melons are good sources of vitamin C.

Selection Tips

1. Count ½ cup cranberries or rhubarb sweetened with sugar substitutes as free foods.
2. Read the Nutrition Facts on the food label. If one serving has more than 15 g of carbohydrate, you will need to adjust the size of the serving you eat or drink.

3. Portion sizes for canned fruits are for the fruit and a small amount of juice.
4. Whole fruit is more filling than fruit juice and may be a better choice.
5. Food labels for fruits may contain the words *no sugar added* or *unsweetened*. This means that no sucrose (table sugar) has been added.
6. Generally, fruit canned in extra light syrup has the same amount of carbohydrate per serving as the *no sugar added* or the juice pack. All canned fruits on the fruit list are based on one of these three types of pack.

One fruit exchange equals 15 g of carbohydrate and 60 calories. The weight includes skin, core, seeds, and rind.

Fruit

Apple, unpeeled, small	1 (4 oz)
Applesauce, unsweetened	½ cup
Apples, dried	4 rings
Apricots, fresh	4 whole (5½ oz)
Apricots, dried	8 halves
Apricots, canned	½ cup
Banana, small	1 (4 oz)
Blackberries	¾ cup
Blueberries	¾ cup
Cantaloupe, small	⅓ melon (11 oz) or 1 cup cubes
Cherries, sweet, fresh	12 (3 oz)
Cherries, sweet, canned	½ cup
Dates	3
Figs, fresh	1½ large or 2 medium (3½ oz)
Figs, dried	1½
Fruit cocktail	½ cup
Grapefruit, large	½ (11 oz)
Grapefruit sections, canned	¾ cup
Grapes, small	17 (3 oz)
Honeydew melon	1 slice (10 oz) or 1 cup cubes
Kiwi	1 (3½ oz)
Mandarin oranges, canned	¾ cup
Mango, small	½ fruit (5½ oz) or ½ cup
Nectarine, small	1 (5 oz)
Orange, small	1 (6½ oz)

Papaya	½ fruit (8 oz) or 1 cup cubes
Peach, medium, fresh	1 (4 oz)
Peaches, canned	½ cup
Pear, large, fresh	½ (4 oz)
Pears, canned	½ cup
Pineapple, fresh	¾ cup
Pineapple, canned	½ cup
Plums, small	2 (5 oz)
Plums, canned	½ cup
Plums, dried (prunes)	3
Raisins	2 tbsp
Raspberries	1 cup
Strawberries	1¼ cup whole berries
Tangerines, small	2 (8 oz)
Watermelon	1 slice (13½ oz) or 1¼ cup cubes

Fruit Juice, Unsweetened

Apple juice/cider	½ cup
Cranberry juice cocktail	⅓ cup
Cranberry juice cocktail, reduced-calorie	1 cup
Fruit juice blends, 100% juice	⅓ cup
Grape juice	⅓ cup
Grapefruit juice	½ cup
Orange juice	½ cup
Pineapple juice	½ cup
Prune juice	⅓ cup

MILK LIST

Different types of milk and milk products are on this list. Cheeses are on the Meat and Meat Substitutes list, and cream and other dairy fats are on the Fat list. Based on the amount of fat they contain, milks are divided into fat-free/low-fat milk, reduced-fat milk, and whole milk. One choice of these includes the following:

Type of Milk	Carbohydrate (g)	Protein (g)	Fat (g)	Calories
Fat-free/low-fat (½% or 1%)	12	8	0-3	90
Reduced-fat (2%)	12	8	5	120
Whole	12	8	8	150

Nutrition Tips

1. Milk and yogurt are good sources of calcium and protein. Check the Nutrition Facts on the food label.
2. The higher the fat content of milk and yogurt, the greater the amount of saturated fat and cholesterol. Choose lower-fat varieties.
3. For those who are lactose-intolerant, look for lactose-reduced or lactose-free varieties of milk. Check the food label for total amount of carbohydrate per serving.

Selection Tips

1. 1 cup equals 8 fluid oz or ½ pint.
2. Look for chocolate milk, rice milk, frozen yogurt, and ice cream on the Sweets, Desserts, and Other Carbohydrates list.
3. Nondairy creamers are on the Free Foods list.

One milk exchange equals 12 g of carbohydrate and 8 g of protein.

Fat-Free and Low-Fat Milk

(0-3 g fat/serving)

Fat-free milk	1 cup
½% milk	1 cup
1% milk	1 cup
Buttermilk, low-fat or fat-free	1 cup
Evaporated fat-free milk	½ cup
Fat-free dry milk	⅓ cup dry
Soy milk, low-fat or fat-free	1 cup
Yogurt, fat-free, flavored, sweetened with nonnutritive sweetener and fructose	⅔ cup (6 oz)
Yogurt, plain, fat-free	⅔ cup (6 oz)

Reduced-Fat

(5 g fat/serving)

2% milk	1 cup
Soy milk	1 cup
Sweet acidophilus milk	1 cup
Yogurt, plain, low-fat	¾ cup

Whole Milk

(8 g fat/serving)

Whole milk	1 cup
Evaporated whole milk	½ cup
Goat's milk	1 cup
Kefir	1 cup
Yogurt, plain (made from whole milk)	¾ cup

SWEETS, DESSERTS, AND OTHER CARBOHYDRATES LIST

You can substitute food choices from this list for a starch, fruit, or milk choice on your meal plan. Some choices will also count as one or more fat choices.

Nutrition Tips

1. These foods can be substituted for other carbohydrate-containing foods in your meal plan, even though they contain added sugars or fat. However, they do not contain as many important vitamins and minerals as the choices on the Starch, Fruit, and Milk lists.
2. When choosing these foods, include foods from the other lists to eat balanced meals.

Selection Tips

1. Because many of these foods are concentrated sources of carbohydrate and fat, saturated fat, and *trans* fat, the portion sizes are often very small.

2. Look for the words *hydrogenated* or *partially hydro-genated* on the ingredient label. The lower down on the list these words appear, the fewer *trans* fats there are.

3. Be sure to check the Nutrition Facts on the food label. It will be your most accurate source of information.

4. Many fat-free or reduced-fat products made with fat replacers contain carbohydrate. When eaten in large amounts, they may need to be counted. Talk with your dietitian to determine how to count these in your meal plan.

5. Look for fat-free salad dressings in smaller amounts on the Free Foods list.

One carbohydrate exchange equals 15 g of carbohydrate, or 1 starch, or 1 fruit, or 1 milk.

Food	Serving Size	Exchanges per Serving
Angel food cake, unfrosted	1/12 cake (about 2 oz)	2 carbohydrates
Brownie, small, unfrosted	2-inch square (about 1 oz)	1 carbohydrate, 1 fat
Cake, unfrosted	2-inch square (about 1 oz)	1 carbohydrate, 1 fat
Cake, frosted	2-inch square (about 2 oz)	2 carbohydrates, 1 fat
Cookie or sandwich cookie with crème filling	2 small (about 2/3 oz)	1 carbohydrate, 1 fat
Cookies, sugar-free	3 small or 1 large (3/4-1 oz)	1 carbohydrate, 1-2 fats
Cranberry sauce, jellied	1/4 cup	1½ carbohydrates
Cupcake, frosted	1 small (about 2 oz)	2 carbohydrates, 1 fat
Doughnut, plain cake	1 medium (1½ oz)	1½ carbohydrates, 2 fats
Doughnut, glazed	3¾-inch across (2 oz)	2 carbohydrates, 2 fats
Energy, sport, or breakfast bar	1 bar (1⅓ oz)	1½ carbohydrates, 0-1 fat
Energy, sport, or breakfast bar	1 bar (2 oz)	2 carbohydrates, 1 fat
Fruit cobbler	½ cup (3½ oz)	3 carbohydrates, 1 fat
Fruit juice bars, frozen, 100% juice	1 bar (3 oz)	1 carbohydrate
Fruit snacks, chewy (pureed fruit concentrate)	1 roll (3/4 oz)	1 carbohydrate
Fruit spreads, 100% fruit	1½ tbsp	1 carbohydrate
Gelatin, regular	½ cup	1 carbohydrate
Gingersnaps	3	1 carbohydrate
Granola or snack bar, regular or low-fat	1 bar (1 oz)	1½ carbohydrates
Honey	1 tbsp	1 carbohydrate
Ice cream	½ cup	1 carbohydrate, 2 fats
Ice cream, light	½ cup	1 carbohydrate, 1 fat
Ice cream, low-fat	½ cup	1½ carbohydrates
Ice cream, fat-free, no sugar added	½ cup	1 carbohydrate
Jam or jelly, regular	1 tbsp	1 carbohydrate
Milk, chocolate, whole	1 cup	2 carbohydrates, 1 fat
Pie, fruit, 2 crusts	1/6 of 8-inch commercially prepared pie	3 carbohydrates, 2 fats
Pie, pumpkin or custard	1/8 of 8-inch commercially prepared pie	2 carbohydrates, 2 fats
Pudding, regular (made with reduced-fat milk)	½ cup	2 carbohydrates
Pudding, sugar-free or sugar-free and fat-free (made with fat-free milk)	½ cup	1 carbohydrate
Reduced-calorie meal replacement (shake)	1 can (10-11 oz)	1½ carbohydrates, 0-1 fat
Rice milk, low-fat or fat-free, plain	1 cup	1 carbohydrate
Rice milk, low-fat, flavored	1 cup	1½ carbohydrates
Salad dressing, fat-free	1/4 cup	1 carbohydrate

= 400 mg or more of sodium per exchange.

Food	Serving Size	Exchanges per Serving
Sherbet, sorbet	½ cup	2 carbohydrates
Spaghetti sauce or pasta sauce, canned	½ cup	1 carbohydrate, 1 fat
Sports drinks	8 oz (1 cup)	1 carbohydrate
Sugar	1 tbsp	1 carbohydrate
Sweet roll or Danish	1 (2½ oz)	2½ carbohydrates, 2 fats
Syrup, light	2 tbsp	1 carbohydrate
Syrup, regular	1 tbsp	1 carbohydrate
Syrup, regular	¼ cup	4 carbohydrates
Vanilla wafers	5	1 carbohydrate, 1 fat
Yogurt, frozen	½ cup	1 carbohydrate, 0-1 fat
Yogurt, frozen, fat-free	⅓ cup	1 carbohydrate
Yogurt, low-fat with fruit	1 cup	3 carbohydrates, 0-1 fat

NONSTARCHY VEGETABLE LIST

Vegetables that contain small amounts of carbohydrate and calories are on this list. Vegetables contain important nutrients. Try to eat at least 2 or 3 vegetable choices each day. In general, one vegetable exchange is:

- ½ cup of cooked vegetables or vegetable juice
- 1 cup of raw vegetables

If you eat 3 cups or more of raw vegetables or 1½ cups of cooked vegetables at one meal, count them as 1 carbohydrate choice.

Nutrition Tips

1. Fresh and frozen vegetables have less added salt than canned vegetables. Drain and rinse canned vegetables if you want to remove some salt.

2. Choose more dark-green and dark-yellow vegetables, such as spinach, broccoli, romaine, carrots, chilies, and peppers.
3. Broccoli, brussels sprouts, cauliflower, greens, peppers, spinach, and tomatoes are good sources of vitamin C.
4. Vegetables contain 1 to 4 g of fiber per serving.

Selection Tips

1. A 1-cup portion of broccoli is a portion about the size of a light bulb.
2. Tomato sauce is different from spaghetti sauce, which is on the Sweets, Desserts, and Other Carbohydrates list.
3. Canned vegetables and juices are available without added salt.
4. Starchy vegetables such as corn, peas, winter squash, and potatoes that contain larger amounts of calories and carbohydrates are on the Starch list.

One vegetable exchange (½ cup cooked or 1 cup raw) equals 5 g of carbohydrates, 2 g of protein, 0 g of fat, and 25 calories.

Foods

Artichoke	Broccoli	Eggplant
Artichoke hearts	Brussels sprouts	Green onions or scallions
Asparagus	Cabbage	Greens (collard, kale, mustard, turnip)
Beans (green, wax, Italian)	Carrots	Kohlrabi
Bean sprouts	Cauliflower	Leeks
Beets	Celery	Mixed vegetables (without corn, peas, or pasta)
	Cucumber	

Mushrooms

Okra

Onions

Pea pods

Peppers (all varieties)

Radishes

Salad greens (endive, escarole, lettuce, romaine, spinach)

Sauerkraut 🧂

Spinach

Summer squash

Tomato

Tomatoes, canned

Tomato sauce 🧂

Tomato/vegetable juice 🧂

Turnips

Water chestnuts

Watercress

Zucchini

🧂 = 400 mg or more sodium per exchange.

MEAT AND MEAT SUBSTITUTES LIST

Meat and meat substitutes that contain both protein and fat are on this list. In general, one meat exchange is as follows:

- 1 oz of meat, fish, poultry, or cheese
- ½ cup of beans, peas, or lentils

Based on the amount of fat they contain, meats are divided into very lean, lean, medium-fat, and high-fat lists. This is done so that you can see which ones contain the least amount of fat. One ounce (one exchange) of each of these includes the following:

Type of Meat	Carbohydrate (g)	Protein (g)	Fat (g)	Calories
Very lean	0	7	0-1	35
Lean	0	7	3	55
Medium-fat	0	7	5	75
High-fat	0	7	8	100

Nutrition Tips

1. Choose very lean and lean meat choices whenever possible. Items from the high-fat group are high in saturated fat, cholesterol, and calories and can raise blood cholesterol levels.
2. Beans, peas, and lentils are good sources of fiber, about 3 g per serving.
3. Some processed meats, seafood, and soy products may contain carbohydrate when consumed in large amounts. Check the Nutrition Facts on the label to see if the amount is close to 15 g. If so, count it as a carbohydrate choice as well as a meat choice.

Selection Tips

1. Weigh meat after cooking and removing bones and fat; 4 oz of raw meat is equal to 3 oz of cooked meat. Some examples of meat portions are as follow:
   - 1 oz cheese = 1 meat choice and is about the size of a 1-inch cube or 4 cubes the size of dice
   - 2 oz meat = 2 meat choices, such as the following: 1 small chicken leg or thigh ½ cup cottage cheese or tuna
   - 3 oz meat = 3 meat choices and is about the size of a deck of cards, such as the following:
     1 medium pork chop
     1 small hamburger
     ½ of a whole chicken breast
     1 unbreaded fish fillet
2. Limit your choices from the high-fat group to three times per week or less.
3. Most grocery stores stock Select and Choice grades of meat. The Select grades of meat are the leanest. The Choice grades contain a moderate amount of fat, and Prime cuts of meat have the highest amount of fat.
4. *Hamburger* may contain added seasoning and fat, but ground beef does not.
5. Read labels to find products that are low in fat and cholesterol (5 g of fat or less per serving).
6. Dried beans, peas, and lentils are also found on the Starch list.
7. Peanut butter, in smaller amounts, is also found on the Fat list.
8. Bacon, in smaller amounts, is also found on the Fat list.
9. Don't be fooled by ground beef packages that say X% lean (e.g., 90% lean). This is the percentage of fat by weight, NOT the percentage of calories from fat. A 3.5-oz patty of this raw ground beef has about half its calories from fat.
10. Meatless burgers are in the Combination Foods list (3 oz of soy-based burger = ½ carbohydrate + 2 very lean meats; 3 oz of vegetable- and starch-based burger = 1 carbohydrate + 1 lean meat).

One exchange equals 0 g of carbohydrate, 7 g of protein, 0-1 g of fat, and 35 calories.

Very Lean Meat and Substitutes List

- One very lean meat exchange is equal to any one of the following items:

  Poultry: Chicken or turkey (white meat, no skin), Cornish hen (no skin) — 1 oz

  Fish: Fresh or frozen cod, flounder, haddock, halibut, trout, lox (smoked salmon); tuna, fresh or canned in water — 1 oz

  Shellfish: Clams, crab, lobster, scallops, shrimp, imitation shellfish — 1 oz

  Game: Duck or pheasant (no skin), venison, buffalo, ostrich — 1 oz

  Cheese with 1 g of fat or less per ounce:
  Fat-free or low-fat cottage cheese — ¼ cup
  Fat-free cheese — 1 oz

Other:

Processed sandwich meats with 1 g of fat or less per ounce, such as deli thin, shaved meats, chipped beef, turkey ham — 1 oz

Egg whites — 2
Egg substitutes, plain — ¼ cup
Hot dogs with 1 g of fat or less per ounce — 1 oz

Kidney (high in cholesterol) — 1 oz
Sausage with 1 g of fat or less per ounce — 1 oz

- Count the following items as one very lean meat and one starch exchange:
  Beans, peas, lentils (cooked) — ½ cup

= 400 mg or more sodium per exchange.

Meal Planning Tips

1. Bake, roast, broil, grill, poach, steam, or boil meat and fish rather than frying.
2. Place meat on a rack so that the fat will drain off during cooking.
3. Use a nonstick spray and a nonstick pan to brown or fry foods.
4. Trim off visible fat or skin before or after cooking.
5. If you add flour, bread crumbs, coating mixes, fat, or marinades when cooking, ask your dietitian how to count it in your meal plan.

One exchange equals 0 g of carbohydrate, 7 g of protein, 3 g of fat, and 55 calories.

Lean Meat and Substitutes List

- One lean meat exchange is equal to any one of the following items:

  Beef: USDA Select or Choice grades of lean beef trimmed of fat, such as round, sirloin, and flank steak; tenderloin; roast (rib, chuck, rump); steak (T-bone, porterhouse, cubed); ground round — 1 oz

  Pork: Lean pork, such as fresh ham; canned, cured, or boiled ham; Canadian bacon; tenderloin, center loin chop — 1 oz

  Lamb: Roast, chop, or leg — 1 oz
  Veal: Lean chop, roast — 1 oz
  Poultry: Chicken, turkey (dark meat, no skin), chicken (white meat, with skin), domestic duck or goose (well-drained of fat, no skin) — 1 oz

  Fish:
  Herring (uncreamed or smoked) — 1 oz
  Oysters — 6 medium

Salmon (fresh or canned), catfish — 1 oz
Sardines (canned) — 2 medium
Tuna (canned in oil, drained) — 1 oz
Game: Goose (no skin), rabbit — 1 oz
Cheese:
4.5%-fat cottage cheese — ¼ cup
Grated Parmesan — 2 tbsp
Cheeses with 3 g of fat or less per ounce — 1 oz
Other:
Hot dogs with 3 g of fat or less per ounce — 1½ oz

Processed sandwich meat with 3 g of fat or less per ounce, such as turkey pastrami or kielbasa — 1 oz
Liver, heart (high in cholesterol) — 1 oz

= 400 mg or more sodium per exchange.

One exchange equals 0 g of carbohydrate, 7 g of protein, 5 g of fat, and 75 calories.

Medium-Fat Meat and Substitutes List
- One medium-fat meat exchange is equal to any one of the following items:

Beef: Most beef products fall into this category (ground beef, meatloaf, corned beef, short ribs, Prime grades of meat trimmed of fat, such as prime rib).	1 oz
Pork: Top loin, chop, Boston butt, cutlet	1 oz
Lamb: Rib roast, ground	1 oz
Veal: Cutlet (ground or cubed, unbreaded)	1 oz
Poultry: Chicken (dark meat, with skin), ground turkey or ground chicken, fried chicken (with skin)	1 oz

Fish: Any fried fish product	1 oz
Cheese with 5 g of fat or less per ounce:	
Feta	1 oz
Mozzarella	1 oz
Ricotta	¼ cup (2 oz)
Other:	
Egg (high in cholesterol, limit to 3 per week)	1
Sausage with 5 g of fat or less per ounce	1 oz
Tempeh	¼ cup
Tofu	4 oz or ½ cup

One exchange equals 0 g of carbohydrate, 7 g of protein, 8 g of fat, and 100 calories.

High-Fat Meat and Substitutes List

Remember that these items are high in saturated fat, cholesterol, and calories and may raise blood cholesterol levels if eaten on a regular basis.
- One high-fat meat exchange is equal to any one of the following items:

Pork: Spareribs, ground pork, pork sausage	1 oz
Cheese: All regular cheeses, such as American 🧂, cheddar, Monterey Jack, Swiss	1 oz

Other:	
Processed sandwich meats with 8 g of fat or less per ounce, such as bologna, pimento loaf, salami	1 oz
Sausage, such as bratwurst, Italian, knockwurst, Polish, smoked	1 oz
Hot dog (turkey or chicken) 🧂	1 (10/lb)
Bacon	3 slices (20 slices/lb)
Peanut butter (contains unsaturated fat)	1 tbsp
• Count the following items as 1 high-fat plus 1 fat exchange:	
Hot dog (beef, pork, or combination) 🧂	1 (10/lb)

🧂 = 400 mg or more sodium per exchange.

FAT LIST

Fats are divided into three groups, based on the main type of fat they contain: monounsaturated, polyunsaturated, and saturated. Monounsaturated and polyunsaturated fats in the foods we eat are linked with good health benefits. Saturated fats and fats called *trans* fatty acids (or *trans* unsaturated fatty acids) are linked with heart disease. In general, one fat exchange is as follows:

- 1 tsp of regular margarine or vegetable oil
- 1 tbsp of regular salad dressing

Nutrition Tips

1. All fats are high in calories. Limit serving sizes for good nutrition and health.

2. Nuts and seeds contain small amounts of fiber, protein, and magnesium.

3. If blood pressure is a concern, choose fats in the unsalted form to help lower sodium intake, such as unsalted peanuts.

Selection Tips

1. Check the Nutrition Facts on food labels for serving sizes. One fat exchange is based on a serving size containing 5 g of fat.

2. The Nutrition Facts on food labels usually list total fat grams and saturated fat grams per serving. When most of the calories come from saturated fat, the food fits into the Saturated Fats list.

3. Occasionally the Nutrition Facts on food labels will list monounsaturated and/or polyunsaturated fats in addition to total and saturated fats. If more than half

---

the total fat is monounsaturated, the food fits into the Monounsaturated Fats list; if more than half is polyunsaturated, the food fits into the Polyunsaturated Fats list.

4. When selecting fats to use with your meal plan, consider replacing saturated fats with monounsaturated fats.

5. When selecting regular margarine, choose those with liquid vegetable oil as the first ingredient. Soft margarines are not as saturated as stick margarines and are healthier choices.

6. Avoid foods on the Fat list (such as margarines) listing hydrogenated or partially hydrogenated fat as the first ingredient because these foods will contain higher amounts of *trans* fatty acids.

7. When selecting reduced-fat or lower-fat margarines, look for liquid vegetable oil as the second ingredient. Water is usually the first ingredient.

8. When used in smaller amounts, bacon and peanut butter are counted as fat choices. When used in larger amounts, they are counted as high-fat meat choices.

9. Fat-free salad dressings are on the Sweets, Desserts, and Other Carbohydrates list and the Free Foods list.

10. See the Free Foods list for nondairy coffee creamers, whipped topping, and fat-free products, such as margarines, salad dressings, mayonnaise, sour cream, cream cheese, and nonstick cooking spray.

One fat exchange equals 5 g of fat and 45 calories.

Monounsaturated Fats List

Avocado, medium	2 tbsp (1 oz)
Oil (canola, olive, peanut)	1 tsp
Olives:	
Ripe (black)	8 large
Green, stuffed	10 large

Nuts:

Almonds, cashews	6 nuts
Mixed (50% peanuts)	6 nuts
Peanuts	10 nuts
Pecans	4 halves
Peanut butter, smooth or crunchy	½ tbsp
Sesame seeds	1 tbsp
Tahini or sesame paste	2 tsp

= 400 mg or more sodium per exchange.

Polyunsaturated Fats List

Margarine:

Stick, tub, or squeeze	1 tsp
Lower-fat spread (30%-50% vegetable oil)	1 tbsp
Mayonnaise:	
Regular	1 tsp
Reduced-fat	1 tbsp
Nuts: walnuts, English	4 halves
Oil (corn, safflower, soybean)	1 tsp

Salad dressing:

Regular	1 tbsp
Reduced-fat	2 tbsp
Miracle Whip salad dressing:	
Regular	2 tsp
Reduced-fat	1 tbsp
Seeds: pumpkin, sunflower	1 tbsp

= 400 mg or more sodium per exchange.

Saturated Fats List

		Cream cheese:	
Bacon, cooked	1 slice (20 slices/lb)	Regular	1 tbsp (½ oz)
Bacon, grease	1 tsp	Reduced-fat	1½ tbsp (¾ oz)
Butter:		Fatback or salt pork	See below*
Stick	1 tsp		
Whipped	2 tsp	Shortening or lard	1 tsp
Reduced-fat	1 tbsp	*Sour cream:*	
Chitterlings, boiled	2 tbsp (½ oz)	Regular	2 tbsp
Coconut, sweetened, shredded	2 tbsp	Reduced-fat	3 tbsp
Coconut milk	1 tbsp		
Cream, half and half	2 tbsp		

*Use a piece 1 inch × 1 inch × ¼ inch if you plan to eat the fatback cooked with vegetables. Use a piece 2 inch × 1 inch × ½ inch when eating only the vegetables with the fatback removed.

= 400 mg or more sodium per exchange.

FREE FOODS LIST

A *free food* is any food or drink that contains less than 20 calories or less than or equal to 5 g of carbohydrate per serving. Foods with a serving size listed should be limited to 3 servings per day. Be sure to spread them out throughout the day. If you eat all 3 servings at one time, it could raise your blood glucose level. Foods listed without a serving size can be eaten whenever you like.

Fat-Free or Reduced-Fat Foods

Cream cheese, fat-free	1 tbsp (½ oz)	Sour cream, fat-free, reduced-fat	1 tbsp
Creamers, nondairy, liquid	1 tbsp	Whipped topping, regular	1 tbsp
Creamers, nondairy, powdered	2 tsp	Whipped topping, light or fat-free	2 tbsp
Mayonnaise, fat-free	1 tbsp	**Sugar-Free Foods**	
Mayonnaise, reduced-fat	1 tsp	Candy, hard, sugar-free	1 candy
Margarine spread, fat-free	4 tbsp	Gelatin dessert, sugar-free	
Margarine spread, reduced-fat	1 tsp	Gelatin, unflavored	
Miracle Whip, fat-free	1 tbsp	Gum, sugar-free	
Miracle Whip, reduced-fat	1 tsp	Jam or jelly, light	2 tsp
Nonstick cooking spray		Sugar substitutes*	
Salad dressing, fat-free or low-fat	1 tbsp	Syrup, sugar-free	
Salad dressing, fat-free, Italian	2 tbsp		

*Sugar substitutes, alternatives, or replacements that are approved by the Food and Drug Administration (FDA) are safe to use. Common brand names include the following:
Equal (aspartame)
Splenda (sucralose)
Sprinkle Sweet (saccharin)
Sweet One (acesulfame K)
Sweet-10 (saccharin)
Sugar Twin (saccharin)
Sweet 'N Low (saccharin)

Drinks

Bouillon, broth, consommé 🧂

Bouillon or broth, low-sodium

Carbonated or mineral water

Club soda

Cocoa powder, unsweetened	1 tbsp
Coffee	
Diet soft drinks, sugar-free	
Drink mixes, sugar-free	
Tea	
Tonic water, sugar-free	

🧂 = 400 mg or more sodium per exchange.

Condiments

Catsup	1 tbsp	Pickles, sweet (bread and butter)	2 slices
Horseradish		Pickles, sweet (gherkin)	¾ oz
Lemon juice		Salsa	¼ cup
Lime juice		Soy sauce, regular or light 🧂	1 tbsp
Mustard		Taco sauce	1 tbsp
Pickle relish	1 tbsp	Vinegar	
Pickles, dill 🧂	1½ medium	Yogurt	2 tbsp

🧂 = 400 mg or more sodium per exchange.

Seasonings*

Flavoring extracts	Spices
Garlic	Tabasco or hot pepper sauce
Herbs, fresh or dried	Wine, used in cooking
Pimento	Worcestershire sauce

*Be careful with seasonings that contain sodium or are salts, such as garlic or celery salt, and lemon pepper.

COMBINATION FOODS LIST

Many of the foods we eat are mixed together in various combinations. These combination foods do not fit into any one exchange list. Often it is hard to tell what is in a casserole dish or prepared food item. This is a list of exchanges for some typical combination foods. This list will help you fit these foods into your meal plan. Ask your dietitian for information about any other combination foods you would like to eat.

Food	Serving Size	Exchanges per Serving
Entrees		
Tuna noodle casserole, lasagna, spaghetti with meatballs, chili with beans, macaroni and cheese 🧂	1 cup (8 oz)	2 carbohydrates 2 medium-fat meats
Chow mein (without noodles or rice) 🧂	2 cups (16 oz)	1 carbohydrate 2 lean meats
Tuna or chicken salad	½ cup (3½ oz)	½ carbohydrate 2 lean meats 1 fat
Frozen Entrees and Meals		
Dinner-type meal 🧂	Generally 14-17 oz	3 carbohydrates 3 medium-fat meats 3 fats
Meatless burger, soy-based	3 oz	½ carbohydrate 2 lean meats
Meatless burger, vegetable- and starch-based	3 oz	1 carbohydrate 1 lean meat
Pizza, cheese, thin crust 🧂	¼ of 12-inch (6 oz)	2 carbohydrates 2 medium-fat meats 1 fat
Pizza, meat topping, thin crust 🧂	¼ of 12-inch (6 oz)	2 carbohydrates 2 medium-fat meats 2 fats
Pot pie 🧂	1 (7 oz)	2½ carbohydrates 1 medium-fat meat 3 fats
Entrée or meal with less than 340 calories 🧂	About 8-11 oz	2-3 carbohydrates 1-2 lean meats
Soups		
Bean 🧂	1 cup	1 carbohydrate 1 very lean meat
Cream (made with water) 🧂	1 cup (8 oz)	1 carbohydrate 1 fat
Instant 🧂	6 oz prepared	1 carbohydrate
Instant with beans/lentils 🧂	8 oz prepared	2½ carbohydrates 1 very lean meat
Split pea (made with water) 🧂	½ cup (4 oz)	1 carbohydrate
Tomato (made with water) 🧂	1 cup (8 oz)	1 carbohydrate
Vegetable beef, chicken noodle, or other broth type 🧂	1 cup (8 oz)	1 carbohydrate

🧂 = 400 mg or more sodium per exchange.

FAST FOODS* LIST

Food	Serving Size	Exchanges per Serving
Burrito with beef 🧂	1 (5 7 oz)	3 carbohydrates 1 medium-fat meat 1 fat
Chicken nuggets 🧂	6	1 carbohydrate 2 medium-fat meats 1 fat
Chicken breast and wing, breaded and fried 🧂	1 each	1 carbohydrate 4 medium-fat meats 2 fats
Chicken sandwich, grilled 🧂	1	2 carbohydrates 3 very lean meats
Chicken wings, hot 🧂	6 (5 oz)	1 carbohydrate 3 medium-fat meats 4 fats
Fish sandwich/tartar sauce 🧂	1	3 carbohydrates 1 medium-fat meat 3 fats
French fries 🧂	1 medium serving (5 oz)	4 carbohydrates 4 fats
Hamburger, regular	1	2 carbohydrates 2 medium-fat meats
Hamburger, large 🧂	1	2 carbohydrates 3 medium-fat meats 1 fat
Hot dog with bun 🧂	1	1 carbohydrate 1 high-fat meat 1 fat
Individual pan pizza 🧂	1	5 carbohydrates 3 medium-fat meats 3 fats
Pizza, cheese, thin crust 🧂	¼ 12-inch (about 6 oz)	2½ carbohydrates 2 medium-fat meats
Pizza, meat, thin crust 🧂	¼ 12-inch (about 6 oz)	2½ carbohydrates 2 medium-feat meats 1 fat
Soft-serve cone	1 small (5 oz)	2½ carbohydrates 1 fat

*Ask at your fast-food restaurant for nutrition information about your favorite fast foods or check websites.

🧂 = 400 mg or more sodium per exchange.

Food	Serving Size	Exchanges per Serving
Submarine sandwich	1 sub (6-inch)	3 carbohydrates 1 vegetable 2 medium-fat meats 1 fat
Submarine sandwich (less than 6 g fat)	1 sub (6-inch)	2½ carbohydrates 2 lean meats
Taco, hard or soft shell	1 (3-3½ oz)	1 carbohydrate 1 medium-fat meat 1 fat

Food Sources of Oxalates

FRUITS

Berries, all
Concord grapes
Currants
Figs
Fruit cocktail
Plums
Rhubarb
Tangerines

VEGETABLES

Baked beans
Beans, green and wax
Beet greens
Beets
Celery
Chard, Swiss
Chives
Collards
Eggplant
Endive
Kale
Leeks
Mustard greens
Okra
Peppers, green
Rutabagas
Spinach
Squash, summer
Sweet potatoes
Tomatoes
Tomato soup
Vegetable soup

NUTS

Almonds
Cashews
Peanut butter
Peanuts

BEVERAGES

Chocolate
Cocoa
Draft beer
Tea

OTHER

Grits
Soy products
Tofu
Wheat germ

Acid and Alkaline Ash Food Groups

ACID ASH

Meat
Whole grains
Eggs
Cheese
Cranberries
Prunes
Plums

ALKALINE ASH

Milk
Vegetables
Fruits (except cranberries, prunes, and plums)

NEUTRAL

Beverages (coffee, tea)

Tyramine-Restricted Diet

GENERAL DIRECTIONS

- Designed for patients on monoamine oxidase inhibitors, drugs that have been reported to cause hypertensive crises when used with tyramine-rich foods. These include foods in which aging, protein breakdown, and putrefaction are used to increase flavor. Studies indicate that as little as 5 to 6 mg of tyramine may produce a response, and 25 mg is a dangerous dose.
- Food sources of other pressor amines such as histamine, dihydroxyphenylalanine, and hydroxytyramine are also avoided.
- Avoid all foods listed. Limited amounts of foods with a lower amount of tyramine, such as yeast bread, may be included in a specific diet.
- Avoid over-the-counter drugs such as decongestants, cold remedies, and antihistamines.

Foods to Avoid	Representative Tyramine Values (μg/g or ml)
Cheeses	
New York State cheddar	1416
Gruyère	516
Stilton	466
Emmentaler	225
Brie	180
Camembert	86
Processed American	50
Wines	
Chianti	25.4
Sherry	3.6
Riesling	0.6
Sauternes	0.4
Beer, ale (varies with brand)	
Highest	4.4
Average	2.3
Least	1.8

ADDITIONAL FOODS TO AVOID

Other aged cheeses
   Blue
   Boursalt
   Brick
   Cheddars (other)
   Gouda
   Mozzarella
   Parmesan
   Provolone
   Romano
   Roquefort
Yeast and products made with yeast
   Homemade bread
   Yeast extracts such as soup cubes, canned meats, and marmite

Italian broad beans with pod (fava beans)
Meat
   Aged game
   Liver
Canned meats with yeast extracts
Fish (salted dried)
   Herring, cod, capelin
   Pickled herring
Other
   Chocolate
   Cream (especially sour cream)
   Salad dressings
   Soy sauce
   Vanilla
   Yogurt

Calculation Aids and Conversion Tables

In 1799 a group of French scientists set up the metric system of weights and measures. Today, with refinements over years of use, it is called the "Système International" (SI). In 1975 the United States Congress passed the Metric Conversion Act, which provides for conversion of our customary British/American system to the simpler metric system used by the rest of the world. We are now in the midst of this conversion, as evidenced by distance signs along highways and labels on many packaged foods in supermarkets. Here are a few conversion factors to help you make these transitions in your necessary calculations.

METRIC SYSTEM OF MEASUREMENT

Like our money system, this is a simple decimal system based on units of 10. It is uniform and used internationally.

Weight Units

1 kilogram (kg) = 1000 grams (gm or g)

1 g = 1000 milligrams (mg)

1 mg = 1000 micrograms (mcg or μg)

Length Units

1 meter (m) = 100 centimeters (cm)

1000 m = 1 kilometer (km)

Volume Units

1 liter (L) = 1000 milliliters (ml)

1 ml = 1 cubic centimeter (cc)

Temperature Units

Celsius (C) scale, based on 100 equal units between 0° C (freezing point of water) and 100° C (boiling point of water); this scale is used entirely in all scientific work.

Energy Units

Kilocalorie (kcal) = Amount of energy required to raise 1 kg water 1° C

Kilojoule (kJ) = Amount of energy required to move 1 kg mass 1 m by a force of 1 newton

1 kcal = 4.184 kJ

BRITISH/AMERICAN SYSTEM OF MEASUREMENT

Our customary system is a confusion of units with no uniform relationships. It is not a decimal system, but rather a collection of different units collected in usage and language over time. It is predominately used in America.

Weight Units

1 pound (lb) = 16 ounces (oz)

Length Units

1 foot (ft) = 12 inches (in)

1 yard (yd) = 3 feet (ft)

Volume Units

3 teaspoons (tsp) = 1 tablespoon (tbsp)

16 tbsp = 1 cup

1 cup = 8 fluid ounces (fl oz)

4 cups = 1 quart (qt)

5 cups = 1 imperial quart (qt), Canada

Temperature Units

Fahrenheit (F) scale, based on 180 equal units between 32° F (freezing point of water) and 212° F (boiling point of water) at standard atmospheric pressure

CONVERSIONS BETWEEN MEASUREMENT SYSTEMS

Weight

1 oz = 28.35 g

2.2 lb = 1 kg

Length

1 in = 2.54 cm

1 ft = 30.48 cm

39.37 in = 1 m

Volume

1.06 qt = 1 L

0.85 imperial qt = 1 L (Canada)

Temperature

Boiling point of water: 100° C; 212° F

Body temperature: 37° C; 98.6° F

Freezing point of water: 0° C; 32° F

Interconversion Formulas

Fahrenheit temperature (°F) = $\frac{9}{5}$ (°C) + 32

Celsius temperature (°C) = $\frac{5}{9}$ (°F) − 32

Approximate Metric Conversions

When You Know	Multiply by	to Find
Weight		
Ounces	28	Grams
Pounds	0.45	Kilograms
Length		
Inches	2.5	Centimeters
Feet	30	Centimeters
Yards	0.9	Meters
Miles	1.6	Kilometers
Volume		
Teaspoons	5	Milliliters
Tablespoons	15	Milliliters
Fluid ounces	30	Milliliters
Cups	0.24	Liters
Pints	0.47	Liters
Quarts	0.95	Liters

Cultural Dietary Patterns and Religious Dietary Practices

Only foods that are specifically associated with these cultural groups are noted. Individuals may also consume typical American foods, as dietary adaptations are common. Assumptions of dietary patterns cannot be made, but knowledge of these unique foods provides a common understanding of the range of possible food choices.

Cultural Dietary Patterns

Culture	Bread, Cereal, Rice, and Pasta Group	Vegetable Group	Fruit Group	Milk, Yogurt, Cheese Group	Meat, Poultry, Fish, Dry Beans, Eggs, and Nuts Groups	Fats, Oils, and Sweets
Native American	Blue corn flour (ground dried blue corn kernels) used to make corn bread, mush dumplings; fruit dumplings (walakshi); fry bread (biscuit dough deep fried); ground sweet acorn; hominy; tortillas; wheat and rye products; wild rice	Artichokes, cacti, chili, mushrooms, nettles, onions, potatoes, pumpkin, squash, sweet potatoes, tomatoes, wild greens, turnips, and yucca	Dried wild berries, cherries and grapes; berries, elderberries, persimmons, plums, and rhubarb	None in traditional diet	Bear, buffalo, deer, elk, moose, rabbit, and squirrel Duck, goose, quail, and wild turkey A variety of fish, legumes, nuts, and seeds	Tallow and lard Maple sugar and pine sugar
Northern European	Barley, hops, oat, rice, rye, and wheat products	Artichokes, asparagus, beets, brussels sprouts, cabbage, carrots, cauliflower, celery, cucumbers, eggplant, fennel, green peppers, kale, leeks, mushrooms, olives, onions, peas, potatoes, radishes, spinach, turnips, and watercress	Apples, apricots, cherries, currants, gooseberries, grapes, lemons, melons, oranges, peaches, pears, plums, prunes, raspberries, rhubarb, and strawberries	Cheese (made from cow, sheep, and goat milk), cream, milk, sour cream, and yogurt	Beef, lamb, oxtail, pork, rabbit, veal, and venison Chicken, duck, goose, pheasant, pigeon, quail, and turkey A wide variety of fish, legumes, and nuts	Butter, lard, margarine, olive oil, vegetable oil, and salt pork Honey and sugar
Southern European	Cornmeal, rice, and wheat products	Arugula, artichokes, asparagus, broccoli, cabbage, cardoon, cauliflower, celery, chicory, cucumber, eggplant, endive, escarole, fennel, kale, kohlrabi, mushrooms, mustard greens, olives, pimentos, potatoes, radicchio, Swiss chard, turnips, and zucchini	Apples, apricots, bananas, cherries, citron, dates, figs, grapefruit, grapes, lemons, medlars, peaches, pears, pineapples, prunes, pomegranates, quinces, oranges, raisins, and tangerines	Cheese (made from cow, sheep, buffalo, and goat milk), and milk	Beef, goat, lamb, pork, and veal Chicken, duck, goose, pigeon, turkey, and woodcock A variety of fish, shellfish, legumes, and nuts	Butter, lard, olive oil, and vegetable oil Honey and sugar

Compiled by Staci Nix for *Williams' basic nutrition & diet therapy*, ed 12, St. Louis, 2005, Mosby. Data from Kittler PG, Sucher KP: *Food and culture*, ed 4, Belmont, Calif, 2004, Brooks/Cole, a division of Thomson Learning; and Grodner M, Long S, DeYoung S: *Foundations and clinical applications of nutrition: a nursing approach*, ed 3, St Louis, 2004, Mosby.

Continued

Cultural Dietary Patterns—cont'd

Culture	Bread, Cereal, Rice, and Pasta Group	Vegetable Group	Fruit Group	Milk, Yogurt, Cheese Group	Meat, Poultry, Fish, Dry Beans, Eggs, and Nuts Groups	Fats, Oils, and Sweets
Central European and Russian	Barley, buckwheat, corn, millet, oats, potato starch, rice, rye, and wheat products	Asparagus, beets, brussels sprouts, cabbage, carrots, cauliflower, celery, chard, cucumbers, eggplant, endive, kohlrabi, leeks, mushrooms, olives, onions, parsnips, peppers, potatoes, radishes, sorrel, spinach, and turnips	Apples, apricots, a variety of berries, currants, dates, grapes, grapefruit, lemons, melons, oranges, peaches, pears, plums, prunes, quinces, raisins, rhubarb, and strawberries	Buttermilk, cheese, cream, milk, sour cream, and yogurt	Beef, boar, hare, lamb, pork, sausage, veal, and venison Chicken, Cornish hen, duck, goose, grouse, partridge, pheasant, quail, squab, and turkey A variety of fish, shellfish, legumes, and nuts	Butter, bacon, chicken fat, flaxseed oil, lard, olive oil, salt pork, and vegetable oil Honey, sugar, and molasses
African American (Southern United States)	Biscuits; corn bread as spoon bread, cornpone, hush puppies, or grits; and rice	Broccoli, cabbage, corn; leafy greens including dandelion greens, kale, mustard greens, collard greens, and turnips. Okra, pumpkin, potatoes, spinach, squash, sweet potatoes, tomatoes, and yams	Apple, banana, berries, fruit juices, peaches, and watermelon	Buttermilk and some cheese	Beef; pork and pork products including scrapple (cornmeal and pork), chitterlings (pork intestines), bacon, pig feet and ears Fried meats and poultry, organ meats (kidney, liver, tongue, and tripe) Fish (catfish, crawfish, salmon, shrimp, and tuna) Frogs, rabbit, squirrel A variety of legumes and nuts	Butter and lard Honey, molasses, and sugar
Mexican	Corn (tortillas, masa harina), wheat, and rice products; sweet bread	Cactus (nopales), calabaza criolla, chili peppers, corn, jicama, onions, peas, plantains, squashes (chayote, pumpkin, etc.) tomatillos, tomatoes, yams, and yucca root (cassava or manioc)	Avocadoes, bananas, cactus fruit, carambola, casimiroa, cherimoya, coconut, granadilla, guanabana, guava, lemons, limes, mamey, mangoes, melon, oranges, papaya, pineapple, strawberries, sugar cane, and zapote	Cheese, flan, sour cream, and milk	Beef, goat, and pork Chicken and turkey Firm-fleshed fish, shrimp, and a variety of legumes	Bacon fat, lard (manteca), salt pork, and dairy cream Sugar and panocha (raw brown cane sugar)
Central American	Corn (tamales, tortillas), rice, and wheat products	Asparagus, beets, cabbage, calabaza, chayote, chili peppers, corn, cucumbers, eggplant,	Apples, avocadoes, bananas, breadfruit, cherimoya, coconut, grapes,	Cheese, cream, and milk	Beef, iguana, lizards, pork, and venison Chicken, duck, and turkey	Butter, lard, vegetable oils, and shortening

	Breads/Cereals	Vegetables	Fruits	Milk Products	Meat/Protein	Fats/Sugars
		hearts of palm, leeks, loroco flowers, onions, pacaya buds, plantains, pumpkin, spinach, sweet peppers, tamatillos, watercress, yams, yucca, and yucca flowers	guava, mameys, mangoes, nances, oranges, papaya, passion fruit, pejibaye, pineapples, prunes, raisins, tamarind, tangerines, and zapote		A variety of fish, shellfish, and legumes	Honey, sugar, and sugar syrup
Caribbean Islands	Cassava bread; cornmeal (surrulitos); oatmeal; rice, and wheat products	Arracacha, arrowroot, black-eyed peas, cabbage, calabaza, callaloo, cassava, chilis, corn, cucumbers, eggplant, malangas, okra, onions, palm hearts, peppers, radishes, spinach, squashes, sweet potatoes, taro, and yams	Acerola cherries, akee, avocadoes, bananas, breadfruit, caimito, cherimoya, citron, coconuts, cocoplum, gooseberries, granadilla, grapefruit, guava, guanabana, jackfruit, kumquats, lemons, limes, mamey, mangoes, oranges, papayas, pineapples, plantains, pomegranates, raisins, sapodilla, sugar cane, and tamarind	Cheese and milk	Beef, goat, and pork; Chicken, turkey, and a variety of fish, shellfish, and legumes	Butter, coconut oil, lard, and olive oil; Sugar cane products
Cuban and Puerto Rican	Rice; starchy green bananas, usually fried (plantain)	Beets, breadfruit, chayote, chili peppers, eggplant, onion, tubers (yucca), white yams (boniato)	Coconuts, guava, mango, oranges (sweet and sour), prune and mango paste	Flan, hard cheese (queso de mano)	Chicken, fish, (all kinds and preparations including smoked, salted, canned, and fresh), shellfish, legumes (all kinds especially black beans), pork (fried), sausage (chorizo), calf brain, beef tongue	Olive and peanut oil, lard; Coconut
South American	Amaranth (corn, rice, quinoa) and wheat products	Ahipa, arracacha, calabaza, cassava, green peppers, hearts of palm, kale, okra, oca, onions, rosella, squash, sweet potatoes, yacon, and yams	Avocado, abiu, acerola, apples, banana, caimito, casimiroa, cherimoya, feijoa, guava, grapes, jackfruit, jabiticaba, lemons, limes, lulo, marmea, mango, melon, olives, oranges, palm fruits, papaya, passion fruit, peaches, pineapple, pitanga, quince, sapote, and strawberries	Cheese and milk	Beef, frog, goat, guinea pig, llama, mutton, pork, and rabbit; Chicken, duck, turkey and a variety of fish, shellfish, and nuts	Palm oil, olive oil, and butter; Sugar cane, brown sugar, and honey

Continued

Cultural Dietary Patterns—cont'd

Culture	Bread, Cereal, Rice, and Pasta Group	Vegetable Group	Fruit Group	Milk, Yogurt, Cheese Group	Meat, Poultry, Fish, Dry Beans, Eggs, and Nuts Groups	Fats, Oils, and Sweets
Chinese	Rice and related products (flour, cakes, and noodles); noodles made from barley, corn, and millet; wheat and related products (breads, noodles, spaghetti, stuffed noodles [won ton] and filled buns [bowl])	Bamboo shoots, cabbage (napa), celery, Chinese turnips (lo bok), dried day lilies, dry fungus (Black Juda's ear); leafy green vegetables including kale, cress, mustard greens (gai choy), chard (bok choy), amaranth greens (yin choy), wolfberry leaves (gou gay), and Chinese broccoli (gai lan); eggplant, lotus tubers, okra, snow peas, stir-fried vegetables (chow yuk), taro roots, white radish (daikon), yams, and yam beans	Apples, bananas, custard apples, coconuts, dates, longan, figs, grapes, kumquats, lime, litchi, mango, muskmelon, oranges, papaya, passion fruit, peaches, persimmons, pineapples, plums, pomegranates, pomelos, tangerines, and watermelon	Milk (cow's, buffalo, and soymilk)	Beef, lamb, and pork Chicken, duck, quail, squab, a large variety of fish and shellfish, in addition to legumes and nuts	Lard; peanut, soy, sesame, and rice oil Honey, rice or barley malt, palm sugar, sorghum sugar, and dehydrated cane juice
Japanese	Rice and rice products, rice flour (mochiko), noodles (comen/soba), buckwheat and millet	Artichoke, asparagus, bamboo shoots (takenoko), burdock (gobo), cabbage (napa), eggplant, horseradish (wasabi), mizuna, mushrooms (shiitake, matsutake, nameko), Japanese parsley (seri), lotus root (renkon), pickled cabbage (kimchee), pickled vegetables, seaweed (laver, nori, wakame, kombu), snow peas, spinach, sweet potato, vegetable soup (mizutaki), watercress, white radish (daikon)	Pear-like apple (nasi), apricots, bananas, cherries, figs, grapefruit (yuzu), kumquats, lemons, limes, persimmons, plums, pineapples, strawberry, and tangerine (mikan)	Milk, butter, and ice cream	Beef, deer, lamb, pork, rabbit, and veal Fish and shellfish including dried fish with bones, raw fish (sashimi), and fish cake (kamaboko) A variety of poultry (chicken, duck, goose, turkey) and legumes (black beans, red beans, soybeans—as tofu, fermented soybean and sprouts)	Lard; soy, sesame, rapeseed, and rice oil Honey and sugar

	Grains/Breads	Vegetables	Fruits	Dairy	Meats/Protein	Fats/Sweets
Korean	Barley, buckwheat, millet, rice, and wheat products	Bamboo shoots, bean sprouts, beets, cabbage, chives, chrysanthemum leaves, cucumber, eggplant, fern, green onion, green pepper, leeks, lotus root, mushrooms, onion, perilla, seaweed, spinach, sweet potato, turnips, water chestnut, watercress, and white radish	Apples, Asian pears, cherries, dates, grapes, melons, oranges, pears, persimmons, plums, and tangerines	Very little, if any, consumption	Beef, oxtail, pork, chicken, pheasant, and a variety of fish, shellfish, legumes, and nuts	Sesame oil and vegetable oil Honey and sugar
Filipino	Noodles, rice, rice flour (mochiko), stuffed noodles (won ton), white bread (pan de sal)	Amaranth, bamboo shoots, beets, burdock root, cassava, Chinese celery, dark green leafy vegetables (malunggay and salvyot), eggplant, garlic, green peppers, hearts of palm, hyacinth bean, kamis, leek, mushrooms, okra, onion, sweet potatoes (camotes), turnips, and root crop (gabi)	Apples, avocado, banana, bitter melon (ampalaya), breadfruit, coconut guavas, jackfruit, limes, mangoes, papaya, pod fruit (tamarind), pomelos, rambutan, rhubarb, star fruit, tangelo (naranghita), and watermelon	White cheese, evaporated cow or goat milk and soymilk	Beef, carabao, goat, pork, monkey, organ meats, and rabbit Fish, dried fish (dilis), egg roll (lumpia), fish sauce (alamang and bagoong) Legumes such as mung beans, bean sprouts, and chickpeas; soybean curd (tofu)	Coconut oil, lard, and vegetable oil Brown and white sugar, coconut, and honey
Pacific Islanders	Rice and wheat products	Arrowroot, bitter melon, burdock root, cabbage, carrot, cassava, daikon, eggplant, ferns, green pepper, horseradish, jute, kohlrabi, leeks, lotus root, mustard greens, green onions, seaweed, spinach, squashes, sweet potato, taro, water chestnuts, and yams	Acerola cherries, apples, apricot, avocado, banana, breadfruit, coconut, guava, jackfruit, kumquat, litchis, loquat, mango, melons, papaya, passion fruit, peach, pear, pineapple, plum, prune, strawberries, and tamarind	Very little, if any, consumption	Beef, pork, chicken, duck, squab, and turkey A variety of fish, shellfish, and legumes	Butter, coconut oil, lard, sesame oil, and vegetable oil Sugar

Continued

Cultural Dietary Patterns—cont'd

Culture	Bread, Cereal, Rice, and Pasta Group	Vegetable Group	Fruit Group	Milk, Yogurt, Cheese Group	Meat, Poultry, Fish, Dry Beans, Eggs, and Nuts Groups	Fats, Oils, and Sweets
South Asian	Rice, wheat, buckwheat, corn, millet, and sorghum products	Agathi flowers, amaranth, artichokes, bamboo shoots, beets, bitter melon, brussels sprouts, cabbage, collard greens, cucumbers, drumstick plant, eggplant, lotus root, manioc, mushrooms, okra, pandanus, plantain flowers, sago palm, spinach, squash, turnips, water chestnuts, water convulus, water lilies, and yams	Apples, apricots, avocados, bananas, coconut, dates, figs, grapes, guava, jackfruit, limes, litchis, loquats, mangoes, melon, nongus, oranges, papaya, peaches, pears, persimmons, pineapple, plums, pomegranate, pomelos, star fruit, sugar cane, tangerines, and watermelon	Milk (evaporated and fermented products), cheese, and milk-based desserts	Beef, goat, mutton, pork, chicken, duck, and a variety of fish, seafood, legumes, and nuts	Coconut oil, ghee, mustard oil, peanut oil, sesame seed oil, and sunflower oil
						Sugar cane, jaggery, and molasses
Jewish (both cultural and religious customs)	Bagel, buckwheat groats (kasha), dumplings made with matzoh meal (matzoh balls or knaidelach), egg bread (challah), noodle or potato pudding (kugel), crepe filled with farmer cheese and/or fruit (blintz), unleavened bread or large cracker made with wheat flour and water (matzoh)	Potato pancakes (latkes); vegetable stew made with sweet potatoes, carrots, prunes, and sometimes brisket (tzimmes); beet soup (borscht)			A mixture of fish formed into balls and poached (gefilte fish); smoked salmon (lox)	Chicken fat

Religious Dietary Practices

	Seventh-Day Adventist	Buddhist	Eastern Orthodox	Hindu	Jewish	Mormon	Moslem	Roman Catholic
Beef		Avoided by most devout		Prohibited or strongly discouraged				
Pork	Prohibited or strongly discouraged	Avoided by most devout		Avoided by most devout	Prohibited or strongly discouraged		Prohibited or strongly discouraged	
All meat	Avoided by most devout	Avoided by most devout	Permitted but some restrictions apply	Avoided by most devout	Permitted but some restrictions apply		Permitted but some restrictions apply	Permitted but some restrictions apply
Eggs/dairy	Permitted but avoided at some observances	Permitted but avoided at some observances	Permitted but some restrictions apply	Permitted but avoided at some observances	Permitted but some restrictions apply			
Fish	Avoided by most devout	Avoided by most devout	Permitted but some restrictions apply	Permitted but some restrictions apply	Permitted but some restrictions apply			
Shellfish	Prohibited or strongly discouraged	Avoided by most devout	Permitted but avoided at some observances	Permitted but some restrictions apply	Prohibited or strongly discouraged			
Meat and dairy at same meal					Prohibited or strongly discouraged			
Leavened foods					Permitted but some restrictions apply			
Ritual slaughter of animals					Practiced		Practiced	
Alcohol	Prohibited or strongly discouraged			Avoided by most devout		Prohibited or strongly discouraged	Prohibited or strongly discouraged	
Caffeine	Prohibited or strongly discouraged						Prohibited or strongly discouraged	Avoided by most devout

Compiled by Staci Nix for *Williams' basic nutrition & diet therapy*, ed 12, St. Louis, 2005, Mosby. Modified from Kittler PG, Sucher KP: *Food and culture*, ed 4, Belmont Calif, 2004, Brooks/Cole, a division of Thomson Learning (www.thomsonrights.com).

absorption Transport of nutrients from the lumen of the intestine across the intestinal wall into the blood (carbohydrates and proteins) or the lymph (fats).

Acceptable Macronutrient Distribution Range (AMDR) The suggested distribution of kcalories across the macronutrients; carbohydrate should provide 45% to 65% of total kcalories, fat should provide 20% to 35% of total kcalories, and protein should provide 10% to 35% of total kcalories.

acculturation The process by which newcomers to a country or region begin to adopt the practices of their neighbors; this term is often used to refer to the adoption of new foods or food patterns by individuals moving to the United States.

achalasia Failure to relax the smooth muscle fibers of the gastrointestinal tract at any point of juncture of its parts; especially failure of the esophagogastric sphincter to relax when swallowing, as a result of degeneration of ganglion cells in the wall of the organ. The lower esophagus also loses its normal peristaltic activity. Also called cardiospasm.

actin Myofibril protein whose synchronized meshing action in conjunction with myosin causes muscles to contract and relax.

adenosine triphosphate (ATP) A high-energy phosphate compound important in energy exchange within the cell. ATP is formed from the nucleotide adenosine with three attached phosphoric acid groups. The splitting off of the terminal phosphate bond (PO_4) to produce adenosine diphosphate (ADP) releases bound energy that is transformed to free energy and available for body work. ATP is then reformed as an energy store for use when needed.

Adequate Intake (AI) The suggested daily intake of a nutrient to meet daily needs and support health; the AI is used when there is not a sufficient amount of research available to develop an RDA; the AI also serves as a guide for intake.

adipocyte A fat cell. All cell names end in the suffix *-cyte,* with the type of cell indicated by the root word to which it is added.

adipose Fat present in fat cells or fatty (adipose) tissue.

admixture A mixture of ingredients that each retain their own physical properties; a combination of two or more substances that are not chemically united or that exist in no fixed proportion to each other.

advance directives Instructions for medical treatment given by a patient while he or she has decisional capacity to do so.

aerobic capacity Milliliters of oxygen consumed per kilogram of body weight per minute; influenced by body composition and fitness level.

aldosterone Potent hormone of the cortex of the adrenal glands, which acts on the distal renal tubule to cause reabsorption of sodium in an ion exchange with potassium. The aldosterone mechanism is essentially a sodium-conserving mechanism but indirectly also conserves water because water absorption follows the sodium reabsorption.

allergens Substances that can produce a hypersensitive reaction in the body; proteins present in milk, eggs, fish, wheat, tree nuts, peanuts, soybeans, and shellfish can result in serious and sometimes fatal reactions in allergic individuals, and the presence of any of these foods must be noted on the food label beginning in 2006.

alpha fetoprotein A fetal antigen in amniotic fluid that provides an early pregnancy test for fetal malformations such as neural tube defect.

alpha-linolenic acid An essential fatty acid for humans; an n-3 polyunsaturated fatty acid.

amenorrhea The absence of menses (menstrual cycle) entirely or no more than three periods in a year; associated with lower than normal estrogen levels in women.

amine An organic compound containing nitrogen. Amino acids and pyridoxine are examples of amines.

amino acid An acid containing the essential element nitrogen (in the amino group NH_2). Amino acids are the structural units of protein and the basic building blocks of body tissue.

aminopeptidase A protein-splitting enzyme that cuts the peptide bond at the amino end of the chain, producing smaller peptide chains and free amino acids.

amniotic fluid The watery fluid within the membrane enveloping the fetus, in which the fetus is suspended.

amphoteric Having opposite characteristics; capable of acting either as an acid or a base or combining with an acid or a base.

ampullae A general term for a flasklike wider portion of a tubular structure; spaces under the nipple of the breast for storing milk.

amyloid A glycoprotein substance having a relation to starchlike structure but more a protein compound; an abnormal complex material forming characteristic brain deposits of fibrillary tangles always found in postmortem examinations of patients with Alzheimer's disease, the only means of definitive diagnosis; found in various body tissues that, when advanced, form lesions that destroy functional cells and injure the organ.

amyotrophic lateral sclerosis (ALS) A progressive neuromuscular disease characterized by the degeneration of the neurons of the spinal cord and the motor cells of the brainstem, causing a deficit of upper and lower motor neurons; death usually occurs in 2 to 3 years.

anabolism Metabolic process for building body tissues.

anaphylactic shock A serious and sometimes fatal hypersensitivity reaction to a drug, food, toxin, chemical, or other allergen; the patient can experience weakness, sweating, and shortness of breath or such life-threatening responses as loss of blood pressure and shock, respiratory congestion, or cardiac arrest.

anastomosis   A surgical joining of two ducts to allow flow from one to the other.

anemia   Condition of abnormally low blood hemoglobin levels caused by too few red blood cells or red blood cells with an abnormally low hemoglobin content.

anorexia nervosa   Extreme psychophysiologic aversion to food resulting in life-threatening weight loss. A psychiatric eating disorder caused by a morbid fear of fat in which a distorted body image is reflected as fat when actually the body is malnourished and thin from self-starvation.

anthropometric   Measurement of the human body to determine height, weight, skinfold thickness, or other dimensions that provide estimates of the relative proportion of body fat and body muscle; such measurements can be used to evaluate health status and risk of chronic disease.

anthropometry   The science of measuring the size, weight, and proportions of the human body.

antidiuretic hormone (ADH)   Water-conserving hormone from posterior lobe of pituitary gland; causes resorption of water by kidney nephrons according to body need.

antimetabolite   A substance bearing a close structural resemblance to one required for normal physiologic functioning that interferes with the utilization of the essential metabolite.

antioxidant   A substance that prevents the formation of free radicals in the cells.

antrum   Lower section of the stomach.

apolipoprotein   A separate protein compound that attaches to its specific receptor site on a particular lipoprotein and activates certain functions, such as protein synthesis of a related enzyme. For example, apolipoprotein C-II is an apolipoprotein of HDL and VLDL that functions to activate the enzyme lipoprotein lipase.

areola   A defined space; a circular area of different color surrounding a central point, such as the darkened pigmented ring surrounding the nipple of the breast.

ariboflavinosis   Group of clinical manifestations of riboflavin deficiency.

arteriosclerosis   Blood vessel disease characterized by thickening and hardening of artery walls, with loss of functional elasticity, mainly affecting the intima (inner lining) of the arteries.

arthroplasty   Plastic surgery of nonfunctioning body joints to form movable joints with replacement metal or plastic materials.

atheroma   A mass of fatty plaque formed in inner arterial walls in atherosclerosis.

atherosclerosis   Common form of arteriosclerosis, characterized by the gradual formation—beginning in childhood in genetically predisposed individuals—of yellow cheeselike streaks of cholesterol and fatty material that develop into hardened plaques in the intima or inner lining of major blood vessels, such as coronary arteries, eventually in adulthood cutting off blood supply to the tissue served by the vessels; the underlying pathology of coronary heart disease.

autonomy   The state of functioning independently, without extraneous influence.

bariatric   Relating to the treatment and the control of obesity and diseases associated with obesity.

basal metabolic rate (BMR)   Amount of energy required to maintain the resting body's internal activities after an overnight fast with the subject awake. See also resting metabolic rate (RMR).

benzphetamine   One of the appetite-suppressant drugs that has been approved for more than 30 years for short-term use but that is regulated by the Drug Enforcement Agency because of potential for addictive abuse; trade name Didrex.

beriberi   A disease of the peripheral nerves caused by thiamin deficiency; characteristics include pain (neuritis), paralysis of the extremities, cardiovascular changes, and edema.

bezoar   A hard ball of hair or vegetable fiber that may develop within the stomach and intestines; can cause an obstruction, requiring removal. Formed because of reduced gastric motility, decreased gastric mixing and churning, and reduced gastric secretions.

bile   A fluid secreted by the liver and transported to the gallbladder for concentration and storage. It is released into the duodenum on entry of fat and acts as an emulsifier to facilitate enzymatic fat digestion.

bilirubin   A reddish bile pigment resulting from the degradation of heme by reticuloendothelial cells in the liver; a high level in the blood produces the yellow skin symptomatic of jaundice.

binge eating   An eating disorder in which individuals consume large amounts of food in a short period of time, but without the purging behavior of bulimia nervosa.

bioavailability   Amount of a nutrient ingested in food that is absorbed and thus available to the body for metabolic use.

blood urea nitrogen (BUN)   The nitrogen component of urea in the blood; a measure of kidney function; elevated levels of BUN indicate a disorder of kidney function.

body composition   The relative sizes of the four body compartments that make up the total body: lean body mass (muscles and organs), fat, water, and mineral (found mostly in bone).

body mass index (BMI)   Body weight in kilograms divided by the height in square meters (kg/m^2). It can be calculated from pounds and inches as 703 times body weight in pounds divided by the height in inches squared. This is the usual measurement to define overweight and obesity.

bolus   Rounded mass of food formed in the mouth and ready to be swallowed.

bradykinesia   Very slow movement.

buffer   Mixture of acid and alkaline components that when added to a solution is able to protect it against large changes in pH, even when strong acids and bases are added. If an acid is added, the alkaline partner reacts to counteract the acidic effect. If a base is added, the acid partner reacts to counteract the alkalizing effect. A solution to which a buffer has been added is called a buffered solution. This process keeps important body fluids at the pH levels required for life.

bulimia nervosa   A psychiatric eating disorder in which cycles of gorging on large quantities of food are followed by self-induced vomiting and use of diuretics and laxatives to maintain a "normal" body weight.

cachexia   A wasting condition marked by weakness, extreme weight loss, and malnutrition.

calcitonin   A polypeptide hormone secreted by the thyroid gland in response to hypercalcemia, which acts to lower both calcium and phosphate in the blood.

calcitriol   Activated hormone form of vitamin D [$1,25(OH)_2D_3$]-1,25-dihydroxycholecalciferol.

calorie   The amount of heat energy needed to raise the temperature of 1 g of water from $14°$ C to $15°$ C. Because this is a small unit, we usually use the term *kilocalorie,* which is 1000 of these small calories, in the study of metabolism. A kilocalorie is the amount of heat required to raise the temperature of 1 kg of water $1°$ C (see also joule).

calorimetry   Measurement of amounts of heat absorbed or given off. Direct method: measurement of the heat produced by a subject enclosed in a small chamber. Indirect method: measurement of heat produced by a subject based on the quantity of nitrogen and carbon dioxide eliminated.

cancer   A malignant cellular tumor with properties of tissue invasion and spreading to other parts of the body.

candidiasis   Infection with the fungus of the genus *Candida,* generally caused by *C. albicans,* so named for the whitish appearance of its small lesions; usually a superficial infection in moist areas of the skin or inner mucous membranes.

capillary fluid shift mechanism   Process that controls the movement of water and small molecules in solution (electrolytes, nutrients) between the blood in the capillary and the surrounding interstitial area. Filtration of water and solutes out of the capillary at the arteriole end and reabsorption at the venule end are accomplished by shifts in balance between the intracapillary hydrostatic blood pressure and the colloidal osmotic pressure exerted by the plasma proteins.

carbohydrate   Compound of carbon, hydrogen, and oxygen; starches, sugars, and dietary fiber made and stored in plants; major energy source in the human diet.

carboxyl (COOH) group   The monovalent radical, COOH, found in organic acids.

carboxypeptidase   A protein-splitting enzyme that cuts the peptide bond at the *carboxyl* (COOH) end of the chain, producing smaller peptide chains and free amino acids.

carcinoma   A malignant new growth made up of epithelial cells, infiltrating the surrounding tissue and spreading to other parts of the body.

cardiac output   Total volume of blood propelled from the heart in a given period; equal to the stroke volume multiplied by the number of beats per the time unit used in the calculation.

carnitine   A naturally occurring amino acid ($C_{17}H_{15}NO_3$) formed from methionine and lysine; carnitine is required to transport long-chain fatty acids into the mitochondria, where they are oxidized for energy.

carotenoids   A group of yellow-red pigments widely distributed in plants that act as antioxidants and protect tissues

from damage caused by free radicals; beta-carotene can be cleaved in the gastric mucosa to form one molecule of vitamin A.

casein hydrolysate formula   Infant formula composed of hydrolyzed casein, a major milk protein, produced by partially breaking down the casein into smaller peptide fragments, making a product that is more easily digested.

catabolism   Metabolic process for breaking down body tissues; the opposite of anabolism.

cheilosis   Cracks and scaly lesions on the lips and mouth resulting from riboflavin deficiency.

chemical bonding   Process of linking chemical elements or groups of elements in a chemical compound.

cholecalciferol   Chemical name for vitamin D in its inactive form. When the inactive cholecalciferol is consumed in food or synthesized in the skin, its first step in activation occurs in the liver and the final step is completed in the kidney to form the active vitamin D hormone *calcitriol,* 1,25-dihydroxycholecalciferol, or $1,25(OH)_2D_3$.

cholecystokinin (CCK)   A peptide hormone secreted by the mucosa of the duodenum in response to the presence of fat. Cholecystokinin causes the gallbladder to contract and propel bile into the duodenum, where it is needed to emulsify the fat and prepare it for digestion and absorption.

cholesterol   A fat-related compound; a sterol ($C_{27}H_{45}OH$) that is normally found in bile and is a principal constituent of gallstones. Cholesterol is synthesized by the liver and is a precursor of various steroid hormones, such as sex hormones and adrenal corticoids. It is found in animal tissues such as meat, egg yolk, and milk fat.

chorea   A wide variety of ceaseless involuntary movements that are rapid, complex, and jerky, yet appear to be well coordinated; characteristic movements of Huntington's disease.

chronologic age   A person's age in years.

chyle   The fat-containing, creamy white fluid that is formed in the lacteals of the intestine during digestion, is transported through the lymphatics, and enters the venous circulation via the thoracic duct.

chylomicrons   Lipoproteins formed in the intestinal wall after a meal that carry food fats into the lymph and then the general circulation for transport to body cells.

chyme   Semifluid food mass in the gastrointestinal tract after gastric digestion.

chymotrypsin   A pancreatic enzyme activated in the intestine from its precursor chymotrypsinogen. It breaks peptide linkages, forming smaller polypeptides and dipeptides.

cirrhosis   Chronic liver disease, characterized by loss of functional cells, with fibrous and nodular regeneration.

cisterna chyli   Cistern or receptacle of the chyle; a dilated sac at the origin of the thoracic duct, which is the common trunk that receives all the lymphatic vessels. The cisterna chyli lies in the abdomen between the second lumbar vertebra and the aorta. It receives the lymph from the intestinal trunk, the right and left lumbar lymphatic trunks, and two descending lymphatic trunks. The chyle, after passing through the cisterna chyli, is carried upward into the chest through the thoracic duct and empties into the venous blood at the point where the left subclavian vein joins the left internal jugular vein. This is the way absorbed fats enter the general circulation.

clinical pathways Clear standards or protocols for patient care that are designed to promote cost efficiency, better outcomes, and faster recovery.

coenzyme A substance that is a necessary partner with a cell enzyme in carrying out a chemical reaction; vitamins and minerals are important coenzymes in energy, lipid, and protein metabolism.

cognitive Pertaining to mental processes such as memory, judgment, and reasoning.

collagen The protein substance of the white fibers of skin, tendon, bone, cartilage, and all other connective tissue.

colloidal osmotic pressure (COP) Pressure produced by the protein molecules in the plasma and in the cell. Because proteins are large molecules, they do not pass through the separating membranes of the capillary cells. Thus they remain in their respective compartments, exerting a constant osmotic pull that protects vital plasma and cell fluid volumes in these compartments.

colon The large intestine extending from the cecum to the rectum.

colostrum Thin yellow fluid first secreted by the mammary gland a few days before and after childbirth, preceding the mature breast milk. It contains up to 20% protein, including a large amount of lactalbumin, more minerals and less lactose and fat than in mature milk, and immunoglobulins representing the antibodies found in maternal blood.

compartment The collective quantity of material of a given type in the body. The four body compartments are *lean body mass* (muscle and vital organs), *bone*, *fat*, and *water*.

complement A complex series of enzymatic proteins occurring in normal serum that interact to combine with and augment (fill out, complete) the antigen-antibody complex of the body's immune system, producing lysis when the antigen is an intact cell; composed of 11 discrete proteins or functioning components, activated by the immunoglobulin factors IgG and IgM.

constipation Difficult or infrequent passage of hard dry stools; fewer than three bowel movements a week.

constitutive proteins Albumin, prealbumin, transferrin. Plasma proteins often used to assess the response to nutrition support. Serum levels are nonspecific and nonsensitive to nutritional status or requirements.

cretinism A congenital disease resulting from absence or deficiency of normal thyroid secretion, characterized by physical deformity, dwarfism, mental retardation, and often goiters.

cruciferous Bearing a cross; botanical term for plants belonging to the botanical family Cruciferae or Brassicaceae, the mustard family, so-called because of crosslike four-petaled flowers; name given to certain vegetables of this family, such as broccoli, cabbage, brussels sprouts, and cauliflower.

cytokines Substances, produced in tissues, that can cause inflammatory changes in tissue cells (e.g., tumor necrosis factor and interleukin-1).

deamination Removal of an amino group (NH_2) from an amino acid.

7-dehydrocholesterol A precursor cholesterol compound in the skin that is irradiated by sunlight to produce cholecalciferol (D_3).

demographic Relating to statistical data describing a population according to age, income, gender, household size, ethnic or cultural group, education, births, or deaths.

diabetes insipidus A condition of the pituitary gland and insufficiency of one of its hormones, vasopressin (antidiuretic hormone); characterized by a copious output of a nonsweet urine, great thirst, and sometimes a large appetite. However, in diabetes insipidus these symptoms result from a specific injury to the pituitary gland, not a collection of metabolic disorders as in diabetes mellitus. The injured pituitary gland produces less vasopressin, a hormone that normally helps the kidneys reabsorb adequate water.

diabetes mellitus A disease defined by a high level of glucose in the blood, which often appears in the urine if it is high enough. There are two general types of diabetes mellitus—(1) type 1, which refers to the disease normally diagnosed in younger individuals (less than 30 years of age) in which the pancreas cannot produce enough insulin and there is thus not enough circulating insulin, and (2) type 2, which refers to the disease normally diagnosed in older people who are often overweight or obese and in which there is more than enough circulating insulin but relatively poor response to this insulin.

dialysis Process of separating crystalloids and colloids in solution by the difference in their rates of diffusion through a semipermeable membrane; crystalloids pass through readily, and colloids pass through only very slowly or not all.

dietary fiber Nondigestible carbohydrates and lignin found in plants; dietary fiber is eaten as an intact part of the plant in which it is found.

Dietary Reference Intake (DRI) The framework of nutrient standards now in place in the United States; the DRIs include the Recommended Dietary Allowance, the Adequate Intake, the Tolerable Upper Intake Level, and the Estimated Average Requirement. They provide reference values for use in planning and evaluating diets for healthy people.

dietetics Management of diet and the use of food; the science concerned with the nutritional planning and preparation of foods and diets.

diethylpropion One of the appetite-suppressant drugs that has been approved for more than 30 years for short-term use but that is regulated by the Drug Enforcement Agency because of potential for addictive abuse; trade name Tenuate.

digestion The process of breaking down food to release its nutrients for absorption and transport to the cells for use in body functions.

dipeptidase Final enzyme in the protein-splitting series that cleaves dipeptides to yield two free amino acids.

disability A mental or physical impairment that prevents an individual from performing one or more gainful activities; not synonymous with handicap, which implies serious disadvantage.

disaccharide Class of compound sugars composed of two molecules of monosaccharide. The three most common disaccharides are sucrose, lactose, and maltose.

distal   Away from the point of origin.

disulfiram   White to off-white crystalline antioxidant; inhibits oxidation of the acetaldehyde metabolized from alcohol. It is used in the treatment of alcoholism, producing extremely uncomfortable symptoms when alcohol is ingested after oral administration of the drug.

dumping syndrome   Constellation of postprandial symptoms that result from rapid emptying of hyperosmolar gastric contents into the duodenum. The hypertonic load in the small intestine promotes reflux of vascular fluid into the bowel lumen, causing a rapid decrease in the circulating blood volume. Rapid symptoms of abdominal cramping, nausea, vomiting, palpitations, sweating, weakness, reduced blood pressure, tremors, and osmotic diarrhea occur. Symptoms of early dumping begin 10 to 30 minutes after eating; late dumping syndrome occurs 1 to 4 hours after a meal. Late dumping is a result of insulin hypersecretion in response to the carbohydrate load dumped into the small intestine. Once the carbohydrate is absorbed, the hyperinsulinemia causes hypoglycemia, which results in vasomotor symptoms such as diaphoresis, weakness, flushing, and palpitations. Individuals who have undergone gastrointestinal surgery resulting in a reduced or absent gastric pouch are more prone to dumping syndrome.

duodenum   The first section of the small intestine entered by food passing through the pyloric valve from the stomach.

dysentery   A general term given to a number of disorders marked by inflammation of the intestines, especially the colon, and accompanied by abdominal pain and frequent stools containing blood and mucus. The cause may be chemical irritants, bacteria, protozoa, or parasites.

dyskinesia   Impairment of the power of voluntary movement.

dyspepsia   Gastric distress or indigestion involving nausea, pain, burning sensations, or excessive gas.

dysphagia   Difficulty in swallowing, commonly associated with obstructive or motor disorders of the esophagus.

dyspnea   Labored, difficult breathing.

eclampsia   Advanced pregnancy-induced hypertension (PIH), manifested by convulsions.

eicosanoids   Long-chain fatty acids composed of 20 carbon atoms.

electrolytes   A chemical element or compound that in solution dissociates as ions carrying a positive or negative charge (e.g., H^+, Na^+, K^+, Ca^{2+}, and Mg^{2+} and Cl^-, HCO_3^-, HPO_4^{2-}, and SO_4^{2-}). Electrolytes constitute a major force controlling fluid balances within the body through their concentrations and shifts from one place to another to restore and maintain balance—*homeostasis.*

elemental formula   A nutrition support formula composed of single elemental nutrient components that require no further digestive breakdown and thus are readily absorbed. Infant formula produced with elemental, ready-to-be-absorbed components of free amino acids and carbohydrate as simple sugars.

emulsifier   An agent that breaks down large fat globules to smaller, uniformly distributed particles. This action is accomplished in the intestine by bile acids, which lower the surface tension of the fat particles. Emulsification increases the surface area of fat, facilitating contact with digestive enzymes.

endemic   Characterizing a disease of low morbidity that remains constantly in a human community but is clinically recognizable in only a few.

endocarditis   Inflammation of the *endocardium,* the serous membrane that lines the cavities of the heart.

endogenous   Originating from within the body; an example is endogenous cholesterol, which is produced by cells in the liver.

energy   The capacity of a system for doing work; available power. Energy is manifest in various forms—motion, position, light, heat, and sound. Energy is interchangeable among these various forms and is constantly being transformed and transferred among them.

energy density   The amount of energy or calories in a food compared with the weight of the food.

enteral   A feeding modality that provides nutrients, either orally or by tube feeding through the gastrointestinal tract.

enterogastrone   A duodenal peptide hormone that inhibits gastric hydrochloric acid secretion and motility.

entitlement program   A government program for which a person is eligible or "entitled" based on income; all persons falling below a certain income level are eligible to receive food stamps.

enzymes   Complex proteins produced by living cells that act as catalysts to speed the rate of chemical reactions. Enzymes facilitate chemical changes in other substances without themselves being changed in the process. Digestive enzymes act on food substances to break them down into simpler compounds. An enzyme is usually named according to the substance (substrate) on which it acts, with the common suffix *-ase;* for example, sucrase is the enzyme that breaks down sucrose to glucose and fructose.

ergogenic   Tendency to increase work output; various substances that increase work or exercise capacity and output.

erythema   Redness of the skin produced by coagulation of the capillaries.

essential fatty acid   A fatty acid required in the diet because the body cannot make it.

essential hypertension   An inherent form of hypertension with no specific discoverable cause and considered to be familial; also called primary hypertension.

ester   A compound produced by the reaction between an acid and an alcohol with elimination of a molecule of water. This process is called esterification. A triglyceride is a glycerol ester, and cholesterol forms esters by combining with fatty acids, largely linoleic acid.

Estimated Average Requirement (EAR)   The average daily intake of a nutrient that will meet the requirement of half of the healthy people of a given age and gender; this standard is used to plan and evaluate intakes of groups, not individuals.

fasciculi   A general term for a small bundle or cluster of muscle, tendon, or nerve fibers.

fatty acid   The building block or structural component of fats.

ferritin Protein-iron compound in which iron is stored in tissues; the storage form of iron in the body.

fetus The unborn offspring in the postembryonic period, after major structures have been outlined; in humans, the growing offspring from 7 to 8 weeks after fertilization until birth.

fistula Abnormal connection between two internal organs, an internal organ and the skin, or an internal organ and a body cavity.

flushing reaction Short-term reaction resulting in redness of neck and face.

food insecurity Limited or uncertain availability of food and the inability to obtain a sufficient supply of nutritionally safe, adequate, and acceptable food through socially acceptable means.

fuel factor The kilocalorie value (energy potential) of food nutrients; the number of kilocalories that 1 g of the nutrient yields when oxidized. The kilocalorie fuel factor is 4 for carbohydrate and protein, 9 for fat, and 7 for alcohol. Fuel factors are used in computing the energy values of foods and diets. (For example, 10 g of fat yields 90 kcal.)

functional fiber Nondigestible carbohydrates isolated from plant foods or manufactured that are added to foods to increase their fiber content.

gastric polyposis An abnormal condition characterized by the presence of numerous polyps in the stomach.

gastrin Hormone secreted by mucosal cells in the antrum of the stomach that stimulates the parietal cells to produce hydrochloric acid. Gastrin is released into the stomach in response to stimulants, especially coffee, alcohol, and meat extracts. When the gastric pH falls below 3, a feedback mechanism cuts off gastrin secretion and prevents excess acid formation.

gastritis Inflammation of the stomach.

gastroesophageal reflux disease (GERD) Describes symptoms that result from reflux of gastric juices, and sometimes duodenal juices, into the esophagus. Symptoms include substernal burning (heartburn), epigastric pressure sensation, and severe epigastric pain. Prolonged and severe GERD can lead to esophageal bleeding, perforation, strictures, Barrett's epithelium, adenocarcinoma, and pulmonary fibrosis (from aspiration). Conservative dietary therapy involves weight reduction; restriction of carbonated beverages, caffeine, fatty foods, peppermint, chocolate, and ethanol; small frequent meals; and wearing of loose clothing to promote symptomatic relief.

geriatrics Branch of medicine specializing in medical problems of older adults.

gerontology Study of the physiologic, biologic, psychologic, and sociologic aspects of the aging process, their effects on individuals, and potential preventive or intervention strategies.

gestation The period of embryonic and fetal development from fertilization to birth; pregnancy.

gingivitis Red, swollen, bleeding gums, most often caused by accumulation of bacterial plaque on the teeth.

glomerulonephritis A form of nephritis affecting the capillary loops in an acute short-term infection. It may progress to a more serious chronic condition leading to irreversible renal failure.

glossitis Swollen, reddened tongue; symptom of riboflavin deficiency.

glucagon A polypeptide hormone secreted by the alpha cells of the pancreatic islets of Langerhans in response to hypoglycemia; has an opposite balancing effect to that of insulin, raising the blood sugar, and thus is used as a quick-acting antidote for the hypoglycemic reaction of insulin. It stimulates the breakdown of glycogen (glycogenolysis) in the liver by activating the liver enzyme phosphorylase and thus raises blood sugar levels during fasting states to ensure adequate levels for normal nerve and brain function.

gluconeogenesis Production of glucose from keto acid carbon skeletons from deaminated amino acids and the glycerol portion of fatty acids.

glyceride Group name for fats; any of a group of esters obtained from glycerol by the replacement of one, two, or three hydroxyl (OH) groups with a fatty acid. Monoglycerides contain one fatty acid; diglycerides contain two fatty acids; and triglycerides contain three fatty acids. Glycerides are the principal constituent of adipose tissue and are found in animal and plant fats and oils.

glycerol An alcohol that is esterified with fatty acids to produce fats and released when fats are hydrolyzed; a colorless, odorless, syrupy sweet liquid.

glycogen A polysaccharide made up of many saccharide (sugar) units. Glycogen is the body storage form of carbohydrate found mostly in the liver, with lesser amounts stored in the muscle.

glycogenesis Synthesis of glycogen from blood glucose.

glycogenolysis Hydrolysis of glycogen to glucose.

glycolysis Cell oxidation of glucose for energy.

goiter Enlargement of the thyroid gland caused by lack of sufficient available iodine to produce the thyroid hormone thyroxine.

gravida A pregnant woman.

growth acceleration Period of increased speed of growth at different points of childhood development.

growth channel The progressive regular growth pattern of children, guided along individual genetically controlled channels, influenced by nutritional and health status.

growth chart grids Grids comparing stature (length), weight, and age of children by percentile; used for nutritional assessment to determine how their growth is progressing. The most commonly used grids are those of the National Center for Health Statistics (NCHS).

growth deceleration Period of decreased speed of growth at different points of childhood development.

growth velocity Rapidity of motion or movement; rate of childhood growth over normal periods of development compared with a population standard.

handicap A mental or physical defect that may or may not be congenital, which prevents the individual from participating in normal life activities; implies disadvantage.

Heimlich maneuver   A first-aid maneuver to relieve a person who is choking from blockage of the breathing passageway by a swallowed foreign object or food particle. Standing behind the person, clasp the victim around the waist, placing one fist under the sternum (breastbone) and grasping the fist with the other hand. Then make a quick, hard, thrusting movement inward and upward.

helix   A coiled structure found in protein. Some are simple chain coils; others are made of several coils, as in a triple helix.

hematuria   The abnormal presence of blood in the urine.

heme iron   Dietary iron from animal sources, from the heme portion of hemoglobin in red blood cells. Heme iron is more easily absorbed and transported in the body than nonheme iron from plant sources, but it supplies the smaller portion of the body's total dietary iron intake.

hemodialysis   Removal of certain elements from the blood according to their rates of diffusion through a semipermeable membrane—e.g., by a hemodialysis machine.

hemoglobin   Oxygen-carrying pigment in red blood cells; a conjugated protein containing four heme groups combined with iron and four long polypeptide chains forming the protein globin, named for its ball-like form; made by the developing red blood cells in bone marrow, hemoglobin carries oxygen in the blood to body cells.

hemolytic anemia   An anemia caused by breakdown of the outer membrane of red blood cells and loss of their hemoglobin.

hemosiderin   Insoluble iron oxide–protein compound in which iron is stored in the liver if the amount of iron in the blood exceeds the storage capacity of ferritin, such as during rapid destruction of red blood cells (malaria, hemolytic anemia).

homeostasis   State of dynamic equilibrium within the body's internal environment; a balance achieved through the operation of various interrelated physiologic mechanisms.

hormones   Internally secreted substances from the endocrine organs that are carried in the blood to another organ or tissue on which they act to stimulate functional activity or secretion. This tissue or organ is called its target tissue.

hydrogenation   Process used to produce margarine and shortening from vegetable oil; when vegetable oils are exposed to hydrogen gas, hydrogen atoms are added at many of the double bonds of the polyunsaturated fatty acids, forming a solid fat.

hydrolysis   Process by which a chemical compound is split into simpler compounds by taking up molecules of water. This process occurs naturally in digestion.

25-hydroxycholecalciferol [25(OH)D$_3$]   Intermediate product formed in the liver in the process of developing the active vitamin D hormone.

hygroscopic   Taking up and retaining moisture readily.

hypercapnia   Excess CO_2 in the blood.

hyperemesis gravidarum   Severe vomiting during pregnancy, which is potentially fatal.

hyperlipoproteinemia   Elevated level of lipoproteins in the blood.

hyperthyroidism   An abnormality of the thyroid gland in which secretion of thyroid hormone is usually increased and is characterized by an elevated plasma level of thyroxin.

hyponatremia   Serum sodium less than 135 mEq/L; a relative excess of body water compared with sodium.

hypovolemia   Abnormally decreased volume of circulating blood in the body.

hypoxemia   Deficient oxygenation of the blood, resulting in hypoxia, reduced O_2 supply to tissue.

iatrogenic   Describes a medical disorder caused by physician diagnosis, manner, or treatment.

icteric   Alternate term for jaundice: nonicteric indicates absence of jaundice; preicteric indicates a state before development of icterus, or jaundice.

immunocompetence   The ability or capacity to develop an immune response, that is, antibody production and/or cell-mediated immunity, after exposure to antigen.

incidence   The number of new cases of a particular condition that develop over time. If among 1000 people, 10 people who were not overweight initially become overweight in 1 year, the incidence rate would be 10 cases per 1000 person-years.

incomplete protein   A protein with a lower amount of one or more of the indispensable amino acids or missing an indispensable amino acid needed to form body proteins.

indispensable (essential) amino acid   An amino acid that the body cannot synthesize or cannot synthesize in sufficient amounts to meet body needs so must be supplied by the diet. The nine indispensable amino acids are histidine, isoleucine, leucine, lysine, methionine, phenylalanine, threonine, tryptophan, and valine. Six amino acids are conditionally indispensable because the body cannot synthesize sufficient amounts under certain conditions.

indole   A compound produced in the intestines by the decomposition of tryptophan; also found in the oil of jasmine and clove.

infarct   An area of tissue necrosis caused by local ischemia, resulting from obstruction of blood circulation to that area.

insulin   Hormone formed in the beta cells of the islets of Langerhans in the pancreas. It is secreted when blood glucose and amino acid levels rise and assists their entry into body cells. It also promotes glycogenesis and conversion of glucose into fat and inhibits lipolysis and gluconeogenesis (protein breakdown). Commercial insulin is manufactured from pigs and cows; new "artificial" human insulin products have recently been made available.

intermittent claudication   A symptomatic pattern of peripheral vascular disease, characterized by the absence of pain or discomfort in a limb, usually the legs, when at rest, which is followed by pain and weakness when walking, intensifying until walking becomes impossible, and then disappearing again after a rest period; seen in occlusive arterial disease.

interstitial fluid   The fluid situated between parts or in the interspaces of a tissue.

intima   General term indicating an innermost part of a structure or vessel; inner layer of the blood vessel wall.

intramural nerve plexus Network of nerves in the walls of the intestine that make up the intramural nervous system, controlling muscle action and secretions for digestion and absorption.

ischemia Deficiency of blood to a particular tissue, resulting from functional blood vessel constriction or actual obstruction walls in atherosclerosis.

jaundice A syndrome characterized by hyperbilirubinemia and deposits of bile pigment in the skin, mucous membranes, and sclera, giving a yellow appearance to the patient.

joule A unit of energy. The International System of Units uses joules in place of calories to refer to food energy, and most nutrition journals require its use instead of calories (1 kcal = 4.184 kilojoules [kJ] often rounded to 4.2 kJ for ease in calculation). A 1000-kcal diet would be equivalent to a 4200 kJ or 4.2 megajoule (MJ) diet.

keratinization The process of creating the protein keratin, a principal constituent of skin, hair, nails, and the matrix forming tooth enamel.

keto acid Amino acid residue after deamination. The glycogenic keto acids are used to form carbohydrates.

kilocalorie The general term *calorie* refers to a unit of heat measure and is used alone to designate the *small calorie*. The *large calorie,* 1000 calories or kilocalorie, is used in the study of metabolism to avoid the use of very large numbers in calculations.

kinetic Energy released from body fuels by cell metabolism and now active in moving muscles and energizing all body activities.

kyphosis Increased, abnormal convexity of the upper part of the spine; hunchback.

labile Easily changed or modified; unstable.

lactase Enzyme that splits the disaccharide lactose, releasing the monosaccharides glucose and galactose.

lactated Ringer's solution Sterile solution of calcium chloride, potassium chloride, sodium chloride, and sodium lactate in water administered to replenish fluid and electrolytes.

lactiferous ducts Branching channels in the mammary gland that carry breast milk to holding spaces near the nipple ready for the infant's feeding.

leptin A peptide of 167 amino acids that is produced primarily in fat cells and released into the blood to circulate as a hormone to the brain to tell the body about long-term regulation of body fat.

life expectancy The number of years a person of a given age, gender, race, or ethnic group can expect to live.

limiting amino acid The indispensable amino acid in a food found in the smallest amount as related to the Reference Amino Acid Pattern.

linoleic acid An essential fatty acid for humans; an n-6 polyunsaturated fatty acid.

lipase Group of fat enzymes that cut the ester linkages between the fatty acids and glycerol in triglycerides (fats).

lipids Chemical group name for fats and fat-related compounds such as cholesterol, lipoproteins, and phospholipids; general group name for organic substances of a fatty nature including fats, oils, waxes, and related compounds.

lipogenesis Synthesis of fat from blood glucose.

lipoprotein Noncovalent complexes of fat with protein. The lipoproteins function as major carriers of lipids in the plasma; this combination of fat surrounded by protein makes possible the transport of fatty substances in a water medium such as plasma.

lumen The cavity or channel within a tube or tubular organ such as the intestines.

lymphoma General term applied to any neoplastic disorder (cancer) of the lymphoid tissue.

macronutrients The three energy-yielding nutrients: carbohydrates, fats, and proteins.

macrosomia Unusually large size.

macular degeneration Destructive changes in the macula, a small spot in the center of the retina required for relay of the visual image; this condition is a major cause of blindness in older adults.

malabsorption and **maldigestion** Malabsorption is a syndrome in which normal products of digestion do not traverse the intestinal mucosa and enter the lymphatic or portal venous branches. Maldigestion, which may be clinically similar to malabsorption, describes defects in the intraluminal phase of the digestive process caused by inadequate exposure of chyme to bile salts and pancreatic enzymes. Clinical symptoms of malabsorption include diarrhea, steatorrhea, and weight loss. Laboratory signs include depressed serum fat-soluble vitamin levels, accelerated prothrombin time, hypomagnesemia, and hypocholesterolemia. Patients with symptoms of malabsorption should have a laboratory work-up to determine the presence and degree of nutrient loss.

malignant melanoma A tumor tending to become progressively worse, composed of melanin (the dark pigment of the skin and other body tissues), usually arising from the skin and aggravated by excessive sun exposure.

maltase Enzyme that splits the disaccharide maltose, releasing two units of the monosaccharide glucose.

median In statistics the middle number in a sequence of numbers such that half are higher and half are lower.

medical foods Specially formulated nutrient mixtures for use under medical supervision to treat various metabolic diseases.

medulla Inner tissue substance of the kidney.

megaloblastic anemia Anemia resulting from faulty production of abnormally large immature red blood cells; caused by vitamin B_{12} or folate deficiency.

menadione A water soluble analogue of vitamin K that is absorbed directly into the portal blood.

menaquinone Form of vitamin K synthesized by intestinal bacteria.

menarche The first menstruation with the onset of puberty.

Ménétrier's disease (giant hypertrophic gastritis) Rare disease characterized by large folds of nodular gastric rugae that may cover the wall of the stomach, causing anorexia, nausea, vomiting, and abdominal distress.

meningitis   Inflammation of the *meninges,* the three membranes that envelop the brain and spinal cord; the cause is a bacterial or viral infection leading to high fever, severe headache, and stiff neck or back muscles.

metabolic syndrome   Multiple metabolic risk factors in one individual: waist circumference greater than 102 cm in men, greater than 88 cm in women; serum triglycerides greater or equal to 150 mg/dL; HDL-cholesterol less than 40 mg/dl in men, less than 50 mg/dl in women; BP greater than or equal to 130/85 mm Hg; FPG (fasting plasma glucose) greater than or equal to 110 mg/dL.

metabolism   Sum of all the various biochemical and physiologic processes by which the body grows and maintains itself (anabolism) and breaks down and reshapes tissue (catabolism) and transforms energy to do its work. Products of these various reactions are called *metabolites.*

metabolites   Any substance produced by metabolism or by a metabolic process.

micellar bile-lipid complex   A combination of bile and fat that carries fat into the wall of the small intestine in preparation for the final stage of absorption into the circulation.

micelle   A particle made up of lipids and bile salts that carries digested lipids into the cells of the intestinal mucosa for absorption; the fat-soluble vitamins are also absorbed as part of this bile-lipid complex.

micronutrients   The two classes of small non–energy-yielding elements and compounds—the minerals and the vitamins. Minerals and vitamins are essential for regulation and control functions in cell metabolism and for building certain body structures.

microvilli   Minute vascular structures protruding from the surface of villi covering the inner surface of the small intestine, forming a "brush border" that facilitates absorption of nutrients.

monosaccharide   Simple single sugar; a carbohydrate containing a single saccharide (sugar) unit. The most common monosaccharides are glucose, galactose, and fructose.

motivation   Forces that affect individual goal-directed behavior toward satisfying needs or achieving personal goals.

mucosa   The mucous membrane constituting the inner surface layer of the gastrointestinal tract, providing extensive nutrient absorption and transport functions.

mucus   Viscous fluid secreted by mucous membranes and glands, consisting mainly of mucin (a glycoprotein), inorganic salts, and water. Mucus lubricates and protects the gastrointestinal mucosa and helps move the food mass along the digestive tract.

myasthenia gravis (MG)   A progressive neuromuscular disease caused by faulty nerve conduction resulting from the presence of antibodies to acetylcholine receptors at the neuromuscular junction.

myelin   Substance made of fat and protein that forms a fatty sheath around the nerve axons; this covering protects and insulates the nerves and facilitates the transmission of neuromuscular impulses.

myofibril   Slender thread of muscle; runs parallel to the long axis of the muscle fiber.

myofilaments   Threadlike filaments of actin or myosin, which are components of myofibrils.

myosin   Myofibril protein whose synchronized meshing action in conjunction with actin causes muscles to contract and relax.

necrosis   Cell death caused by progressive enzyme breakdown.

neoplasm   Any new tissue growth that is abnormal, uncontrolled, and progressive.

neoplastic   Describing abnormal growth of tissue, usually associated with the formation of tumors.

nephron   Microscopic anatomic and functional unit of the kidney that selectively filters and resorbs essential blood factors, secretes hydrogen ions as needed for maintaining acid-base balance, and then resorbs water to protect body fluids and forms and excretes a concentrated urine for elimination of wastes. The nephron includes the renal corpuscle (glomerulus), the proximal convoluted tubule, the loop of Henle, the distal convoluted tubule, and the collecting tubule, which empties the urine into the renal medulla. The urine passes into the papilla and then to the pelvis of the kidney. Urine is formed by filtration of blood in the glomerulus and by the selective reabsorption and secretion of solutes by cells that constitute the walls of the renal tubes. There are approximately 1 million nephrons in each kidney.

nephropathy   Disease of the kidneys; in diabetes, renal damage associated with functional and pathologic changes in the nephrons, which can lead to glomerulosclerosis and chronic renal failure.

neuropathy   General term for functional and pathologic changes in the peripheral nervous system; in diabetes, a chronic sensory condition affecting mainly the nerves of the legs, marked by numbness from sensory impairment, loss of tendon reflexes, severe pain, weakness, and wasting of muscles involved.

niacin equivalent (NE)   A measure of the total dietary sources of niacin; 1 NE equals 1 mg of niacin or 60 mg of tryptophan.

night blindness   Inability to see well in diminished light, resulting from vitamin A deficiency.

nitrogen balance   The metabolic balance between nitrogen intake in dietary protein and nitrogen output in urinary nitrogen compounds such as urea and creatinine; 6.25 g dietary protein contains 1 g of nitrogen.

nonheme iron   The larger portion of dietary iron, including all the plant food sources and 60% of the animal food sources. This form of iron is not part of a heme complex and is less easily absorbed.

nonnutritive sweetener   A substance with sweetening power that is not efficiently absorbed by the body or cannot be metabolized to provide energy; these substances are used in small amounts and in most cases the kcalories added to the food product are negligible.

nulligravida   A woman who has never been pregnant.

nutrients Substances in food that are essential for energy, growth, normal body function, and maintenance of life.

nutrition The sum of the processes involved in taking in food, releasing the nutrients it contains, and assimilating and using these nutrients to provide energy and maintain body tissue; a foundation for life and health.

nutrition science The body of scientific knowledge developed through controlled research that relates to all aspects of nutrition—national, international, community, and clinical.

obesity An excess amount of body fat. Operationally it is usually defined as a body mass index (BMI) of 30 kg/m^2 or greater, which uses height and weight. Three subclasses of obesity are defined as follows:

- Class 1 = BMI 30-34.9 kg/m^2
- Class 2 = BMI 35-39.9 kg/m^2
- Class 3 = BMI ≥40 kg/m^2

oligosaccharides Intermediate products of polysaccharide digestion that contain from 3 to 10 glucose units.

oliguria Secretion of a very small amount of urine in relation to fluid intake.

oncogene Any of various genes that, when activated as by radiation or a virus, may cause a normal cell to become cancerous; viral genetic material carrying the potential of cancer and passed from parent to offspring.

organic Carbon-based chemical compounds.

orlistat Drug (trade name Xenical) that partially blocks pancreatic lipase, thus decreasing digestion of dietary fat. It is available by prescription and over the counter.

osmolality The ability of a solution to create osmotic pressure and determine the movement of water between fluid compartments; determined by the number of osmotically active particles per kilogram of solvent; serum osmolality is 280 to 300 mOsm/kg.

osmolarity The number of millimoles of liquid or solid in a liter of solution; parenteral nutrition solutions given by central vein have an osmolarity around 1800 mOsm/L; peripheral parenteral solutions are limited to 600 to 900 mOsm/L (dextrose and amino acids have the greatest impact on a solution's osmolarity).

osteodystrophy Defective bone formation.

osteopenia Below-normal level of bone mineral density, which increases the risk of stress fractures; the bone thinning is not as severe as that found in osteoporosis.

osteoporosis Abnormal loss of bone mineral and matrix leading to porous, fragile bone tissue with enlarged spaces that is prone to fracture or deformity; common disease of aging in both older men and women.

overweight A weight above the upper limit of some arbitrarily set standard (see also *obesity*).

palliative Care affording relief but not cure; useful for comfort when cure is still unknown or obscure.

palmar grasp Early grasp of the young infant, clasping an object in the palm and wrapping the whole hand around it.

pancreas Gland located near the duodenum and small intestine that has two sets of cells: (1) acinar cells, which secrete digestive enzymes into the intestine, and (2) beta cells, which produce and secrete insulin into the blood.

pandemic A widespread epidemic, distributed through a region, a continent, or the world.

pantothenic acid A member of the B vitamin complex widely distributed in nature and throughout body tissues; it functions as a part of coenzyme A, important in lipid and carbohydrate metabolism.

paradigm A pattern or model serving as an example; a standard or ideal for practice or behavior based on a fundamental value or theme.

parasite An organism that lives on or in an organism of another species, known as the host, from whom all life cycle nourishment is obtained.

parenchymal cells Functional cells of an organ, as distinguished from the cells constituting its structure or framework.

parenteral A mode of feeding that does not use the gastrointestinal tract, but instead provides nutrition by intravenous delivery of nutrient solutions.

paresthesia Abnormal sensations such as prickling, burning, and crawling of skin.

parity The condition of a woman with respect to having borne viable offspring.

pathology The science of disease. Changes that reflect disease can be in organs (liver disease), tissues (skin disease), cells, or parts of cells.

pathophysiologic Term referring to the processes by which the disease develops.

pepsin A gastric enzyme specific for proteins. Pepsin breaks large protein molecules into shorter chain polypeptides, proteases, and peptones. Gastric hydrochloric acid is necessary to activate pepsin.

peptide bond The characteristic joining of amino acids to form proteins. Such a chain of amino acids is termed a peptide. Depending on the number of amino acid units, it may be a dipeptide or a large polypeptide.

percentile One of 100 equal parts of measured series of values; rate or proportion per hundred.

peristalsis A wavelike progression of alternate contraction and relaxation of the muscle fibers of the gastrointestinal tract.

peritoneal dialysis Dialysis through the peritoneum into and out of the peritoneal cavity.

peritoneum A strong smooth surface—a serous membrane—lining the abdominal/pelvic walls and the undersurface of the diaphragm, forming a sac enclosing the body's vital visceral organs within the peritoneal cavity.

pernicious anemia A chronic macrocytic anemia caused by absence of intrinsic factor necessary for the absorption of cobalamin (B$_{12}$); it is treated with intramuscular injections of vitamin B$_{12}$.

phendimetrazine One of the appetite-suppressant drugs that has been approved for more than 30 years for short-term use but that is regulated by the Drug Enforcement Agency because of potential for addictive abuse; trade names Adipost, Anorex-SR, Appecon, Bontril PDM, Bontril Slow-Release, Melfiat, Obezine, Phendiet, Plegine, Prelu-2, and Statobex.

phentermine   One of the appetite-suppressant drugs that has been approved for more than 30 years for short-term use but that is regulated by the Drug Enforcement Agency because of potential for addictive abuse; trade names Adipex-P, Fastin, Ionamix, Obenix, Obephen, Oby-Cap, Oby-Trim, Panshape M, Phentercot, Phentride, Pro-Fast HS, Pro-Fast SA, Pro-Fast SR, Teramine, and Zantryl.

phospholipid   A class of fat-related substances that contain phosphorus, fatty acids, and a nitrogenous base. The phospholipids are important components of cell membranes, nerve tissues, and lipoproteins.

photosynthesis   Process by which plants containing chlorophyll are able to manufacture carbohydrate by combining CO_2 from air and water from soil. Sunlight is used as energy; chlorophyll is a catalyst.

$$6\,CO_2 + 6\,H_2O + Energy + Chlorophyll \rightarrow$$
$$C_6H_{12}O_6 + 6\,O_2$$

phylloquinone   A fat-soluble vitamin of the K group found in green plants or prepared synthetically.

physiologic age   Rate of biologic maturation in individual adolescents that varies widely and accounts more for wide and changing differences in their metabolic rates, nutritional needs, and food requirements than does chronologic age.

pincer grasp   Later digital grasp of the older infant, usually picking up smaller objects with a precise grip between thumb and forefinger.

placenta   Special organ developed in early pregnancy that provides nutrients to the fetus and removes metabolic waste.

plaque   Thickened deposits of fatty material, largely cholesterol, within the arterial wall that eventually may fill the lumen and cut off blood supply to the tissue served by the damaged vessel.

portal   An entryway, usually referring to the portal circulation of blood through the liver. Blood is brought into the liver via the portal vein and moves out via the hepatic vein.

potential   Energy existing in stored fuels and ready for action but not yet released and active.

poverty line   The minimum amount of income required to provide food, clothing, shelter, and other basic necessities for a family of a given size and composition; this index is calculated by government economists and used to determine eligibility for various government programs such as food stamps or free or reduced-cost school lunches.

prebiotics   Nondigestible food products that promote growth of symbiotic bacterial species already present in the colon.

precursor   A substance from which another substance is derived.

prediabetes   A condition also known as *impaired glucose tolerance* and defined as a fasting glucose between 100 and 126 mg/dl and a blood glucose between 140 and 199 mg/dl 2 hours after ingestion of 75 g of glucose.

pressure sores   Long-term bed-bound or immobile patients risk the development of pressure sores at points of bony protu-berances, where prolonged pressure of body weight in one position cuts off adequate blood circulation to that area, causing tissue death and ulceration.

prevalence   This term relates the number of individuals with a particular condition at a particular time to the total number of people. If 10 people were overweight in a population of 1000, this would indicate a prevalence of 1%.

primigravida   A woman who is pregnant for the first time.

probiotics   Microbial foods or supplements that can be used to modify or reestablish intestinal flora and improve health of the host.

proenzyme   An inactive precursor converted to the active enzyme by the action of an acid or other enzyme.

programming   The mechanism(s) through which adaptations to nutrient supplies during gestation result in permanent changes in organ and body system structures and functions, potentially leading to chronic disease risk.

prostaglandins   Group of naturally occurring substances derived from long-chain fatty acids that have multiple local hormonelike actions; they regulate gastric acid secretion, blood platelet aggregation, body temperature, and tissue inflammation.

prostration   Extreme exhaustion.

protein balance   The balance between the building up (anabolism) and the breaking down (catabolism) of body tissues, necessary to maintain positive growth and maintenance.

proteinuria   The presence of an excess of serum proteins, such as albumin, in the urine.

prothrombin   Blood-clotting factor synthesized in the liver from glutamic acid and CO_2; catalyzed by vitamin K.

public health nutritionist   A professional nutritionist who has completed an academic program and special graduate study (MPH, DrPH) in a school of public health accredited by the American Association of Public Health and is responsible for nutrition components of public health programs in varied community settings—county, state, national, international.

pulmonary edema   Accumulation of fluid in tissues of the lung.

pyrosis   Heartburn.

radiation   A highly controlled treatment for cancer, using radioactive substances in limited, controlled exposure to kill cancerous cells.

raffinose   A colorless crystalline trisaccharide composed of galactose and sucrose joined by bonds that human enzymes cannot break; raffinose is found in legumes and in the intestine is attacked by bacteria, producing the gas associated with eating these foods.

Recommended Dietary Allowance (RDA)   The average daily intake of a nutrient that will meet the requirement of nearly all (97% to 98%) healthy people of a given age and gender. The RDAs are established and reviewed periodically by an expert panel of nutrition scientists and amended as needed based on new research. When planning diets it is best to aim for this level of intake.

registered dietitian (RD)   A professional dietitian who has completed an accredited academic program and 900 hours of postbaccalaureate supervised professional practice and has passed the National Registration Examination for Dietitians administered by the Commission on Dietetic Registration.

renal solute load Collective number and concentration of solute particles in a solution carried by the blood to the kidney nephrons for excretion in the urine. The particles are usually nitrogenous products from protein metabolism and the electrolyte sodium.

renin-angiotensin-aldosterone mechanism Three-stage system of sodium conservation, hence control of water loss, in response to diminished filtration pressure in the kidney nephrons: (1) pressure loss causes kidney to secrete the enzyme renin, which combines with and activates angiotensinogen from the liver; (2) active angiotensin stimulates the adjacent adrenal gland to release the hormone aldosterone; and (3) aldosterone causes reabsorption of sodium from the kidney nephrons and water follows.

replication Making an exact copy; to repeat, duplicate, or reproduce. In genetics, replication is the process by which double-stranded deoxyribonucleic acid (DNA) makes copies of itself with each separating strand synthesizing a complementary strand. Cell replication is the process by which living cells under gene control divide to produce exact copies of themselves a programmed number of times during the life span of the organism. Cultured cell lines reproduced in the laboratory are used to study the aging process.

resting metabolic rate (RMR) Amount of energy required to maintain the resting body's internal activities when in a comfortable environmental temperature and awake. Because of small differences in measuring techniques, an individual's RMR and BMR (basal metabolic rate) may differ slightly. In practice, however, RMR and BMR measurements are used interchangeably.

retinal The aldehyde form of retinol (vitamin A) derived from the enzymatic splitting of carotene in the intestinal wall. In the retina of the eye, retinal combines with opsins to form visual pigments. In the rods it forms rhodopsin (visual purple), and in the cones it forms the pigments responsible for color vision.

retinol Chemical name for vitamin A derived from its function in the retina of the eye producing light-dark adaptation.

retinol activity equivalent (RAE) Unit of measure for dietary sources of vitamin A, including both preformed retinol and the precursor provitamins beta-carotene, alpha-carotene, and beta cryptoxanthin.

retinopathy Noninflammatory disease of the retina—the visual tissue of the eye—characterized by microaneurysms, intraretinal hemorrhages, waxy yellow exudates, "cotton wool" patches, and macular edema; a complication of diabetes that may lead to proliferation of fibrous tissue, retinal detachment, and blindness.

retrovirus Any of a family of single-strand RNA viruses having an envelope and containing a reverse coding enzyme that allows for a reversal of genetic transcription from RNA to DNA rather than the usual DNA to RNA, the newly transcribed viral DNA then being incorporated into the host cell's DNA strand for the production of new RNA retroviruses.

rooting reflex A reflex in a newborn in which stimulation of the side of the cheek or the upper or lower lip causes the infant to turn its mouth and face to the stimulus.

rule of nines Describes the percentage of the body surface represented by various anatomic areas. For example: each upper limb, 9%; each lower limb, 18%; anterior and posterior trunk, each 18%; head and neck, 9%; and perineum and genitalia, 1%.

sarcoma A tumor, usually malignant, arising from connective tissue.

saturated Term used for a substance that is united with the greatest possible number of other atoms or chemical groups through solution, chemical combination, or the like. A fatty acid is saturated if all available chemical bonds of its carbon chain are filled with hydrogen. If one bond remains unfilled, it is a monounsaturated fatty acid. If two or more bonds remain unfilled, it is a polyunsaturated fatty acid. A fat is saturated if the majority of fatty acids making up its structure are saturated.

scurvy A hemorrhagic disease caused by lack of vitamin C; physical changes include diffuse tissue bleeding, painful and swollen limbs and joints, swollen and bleeding gums, loosening of teeth, and poor wound healing.

seborrheic dermatitis Greasy scales and crusts that appear on the skin in riboflavin deficiency; they are most likely to occur in the moist folds of the body.

secretin Hormone produced in the mucous membrane of the duodenum in response to the entrance of acid contents from the stomach into the duodenum. Secretin in turn stimulates the flow of pancreatic juices, providing needed enzymes and the proper alkalinity for their action.

sepsis Presence in the blood or other tissues of pathogenic microorganisms or their toxins; conditions associated with such pathogens.

serosa Outer surface layer of the intestines interfacing with the blood vessels of the portal system going to the liver.

sibutramine A newer appetite-suppressant drug that has been approved for long-term use but that is still regulated by the Drug Enforcement Agency because of potential for addictive abuse (trade name Meridia).

solutes Particles of a substance in solution; a solution consists of a substance and a dissolving medium (solvent), usually a liquid.

somatostatin A hormone formed in the delta cells of the pancreatic islets of Langerhans and the hypothalamus. It is a balancing factor in maintaining normal blood glucose levels by inhibiting insulin and glucagon production in the pancreas as needed.

sphincter A circular band of muscle fibers that constricts a passage or closes a natural opening in the body (e.g., lower esophageal sphincter, pyloric sphincter).

spina bifida A congenital defect in the fetal closing of the neural tube to form a portion of the lower spine, leaving the spine unclosed and the spinal cord open in various degrees of exposure and damage.

steroids Group name for lipid-based sterols including hormones, bile acids, and cholesterol.

stigma   A mark or identification marking. In this context it is an increased body fat that is obvious to the viewer and that elicits emotional feelings, which are usually negative.

stomatitis   Inflammation of the oral mucosa, especially the buccal tissue lining the inside of the cheeks, but it also may involve the tongue, palate, floor of mouth, and the gums.

stroke volume   The amount of blood pumped from a ventricle (chamber of the heart releasing blood to body circulations) with each beat of the heart.

substrate   The specific organic substance on which a particular enzyme acts to produce a new metabolic product.

sucrase   Enzyme that splits the disaccharide sucrose, releasing the monosaccharides glucose and fructose.

sugar alcohol   An alcohol formed from a simple sugar; many sugar alcohols are used as sweetening agents by food manufacturers because they do not react with bacteria in the mouth to form dental caries.

supine   Lying down.

synergism   The joint action of separate agents in which the total effect of their combined action is greater than the sum of their separate actions (adjective: synergistic).

synosheath   Protective pliable connective tissue surrounding the bony collagen mesh and fluid that come together in the synovial area between major bone heads in joints, which allows normal padded and lubricated joint movement and motion.

synthesis   The making of a substance or compound by the body.

synthesize   To form new compounds in the body for use in building tissues or carrying out metabolic or physiologic functions.

tactile   Pertaining to the touch.

taurine   A sulfur-containing amino acid, $NH_2(CH_2)_2 \cdot SO_2OH$, formed from the indispensable amino acid methionine. It is found in lung and muscle tissues and in bile and breast milk.

thermic effect of food (TEF)   Body heat produced by food; the amount of energy required to digest and absorb food and transport nutrients to the cells. This work accounts for about 10% of the day's total energy (kcalorie) requirement.

thiamin pyrophosphate (TPP)   Activating coenzyme form of thiamin key in carbohydrate metabolism.

tocopherol   Chemical name for vitamin E; it functions as an antioxidant to preserve structural membranes and other tissues with a high content of polyunsaturated fatty acids.

Tolerable Upper Intake Level (UL)   The highest amount of a nutrient that can be safely consumed with no risk of toxicity or adverse effects on health; this standard can be used when evaluating dietary supplements or reviewing total nutrient intake from food and supplements; intakes exceeding the UL usually occur from the use of concentrated dietary supplements, not intake from food.

total fiber   Dietary fiber plus functional fiber; the total amount of fiber in an individual's diet from all sources.

trans fatty acids   Fatty acids that have been hydrogenated to be used in margarine and in the food industry; have been shown to increase LDL cholesterol and lower HDL cholesterol.

triglyceride   Chemical name for fat that indicates the structure of three fatty acids attached to a glycerol base. A neutral fat synthesized from carbohydrate and stored in adipose tissue; it releases free fatty acids into the blood when hydrolyzed by enzymes.

trypsin   A pancreatic enzyme activated in the intestine from its precursor trypsinogen; it acts on proteins and polypeptides to yield smaller peptides and dipeptides.

vagotomy   Cutting of certain branches of the vagus nerve, performed with gastric surgery, to reduce the amount of gastric acid secreted and lessen the chance of recurrence of a gastric ulcer.

valence   Power of an element or a radical to combine with or to replace other elements or radicals. Atoms from various elements combine in definite proportions. The valence number of an element is the number of atoms of hydrogen with which one atom of the element can combine.

vasoactive   Having an effect on the diameter of blood vessels.

vasopressin   Alternative name of antidiuretic hormone (ADH).

villi   Small protrusions from the surface of a membrane; fingerlike projections covering mucosal surfaces of the small intestine.

virus   Minute infectious agent, characterized by lack of independent metabolism and by the ability to reproduce with genetic continuity only with living host cells. They range in decreasing size from about 200 nanometers (nm) down to only 15 nm. (A nanometer is a linear measure equal to one billionth of a meter; it is also called a millimicron.) Each particle (virion) consists basically of nucleic acids (genetic material) and a protein shell, which protects and contains the genetic material and any enzymes present.

visceral   Referring to the organs in the abdominal cavity.

viscous   Sticky; physical property of a substance dependent on the friction of its component molecules as they slide by one another; viscosity.

VO_2max   Maximal uptake volume of oxygen during exercise; used to measure the intensity and duration of exercise a person can perform.

Zollinger-Ellison syndrome   A condition characterized by severe peptic ulceration, gastric hypersecretion, elevated serum gastrin, and gastrinoma of the pancreas or the duodenum. Total gastrectomy may be necessary.

INDEX

Page numbers followed by b indicate boxed material (numbered and unnumbered); f, figures; t, tables.